DULCAN'S TEXTBOOK OF

CHILD AND ADOLESCENT PSYCHIATRY

SECOND EDITION

DULCAN'S TEXTBOOK OF
CHILD AND ADOLESCENT PSYCHIATRY

SECOND EDITION

Edited by

Mina K. Dulcan, M.D.

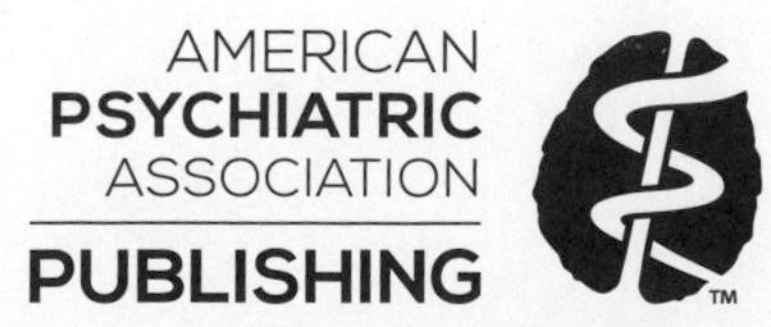

Note: The authors have worked to ensure that all information in this book is accurate at the time of publication and consistent with general psychiatric and medical standards. As medical research and practice continue to advance, however, therapeutic standards may change. Moreover, specific situations may require a specific therapeutic response not included in this book. For these reasons and because human and mechanical errors sometimes occur, we recommend that readers follow the advice of physicians directly involved in their care or the care of a member of their family.

Books published by American Psychiatric Association Publishing represent the findings, conclusions, and views of the individual authors and do not necessarily represent the policies and opinions of American Psychiatric Association Publishing or the American Psychiatric Association.

If you wish to buy 50 or more copies of the same title, please go to www.appi.org/special discounts for more information.

Manufactured in the United States of America on acid-free paper
19 18 17 16 15 5 4 3 2 1
Second Edition

Typeset in Palatino LT and Helvetica Neue LT.

American Psychiatric Association Publishing
1000 Wilson Boulevard
Arlington, VA 22209-3901
www.appi.org

Library of Congress Cataloging-in-Publication Data

Dulcan's textbook of child and adolescent psychiatry / edited by Mina K. Dulcan. — Second edition.
p. ; cm.
title: Textbook of child and adolescent psychiatry
Includes bibliographical references and index.
ISBN 978-1-58562-493-5 (hc : alk. paper)
I. Dulcan, Mina K., editor. II. American Psychiatric Association, issuing body. III. Title: Textbook of child and adolescent psychiatry.
[DNLM: 1. Mental Disorders. 2. Adolescent. 3. Child. 4. Infant. WS 350]
RJ499
618.92'89—dc23

2015012547

British Library Cataloguing in Publication Data
A CIP record is available from the British Library.

Contents

Part I

Assessment and Diagnosis

Part II

Neurodevelopmental and Other Psychiatric Disorders

Part III

Disorders Affecting Somatic Function

Part IV

Special Topics

Part V

Somatic Treatments

Part VI

Psychosocial Treatments

Part VII
Consultation

Contributors

Sarah Armstrong, M.D., FAAP
Associate Professor, Departments of Pediatrics and Community and Family Medicine, Duke University, Durham, North Carolina

L. Eugene Arnold, M.D., M.Ed.
Professor Emeritus of Psychiatry, Ohio State University, Columbus, Ohio

Miya R. Asato, M.D.
Associate Professor of Pediatrics and Psychiatry, Children's Hospital of Pittsburgh of UPMC, Pittsburgh, Pennsylvania

Deborah C. Beidel, Ph.D., ABPP
Pegasus Professor of Psychology and Medical Education, University of Central Florida, Orlando, Florida

Gail A. Bernstein, M.D.
Endowed Professor in Child and Adolescent Anxiety Disorders, and Head, Program in Child and Adolescent Anxiety and Mood Disorders, University of Minnesota Medical School, Minneapolis, Minnesota

Joseph Biederman, M.D.
Chief, Clinical and Research Programs in Pediatric Psychopharmacology and Adult ADHD, Massachusetts General Hospital, and Professor of Psychiatry, Harvard Medical School, Boston, Massachusetts

Boris Birmaher, M.D.
Professor of Psychiatry, University of Pittsburgh Medical Center, Pittsburgh, Pennsylvania

David A. Brent, M.D.
Academic Chief, Western Psychiatric Institute and Clinic; Endowed Chair, Suicide Studies, and Director, Services for Teens at Risk, University of Pittsburgh Medical Center, Pittsburgh, Pennsylvania

Oscar G. Bukstein, M.D., M.P.H.
Medical Director, DePelchin Children's Center, Houston, Texas

Sharon Cain, M.D.
Professor, Department of Psychiatry and Behavioral Sciences, Director, Division of Child and Adolescent Psychiatry, and Director, Child and Adolescent Psychiatry Residency Program, University of Kansas School of Medicine, Kansas City, Kansas

Gabrielle A. Carlson, M.D.
Professor of Psychiatry and Pediatrics, Stony Brook University, Stony Brook, New York

Anil Chacko, Ph.D.
Associate Professor, Department of Applied Psychology, New York University, New York, New York

Meredith R. Chapman, M.D.
Assistant Professor, UT Southwestern Medical Center, Dallas, Texas

Diane Chen, Ph.D.
Instructor of Psychiatry and Behavioral Sciences, Northwestern University Feinberg School of Medicine, and Medical Psychologist, Division of Adolescent Medicine, Ann & Robert H. Lurie Children's Hospital of Chicago, Chicago, Illinois

Judith A. Cohen, M.D.
Professor of Psychiatry, Drexel University College of Medicine, Allegheny General Hospital, Pittsburgh, Pennsylvania

Sucheta D. Connolly, M.D.
Professor of Clinical Psychiatry, University of Illinois at Chicago, Chicago, Illinois

Christoph U. Correll, M.D.
Professor of Psychiatry and Molecular Medicine, Hofstra North Shore Long Island Jewish School of Medicine, Zucker Hillside Hospital, Glen Oaks, New York

Paul Croarkin, D.O.
Assistant Professor, Mayo Clinic, Rochester, Minnesota

Steven P. Cuffe, M.D.
Professor and Chair, University of Florida College of Medicine, Jacksonville, Florida

Lisa M. Cullins, M.D.
Director, Outpatient Psychiatry Clinic, Associate Training Director, Adolescent Psychiatry Fellowship Program, and Assistant Professor of Psychiatry and Pediatrics, Children's National Medical Center, George Washington University School of Medicine, Washington, DC

Eric Daleiden, Ph.D.
Chief Operating Officer, PracticeWise, LLC, Satellite Beach, Florida

Arman Danielyan, M.D.
John Muir Health, Concord, California

Nina de Lacy, M.D., M.B.A.
Fellow, Child and Adolescent Psychiatry, University of Washington, Seattle Children's Research Institute Center for Integrative Brain Research, Seattle, Washington

Mary Lynn Dell, M.D., D.Min.
Director of Psychosomatic Medicine and Professor of Clinical Psychiatry and Pediatrics, Nationwide Children's Hospital and Ohio State University, Columbus, Ohio

Chirag V. Desai, M.D.
Assistant Professor and Associate Director, Psychiatry Residency Program, University of Florida College of Medicine, Jacksonville, Florida

Mina K. Dulcan, M.D.
Head, Child and Adolescent Psychiatry, Ann & Robert H. Lurie Children's Hospital of Chicago, and Professor, Psychiatry and Behavioral Sciences and Pediatrics, Northwestern University Feinberg School of Medicine, Chicago, Illinois

Kamryn T. Eddy, Ph.D.
Assistant Professor of Psychology, Department of Psychiatry, Harvard Medical School, Massachusetts General Hospital, Boston, Massachusetts

Graham J. Emslie, M.D.
Professor of Psychiatry and Pediatrics, UT Southwestern, Dallas, Texas

Robert L. Findling, M.D., M.B.A.
Professor of Psychiatry and Pediatrics, Child and Adolescent Psychiatry, Johns Hopkins University, Baltimore, Maryland

Mary A. Fristad, Ph.D., ABPP
Professor, Psychiatry and Behavioral Health, Psychology, and Nutrition, Ohio State University, Columbus, Ohio

Daniel A. Geller, M.B.B.S., FRACP
Associate Professor, Harvard Medical School, and Director, Pediatric OCD Program, Massachusetts General Hospital, Boston, Massachusetts

Lisa L. Giles, M.D.
Assistant Professor of Pediatrics and Psychiatry, Primary Children's Hospital, Salt Lake City, Utah

Mary Margaret Gleason, M.D.
Associate Professor, Psychiatry and Pediatrics, Tulane University School of Medicine, New Orleans, Louisiana

Tina R. Goldstein, Ph.D.
Associate Professor, Psychiatry, Western Psychiatric Institute and Clinic, University of Pittsburgh Medical Center, Pittsburgh, Pennsylvania

Karen R. Gouze, Ph.D.
Director of Training in Psychology, Ann & Robert H. Lurie Children's Hospital,

and Professor of Psychiatry and Behavioral Sciences, Feinberg School of Medicine, Northwestern University, Chicago, Illinois

Barbara L. Gracious, M.D.
Associate Professor of Clinical Psychiatry and Nutrition, Ohio State University College of Medicine, and Jeffrey Research Fellow, Research Institute at Nationwide Children's Hospital, Columbus, Ohio

Meredith L. Gunlicks-Stoessel, Ph.D.
Assistant Professor, Department of Psychiatry, University of Minnesota, Minneapolis, Minnesota

John Hamilton, M.D.
Staff Psychiatrist, Harvard University Health Services, Cambridge, Massachusetts

Marco A. Hidalgo, Ph.D.
Assistant Professor of Psychiatry and Behavioral Sciences, Northwestern University Feinberg School of Medicine, and Medical Psychologist, Division of Adolescent Medicine, Ann & Robert H. Lurie Children's Hospital of Chicago, Chicago, Illinois

Anna Ivanenko, M.D., Ph.D.
Associate Professor of Clinical Psychiatry and Behavioral Sciences, Feinberg School of Medicine, Northwestern University, Division of Child and Adolescent Psychiatry, Ann & Robert H. Lurie Children's Hospital of Chicago, Chicago, Illinois

Iliyan Ivanov, M.D.
Associate Professor, Icahn School of Medicine at Mount Sinai, New York, New York

Shabnam Javdani, Ph.D.
Assistant Professor, Department of Applied Psychology, New York University, New York, New York

Poonam Jha, M.D.
Assistant Professor of Psychiatry and Behavioral Sciences, Northwestern University Feinberg School of Medicine, Chicago, Illinois

Kyle P. Johnson, M.D.
Associate Professor, Department of Psychiatry and Pediatrics, Oregon Health & Science University, Portland, Oregon

Paramjit T. Joshi, M.D.
Endowed Professor and Chair, Department of Psychiatry and Behavioral Sciences, Children's National Medical Center, George Washington University School of Medicine, Washington, DC

Nina M. Kaiser, Ph.D.
Assistant Clinical Professor, University of California, San Francisco, San Francisco, California

Bryan H. King, M.D., M.B.A.
Professor and Vice Chair of Psychiatry and Behavioral Sciences; Director, Seattle Children's Autism Center; and Director of Child and Adolescent Psychiatry, University of Washington and Seattle Children's Hospital, Seattle, Washington

Ian Kodish, M.D., Ph.D.
Assistant Professor, Department of Psychiatry and Behavioral Sciences, University of Washington, Seattle, Washington

Robert A. Kowatch, M.D., Ph.D.
Professor of Psychiatry, Ohio State Wexner University Medical Center, Nationwide Children's Hospital, Columbus, Ohio

Anlee D. Kuo, J.D., M.D.
Assistant Clinical Professor, Department of Psychiatry, University of California San Francisco, San Francisco, California

John V. Lavigne, Ph.D., ABPP
Professor of Psychiatry and Pediatrics, Ann & Robert H. Lurie Children's Hospital of Chicago, Chicago, Illinois

Esther S. Lee, M.D.
Clinical Instructor, Child and Adolescent Psychiatry, Johns Hopkins University, Baltimore, Maryland

Daniel Le Grange, Ph.D.
Professor of Psychiatry, UCSF School of Medicine, San Francisco, California

Scott Leibowitz, M.D.
Assistant Professor of Psychiatry and Behavioral Sciences, Department of Child and Adolescent Psychiatry and Division of Adolescent Medicine, Ann & Robert H. Lurie Children's Hospital of Chicago, Northwestern University Feinberg School of Medicine, Evanston, Illinois

W. David Lohr, M.D.
Clinical Co-Director, University of Louisville Autism Center at Kosair Charities, Assistant Professor of Child Psychiatry, Department of Pediatrics, and Associate of Department of Psychiatry, University of Louisville School of Medicine, Louisville, Kentucky

Kelly Walker Lowry, Ph.D.
Assistant Professor, Ann & Robert H. Lurie Children's Hospital of Chicago and Northwestern University, Chicago, Illinois

Joan Luby, M.D.
Samuel and Mae S. Ludwig Professor of Child Psychiatry, Department of Psychiatry, Washington University School of Medicine, St. Louis, Missouri

Anthony P. Mannarino, Ph.D.
Professor of Psychiatry, Department of Psychiatry, Drexel University College of Medicine, Allegheny General Hospital, Pittsburgh, Pennsylvania

D. Richard Martini, M.D.
Professor of Pediatrics and Psychiatry, Primary Children's Hospital, Salt Lake City, Utah

Taryn L. Mayes, M.S.
Faculty Associate, UT Southwestern Medical Center, Dallas, Texas

Jon M. McClellan, M.D.
Professor, Department of Psychiatry, University of Washington, Seattle, Washington

Amy N. Mendenhall, Ph.D., M.S.W.
Assistant Professor and Director, Center for Children and Families, University of Kansas School of Social Welfare, Lawrence, Kansas

Stephanie E. Meyer, Ph.D.
Los Angeles, California

Edwin J. Mikkelsen, M.D.
Associate Professor of Psychiatry, Harvard Medical School, Boston, Massachusetts

Laura Mufson, Ph.D.
Professor of Medical Psychology, Columbia University College of Physicians and Surgeons and New York State Psychiatric Institute, New York, New York

Helen B. Murray, B.A.
Massachusetts General Hospital, Boston, Massachusetts

Kathleen Myers, M.D., M.P.H., M.S.
Professor, University of Washington and Seattle Children's Hospital, Seattle, Washington

Paul Nagy, M.S., LPC, LCAS, CCS
Assistant Professor, Department of Psychiatry and Behavioral Sciences, Duke University, Durham, North Carolina

Neha Navsaria, Ph.D.
Assistant Professor of Psychiatry, Washington University School of Medicine, St. Louis, Missouri

Eve-Lynn Nelson, Ph.D.
Director, Center for Telemedicine & Telehealth, and Professor, Pediatrics, University of Kansas Medical Center, Fairway, Kansas

Jeffrey H. Newcorn, M.D.
Associate Professor of Psychiatry and Pediatrics, Icahn School of Medicine at Mount Sinai, New York, New York

John D. O'Brien, M.D.
Clinical Professor of Psychiatry, Mount Sinai School of Medicine, New York, New York

Caroly Pataki, M.D.
Clinical Professor of Psychiatry and Biobehavioral Sciences, David Geffen School of Medicine at UCLA, Los Angeles, California

Theodore A. Petti, M.D., M.P.H.
Professor, Rutgers Robert Wood Johnson Medical School, Piscataway, New Jersey

Linda J. Pfiffner, Ph.D.
Professor of Psychiatry, University of California, San Francisco, San Francisco, California

Karen Pierce, M.D.
Clinical Associate Professor, Northwestern Feinberg School of Medicine, Chicago, Illinois

Sigita Plioplys, M.D.
Professor of Psychiatry, Ann & Robert H. Lurie Children's Hospital of Chicago, Chicago, Illinois

Steven R. Pliszka, M.D.
Professor and Chair, Department of Psychiatry, University of Texas Health Science Center at San Antonio, San Antonio, Texas

Yann Poncin, M.D.
Assistant Professor, Child Study Center, Yale School of Medicine, New Haven, Connecticut

Mark A. Reinecke, Ph.D., ABPP, ACT
Professor of Psychiatry and Behavioral Sciences, Northwestern University, Chicago, Illinois

Barry Sarvet, M.D.
Clinical Professor, Tufts University School of Medicine, Baystate Medical Center, Springfield, Massachusetts

John B. Sikorski, M.D.
Clinical Professor, Child and Adolescent Psychiatry Division and the Psychiatry and the Law Program, University of California San Francisco, San Francisco, California

Cathy A. Southammakosane, M.D.
Assistant Professor of Psychiatry and Pediatrics, Children's National Medical Center, George Washington University School of Medicine, Washington, DC

Thomas J. Spencer, M.D.
Associate Professor of Psychiatry, Harvard Medical School; Associate Chief, Clinical and Research Program, Pediatric Psychopharmacology and Adult ADHD, Massachusetts General Hospital, Boston, Massachusetts

Liza M. Suárez, Ph.D.
Clinical Assistant Professor of Psychology in Psychiatry, University of Illinois at Chicago, Chicago, Illinois

L. Read Sulik, M.D.
Chief Integration Officer, PrairieCare/PrairieCare Institute; Clinical Associate Professor, Department of Psychiatry, University of Minnesota, Minneapolis, Minnesota

Peter E. Tanguay, M.D.
Ackerly Endowed Chair in Child and Adolescent Psychiatry (Emeritus), Department of Psychiatry and Biobehavioral Sciences, Division of Child and Adolescent Psychiatry, University of Louisville School of Medicine, Louisville, Kentucky

Lenore Terr, M.D.
Clinical Professor of Psychiatry, University of California San Francisco, San Francisco, California

Christopher R. Thomas, M.D.
Robert L. Stubblefield Professor of Child Psychiatry, Department of Psychiatry and Behavioral Sciences, University of Texas Medical Branch at Galveston, Galveston, Texas

Karen Toth, Ph.D.
Research Scientist, Seattle Children's Research Institute, Seattle, Washington

Kenneth E. Towbin, M.D.
Chief, Clinical Child and Adolescent Psychiatry, Mood and Anxiety Disorders Program, Emotion and Development Branch, NIMH-IRP, National Institute of Mental Health, U.S. Department of Health and Human Services; Clinical Professor, Psychiatry and Behavioral Sciences, George Washington University School of Medicine, Washington, DC

Andrea M. Victor, Ph.D.
Clinical Director, Chicago Neurodevelopmental Center, Northbrook, Illinois

Froma Walsh, Ph.D.
Mose and Sylvia Firestone Professor Emerita, University of Chicago, Chicago, Illinois

Heather J. Walter, M.D., M.P.H.
Professor of Psychiatry and Pediatrics, Boston University School of Medicine, Boston, Massachusetts

Richard Wendel, Ph.D.
Associate Professor of Clinical Psychiatry and Behavioral Sciences, Feinberg School of Medicine, Northwestern University, Chicago, Illinois

Timothy E. Wilens, M.D.
Chief, Division of Child and Adolescent Psychiatry, and Director, Center for Addiction Medicine, Massachusetts General Hospital; Associate Professor of Psychiatry, Harvard Medical School, Boston, Massachusetts

Kyle Williams, M.D.
Director, Pediatric Neuropsychiatry and Immunology Clinic, Massachusetts General Hospital; Instructor, Department of Psychiatry, Harvard Medical School, Boston, Massachusetts

Joseph Woolston, M.D.
Albert J. Solnit Professor of Pediatrics and Child Psychiatry, Child Study Center, Yale School of Medicine, New Haven, Connecticut

Eric Youngstrom, Ph.D.
Professor of Psychology and Psychiatry, University of North Carolina at Chapel Hill, Chapel Hill, North Carolina

Alexandra D. Zagoloff, Ph.D.
Assistant Professor, University of Minnesota Medical School, Minneapolis, Minnesota

Charles H. Zeanah, M.D.
Mary Peters Sellars-Polchow Chair in Psychiatry, Professor of Psychiatry and Pediatrics, and Vice-Chair for Child and Adolescent Psychiatry, Tulane University School of Medicine, New Orleans, Louisiana

Frank Zelko, Ph.D.
Associate Professor of Psychiatry and Behavioral Sciences, Northwestern University Feinberg School of Medicine, Chicago, Illinois

Disclosure of Interests

The following contributors to this book have indicated a financial interest in or other affiliation with a commercial supporter, a manufacturer of a commercial product, a provider of a commercial service, a nongovernmental organization, and/or a government agency, as listed below:

L. Eugene Arnold, M.D. *Grants/contracts:* CureMark, Forest, Lilly, Shire, Novartis, Noven, Young Living. *Consultant/advisor:* Tris Pharma, Biomarin, Roche, Seaside Therapeutics, Shire, Noven.

Miya R. Asato, M.D. *Grants:* Health Resources and Services Administration.

Gail A. Bernstein, M.D. *Grants:* NIMH, NSF, Genentech Foundation.

Joseph Biederman, M.D. *Grants:* Department of Defense, AACAP, Alcobra, Forest Research Institute, Ironshore, Lundbeck, Magceutics, Merck, PamLab, Pfizer, Shire Pharmaceuticals, SPRITES, Sunovion, Vaya Pharma/Enzymotec, NIH. *Honoraria:* MGH Psychiatry Academy. *U.S. patent pending:* provisional number 61/233,686 through MGH corporate licensing. *Royalties:* Ingenix, Prophase, Shire, Bracket Global, Sunovion, Theravance.

Boris Birmaher, M.D. *Grants:* NIMH. *Royalties:* Books and chapters.

David A. Brent, M.D. *Grants:* NIMH. *Royalties:* Guilford Press, ERT. *Editor:* UpToDate Psychiatry. *Honoraria:* presentations for continuing medical education events.

Oscar G. Bukstein, M.D., M.P.H. *Royalties:* Routledge Press.

Sharon Cain, M.D. *Research support:* Pfizer.

Judith A. Cohen, M.D. *Royalties:* Guilford Press.

Sucheta D. Connolly, M.D. *Grants:* NIMH, SAMHSA.

Christoph U. Correll, M.D. *Grants:* NIMH; American Academy of Child and Adolescent Psychiatry, Bristol-Myers Squibb, Janssen/Johnson and Johnson, Novo Nordisk A/S, Otsuka, Thrasher Foundation. *Consultant/advisor:* Actelion, Alexza Pharmaceuticals, AstraZeneca, Bristol-Myers Squibb, Eli Lilly, Genentech, Gerson Lehrman Group, Intracellular Therapies, Janssen/Johnson and Johnson, Lundbeck, Medavante, Medscape, Merck, NIMH, Otsuka, Pfizer, ProPhase, Roche, Sunovion, Supernus, Takeda, Vanda. *Speakers bureau:* Merck. *Expert testimony:* Janssen.

Paul Croarkin, D.O., MCSC *Grants:* Pfizer, NIMH (K23 MH100266), Brain and Behavior Research Foundation, Mayo Foundation. *In-kind support:* Neuronetics, Assurex.

Eric Daleiden, Ph.D. *Co-owner:* PracticeWise.

Nina de Lacy, M.D., M.B.A. *Grants:* American Psychiatric Foundation/Janssen Pharmaceuticals Resident Psychiatric Research Scholars Award.

Mary Lynn Dell, M.D. *Royalties:* Abingdon Press, Oxford University Press.

Graham J. Emslie, M.D. *Grants:* Duke University, Forest Laboratories. *Consultant:* Alkermes, Allergan, NCS Pearson (previously BioBehavioral Diagnostics), Bristol-Myers Squibb, INC Research, Lundbeck, Pfizer (replacement for Wyeth).

Robert L. Findling, M.D., M.B.A. *Grants:* Alcobra, AstraZeneca, Bristol-Myers Squibb, CogCubed, Forest, GlaxoSmithKline, Johnson & Johnson, Lilly, Lundbeck, Merck, National Institutes of Health, Neurim, Novartis, Otsuka, Pfizer, Purdue, Rhodes, Roche, Shire, Stanley Medical Research Institute, Sunovion, Supernus. *Consultant:* Bracket, Bristol-Myers Squibb, Cognition Group, Coronado Biosciences, Dana Foundation, Elsevier, Forest, GlaxoSmithKline, Guilford Press, Jubilant Clinsys, Kempharm, Lilly, Lundbeck, Merck, National Institutes of Health, Novartis, Noven, Otsuka, Pfizer, Physicians Postgraduate Press, Roche, Shire, Sunovion, Supernus, Transcept, Validus, WebMD. *Speakers' bureau:* American Academy of Child & Adolescent Psychiatry, American Physicians' Institute, Shire. *Royalties:* American Psychiatric Association Press, Johns Hopkins University Press, Oxford University Press, Sage.

Mary A. Fristad, Ph.D., ABPP *Royalties:* American Psychiatric Association Press, Guilford Press, Child & Family Psychological Services.

Tina R. Goldstein, Ph.D. *Research support:* NIMH, National Institute on Drug Abuse, National Institute of Child Health and Human Development, Pittsburgh Foundation. *Royalties:* Guilford Press.

Meredith L. Gunlicks-Stoessel, Ph.D. *Grants:* NIMH.

Iliyan Ivanov, M.D. *Board member:* Data Safety Monitoring board for Lundbeck. *Travel support:* NIDA, AACAP, UKAAN, APSARD.

Bryan H. King, M.D., M.B.A. *Research support*: Roche.

Anthony P. Mannarino, Ph.D. *Royalties:* Guilford Press.

Stephanie E. Meyer, Ph.D. *Grants:* Forest Research Institute.

Laura Mufson, Ph.D. *Royalties:* Guilford Press.

Paul Nagy, M.S., LPC, LCAS, CCS *Speakers bureau:* Alkermes.

Jeffrey H. Newcorn, M.D. *Consultant/advisor/research support:* Alcobra, Biobehavioral Diagnostics, GencoSciences, Lupin, Ironshore, Neurovance, Shide, Sunovion.

Steven R. Pliszka, M.D. *Research support:* Shire Laboratories, Purdue Pharmaceutical.

Thomas J. Spencer, M.D. *Research support:* Shire Laboratories, Alcobra, Sunovion, VayaPharma, FDA, Department of Defense. *Consultant:* Alcobra, Heptares, Impax, Ironshore, Lundbeck Inc., Shire Laboratories, Sunovion, VayaPharma. *Advisory board:* Alcobra. Royalties: MGH Corporate Sponsored Research and Licensing. *U.S. patent pending:* provisional number 61/233,686 through MGH corporate licensing.

Liza M. Suárez, Ph.D. *Grants:* SAMHSA.

Timothy E. Wilens, M.D. *Grants:* NIH (NIDA). *Consultant:* Euthymics/Neurovance, NIH (NDA), Ironshore, TRIS, U.S. National Football League (ERM Associates), U.S. Minor/Major League Baseball, Bay Cove Human Services. *Royalties:* Guilford Press, Before School Functioning Questionnaire. *Licensing agreement:* Ironshore.

Kyle A. Williams, M.D. *Research support:* Grifols Therapeutics.

Alexandra D. Zagoloff, Ph.D. *Grants:* NIMH.

The following contributors have indicated that they have no financial interests or other affiliations that represent or could appear to represent a competing interest with their contributions to this book:

Deborah C. Beidel, Ph.D.; Gabrielle A. Carlson, M.D.; Meredith R. Chapman, M.D.; Diane Chen, Ph.D.; Steven P. Cuffe, M.D.; Armam Danielyan, M.D.; Chirag V. Desai, M.D.; Mina K. Dulcan, M.D.; Kamryn T. Eddy, Ph.D.; Daniel A. Geller, M.B.B.S., FRACP; Lisa Giles, M.D.; Mary Margaret Gleason, M.D.; Karen R. Gouze, Ph.D.; Barbara L. Gracious, M.D.; John Hamilton, M.D.; Marco A. Hidalgo, Ph.D.; Anna Ivanenko, M.D., Ph.D.; Poonam Jha, M.D.; Kyle P. Johnson, M.D.; Paramjit T. Joshi, M.D.; Nina M. Kaiser, Ph.D.; Ian Kodish, M.D., Ph.D.; Robert A. Kowatch, M.D., Ph.D.; Anlee D. Kuo, J.D., M.D.; John V. Lavigne, Ph.D., ABPP; Esther S. Lee, M.D.; Daniel Le Grange, Ph.D.; Scott Leibowitz, M.D.; W. David Lohr, M.D.; Kelly Walker Lowry, Ph.D.; Joan Luby, M.D.; D. Richard Martini, M.D.; Taryn L. Mayes, M.S.; Jon M. McClellan, M.D.; Amy N. Mendenhall, Ph.D., M.S.W.; Edwin J. Mikkelsen, M.D.; Helen B. Murray, B.A.; Kathleen Myers, M.D., M.P.H., M.S.; Neha Navsaria, Ph.D.; Eve-Lynn Nelson, Ph.D.; John D. O'Brien, M.D.; Caroly Pataki, M.D.; Darshan A. Patel, M.D.; Theodore A. Petti, M.D., M.P.H.; Linda J. Pfiffner, Ph.D.; Sigita Plioplys, M.D.; Karen Pierce, M.D.; Yann Poncin, M.D.; Barry Sarvet, M.D.; John B. Sikorski, M.D.; Cathy A. Southammakosane, M.D.; L. Read Sulik, M.D.; Peter E. Tanguay, M.D.; Lenore Terr, M.D.; Christopher R. Thomas, M.D.; Karen Toth, Ph.D.; Kenneth E. Towbin, M.D.; Andrea M. Victor, Ph.D.; Froma Walsh, Ph.D.; Heather J. Walter, M.D., M.P.H.; Richard Wendel, Ph.D.; Joseph Woolston, M.D.; Charles H. Zeanah, M.D.; Frank Zelko, Ph.D.

Preface to the Second Edition

It is difficult to believe that I wrote the Preface for the first edition of this textbook 6 years ago. I greatly appreciate all of the feedback I have received. This edition has been fully updated for DSM-5, as well as the latest in clinically relevant research. It is in the new, more efficient and focused American Psychiatric Association Publishing textbook format. This book is more compact and about 30% shorter than the previous edition. The number of chapters has been reduced from 65 to 49, retaining those that are most relevant to clinical work, reflecting the latest in both art and science. Several chapters each combine material from two chapters in the first edition. This text aims to communicate the clinical art and wisdom of child psychiatry, tied firmly to the science of our clinical disciplines. Each chapter highlights what we know about evidence-based practices in assessment and treatment, covering the most important topics in an even more efficient format for the mental health professional in training or the clinician seeking an update. Like its predecessor, this book is designed to be used as a core text for child and adolescent psychiatry fellowship training as well as a reference for practicing child and adolescent psychiatrists, pediatricians, family physicians, general psychiatrists, child neurologists, psychologists, advanced practice nurses, and psychiatric social workers. As trainees and clinicians are increasingly mobile, access to the full-text electronic version of this book via Psychiatry Online (available at www.psychiatryonline.org) is a great bonus. A study guide with questions and answers based on this text is in the planning stages for publication by American Psychiatric Association Publishing as a companion volume.

Chapters are organized by sections that include assessment, categories of diagnoses, and types of treatment, as well as special topics and consultation. The six chapters in "Part I: Assessment and Diagnosis" address the clinical aspects of evaluating youth ranging in age from infancy to late adolescence, as well as the neurological aspects of assessment. "Part II: Neurodevelopmental and Other Psychiatric Disorders" (12 chapters) and "Part III: Disorders Affecting Somatic Function" (5 chapters) cover the key DSM-5 psychiatric disorders seen in children and adolescents. These chapters have a consistent structure that includes definition and clinical description, diagnosis, epidemiology, comorbidity, etiology and risk factors, prevention, course and prognosis, evaluation, and the variety of treatments. "Part IV: Special Topics" includes 10 chapters on evidence-based practice, child abuse and neglect, cultural and religious issues, suicide, gender dysphoria and nonconformity, aggression and violence, psychiatric emergencies, family transitions, legal and ethical issues, and telemental health. There are two sections on treatments: "Part V: Somatic Treatments," with 5 psychopharmacology chapters, and "Part VI: Psychosocial Treatments," which comprises 9 chapters on the range of psychosocial treatments that focus on individuals, families, therapeutic milieus, and systemic models of care. With the increasing emphasis on taking mental health care beyond the clinician's office, "Part VII: Consultation" has chapters related to schools and to primary care. Each chapter in the book ends with summary points—5 to 10 key learning points or "take-home messages." In addition, the book contains "Additional Resources," with sections on "Selected Books for Professionals" and "Web Sites for Professionals, Patients, and Families."

Of the 49 chapters in this book, 2 chapters have all new authors for this edition. Many chapters have added or changed junior authors, keeping the same senior author. The authors represent the expertise of a variety of child mental health disciplines. The chapter authors exceeded my high expectations and responded patiently to my detailed copyediting and content suggestions. The most difficult part both for the authors and for me was to distill their great knowledge and expertise into the even more limited number of pages possible in this volume.

I remain grateful for what I have learned in close to 40 years in academic child and adolescent psychiatry as a teacher, clinician, administrator, researcher, and editor. I find that I still refer to the wisdom of Peter B. Henderson, M.D., and Richard L. Cohen, M.D., as well as many other teachers. I have learned so much from my local and national colleagues from child and adolescent psychiatry, psychology, and social work and my residents and fellows (many of whom are now experts and academic leaders). The children and parents who have been my patients and advisors have been unfailingly generous with their experience and insights.

Onward and upward!

Mina K. Dulcan, M.D.

Ann & Robert H. Lurie
Children's Hospital of Chicago
Northwestern University
Feinberg School of Medicine
Chicago, Illinois

Additional Resources

Selected Books for Professionals

Dulcan MK, Ballard R: Helping Parents and Teachers Understand Medications for Behavioral and Emotional Problems: A Resource Book of Medication Information Handouts, 4th Edition. Washington, DC, American Psychiatric Publishing, 2015

Haddad F, Gerson R: Helping Kids in Crisis: Managing Psychiatric Emergencies in Children and Adults. Washington, DC, American Psychiatric Publishing, 2015

Klykylo WM, Bowers R, Weston C, Jackson J: Green's Child and Adolescent Clinical Psychopharmacology, 5th Edition. Philadelphia, PA, Lippincott Williams & Wilkins, 2014

Manassis K: Case Formulation with Children and Adolescents. New York, Guilford, 2014

McVoy M, Findling RL: Clinical Manual of Child and Adolescent Psychopharmacology, 2nd Edition. Washington, DC, American Psychiatric Publishing, 2013

Petti TA, Salguero C (eds): Community Child and Adolescent Psychiatry: A Manual of Clinical Practice and Consultation. Washington, DC, American Psychiatric Publishing, 2006

Shaw RJ, DeMaso DR: Clinical Manual of Pediatric Psychosomatic Medicine: Mental Health Consultation with Physically Ill Children and Adolescents. Washington, DC, American Psychiatric Publishing, 2006

Web Sites for Professionals, Patients, and Families

American Academy of Child and Adolescent Psychiatry (AACAP)

www.aacap.org

Includes "Facts for Families," brief information sheets on a wide variety of topics in child and family development and mental health, resource centers, and practice guidelines

American Academy of Pediatrics

www.aap.org

American Psychiatric Association

www.healthyminds.org

Autism Society of America

www.autism-society.org

Canadian Alliance for Monitoring Effectiveness and Safety of Antipsychotic Medications in Children (CAMESA)

www.camesaguideline.org

Center for Mental Health Services (CMHS)

Information on child and adolescent mental health and on family mental health resources

www.mentalhealth.gov

Child Mind Institute

www.childmind.org

Children and Adults with Attention-Deficit/Hyperactivity Disorder (CHADD)

www.chadd.org

National Alliance on Mental Illness (NAMI)

www.nami.org

National Institute of Mental Health (NIMH)

www.nimh.nih.gov

National Resource Center on AD/HD

A cooperative venture of CHADD and the Centers for Disease Control and Prevention

www.help4adhd.org

Parents Medication Guide

Resources developed by the American Psychiatric Association and the American Academy of Child and Adolescent Psychiatry on the following:

- Attention-deficit/hyperactivity disorder (also in Spanish)
- Bipolar disorder
- Depression

www.parentsmedguide.org

The Annenberg Foundation Trust at Sunnylands Adolescent Mental Health Initiative

MindZone—a mental health site for teenagers

Downloadable concise guides for teens, parents, and counselors on psychiatric disorders in youth. Spanish language versions available

www.copecaredeal.org

The Balanced Mind Parent Network (a program of the Depression and Bipolar Support Alliance)

http://www.thebalancedmind.org/

National Tourette Syndrome Association

www.tsa-usa.org

Acknowledgments

The Osterman Chair of Child Psychiatry at the Ann & Robert H. Lurie Children's Hospital of Chicago (the new name for our newly built hospital, to which we moved in 2012 from the very old Children's Memorial Hospital) provided essential support for my work on this book. My husband, Richard Wendel, not only coauthored a chapter from his expertise in family therapy but also cheerfully interrupted his own academic work whenever a screech from my adjacent study signaled a need for his assistance when I was frustrated with the computer or a contributor. The American Psychiatric Association Publishing team, as always, joined in the effort to produce the best possible book. Bob Hales and John McDuffie prodded me to consider a new edition of this book sooner rather than later. Greg Kuny, Managing Editor, Books, provided scheduling structure and wise advice. Carrie Farnham, Senior Editor, Books, edited with care, wisdom, and restraint. Most of all, the chapter authors were generous with their expertise, energetic regarding updating their content to the cutting edge, and patient with the restrictions on length and my detailed editing. They received my reminders and responded (mostly promptly). I have learned a great deal in this process, which is one of the best reasons to edit such a book. I am deeply grateful.

Acknowledgments

PART I

Assessment and Diagnosis

CHAPTER 1

The Process of Assessment and Diagnosis

John D. O'Brien, M.D.

The purpose of a psychiatric evaluation is to answer several fundamental questions. The first is: Does this child or adolescent have one or more psychiatric disorders? If the answer is yes, the next question confronting the clinician is: What is the disorder(s)? (Do the symptoms and their patterns fit a known recognizable clinical syndrome or diagnosis?) The next question is: How did this disorder come to be? (What are the factors—biological, psychological, and social—that have influenced this child or adolescent and his family to be in their current state and present for evaluation?) The final fundamental question for the evaluation is: What is the recommended treatment (if any)?

These are very complex questions and require the collecting, sifting, and prioritizing of data from many sources. While there are several supplemental ways to gather information about a child and his family (e.g., agency reports, questionnaires, rating scales), the clinical interview of both the parents and the child is the primary source of information that will be used to come to a diagnosis, formulate a case, and provide a treatment plan. This chapter focuses on the process of assessment, diagnosis, and treatment planning. The direct interview of the child at various ages is covered in Chapter 2, "Assessing Infants and Toddlers"; Chapter 3, "Assessing the Preschool-Age Child"; Chapter 4, "Assessing the Elementary School–Age Child"; and Chapter 5, "Assessing Adolescents."

Some general comments must be kept in mind regarding the assessment process, which is too often focused on what is wrong with the child. It is essential to also look at the strengths and assets of the child, the family, and their environment. What are the factors that help to facilitate a child's normal developmental trajectory? Often a parent will come in with a litany of complaints about the child. It is important for the clinician to listen carefully but then to ask a question such as "What are the things your child does well?" or "What about your child makes you proud?"

No assessment is complete without including an evaluation of the impairment caused by the syndrome—often referred to as *severity.* This level of impairment or severity needs to be ascertained to answer the question of whether intervention is needed and, if so, what kind of intervention and in what time frame. For example, for the symptom of aggression, is the aggression at home, at school, and/or on the playground? Is the aggression toward the self, others, or both? How has this symptom affected the patient's relationships with family, peers, and so forth? The answers to these questions not only give the clinician a picture of the impact caused by the symptom but also point the way to various interventions. Severity often influences clinical decision making in assessing the urgency of intervention. Is the aggression affecting safety of self or others? If so, the clinician needs to act quickly to prevent harm.

The evaluation of any child requires the use by the clinician of a *developmental framework.* The clinician, through his or her knowledge of development, has in mind an idea of what the average expectable child will be like at any given age. The child's developmental profile will be compared with a developmental standard as the clinician seeks to discover if this child's behavior or degree of competence in any particular area differs significantly from that of the child's peers. The pediatrician uses height and weight charts to assess a child's physical growth. The psychiatric clinician does not have such specifics but applies the same process of evaluation of normality and deviation from it. The developmental perspective brings the clinician back to the aforementioned issue of impairment: How do the present impairments caused by the child's symptoms affect the developmental tasks of the child and the acquisition of new skills? Finally, do the current adaptation and set of problems reflect a disorder rooted in earlier developmental periods, and/or how will this current status affect later development? While these questions are paramount in the mind of the clinician, these are the same questions that parents will ask, particularly with regard to future functioning.

Comparison of Adult Assessment With Child Assessment

Sullivan (1954) defined an adult psychiatric interview as

> a situation of primarily *vocal* communication in a *two-group,* more or less *voluntarily integrated,* on a progressively unfolding *expert-client* basis for the purpose of elucidating *characteristic patterns of living* of the subject person, the patient or client, which patterns he experiences as particularly troublesome or especially valuable, and in the revealing of which he expects to derive *benefit.* (p. 4)

The prime source of information in the evaluation of an adult is the person himself. There are some exceptions to this, particularly in the geriatric population, where other informants, especially caregivers, are needed. It would be quite unusual for a psychiatrist to request information from the employer of an adult patient. However, multiple sources, especially the parents, constitute the field for data collection with children. At the very least, Sullivan's "two-group" becomes a three-group or a four-group (in intact families). Teachers, guidance counselors, and foster care workers all contribute essential data. In an overwhelming majority of child assessments, information from the school is needed regarding not only academic status but also social relatedness to peers and adults. A child psychiatrist sees contacting the school and other agencies as a necessary and vital part of a complete evaluation. Children are strongly affected by their environment, and the evaluation needs to take that into account.

The interchange between psychiatrist and adult patient is generally verbal, with some data gathered from nonverbal communication. While this is true for most adolescents, the younger the child, the more central is the role of play in the evaluation process. How a child plays and what he plays is a window to the child and his world. In the assessment of the infant or preschool child, there is less emphasis on verbal production, and the clinician needs to be well versed in the popular toys, video games, and so forth that form an important part of a child's life.

The issue of *volitional participation* is another area of difference. Children are brought to the evaluation; they rarely seek it out. Infants and children are brought because, in general, their behavior is bothersome to others, not necessarily to themselves. An old-fashioned example illustrates this point. If Johnny puts Mary's pigtail in the inkwell, who has the problem? If the individual does not see himself as having a problem, the person certainly will not seek help.

The concept of the psychiatrist as expert is not easily grasped by a child. Adults generally see the psychiatrist as someone from whom they can benefit, even though they may approach the process with trepidation. Generally, when children come to see a doctor, they have two associations—needles and white coats. As a result, this issue has to be dealt with in preparing the child for evaluation. Most children do not see the doctor as particularly helpful. In fact, children are wary of the experience and often see the psychiatrist as an annoyance—someone who takes them away from their baseball game, video game, and so forth. The usual positive expectations that provide motivation for the initial phases of adult evaluation are absent with children. Thus, the child and adolescent psychiatrist has to work much harder to establish rapport and a working relationship with the child, who often regards him or her with suspicion or even as an agent of the parents or the school. The primary purpose of the initial phase of an assessment is to put the child at ease, present to him in language he is able to understand the purpose of the assessment and why he is there, and establish a working relationship. It must be emphasized that the evaluation is a collaboration among the parents, the child, and the psychiatrist. All three parties work together to facilitate the psychiatric evaluation.

Data Collection

The assessment of children and adolescents must be multifaceted. The clinician assesses multiple domains and dimensions of functioning, regardless of the reason for referral. Information is gathered about various situations from diverse informants, using multiple methods.

In addition to focusing on the nature and type of the specific referral problem, the clinician should assess all areas of the child's functioning and various dimensions of the child's capabilities, including cognitive abilities and interpersonal relationships (home and peers). The clinician should also assess for other symptoms that may be comorbid with the presenting problem.

Information concerning child and adolescent functioning in four different areas (home, school, with peers, with himself) needs to be gathered:

1. How does the child function at home? This information can be obtained from parents, the child himself, babysitters, siblings, grandparents, and so forth.
2. The school is the child's workplace, where he spends much time. Again, the clinician looks to the child and parents. However, teachers, guidance counselors, and principals are the main sources of information in this area, with parental consent for contact. Not only does the clinician get data regarding academic progress from the school, but the school can give valuable information regarding the child's peer relationships and relationships with those in authority.
3. The clinician gets data on peer relationships from parents, children themselves, and school reports. An opportunity to actually observe the child with peers provides uniquely valuable information. Peers have a great deal of knowledge about other children, but it is difficult to tap this source of information without breaking confidentiality. Knowledge about current and past relationships is crucial in assessing a child's social and interpersonal competence.
4. All too frequently neglected is how the child views himself. Collateral information can be gathered from parents and the school, but the major source of data is the child himself. Often the child's view of himself cannot be assessed directly. The clinician must use indirect means, such as drawings, dreams, and fantasy questions.

What are the tools or instruments that the clinician uses to view these four domains? What do clinicians do in the clinical setting to complete an assessment? They use some or all of the following: an interview with the parents and/or significant others; observation and interview of the child; family interviews; behavioral ratings by parents, teachers, the child, and significant others; physical examination; neurological examination; psychological and neuropsychological testing; and various biological and laboratory measures.

The relative value of each of these components in evaluating a particular child varies with the child's age, developmental state, and presenting problems. Interviews with the parents, observation of and interviews with the child, and use of behavioral rating scales in different settings are essential for any psychiatric assessment done today. Each element can provide unique information. In certain cases, specialized psychological testing, laboratory measures, and physical and neurological exams may add useful information. The important point is that sufficient data be collected to assess all areas of current functioning of the child and that, on the basis of a developmental history, functioning from birth to the present be assessed.

Beginning the Process

The initial contact for the evaluation most likely begins with a telephone call from the parents, who may be acting on their own or in conjunction with or at the behest of an agency, such as the school. This initial contact is important because it sets a tone for the evaluation process to come. The person taking the call must remember that parents have many emotions related to this call, most commonly anxiety. The usual identifying data are taken about *both* the parents and the child. In some instances, who has custody of the child and who can give permission for the evaluation to take place become an issue. This is particularly true for children in foster care and in divorce situations. A brief history of the reason for the referral is then taken. Obviously, the information gatherer needs to assess if the presenting problem constitutes an emergency and, if so, deal with that issue. (Emergencies are discussed in Chapter 30, "Psychiatric Emergencies.") The contact person explains to the parent in as succinct and clear a way as possible the process of the evaluation. Depending on a variety of factors, such as age and clinic policy, the parents may be seen first. For adolescents, the identified patient may be seen initially. In some instances the family as a whole will be seen. Whatever the process, it should be clearly explained. A general description of what will happen in each part of the evaluation is discussed, such as that the parents will be seen by the clinician to gather their ideas about the problem and a developmental history. Some estimate of the length of each session and a summary of who is expected to be there are given. If previous evaluations have been done or there is pertinent current collateral information, parents are asked to either send it in advance or bring it with them. When school problems are at issue, report cards, special education evaluations, results of psychological testing, and so forth need to be included. It is helpful if previous data can be reviewed prior to the first meeting. Finally, payment, such as fees, insurance coverage, authorization, or other issues, needs to be discussed. Thoroughness and directness are necessary so that parents can be prepared for the process. It is important to ask if there are any questions and to inform the parents whom to contact with questions or additional information. Although this process may be lengthy, such completeness at the beginning saves time later and facilitates forming an alliance with parents that is crucial to the successful completion of the evaluation.

The Parent Interview

The purposes of the parental interview include gathering data about the current problem; determining what interventions, if any, have been previously tried; and taking a detailed developmental history. The clinician aims to assess parental understanding of the problem and ex*pectations of the assessment, as well as parenting strengths and weaknesses. For treatment planning, it is important to get a sense of how the parents might view treatment recommendations. For example, some parents may strenuously object to the use of medication. The parental interview also serves to gather information that may help the clinician in approaching the child, such as favorite activities, interests, and strengths. Finally, the parent interview gives the clinician an opportunity to determine what preparation, if any, the parents have given to the child for the evaluation and, if necessary, to recommend other approaches that may facilitate the child's participation. This process also gives clues to how the child is perceived in the family and the degree of thoughtfulness and caring the parents show their offspring.

It is extremely important to ascertain what the parents want from the evaluation and immediately deal with inappropriate expectations. The parents, child, referring agency, and so forth likely have different goals for the process.

Case Example 1

A mother of a 9-year-old boy, Evan, sought evaluation because she felt the visitation schedule set out in the divorce settlement was a burden for her son and was affecting his schoolwork. I made it clear from the beginning that I would not get involved in revisiting the divorce agreement or testify in court. The mother herself was a lawyer. She agreed to my focus and said this is what she wanted. After much work evaluating the mother and her husband, Evan's father, and Evan alone and with each parent and discussions with the school, I proposed a plan that I felt would put the least onus on the child. The mother immediately rejected it. It became clear that her real purpose was to change the custody judgment and show her ex-husband to be a poor father (which was not the case). When the plan was not to her liking, she revealed her real reason for the evaluation and refused to pay for the last session. Even though what I would do was initially made clear, she had a very different expectation. Every effort should be made at the very outset to have a frank discussion of what the evaluation is for and what can or cannot be accomplished.

It is important to make it clear to the parents that this is not treatment but an evaluation and that the evaluation may or may not lead to intervention. The clinician needs to focus on getting the data, formulating the data, arriving at a diagnosis, and establishing a treatment plan (which may or may not involve the evaluating clinician). An alliance with the parents and child not only will form the basis for a good evaluation but also will set the groundwork for whatever future work may be needed.

The confidentiality of the sessions between the child and the clinician needs to be discussed up front with the parents and child. Parents are reminded that unless there is an overriding reason (such as a danger to self or others), the specifics of the interactions between the clinician and child are confidential. However, what is said between the parents and the therapist may be brought up with the child. It is not uncommon for parents to come to the clinician after the first session and ask how it went or if the child did or said this or that. The clinician might share in advance with the parents that they may be curious about the session but details will not be reported back to them unless, for example, there is a safety concern.

Preparation of the Child for the Interview

The parents' preparation of the child for the interview can be crucial for its success or failure.

Case Example 2

A parent sought consultation regarding her teenage son, James, who was presenting with a somatic symptom. It was a very complicated case, and the mother had not told her son she was seeking an evaluation. I discussed with her in great detail how to present to James the need and reason for evaluation. He had been seen by other medical subspecialists, so she asked if she could tell him it was another medical evaluation (as opposed to a psychiatric one). I told her that would not work because James would feel deceived and tricked, which would negatively affect the process. I reinforced with her what I had said previously. James arrived promptly and we began speaking. I explained who I was and

> what I intended to do. He jumped up and said that he thought I was another type of specialist and that he certainly did not need to see a shrink, and ran from the room. His mother then confessed she had lied to James about my specialty and the purpose of the session. Despite strenuous efforts, he would not continue the evaluation.

Obviously, how the parents approach this issue will depend on the age of the child, the purpose of the evaluation, and the parent-child relationship. The idea that the child has nothing to fear from the evaluation and the doctor (e.g., no needles) needs to be conveyed by the parents and later the clinician. The best way to do this is a forthright discussion of the symptom or issue at hand. The parents can say that the clinician works with children who have troubles at home, at school, or with other children. He or she is an expert in children's troubles. He or she is a talking doctor and may also play and draw. This direct approach works well with most children. With younger children, the clinician is quite concrete about the problem and its consequences. With adolescents, it is helpful to discuss the effect the symptom has on their social and psychological lives.

Other Sources of Data

The clinician should obtain (with permission) information from others in the child's community. This information gives other viewpoints about the child. Bringing this information back to the interview with parents, child, or family may stimulate further disclosure and discussion essential to diagnosis and treatment. Asking parents what they think and how they feel about the various reports provides data on how they see the problem, their defensive maneuvers (denial, blaming, and so forth), their motivation for change, and how they may view treatment recommendations.

The most important of these "outside" reports is the school report. Teachers spend long periods of time with the child, and they observe the child's response to work demands and learning. They are able to compare the child with same-age peers. The school is also the natural setting for interactions with other children. At school, the child's behavior and symptoms can be different from anywhere else. The behavior in school must be compared with the behavior at home and in the clinician's office (on a one-to-one basis). Another important source of information is the pediatrician, who often contributes both a medical perspective and a longitudinal view of the child's and family's development. Particularly important is whether the pediatrician had seen the need for and recommended psychiatric evaluation and how that recommendation had been presented and received. Data also can be gathered from other agencies, such as child welfare or protective services, foster care, and courts.

The clinician should remember to get information about hobbies, group activities, and athletics. These can help the clinician understand how the child organizes his life and follows rules, what his capacity to function as a team member is, what his competitive strategies are, and how he sees himself in relation to others. The child's willingness to accept delays, capacity to persevere, ability to organize a project, and creativity can be estimated from these activities.

Family Assessment

Some clinicians prefer to have a family interview as a part of the assessment process. This can be helpful in many ways, particularly if it is the initial contact beginning the evaluation. With the family together, the clinician can clarify why the child is being brought for evaluation and inform everyone about the evaluation process. On the other hand, such a meeting can be held at any time during the evaluation process or not at all. The Group for the Advancement of Psychiatry (1973) listed eight major reasons for a family interview: to establish

> the nature of the family as a unit (stable, cohesive, divisive, close, distant), the family capacity for cooperation with treatment plans, the psychological-mindedness of members of the family, the capacity for communication among family members, the degree of mental health or ill health of the family as a unit or in terms of the individual members, the role of the child's disorder in the psychic economy of the family (secondary gain, or family misuse of the child's disorder), the relationship of the family to the community (distant, isolated, involved) and the subcultural values dominant in the family. (p. 556)

In a family interview, the clinician is able to glimpse the ways the members of the family live with each other. Whether or not the family interactions contribute to the child's problems, they can be helpful or detrimental to a treatment proposal. Family members other than the identified patient may suffer from stressful interactions within the family or may be negatively affected by the child's symptoms. This is particularly true of siblings in a family with a developmentally disabled or chronically physically or emotionally ill child. Finally, in any family assessment interview, the clinician needs to establish that the group is embarking on an effort to find real solutions to real problems and not to assign blame.

Formulation

One of the most crucial phases of the evaluation process is the *formulation,* which is too often misunderstood or neglected. A common error is to simply repeat the history instead of constructing a formulation of a case. As Jellinek and McDermott (2004) stress, "The presence of symptoms is only a starting point, not sufficient by itself for us to understand the context, feelings or behavior behind them" (p. 914). Formulations are typically organized in one of two ways: using a biopsychosocial approach or a shortened form of a temporal axis (Ebert et al. 2000, pp. 520–521). In the biopsychosocial model, those variables that influence the child and family to present in their current state are grouped into three categories: biological, psychological, and social. Biological factors include, but are not limited to, genetic factors, pregnancy and birth factors, and medical illnesses. Some examples of psychological factors are the child's and family's level of development, self-esteem, and ego defenses. Social variables include family functioning, spiritual and cultural issues, and peers. Ebert et al. (2000) suggest another viewpoint—that of looking at factors along a time axis grouped as predisposing, precipitating, perpetuating, and prognostic. *Predisposing factors* are genetic heritability, intrauterine or perinatal insults, neglect, and so forth. *Precipitating factors* are defined as stressors (e.g., physical illness, loss, divorce) that test the coping mechanisms and cause signs and symptoms to occur. *Perpetuating factors* (e.g., continuous trauma, parental style) are those that reinforce symptomatology. *Prognostic factors* are those that influence a child's symptom future, duration of illness, severity of illness, time of onset of illness, and so forth. Regardless of which system the clinician uses, "a formulation is necessary to sift, prioritize, and integrate the data for treatment planning" (Jellinek and McDermott 2004, p. 913).

The formulation leads to a differential diagnosis wherein the clinician considers the most likely diagnoses and chooses one or more that are consistent with the data. The purpose of the entire process is to make treatment recommendations tailored for the child and the family.

Treatment Planning

According to the Group for the Advancement of Psychiatry (1973), "Differential treatment planning consists of selecting, in order of priority, curative, corrective, ameliorative or palliative approaches to the child patient, his family, and, when needed, his extended environment. Such planning takes the fullest advantage of the available assets of the child, his family and the community" (p. 546). Looney (1984) makes the case for treatment planning:

> The skillful matching of a child's problems with appropriate interventions is as important as either an accurate assessment of the nature of those problems or a skillful application of any modality of treatment. A misalignment of a child's constellation of problems with an array of therapeutic interventions even if those interventions are artfully administered, may lead to an unsatisfactory outcome. (p. 529)

Treatment planning is done by the clinician or clinical team after the formulation and differential diagnosis. The clinician has found a set of problems that besets the child, family, and/or community, as well as assets or strengths that can be used to help alleviate these problems. Both behavioral and psychodynamic paradigms are useful. In child work, a combination is usually done. These problems and interventions then need to be put in terms understandable to the family and child.

Ebert et al. (2000, pp. 523–524) have put forth a highly structured approach to treatment planning, which is called *goal-directed treatment planning.* This approach emphasizes *pivotal foci,* which are "factors external or internal that activate, reinforce or perpetuate psychopathology." *Goals* are the aims a clinician wants to achieve. A goal is a focus preceded by a verb. For example, a focus might be depressed mood (the problem) preceded by a verb (e.g., alleviate depressed mood). There may be a variety of goals, which lead to different verbs, such as reduce the frequency or intensity of, stabilize, or facilitate. To these are added *objectives,* which are things "the patient will be able to do or exhibit at the end of that stage of treatment." For Ebert's group, the objective is stated in behavioral terms (e.g., the child will be able to not fight or to hold his temper). Finally, "for each goal, the clinician selects a therapy or set of therapies, according to the following criteria: most empirical support, resource availability (i.e., clinical resource, time, finances), least risk, greatest economy (i.e., time, expense) and appropriateness to family values and intervention style" (Ebert et al. (2000). As treatment progresses, the goals are monitored and revised as necessary.

In summary, the process is to 1) identify the problems and determine 2) what changes in the problems the clinician wishes to see, 3) the order in which the clinician needs to deal with them, and 4) the interventions most appropriate not only to the problem but to this child and his family.

The order of interventions must be considered. Obviously, the acuity of a situation or safety issues will determine what is to be addressed first. However, in most cases the problems are semiacute or chronic. In some cases, a child may be so depressed that medication may be needed first before the child can use any type of psychotherapy. Or in the reverse case, the clinician may need to start with psychotherapy to form an alliance with the child so that he may become more disposed to take medication. In conjunction with the child and the family, the clinician may choose a problem of lesser severity to work on initially because it is more amenable to timely intervention. Thus, the clinician has an experience of success to build on to approach more complex issues. Looney (1984) sees treatment planning as having two basic steps:

> The first is to formulate the problems and to state them in a commonsense manner so that they can be understood by the child and those referring the child for treatment. In addition, problems should be formulated in such a way that points of intervention and a reasonable order of progression of treatment are clear. The second step is to choose treatment modalities which would be most powerful, most rapid, least restrictive and most cost effective. (p. 530)

Supported by this process of thinking, the clinician approaches the next evaluation phase.

Interpretative or Feedback Interview

The purpose of the interpretive or feedback interview is to inform the parents and child what has been found and what the clinician, with their help, would recommend to address the issues for which they came. This process often is more complicated than in adult psychiatry, where the clinician generally has one patient. In the evaluation of a child, both parents and child need to hear and understand what the clinician says, and their participation in the process needs to be encouraged and enlisted. Also, the issues for which they came may be the tip of the iceberg and may lead to discovery of other problems that were not initially apparent. For example, a child's fighting behavior in school may be a reaction to the loss of a beloved grandparent, with subsequent depression. This sequence needs to be identified and explained.

For the parents, it is useful to start with a summary of what has been done in the assessment process and proceed from there to the findings. It is very important to put the findings in language that is understood by the parents, and it is helpful to give concrete examples from the history as well as the interview to illustrate and support conclusions drawn. Parents may need help to understand that human behavior, especially children's behavior, is shaped by many interacting variables, not a single cause, and because of this complexity, multiple interventions may be needed.

For many, "the evaluation is a crisis for the family, for though they may be aware that something has been wrong for a long time, the diagnosis…confronts them with the reality" (O'Brien et al. 1992, p. 113). Often, the presentation of the results precipitates a state of anxiety akin to an acute stress reaction. There is shock, and even numbness and loss of focus. The clinician needs to be as supportive as possible, explaining what the diagnosis means, how it affects present functioning, what factors contributed to the genesis of the problem, and what needs to be done. The clinician may have to repeat these points several times, because the emotional state of the parents affects their ability to process the information.

Often guilt and anger come to the fore. Parents may ask what they did wrong. At this time, the clinician returns to the statement that behavior is multidetermined. Parents may blame each other or the school. Under these circumstances, emphasis is put on the future, not the past. How can we alter relationships and attitudes to change the situation? Often it is necessary to allow parents to ventilate their feelings about the evaluation and their present situation: "It is not uncommon for the anxiety of making the unknown known to further solidify previous unhealthy patterns. Thus, an overprotective parent may become more intrusive and overinvolved in the child's life. This tendency should be discussed with the parents and examples in their behavior pointed out" (O'Brien et al. 1992, p. 115).

The interview needs to focus on collaboration among the various participants. What is *each participant*—parent(s), child, clinician, agencies, and so forth—going to do to address the issue? Obviously, major emphasis here will be on the family, child, and clinician. While the clinician addresses problems, the clinician should include the positive aspects of the child and family and how these can be used to deal with the problems and form a treatment plan.

The clinician shares with the family the process of treatment planning. What are the family's thoughts about the goals and objectives, and how realistic and applicable are they to the family situation? The more active the parents are in setting up the treatment, the more likely they are to participate in the treatment process and facilitate their child's participation.

A major objective of the feedback session is to help parents realistically appraise their situation and their child. This is especially true for children who have a developmental disability or a chronic illness. In these circumstances, parents need to reevaluate the child and their expectations of the child (O'Brien et al. 1992). For these parents, "the primary issue that has to be worked through is the loss and subsequent mourning of the idealized child" (O'Brien et al. 1992, p. 113).

The clinician should always ask the parents for their understanding of what has been said and how they feel about it. This gives the clinician a chance to see how much the parents heard and understood and to correct any distortions. Parents are urged to go home and discuss the recommendation together and, depending on the age of the child, with the child. Parents are encouraged to ask questions now and in the future. They are given the clinician's telephone number in case they have questions or concerns.

How the clinician talks with the child about the findings is related to the age of the child. With preschoolers, the emphasis is on helping do something or attain something, and considerable assistance is needed from the parents. With school-age children, the clinician deals with concrete issues, such as "help you learn better at school" or "help you get along better with other children." With this age group, the clinician may say, "You came here because of this issue, and this is how we intend to help you with the problem." With early school-age children, the clinician focuses on behavior and doing things. With later school-age children, the clinician can introduce concepts of emotions and inner emotional states (e.g., "We want to help you be happier and less sad"). With adolescents, the clinician addresses a mixture of behavior and feelings, particularly about the self (e.g., "We want you to feel less depressed and feel better about yourself"). Parents need to be told how the child is being approached so they can reinforce the process in the home.

A study by Yeh and Weisz (2001) raises an important point that needs to be considered in any assessment of a child and his family. According to their study, "more than 60% of the parent-child pairs failed to agree on even a single problem for which the child needed help" (p. 1022). Yeh and Weisz suggest that "it may be wise for clinicians to assess parent and child concerns independently and then bring parents and child together to formulate joint goals" (p. 1024). They caution that "whatever the response of therapists and clinics, our findings suggest that parent-child discrepancies in perceived problems can be so pronounced at the beginning of clinic care that it would be unwise to leave them unassessed and unaddressed" (pp. 1024–1025).

When communicating information to others, the clinician should be judicious. No information can be shared without parental (and sometimes adolescent) permission. It is wise for the clinician to summarize what he or she intends to say and even to show parents the reports that will be sent. A large percentage of referrals come at the behest of the school or indicate at least some difficulty at school. Information should be given that relates to school functioning only. Personal issues such as family history of mental illness or marital strife are not shared with school personnel. How to help the child academically, such as small class size, extra time to complete tasks, and sitting near the teacher, should be addressed. Some suggestions related to social interchanges and peer relationships may also be warranted. Information sent to the school is subject to distribution and discussion with numerous people and needs to be given with great care.

Feedback to pediatricians, again with parental knowledge and consent, should be prompt and specific to the question asked and should not be a detailed description, especially about personal issues. What the clinician sees as the problem and what he or she intends to do and how he or she intends to do it should be the focus rather than how things came to be the way they are. Obviously, if the clinician is working closely with a pediatrician on a problem such as nonadherence in a child with diabetes, parents and child need to know that there will be continuous and in-depth exchange of information with the pediatrician but certain information will not be shared.

In working with any agency, parents need to know what the clinician feels are the goals for that agency, such as a more appropriate class or supervised visitation for relatives, and the best way to approach the agencies and work with them. The clinician and parents need to discuss how these goals will affect the child and the treatment plan. Thus, clinician and parents form an alliance to promote change for the child in his environment.

There is a very high rate of dropout in the treatment of children, adolescents, and their families. Establishing an accurate diagnosis through a complete evaluation and formulation and forming an alliance with parents and child through the process of evaluation are the surest ways of helping parents and child enter into treatment positively. A helpful experience in the evaluation process will motivate parents and child to follow through on the treatment that is recommended and bodes well for its success.

Summary Points

- The purpose of a psychiatric evaluation of a child (or adolescent) is to ascertain if the child has a psychiatric disorder and what the next step(s) should be. A child may present with a set of symptoms that may be reactions to environmental circumstances, either familial or school. Who is the patient? is an important question in the evaluation.
- Any evaluation must proceed from a developmental framework.
- A psychiatric evaluation of a child is different from that of an adult.
- Data must be collected from multiple sources, detailing the child's functioning at home, in school, with peers, and alone.
- The child and parental interviews, behavioral ratings, and a recent physical exam form the core of every evaluation. Psychological testing and the like may be needed in specialized cases (see Chapters 2–6 in this textbook).
- The process begins with the first telephone call, and the importance of that tone-setting interchange cannot be overestimated.
- The parental interview has many purposes, chief among which is collecting data (regarding present, past, and expectations) and helping parents prepare the child for his interview. The parental interview gives the clinician the opportunity to form an alliance with the parents, which is crucial to forming an alliance with the child and for involvement in future treatment, if needed.
- The formulation categorizes the biological, social, and psychological factors critical to the genesis of, sustaining of, and future of the psychiatric syndrome.
- Treatment planning matches the problems of child and family with the appropriate interventions in a timely, cost-effective way.
- The feedback interview presents to parents and child what was found and invites their participation in the process. This interview sets the groundwork for building on the alliances formed throughout the evaluation so that treatment flows naturally and smoothly from the evaluation.

References

Ebert MH, Loosen PT, Nurcombe B: Current Diagnosis and Treatment in Psychiatry. New York, McGraw-Hill, 2000

Group for the Advancement of Psychiatry: From diagnosis to treatment: an approach to treatment planning for the emotionally disturbed child. Rep Group Adv Psychiatry 8(87):517–662, 1973 4742034

Jellinek MS, McDermott JF: Formulation: putting the diagnosis into a therapeutic context and treatment plan. J Am Acad Child Adolesc Psychiatry 43(7):913–916, 2004 15213593

Looney JG: Treatment planning in child psychiatry. J Am Acad Child Psychiatry 23(5):529–536, 1984 6481025

O'Brien JD, Pilowsky D, Lewis O: Psychotherapies With Children and Adolescents: Adapting the Psychodynamic Process. Washington, DC, American Psychiatric Press, 1992

Sullivan HS: The Collected Works of Harry Stack Sullivan, Vol 1: The Psychiatric Interview. Edited by Perry HS, Gawel ML. New York, WW Norton, 1954

Yeh M, Weisz JR: Why are we here at the clinic? Parent-child (dis)agreement on referral problems at outpatient treatment entry. J Consult Clin Psychol 69(6):1018–1025, 2001 11777105

CHAPTER 2

Assessing Infants and Toddlers

Mary Margaret Gleason, M.D.
Charles H. Zeanah, M.D.

Considerable evidence supports the importance of experiences in early childhood that provide the foundation for development across multiple developmental domains. Increasingly, opportunities for early intervention include attention to the mental health needs of infants and toddlers. Early intervention programs provide opportunities for collaboration among mental health, health, and developmental specialists to formulate an understanding of the clinical concerns and strengths. Infant and early childhood psychiatry is a strength-based, prevention-focused subspecialty of child and adolescent psychiatry and one component of the interdisciplinary field of infant mental health. Focused on early identification of risk and resilience factors and mental health disorders in infants, young children, and their families, clinical practice in early childhood mental health requires a specialized assessment approach somewhat different from that used with older children and adolescents.

The practice of "infant mental health," a field that includes care of children up to age 5 or 6 years, explicitly focuses on the emotional well-being of a young child embedded in a complex set of contexts, including the child's neurobiological endowment as well as the larger family, social, and cultural contexts in which the child develops. This approach to families is founded on an empirical base that demonstrates the importance of prenatal factors, developmental level, quality of relationships, and cumulative exposure to risk and protective factors in young children's current and future functioning (Shonkoff et al. 2012). In the last decade, the empirical base highlighting the biological processes that underlie the links between early experiences and developmental trajectory has grown exponentially. We have long known that infancy and toddlerhood are characterized by extraordinarily rapid development. During early childhood, rates of synaptogenesis are as high as 700 per second in the early years, brain volume reaches 80% of adult size by 36 months of life, and children demonstrate rapid progress through observable physical and emotional developmental milestones (Nelson and Bosquet 2000; Shonkoff et al. 2012). Increasingly, research shows that prenatal and early experiences are linked to measurable differences at the genetic, hormonal, and brain region volume levels, with indications that these markers of adversity are associated with later psychopathology and other adverse health outcomes (Drury et al. 2012; Essex et al. 2013; Luby et al. 2012; Monk et al. 2012; Zalewski et al. 2012).

Relational Approach to Assessing Infants and Toddlers: Rationale and Implications

In the clinical practice of infant and early childhood mental health, the primary focus of assessment is the young child's important caregiving relationships. In isolation, the individual characteristics of the infant or toddler have limited predictive value for the child's future development. The child's important caregiving relationships, on the other hand, are far more predictive of subsequent outcomes (Shonkoff et al. 2012). Infants who develop a secure attachment relationship with a primary caregiver during the first year of life are more likely to have positive relationships with peers, to be liked by their teachers, to perform better in school, and to be more resilient in the face of stress or adversity as preschoolers and later. Infants who develop an insecure attachment relationship, in contrast, are at risk for a more troublesome trajectory. Furthermore, secure attachments buffer stress (Tharner et al. 2012) and are especially protective in more extreme conditions (McGoron et al. 2012). The infant-caregiver relationship can serve as a buffer against adversity or can compound other risk factors. Because of the importance of the infant-caregiver relationship, any factors that affect this relationship strongly influence the emotional functioning of the young child. Clinical assessment and treatment focus on systematically identifying and addressing influential patterns in young children's caregiving relationships.

A second reason for a relational focus is that through the caregiving relationships, infants begin to understand the social world, learn how to interact with others, and begin to develop a sense of competence and self-worth. A disturbed relationship may adversely affect a child's social and relational development by changing these experiences. Additionally, even when a young child's development is at risk because of factors outside of the caregiving relationship, intervening through the infant-caregiver relationship may be the most effective means of buffering the child against the risks.

Third, environmental risks exert their effect on the young child primarily through the caregiving relationship. Poverty, for example, is a well-known risk factor in young children, but it means little to an infant to be poor except as poverty is experienced through the infant's primary caregiving relationships (Conradt et al. 2013; Knitzer and Perry 2012).

Fourth, intrinsic risk factors and biological processes can be moderated by the infant's caregiving relationships. For example, the quality of the caregiving relationship predicts cognitive outcomes in infants born preterm (Bergman et al. 2010; Treyvaud et al. 2009).

Young children construct relationships with their caregivers on the basis of experiences they have had with them. There is no evidence that children during the first 18–24 months of life can even imagine what they have not experienced directly. On the basis of experience, young children may develop different kinds of relationships with different caregivers, as has been demonstrated in attachment research in which young children are found simultaneously to have different types of attachments to different caregivers.

A child may have qualitatively different relationships with different caregiving adults. During a clinical assessment, the clinician always considers the possibility that a described or observed pattern of behaviors or symptoms is relationship-specific. The more consistently a child's oppositional behavior, for example, is observed in different important relationships, the more confident the clinician can be that the problem is pervasive and not relationship-specific. In clinical practice, however, it is not uncommon for symptomatic behavior observed in young children to be relationship-specific and require interventions focused at one or more components of the relationship. Relationship-focused interventions may target the caregiver's perceptions of the child, the caregiver's interactive behavior with the child, and the child's behaviors with the caregiver. A comprehensive relationship assessment will examine each of these components of the assessment as described later in this chapter (see section "Comprehensive Assessment").

The final implication of this model is that clinically significant problems may derive primarily from within the child, primarily from within the parent, or from the unique pattern of interactions between the two. In most cases, all of these sources contribute to some degree. In most cases, the intervention implemented will most likely use the parent-child relationship as a primary vehicle for change.

Diagnostic Issues Regarding Disorders of Early Childhood

The consideration of diagnoses in infants and toddlers is fraught with controversy. In most of medicine, diagnosis is a primary determinant of treatment planning. From a clinical perspective, systematic use of diagnostic nosologies promotes clear communication across providers and with families. Systematic use of these diagnoses in clinical settings can also facilitate clinical research that can inform further refinement of the criteria.

Diagnosis in early childhood warrants further consideration. First, most major diagnostic systems focus on the individual and do not provide mechanisms to incorporate relationship factors into the diagnostic approach. Second, in this age group, interventions may be implemented to target risk status rather than for fully developed psychiatric diagnoses. Among early childhood mental health clinicians, there are providers who are reluctant to apply a diagnosis to an infant or young child because of stigma or limited predictive value or because an individual diagnosis does not include the caregiving contextual factors. Last, the empirical evidence for the validity of diagnoses in this age group is variable and, for some diagnoses, quite limited. Despite efforts to address developmental issues in DSM-5 (American Psychiatric Association 2013), few diagnoses in DSM have been validated in infants and toddlers.

The early childhood mental health community has made efforts to address the developmental specificity of diagnoses in young children. The American Academy of Child and Adolescent Psychiatry's Task Force on Research Diagnostic Criteria developed the Research Diagnostic Criteria: Preschool Age (RDC:PA) to increase consistency of application of diagnoses in research settings (Task Force on Research Diagnostic Criteria: Infancy Preschool 2003). This nosology applied evidence-based modifications to the DSM-IV criteria (American Psychiatric Association 1994). Zero to Three has published two editions of Diagnostic Criteria 0–3 (DC:0–3), and a third edition is scheduled for publication in 2016 to provide an empirically derived system of diagnosis for the youngest patients (Zero to Three Diagnostic Classification Task Force 1994, 2005). This multiaxial system includes explicit attention to the primary caregiving relationship.

A few efforts to examine the validity and use of the DC:0–3 system have been reported. Studies that compared DC:0–3R diagnoses to those of the ICD or DSM systems, for example, have reported high concordance (Dunst et al. 2006). To facilitate implantation of these developmentally specific criteria, a number of states and local entities, including Colorado, Indiana, Florida, Washington, Michigan, and Maine, have approved the use of "crosswalks" from the DC:0–3R system to the ICD system to allow clinicians to apply the developmentally appropriate diagnosis and receive reimbursement for the care they provide (Zero to Three 2007). Such innovations are necessary to ensure that young children have adequate access to care in systems where diagnosis can drive reimbursement.

In all nosologies, rigorous use of all axes in the multiaxial system is necessary, as the other axes may be as or more important than the Axis I diagnosis. Although the DSM-5 nosology does not include the traditional five axes, attention to developmental status (formerly Axis II), medical or biological conditions (formerly Axis III), environmental factors (formerly Axis IV), and the child's level of functioning or impairment (formerly Axis V) contribute to the understanding of the child and family. The DC:0–3R system includes a relationship classification axis (Axis II) and a social-emotional functioning axis (Axis V). Regardless of the classification system applied, caregiver-child relationship qualities, biological factors, environmental and family stressors and strengths, and child functioning all must be considered in the clinical formulation and treatment planning.

Assessment Settings

Assessments of infants and toddlers can occur in a number of different settings. In all clinical settings, collaboration and cross-specialty education for providers are important components of infant mental health services. Sometimes, assessments occur within an office-based mental health setting, where the child psychiatrist may be a solo practitioner (who collaborates with colleagues who work in different settings) or part of a clinical team. Increasingly, other clinical settings, such as early intervention programs, pediatric primary care practices, inpatient pediatric units, juvenile court settings, child care centers, child protection services, or homeless shelters, can include infant mental health services. New or enhanced federal funding programs such as the Substance Abuse and Mental Health Services Administration's Project LAUNCH, the Affordable Health Care Act's maternal infant and early childhood home visiting programs, and quality child care initiatives highlight mental health or social-emotional well-being in very young children and promote the implantation of infant and early childhood mental health in nontraditional settings (The White House 2014). In nontraditional settings, the infant mental health assessment may be focused in the context of a larger comprehensive team evaluation or may respond to a specific clinical consultation question and may not require a comprehensive assessment. The setting and specific question usually guide the approach to assessing infants and toddlers.

Wherever the assessment takes place, attention to the physical environment can facilitate the therapist-parent relationship, even before the clinician sees the family. Waiting rooms and offices with child-size furniture and child activities (e.g., culturally appropriate reading material and baby books as well as parenting-focused magazines) may help the family feel welcome even before the assessment begins. Additionally, an office that supports breastfeeding (e.g., by having a breastfeeding room) may help families of breastfeeding infants feel comfortable and may facilitate this healthy practice.

Goals of Infant Mental Health Assessments

The first step in the assessment is to create a warm and welcoming environment for families and, early in the assessment, to develop a shared understanding of the goals and process of the assessment. Stigma can affect all patients seen in child psychiatry practice, but its impact may be especially strong in early childhood. A first step in addressing these concerns may be to acknowledge some of the spoken or unspoken concerns a parent may have about the referral. Parents may be concerned that they are "bad parents" or that the referral indicates concerns that the infant is irremediably disordered. For example, it is not uncommon for low-resource parents to be concerned that an early childhood mental health referral may result in losing custody of the child. Addressing these fears explicitly can be a useful step toward developing a collaborative relationship with the parents.

The clinician-parent relationship is central to the assessment and treatment process. A trusting relationship is necessary for the parent to share openly his or her observations and perceptions of the child, a primary source of the clinical history. In addition, aspects of the clinician-parent relationship may serve as models for ongoing development of the infant-caregiver relationship, especially for parents who have not experienced nurturing, consistent, warm relationships in the past.

Through the assessment, the clinician aims to understand the factors affecting a child's emotional and relationship development, in order to intervene early, reduce current distress and impairment, and positively influence the child's developmental trajectory. Assessments of infants and toddlers should provide sufficient information to develop a biopsychosocial formulation, with a specific focus on the parent-child relationship. The assessment of the relationship is used to understand the strengths and risks conveyed through the relationship and to identify the modalities that will be best suited for treating the dyad.

Comprehensive Assessment

Assessment of infants and toddlers ought to include multiple appointments, using multiple informants, and multiple modes of assessment, including formal and informal observational and history collection procedures (Table 2–1). Including the infant or toddler in most appointments can allow for extensive, informal observations of parent-child interactions and reduces the parent's need for child care during the appointments.

As in all psychiatric interviews, open-ended questions provide useful information. Questions about the child's personality and strengths can be a nonthreatening way to begin the interview, emphasize a strength-based perspective, and provide the clinician with a sense of the parent's ability to describe both the positive attributes and the concerning behaviors of the child.

History of Presenting Problem

In taking the history of present illness, clinicians try to understand the chief complaint in detail, with attention to the child's behavior, the context and potential environmental influences of the behavior, and the parent's reaction (internal and external) to the behavior. Parental responses to a child's behaviors have the potential to help the child regulate behaviors or may exacerbate the pattern. The parent's attribution of meaning to a behavior is crucial. For example, although a 24-month-old's tantrums may seem developmentally appropriate to the clinician, they become an important clinical focus if the parent perceives the child as an aggressor or believes that these behaviors mean the child will follow the path of a psychiatrically disturbed relative.

Review of Systems

A review of psychological and regulatory systems is critical in placing the chief complaint in context. It is helpful to understand the child's self-regulatory skills, including emotional regulation as well as biological processes such as sleep and feeding. These regulatory processes may be the most prominent patterns in young infants. In older toddlers, overall mood and patterns of mood changes, fears, activity level, impulsivity, aggression, and social interactions also contribute to the understanding of the child's emotional functioning. In the interview, it is useful to explore factors in the parent-child relationship, including 1) the child's developing attachment behaviors, such as seeking comfort in times of distress or new situations, as well as experiences of mutual enjoyment, and 2) the parent's expectations and hopes for the child. See section "Formal Assessment Procedures" later in this chapter for more information.

Throughout the interview, the clinician attends to the parent's tone, his or her ability to consider events from the child's perspective or to recognize the child's needs, and the parent's sense of the child as having strengths as well as the problem that brought the family to the evaluation. When two parents are present, observing the way that the parents share the time in the interview and negotiate disagreements and the similarities and differences in the parents' internal working model or perception of

TABLE 2–1. Key elements of the infant-toddler assessment

History (from all available sources)	Child observations	Parent-child interactions	Structured assessment tools
History of presenting problem	Dysmorphic features	Tone of interactions	Parent perception
Review of systems	Size for age	Pacing of interactions	Interview (e.g., Working Model of the Child Interview)
Medical history	Regulatory capacity	Mutual engagement and reciprocity	Structured parent-child interaction (e.g., Crowell procedure)
Developmental history	Behavior with parent vs. examiner	Conflict	Behavior/emotion checklists
Family history	Activity level	Parent responsivity to child	Structured psychiatric interviews
Social history	Patterns of play	Separation and reunion (if developmental age is at least 7 months)	Questionnaires/interviews regarding competence
	Vocalization	Child use of parent for help	

the child yields important information about family functioning.

Medical History

A child's medical history can provide important information about biological influences on development and behavior, as well as events that could affect the infant's and family's emotional development. It is useful to begin the history in the preconception period. Pregnancy planning, including unwanted pregnancies, difficulty conceiving, and pregnancy losses, may influence a parent's expectations about a child. When a mother did not plan or want to be pregnant, it can be useful to understand what influenced her decision (or nondecision) to continue the pregnancy and whether she changed her mind during the pregnancy. For families who have adopted or used reproductive assistive technology or surrogates, it is important to understand these decisions as well. These topics can be included in other parts of the history but often can be easily incorporated into the medical history.

Illnesses during pregnancy, infections, substance use, exposure to violence, and maternal psychopathology all may influence fetal growth and can influence later development (Koren et al. 1998; Yehuda et al. 2005). A history of prematurity, particularly if it necessitated a stay in the neonatal intensive care unit, may have implications for the child's development and may be an early trauma impacting the parent-child relationship (Muller-Nix and Forcada-Guex 2009; Vanderbilt and Gleason 2010). In addition to major medical events or hospitalizations, it is useful to explore any history of colic, failure to thrive, elevated serum lead levels, pica, head trauma, or other central nervous system events that may be related to the infant's or toddler's presentation (Coolbear and Benoit 1999; Lidsky and Schneider 2006)

Developmental History

Every child seen for an infant psychiatry assessment warrants an assessment of developmental milestones to understand the child in the context of his or her developmental pattern in relation to the chronological age. Standardized measures, such as the Ages and Stages Questionnaire (Squires and Bricker 2009), may be useful adjuncts to this clinical evaluation. The Centers for Disease Control and Prevention also has free, clinically useful, albeit not validated, developmental checklists and handouts for parents (http://www.cdc.gov/ncbddd/childdevelopment). Clinicians with less familiarity with typical development may use a low threshold for requesting a formal assessment of a child's development, as developmental status may greatly influence the clinical presentation.

Attention to atypical development that could indicate autism spectrum disorder patterns is warranted in assessing very young children. The DSM-5 criteria for autism spectrum disorder include two main categories—persistent deficits in social communication and interactions and repetitive patterns or sensory hypo- or hyper-reactivity (American Psychiatric Association 2013). In very young children, observations of reciprocity by eye contact and joint attention, gestural communication, ability to participate in social interactions, and (in older children) representational play are particularly important. Because of the powerful effects of evidence-based interventions on this neurodevelopmental disorder, vigilance for signs of autism spectrum disorder is warranted.

Family History

The family psychiatric history can be of particular importance in the infant psychiatry assessment. It can be helpful to draw a multiple-generation genogram to clarify the relationships among family members, provide an opportunity to learn more about the parents' early caregiving environments, and identify potential genetic influences as well as patterns of relationships among family members. When parents or other adults in the household have histories of psychiatric disorders, a sensitive exploration of their current symptoms and how the symptoms influence the child or the parent's caregiving style is warranted. Furthermore, when family histories are positive for certain disorders, parents may fear that the child's behavior problems are reflective of those disorders.

Social History

As noted earlier, the context of early childhood development is the primary caregiving relationship. This relationship exists within a larger social context, with factors that can support or impair a child's social and emotional development. Thus, the social history in infant psychiatry ought to include attention to household members, extended family, cultural or spiritual influences, and community factors, including support systems or early adversity. Support systems are varied and may include extended family, a faith community, or a supportive neighborhood or educational setting (Lieberman et al. 2005). The definition of early adversity is broad and may include the events measured in the Adverse Childhood Experiences Study (child abuse or neglect, family violence, caregiver incarceration, caregiver psychopathology, parental separation) but may also include parental history of abuse, institutional care, natural or man-made community disasters, community violence, and even prenatal exposures to adversity (Drury et al. 2012; Felitti et al. 1998; Hunter et al. 2011). A growing literature demonstrates that the long-lasting sequelae of these experiences, likely through epigenetic changes, predict measurable biological differences, cognitive problems, and psychiatric disorders into adolescence (Tyrka et al. 2013). Family violence, including partner violence and child abuse, is a particularly important influence that may be ongoing and may not be shared spontaneously.

Because perspectives on parenting and parent-child relationships may differ across cultures, even within ethnic groups, it can be useful to explore the family's expectations about the parent-child relationship and the types of interactions that are culturally acceptable or optimal. Understanding these expectations facilitates a collaborative therapeutic process with the parent.

Finally, the impact of community factors, parents' perceptions of safety within the home and community, and the degree to which the parents feel they can meet the basic needs of their family can be strong influences on the clinical presentation and appropriate interventions. Some clinical infant mental health programs include intensive case management to meet the family's basic needs, with the recognition that a family may not be able to participate in needed therapy if the parents' primary concern relates to having enough food to feed their children or threats of eviction.

Observations

In any infant psychiatry assessment, observations of parent-child interactions and clinician interactions with the child are important components of the evaluation. Observing the infant and parent-child interactions while taking the history allows the clinician to examine unscripted interactions and behaviors. Additionally, it can be useful for clinicians to observe a specific activity in all assessments, such as a feeding of a young infant or a free-play period with toddlers. Observations of infants include noting the infant or young child's appearance, including the presence of stigmata of genetic syndromes that may influence behavior or development, such as fragile X, or those associated with prenatal teratogenic exposures such as alcohol. Behavioral observations of infants and toddlers include level of activity; vocalizations or verbalizations; reciprocity; regulatory capacity (level of arousal, ability to reorganize after limit setting or frustration); and, in toddlers, patterns of play and aggressive behaviors. Observable patterns of emotional development are described in Table 2–2.

Domains of parent-child interactions that can be observed informally include the child's use of the parent for assistance, joy sharing, comfort seeking, and play, as well as the parent's anticipation of the infant's needs, responsiveness to the child's cues, ability to structure the interactions to match the child's developmental needs, level of engagement in the interaction, and overall enjoyment of the child. While observing dyadic play, the evaluator can note the level of mutual engagement, shared attention, reciprocity, and, with verbal children, shared representational play themes. The tone of the interaction and the dyad's comfort together, as well as the nature of affective interactions, also reflect the quality of the relationship.

With children whose developmental age is at least 7–9 months, it can be informative to negotiate a separation and reunion during the evaluation to provide an indicator of how the dyad reconnects following a brief separation. Once a child reaches 7–9 months of developmental age, separation activates the child's attachment system, which is manifested by separation anxiety and separation distress. Parents can demonstrate sensitivity by preparing a child for the separation. However, the information most reflective of the quality of the attachment is the dyad's ability to resolve separation distress together during the reunion (Thomas et al. 1997; Zeanah et al. 2000)—that is, whether the child appears to have a strategy for using the parent to resolve her distress, such as seeking proximity to the parent.

Formal Assessment Procedures

Parent-Child Relationship Assessments

A number of structured procedures can augment informal clinical history and observations. In this section, we present selected examples of structured interviews and observational procedures that can be used in clinical settings.

The working model of the child interview is an approximately 1-hour interview focused on a parent's understanding of his or her child and of the relationship they share (available at www.infantinstitute.com/training.htm). During this interview, the parent is asked about the child's personality and the relationship he or she has with the child. The content of the parent's responses can be useful information about the parent's experience of the infant or toddler. Additionally, and often more saliently, a clinician can learn about the parent's internal representation of the child by

TABLE 2–2. Observable patterns of emotional development in clinically salient developmental epochs

Domains	Birth to 2 months	2–7 months	7–18 months	18–36 months
Social	Quiet, alert state evident for minutes at a time	Social smiling Sustained eye-to-eye contact	Stranger wariness Separation protest from attachment figures Social referencing	Awareness of relationship to group More emphasis on personal possessions
Emotional	Crying, peaking at 6 weeks cross-culturally and then waning	Joy, fear, surprise apparent	Affective attunement Greater differentiation of affective states	Moral emotions: shame, guilt, pride
Communicative	Crying indicating distress	Responsive cooing	Intentional communication; some protowords and some words	Expressive language blossoms
Play		Exploratory	Parallel play (12–24 months)	Early representational play (24–36 months)
Gross motor	Improved tone	Rolling over (3–4 months) Sitting independently (6–8 months)	Walking (12–15 months)	Running (1½–2 years); jumping (2½–3 years)
Fine motor		Grasping with one hand (6 months)	Pincer grasp (7–9 months); transfer of objects from one hand to the other (12 months)	Development of hand dominance; ability to stack two blocks at 18 months and eight blocks at 30 months, to scribble spontaneously, and to copy a circle (36 months)
Growth	Regaining of birth weight by 2 weeks	Doubling of birth weight by 4–6 months	Tripling of birth weight at 1 year	Quadrupling of birth weight at 2 years

attending to the characteristics of the narrative itself, including affective tone, level of emotional involvement, coherence of the responses, and the balance of the parent's positive and negative descriptions about the child (Zeanah and Benoit 1995). The interview can be videotaped for further review. When the interview is formally coded for research purposes, parental representation differentiates between clinically referred and non–clinically referred infants (Benoit et al. 1997). Additionally, parents who present balanced representations of their child in the interview are likely to have children who have a secure attachment relationship with the parent, based on the Strange Situation Procedure (Zeanah et al. 1994). Importantly, the interview has been rigorously evaluated in research (Vreeswijk et al. 2012), and it has also been used extensively in clinical settings (Zeanah and Benoit 1995).

The insightfulness assessment (IA) specifically measures a parent's ability to take the infant's perspective (Oppenheim and Koren-Karie 2002). In this procedure, parents are interviewed after reviewing a video of themselves interacting with their child in a structured set of interactions. The interview focuses on the parent's understanding of what the child was feeling and how the parent felt during the video replay. Coding of the interview again focuses on the quality and coherence of the parent's narrative, yielding four groups: positively insightful, one-sided, disengaged, and mixed. The validity of the IA has been demonstrated by associations with child attachment classification, maternal observed sensitivity, and even child theory of mind skills 3 years later (Oppenheim and Koren-Karie 2013). Insightfulness on the IA has been demonstrated to change with dyadic interventions and is associated with improvement in child signs of internalizing and externalizing problems (Oppenheim et al. 2004).

The Circle of Security treatment model includes an interview developed specifically for use in that clinical intervention model. Derived from the Adult Attachment Interview and the Parent Development Interview, the Circle of Security Interview also includes questions about the parent's experience of participating in the Strange Situation procedure (Cooper et al. 2009). From the interview, clinicians can identify the parent's primary defensive strategy or "core sensitivity" from one of three categories: esteem sensitive, safety sensitive, and separation sensitive. This interview may be helpful for clinicians hoping to understand when a parent may feel uncomfortable in the relationship with the child.

Parent-child relationships can also be assessed using observational approaches. In the Crowell procedure (Crowell and Feldman 1988), the parent and child (of at least 6 months developmental age) are observed in a series of activities including free play, cleanup, a bubbles sequence, and four puzzle tasks, as well as a separation and reunion. The procedure provides a standardized method of assessing a number of domains of the parent-child relationship including reciprocal emotions, protection and safety, comforting and comfort seeking, teaching and learning, play, discipline and response to limits, and parental structure and child's self-regulation. The assessment can provide more depth of understanding of the dyad's interactions, capacity for joy, and ability to negotiate stressful situations. The process of separation and reunion provides valuable information about how the child uses the parent for comfort during a mild relationship stressor.

For younger infants (3–6 months), the still-face paradigm can also provide valuable information about dyadic emotional regulation. The procedure includes three phases: a naturalistic interaction, a 3-minute period when the parent maintains a nonreactive ("still") facial expression, and a 3-minute reengagement period when the parent interacts as usual. Responses to the still-face procedure correlate with maternal internal representation of the infant (Rosenblum et al. 2002) and predict future attachment classification. Clinically, the still-face paradigm may provide an opportunity to observe mutual regulatory capacities of an infant and parent.

Measures of Infant or Toddler Functioning

Diagnostic Interviews

Structured interviews may provide a systematic approach to assessing parent report of toddler symptoms and yield information to guide application of diagnoses. These interviews also provide critical information about the level of impairment associated with a child's symptoms and the degree to which a family has accommodated the child's symptoms. As with any single tool, the information provided by systematic interviews can add to the clinical impression and be incorporated into the diagnostic formulation, but these interviews do not, independently, provide sufficient information to make a diagnosis. All parent report measures provide information about the parent's experience and observations of the child and therefore are considered within the context of a larger assessment.

The Preschool Age Psychiatric Assessment (PAPA) was the first comprehensive interview tested for use in young children (Egger and Angold 2006). The PAPA is an interviewer-based psychiatric diagnostic interview focusing on children ages 2–5 years. The interview includes assessment of the symptoms included in DSM-IV, RDC:PA, DC:0–3R, and ICD-10, as well as behavioral patterns applicable to young children but not included in these nosologies. Importantly, the interview examines systematically the impairment associated with the child's symptoms in a number of functional domains. The PAPA has shown similar test-retest reliability as other diagnostic interviews, and outcomes correlate with the Child Behavior Checklist results (Egger et al. 2006). The PAPA was developed as a research tool and in its entirety may not be appropriate for clinical settings, although efforts to create an electronic version may facilitate its clinical use.

The Diagnostic Infant Preschool Structured Interview is a respondent-based interview of parents of children 18–60 months (Scheeringa and Haslett 2010). Like the PAPA, the interview includes symptoms from the RDC:PA and DSM-IV. It also explores the degree to which parents have accommodated their children's behavioral patterns. Test-retest reliability is similar to that of the PAPA, and most symptom scales show meaningful correlation with the Child Behavior Checklist scales and diagnostic categories. The interview is intended to provide an efficient approach to the early childhood diagnostic interview and includes diagnostic algorithms in each module.

Caregiver-Report Checklists

Parent or child care provider report measures can be useful ways of assessing the level of reported symptoms (Table 2–3). Validated, normed measures allow comparison of the child's symptom level with larger populations. Additionally, when completed by more than one reporter, these measures can be used to develop a multidimensional picture about the child in more than one context or relationship. Clinicians can also use these measures to track the symptoms or strengths across time. Although they are useful adjuncts to the clinical assessment, adult report checklists share a number of limitations. Most notably, they reflect the specific subjective experiences and perceptions of the reporter. The best studied influence on parent report measures is maternal depression. Maternal depression is associated with higher levels of reported symptoms than concurrent reports by child care providers, but also higher levels of clinician-observed symptoms in play, especially when mothers have comorbid psychopathology (Carter et al. 2001; Chilcoat and Breslau 1997; Dawson et al. 2003). Researchers and clinicians postulate that maternal depression may influence child behaviors within the relationship and child development in multiple domains, as well as parental sensitivity to challenging child behaviors. It is likely that a myriad of other factors beyond depression also influence reporting patterns. Thus, these checklists are best considered within the context of the complete assessment.

Table 2–3 presents the psychometric properties of selected validated measures that can be used to identify young children with mental health concerns. The measures have used various "gold standards" to demonstrate validity, with some using other parent report checklists like the Child Behavior Checklist as the gold standard and others using diagnostic interviews. Parent report measures of infants' mental health, compared with toddlers', demonstrate lower indices of validity, and the selection of the gold standard marker against which to demonstrate a mental health concern in infants under 12 months remains a challenge (de Wolff et al. 2013). Reports of infant mental health patterns, even more than toddler mental health patterns, can be considered only in the context of the parent-child relationship, and measures that do not assess some aspect of this relationship will likely be inadequate.

Parent Screening

Some clinical problems within the infant-parent relationship may stem from parent distress or psychopathology. Structured tools such as the Edinburgh Postnatal Depression Scale (Cox et al. 1987) and the Patient Health Questionnaires (PHQ-2 and PHQ-9) are effective in identifying parental depression (Olson et al. 2006). The Parenting Stress Index—Short Form (Haskett et al. 2006) may be helpful in assessing parental distress, regardless of the etiology. Although maternal depression may be the best studied form of parental psychopathology in the context of infant and early childhood well-being (Dawson et al. 2003; Seifer et al. 2001), maternal conditions comorbid with depression are the strongest predictor of adverse early childhood outcome (Carter et al. 2001). An expanding literature highlights the biological effects of prenatal and antenatal exposure to parental stressors on infant and later development, increasing the importance of identifying these risks early in young children's lives (O'Connor et al. 2014).

TABLE 2–3. Selected measures of early childhood symptoms

Measure	Ages, months	Domains	Format	Number of items	Validity	Reliability	Special characteristics
Ages & Stages Questionnaires: Social-Emotional (Squires et al. 2002)[a]	6–60	Self-regulation, compliance, communication, adaptive functioning, autonomy, affect, and interaction with people	3-point Likert scale Different forms for each age group (months): 6, 18, 24, 30, 36, 48, 60	22–36	Sensitivity in predicting a positive score on the CBCL and Vineland Social-Emotional Early Childhood Scales, or a known diagnosis: 71%–85% Specificity: 90%–98% In children under 18 months, no correlation with observed infant interactive behavior; high correlation with maternal distress and psychological symptoms (Salomonsson and Sleed 2010)	Excellent test-retest reliability after 1–3 weeks (r=0.91)	Screening measure; includes strength-based items; validity using broadly defined
Child Behavior Checklist 1½–5 (Achenbach and Rescorla 2000)[b]	18–60	Internalizing, externalizing, and total problems	3-point Likert scale	99	Higher scores in clinically referred children than in non–clinically referred children (effect size=0.3); 77% referred sample vs. 26%	1-week test-retest reliability: mean=0.85 (parent report), 0.81 (teacher report)	Computer scoring system; validated teacher rating form
Early Childhood Screening Assessment (Gleason et al. 2010)[c]	18–60	Internalizing, externalizing, relationship, parent depression and distress	3-point Likert scale	40 (36 child-focused, 4 parent-focused)	Sensitivity 86% predicting DIPA diagnosis; specificity 83%; Strong correlations with CBCL and moderate with BITSEA	Test-retest reliability: Spearman's ρ=0.81	Includes parent depression and distress items and opportunity to indicate concern about individual items

TABLE 2–3. Selected measures of early childhood symptoms *(continued)*

Measure	Ages, months	Domains	Format	Number of items	Validity	Reliability	Special characteristics
Infant-Toddler Social and Emotional Assessment and Brief Infant-Toddler Social and Emotional Assessment (Briggs-Gowan and Carter 2002)[d]	12–36	Internalizing, externalizing, dysregulation, and competence	3-point Likert scale	166 (42 for BITSEA)	Correlation with CBCL total problem scores: $r=0.47$ (internalizing problems); $r=-0.67$ (externalizing problems) Correlation with observer ratings $r=0.20$–0.31	Mean 1-month test-retest reliability: $r=0.82$–0.90 for domains	Includes strengths; BITSEA screener (a companion measure) available
Survey of Well-being of Young Children: Baby Pediatric Symptom Checklist and Preschool Pediatric Symptom Checklist (Sheldrick et al. 2012)[e]	0–18 (BPSC), 18–60 months (PPSC)	BPSC: irritability, inflexibility, and difficulty with routines PPSC: externalizing, internalizing, attention problems, and parenting challenges	3-point Likert Scale	BPSC: 12 PPSC: 18	BPSC correlates at low-moderate levels with ASQ:SE, PHQ-2, and difficult child on PSI PPSC predicting clinical range CBCL scale Sensitivity: 0.75–0.89; specificity: 0.77	Test-retest reliability=0.71–0.75	Part of larger system of primary care screening; ease of use, free

Note. ASQ:SE=Age & Stages Questionnaires: Social-Emotional; BITSEA=Brief Infant-Toddler Social and Emotional Assessment; BPSC=Baby Pediatric Symptom Checklist; CBCL=Child Behavior Checklist; DIPA=Diagnostic Interview for the Preschool Age; PHQ-2: Patient Health Questionnaire–2; PPSC=Preschool Pediatric Symptom Checklist; PSI=Parenting Stress Index.

[a]Purchasing information: www.brookespublishing.com/store/books/squires-asqse/index.htm.

[b]Purchasing information: www.aseba.com.

[c]Free download information: http://www.infantinstitute.org/measures-manuals/.

[d]Purchasing information: http://pearsonassess.com.

[e]Free download information: theswyc.org.

Summary Points

- The quality of the primary caregiving relationship is the strongest determinant of early childhood development.
- Use of systematic developmentally sensitive approaches to diagnosis in infancy and early childhood can assist with communication across providers and with consistency across patients and may provide important data to allow the field to progress.
- Although assessment can take place in a variety of settings, every effort should be made to help a family feel comfortable by creating a welcoming physical environment and to help parents feel comfortable seeking mental health treatment.
- Assessment is never a single event: it takes place over multiple appointments, with multiple informants, using multiple forms of information gathering.
- Assessment in infancy and early childhood includes not only the usual components of a psychiatric assessment but also attention to parent-child interactions and the parent's perception of the child.
- Structured assessments can provide useful information to supplement a thorough clinical history and observation.

References

Achenbach T, Rescorla L: Manual for the ASEBA Preschool Form. Burlington, University of Vermont, 2000

American Psychiatric Association: Diagnostic and Statistical Manual of Mental Disorders, 4th Edition. Washington, DC, American Psychiatric Association, 1994

American Psychiatric Association: Diagnostic and Statistical Manual of Mental Disorders, 5th Edition. Arlington, VA, American Psychiatric Association, 2013

Benoit D, Parker KC, Zeanah CH: Mothers' representations of their infants assessed prenatally: stability and association with infants' attachment classifications. J Child Psychol Psychiatry 38(3):307–313, 1997 9232477

Bergman K, Sarkar P, Glover V, et al: Maternal prenatal cortisol and infant cognitive development: moderation by infant-mother attachment. Biol Psychiatry 67(11):1026–1032, 2010 20188350

Briggs-Gowan M, Carter AS: Brief Infant Toddler Social Emotional Assessment (BITSEA) Manual Version 2.0. New Haven, CT, Yale University, 2002

Carter AS, Garrity-Rokous FE, Chazan-Cohen R, et al: Maternal depression and comorbidity: predicting early parenting, attachment security, and toddler social-emotional problems and competencies. J Am Acad Child Adolesc Psychiatry 40(1):18–26, 2001 11195555

Chilcoat HD, Breslau N: Does psychiatric history bias mothers' reports? An application of a new analytic approach. J Am Acad Child Adolesc Psychiatry 36(7):971–979, 1997 9204676

Conradt E, Measelle J, Ablow JC: Poverty, problem behavior, and promise: differential susceptibility among infants reared in poverty. Psychol Sci 24(3):235–242, 2013 23361232

Coolbear J, Benoit D: Failure to thrive: risk for clinical disturbance of attachment? Infant Ment Health J 20(1):87–104, 1999

Cooper G, Hoffman GT, Powell B: Circle of Security: COS-P facilitator DVD manual 5.0. Spokane, WA, Marycliff Institute, 2009

Cox JL, Holden JM, Sagovsky R: Detection of postnatal depression. Development of the 10-item Edinburgh Postnatal Depression Scale. Br J Psychiatry 150:782–786, 1987 3651732

Crowell JA, Feldman SS: Mothers' internal models of relationships and children's behavioral and developmental status: a study of mother-child interaction. Child Dev 59(5):1273–1285, 1988 2458891

Dawson G, Ashman SB, Panagiotides H, et al: Preschool outcomes of children of depressed mothers: role of maternal behavior, contextual risk, and children's brain activity. Child Dev 74(4):1158–1175, 2003 12938711

de Wolff MS, Theunissen MHC, Vogels AGC, Reijneveld SA: Three questionnaires to detect psychosocial problems in toddlers: a comparison of the BITSEA, ASQ:SE, and KIPPPI. Acad Pediatr 13(6):587–592, 2013 24238686

Drury SS, Theall K, Gleason MM, et al: Telomere length and early severe social deprivation: linking early adversity and cellular aging. Mol Psychiatry 17(7):719–727, 2012 21577215

Dunst CJ, Storck A, Snyder D: Identification of infant and toddler social-emotional disorders using the DC: 0–3 diagnostic classification system. Cornerstones 2:1–21, 2006

Egger HL, Angold A: Common emotional and behavioral disorders in preschool children: presentation, nosology, and epidemiology. J Child Psychol Psychiatry 47(3–4):313–337, 2006 16492262

Egger HLM, Erkanli A, Keeler G, et al: Test-retest reliability of the Preschool Age Psychiatric Assessment (PAPA). J Am Acad Child Adolesc Psychiatry 45(5):538–549, 2006 16601400

Essex MJ, Boyce WT, Hertzman C, et al: Epigenetic vestiges of early developmental adversity: childhood stress exposure and DNA methylation in adolescence. Child Dev 84(1):58–75, 2013 21883162

Felitti VJ, Anda RF, Nordenberg D, et al: Relationship of childhood abuse and household dysfunction to many of the leading causes of death in adults: the Adverse Childhood Experiences (ACE) Study. Am J Prev Med 14(4):245–258, 1998

Gleason MM, Zeanah CH, Dickstein S: Recognizing young children in need of mental health assessment: development and preliminary validity of the early childhood screening assessment. Infant Ment Health J 31(3):335–357, 2010

Haskett ME, Ahern LS, Ward CS, et al: Factor structure and validity of the parenting stress index-short form. J Clin Child Adolesc Psychol 35(2):302–312, 2006 16597226

Hunter AL, Minnis H, Wilson P: Altered stress responses in children exposed to early adversity: a systematic review of salivary cortisol studies. Stress 14(6):614–626, 2011 21675865

Knitzer J, Perry DF: Poverty and infant and toddler development, in Handbook of Infant Mental Health, 3rd Edition. Edited by Zeanah CH. New York, Guilford, 2012, pp 135–152

Koren G, Pastuszak A, Ito S: Drugs in pregnancy. N Engl J Med 338(16):1128–1137, 1998 9545362

Lidsky TI, Schneider JS: Adverse effects of childhood lead poisoning: the clinical neuropsychological perspective. Environ Res 100(2):284–293, 2006 16442997

Lieberman AF, Padron E, Van Horn P, et al: Angels in the nursery: the intergenerational transmission of benevolent parental influences. Infant Ment Health J 26(6):504, 2005

Luby JL, Barch DM, Belden A, et al: Maternal support in early childhood predicts larger hippocampal volumes at school age. Proc Natl Acad Sci USA 109(8):2854–2859, 2012

McGoron L, Gleason MM, Smyke AT, et al: Recovering from early deprivation: attachment mediates effects of caregiving on psychopathology. J Am Acad Child Adolesc Psychiatry 51(7):683–693, 2012 22721591

Monk C, Spicer J, Champagne FA: Linking prenatal maternal adversity to developmental outcomes in infants: the role of epigenetic pathways. Dev Psychopathol 24(4):1361–1376, 2012 23062303

Muller-Nix C, Forcada-Guex M: Perinatal assessment of infant, parents, and parent-infant relationship: prematurity as an example. Child Adolesc Psychiatr Clin N Am 18(3):545–557, 2009 19486837

Nelson CA, Bosquet M: Neurobiology of fetal and infant development: implications for infant mental health, in Handbook of Infant Mental Health. Edited by Zeanah CH. New York, Guilford, 2000, pp 37–59

O'Connor TG, Monk C, Fitelson EM: Practitioner review: maternal mood in pregnancy and child development—implications for child psychology and psychiatry. J Child Psychol Psychiatry 55(2):99–111, 2014 24127722

Olson AL, Dietrich AJ, Prazar G, et al: Brief maternal depression screening at well-child visits. Pediatrics 118(1):207–216, 2006 16818567

Oppenheim D, Koren-Karie N: Mothers' insightfulness regarding their children's internal worlds: the capacity underlying secure child-mother relationships. Infant Ment Health J 23(6):593–605, 2002

Oppenheim D, Koren-Karie N: The insightfulness assessment: measuring the internal processes underlying maternal sensitivity. Attach Hum Dev 15(5–6):545–561, 2013 24299134

Oppenheim D, Goldsmith D, Koren-Karie N: Maternal insightfulness and preschoolers' emotion and behavior problems: reciprocal influences in a therapeutic preschool program. Infant Ment Health J 25(4):352–367, 2004

Rosenblum KL, McDonough S, Muzik M, et al: Maternal representations of the infant: associations with infant response to the still face. Child Dev 73(4):999–1015, 2002 12146751

Salomonsson B, Sleed M: The Ages & Stages Questionnaire: Social-Emotional: a validation study of a mother-report questionnaire on a clinical mother-infant sample. Infant Ment Health J 31(4):412–431, 2010

Scheeringa MS, Haslett N: The reliability and criterion validity of the Diagnostic Infant and Preschool Assessment: a new diagnostic instrument for young children. Child Psychiatry Hum Dev 41(3):299–312, 2010 20052532

Seifer R, Dickstein S, Sameroff AJ, et al: Infant mental health and variability of parental depression symptoms. J Am Acad Child Adolesc Psychiatry 40(12):1375–1382, 2001 11765282

Sheldrick RC, Henson BS, Merchant S, et al: The Preschool Pediatric Symptom Checklist (PPSC): development and initial validation of a new social/emotional screening instrument. Acad Pediatr 12(5):456–467, 2012 22921494

Shonkoff JP, Garner AS, Committee on Psychosocial Aspects of Child and Family Health, et al: The lifelong effects of early childhood adversity and toxic stress. Pediatrics 129(1):e232–e246, 2012 22201156

Squires J, Bricker D: Ages & Stages Questionnaires, Third Edition (ASQ-3). Baltimore, MD, Brookes, 2009

Squires J, Bricker D, Twombly ES, et al: Ages & Stages Questionnaires: Social-Emotional. Baltimore, MD, Brookes, 2002

Task Force on Research Diagnostic Criteria: Infancy Preschool: Research diagnostic criteria for infants and preschool children: the process and empirical support. J Am Acad Child Adolesc Psychiatry 42(12):1504–1512, 2003 14627886

Tharner A, Luijk MPCM, van IJzendoorn MH, et al: Infant attachment, parenting stress, and child emotional and behavioral problems at age 3 years. Parenting 12(4):261–281, 2012

The White House: Education: Knowledge and Skills for the Jobs of the Future. Washington, DC, The White House, 2014. Available at: www.whitehouse.gov/issues/education/early-childhood. Accessed July 7, 2014.

Thomas JM, Benham AL, Gean M, et al: Practice parameters for the psychiatric assessment of infants and toddlers (0–36 months). J Am Acad Child Adolesc Psychiatry 36(10 suppl):21S–36S, 1997 9334564

Treyvaud K, Anderson VA, Howard K, et al: Parenting behavior is associated with the early neurobehavioral development of very preterm children. Pediatrics 123(2):555–561, 2009 19171622

Tyrka AR, Burgers DE, Philip NS, et al: The neurobiological correlates of childhood adversity and implications for treatment. Acta Psychiatr Scand 128(6):434–447, 2013 23662634

Vanderbilt D, Gleason MM: Mental health concerns of the premature infant through the lifespan. Child Adolesc Psychiatr Clin N Am 19(2):211–228, vii–viii, 2010 20478497

Vreeswijk CMJM, Maas AJBM, van Bakel HJA: Parental representations: a systematic review of the Working Model of the Child Interview. Infant Ment Health J 33(3):314–329, 2012

Yehuda R, Engel SM, Brand SR, et al: Transgenerational effects of posttraumatic stress disorder in babies of mothers exposed to the World Trade Center attacks during pregnancy. J Clin Endocrinol Metab 90(7):4115–4118, 2005 15870120

Zalewski M, Lengua LJ, Kiff CJ, et al: Understanding the relation of low income to HPA-axis functioning in preschool children: cumulative family risk and parenting as pathways to disruptions in cortisol. Child Psychiatry Hum Dev 43(6):924–942, 2012 22528032

Zeanah CH, Benoit D: Clinical applications of a parent perception interview in infant mental health. Child Adolesc Psychiatr Clin N Am 4(3):539–554, 1995

Zeanah CH, Benoit D, Hirschberg L, et al: Mothers' representations of their infants are concordant with infant attachment classifications. Developmental Issues in Psychiatry and Psychology 1:9–18, 1994

Zeanah CH, Larrieu JA, Valliere J, et al: Infant-parent relationship assessment, in Handbook of Infant Mental Health, Edited by Zeanah CH. New York, Guilford, 2000, pp 222–235

Zero to Three: DC: 0-3R: Crosswalk development and use in professional development and reimbursement. Washington, DC, Zero to Three, 2007. Available at: http://main.zerotothree.org/site/DocServer/DC_0-3R_notes.pdf?docID=5509. Accessed October 15, 2014.

Zero to Three Diagnostic Classification Task Force: Diagnostic Classification of Mental Health and Developmental Disorders of Infancy and Early Childhood. Arlington, VA, Zero to Three Press, 1994

Zero to Three Diagnostic Classification Task Force: Diagnostic Classification of Mental Health and Development Disorders of Infancy and Early Childhood: DC:0-3R. Washington, DC, Zero to Three Press, 2005

CHAPTER 3

Assessing the Preschool-Age Child

Neha Navsaria, Ph.D.
Joan Luby, M.D.

It is necessary to use specialized techniques to conduct a developmentally valid mental health assessment of the preschool-age child (ages 2–6 years). The standard approaches used for older children and adolescents will not be sufficient to obtain an age-appropriate and clinically meaningful assessment. Significant developmental differences between a preschool- and school-age child require a tailored approach to obtaining a history and eliciting a mental status examination. The most fundamental principle is that the preschool child does not function as a psychologically autonomous individual and remains inextricably tied to the primary caregiver for adaptive and emotional functioning. This idea was succinctly expressed by Winnicott (1965), whose famous phrase "There is no such thing as a baby" emphasized the importance of the dyad very early in life. This adage remains applicable during the preschool period, despite the important developmental transitions in the primary relationship. Therefore, the caregiver-child dyad is the most meaningful unit of observation or assessment. This means that, whenever possible, the mental status exam of a preschool child should be conducted with the child and caregiver together rather than with the child individually. While an individual play interview of the preschooler alone may be necessary in some circumstances (e.g., with preschoolers without the benefit of primary caregivers), observation of the child with the caregiver present is generally the most appropriate method.

The second developmentally driven principle is that the mental status exam of the preschooler must be conducted in the context of play. While this may seem an obvious component of any child assessment, it is essential to a valid preschool mental status exam. The facilitation and interpretation of play during the mental status exam will be discussed in more detail later in this chapter. Both the availability of age-appropriate toys to facilitate representational play, if the child is capable, and the examiner's willingness and ability to engage the child in play are essential. Concretely, this means the examiner should not wear a white coat or carry a chart or examination tools. The examiner should be able to adopt a playful posture, which often involves sitting on the floor, following the child's play, and assuming a more imaginative and whimsical demeanor. Clinicians unwilling or unable to engage in elaborate play will not be well suited to work with preschoolers.

Another key principle of preschool assessment is that because of significant state- and relationship-related variation in the mental status of the young child, it is necessary to observe a preschooler on more than one occasion and, ideally, with more than one caregiver. For this reason, assessments are best done over a series of several sessions on different days and, whenever possible, with different caregivers. In general, this requires an extended evaluation conducted over several days or weeks. While this is more cumbersome to schedule, changes in the child's behavior, evident within relationships and over time, are often invaluable in deriving an accurate diagnosis.

Socioeconomic and social pressures make such a comprehensive multisession assessment challenging. Insurance carriers or families are resistant to paying for the number of sessions required to conduct an appropriate assessment. It is inconvenient for families to schedule and attend multiple sessions and successfully involve multiple caregivers in the assessment process. However, it is critical that the clinician take a firm stance about the need for this kind of evaluation in order to obtain a valid diagnosis. More harm than good can come from conducting an assessment that is abbreviated and insufficient. Appropriate assessment and intervention during the preschool years can potentially offset negative social and economic outcomes for children and families. For example, early childhood interventional programs have been shown to have benefits for reducing crime, raising earnings, and promoting education and improved adult health (Campbell et al. 2014; Heckman 2011). The potential for greater efficacy for early intervention may prove that these techniques are cost-effective from a societal point of view.

Format of a Preschool Assessment

On the basis of the principles just described, a standard format for a preschool mental health assessment has been established in the Washington University School of Medicine Infant/Preschool Mental Health (WUSM IPMH) clinic. This format has been used successfully for nearly two decades; however, many variations on this format have been used in other clinics and may prove more feasible and equally useful. The WUSM IPMH clinic format (Table 3–1) is an example of one approach that incorporates all of the principles outlined earlier. The preschool assessment is conducted in four 50-minute sessions over 4 consecutive weeks. In the first session, all primary caregivers (both parents, or parent and grandparent, if available) are asked to come in without the child to obtain a comprehensive history. This information is more expediently obtained when the child is not present, and unlike in the assessment of the adolescent, there is little risk of damaging the rapport with the preschool child when caregivers are interviewed before the child.

TABLE 3–1. Washington University School of Medicine Infant/Preschool Mental Health clinic assessment paradigm

Session 1	Complete emotional, psychological, family, and developmental history of child obtained from caregivers
Session 2	Free-play observation with secondary caregiver
Session 3	Semistructured observation with primary caregiver: shared snack, mildly challenging cognitive task, dyadic play, and then separation and reunion
Session 4	Review of observations/findings, biopsychosocial formulation, differential diagnosis, and treatment plan with caregivers

The mental health history of the preschool child includes all of the components of a standard mental health history, such as chief complaint and history of present illness, as well as family and medical histories. In addition, detailed social and developmental histories are required. The developmental history includes milestone achievement in the following domains: motor, language, cognitive, sensory, social, and emotional. Details about eating and sleeping patterns are pertinent to the child's adaptation. Information about bedtime routines and rituals—for example, whether the child sleeps alone or with parents, or whether the child can self-soothe during awakenings or requires comfort from caregivers—is important. Eating habits, such as limitations in the child's food repertoire, ability to sit down for family mealtimes, and food refusal, may be a chief complaint or a complaint related to other behavioral and emotional problems. Information about family eating habits and parental expectations for eating is relevant to this domain.

Details of pregnancy and perinatal history—both medical and psychological—are essential and are often relevant to the chief complaint and current mental state. Premature birth or extended hospital stays may influence both development and the early relationship between parent and child. Exposure to drugs or alcohol in utero is of obvious relevance. Details of the maternal mental status during the perinatal period may be relevant to the presenting problems, as maternal mental illness or psychosocial stressors could impair parent-child relationship development. As has been elaborated so eloquently by Selma Fraiberg (1980) and others, the primary caregivers' internal working models of the child, as well as their expectations of the child, are often key contributors to the child's symptoms and the family's reaction and coping. Open-ended questions about the parents' own experiences of being parented, as well as their expectations of the child and attributions about the etiology of the child's presenting problems, should be explored. The psychiatric history of the preschooler should also include questions about parental discipline and parenting practices. Information should be obtained from all relevant caregivers. This will ensure a less biased understanding of the child's symptomatology and avoid one caregiver assuming the role as "spokesperson" for the child's behaviors.

Detailed information about the child's play is essential for the evaluation of a preschooler, including questions about the child's favorite toys, typical spontaneous play themes, and preferred play activities. Parents are likely to provide general descriptions of their child's play, and probing is often required. It is often useful for the clinician to ask the parents to walk him or her through the child's typical play activity. The capacity for symbolic or representational versus sensorimotor or mechanical play is important. When symbolic play is present, the complexity may illustrate the child's cognitive capacities. Perhaps more importantly, the thematic content of symbolic play may elucidate the preschooler's internal preoccupations. Information about the child's ability to enjoy play and his or her affective range during play is also important. The preschooler's interest in and capacity for parallel or interactive play with same-age peers, siblings, and others are also key components of the mental health assessment (Table 3–2).

When the focus is on the presence or absence of specific symptoms of disorders in DSM-5 (American Psychiatric Association 2013), it is critical to ask caregivers detailed questions about age-appropriate manifestations of symptom states. The clinician must "translate" DSM-5 symptom criteria to address the life experiences and developmental abilities of the preschool-age child. Several structured psychiatric interviews are now available that have been designed for the research assessment of preschool children. The Preschool Age Psychiatric Assessment (PAPA; Egger et al. 1999, 2006) is a comprehensive interview with established reliability that includes symptoms from DSM-IV (American Psychiatric Association 1994) as well as commonly occurring symptoms that arise in young children that are not included in the DSM system. The Disruptive Behavior Diagnostic Observation Schedule (DB-DOS; Wakschlag et al. 2008) is an observational method of assessing preschool disruptive behavior. It has established validity and characterizes preschool disruptive behaviors into two subtypes. A preschool version of the Schedule for Affective Disorders and Schizophrenia—the Schedule for Affective Disorders and Schizophrenia for School-Age Children, Present and Lifetime Version (K-SADS-PL; Birmaher et al. 2009)—is also available. While structured interviews specifically designed for clinical use are not yet available, a review of these measures may be useful to the clinician for ideas about how to assess preschool age–appropriate symptom states.

Obtaining collateral information from multiple contexts—for example, from preschool, day care, home, and another family member's home—is a key feature of the assessment of the young child. The need for approaches that combine reports from multiple informants across contexts has been empirically supported (Kraemer et al. 2003). Environment-specific behaviors may be important in understanding the nature of the presenting complaints. For example, the preschool child who is adjusting to a new preschool may act withdrawn or distressed according to the teacher but appear happy and engaged at home. Some DSM-5 diagnoses, such as attention-deficit/hyperactivity disorder (ADHD), require impairment in at least two settings for diagnosis. For example, if a child becomes hyperactive only at a grandparent's house when multiple peers are present, the problem may not represent clinical psychopathology. It may be useful to have multiple informants complete standardized behavioral measures on the child.

Preparing the Preschooler for the Play Evaluation

Once a comprehensive history has been obtained, play assessment sessions are

TABLE 3–2. Developmental observation of play in young children

Type	Approximate age range	Description	Examples
Sensorimotor play I	0–12 months	Engages in play activities in which child gains the pleasure of being the cause of action	Mouthing, banging, dropping and throwing toys or other objects
Sensorimotor play II	6–12 months	Develops ability to combine different sensorimotor action patterns into play to explore characteristics of objects	Moving parts, poking, pulling
Functional play	12–18 months	Uses objects in a way that demonstrates understanding and exploration of their use or function	Pushes car, touches comb to hair, puts telephone to ear, places pretend food on plate
Early symbolic play	18 months and older	Begins pretend play with increasing complexity. Makes transition from sensorimotor patterns to mental operations/representations.	Pretends to sleep/eat and pretends with others. "Feeds" mother or doll; one object represents another (e.g., a block becomes a car); pretend cooking or eating.
Complex symbolic play	30 months and older	Develops play themes with greater imaginative depth, richness, organization, and logical sequence. Puts together details of scenes that were previously demonstrated in isolation. As complexity increases, develops abilities to alter reality rather than reproduce it, anticipate outcomes, and adapt actions in the play context.	Reenacts a tea party; washes and dresses a doll; describes elaborate themes/stories of characters who live in a dollhouse and what they do over a period of time
Play themes and content	Throughout childhood	The way the child uses playroom environment. The degree to which the child can synthesize and integrate different elements into his or her own personality. The range and depth of themes provide an initial picture of certain aspects of child's internal life	May take it all in at the beginning, move around and develop a few themes, and finally weave together different themes. Might move into one corner and stay there for the majority of the session. May repeat one theme for the entire session.

Source. Casby 2003; Greenspan 2003; Thomas et al. 1997.

the next step. At the completion of the session in which the history was obtained, it is very important to instruct the parents on how to prepare the child for the play session. If the child comes to the session with a basic knowledge of the purpose of the encounter, the evaluation is likely to be far more fruitful and productive. The most important first step in the assessment as well as the therapeutic process is to inform the child about the assessment and the reasons for it in a nonjudgmental way, using clear, simple, and understandable language. The clinician should encourage the parents to be as honest as possible with the child about the nature of the concern. This may be the first time that caregivers engage in a direct and candid exchange with the child about the problem. It is important for parents to communicate that they are visiting the doctor so both the child and parent can get guidance on managing the child's feelings and behaviors. In this way, the child does not feel like the targeted individual with the "problem," thus reducing feelings of shame, anxiety, or embarrassment. It is also important to make sure the child understands that the assessment will involve play and not any frightening or painful medical examinations or procedures. Using the term "play doctor" can be helpful. To avoid unnecessary anticipatory anxiety, and in keeping with limitations in the young child's sense of time, it may be most sensible to inform the child about the evaluation on the day prior. Further, it is also useful for both the parents and the clinician to disclose to the child that they have already met to share information about the child, the family, and the nature of the problem.

Dyadic Play Assessment and Mental Status Examination

Part I: Dyadic Free-Play Session

The child's experience of the first encounter in the clinical setting is important to set the stage for the evaluation, as well as his or her general feelings and attitudes about mental health treatment. For this reason, it is important to conduct a free-play session prior to any structured tasks that may involve minor stressors (detailed in the next subsection). At the onset of the session, it is important for the clinician to communicate two basic principles. The first is to explain to the child the purpose of the session and to disclose what the therapist knows from meeting with the parent about the nature of the child's problems. The second is that the child may play with the toys however he or she would like. Since this session is conducted in a dyadic format with both the parent and clinician present in the playroom, it is imperative that the parent also be given instructions to play with the child "as you normally would at home." It is often necessary to redirect parents' natural attempts to engage in conversational exchanges with the therapist. This will derail the parent-child dyadic interaction, which is the central purpose of this session. Advise parents that there will be another time to ask questions and relay further details of history. In general, since the free-play session is thought to be less demanding than the semistructured play session, it should be conducted when feasible with a secondary caregiver. The semistructured observation that follows is both more stressful and comprehensive and therefore more appropriate for the child and primary caregiver.

The role of the examiner in this dyadic free-play observation is to serve as a "participant-observer" in the play. That is, the examiner should be prepared to respond to any bids from the child to engage in play. The examiner, though, should follow and not lead the child's play. This requires a delicate balance of acting in a spontaneous and playful fashion while also seeking direction and narration from the child to inform his or her role in play. The primary purpose of the dyadic free-play session is to observe the child in play with the caregiver. The examiner should be cautious not to overshadow the parent in play while being participatory. The examiner should respond fully if preferentially engaged by the child. It is necessary for the examiner to sit on the floor or at a table with the parent and child and to be fully attentive to the child and refrain from taking notes or charting.

It may be useful to enact a brief separation between parent and child midway through the free-play session. This allows observation of how the parent separates from the child, how the child responds to this separation, and how the parent and child reunite. Further, during the brief period that the parent is out of the room, the examiner has the opportunity to engage the child in individual play. In the event that the preschooler is highly resistant to the separation and/or expresses an intense emotional response, the attempt to separate the dyad can be abandoned (as important aspects of the dyadic relationship will have already been illuminated). The examiner should not give the parent detailed instructions about how to warn the child he or she is leaving but rather should leave it to the parent to do "what you think is best."

Part II: Semistructured Play Session

In keeping with the need to observe the preschooler on more than one occasion and with more than one caregiver, a second session is recommended with the primary caregiver. A semistructured format, in which the dyad is observed performing specific tasks, provides another useful method of observation for the preschool assessment. Observing the dyad sharing a snack, performing a mildly stressful structured cognitive task under time pressure, during a brief separation and reunion, and during free play are all useful exercises in the clinical setting. In contrast to Part I, the room setup should be minimal: a table with two chairs and no toys to limit a child's distractibility and assess his or her behaviors in a less stimulating environment. The clinician will bring the toys and activities into the room as each task begins to elicit specific kinds of behaviors and interactions.

Several standardized semistructured interviews, originally developed for research, are now available and may be useful in the clinical setting. In one such interview, the Parent-Child Early Relational Assessment (PCERA; Clark 1985), the clinician observes, through a one-way mirror, the dyad performing several tasks. The primary caregiver and child share a snack and then perform a structured task in which block designs are made from sample cards. Next, they engage in free play, and, lastly, a brief separation and reunion is enacted. This interview provides an interesting and varied format in which the quality of the parent-child relationship, parenting, and the child's behaviors toward the caregiver are observed. The Crowell procedure (Crowell and Fleischmann 1993) is a similar interview that adds blowing bubbles to specifically elicit affect in the child. Other similar useful dyadic observational assessments include the Teaching Task (Egeland et al. 1995), in which tasks of escalating difficulty are performed by the dyad while parent-child interactions are observed and videotaped for later review.

Another useful clinical component of the semistructured interview is the review of a video of the interaction. The review at a later point often leads the clinician to detect important interactions that might be missed during the live observation. The video is also a useful teaching tool, with appropriate written consent from the child's legal guardian. Furthermore, video review can be used as part of a feedback session with parents to elucidate the child's behaviors and parent-child interactional patterns. There is evidence to suggest that showing video interactions to caregivers can enhance parental attitudes toward sensitivity and discipline. Protocols with proven effectiveness are the Video-feedback Intervention to promote Positive Parenting and Sensitive Discipline (VIPP-SD; Van Zeijl et al. 2006) and the Modifying Attributions of Parents (MAP; Bohr et al. 2008) intervention.

Providing Feedback and Recommendations to Caregivers

The final session of the evaluation consists of meeting with the child's caregivers and reviewing the clinician's observations, formulation, and recommendations. A clinician should be careful to not minimize the importance of this session, as it should not be assumed that all parents would fully accept or understand the diagnosis and follow through with the recommended plan. The likelihood of parents' receptiveness increases the more a clinician approaches this session in a collaborative manner. Greenspan (2003) makes a number of suggestions on ways to provide feedback to caregivers: 1) let the parents begin by presenting their concerns, to assess whether they remain the same or have changed; 2) focus on and address any parental resistance; 3) serve as a collaborator by helping parents integrate their earlier perceptions of their child with one arising from the evaluation; 4) refer to observations of the child in a developmental context (i.e., referencing age-level anchors, attachment disruptions) in order to present information in a nonthreatening way; and 5) acknowledge any ambivalence displayed by the parent.

Given the emphasis of parent-child relational qualities in these assessments, it is likely that some feedback will pertain to parenting styles. Providing supportive yet honest feedback on parenting skills can be challenging. When discussing parent-child interactions, the clinician should

- Refrain from statements that are critical or judgmental
- Align with the parent and present the feedback in the context of the mismatch between parent behaviors and the child's developmental and emotional needs
- Explore how the parenting style may have emerged (i.e., lack of knowledge on parenting skills, negative attributions, unhealthy parenting models)
- Identify the parent's intended goals (likely to reduce negative behaviors) and how the parent's response can serve to increase the unwanted behavior rather than reduce it
- Conclude by suggesting alternative approaches, making sure to connect possible child behavioral outcomes

back to the parent's original intended goal

In this way, parents can experience the final session as collaborative.

Clinical Threshold: Differentiation From Developmental Norms

One of the challenges of the mental health assessment of preschoolers is making the distinction between developmentally normative behavioral extremes and clinically significant psychopathology. A comprehensive understanding of the rapid changes in social and emotional development that characterize the preschool period is required. For example, the preschooler's normal growing sense of autonomy commonly referred to as the "terrible twos" may mimic clinical oppositional behavior. Defiance or temper tantrums may bring caregivers to seek clinical attention although these behavioral patterns may be developmentally appropriate. Belden et al. (2008) have shown that the frequency, intensity (e.g., hits others, breaks items), duration (e.g., tantrums lasting longer than 20 minutes), and functional impairment across contexts (e.g., home, school, day care) are key factors in distinguishing normative from pathological temper tantrums.

Knowledge of developmental milestones, including gross and fine motor development and receptive and expressive language development, as well as social and emotional development, is essential for the assessment of the preschooler. The preschooler's developmental functioning in all of these domains can be ascertained through play observation. Markers of various stages of play development are summarized in Table 3–2.

When the clinician is making interpretations about developmental capacities, the distinction between delayed development and altered development should be noted. For example, does the 3-year-old display behaviors of a healthy 18-month-old (delayed), or do these behaviors deviate from the normal developmental trajectory (altered)? Delays in play skills may signal cognitive and/or social reciprocity deficits characteristic of developmental delays or autistic spectrum disorders. When significant cognitive delay is detected, organic and metabolic disorders must be ruled out. A neurological exam and an organic workup, as well as referral to a geneticist and other specialists during both assessment and treatment, may be indicated (see Chapter 6, "Neurological Examination, Electroencephalography, Neuroimaging, and Neuropsychological Testing").

Furthermore, developmental studies have demonstrated that preschoolers are more cognitively and emotionally competent than previously assumed. For example, it is not uncommon for 4-year-olds to personify or attribute human qualities to other organisms (Siegler et al. 2003), as in "my goldfish says he is hungry." Also characteristic of the preschool period—and often reviewed in textbooks of development—is Piaget's concept of egocentrism evident in the preschooler's inability to understand another's viewpoint (for review, see Shaffer 2002). In the assessment of the preschooler, the clinician must consider the range of individual variations that may be based on environment, context, or temperament. Texts that elaborate on developmental norms and their variations specific to this age group may be helpful for review (Shaffer 2002; Siegler et al. 2003).

Accessing the Preschool Child as Informant in the Assessment

The clinician must use different strategies to access the internal emotional state of the preschooler than the direct interview methods used with older children and adults. Direct approaches may even be counterproductive, causing the child to become more inhibited. A normally developing preschooler is unlikely to possess the verbal sophistication or insight to answer direct questions about emotional issues. Furthermore, a preschooler may fear reprisal or believe that negative feelings are not acceptable. Shorter attention span and greater suggestibility also limit the usefulness of direct questions. Several age-appropriate specialized assessment techniques, designed primarily for research, have been developed to adapt to these issues. Some of these techniques may also be fruitful when used in a clinical assessment.

Both direct and indirect methods for the assessment of the child's internal emotional state have been developed. The Berkeley Puppet Interview (BPI; Ablow and Measelle 1993) is a reliable and validated interview for young children that has been widely used in developmental research (Measelle et al. 1998). The BPI uses two puppets that make discrepant emotional statements, one of which the child selects as more representative of his or her own feelings. While a young child's self-report is being accessed, the child is able to displace his or her emotion to the puppet, making the interview less confrontational. Preschoolers' reported depressive and anxiety symptoms on the BPI have been shown to correlate with both teacher and parent ratings (Luby et al. 2007).

A more indirect, but potentially richly informative, semiprojective method that has been used in developmental research is the narrative story stem. One form of this approach that has been used in clinical populations is the MacArthur Story Stem Battery (Bretherton et al. 2003). This instrument contains emotionally evocative story stems that the child completes. Another method that uses the narrative approach is the Parent-Child Interaction Assessment–II (PCIA-II; Holigrocki RJ, Kaminski PL, Frieswyk SH: "PCIA-II: Parent-Child Interaction Assessment Version II," unpublished manuscript, University of Indianapolis, 2002 [update of PCIA Tech. Rep. No. 99-1046, Topeka, KS, Child and Family Center, The Menninger Clinic]). This protocol relies on a set of videotaped dyadic interactions in the context of a structured story stem play activity focused on a staged visit to the zoo. Story completions may be a useful play assessment method in the clinical setting. Oppenheim et al. (1997) examined children's representations of their caregivers interpreted through narrative completion and found significant correlations between low levels of psychological distress and children's perception of caregivers as "positive" or "disciplinary." Belden et al. (2007) have also shown that narratives distinguish clinically referred from healthy preschoolers by their perceptions and representations of their caregivers.

Mental Status Examination of the Preschool Child

As noted in this chapter, observation of the preschool child in play is essential to the mental status exam. In addition to the thematic content of play, a number of other mental status observations can be made. Observation of the preschooler should include general appearance and initial behavior on greeting the examiner, including cooperativeness, eye contact, social engagement, and social referencing. The assessment of developmental functioning during play is also feasible. Speech and all of its components, including articulation, prosody, rate, volume, and the presence of unique presentations such as echolalia, should be noted. Fine and gross motor skills can also be observed as the child moves around the playroom and manipulates the toys.

Flow of play, including perseveration or repetition of phrases or play themes as well as disorganization in play, may inform the differential diagnosis. Observation of the complexity and thematic content of play is essential. The clinician may note the child's preferences, including isolative, repetitive, violent, or aggressive themes in play, as well as how play figures behave toward each other. The clinician's ability to tolerate negative play themes is critical. Unless the child is harming himself or others or damaging property, the clinician should let the child's play themes unfold without interference. The child's ability to sustain attention to play is also of interest. The clinician, who serves as a participant-observer, may engage in descriptive commenting by making brief narrative comments about the child's play such as "The family is going together into the house" as a neutral and nonleading way to express interest in the play. The clinician may unobtrusively wonder about the play to help facilitate an understanding of what the child is enacting, by stating questions such as "I wonder why that baby is crying?" However, it is important for the clinician to refrain from leading the play or asking questions that require an answer from the child.

Furthermore, the mental status exam of a preschooler includes observation of the child's interaction with the primary caregiver as well as with the clinician. The child's ability to engage the caregiver and the caregiver's response are both noteworthy. The addition of a structured or mildly stressful task, as outlined earlier (see subsection "Part II: Semistructured Session"), can help elicit how child and caregiver interact under a variety of specific conditions. Significant qualities of the parent-child relationship and the child's relationship to the clinician are summarized in Table 3–3. Key features of the mental status exam, such as mood and affect, can be gleaned during the series of play observations. As outlined earlier, several methods to access the child's internal emotional state, in addition to observation of dyadic free play, may be useful in the clinical evaluation.

The Infant and Toddler Mental Status Exam (ITMSE; Thomas et al. 1997) is a useful guide for the clinician, reflecting modifications of the adult mental status exam pertinent to the infant and young child, including attention to the child's sensory and state regulation. While the ITMSE has not undergone empirical testing, it was designed by a highly experienced infant and preschool clinician and may be a useful clinical guide. The Caregiver-Child Social/Emotional Relational Rating Scale (CCSERRS; McCall et al. 2010) is a newer measure that emphasizes specific social and emotional aspects to parent and child interactions and relationships. The CCSERRS can serve as a practical instrument during the observation process as it was designed to assess dimensions that cover the range of caregiver-child interactions, but it can be administered in a relatively short period of time in a variety of situa-

TABLE 3–3. Qualities of the parent-child dyad and relatedness to the examiner

Term	Description
Attachment	Level of attachment. Observe reaction to separation and reunion. Note levels of comfort seeking, asking for and accepting help, cooperating, exploring and controlling behavior. Does the child use the parent as a "secure base" to explore? Abused and neglected children may display disrupted attachments: fearfulness, clinginess, overcompliance, hypervigilance, and impulsive overactivity and defiance; restricted, hyperactive, and distractible exploratory behavior; and indiscriminate affection and comfort seeking.
Attunement	Extent to which the caregiver paces interactions based on the child's behavior, signals, and communication. Does the caregiver provide empathic verbalizations or facial expressions? Is there shared joy and excitement? Does caregiver modulate response to the child's behavior? Is there a pattern of responding *to* rather than *at* the child?
Caregiver affect	Level of physical or verbal affection expressed toward the child. Is the parent nurturing, warm, loving, and expressive? Or is there negative affect present: harsh, hostile, critical, and blaming? Does the caregiver express positive emotion and enthusiasm to the child's accomplishments? Is the caregiver expressionless or mechanical? How does the caregiver's affect change over time?
Caregiver disciplinary control	The manner and extent by which limits are enforced. Observe level of supportive and empathic guidance in managing the child. Does the caregiver change the child's behavior in a positive and supportive way? Or is he or she intrusive, controlling, and demanding of obedience? Can the caregiver explain a rule/consequence and calmly redirect behavior?
Caregiver support	Ability to regulate the child's emotional responses. Note the extent to which a caregiver is sympathetic or empathetic with a child who is having difficulty.
Caregiver/child-directed behaviors	The manner in which the caregiver facilitates autonomous play in the child. Does caregiver ask what the child wants to do and how, or does he or she talk at the child and teach an activity? Observe the extent to which the caregiver interferes with the child's stream of behavior and the role played by parent during play. Is there an appropriate balance of the caregiver modeling use of an object/showing the child what to do versus letting the child lead and structure the play?
Child affect	Child's capacity for affective involvement with the parent. Note whether the child demonstrates negative affect but appears to modulate emotions appropriately. Does the child match emotions to the caregiver's emotions or situation? How does the child's affect change over time?

TABLE 3–3. Qualities of the parent-child dyad and relatedness to the examiner *(continued)*

Term	Description
Engagement	Caregiver willingness and ability to engage the child (verbally and nonverbally). Does he or she look the child in the eye when interacting, listen attentively when the child speaks, or get at the level of the child (kneels, sits on floor)? Note the level of harmony during play and the extent of the child's physical, verbal, and eye contact with the caregiver. How does the child engage or initiate play with the parent? Is there active avoidance by the child? Observe the child's level of comfort with being held or "molding" into the caregiver's body. Does child check back? Bring toys to show to play with together or near the caregiver? Does the child express positive anticipation when the caregiver attends to him or her?
Relatedness to examiner	How the child treats the examiner as a person; how the examiner's relationship with the child develops and how differentiated it is (from the caregiver's relationship with the child). How does the child greet you? Is the child eager to come with you, or does he or she cling to the caregiver? Is there caution and apprehension present, yet a willingness to follow you? Does the child slowly warm up to you? The child may watch the examiner while staying close to the caregiver before engaging. The child may initially show constriction of affect, vocalization, or play. How does the child negotiate your relationship? Is the child controlling? Is there a mechanical or distant quality to the relationship? Does the child regard you as an object in the room?

Source. Greenspan 2003; McCall et al. 2010; Thomas et al. 1997.

tions and does not require extensive coder training, manuals, or materials.

Cultural Context of the Preschool Assessment

The comprehensive evaluation of a preschool child involves not only relational and contextual assessment, as emphasized thus far in this chapter, but also a consideration for the cultural context of the preschooler and his or her family. Several authors have emphasized the need for a culturally sensitive evaluation (Garcia-Coll and Meyer 1993). Borrowing from an ecological systems model (Bronfenbrenner 1992), this context should include an understanding of the child in relation to the family, home, school, community, and society. Therefore, culture should not be defined only by race and ethnicity but should include other cultural contexts such as poverty, trauma, and the child welfare system.

Play is influenced by a number of variables, including cultural values, family relationships, child-rearing practices, toy familiarity, developmental expectations, and life experiences (Hwa-Froelich 2004). There are cultural differences in the frequency and content of play as well as caregiver-child interactions (Jent et al. 2011). For example, some families may value academic components of play over pretend play (Farver and Shin 1997). Other families, depending on their values and life experiences, may emphasize individualism and self-reliance, preferring more child-directed play. For collectivistic families, early choice making may be discouraged because of the emphasis on child obedience and respect (Johnston and Wong 2002). These dynamics could lead to seemingly restrained play that is more parent driven. Furthermore, collectivistic societies often rely on the extended family or community to engage children in play activity. Parents in these societies may appear to place less importance on one-to-one playtime, when in reality, they expect the child has other adults and children involved in their play. Young children in impoverished homes might have limited access to toys and play opportunities. This outcome is relevant to recent refugee and immigrant families, children of teen mothers, children fostered by relatives, families who cannot meet basic needs, and homeless families or those who move repeatedly (Nwokah et al. 2013). Many parents living in poverty and those with limited education do not understand the benefits of age-appropriate play and are likely not aware of what is developmentally appropriate because of a lack of role models (Nwokah et al. 2013). These factors influence what is observed during an assessment.

Lewis (2000) emphasizes the importance of the clinician's own awareness of personal theories and beliefs about childhood as well as the role of the caregiver. It is important for the clinician to engage in the practice of awareness and reflection in order to prevent judgment and bias from affecting the outcome of the evaluation and inform diagnosis and interventions in a culturally competent manner.

Differential Diagnosis in Preschoolers: Review of DSM-5 Preschool Disorders

A wide variety of psychopathological symptoms and categorical DSM-5 disorders may present in the preschool period. These include ADHD, oppositional defiant disorder (ODD), and, more rarely, conduct disorder. Mood disorders, including major depressive disorder, and anxiety disorders, such as separation anxiety disorder and generalized anxiety disorder, as well as obsessive-compulsive disorder, may also arise in preschool children. Specific phobias may be common, although they are relatively less impairing and therefore not often clinically significant. There is some evidence that bipolar disorder may very rarely appear as early as age 3 years; however, this remains an area in which further research is needed to inform the validity of this diagnosis in preschoolers. Sleep disorders and feeding disorders are also relatively common primary or secondary presenting problems.

Over the last decade, there has been an emerging body of empirical data investigating the nosology and validity of several DSM disorders among preschoolers. The diagnosis of ODD has been well studied with established validity in preschoolers. DSM-IV ADHD and conduct disorder have also been well validated, and little modification was made for current DSM-5 criteria. There is also a substantial body of support for the diagnosis of major depressive disorder (for review, see Luby 2010). Posttraumatic stress disorder has also been well studied, and findings have resulted in age-adjusted criteria in DSM-5 (fewer numbing and avoidance symptoms). There has been significant progress in the nosology and validity of attachment disorders with recent changes in DSM-5. Sleep disorders (see Chapter 23, "Sleep Disorders") and feeding disorders (Chatoor and Ammaniti 2007) have also been investigated in young children but are not well integrated into the current DSM system.

The presence of functional impairment is key to crossing the clinical threshold, as defined by DSM. However, impairment is more difficult to detect in a preschool-age child who does not function autonomously and may not be in structured preschool settings. The assessment of impairment must consider not only the individual functioning of the child but also the effect his or her symptoms is having on the functioning of the family system (e.g., the mother cannot maintain a job because her preschool child has been expelled from several day care centers for aggression). Excessive fears that delay acquisition of developmental capacities (e.g., preschool child will not separate from mom and hence cannot start school or learn to sleep alone) should be considered in the assessment of impairment (Carter et al. 2004).

Overall, studies suggest that preschool diagnoses (ODD, ADHD, major depressive disorder) persist into school age and therefore warrant early intervention (Bufferd et al. 2012; Keenan and Wakschlag 2002; Lahey et al. 2004; Luby et al. 2014). The finding of longitudinal stability is also pertinent to nosology and supports the validity of these early-onset disorders. ADHD diagnosed in 4- to 6-year-old preschoolers persisted 3 years later into elementary school age (Lahey et al. 2004). Stability of preschool diagnoses was found to be related to a number of factors, including low family cohesion, socioeconomic status, maternal support, and negative life events (Bufferd et al. 2012; Lavigne et al. 1998).

Psychotic disorders are extremely rare at this early age. The assessment of psychosis in the preschooler is a challenge, given the limited capacity for expressive language, as well as the developmentally normative confusion between fantasy and reality. Preschool studies of psychosis are essentially limited to case reports (Beresford et al. 2005). Nonetheless, it is essential for the preschool clinician to thoroughly investigate any behaviors suggestive of psychosis, which might include bizarre or disorganized play or descriptions of hallucinatory experiences. Assessment should rule out delirium, exposure to toxins or psychoactive substances, and (in an acute setting) febrile status. Hallucinations should be distinguished from normative phenomena such as imaginary companions, illusions, and elaborate fantasies common among preschoolers (Sosland and Edelsohn 2005). The family history may help inform the differential diagnosis on the basis of the finding that psychotic and mood disorders (in which psychotic symptoms may arise) are often familial.

Characteristics of Preschool Clinic Samples

Clinicians can anticipate a wide variety of referrals to a preschool mental health clinic, although externalizing disorders (ADHD and ODD) predominate (Hooks et al. 1988; Lee 1987; Luby and Morgan 1997). A substantial minority present with internalizing disorders, defined as depressive and anxiety disorders, followed in prevalence by somatic disorders, including sleep and eating disorders, along with enuresis and encopresis (Luby and Morgan 1997). More than a third present with developmental disorders. One clinically referred sample found 13% present with autism spectrum disorders. Boys present more frequently than girls for evaluation, and externalizing symptoms, including aggression and oppositionality, are more common reasons for seeking care (Hooks et al. 1988; Lee 1987). Language delays are associated with higher rates of externalizing psychopathology. While the disruption of externalizing disorders prompts caregivers to seek care, the impact of internalizing symptoms may be even more distressing to the child and family. Many children have both types of symptoms.

Summary Points

- A comprehensive assessment of a preschool-age child is ideally completed over several sessions on different days, with more than one caregiver.
- Use of both unstructured and semistructured observation is most informative.
- Observation of dyadic play is essential to the preschool evaluation.
- When the clinician is providing feedback to parents, a collaborative approach is necessary to increase the likelihood of follow-through with recommendations.
- While disruptive behavior is the most common reason for seeking mental health assessment in the preschool period, it is also necessary to carefully assess for the presence of internalizing symptoms.
- Mental health disorders in preschoolers have been shown to be impairing, and many have demonstrated longitudinal stability.

References

Ablow JC, Measelle JR: The Berkeley Puppet Interview. Berkeley, University of California, Berkeley, 1993

American Psychiatric Association: Diagnostic and Statistical Manual of Mental Disorders, 4th Edition. Arlington, VA, American Psychiatric Association, 1994

American Psychiatric Association: Diagnostic and Statistical Manual of Mental Disorders, 5th Edition, Arlington, VA, American Psychiatric Association, 2013

Belden AC, Sullivan JP, Luby JL: Depressed and healthy preschoolers' internal representations of their mothers' caregiving: associations with observed caregiving behaviors one year later. Attach Hum Dev 9(3):239–254, 2007 18058432

Belden AC, Thomson NR, Luby JL: Temper tantrums in healthy versus depressed and disruptive preschoolers: defining tantrum behaviors associated with clinical problems. J Pediatr 152(1):117–122, 2008 18154912

Beresford C, Hepburn S, Ross RG: Schizophrenia in preschool children: case reports with longitudinal follow up at 6 and 8 years. Clin Child Psychol Psychiatry 10:429–439, 2005

Birmaher B, Ehmann M, Axelson DA, et al: Schedule for Affective Disorders and Schizophrenia for School-Age Children (K-SADS-PL) for the assessment of preschool children: a preliminary psychometric study. J Psychiatr Res 43(7):680–686, 2009 19000625

Bohr Y, Dhayanandhan B, Armour L, et al: Mapping parent-infant interactions: a brief cognitive approach to the prevention of relationship ruptures and infant maltreatment (the MAP method). IMPrint 51:2–7, 2008

Bretherton I, Oppenheim D, Emde RN, et al: The MacArthur Story Stem Battery, in Revealing the Inner Worlds of Young Children: The MacArthur Story Stem Battery and Parent–Child Narratives. Edited by Emde RN, Wolf DP, Oppenhem D. New York, Oxford University Press, 2003, pp 381–396

Bronfenbrenner U: Ecological Systems Theory in Six Theories of Child Development. Edited by Vasta R. Philadelphia, PA, Jessica Kingsley, 1992, pp 187–250

Bufferd SJ, Dougherty LR, Carlson GA, et al: Psychiatric disorders in preschoolers: continuity from ages 3 to 6. Am J Psychiatry 169(11):1157–1164, 2012 23128922

Campbell F, Conti G, Heckman JJ, et al: Early childhood investments substantially boost adult health. Science 343(6178):1478–1485, 2014 24675955

Carter AS, Briggs-Gowan MJ, Davis NO: Assessment of young children's social-emotional development and psychopathology: recent advances and recommendations for practice. J Child Psychol Psychiatry 45(1):109–134, 2004 14959805

Casby MW: The development of play in infants, toddlers, and young children. Communication Disorders Quarterly 24:163–174, 2003

Chatoor I, Ammaniti M: Classifying feeding disorders of infancy and early childhood, in Age and Gender Considerations in Psychiatric Diagnosis: A Research Agenda for DSM-IV. Edited by Narrow WE, First MB, Sirovatka PJ. Washington, DC, American Psychiatric Association, 2007, pp 227–242

Clark R: The Parent-Child Early Relational Assessment, Manual and Instrument. Madison, University of Wisconsin Department of Psychiatry, 1985

Crowell J, Fleischmann MA: Use of structured research procedure in clinical assessments of infants, in Handbook of Infant Mental Health, 2nd Edition. Edited by Zeanah CH. New York, Guilford, 1993, pp 210–221

Egeland B, Weinfeld N, Hiester M, et al: Teaching Tasks Administration and Scoring Manual. Minneapolis, University of Minnesota Institute of Child Development, 1995

Egger HL, Ascher BH, Angold A: The Preschool Age Psychiatric Assessment, Version 1.1. Durham, NC, Center for Developmental Epidemiology, Department of Psychiatry and Behavioral Sciences, Duke University Medical Center, 1999

Egger HL, Erkanli A, Keeler G, et al: Test-retest reliability of the Preschool Age Psychiatric Assessment (PAPA). J Am Acad Child Adolesc Psychiatry 45(5):538–549, 2006 16601400

Farver JA, Shin YL: Social pretend play in Korean- and Anglo-American preschoolers. Child Dev 68(3):544–556, 1997 9249965

Fraiberg S (ed): Clinical Studies in Infant Mental Health. New York, Basic Books, 1980

Garcia-Coll CT, Meyer EC: The sociocultural context of infant development, in Handbook of Infant Mental Health. Edited by Zeanah CH. New York, Guilford, 1993, pp 56–69

Greenspan SI: The Clinical Interview of the Child. Washington, DC, American Psychiatric Publishing, 2003

Heckman JJ: The economics of inequality: the value of early childhood education. Am Educ 35(1):31–35, 2011

Hooks MY, Mayes LC, Volkmar FR: Psychiatric disorders among preschool children. J Am Acad Child Adolesc Psychiatry 27:623–627, 1988

Hwa-Froelich DA: Play assessment for children from culturally and linguistically diverse backgrounds. Perspectives on Communication Disorders and Sciences in Culturally and Linguistically Diverse Populations 11(2):5–9, 2004

Jent JF, Niec LN, Baker SE: Play and interpersonal processes, in Play in Clinical Practice: Evidenced-Based Approaches. Edited by Russ SW, Niec LN. New York, Guilford, 2011, pp 23–47

Johnston J, Wong MYA: Cultural differences in beliefs and practices concerning talk to children. J Speech Lang Hear Res 45(5):916–926, 2002

Keenan K, Wakschlag LS: Can a valid diagnosis of disruptive behavior disorder be made in preschool children? Am J Psychiatry 159(3):351–358, 2002 11869995

Kraemer HC, Measelle JR, Ablow JC, et al: A new approach to integrating data from multiple informants in psychiatric assessment and research: mixing and matching contexts and perspectives. Am J Psychiatry 160(9):1566–1577, 2003 12944328

Lahey BB, Pelham WE, Loney J, et al: Three-year predictive validity of DSM-IV attention deficit hyperactivity disorder in children diagnosed at 4–6 years of age. Am J Psychiatry 161(11):2014–2020, 2004 15514401

Lavigne JV, Arend R, Rosenbaum D, et al: Psychiatric disorders with onset in the preschool years: II. Correlates and predictors of stable case status. J Am Acad Child Adolesc Psychiatry 37(12):1255–1261, 1998 9847497

Lee BJ: Multidisciplinary evaluation of preschool children and its demography in a military psychiatric clinic. J Am Acad Child Adolesc Psychiatry 26(3):313–316, 1987 3597286

Lewis ML: The cultural context of infant mental health: the development niche of infant-caregiver relationships, in Handbook of Infant Mental Health, 2nd Edition. Edited by Zeanah CH. New York, Guilford, 2000, pp 91–107

Luby JL: Preschool depression: the importance of identification of depression early in development. Curr Dir Psychol Sci 19(2):91–95, 2010 21969769

Luby JL, Morgan K: Characteristics of an infant/preschool psychiatric clinic sample: implications for clinical assessment and nosology. Infant Ment Health J 18(2):209–220, 1997

Luby JL, Belden A, Sullivan J, et al: Preschoolers' contribution to their diagnosis of depression and anxiety: uses and limitations of young child self-report of symptoms. Child Psychiatry Hum Dev 38(4):321–338, 2007 17620007

Luby JL, Gaffrey MS, Tillman R, et al: Trajectories of preschool disorders to full DSM depression at school age and early adolescence: continuity of preschool depression. Am J Psychiatry 171(7):768–776, 2014 24700355

McCall RB, Groark CJ, Fish L: A Caregiver-Child Social/Emotional and Relationship Rating Scale (CCSERSS). Infant Ment Health J 31(2):201–219, 2010 20556236

Measelle JR, Ablow JC, Cowan PA, et al: Assessing young children's views of their academic, social, and emotional lives: an evaluation of the self-perception scales of the Berkeley Puppet Interview. Child Dev 69(6):1556–1576, 1998 9914640

Nwokah E, Hsu H, Gulker H: The use of play materials in early intervention: the dilemma of poverty. American Journal of Play 5(2):187–218, 2013

Oppenheim D, Emde RN, Warren S: Children's narrative representations of mothers: their development and associations with child and mother adaptation. Child Dev 68(1):127–138, 1997 9084129

Shaffer DR: Developmental Psychology, Childhood and Adolescence, 6th Edition. Belmont, CA, Wadsworth/Thompson Learning, 2002

Siegler R, DeLoache J, Eisenberg N: How Children Develop. New York, Worth, 2003

Sosland MD, Edelsohn GA: Hallucinations in children and adolescents. Curr Psychiatry Rep 7(3):180–188, 2005 15935131

Thomas JM, Benham AL, Gean M, et al: Practice parameters for the psychiatric assessment of infants and toddlers (0–36 months). J Am Acad Child Adolesc Psychiatry 36(10 suppl):21S–36S, 1997 9334564

Van Zeijl J, Mesman J, Van IJzendoorn MH, et al: Attachment-based intervention for enhancing sensitive discipline in mothers of 1- to 3-year-old children at risk for externalizing behavior problems: a randomized controlled trial. J Consult Clin Psychol 74(6):994–1005, 2006 17154730

Wakschlag LS, Briggs-Gowan MJ, Hill C, et al: Observational assessment of preschool disruptive behavior, part II: validity of the disruptive behavior diagnostic observation schedule (DB-DOS). J Am Acad Child Adolesc Psychiatry 47(6):632–641, 2008 18434925

Winnicott DW: The Maturational Process and the Facilitating Environment: Studies in the Theory of Emotional Development. New York, International Universities Press, 1965

CHAPTER 4

Assessing the Elementary School-Age Child

Poonam Jha, M.D.

School-age children are defined as children ages 6–12 years. This chapter contains a framework for the evaluation process, highlighting the critical components and identifying special considerations when working with a school-age child. Children may be evaluated in many settings: the emergency room, a pediatric hospital room, a school, or an outpatient psychiatric clinic, among others. The goals of assessment differ with the setting. The focus of this chapter is on the outpatient clinic setting, where the goal is to perform a comprehensive evaluation.

Assessment Process

Work flow varies according to the clinical setting. Consent to evaluate and treat must be obtained from the parent prior to starting the evaluation. In this chapter, "parent" will refer to the parent(s) or legal guardian(s). The assessment process can often begin prior to formally meeting with the family. If possible, it is valuable for the clinician to observe the informal interactions and behavior of the child and family in the waiting area prior to introducing himself or herself. The clinician may note the child's level of activity, curiosity in a new setting, social interactions with other children and adults, and level of impulse control. Additionally, it may be valuable for the clinician to watch the parents' level of interest in and supervision of the child, how the parents attend to the child's needs, and how they manage frustrations that may arise.

The next step is for the clinician to introduce himself or herself and describe the evaluation process to the child and parent. Most families have some level of distress when seeking help for mental health challenges, because of the severity of problems and their impact on the family and/or because of shame or embarrassment regarding seeking mental health help. The clinician must make an effort to place the family at ease. This can best be accomplished with a neutral, nonjudgmental, and calm demeanor. An office that is comfortable for adults and welcoming to the child can help make the family feel more at ease. This may include comfortable seating, placement of furniture to facilitate direct eye contact, and age-appropriate toys for the child. School-age children begin to understand and gravitate toward games with rules (e.g., board games, puzzles). At this age, children still engage in imaginative play; thus, having dolls, action figures, and building blocks available is useful. Paper and drawing supplies are especially helpful to provide an activity for the child and a means of communicating and assessing the child's motor, writing, and artistic skills. It is also important for the clinician to be aware that most school-age children are accustomed to going to pediatrician offices, where they are physically examined and administered vaccinations. That experience can be intimidating for the child. It is helpful to clarify at the beginning that the purpose of this particular doctor's visit is to talk and that there will be no shots given at the visit.

There is clinician variation in structuring the initial appointment. Some clinicians prefer to meet with the parent and child together, while others prefer to first meet with the parent alone. Meeting with the family together helps all to feel that their input is equally valued. The child may be confused about the appointment, and meeting with the caregivers alone initially may arouse suspicions of what is being discussed. Ultimately, separate meetings with the child and parent are necessary. It is important to ascertain the main reason for seeking help. However, for school-age children, the concept of meeting with a professional to address emotional or behavioral problems may be hard to understand. Thus, it is often worth spending a few minutes to "get to know one another." Asking nonthreatening questions that children often hear is an effective method of placing the child at ease and conveying that his or her input is important. Examples are questions about age, grade level, family members' names, pets, interests, hobbies, and friends. The responses can also provide information pertinent to social history and mental status.

After the ice is broken, it is important to discuss confidentiality and its limits with mandatory reporting. Seeking mental health treatment can create much anxiety in families because of concerns of what will be shared with schools, employers, and other providers. A child may be told the following: "Kevin, what you share with me is very important, and I cannot share any of the information with anyone else unless I think it is important and I have your parents' permission. But there may be other times when I am worried about your safety or the safety of other people around you, and I may share information with people who can help." It is equally important that parents are informed of the confidentiality rules so that they understand that if they share information regarding safety, then steps to inform protective agencies may be necessary.

The clinician's understanding of the child should not be limited to the individual child and family. The child functions in other important domains: school, social relationships, leisure activities, and so forth. Also, it is important to gather information regarding any previous evaluations or psychiatric treatment and the experiences that accompanied that treatment. Gathering collateral information both provides a more comprehensive picture and corrects inaccurate reports. People, especially young children, have only modestly accurate recall of events (Edelbrock et al. 1985;

Henry et al. 1994). Also, often there is little agreement in reporting of events among children, caregivers, and teachers (Herjanic and Reich 1982). Sharing with other people will require verbal and written consent to communicate information. Most of the time, people willingly agree to communication with other pertinent parties such as teachers, previous providers, pediatricians or other medical doctors, and relatives. However, some parents opt to either limit communication to specific types of information or to not share any information at all. These preferences must be honored, and perhaps as the working relationship grows, they can be revisited.

While each clinician varies in his or her evaluation practice, most comprehensive evaluations cannot be completed in a single 1-hour session. Optimally, most evaluations are completed after several 1-hour sessions. This should be explained to the family at the beginning of the evaluation to help them understand what to expect. Exceptions may occur when the acuity of the presentation warrants more expedient progression to the treatment phase. Also and unfortunately, payers are increasingly dictating time constraints.

Assessment Components

The components of the psychiatric evaluation of a school-age child are outlined in Table 4–1. Developmental factors influence the conduct of the interview. When the clinician is assessing the chief complaint, it is helpful to ask the child what he or she was told about the meeting. This may help shed light on the child's awareness of problems or the child's level of compliance (often, oppositional children will deny existence of any problems). Much of the first session consists of gathering information from the parents. School-age children can contribute most usefully to the history of the present illness, review of psychiatric and medical symptoms, and certain components of the social history.

When the clinician is assessing the history of the presenting illness, an effective strategy is to ask what led the family to seek out mental health treatment. Asking the family such questions as "What has concerned you regarding Jocelyn? Why are you seeking out treatment now? How were you referred to this practice?" can help initiate the discussion regarding pertinent concerns. Broader general questions should be followed by more directed questions. Asking about intensity, frequency, duration, time of onset, triggers, ameliorators, associated symptoms, timing patterns, and responses by others can yield significant information. Understanding whether the concerning symptoms are pervasive/limited or acute/chronic is important. Asking about stressors or recent changes (e.g., relative's illness/death, school change, parental separation, involvement with traumatic event, family move, birth of sibling, parental marriage) also can yield helpful information.

When the clinician is conducting the psychiatric review of symptoms, some areas should be covered, even if they do not pertain to the chief complaint. Disorders that commonly affect school-age children include anxiety disorders (i.e., separation anxiety disorder, social anxiety disorder, selective mutism, specific phobia); attention-deficit/hyperactivity disorder (ADHD); disruptive, impulse-control, and conduct disorders (i.e., oppositional defiant disorder, conduct disorder); learning disorders, autism spectrum disorders, or social concerns; trauma- and stressor-related disorders,

TABLE 4–1. Outline for psychiatric evaluation of the elementary school-age child

I. Chief complaint
   a. What the child says
   b. What the parent says

II. History of present illness
   a. Main concerning symptoms
   b. Timeline of symptoms
   c. Onset, duration, severity, frequency of symptoms
   d. Triggers or ameliorators of symptoms

III. Psychiatric review of symptoms
   a. Learning problems, attentional problems
   b. Anxiety symptoms of separation anxiety, selective mutism, social anxiety, specific phobia, generalized anxiety disorder
   c. Mood symptoms of major depression, bipolar disorder, disruptive mood dysregulation disorder
   d. Behavioral problems of oppositional defiant disorder, conduct disorder
   e. Neurovegetative symptoms of sleep, appetite, concentration, toileting
   f. Tics
   g. History of traumatic events

IV. Past psychiatric history
   a. Past evaluation, treatment history
   b. Use of emergency room, partial hospital programs, inpatient hospitalizations
   c. Therapy history, in mental health facility, school-based clinic, or spiritual guidance center
   d. Medication trials, including those that may have been prescribed by the primary care physician
   e. History of suicide ideation, attempts, or near attempts; nonsuicidal self-injurious ideation or behaviors; homicidal ideation or attempts; serious physical aggression

V. Past medical history
   a. Chronic medical problems
   b. Recent acute illnesses
   c. Hospitalizations
   d. Head injuries/loss of consciousness
   e. Seizures
   f. Surgeries
   g. Cardiac pathology

VI. Medications/allergies
   a. Current prescribed medications
   b. Current over-the-counter medications (vitamins, supplements, herbal remedies)
   c. Medication allergies/sensitivities

VII. Developmental history
   a. Maternal history of medical problems, medication use, toxin exposure, gestational complications
   b. Delivery history (full-term gestation, spontaneous delivery, route of delivery, birth weight, Apgar scores)
   c. Perinatal, postnatal complications
   d. Developmental milestone achievement
   e. Temperament of the child

TABLE 4–1. Outline for psychiatric evaluation of the elementary school-age child *(continued)*

VIII. Educational history
  a. History of early intervention or early childhood programming
  b. Day care/preschool assessment: behaviors, level of activity, social assessment, language and learning
  c. School history: retention, school changes
  d. School records: report cards, behavior reports, standardized testing scores
  e. Special education: 504 plan, IEP
  f. History of attendance, academics, behavior, social interactions

IX. Family medical history
  a. Major medical problems
  b. History of genetic disorders, thyroid disease, cardiac pathology (especially of functional and structural abnormalities, history of early sudden death), seizures, headaches

X. Family psychiatric history
  a. Major psychiatric problems in blood-related relatives
  b. Learning problems, emotional problems, behavioral problems, personality problems
  c. Substance use
  d. Completed or attempted suicide
  e. Medication treatment and response

XI. Social history
  a. Child's living situation: location/neighborhood, type of home, who lives in the home
  b. Family structure in the home
  c. Parental relations: marital status, nature of their relationship, custody parameters
  d. If present, stepparents or parental significant others
  e. Parental attitudes on parenting
  f. Parental employment
  g. Family financial status
  h. Siblings' ages and nature of relations
  i. Other caretakers
  j. Child's attitude towards parents, siblings, caretakers
  k. Friendships, peer group
  l. Child's skills, interests, hobbies
  m. History of child welfare involvement
  n. Parental legal involvement
  o. If in foster care, nature of foster placement(s), agency involvement, case worker involvement
  p. History of foster placement: when removed, why removed, how many placements

XII. Abuse and risk assessment
  a. Abuse reported by parent
  b. Abuse reported by child (separately assessed)
  c. Harm in home: domestic violence, physical abuse, presence of firearms, neglectful caregivers, substance-using caregivers
  d. Child's report of suicidal ideation, plans, intentions, past attempts, past behaviors to prepare or near attempts
  e. Significant physical aggression

Note. IEP=individualized education program.

including adjustment disorders; mood disorders, including depression and disruptive mood dysregulation disorder; and elimination disorders (Kessler et al. 2005).

Assessing the past psychiatric history includes reviewing past evaluations and treatment, whether these occurred in a mental health setting or with a pediatrician or school-based clinician. Suicidal thinking and behaviors do exist in this age group. It is therefore imperative to evaluate for past and current history of suicidal ideation and suicide plans/attempts, as well as nonsuicidal self-injurious ideation and behaviors (Tishler et al. 2007). Inquiry regarding suicidal thinking and behavior does not cause a child to adopt this thinking and behavior (Greene 1994). Far more harm is possible if this line of questioning is excluded.

Substance use assessment is not commonly performed with this age group, although use of tobacco or inhalants can start in the preteen years. Exposure to substance-using parents can be a predictor of substance use and mood and anxiety problems, as well as poor self-concept in children (Merikangas et al. 1998). Therefore, understanding parental substance use is important, and substance use should be assessed privately with the parent.

Medical history is important to assess. Mood and anxiety symptoms can have somatic manifestations in this age group. If there are somatic complaints, it is important to ascertain that a thorough medical evaluation was conducted. Some medical conditions, such as thyroid disease and hematological abnormalities, can be accompanied by psychiatric symptoms. Further, prescription of psychotropic medication can affect some organ systems; thus, having a baseline understanding of the child's health is imperative. Neurological review, including history of head injuries, loss of consciousness, and seizures, is important (see Chapter 6, "Neurological Examination, Electroencephalography, Neuroimaging, and Neuropsychological Testing"). A thorough patient and family cardiac history is important as a precaution for subsequent medication prescription. A review of all current medications is necessary.

Knowing the family medical history, notably for cardiac disease, thyroid disease, and neurological disease, can help in evaluating the child's risk for these medical diseases. Family psychiatric illness and substance use history are very important to ascertain. In addition to knowing what genetic predispositions the child has, being aware of family members' mental health and how difficulties such as parental depression, parental substance use, sibling depression, and sibling disruptive behavior affect the family helps inform the clinician regarding the child's life (Ramchandani and Stein 2003).

The gathering of social history focuses on understanding family relationships. School-age children are not autonomous for many functions, and their lives are still intertwined with their caregivers. What does the caregiver think are the child's strengths and skills? At this age, peers begin to have increasing importance in the child's life. Friendships test a child's ability to socially navigate in the world. Assessing the quality of the friendships is important. Other important aspects of social history include legal issues such as social service involvement, custody issues, and parental criminal history. Assessing for past and/or current history of abuse of the child or other family members is an important topic that may be difficult to discuss but is necessary.

Educational history may have already been reviewed, as educational concerns are often the main reason for seeking help. School-age children may demonstrate symptoms that were tolerated by family members and accommodated in the home setting. School entry can uncover behavioral problems, learning problems, social problems, and anxiety. Knowing the school's response to the child's problems is also important. What services or evaluation has the child received?

Developmental history is important to review. Understanding the child's temperament can help in identifying risk factors for anxiety or disruptive behavior disorders. In utero toxin exposure can help explain problems in learning or behavior. Attainment of motor, speech, and toileting skills is important to ascertain.

It is important to interview the child and parent separately. Certain topics should be discussed in the absence of the child or the parent. It is critical to ask about possible abuse privately with the child and with the parents. Children may find it more difficult to discuss abuse in the presence of others, because of shame, fear of consequences, or guilt. Meeting with the child alone is also an opportunity to ask the child about his or her self-esteem. The child's self-esteem can be assessed by asking about friendships and hobbies. In discussing relations between parents, family history of mental illness, and discipline practices, it is best to interview the parent alone. Often parents also welcome the opportunity to expand on other issues in the absence of their child. During the joint portion of the session, for families with poor boundaries it is the clinician's role to halt discussion of sensitive topics if inappropriate content is being shared in the presence of the child. This helps promote a comfortable evaluation process and models for parents appropriate topics to discuss in the presence of the child.

Typical Developmental Features of the School-Age Child

To effectively assess a school-age child, the clinician needs to understand the tasks that typically are completed in this stage. Table 4–2 summarizes normal developmental milestones of the school-age child. School-age children become aware of rules, and such awareness may lead to cognitive rigidity at times. Typically, children have attained a better understanding of space and time. They can manage their personal grooming, and they are able to help do basic household chores. Children in this stage are typically eager to learn, and self-esteem begins to build with accomplishments gained in school, home, and pleasurable activities. Children who have impaired learning (intellectual disability, learning disorders, attentional problems) may be at risk for low self-esteem.

Many theorists have described emotional development. Erik Erikson described children ages 5–12 years as meeting the challenge of achieving competence (Erikson 1950). In this stage, children become much more active in learning and other activities. In most societies, they begin to spend a majority of time in school, and they use learning activities to build a sense of accomplishment. If they fail to make such achievements, then children may struggle with a sense of inferiority or low self-esteem.

Social development also is a significant task for school-age children. They begin to move from the world restricted to their primary caretakers to a world occupied by peers and teachers. Increasingly, children engage in social activities independent of their parents and begin to identify best friends and friend

TABLE 4–2. Assessing the elementary school-age child: typical developmental features

Developmental facet	Description
Cognitive	Can carry out concrete operations: conservation and classification Understands that others think differently Appreciates rules Grasps time and space better
Emotional	Strives for competence: mastery leads to good self-esteem; lack of mastery leads to low self-esteem, hopelessness, easy frustration, resistance to trying novel things Has fewer outbursts due to ability to delay gratification
Moral	Understands right and wrong based on internal principles Begins to build empathy and taking perspective of others
Self-view	Is informed by internal evaluation and evaluation by others Has comparative awareness Defines himself or herself by physical appearance, possessions, and activities Is more self-conscious about differences
Social	Begins to engage more independently from parents in activities with peers May identify best friend and friend group Participates in team activities
Family	Is more independent of family routines; however, still values family time and parental views Parents are no longer sole authority Begins to compare parents with other adults May grow attachments to nonparental adults (teachers, coaches)

groups. They begin to value what peers think of them. This grouping of children may lead to a sense of exclusion. Inability to form and maintain friendships may be a source of low self-worth (Davies 2011). Children also begin to have empathy and the ability to take the perspective of others (Kohlberg 1970). On the other hand, children at this age can be critical and may impulsively say or do things that are not kind.

Speaking With the School-Age Child

Children of this age often have the language skills to communicate, leading the listener to believe that they can converse like an adult. However, their cognitive abilities are not as mature as an adult's, as they lack the higher and more complex mental processes. When speaking with children in this age range, the clinician should consider certain principles. Mature communication integrates language skills, cognitive skills, and social skills. Such things as turn-taking, use of facial and body gestures, nonverbal language, inferences, and abstract concepts may not be fully understood by children in this age group, especially the younger ones. Older children in this age group begin to understand abstract ideas, approximately at ages 9–10 years (Caplan and Bursch 2013).

School-age children generally do not spontaneously discuss many of the matters that are important to review during a psychiatric assessment. Additionally, they often do not expand on questions. Children typically use short sentences. Children's lack of elaborate responses is indicative not of their unwillingness to speak, rather, their tendency to be terse. It is the clinician's job to guide them to expand. A general rule of asking children questions is to avoid "why" questions. Asking about cause requires analytical thinking that is beyond many children's abilities. Instead, using questions with "what," "where," and "how" are more effective. For example, "Why did you hit your brother?" usually will yield an "I don't know" response. Instead, asking "What happened to make you hit your brother?" "What did your brother do to make you hit him?" or "What did you feel when you hit your brother?" typically will yield a more informative response.

While older children begin to master time constructs, children typically are poor historians in regard to onset and duration. It is more useful to ask children about events in relation to recognizable markers. For example, "You told me you have been feeling sad. Were you feeling sad back when it was still summer vacation?" instead of asking "For how many weeks have you been feeling sad?"

Children in this age group generally have poor working memories. Therefore, questions should be limited in not only types of words (vocabulary that is age appropriate) but also quantity of words. Asking "How old is your brother, Ralph?" will be better than requesting "Tell me the ages of your brothers and sisters, Ralph, Simon, Lucy, and Lena." Mixing open-ended and more directive questions is important. Asking too many directed questions sequentially may lull the child into responding with the same, automatic response (for example, answering yes or no repeatedly). Giving choices of response is a good strategy, but with too many choices, children may simply choose the last option because that is what they remember. When offering choices, the clinician should allow time for a response after each option.

When a child struggles to communicate verbally or has difficulty with using words to describe emotional states or sensitive issues, using pictures or toys can be helpful. Children may be more comfortable displacing the story onto a picture, puppets, or figurines/dolls. For children with selective mutism, trauma-related symptoms, or communication disorders, these strategies can be especially helpful. Having the child draw with or without instruction each has advantages. With instruction (such as asking the child to draw her family), drawing allows the child to demonstrate her ability to hear, process, and comprehend what is being asked. It also demonstrates her level of compliance. Without instruction (asking the child to draw whatever she pleases), drawing allows an entry into her thoughts and serves as the basis for further inquiry.

Mental Status Examination

The mental status exam of the school-age child should be assessed through the developmental lens (Table 4–3). It is important for the clinician, in gauging appearance, to assess size relative to chronological age. Height and weight abnormalities can be the source of social ostracism. Facial or body dysmorphisms can suggest genetic abnormalities or in utero toxin exposure. Hygiene, grooming, and appropriateness of clothes can be reflective of adequate parental care. Presence of scars can be indicative of abuse or self-harmful behavior. The

TABLE 4–3. Mental status examination of the elementary school-age child

- Appearance
  - Size, dysmorphic features, scars
  - Grooming, hygiene, clothing
- Behavior
  - Level of cooperation
  - Ability to transition
  - Level of flexibility
- Relatedness to others
  - Interactions with parents
  - Interactions with examiner
- Speech
  - Rate, rhythm, tone, volume, prosody
- Motor exam
  - Gait, abnormal movements, tics, tremors, stereopathies
- Mood
  - Child's description, in his or her own words
- Affect: Examiner's assessment of
  - Quality of mood
  - Stability of mood
  - Intensity of mood
  - Appropriateness of mood
  - Range of mood
- Thought process
  - Organization of thought, coherence of thoughts
- Thought content
  - Presence of psychiatric symptoms
  - Presence/absence of suicidal thinking
  - Presence/absence of homicidal thinking
- Perceptual exam
  - Child's description of hallucinations
  - Clinician's observation of organization of behavior
- Cognitive exam
  - Orientation
  - Attention
  - Memory
  - Calculation
  - Reading Skills
  - Writing Skills
  - Fund of Knowledge
- Impulse control
  - Per history and presentation
- Insight
  - Child's awareness of symptoms
- Judgment
  - Per history and presentation

behavior examination can be very informative in many domains. How readily does the child engage with the interview? Sustained inhibition may reflect anxiety. A child who is overly familiar may demonstrate behaviors suggestive of poor attachment. A child who is aloof may demonstrate symptoms suggestive of autism spectrum disorder. Relatedness to others is assessed by observation. How do the child and parent interact? Do they appear to have a bond? Is the parent overly passive or harsh? Is the child comfortable or tense? How does the parent respond to the child's confusion, the child's disruptive behaviors, or the child's anxiety? How does the child interact with the examiner? Is she cooperative, indifferent, disrespectful, overly familiar, or friendly? Speech assessment is noteworthy for communication difficulties of expression and comprehension. Does the child have understandable speech? Are there fluency difficulties? Does the child seem to understand words appropriate for her developmental age? The motor exam is also very pertinent for the school-age child. How active is the child in the office setting? Is the child able to inhibit impulses? Does the child have abnormal movements, repetitive movements, tics, stereopathies, or motor compulsions? Mood is described on the basis of direct questioning. For children in the younger cohort, examples or pictures may be useful. Affect is based on the examiner's assessment of the appropriateness to situation, stability, range, and quality. Thought processes of these children are typically concrete. Linear and organized thoughts are to be expected in this age group. Thought content is notable for ability to distinguish fantasy from reality, especially in the older cohort. Suicidal and homicidal thinking are critical to include in describing thought content. Perceptual examination assesses for the child's awareness of reality. Is he able to distinguish fantasy thoughts from reality-based experiences? While truly psychotic symptoms are rare in this age group, it is important to assess the child for such symptoms. If psychotic symptoms are endorsed, then more thorough attention should be placed on looking for trauma-reactive symptoms or mood symptoms, conditions in which hallucinations are more commonly seen. Delirium from medical conditions or substances also should be considered. The cognitive exam has many subcomponents, including orientation, attention, memory, fund of knowledge, writing/reading/calculation ability, and judgment. How does the child do with reading, writing, and simple calculations? Insight may be age-limited in the younger age cohort, but children in this age group begin to have awareness of situations. Judgment can be assessed by either asking about hypothetical questions or gleaning from the history.

Assessment Tools

While the clinical interview and observation are the best ways of collecting information to determine diagnosis, they can be supplemented with semi-structured or structured interviews. Examples of such interviews include the Schedule for Affective Disorders and Schizophrenia for School-Age Children (K-SADS), National Institute of Mental Health Diagnostic Interview Schedule for Children (DISC), Anxiety Disorders Interview Schedule (ADIS), Diagnostic Interview for Children and Adolescents (DICA), Children's Interview for Psychiatric Syndromes (ChIPS), Child and Adolescent Psychiatric Assessment (CAPA), and Children's Yale-Brown Obsessive Compulsive Scale (CY-BOCS)

(Carlisle and McClellan 2010). The advantage of using such instruments is to elicit symptoms in a standardized and comprehensive format. Many instruments have diagnostic algorithms. The disadvantages include need for training, cost, lengthy administration time, and possible delay of procession to treatment (Carlisle and McClellan 2010).

Rating scales can be used to detect symptoms and impairment. The scales can be broadband or category specific. Commonly used broadband rating scales for this age group include the Child Behavior Checklist (CBCL), the Behavior Assessment System for Children (BASC), and the Children's Symptom Inventory (CSI). Examples of rating scales specific for externalizing disorders include Conners Rating Scale (CSR) and the Vanderbilt ADHD Diagnostic (VAD) rating scales. Examples of rating scales specifically for internalizing disorders are the Children's Depression Inventory (CDI), Children's Depression Rating Scale (CDRS), Beck Depression Inventory (BDI), Multidimensional Anxiety Scale for Children (MASC), Screen for Child Anxiety Related Disorders (SCARED), Young Mania Rating Scale (YMRS), Child PTSD Symptom Scale (CPSS), and Trauma Symptom Checklist for Children (TSCC; Leary et al. 2010). Selected rating scales should be routinely administered to enhance the diagnostic process as well as to gauge treatment response. They are typically brief and easy to administer. They can also provide an avenue to collect data from other informants (e.g., teachers, other family members) (Leary et al. 2010).

Direct information gathering from other people (with the family's consent) can also prove to be valuable. Such people may include other important family members; caregivers; teachers; school-based psychologists, social workers and case workers; and coaches. Other clinicians who can give important information include other mental health providers, pediatricians, pediatric specialists, and child welfare workers.

For a thorough evaluation, a medical examination within the past year is critical, followed by consulting with the pediatrician on whether further medical and diagnostic testing is necessary. When there is suspicion of an underlying medical cause, appropriate next steps can include laboratory, imaging, or procedural testing or referral to the corresponding specialists. A common concern with children in this age group is learning and academic lag. To fully assess for learning-based disorders, psychological testing should be pursued. For problems related to language and speech, referral to a speech and language pathologist should be considered.

Common Problems and Disorders in the School-Age Child

School entry is a major transition. For children who have not had formal early childhood education (preschool), it can be especially challenging. Children must learn to feel confident without being near their parents. Separation anxiety is common in this age group. School also imposes many tasks and responsibilities (e.g., being on time, doing school work, turning in assignments, taking tests, following classroom rules) that can call attention to a child with underlying generalized anxiety. Being in a large group setting and being expected to participate and interact with others are common social tasks for school-age children.

The learning challenges with formal education, especially when children are compared with same-age peers, can uncover primary learning problems, language problems, or attentional problems. The structure of the classroom, with many routines and rules, may be a challenge for children with hyperactivity, poor impulse control, or compliance problems. For these reasons, it is not uncommon to see diagnoses of learning disorders, speech and language disorders, and ADHD.

School cultivates social interactions, and children must learn to navigate in this world. Children with social anxiety disorder may have newly uncovered difficulties. Children with autism spectrum disorder typically are identified prior to school age. However, children with more subtle signs of the disorder may not be identified until they are in school, where their peculiar ways of interacting are not tolerated by their peers. School problems such as teasing and bullying are common. Bullying can have catastrophic results (e.g., suicide, homicide) and must be taken seriously (Klomek et al. 2009). Cyberbullying done by older school-age children has magnified the problem. Questions regarding the child's involvement with social media sites and online activities are critical to review.

Mood disorders, including major depressive disorder and bipolar disorder, are not common in prepubescent children. Nonetheless, children in this age group are not fully immune to these disorders. Children who are lagging in meeting the challenges of school (academically, socially) may be vulnerable to the development of depression. The emergence of symptoms of bipolar disorder in this age group is uncommon, but special attention should be given to children who present with symptoms of sustained mood changes with family history of mood and psychotic disorders. Disruptive mood dysregulation disorder (DMDD), first described in DSM-5 (American Psychiatric Association 2013), is a condition with onset of symptoms prior to age 10. DMDD describes children with chronic irritability and recurrent temper tantrums, complaints that often lead families to seek psychiatric care (Copeland et al. 2013).

Tic disorders may also be observed in this age group. Transient tics are common and peak in this age range. Help may be sought out if these tics persist or cause significant impairment.

While not specific to this age group, trauma-related symptoms should also be assessed. Children in this age group may present differently than the classic posttraumatic stress disorder (PTSD) symptom presentation as described in DSM-5. Using the developmental lens, children with PTSD may present with somatic complaints (e.g., recurrent headaches, stomachaches), regression in skills, increase in clinginess, onset of separation anxiety, school academic decline, social changes, sleep disturbance, behavioral problems, or increased level of anxiety (Perrin et al. 2000).

Assessment: Formulation and Treatment Planning

Once all the information has been gathered, the clinician must synthesize a biopsychosocial formulation (see Chapter 1, "The Process of Assessment and Diagnosis"). The findings should be presented to the family in a direct and neutral manner. Often families have much apprehension, guilt, and anxiety about psychiatric illnesses. Typically, meeting with the child and parent together is appropriate to present the findings. It is best to present, and often lead with, the strengths of the child and family and, where appropriate, to highlight domains where psychopathology is absent. When the clinician is discussing the diagnostic conclusions, it is best not only to list the symptoms but also to explain the possible factors that have contributed to the symptoms. While it is difficult to raise topics such as family relations as contributors, it is important to do so, as the explanation can help justify the recommended interventions, such as parental guidance or family therapy. Medication may also be a topic to address for certain children. Making the decision to medicate a child in this age group can be a difficult one, requiring extra sensitivity when medication options are being proposed.

Conclusion

Mental health problems in school-age children are not uncommon. Therefore, it is an opportunity to tend to the mental health needs of the families who present for mental health services. Understanding the child's developmental challenges and the common areas of problems and knowing how to communicate with a school-age child are critical skills needed in order to effectively evaluate and treat the child and family.

Summary Points

- Mental health problems are significant in school-age children and can affect the child's emotional, cognitive, and social development.
- Common problems include anxiety, learning and attention problems, behavioral problems, and social problems.
- The assessment of the school-age child should include multiple informants.
- When interviewing the school-age child, the clinician must use developmentally appropriate language and communication skills.
- School-age children should be interviewed alone during part of the assessment.
- School-age children may develop problems because of an inability to meet developmental tasks, and therefore understanding typical social, emotional, and cognitive developmental tasks is important.

References

American Psychiatric Association: Diagnostic and Statistical Manual of Mental Disorders, 5th Edition. Arlington, VA, American Psychiatric Association, 2013

Caplan R, Bursch B: How Many More Questions? Techniques for Clinical Interviews of Young Medically Ill Children. New York, Oxford University Press, 2013, pp 3–27

Carlisle L, McClellan JM: Diagnostic interviews, in Dulcan's Textbook of Child and Adolescent Psychiatry. Edited by Dulcan MK. Washington, DC, American Psychiatric Publishing, 2010, pp 79–88

Copeland WE, Angold A, Costello EJ, et al: Prevalence, comorbidity, and correlates of DSM-5 proposed disruptive mood dysregulation disorder. Am J Psychiatry 170(2):173–179, 2013 23377638

Davies D: Child Development, a Practitioner's Guide, 3rd Edition. New York, Guilford, 2011, pp 380–392

Edelbrock C, Costello AJ, Dulcan MK, et al: Age differences in the reliability of the psychiatric interview of the child. Child Dev 56(1):265–275, 1985 3987406

Erikson EH: Childhood and Society. New York, WW Norton, 1950

Greene DB: Childhood suicide and myths surrounding it. Soc Work 39(2):230–232, 1994 8153764

Henry B, Moffitt TE, Caspi A, et al: On the "remembrance of things past": a longitudinal evaluation of the retrospective method. Psychol Assess 6(2):92–101, 1994

Herjanic B, Reich W: Development of a structured psychiatric interview for children: agreement between child and parent on individual symptoms. J Abnorm Child Psychol 10(3):307–324, 1982 7175040

Kessler RC, Berglund P, Demler O, et al: Lifetime prevalence and age-of-onset distributions of DSM-IV disorders in the National Comorbidity Survey Replication. Arch Gen Psychiatry 62(6):593–602, 2005 15939837

Klomek AB, Sourander A, Niemelä S, et al: Childhood bullying behaviors as a risk for suicide attempts and completed suicides: a population-based birth cohort study. J Am Acad Child Adolesc Psychiatry 48(3):254–261, 2009 19169159

Kohlberg L: Stages of moral development as a basis for moral education, in Moral Education. Edited by Beck CM, Sullivan E. Toronto, ON, Canada, University of Toronto Press, 1970, pp 23–92

Leary A, Collett B, Myers K: Rating scales, in Dulcan's Textbook of Child and Adolescent Psychiatry. Edited by Dulcan MK. Washington, DC, American Psychiatric Publishing, 2010, pp 89–110

Merikangas KR, Dierker LC, Szatmari P: Psychopathology among offspring of parents with substance abuse and/or anxiety disorders: a high-risk study. J Child Psychol Psychiatry 39(5):711–720, 1998 9690934

Perrin S, Smith P, Yule W: The assessment and treatment of posttraumatic stress disorder in children and adolescents. J Child Psychol Psychiatry 41:277–289, 2000 10784075

Ramchandani P, Stein A: The impact of parental psychiatric disorder on children. BMJ 327(7409):242–243, 2003 12896914

Tishler CL, Reiss NS, Rhodes AR: Suicidal behavior in children younger than twelve: a diagnostic challenge for emergency department personnel. Acad Emerg Med 14(9):810–818, 2007 17726127

CHAPTER 5

Assessing Adolescents

Steven P. Cuffe, M.D.
Chirag V. Desai, M.D.

The psychiatric assessment of adolescents is a complex, challenging, and multifaceted task. In many ways, this assessment is more similar to assessment of adults than is the assessment of younger children. Adolescents are able to give historical information, verbalize feelings, and be introspective. Many are able to think abstractly. However, clinicians assessing adolescents should be aware that adolescents are not just younger adults. Adolescents live in a complex web of interdependent relationships within their family, peer group, school, agencies (e.g., social services, juvenile justice), and broader community and cultural groups. The assessment of adults typically relies to a great degree on an individual adult's report of symptoms and problems. Many times the only source of information is the adult being evaluated. To do this with adolescents would be a grave mistake. Developmental considerations are critically important in the assessment of adolescents, particularly when gauging their physical and emotional maturation. The brain continues to develop into the early 20s, especially the areas involved in executive functions such as inhibition, impulse control, and critical decision making (see, e.g., Lebel and Beaulieu 2011). Developmental immaturity of the brain places adolescents at much higher risk for multiple problems, including violence and aggression, substance abuse, motor vehicle accidents, and risky sexual behavior.

Psychosocial developmental issues are also prominent in adolescents. Adolescents' development of a sense of self and identity is intimately connected with their striving for autonomy. Relationships with parents and family issues are pivotal in this process. The goal of parenting adolescents is to allow them to grow in independence and increase their decision-making authority within the context of a safe "container," with appropriate limits established by loving and supportive parents. Either absent/neglectful or overbearing and restrictive parenting styles can contribute to the development of problem behaviors in adolescents. Similarly, an adolescent's peer and community groups can have a strong influence on the developing sense of identity (belonging) and subsequent behavior and choices. Emerging sexuality plays out in this context, as does experimentation with other "adult" behaviors such as substance use and driving habits. Adolescents' relationships with peers have been strongly influenced by the rapid changes in so-called social media that are ubiquitous among teens, allowing almost constant contact with friends and acquaintances. Participation in social media can have both positive and negative effects on an adolescent. Inquiry into a teen's use of social media should be a part of the assessment (see Case Example 3).

Although there are some circumstances in which an assessment can or must be brief (hospital consults, emergency room evaluations, and so forth), in this chapter we focus on how to conduct a thorough assessment of an adolescent. The clinician begins the assessment seeking to understand the adolescent's problems and symptoms within his or her genetic, developmental, family, peer, and community/cultural context. To accomplish this, a comprehensive assessment plan must be developed. Information from different sources must be obtained. Adolescents and parents have at best only modest agreement in their reporting of behaviors and symptoms (Cantwell et al. 1997; King and American Academy of Child and Adolescent Psychiatry 1995; Kramer et al. 2004). Parents tend to report more accurately on externalizing symptoms and behaviors, and adolescents tend to report more accurately on internalizing symptoms (Cantwell et al. 1997). Information from school and other agencies involved with the adolescent is also important.

Table 5–1 lists the elements involved in a comprehensive evaluation. The amount of time it takes to collect the information, establish relationships with parents and the adolescent (and other family members if needed), develop a case formulation and treatment plan, and present the plan to the parents and adolescent is highly variable and may range from a single 1 hour visit to many hours over multiple weeks. Clinicians from a variety of mental health and health care disciplines may perform these functions, with greater expertise (including the involvement of a child and adolescent psychiatrist) for more complex problems.

Prior to beginning the assessment, it is important to understand how the adolescent has been referred for treatment. Did the parents self-refer? Was the school or the juvenile court involved? Do the parents or the adolescent believe there is a problem, or are they only following through on a forced assessment?

Deciding whom to interview may be complicated. Legal and family issues are important to discern. Are both parents available and do they maintain their parental rights? Are they both involved in important aspects of the child's life? Are divorce and custody issues involved? Are other adult caregivers taking primary roles in the care of the child? Establishing custody or guardianship is an important prerequisite to beginning an assessment. For children, usually the noncustodial parent has the right to participate in medical assessment and treatment but not to begin a treatment process unless it is emergent. Since laws vary between states, it is also critical for the clinician to know the legal age for consent for medical treatment in the relevant state. Many states have enacted laws allowing minors older than age 14 or 16 to consent to most medical treatment (see Chapter 32, "Legal and Ethical Issues").

TABLE 5–1. Elements of a comprehensive assessment

Parent interview
Adolescent interview
Interview with teachers as appropriate (could be by phone)
Family interview as appropriate
Interviews with other family members as needed (siblings, grandparents, other caretakers)
Medical records from primary and specialty care
Prior mental health treatment records
School records
Records from other involved agencies (e.g., social services, juvenile justice)
Standardized measures (rating scales, symptom checklists, diagnostic interviews) as needed to assess problem behaviors or symptoms
Psychological testing as indicated and available

Involving as many informants as possible provides the broadest data set from which to base the diagnostic assessment and proposed treatment plan. Mothers and fathers frequently have divergent views about the adolescent's problems and their underlying causes (Chess et al. 1966; Youngstrom et al. 2000). Whenever possible, both parents should be involved. They can be interviewed with the child, as a couple, or separately. Many times a combination of formats is best. Other primary caregivers can be included with the permission of the legal guardian. Data from rating scales, standardized diagnostic interviews, or psychological testing can also be helpful in establishing the correct diagnosis and an accurate problem list, leading to a plan of treatment.

Beginning the Assessment

The first decision is whom to invite to the initial interview. Since autonomy issues and struggles for separation are frequently important issues, the way the initial interview is handled can have a significant effect, positive or negative, on the outcome of the assessment process. If the parent is seen first, the adolescent may see the clinician in the role of agent of the parent. Resistance and oppositional behavior from the adolescent are a frequent result. On the other hand, the clinician can choose to see the adolescent first. However, the adolescent may have little to say, so the result may be a quick session with little accomplished. The key is to engage both the adolescent and the parent in the assessment in a way that promotes a positive connection and thus a promising beginning to treatment.

In most cases, starting the initial assessment with parent(s) and adolescent together can be productive. How long to continue this interview is a decision based on the interaction of the parties. At a minimum, this allows the clinician to assess the relationship between the adolescent and the parent(s). An introduction to the problems causing the referral gives the clinician information on which to base the interview with the adolescent alone. The level of resistance and oppositional behavior can be seen. In order to minimize the perception of the clinician as solely a parental agent, this interview may be short and quickly transition to the adolescent alone. Maintaining this interview in the face of significant oppositional behavior can be counterproductive, as illustrated below.

Case Example 1

A clinician was administering a diagnostic interview to a 15-year-old girl, Gina, referred to the outpatient clinic for assessment. The goal of the first part of the interview was to obtain consent from the parent and assent from the adolescent for participating in the assessment. Gina was close-mouthed during the entire discussion. When it came time for her to sign the form, she refused. The clinician spent much time trying to convince Gina that it would be in her best interest to participate. Still, Gina dug her heels in even further. The mother and clinician both became frustrated and were at the point of terminating the interview. It was clear that Gina could not accept any possibility of giving her mother what she wanted. There was anger and defiance in her manner, and the initial interview was about to end in failure. A child and adolescent psychiatrist whose role was to observe decided to knock on the door. He spoke to the clinician and recommended she ask the mother to leave the room so the clinician could speak to Gina alone. He further recommended she focus not on the task of assenting to the evaluation but on getting a rapport established with Gina by getting her to talk about something, anything, about herself and her life. As soon as the mother left the room, Gina began to soften. Soon she was talking about her life at home, school, and with friends. Within a few minutes, she readily signed the assent-to-treatment form, and the interview proceeded without further incident. Understanding when and how to involve the various parties in the assessment process can be critical to the success of the initial interview.

In the beginning of the assessment process, it is vital that both parent and adolescent understand the structure and process of the evaluation. Confidentiality issues must be explained to both the parent and the adolescent. In order for adolescents to feel comfortable providing details about their life, symptoms, actions, and feelings, they need to know how much of what they disclose will be communicated to a parent. If adolescents assume that everything they say will be communicated directly to the parent, this is likely to block the flow of information. However, some teens will assume that everything will be kept confidential, causing difficulties when significant issues need to be disclosed to parents. Conversely, parents often think it is their right to know every detail divulged by the adolescent in the interview because they are bringing their underage child for assessment, and they are paying for it too. Coming to an understanding of just how confidentiality is handled will avoid some uncomfortable situations and allows for a much easier first interview with the adolescent. It is important to share at the beginning of the assessment the limits of confidentiality posed by disclosures of abuse and neglect and the legal "duty to report" such incidents to authorities (see Chapter 32). Laws vary by state, and all clinicians need to understand the laws under which they practice.

What is the proper balance between confidentiality for the adolescent and sufficient communication with the parent? In order to facilitate communication by the adolescent, he or she should feel that the clinician is, at least in part, his or her advocate. Parents should be told the clinician will give them the overview of problems and diagnoses, without specific details of statements and behaviors reported by the adolescent, *unless the adolescent would be at risk of harm* if the parents were not informed. In cases of suicidal behaviors, dangerous sexual behaviors (multiple partners and/or unprotected sex), dangerous driving behaviors, and the like, the safety of the adolescent takes precedence over confidentiality. Where the line is drawn is up to the individual practitioner; however, it would be wise to give some examples of the limits of confidentiality for both the parent and the child. Parents can, at times, have unreasonable expectations.

Case Example 2

During the assessment of Jordan, an adolescent boy, it became clear that substance abuse was a problem. His drug use involved marijuana and alcohol predominantly but also experimentation with cocaine on two occasions. Jordan asked that his limited cocaine use not be disclosed to his mother. The clinician agreed to this since he felt Jordan was accurately reporting his use, and he knew that random drug screenings would be recommended as part of the treatment—therefore, more extensive and dangerous use would be uncovered. When during the course of the treatment Jordan disclosed his limited cocaine use to his mother, she became outraged that she had not been informed and demanded that her son be hospitalized. The clinician explained that his cocaine use was neither at a level that placed him at risk of harm nor at a level warranting hospitalization. She responded with a question, "Can the ingestion of cocaine kill you?"

Case Example 3

In the process of completing an evaluation of a 14-year-old boy named Alex, a clinician met with his mother to gather collateral history. At one point in the interview, she showed the clinician several printed copies of a Facebook page showing recent evidence of Alex engaging in high-risk behaviors such as substance abuse and references to sexual activity. She asked the clinician to address these issues directly with Alex while she was present in the interview.

These vignettes illustrate some common issues that can arise in the course of assessing adolescents. Setting the appropriate boundaries for an assessment can aid in rapport building with the adolescent and help avoid the pitfall of becoming solely the parental agent.

Case Example 3 also illustrates the pervasive influence of social media on today's youth. The role of social media has been revolutionary in changing entertainment, social interactions, and communication styles for adolescents (and adults). There are a variety of new and constantly evolving platforms, including but not limited to Facebook, Twitter, Snapchat, Instagram, and Tumblr, which teens routinely access, often having several simultaneous accounts for various functions. More than 60% of 13- to 17-year-olds have at least one profile on a social networking site, many spending more than 2 hours per day on social networking sites (O'Keeffe et al. 2011). As with any new technology, there are benefits as well as risks to use of social media. Teens may use these sites to continue off-line socialization and engage in a sense of community with peers with similar interests or to project idealized images of themselves, and they may even use them as part of their educational curriculum in schools. Unfortunately, other online behaviors can also negatively affect teens and their families in the form of compulsive use, cyberbullying, or "sexting" (sending sexually explicit messages or images through digital media). While parents often feel ill equipped or inadequate to keep pace with evolving technology that their children navigate with ease, it is imperative for parents to be able to safely monitor their child's online presence and set appropriate limits with regard to time spent on social media as well as with the degree of personal information shared. Often, this is a source of conflict among teens and parents. Use of and conflicts surrounding social media use should be part of an assessment and often become issues to address in treatment.

After dealing with confidentiality issues, the clinician should explain in general terms the structure anticipated in the first session: usually a joint interview to start, and then individual meetings with the adolescent and parent(s) to flesh out the presenting problems and history.

The Adolescent Interview

Most adolescents are brought for evaluation at least in part against their will. As a matter of fact, there is a significant decrease in the proportion of adolescents who receive an evaluation or treatment for psychiatric disorders as they age. As youth progress through adolescence, they are less likely to receive mental health evaluation or treatment (Cuffe et al. 2001). Many youth are forced into treatment by parents, social service agencies, schools, courts, and probation officers. How can an adolescent in such a position be successfully engaged?

An evidence-based approach that has been successfully used in adolescents, particularly teens with substance abuse, is called *motivational interviewing* or *motivational enhancement therapy* (see Chapter 45, "Motivational Interviewing"). Motivational interviewing focuses on the person's interests, concerns, and goals, and thus likely provides the adolescent with a more positive experience. This enhances the interviewer's role as an advocate for the adolescent rather than an agent of the parent. Motivational interviewing specifically focuses on the resolution of ambivalence, guiding the person toward positive change. The interviewer elicits from the adolescent thoughts about change, reinforces them, and deals with resistance in ways intended to reduce it.

In the first individual meeting with the adolescent, the key dialectic on which to focus is between rapport building and data collection. Both need to be accomplished. However, excessive focus on data collection can impede rapport building. In most cases, collecting data from the adolescent on the chief complaint and history of the present illness is off-putting and may result in impairing both rapport and data collection. The primary focus at the start of the interview is to begin to understand the adolescent's interests and strengths. This approach can break the ice for collecting data later in the interview.

After initial rapport building, the discussion of the adolescent's perception of why he or she has been brought for evaluation can proceed. It is important to try to elicit the adolescent's ideas as distinct from the parents' views. What does the adolescent see as the real problems? How would he or she like to see change in himself or herself and the family? This approach can begin to show that the clinician is interested and that the adolescent's ideas are important. The clinician should elicit ideas about problems in the family, in the adolescent, and in the adolescent's peer relationships and school functioning. The interviewer should begin with open-ended questions in order to obtain as broad and complete an idea as possible about the adolescent's views. Follow-up questions can be

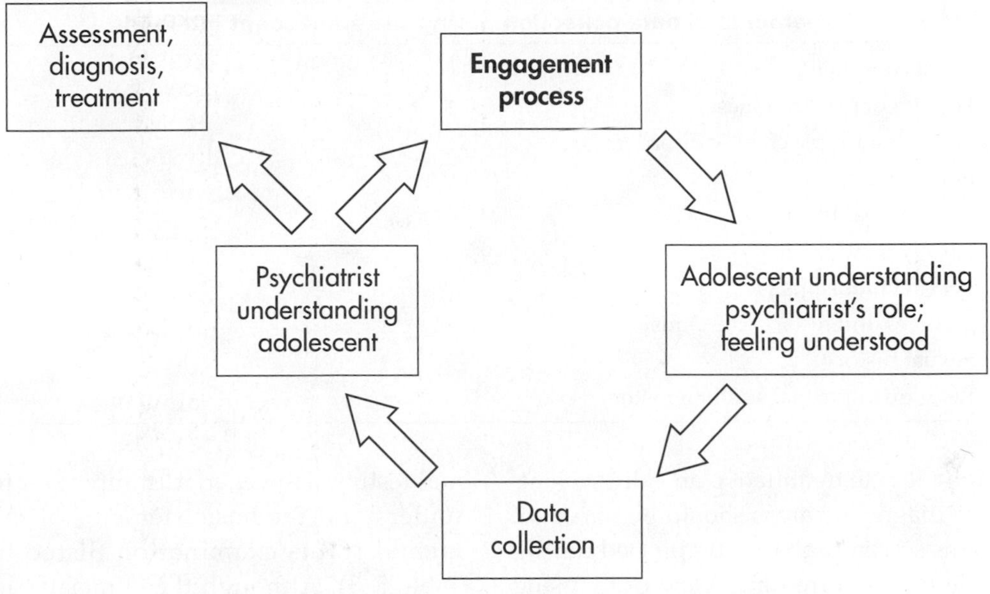

FIGURE 5–1. Adolescent interview.
Source. Adapted from Shea SC (ed): *Psychiatric Interviewing: The Art of Understanding.* Philadelphia, PA, W.B. Saunders, 1988, p. 8.

more focused and specific to elaborate topics. The interview should feel more like a conversation than a question-and-answer session.

Frequently, an adolescent may deny any problems or shrug and say "I don't know" when asked for ideas about problems. This is often a sign that the adolescent is not yet engaged. The interviewer may have to spend more time in the engagement process, perhaps using some motivational enhancement techniques, in order to move forward. The interview can be conceived as a cycle (Figure 5–1), consisting of the following elements:

1. The clinician engages the adolescent and seeks to understand his or her concerns, fears, and hopes.
2. The clinician conveys this understanding to the adolescent.
3. The adolescent begins to feel understood and to see the clinician as an ally, leading to the clinician's improved ability to collect accurate data.
4. The clinician uses data collection to increase understanding of the patient's problems.
5. The clinician conveys this increased understanding to improve engagement with the adolescent.

Table 5–2 lists the elements of data that should be obtained during the course of one or more interviews with the adolescent. The history of present illness includes the timing, onset, severity, and variability of symptoms, including whether the adolescent has experienced a similar episode or episodes in the past. Comorbid psychiatric disorders should always be investigated. Comorbid diagnoses are extremely common in children and adolescents (Angold et al. 1999; Lewinsohn et al. 1995). One of the most common mistakes inexperienced interviewers make is to prematurely home in on a diagnosis. This often excludes other diagnoses from consideration and results in an incomplete evaluation and

TABLE 5–2. Elements of data collection during the adolescent interview

Chief complaint
History of present illness
Screening for psychiatric disorders
Substance use
Educational history
Family relationships
Peer relationships
Hobbies, interests, sports, music
Sexual history
Religious, spiritual, cultural history

inadequate treatment plan. All psychiatric diagnostic areas should be screened. This screen can be accomplished during the unstructured interview or by using structured diagnostic instruments or rating scales (discussed in the section "Standardized Measures" later in this chapter). If not explicitly determined during the history of present illness, an assessment of suicidal and homicidal ideation, planning, and intent should be obtained, in addition to other dangerous or risky behaviors.

The interview should end with a brief discussion with the adolescent of the clinician's initial impressions and a review with the adolescent of how the interview with parents will be conducted, what areas will be covered, and how confidentiality will be handled. If there are areas the psychiatrist feels must be reported to the parent from the first adolescent interview, these should be discussed.

Mental Status Examination

The mental status examination is an important element of any assessment. Many aspects of the mental status examination can be done during the course of the interview, reducing the need for formal testing. However, it is important to understand the basic elements of the mental status examination (listed in Table 5–3). Although the clinician can often get a sense of the level of cognitive functioning from the interview, the astute clinician looks in the history for areas of strength or weakness that may not be apparent in the interview.

The Parent Interview

The clinician should have multiple goals for the initial parent interview. First and foremost, this interview provides an opportunity for the clinician to establish a relationship with the parent(s) that sets the stage for the ongoing treatment of the adolescent and, possibly, for the success or failure of that treatment. Absent a positive, collaborative relationship with an adolescent's parent, treatment is arduous at best.

A second goal of the interview is to understand the presenting problems from the parent's point of view. This is best done without the presence of the adolescent. The adolescent has likely heard about his or her problems many times in the past. Hearing the recitation of problems in front of a stranger often creates a hostile, antagonistic, and resis-

TABLE 5–3. Elements of the mental status examination

Attitude and behavior
Hygiene and style of dress
Speech: fluency, rate, rhythm, prosody
Motor: gait, coordination, abnormal movements
Orientation: person, place, time, circumstance
Affect (perceived by interviewer)
Mood (reported by adolescent)
Suicidal or homicidal ideation, plan, intent
Thought content: obsessions, delusions, looseness of associations
Perceptions: auditory, visual, tactile, olfactory hallucinations
Memory: immediate, recent, remote
Intellectual functioning: calculations, geography, presidents, and so forth
Abstraction: proverbs, similarities
Judgment
Insight

tive response from the adolescent. In addition, many parents will not frankly discuss their concerns about the adolescent in the presence of their child. It is important to remember that information from the parent about the adolescent's current problems and functioning is frequently not complete and is sometimes not accurate. Some parents may deny a particular problem or be unable to accurately recall certain events (Chess et al. 1966). A secondary goal of the parent interview is thus to try to gain insight into the validity of the parent's report.

Data collection is a third primary aim of the parent interview. The present illness should be thoroughly explored from the parent's perspective. Similar to the adolescent interview, a screening for other psychiatric disorders should be completed with the parents. Following discussion of the present illness, clinicians should explore historical information about both the child and the family. Table 5–4 lists the data elements parents can provide. This interview provides depth for the clinician's understanding of the child's and family's problems. How did the problems develop? Creating a timeline of important events in the family's and child's life, including the development of psychiatric symptoms, can aid in the understanding of the patient and family. If, during the course of the parent interview, information is obtained that one or both parents have experienced psychiatric or emotional problems, the clinician should strongly consider individual interviews with each parent to further explore how these problems may have affected the adolescent. From child abuse and domestic violence to anxiety, depression, or psychotic disorders, parental emotional problems may have an immense impact on a developing child (Cuffe et al. 2005). Absence or unavailability of a parent may cause anxiety, particularly separation fears, in the child. Divorce, separations, and the deaths of important family members should all be explored. A thorough family history of mental disorders should be obtained. In complex families, a family genogram, a diagram of the family history and relationship patterns of three or more generations of

TABLE 5–4. Elements of data collection from parents

- Parental history
  - Significant relationship issues
  - Current family stresses
  - Style of discipline
- Developmental history of the identified patient
  - Problems during pregnancy
    - Perinatal problems
    - Birth and delivery
  - Developmental milestones
    - Attachment/separation problems
    - Feeding problems
    - Motor development
    - Language development
    - Play
    - Peer relationships
  - Educational history: learning disabilities?
- Sibling relationships
  - Birth order
  - Relationship with siblings
  - Physical or emotional problems of siblings
- Family history of mental illness
  - Examination of each parent may be needed

family members (Hartman 1995; McGoldrick et al. 2008), is a helpful tool for organizing this information. More detailed information on parental history and functioning can be useful to obtain during the course of the evaluation and treatment. These elements may include a history of the parents' relationship; whether the patient's birth was planned; reactions to the pregnancy; and parent education level, employment, and financial situation. Conversely, it is also important for the clinician to try to understand how this child has affected the family. A child with serious emotional or behavioral problems can distort and impair the functioning of an otherwise healthy family. In some cases, the family's functioning improves once the impaired child is out of the home (Hechtman 1996).

At the conclusion of the initial interview with the parents, the clinician should provide to the parents an initial view of the strengths and weaknesses of their child and tell them how the evaluation will proceed. This presentation of initial findings is another time when the clinician can engage the parents in collaboration and further develop an alliance.

Family Assessment

The family assessment has already begun with the parent interview. In uncomplicated cases, there may be no need to interview each family member or see the entire family as a group. As a minimum requirement, the family assessment must include an observation of the child's interaction with caretakers (Josephson and AACAP Work Group on Quality Issues 2007). If there are clear indications that family interaction patterns, discipline style, or structure promote, precipitate, or perpetuate the adolescent's psychiatric or behavioral problems, a more thorough family evaluation should be undertaken. At this point, the assessment goals expand to include the meaning and function of the symptom in relation to the family (Josephson and AACAP Work Group on Quality Issues 2007).

For example, a family living in a small town once consulted the lead author about their teenage daughter. The girl was acting out and oppositional. During the initial interview with her, she expressed anger at having to live in such a small town (she and her family had recently moved from a large city). During the initial parent interview, it became clear that the daughter was acting out her mother's fury at her husband for having moved her to this town. The focus of the treatment, in order to be successful, had to include the treatment of the family to deal with this dynamic.

When a thorough evaluation of the family is indicated, the evaluation should adequately inform the clinician about the family's structure, communication, belief systems, and regulatory processes (Josephson and AACAP Work Group on Quality Issues 2007; see also Chapter 42, "Family-Based Assessment and Treatment"). *Family structure* refers to the important relationships and boundaries within families and the transactional patterns that exist within these relationships (Minuchin 1974). Boundaries should exist between generational elements in the family, such as between parent and child. Elements of family structure include its ability to change and adapt to new circumstances (adaptability) and the degree of cohesion among the members of the family. Is there a correct balance between autonomy of family members and closeness or connectedness among family members? Is the family enmeshed or disorganized and chaotic? Do healthy family boundaries exist, or is there evidence of boundary violations? Has the family been able to adapt to changes such as childbirth, divorce, or the death of a family member? Are the family rules and discipline clear and consistent?

Family communication refers not only to the ability to communicate clearly and effectively both facts and emotional content but also to the ability to problem solve. Are family members able to identify problems, negotiate conflicts, and resolve issues in a way that enhances family functioning? Do family members feel part of the process, or is the decision making authoritarian? *Family beliefs* often influence the way in which families make decisions and function. Family beliefs are ideas about reality that are shared among family members and denote a kind of family memory system (Josephson and AACAP Work Group on Quality Issues 2007). Family beliefs often guide decision making. They may be healthy and promote positive action (family members protect each other in times of stress) or may be unhealthy (e.g., men are alcoholic and abusive). These beliefs may show a generational pattern of continuity.

The final element of family functioning, *family regulatory processes,* refers to the ability of the family to meet the developmental needs of the children and promote healthy growth and development. Are family members able to nurture and support the children? At the conclusion of the family assessment, the clinician should be able to incorporate the family's strengths and problems into an overall formulation of the identified patient and be able to understand the reciprocal effects of the adolescent and the family on each other.

Standardized Measures

Psychological testing and standardized instruments that rate symptoms and behaviors can supplement data from the clinical interview and observations of the adolescent and family. In this section we briefly mention diagnostic interviews and symptom rating scales. Diagnostic interviews are generally modular and can be used to assess symptoms of a particular diagnostic category or to broadly screen across all diagnostic areas. It is important to note that these measures cannot replace the clinical interview but rather should be used to help focus the clinical interview on areas of concern. Compared with earlier developmental periods, adolescence may be an optimal time for structured interviews. The adolescent is cognitively capable of completing the interviews in either a computer or an interview format. Adolescents may also be more open and responsive in the less personal computer-administered format.

Diagnostic interviews allow a comprehensive assessment of psychiatric diagnoses and are of two primary types: interviewer-based and respondent-based interviews. The Schedule for Affective Disorders and Schizophrenia for School-Age Children (K-SADS; Ambrosini 2000; Chambers et al. 1985) and the Child and Adolescent Psychiatric Assessment (CAPA; Angold and Costello 2000) are examples of interviewer-based diagnostic interviews. These are semistructured interviews that allow the interviewer to make judgments during the interview. They require a clinician or highly trained interviewer and thus are more expensive to administer. Respondent-based interviews, such as the National Institute of Mental Health Diagnostic Interview Schedule for Children, Version IV (DISC-IV; Shaffer et al. 2000), are highly structured and use trained lay interviewers. The interviewer follows a predetermined script and is not allowed to deviate from the script or interpret the subject's response. The DISC-IV has also been formatted for computer administration and has a special program for adolescents to self-administer the interview (Voice DISC-IV; Lucas 2003; Shaffer et al. 2000).

Rating scales screen for problem symptoms or behaviors using parent, adolescent, or teacher reports. They should be used to help focus the clinician on problem areas to explore. These instruments generally compare responses for the individual being assessed with standardized population norms. Rating scales may be broadband scales assessing problems across broad dimensions of behavior, such as the Child Behavior Checklist (CBCL; Achenbach and Rescorla 2001) and the Behavior Assessment System for Children (BASC; Kamphaus et al. 2007), or narrowband scales focused on a dimension of behavior, such as depression or attention-deficit/hyperactivity. Rating scales place subjective reports from parents, teachers, or adolescents into a more objective form by comparing their responses with those of a normative population. This allows the clinician to better understand how deviant the adolescent's behavior is from that of other adolescents.

Presenting the Findings

At the conclusion of any assessment, whether it is a single interview or a highly complex assessment involving multiple interviews, the clinician analyzes the data obtained and uses his or her diagnostic skill and clinical acumen to develop an understanding of the problems and strengths of the adolescent and family. Using a biopsychosocial framework, the clinician should understand the predisposing, precipitating, perpetuating, and protective factors at work in the case and develop a treatment plan to address those areas. Next, the clinician must convey the assessment and recommended plan to the adolescent and parents. The presentation of the findings is a critical aspect of the assessment process (Group for the Advancement of Psychiatry 1957) and should be done with care and empathy for those receiving the results. Coming for a psychiatric evaluation is difficult, and both the adolescent and parents may be anxious about the results, fearing that each will be identified as the cause of the problem. Parents feel guilty and fear their "failings as parents" will be exposed, while the adolescent is braced for more blows to his or her self-esteem. It is important, therefore, to be supportive and reassuring during this discussion (Cox 1994). In order to maintain and enhance the relationship with the adolescent, it is often best to meet with the adolescent first to let him or her hear the results. The adolescent can then respond without having to deal with the complicated relationships that may exist with parents. Following this, the clinician can meet with the parents, with or without the adolescent's presence.

The first part of the presentation should always focus on the strengths of both the adolescent and the parents. The psychiatrist might say, for example, "Mike is a bright and engaging boy...very creative and funny. He has a lot going for him." Beginning this way helps to set everyone at ease. The important thing to keep in mind is that the positive attributes must reflect reality. The clinician may also want to highlight problems not found, which the parents or adolescent may have feared. Next, the clinician begins to discuss the problem areas uncovered during the assessment. It is important to convey not only what symptoms and diagnoses have been found but also a formulation of how the problems developed and are perpetuated. The clinician must not shy away from discussing parental or family factors. While it is important not to make the parents feel they are solely to blame for their child's problems, it is equally important that family and social issues are acknowledged and discussed frankly.

Finally, the clinician presents the proposed plan for treatment. This should be done in a manner that encourages discussion and collaboration. In addition, the clinician should incorporate the strengths of the child and family into the discussion of the plan of treatment and prognosis. This allows the session to end on a positive and hopeful note. In this way, the discussion of the problems and difficulties are "sandwiched" between discussions of the positive attributes of the child and family, allowing the family to feel understood and supported at the end of the assessment and, hopefully, setting the stage for a positive working relationship to begin the treatment.

Summary Points

- Adolescents must be assessed from a developmental perspective that includes family, school, peer, and community assessments.
- Reports from adolescents, mothers, fathers, teachers, and other caregivers show only modest agreement. Information should be collected from multiple sources.
- Confidentiality and consent to treatment should be explicitly discussed at the onset of the evaluation.
- Oppositional behavior is frequent among adolescents forced to participate by parents, school, or the legal system.
- Motivational interviewing is a promising tool to enhance the engagement of adolescents in the assessment and treatment process.
- Family assessment is crucial, and the adolescent should, at a minimum, be observed interacting with caregiver(s).
- Symptom or behavior rating scales make parent, teacher, and youth reports more objective by comparing responses with a normative population.
- Assessment of adolescents should result in a formulation of the biological, psychological, social, cultural, and spiritual factors predisposing, precipitating, and perpetuating the development of psychopathology in the adolescent and family.
- Presentation of the findings of the assessment should emphasize the strengths of the adolescent and family, in addition to the problems or weaknesses, and should be done in an empathic, supportive manner.

References

Achenbach TM, Rescorla LA: Manual for ASEBA School-Age Forms and Profiles. Burlington, University of Vermont, Research Center for Children, Youth, and Families, 2001

Ambrosini PJ: Historical development and present status of the Schedule for Affective Disorders and Schizophrenia for School-Age Children (K-SADS). J Am Acad Child Adolesc Psychiatry 39(1):49–58, 2000 10638067

Angold A, Costello EJ: The Child and Adolescent Psychiatric Assessment (CAPA). J Am Acad Child Adolesc Psychiatry 39(1):39–48, 2000 10638066

Angold A, Costello EJ, Erkanli A: Comorbidity. J Child Psychol Psychiatry 40(1):57–87, 1999 10102726

Cantwell DP, Lewinsohn PM, Rohde P, et al: Correspondence between adolescent report and parent report of psychiatric diagnostic data. J Am Acad Child Adolesc Psychiatry 36(5):610–619, 1997 9136495

Chambers WJ, Puig-Antich J, Hirsch M, et al: The assessment of affective disorders in children and adolescents by semistructured interview. Test-retest reliability of the Schedule for Affective Disorders and Schizophrenia for School-Age Children, Present Episode Version. Arch Gen Psychiatry 42(7):696–702, 1985 4015311

Chess S, Thomas A, Birch HG: Distortions in developmental reporting made by parents of behaviorally disturbed children. J Am Acad Child Psychiatry 5(2):226–234, 1966 5908286

Cox AD: Interviews with parents, in Child and Adolescent Psychiatry: Modern Approaches. Edited by Rutter M, Taylor E,

Hersov L. Oxford, UK, Blackwell Scientific, 1994, pp 34–50

Cuffe SP, Waller JL, Addy CL, et al: A longitudinal study of adolescent mental health service use. J Behav Health Serv Res 28(1):1–11, 2001 11329994

Cuffe SP, McKeown RE, Addy CL, et al: Family and psychosocial risk factors in a longitudinal epidemiological study of adolescents. J Am Acad Child Adolesc Psychiatry 44(2):121–129, 2005 15689725

Group for the Advancement of Psychiatry: The Diagnostic Process in Child Psychiatry (Rep No 38). New York, Group for the Advancement of Psychiatry, 1957

Hartman A: Diagrammatic assessment of family relationships. Fam Soc 76(2):111–122, 1995

Hechtman L: Families of children with attention deficit hyperactivity disorder: a review. Can J Psychiatry 41(6):350–360, 1996 8862854

Josephson AM, AACAP Work Group on Quality Issues: Practice parameter for the assessment of the family. J Am Acad Child Adolesc Psychiatry 46(7):922–937, 2007 17581454

Kamphaus RW, VanDeventer MC, Brueggemann A, et al: Behavior Assessment System for Children, in The Clinical Assessment of Children and Adolescents: A Practitioner's Handbook. Edited by Smith SR, Handler L. Mahwah, NJ, Lawrence Erlbaum Associates, 2007, pp 311–326

King RA, American Academy of Child and Adolescent Psychiatry: Practice parameters for the psychiatric assessment of children and adolescents. J Am Acad Child Adolesc Psychiatry 34(10):1386–1402, 1995 7592276

Kramer TL, Phillips SD, Hargis MB, et al: Disagreement between parent and adolescent reports of functional impairment. J Child Psychol Psychiatry 45(2):248–259, 2004 14982239

Lebel C, Beaulieu C: Longitudinal development of human brain wiring continues from childhood into adulthood. J Neurosci 31(30):10937–10947, 2011 21795544

Lewinsohn PM, Rohde P, Seeley JR: Adolescent psychopathology: III. The clinical consequences of comorbidity. J Am Acad Child Adolesc Psychiatry 34(4):510–519, 1995 7751265

Lucas CP: Use of structured diagnostic interviews in clinical child psychiatric practice, in Standardized Evaluation in Clinical Practice (Review of Psychiatry, Vol 22). Edited by First MB. Washington, DC, American Psychiatric Publishing, 2003, pp 75–101

McGoldrick M, Gerson R, Petry S: Genograms: Assessment and Intervention, 3rd Edition. New York, WW Norton, 2008

Minuchin S: Families and Family Therapy. Cambridge, MA, Harvard University Press, 1974

O'Keeffe GS, Clarke-Pearson K, Council on Communications and Media: The impact of social media on children, adolescents, and families. Pediatrics 127(4):800–804, 2011 21444588

Shaffer D, Fisher P, Lucas CP, et al: NIMH Diagnostic Interview Schedule for Children Version IV (NIMH DISC-IV): description, differences from previous versions, and reliability of some common diagnoses. J Am Acad Child Adolesc Psychiatry 39(1):28–38, 2000 10638065

Youngstrom E, Loeber R, Stouthamer-Loeber M: Patterns and correlates of agreement between parent, teacher, and male adolescent ratings of externalizing and internalizing problems. J Consult Clin Psychol 68(6):1038–1050, 2000 11142538

CHAPTER 6

Neurological Examination, Electroencephalography, Neuroimaging, and Neuropsychological Testing

Sigita Plioplys, M.D.
Miya R. Asato, M.D.
Frank Zelko, Ph.D.

The Neurological Examination

Despite advances in neuroimaging, genetics, and biochemical evaluations, there is no substitution for the clinical art of history taking and a thorough neurological examination.

Chief Complaint

While many patients and families may be able to articulate a specific symptom or problem(s), others may only be able to define a functional difficulty that may point to a neurological symptom, such as clumsiness in a child with hypotonia or ataxia, or inattention in a child with absence epilepsy. The clinician should elicit historical information to define the problem as

- Acute or chronic
- Static or progressive
- Focal or generalized/systemic

The examination findings will point toward localization.

Case Example 1

John is an 8-year-old boy with a history of premature birth and associated hypoxic ischemia resulting in spastic diplegia and mild intellectual disability presents with a 4-week history of sudden jerking of the extremities. These events occur in the awake state only and involve a quick jerk of the arms and legs and a stiffening of the trunk without alteration in level of consciousness prior to, during, or after the event. The events occur singly at random times. He is easily distractible and fidgety and has significant difficulties sustaining attention, following directions, and learning. The remainder of his history and review of systems is unremarkable.

The events in question are episodic and represent either an epileptic or a nonepileptic phenomenon. Because of the symmetric nature of the event, bilateral involvement of the motor cortex or basal ganglia may be a possibility. Extremity jerking can also originate from the brainstem or spinal cord. Relevant findings on the examination and diagnostic testing will be essential to finalize localization and determine whether the events are tics, epileptic myoclonus, spinal myoclonus, and/or a sign of a more disseminated brain disease, such as central nervous system (CNS) infection or demyelinating conditions.

General Guidelines and Developmental Aspects

A significant proportion of the neurological examination can be obtained by simply observing and speaking with the child or adolescent, and guidelines are included in Table 6–1. The younger the child, the less the neurological examination resembles the examination of an adult.

The *mental status examination* needs to assess level of alertness, consciousness, speech and language, social skills, and affect. Depending on the age of the patient, assessments of specific cognitive skills (calculation, reading, recall) may also be included.

Cranial nerve assessment is easily observed during the interview. Any asymmetry should be further evaluated during the extremity motor examination to elucidate whether this represents only facial involvement or the whole body and whether this would localize to the peripheral nerve, brainstem, or contralateral motor cortex. For a patient with suspected weakness in the oral or facial muscles, observing the patient chew or swallow is helpful. Ocular muscle weakness due to neuromuscular junction disorders such as myasthenia gravis can be assessed by testing eye muscle strength needed to maintain upgaze and a history of drooping eyelids.

The *sensory examination* can be challenging and is the least objective part of the examination in nonverbal and/or young patients. The *motor examination* typically consists of assessment of muscle tone and strength. However, children younger than 4 years typically cannot understand directions adequately for a formal muscular strength assessment. In such patients, having the patient perform different tasks will give at a minimum an idea of how the muscles oppose gravity and whether the patient can withstand the resistance of his or her own body (e.g., getting up from the prone position on the floor). Major motor developmental milestones in children include attainment of walking around 12–17 months, running before age 2 years, and hopping on one foot by age 4 years. Hand dominance prior to age 1 year can be a sign of weakness of the contralateral extremity. For evaluation of patients with chronic problems, documentation of functional abilities from one visit to the next can be a useful marker of clinical progression, such as increased difficulty getting up from a chair in a patient with muscular dystrophy who is having increased proximal muscle weakness.

For patients with motor limitations, localization of the presenting problem is

TABLE 6–1. Elements of the neurological examination based on observation

Examination component	Observation questions
Mental status	• How engaged and oriented is the patient to the environment, people, and presenting concern? • Is he or she able to articulate and speak coherently and understand language? • Does the speech have regular rate and prosody? • What is the mood and affect of the patient? Does he or she make good eye contact? • Does the patient pay attention and show age-appropriate fund of knowledge?
Cranial nerves	• Is the face symmetric with a good range of facial expression? • Is there any eyelid or facial drooping?
Motor	• What is the sitting posture of the patient? • Are there any gross or fine movement abnormalities, asymmetry? • Can he or she get up and down from the chair without using the armrests (i.e., good proximal muscle strength)?
Sensory	• Does the patient have a high-stepping gait, sometimes seen in sensory neuropathies (Friedrich's ataxia, vitamin B_{12} deficiency)?
Cerebellar	• Are there any tremors, ataxia, or clumsiness?
Gait	• Is there any toe walking (a potential sign of lower-extremity spasticity) or asymmetry of arm swing while walking (a potential sign of mild limb paresis)?

necessary to differentiate whether the motor weakness is due to an upper or a lower motor neuron lesion (Table 6–2). Since motor and muscle tone pathways share many of the same neuroanatomical pathways, weakness may often be accompanied by alterations in muscle tone. *Deep tendon reflexes* could point to either upper or lower motor neuron deficits, as noted in Table 6–2.

Coordination assessment may be accomplished by holding toys so the patient has to reach across the midline to reach them; any tremors, dysmetria, or dyscoordination may be noted. Having the patient kick an imaginary ball to assess gross motor lower extremity coordination or walk on an imaginary tightrope to assess tandem gait is a nonthreatening way to perform this part of the examination. By age 3 years, children are able to stand on one foot; by age 4 years, children are able to hop on one foot, and by age 6 years, they can perform tandem gait.

Gait should be assessed in all patients, as observation of the trunk and limbs is important. If the patient wears any splints or uses any assistive devices, he or she should ideally be observed both with and without them. The examiner should note whether there is any asymmetry, particularly in shifting from leg to leg; how the foot makes contact with the walking surface (e.g., flat-footed, slapping, or walking on toes); and whether there are any associated unusual movements, such as posturing of the upper extremities in patients with hemiparesis. These abnormalities can often be accentuated during running.

The *general physical examination* is also relevant, as many conditions can have multisystem effects. Starting with

TABLE 6–2. Localization of weakness

	Upper motor neuron	Lower motor neuron
Character of weakness	Spastic paralysis with muscle hypertonia	Flaccid paralysis with hypotonia
Mental status	Encephalopathy, developmental delay, intellectual disability, and seizures	Generally preserved
Distribution	Asymmetric if due to cortical lesion	Usually bilateral
DTRs	Increased	Decreased or absent
Other findings	Babinski reflex positive	Babinski reflex not present Muscle fasciculations and fibrillations

Note. DTR=deep tendon reflex.

growth assessment, the examiner should note the patient's height, weight, and head circumference. Growth retardation affecting all parameters or just the head can be seen in genetic syndromes or congenital infections. Likewise, large head circumference (greater than the 98th percentile) should be investigated further to rule out whether there is an expansive process causing rapid head enlargement, such as hydrocephalus.

Dysmorphic features in conjunction with developmental or neurological problems may point to a clinical syndrome. Cleft lip and palate and aortic arch defects can signify midline brain structural abnormalities. The cardiac and renal systems can be involved in multisystem conditions such as myotonic dystrophy. Because both the brain and skin have embryological origins in the ectoderm, clues to neurological disease can be found in the skin examination, such as café au lait spots and axillary freckling in neurofibromatosis type 1.

Neurological Differential Diagnosis Guided by the History and Examination

The initial differential diagnosis should focus on broad etiologic categories, such as vascular, metabolic, epileptic, infectious, traumatic, toxic, congenital, or neoplastic. Knowledge of the full medical history and review of systems are essential to frame the chief complaint and the findings on the physical examination to determine whether they fall into a clinically recognizable syndrome.

Case Example 2

Rose, a 3-year-old girl with features of autism and global developmental delay, presents with staring spells, typically occurring at school and lasting 30–60 seconds. During this time, she is unresponsive and picks at her clothes. She seems tired afterward. Her physical examination is otherwise unremarkable, except for a red papular rash on her cheeks and one hypopigmented macule on her back measuring 5 centimeters. Her neurological examination is notable only for limited verbal communication skills and eye contact and some clumsiness in rapidly alternating movements.

The events under question are associated with alteration in consciousness, stereotypic movements, and fatigue after the event, suggestive of seizures. The examination findings are remarkable for possible neurocutaneous stigmata on the cheeks, possibly representing adenoma sebaceum, also known as *facial angiofibromas.* The hypopigmented macule could represent an ash leaf spot. Taken together, the two skin findings, preexisting autism, and events concerning for seizures may be representative of tuberous sclerosis. With this possible diagnosis in mind, localization of the paroxysmal events would most likely be central in origin, given that intracranial tubers can cause seizures that may be identified with electroencephalography and neuroimaging.

Electroencephalography

Electroencephalography (EEG) is an important part of the neurological evaluation in CNS disorders. EEG interpretation is optimally performed by a neurologist with experience in pediatric EEG who can provide interpretation in light of the patient's developmental and clinical status.

The electroencephalographic waves are recorded from surface electrodes and ideally document the patient in the awake, drowsy, and light sleep states. Each electroencephalographic channel measures the electropotential difference between the two points where the channel is applied on the scalp (for more details, see Wylie et al. 2011).

Indications for EEG include diagnostic evaluation of seizures, seizure-like paroxysmal episodes, assessment of the adequacy of antiepileptic treatment, and altered mental status. Examination of the electroencephalographic background waves and their ongoing rhythm provides the baseline electroencephalographic state of the patient. The electroencephalographic waves are highly influenced by the state of alertness—whether the patient is alert, drowsy, or asleep—and the child's age, medications, structural brain lesions, and disease states. Typical rhythms are classified according to their frequency as delta (1–3/second), theta (4–7/second), alpha (8–12/second), and beta (13–20/second). Delta waves can be seen in deeper stages of sleep and also in pathological states such as encephalopathy. Alpha is the predominant wave pattern while one is awake with the eyes closed, best seen in the posterior head leads. Beta waves can be seen during sleep states, particularly in infants and children, and also in patients receiving medications such as benzodiazepines. Theta waves can be seen during awake states in children, although they are more common in drowsy states.

Patients with epilepsy may not consistently demonstrate seizures or epileptiform activity on routine electroencephalographic recordings, although with repeated and prolonged video EEG studies and under sleep deprivation, epileptiform interictal activity can be captured.

Not all epileptiform activity signifies epilepsy. If epileptic discharges are found on the electroencephalogram of an otherwise normal child, correlation of the electroencephalographic findings to the clinical scenario is crucial. For example, high-amplitude slowing in school-age children is a normal phenomenon, whereas spike and slow-wave discharges induced by either hyperventilation or photic stimulation are pathological and represent an increased possibility of seizures.

Compared with psychiatrically healthy control subjects, patients with psychiatric diagnoses, such as attention-deficit/hyperactivity disorder (ADHD), have increased incidence of epileptiform abnormalities and risk for development of seizures (Hesdorffer et al. 2004). Patients with migraine also have been reported to have epileptiform abnormalities (Gronseth and Greenberg 1995), which may account in part for the common co-occurrence of both disorders (Andermann and Andermann 1987).

Clinical Indications for Electroencephalography Use in Child Psychiatry

Altered Mental Status

An electroencephalogram may be indicated to rule out nonconvulsive seizures. CNS infections, such as herpes encephalitis manifesting with altered mental status, can have either generalized or lateralizing periodic epileptiform discharges that are not due to primary epilepsy but signify the ongoing disease process. Given increased recognition of a type of autoimmune encephalitis, anti-*N*-methyl-D-aspartate receptor (NMDAR) encephalitis, EEG along with other diagnostic testing should be considered in patients with new onset of acute psychiatric symptoms with concurrent neurological features such as seizures, abnormal movements, or tic-like facial dyskinesias (Armangue et al. 2013). Patients who are in the postictal state may present similarly and may demonstrate generalized or focal slowing on EEG. In general, the degree of slowing on the electroencephalogram correlates with the severity of the alteration of consciousness.

Loss of Language or Other Acquired Skills

Alterations of previously acquired skills may be due to epileptic processes, such as Landau-Kleffner syndrome, autoimmune CNS disorders, or electrical status epilepticus of slow-wave sleep, in which continuous spike and slow-wave discharges predominate in at least 85% of slow-wave sleep time. Landau-Kleffner syndrome is characterized by sudden or gradual acquired aphasia, predominantly affecting receptive language. In such presentations, overnight sleep EEG facilitates diagnosis.

Paroxysmal Events

Paroxysmal nonepileptic events that occur in childhood and adolescence are listed by differential diagnosis in Table 6–3.

Events that are suspected to be seizures should be investigated with video EEG. Alternatively, an ambulatory EEG via a portable electroencephalographic recording device can offer extended monitoring for a patient with limited access to telemetry. All clinical events in question should be noted and documented by the patient and/or family. The goal is correlation of observed episodic events with electroencephalographic findings.

Neurodevelopmental Disabilities

Patients with intellectual disability and/or autism pose the greatest diagnostic challenge, because of frequent baseline electroencephalographic abnormalities and limited cognitive and verbal abilities. The predictive value of epileptiform electroencephalographic findings and the higher risk for seizures in this clinical population continue to be studied; thus, electroencephalographic abnormalities may not actually represent seizures and may not necessarily indicate a need for treatment. The improvement of the events under question with antiepileptic medications is not a reliable diagnostic test for seizures, as this type of treatment may represent a placebo effect or may be due to the drug's mood-stabilizing properties. Both epilepsy and nonepileptic events are common in this population. Staring episodes, rage attacks, and repetitive movements should be investigated with EEG before a diagnosis of

TABLE 6–3. Paroxysmal nonepileptic events in children and adolescents

Altered responsiveness
Syncope
Migraine and equivalents
Toxic ingestion
Falling with unresponsiveness
Syncope (vasovagal or neurocardiogenic)
Craniocervical junction disorders
Chiari type I malformation
Organized repetitive movements
Tics
Stereotypic behaviors
Paroxysmal torticollis
Psychogenic myoclonus
Psychogenic nonepileptic seizures
Disorganized movements
Psychogenic nonepileptic seizures
Chorea (Sydenham, toxic, stroke related)
Paroxysmal dyskinesia
Dystonia
Staring
Daydreaming
Inattention
Stereotypic behaviors
Nocturnal events
Head banging, sleepwalking, and sleep talking
Night terrors and nightmares
Narcolepsy and cataplexy
Periodic leg movements

epilepsy is made and treatment with antiepileptic medications is started.

Neuroimaging

Significant progress in neuroimaging has advanced understanding of the structure and function of the brain and has further supported the neurodevelopmental model of pediatric psychiatric disorders (Marsh et al. 2008).

Review of Neuroimaging Methods

In this section, we discuss basic theoretical and technical principles underlying neuroimaging testing. For detailed review of specific technological characteristics and interpretation of neuroimaging data, see discussions by Hess and Barkovich (2012) and Tortori-Donati et al. (2005).

Computed Tomography

Currently, the main indications for computed tomography (CT) of the brain are urgent evaluations of CNS trauma, acute brain hemorrhage, and increased intracranial pressure, or when magnetic resonance imaging (MRI) is not available or is contraindicated (for review, see Wycliffe et al. 2006). CT may be superior to MRI in detecting small areas of calcification.

Magnetic Resonance Imaging

MRI has an extremely high safety profile and does not expose patients to radiation. Thus, it is the first choice for neuroimaging in the pediatric population. MRI uses magnetic fields and radiofrequency pulses to obtain images of body organs (for review, see Hess and Barkovich 2012). MRI provides high resolution and discrimination of white and gray matter and cerebrospinal fluid, and it presents exquisite details of cortical and subcortical architecture as well as other brain structures (Durston et al. 2001; Giedd 2004).

Functional MRI (fMRI) measures the blood oxygen level–dependent signal (BOLD), which represents functional use of energy by brain tissue during cognitive, sensory, and motor tasks (for review, see Ernst and Rumsey 2000). Changes in oxygen concentration are detected within seconds after the initiation of the task. Clinically, fMRI is most commonly used to preoperatively evaluate patients with epilepsy to determine hemispheric language dominance and for surgical planning (Cascio et al. 2007).

Magnetic Resonance Spectroscopy

Magnetic resonance spectroscopy (MRS) provides information on biochemical brain functions by measuring the concentration and distribution of several metabolites, such as creatine, choline, and *N*-acetyl aspartate (NAA) (for review, see Hess and Barkovich 2012). Creatine is an indicator of the brain's bioenergetic metabolism, choline is a marker of neuronal structural integrity, and NAA is a marker of neuronal functioning. In children, MRS is used for the assessment of metabolic, mitochondrial, and neurodegenerative disorders; identification of epileptic focus; and preoperative evaluation of brain tumors (Wycliffe et al. 2006). Although the exact relationship between the concentration of a particular metabolite and psychopathology is not clear, MRS has been extensively used as a research tool in ADHD and mood and anxiety disorders. MRS can measure concentrations of excitatory and inhibitory neurotransmitters, such as glutamate, glutamine, and γ-aminobutyric acid (GABA).

Diffusion Tensor Imaging

Diffusion tensor imaging (DTI) measures the net movement (diffusion) of water molecules in the brain and is a readily available MRI method for visualizing and quantifying brain white matter (Cascio et al. 2007). DTI provides three-dimensional maps of the white matter microstructure and spatial organization in the hemispheres by showing water diffusion along the white matter tracts. Clinically, DTI is used for early assessment of tumors as well as in ischemic and traumatic brain injury (Hess and Barkovich 2012). As a research tool, DTI is a primary method to investigate neural connectivity in normal and clinical conditions, such as language and learning disorders, autism, ADHD, and schizophrenia (Ashtari et al. 2007; Barnea-Goraly et al. 2005).

Positron Emission Tomography and Single-Photon Emission Computed Tomography

Positron emission tomography (PET) and single-photon emission computed tomography (SPECT) use radioactive isotopes to measure cerebral blood flow; metabolism of glucose, oxygen, and proteins; and function of neurotransmitters in the brain (Hess and Barkovich 2012). Clinically, PET and SPECT are most useful in identification of focal epileptogenic brain regions in patients with seizures and with or without structural MRI or electroencephalographic abnormalities (Wycliffe et al. 2006). Although modern radioactive isotopes have a very short radioactive half-life (2–20 minutes for oxygen-15 and carbon-11) and produce minimal radiation (Wycliffe et al. 2006), ethical considerations of patient exposure to radiation have limited use of PET and SPECT in clinical child psychiatry.

Neuroimaging of Brain Development

Neuroimaging data on longitudinal brain development are available from the National Institute of Mental Health (NIMH) pediatric brain MRI project of children and youth with normal development and those with psychopathology (Almli et al. 2007; Giedd et al. 1999, 2006; Lenroot and Giedd 2006). Normative pediatric samples demonstrate that total brain volume reaches adult size by age 5–8 years and remains stable until about age 20 years (Lenroot and Giedd 2006). Different brain structures mature at different times (Thompson et al. 2005). Phylogenetically older brain areas, such as the olfactory, visual, or somatosensory cortex, appear to mature first, followed by the temporal, parietal, and finally prefrontal cortex (Casey et al. 2000; Gogtay et al. 2004). Maturation of white matter is an intense process during the first 2 years of life (Zhang et al. 2005) but also continues throughout adolescence (Barnea-Goraly et al. 2005; Mukherjee et al. 2002; Schneider et al. 2004).

In typically developing populations, total cerebral volume, specifically, the volume of prefrontal and subcortical gray matter, may explain variance in IQ (Shaw et al. 2006). However, the relationship between brain size and intellectual functions cannot be directly interpreted because of complex anatomical, chemical, and electrophysiological interactions in the distributed neural networks (Giedd 2001; Lenroot and Giedd 2006). Furthermore, several disorders associated with intellectual disability, such as fragile X, Turner, Down, Williams, velocardiofacial, Cohen, and Sotos syndromes, may not necessarily exhibit reliable changes in whole brain volume. In such cases, imaging studies of the specific brain regions of interest may be more informative to investigate the pathogenesis and guide treatment targets.

Imaging data demonstrate the associations between brain maturation and improved cognitive abilities (Casey et al. 2000; Shaw et al. 2006; Zhang et al. 2005). For example, fMRI studies have shown that cortical activation changes from a more diffuse, nonspecific pattern in younger children to more focal and defined in older children (Durston et al. 2006). The strength of hemispheric language lateralization continues to increase into adulthood, although primary language dominance is reached before age 7–8 years (Holland et al. 2001; Lee et al. 1999). Increased white matter maturation in the frontostriatal and frontotemporal cortex is associated with improved language, semantic memory, and executive function performance (Ashtari et al. 2007). Developmental changes in the white and gray matter structures may be associated with enhanced neuronal connectivity and cortical differentiation.

Clinical Applications in Child Psychiatry

Neuroimaging has become an essential clinical diagnostic tool in pediatric neurology, but in today's child psychiatry, its primary application is still in research. The use of any neuroimaging testing to diagnose or suggest treatment for psychiatric disorders in children is unsupported by clinical or scientific data and is further complicated by ethical considerations (Zametkin et al. 2005).

High-quality neuroimaging studies in children may be challenging to obtain. Young age and developmental delay often limit understanding and compliance with the procedures necessary for accurate testing. Impulsivity, hyperactivity, anxiety, and fear may also impair testing; thus, sedation is necessary for most MRI studies in children younger than 8 years, unless an audiovisual system is available for the child's entertainment during the procedure (Hess and Barkovich 2012). Sedation, however, impairs participation in the cognitive task; thus, it is not compatible with functional MRI testing. Any sedation should be administered and monitored by a trained physician under the American Academy of Pediatrics Committee on

Drugs (1992) guidelines for monitoring and management of pediatric patients during and after sedation for diagnostic and therapeutic procedures.

In clinical child psychiatry practice, neurology consultation and neuroimaging are indicated for patients with new neurological symptoms or deterioration of previously stable neurological functioning and in some cases of suspected child abuse or inconsistent history of a traumatic event. It is the child neurologist's role to determine the specific imaging modality. In psychiatric patients, neuroimaging may be used to rule out systematic or CNS disorders that potentially contribute to psychopathology, such as first-episode psychosis. MRI scans should be ordered in the evaluation of movement disorders of uncertain etiology, anorexia nervosa (to rule out a pituitary tumor), and severe treatment-resistant mood and psychotic disorders (Giedd 2001).

Neuropsychological Testing

Neuropsychological testing is used to characterize in detail the cognitive functioning of a patient compared with same-age peers. The composition of neuropsychological testing varies with the age and developmental status of the patient, but a common core is a measure of general cognitive development or intelligence. In the analysis of neuropsychological testing results, subcomponents of intellectual ability such as verbal comprehension, perceptual organization, working memory, and processing speed are considered in relation to other domains of cognitive functioning such as receptive and expressive language, visuographic and visuoconstructional ability, verbal and visual memory, attention, executive skills, fine motor dexterity, and academic achievement (Baron 2004). A list of domains and measures commonly employed in neuropsychological assessment is provided in Table 6–4.

The patient's profile of strengths and weaknesses in these domains is the focus of interpretation in a neuropsychological evaluation report. While this profile may be of some use in localization of cerebral dysfunction, it often does not have high diagnostic specificity. For example, disruptions of attention, processing speed, and executive skills are common to a number of neurological, psychiatric, and general medical disorders. However, the profile can assist in differential diagnosis and monitoring a patient's cognitive status over time.

Neuropsychological testing also affords the opportunity to observe a patient's response to challenge and other performance-related behaviors closely over a time period of several hours. Cognitive test results are considered in the context of these behaviors and other sources of information about the patient's behavioral and emotional status. However, in the controlled testing environment, which carefully structures tasks and limits external distractors, functional deficits observed in a patient's everyday life (e.g., absentmindedness) are sometimes not seen.

While long, comprehensive, multihour neuropsychological evaluations are common, short evaluation formats can effectively address questions such as declining memory or mental status changes in populations such as cancer survivors (Krull et al. 2008). However, such short formats trade efficiency for detailed information relevant to academic and rehabilitation interventions.

Given the cost and time demands, the decision to refer a patient for neuropsy-

TABLE 6–4. Cognitive domains and examples of measures used in neuropsychological assessment

Cognitive domain	Examples of measures
General intellectual ability	Wechsler Scales of Intelligence Stanford-Binet Intelligence Scale Differential Ability Scales
Receptive/expressive language	Clinical Evaluation of Language Fundamentals Peabody Picture Vocabulary Test Expressive Vocabulary Test
Visuographic/visuoperceptual	Beery Developmental Test of Visual Motor Integration Rey-Osterrieth Complex Figure test
Memory/learning	Children's Memory Scale Wide Range Assessment of Memory and Learning California Verbal Learning Test
Executive functions	Delis-Kaplan Executive Function System Wisconsin Card Sorting Test
Sustained attention/effort	Conners' Continuous Performance Test Tests of Variables of Attention
Academic mastery	Woodcock-Johnson Scales of Achievement Wechsler Individual Achievement Test
Fine motor dexterity/speed	Grooved Pegboard Test

chological testing should consider the question of whether the patient's care is likely to be significantly enhanced by an evaluation's results. The timing of a referral can also be important. Results of testing during a period of acute distress may not be generalizable to a patient's general functioning. Furthermore, because of practice effects, many cognitive measures cannot be readministered within a given time period without compromised validity. For example, it is not advisable to repeat intelligence and memory tests in less than 6 months, and longer test-retest intervals are generally preferred.

Indications for Neuropsychological Testing

- Resolve question of intellectual deficiency
- Clarify lack of response to educational or therapeutic intervention
- Identify areas of cognitive dysfunction that may be related to a medical or neurological disorder, including localized structural or physiological abnormality
- Determine the functional significance of a known brain abnormality
- Examine the cognitive basis of functional complaints (e.g., poor memory)
- Evaluate deterioration of cognitive functioning or document changes in functioning over time
- Assess prognosis for deterioration or improvement in functioning in relation to treatment (e.g., epilepsy surgery)

Contraindications for Neuropsychological Testing

- Patient is acutely ill and mental status is unstable
- Uncontrolled (but treatable) ADHD or other psychiatric disorder is present

- Patient is in the midst of medication change having potential cognitive effects
- Similar evaluation has recently been completed or is in process (e.g., at school)

Summary Points

- The three most important indications for a neurological evaluation in children with psychiatric problems are
  1. Neurological signs and symptoms, suggestive of an acute or chronic (static or progressive) CNS lesion
  2. Episodic signs or symptoms suggestive of seizures
  3. Objective loss of previously well developed skills (not just declining grades), suggesting a degenerative CNS process
- The chief complaint, history, and physical examination all provide valuable clues for generating the differential diagnosis and guiding the neurological evaluation. The discerning clinician should try to fit constellations of findings into a clinical syndrome that encapsulates the presenting problem.
- Abnormal electroencephalographic patterns, such as generalized slowing or global suppression, often correlate with encephalopathic states. Specific electroencephalographic discharges, such as spikes, suggest an epileptogenic process.
- Epileptiform electroencephalographic discharges may specify seizure localization; however, some epileptic discharges may not be detected by surface electrodes and may require more in-depth evaluation.
- Some children and adolescents with psychiatric diagnoses and neurodevelopmental disorders, especially autism, often have electroencephalographic abnormalities that do not necessarily imply epilepsy. While epileptiform electroencephalographic findings may indicate an elevated risk for seizures, in the absence of clinical seizures, treatment of abnormal electroencephalographic findings with antiepileptic medications is not indicated. Electroencephalographic abnormalities should be considered in the context of the clinical neuropsychiatric picture.
- The relationship between brain size, microstructure, and function is a complex developmental process due to anatomical, physiological, and functional interactions in distributed neural networks.
- The use of neuroimaging tests to diagnose or suggest treatment for primary pediatric psychiatric disorders is still unsupported by clinical and scientific data, in addition to there being ethical considerations. Such tests are primarily used in research of the underlying neurobiological factors of psychiatric disorders.
- Brain abnormalities in youth with primary psychiatric disorders should be interpreted with consideration of comorbidities with neurological and genetic disorders.

- Neuropsychological testing adds valuable information regarding cognitive abilities, allowing them to be monitored over time. It can also assist in determining the functional impact of an identified brain structural or physiological abnormality on cognition, to assess prognosis for surgical outcome and educational attainment, and to inform educational and rehabilitative interventions.
- Neuropsychological testing should be driven by a clinical question, the answer to which will enhance clinical care, and it should be carefully planned to ensure accurate assessment and interpretation.

References

Almli CR, Rivkin MJ, McKinstry RC, et al: The NIH MRI study of normal brain development (Objective-2): newborns, infants, toddlers, and preschoolers. Neuroimage 35(1):308–325, 2007 17239623

American Academy of Pediatrics Committee on Drugs: Guidelines for monitoring and management of pediatric patients during and after sedation for diagnostic and therapeutic procedures. Pediatrics 89(6 Pt 1):1110–1115, 1992 1594358

Andermann E, Andermann FA: Migraine-epilepsy relationships: epidemiological and genetic aspects, in Migraine and Epilepsy. Edited by Andermann FA, Lugaresi E. Boston, MA, Butterworths, 1987, pp 281–291

Armangue T, Titulaer MJ, Málaga I, et al: Pediatric Anti-NMDAR encephalitis—clinical analysis and novel findings in a series of 20 patients. J Pediatr 162(4):850–856, 2013 23164315

Ashtari M, Cervellione KL, Hasan KM, et al: White matter development during late adolescence in healthy males: a cross-sectional diffusion tensor imaging study. Neuroimage 35(2):501–510, 2007 17258911

Barnea-Goraly N, Menon V, Eckert M, et al: White matter development during childhood and adolescence: a cross-sectional diffusion tensor imaging study. Cereb Cortex 15(12):1848–1854, 2005 15758200

Baron IS: Neuropsychological Evaluation of the Child. New York, Oxford University Press, 2004

Cascio CJ, Gerig G, Piven J: Diffusion tensor imaging: application to the study of the developing brain. J Am Acad Child Adolesc Psychiatry 46(2):213–223, 2007 17242625

Casey BJ, Giedd JN, Thomas KM: Structural and functional brain development and its relation to cognitive development. Biol Psychol 54(1–3):241–257, 2000 11035225

Durston S, Hulshoff Pol HE, Casey BJ, et al: Anatomical MRI of the developing human brain: what have we learned? J Am Acad Child Adolesc Psychiatry 40(9):1012–1020, 2001 11556624

Durston S, Davidson MC, Tottenham N, et al: A shift from diffuse to focal cortical activity with development. Dev Sci 9(1):1–8, 2006 16445387

Ernst M, Rumsey J: Functional Neuroimaging in Child Psychiatry. Cambridge, UK, Cambridge University Press, 2000

Giedd JN: Neuroimaging of pediatric neuropsychiatric disorders: is a picture really worth a thousand words? Arch Gen Psychiatry 58(5):443–444, 2001 11343522

Giedd JN: Structural magnetic resonance imaging of the adolescent brain. Ann N Y Acad Sci 1021:77–85, 2004 15251877

Giedd JN, Blumenthal J, Jeffries NO, et al: Brain development during childhood and adolescence: a longitudinal MRI study. Nat Neurosci 2(10):861–863, 1999 10491603

Giedd JN, Clasen LS, Lenroot R, et al: Puberty-related influences on brain development. Mol Cell Endocrinol 254–255:154–162, 2006 16765510

Gogtay N, Giedd JN, Lusk L, et al: Dynamic mapping of human cortical development during childhood through early adulthood. Proc Natl Acad Sci USA 101(21):8174–8179, 2004 15148381

Gronseth GS, Greenberg MK: The utility of the electroencephalogram in the evaluation of patients presenting with headache: a review of the literature. Neurology 45(7):1263–1267, 1995 7617180

Hesdorffer DC, Ludvigsson P, Olafsson E, et al: ADHD as a risk factor for incident unprovoked seizures and epilepsy in children. Arch Gen Psychiatry 61(7):731–736, 2004 15237085

Hess CP, Barkovich AJ: Techniques and methods in pediatric neuroimaging, in Pediatric Neuroimaging, 5th Edition. Edited by Barkovich AJ, Raybaud C. Philadelphia, PA, Lippincott Williams and Wilkins, 2012, pp 1–19

Holland SK, Plante E, Weber Byars A, et al: Normal fMRI brain activation patterns in children performing a verb generation task. Neuroimage 14(4):837–843, 2001 11554802

Krull KR, Okcu MF, Potter B, et al: Screening for neurocognitive impairment in pediatric cancer long-term survivors. J Clin Oncol 26(25):4138–4143, 2008 18757327

Lee BC, Kuppusamy K, Grueneich R, et al: Hemispheric language dominance in children demonstrated by functional magnetic resonance imaging. J Child Neurol 14(2):78–82, 1999 10073427

Lenroot RK, Giedd JN: Brain development in children and adolescents: insights from anatomical magnetic resonance imaging. Neurosci Biobehav Rev 30(6):718–729, 2006 16887188

Marsh R, Gerber AJ, Peterson BS: Neuroimaging studies of normal brain development and their relevance for understanding childhood neuropsychiatric disorders. J Am Acad Child Adolesc Psychiatry 47(11):1233–1251, 2008 18833009

Mukherjee P, Miller JH, Shimony JS, et al: Diffusion-tensor MR imaging of gray and white matter development during normal human brain maturation. AJNR Am J Neuroradiol 23(9):1445–1456, 2002 12372731

Schneider JFL, Il'yasov KA, Hennig J, et al: Fast quantitative diffusion-tensor imaging of cerebral white matter from the neonatal period to adolescence. Neuroradiology 46(4):258–266, 2004 14999435

Shaw P, Greenstein D, Lerch J, et al: Intellectual ability and cortical development in children and adolescents. Nature 440(7084):676–679, 2006 16572172

Thompson PM, Sowell ER, Gogtay N, et al: Structural MRI and brain development. Int Rev Neurobiol 67:285–323, 2005 16291026

Tortori-Donati P, Rossi A, Biancheri R: Pediatric Neuroradiology. Berlin, Springer-Verlag, 2005

Wycliffe ND, Thompson JR, Holshouser BA, et al: Pediatric Neuroimaging in Pediatric Neurology: Principles and Practice, 4th Edition. Edited by Swaiman KF, Ashwal S, Ferriero DM. Philadelphia, PA, Mosby Elsevier, 2006

Wylie E, Cascino GD, Gidal BE, et al (eds): The Treatment of Epilepsy: Principles and Practice, 5th Edition. Philadelphia, PA, Lippincott Williams and Wilkins, 2011

Zametkin AJ, Schroth E, Faden D: The role of brain imaging in the diagnosis and management of ADHD. The ADHD Report 13(5):11–14, 2005

Zhang L, Thomas KM, Davidson MC, et al: MR quantitation of volume and diffusion changes in the developing brain. AJNR Am J Neuroradiol 26(1):45–49, 2005 15661698

PART II

Neurodevelopmental and Other Psychiatric Disorders

CHAPTER 7

Intellectual Disability

Karen Toth, Ph.D.
Nina de Lacy, M.D., M.B.A.
Bryan H. King, M.D., M.B.A.

On October 5, 2010, a bill known as "Rosa's Law" (P.L. 111-256) was signed into legislation, thereby stripping the terms "mental retardation" and "mentally retarded" from federal health, education, and labor policy and replacing them with the terms "intellectual disability" and "individual with an intellectual disability." This legislation reflects a change in terminology that had already taken place in research, medical, and educational professions as well as advocacy groups. In fact, in 2007, the American Association on Mental Retardation, the oldest interdisciplinary professional association, since 1910, and leader in the terminology and classification of intellectual disability, became the American Association on Intellectual and Developmental Disabilities (AAIDD). In May 2013, with the publication of DSM-5 (American Psychiatric Association 2013), the term *intellectual disability* (ID) replaced *mental retardation* for the first time in DSM, and the language used to define ID became more closely aligned with that of the AAIDD. (The terminology proposed for ICD-11, anticipated to be released in 2015, is *intellectual developmental disorders.*) For example, among other revisions reflected in DSM-5, severity levels are now classified by adaptive functioning rather than IQ, and IQ criteria are based on approximate rather than absolute cutoffs (e.g., 65–75 rather than 70). As such, there is a greater recognition of the importance of clinical judgment in diagnosing ID than ever before.

Adaptive functioning includes abilities in three domains: *conceptual,* which refers to language, reading, writing, math, reasoning, knowledge, and memory; *social,* as in empathy, social judgment, interpersonal communication skills, and the ability to follow rules and to make and retain friendships; and *practical,* or self-management in areas such as personal care, job responsibilities, money management, recreation, and organizing school and work tasks.

Definition, Clinical Description, and Diagnosis

The AAIDD has been responsible for defining ID and providing diagnostic criteria since 1910. Currently, as in DSM, the AAIDD defines ID by significant limitations in intellectual functioning and adaptive behavior, which includes conceptual, social, and practical skills and origination prior to age 18. However, in contrast to DSM, the AAIDD emphasizes strengths over limitations and supports based on severity rather than severity levels alone. In defining and assessing ID, the AAIDD emphasizes the following factors: the community environment typical of the individual's peers and culture; linguistic diversity and cultural differences in the way people communicate, move, and behave; the individual's strengths; and the use of personalized supports provided over a sustained period to improve level of life functioning. The American Association on Mental Retardation proposed in 1992 the following classification system for individuals with intellectual disabilities; this system contrasts with the DSM use of severity levels (American Association on Mental Retardation 1992):

- *Intermittent support:* Higher-functioning individuals who require little intervention to function, except during times of uncertainty or stress (mild ID under the old system of classification)
- *Limited support:* Individuals who may require additional support to navigate through everyday situations (moderate disability)
- *Extensive support:* Individuals who rely on around-the-clock daily support to function (severe disability)
- *Pervasive support:* Individuals who require daily interventions and lifelong support to help them function in every aspect of daily routines (profound disability)

The DSM-5 diagnostic criteria and severity levels for ID are summarized in Table 7–1.

Differential Diagnosis

Neurocognitive disorders are differentiated from ID by a loss of cognitive function. When the onset of an ID occurs after a period of normal functioning or after age 18 years, the diagnosis is often dementia. Major neurocognitive disorder can co-occur with ID, and in these cases both diagnoses may be given. For example, in trisomy 21 (Down syndrome [DS]), it is common for individuals to develop dementia. Learning and communication disorders (see Chapter 9, "Neurodevelopmental Disorders: Specific Learning Disorder, Communication Disorders, and Motor Disorders") are diagnosed when there is impairment in a specific communication and/or learning domain but not general impairment in intellectual and adaptive functioning. Communication and learning disorders can co-occur with ID, and both diagnoses can be given when full criteria are met for each. It is common for individuals with autism spectrum disorders (Chapter 8, "Autism Spectrum Disorders") to also meet criteria for ID. Historically, comorbidity rates were 70%–75%; epidemiological studies now indicate rates of 40%–55% (Chakrabarti and Fombonne 2001).

TABLE 7–1. Summary of DSM-5 diagnostic criteria and severity classifications for intellectual disability

DIAGNOSTIC CRITERIA

A. Intellectual function	B. Adaptive function	C. Onset
Deficits in intellectual function, such as reasoning, problem solving, planning, abstract thinking, judgment, academic learning, and learning from experience, confirmed by both clinical assessment and individualized, standardized intelligence testing.	Deficits in adaptive functioning that result in failure to meet developmental and sociocultural standards for personal independence and social responsibility. Without ongoing support, the adaptive deficits limit functioning in one or more activities of daily life, such as communication, social participation, and independent living across multiple environments, such as home, school, work and community.	Onset of intellectual and adaptive deficits during the developmental period.

SEVERITY

Severity level (% children)	Conceptual domain	Social domain	Practical domain
Mild (85%)	For preschool children, there may be no obvious conceptual differences. For school-age children and adults, there are difficulties in learning academic skills involving reading, writing, arithmetic, time, or money, with support needed in one or more areas to meet age-related expectations. In adults, abstract thinking, executive function (i.e., planning, strategizing, priority setting, and cognitive flexibility), and short-term memory, as well as functional use of academic skills (e.g., reading, money management), are impaired. There is a somewhat concrete approach to problems and solutions compared with age-mates.	Compared with typically developing age-mates, the individual is immature in social interactions. For example, there may be difficulty in accurately perceiving peers' social cues. Communication, conversation, and language are more concrete or immature than expected for age. There may be difficulties regulating emotion and behavior in age-appropriate fashion; these difficulties are noticed by peers in social situations. There is limited understanding of risk in social situations; social judgment is immature for age, and the person is at risk of being manipulated by others (gullibility).	The individual may function age-appropriately in personal care. The individual needs some support with complex daily living tasks in comparison to peers. In adulthood, supports typically involve grocery shopping, transportation, home and child-care organizing, nutritious food preparation, and banking and money management. Recreational skills resemble those of age-mates, although judgment related to well-being and organization around recreation requires support. In adulthood, competitive employment is often seen in jobs that do not emphasize conceptual skills. The individual generally needs support to make health care and legal decisions, and to learn to perform a skilled vocation competently. Support is typically needed to raise a family.

TABLE 7–1. Summary of DSM-5 diagnostic criteria and severity classifications for intellectual disability *(continued)*

SEVERITY *(continued)*

Severity level (% children)	Conceptual domain	Social domain	Practical domain
Moderate (10%)	All through development, the individual's conceptual skills lag markedly behind those of peers. For preschoolers, language and pre-academic skills develop slowly. For school-age children, progress in reading, writing, mathematics, and understanding of time and money occurs slowly across the school years and is markedly limited compared with that of peers. For adults, academic skill development is typically at an elementary level, and support is required for all use of academic skills in work and personal life. Ongoing assistance on a daily basis is needed to complete conceptual tasks of day-to-day life, and others may take over these responsibilities fully for the individual.	The individual shows marked differences from peers in social and communicative behavior across development. Spoken language is typically a primary tool for social communication but is much less complex than that of peers. Capacity for relationships is evident in ties to family and friends, and the individual may have successful friendships and sometimes romantic relations in adulthood. However, the individual may not perceive or interpret social cues accurately. Social judgment and decision-making abilities are limited, and caretakers must assist with life decisions. Friendships with typically developing peers are often affected by communication or social limitations. Significant social and communicative support is needed in work settings for success.	The individual can care for personal needs involving eating, dressing, elimination, and hygiene as an adult, although an extended period of teaching and time is needed for the individual to become independent in these areas, and reminders may be needed. Similarly, participation in all household tasks can be achieved by adulthood, although extended teaching and ongoing supports for adult-level performance are needed. Independent employment in jobs that require limited conceptual and communication skills can be achieved, but considerable support from co-workers and others is needed to manage social expectations, job complexities, and responsibilities such as scheduling, transportation, health benefits, and money management. A variety of recreational skills can be developed but require supports and learning opportunities over an extended period. Maladaptive behavior is present in a significant minority and causes social problems.

TABLE 7–1. Summary of DSM-5 diagnostic criteria and severity classifications for intellectual disability *(continued)*

SEVERITY *(continued)*

Severity level (% children)	Conceptual domain	Social domain	Practical domain
Severe (5%)	Attainment of conceptual skills is limited. The individual generally has little understanding of written language or of concepts involving numbers, quantity, time, and money. Caretakers provide extensive supports for problem solving throughout life.	Spoken language is quite limited in vocabulary and grammar. Speech may be single words or phrases and may be supplemented through augmentative means. Communication is focused on the here and now. Language is used for social communication more than explication. The individual understands simple speech/gestures. Relationships with familiar others are a source of pleasure and help.	The individual requires support for all activities of daily living (e.g., meals, dressing, bathing, and elimination), requires supervision at all times, and cannot make responsible decisions regarding well-being of self or others. In adulthood, tasks at home, recreation, and work require ongoing support/assistance. Skill acquisition in all domains involves long-term teaching and support. Maladaptive behavior, including self-injury, is present in a significant minority.

TABLE 7–1. Summary of DSM-5 diagnostic criteria and severity classifications for intellectual disability *(continued)*

SEVERITY *(continued)*

Severity level (% children)	Conceptual domain	Social domain	Practical domain
Profound (<1%)	Conceptual skills generally involve the physical world rather than symbolic processes. The individual may use objects in goal-directed fashion for self-care, work, and recreation. Certain visuospatial skills, such as matching and sorting based on physical characteristics, may be acquired. However, motor and sensory impairments may prevent functional use of objects.	The individual has very limited understanding of symbolic communication in speech or gesture. He or she may understand some simple instructions or gestures. The individual expresses his or her own desires and emotions largely through nonverbal, nonsymbolic communication. The individual enjoys relationships with familiar others, and initiates and responds to social interactions through gestural and emotional cues. Sensory and physical impairments may prevent many social activities.	The individual is dependent on others for all aspects of daily physical care, health, and safety, although he or she may participate in some of these activities as well. Individuals without severe physical impairments may assist with daily work tasks at home, like carrying dishes to the table. Simple actions with objects may be the basis of participation in some vocational activities with high levels of support. Recreational activities may involve music, movies, walks, or participating in water activities, all with support. Physical and sensory impairments are frequent barriers to home, recreational, and vocational activities. Maladaptive behavior is present in a significant minority.

Assessment of Intellectual and Adaptive Function

A comprehensive assessment of functioning—cognitive, adaptive, sensory, motor, and other domains (such as sleep, mood, and self-injurious behavior)—is critical to making an accurate diagnosis of ID and ensuring that the most appropriate available treatments and supports are provided. Genomewide microarray-based comparative genomic hybridization (aCGH), metabolic testing, and neuroimaging may play a role in this evaluation and are useful in identifying underlying genetic syndromes and behavioral phenotypes. The first step in establishing the diagnosis is to obtain an appropriate and valid assessment of intellectual and adaptive functioning.

While intelligence tests are a necessary component of the diagnostic process, there are a number of potential problems in using standardized, norm-referenced tests with individuals with ID. Standardized intelligence tests are of particularly limited value in assessing individuals with severe and profound ID. These individuals have difficulty understanding and following verbal directions and are often not able to display their knowledge within the parameters of most standardized tests, which have rigid administration and scoring procedures. Standardized tests also have a small number of items at the extreme ends of ability, further restricting the sampling of abilities of individuals with severe and profound ID. However, individual items on these tests, as well as behaviors observed during testing, may provide useful information about an individual's current abilities, and the test scores themselves provide a general index of the individual's current developmental level.

Table 7–2 includes standardized instruments that are especially well suited for evaluating children with intellectual disabilities.

Table 7–3 provides information on psychometrically sound infant and toddler measures, which do not provide a true IQ score but are useful for establishing the presence of early developmental delays, informing treatment approaches, and tracking progress over time. These measures provide normative comparisons.

Along with a measure of intellectual function, a valid assessment of adaptive behavior is required for the diagnosis of ID. A number of factors can influence the assessment of adaptive behavior (as well as the reliability and validity of scores obtained), including the scale used; the child's age and sex; the informant (expectancies, recall ability, response bias); the examiner; the setting (school, home); and reasons for the evaluation (diagnosis, placement). Table 7–4 provides a short list of reliable, standardized measures of adaptive behavior.

Communication of the Diagnosis

The initial evaluation of the child for an ID is a stressful and emotionally significant time for parents. This experience can greatly influence the family's willingness to seek and use resources needed for optimal outcomes for their child. During the evaluation phase, the clinician should provide clear information about the type of testing that will take place and why, inquire about the family's expectations, and solicit their questions and reactions to the assessment process. In presenting results, can-

TABLE 7–2. Standardized measures of intelligence for use with children with intellectual disabilities

Test	Age range	Strengths	Limitations
Stanford-Binet Intelligence Scales, 5th Edition (SB5; Roid 2003)	2 years to 85+ years	Excellent standardization, reliability, and validity; clear scoring criteria	Different batteries for different age ranges; difficult to score; long administration time
Wechsler Preschool and Primary Scale of Intelligence, 4th Edition (WPPSI-IV; Wechsler 2012)	2 years, 6 months to 7 years, 3 months	Excellent psychometric properties; useful diagnostic information	Limited floor for children with significant delays; long administration time
Wechsler Intelligence Scale for Children, 5th Edition (WISC-V; Wechsler 2014)	6 years to 16 years, 11 months	Excellent standardization, reliability, and validity	Insufficient floor for the severely disabled; verbal responses can be difficult to score
Kaufman Assessment Battery for Children, 2nd Edition (K-ABC-II; Kaufman and Kaufman 2004)	3–18 years	Norms for children with developmental disabilities; provides a composite mental processing score for nonverbal children	Relies heavily on short-term memory and attention, making it less effective for children with these difficulties; limited subtests for very young children
Differential Ability Scales, 2nd Edition (DAS-II; Elliott 2006)	2 years, 6 months to 17 years, 11 months	Clinical samples were expanded to include children with a variety of special needs; engaging	Certain subtests rely on complex verbal instructions, making it less useful for children with these delays
Leiter International Performance Scale—Revised (Leiter-R; Roid and Miller 1997)	2 years to 20 years, 11 months	Useful for nonverbal individuals and for treatment planning	Measures only nonverbal problem-solving and reasoning abilities
Universal Nonverbal Intelligence Test (UNIT; Bracken and McCallum 1998)	5 years to 17 years, 11 months	Useful for nonverbal individuals and for treatment planning	Measures only nonverbal problem-solving and reasoning abilities

TABLE 7–3. Standardized measures of development for use with infants and toddlers

Test	Age range	Strengths	Limitations
Bayley Scales of Infant and Toddler Development, 3rd Edition (Bayley III; Bayley 2005)	1 year to 3 years, 6 months	Provides separate indices for motor and cognitive abilities	Valid administration requires considerable experience; best for children without motor, language, or attentional difficulties
Mullen Scales of Early Learning: AGS Edition (Mullen 1995)	0 years to 5 years, 8 months	Provides separate indices for receptive and expressive language	Very few items at the lowest end of the age range limits usefulness with toddlers with language/motor delays

TABLE 7–4. Measures of adaptive functioning

Measure	Age range	Strengths	Limitations
Adaptive Behavior Assessment System, 2nd Edition (ABAS-II; Harrison and Oakland 2003)	0–89 years	Assesses conceptual, social, and practical aspects of adaptive behavior, as well as 10 adaptive skill areas.	Ratings depend on informant's ability to accurately interpret items and provide information on current functioning.
Vineland Adaptive Behavior Scales, 2nd Edition: Survey, Caregiver, Expanded Forms (Sparrow et al. 2005)	0 years to 18 years, 11 months	Addition of early childhood items in this new edition improves classification of children with moderate to profound ID.	Versions are available only for children/adolescents; some items rely on information the informant may not possess.
Vineland Adaptive Behavior Scales, 2nd Edition: Teacher Form (Sparrow et al. 2005)	3 years to 21 years, 11 months	Assesses adaptive behavior in school, preschool, or structured day care setting.	Ratings depend on ability to accurately interpret items; no version for 0–3.
Diagnostic Adaptive Behavior Scale (DABS; American Association on Intellectual and Developmental Disabilities 2015)	4–21 years	Focuses on the critical "cut-off area" for the purpose of ruling in or out a diagnosis of ID or related disability.	Available only for children age 4 years or older.
Battelle Developmental Inventory, 2nd Edition (BDI-2; Newborg 2004)	0 years to 7 years, 11 months	Combines structured test items with interview items and observational data; allows for assessing children with physical handicaps.	Available only for children younger than 8 years; ratings depend heavily on informant's ability to provide accurate information.
Scales of Independent Behavior—Revised (SIB-R; Bruininks et al. 1996)	0–80+ years	Expanded items for infant and geriatric populations; Support Score predicts level of support needed.	Ratings depend on informant's ability to accurately interpret items and provide information.

dor and truthfulness are essential, and technical and diagnostic terms should be introduced and explained in terms the family can understand. Most importantly, communication of results should always reflect strengths as well as challenges in the child's functioning. Finally, it is helpful if a written report of these results includes additional sources of information, resource and referral information, and appropriate treatment recommendations. There may be specific criteria for eligibility for services in a state's Developmental Services system that may be very helpful to address in an evaluation summary report.

Epidemiology

ID is one of the most common neuropsychiatric disorders in children and adolescents, especially among children under age 15 years. Approximately 30% more males than females are diagnosed with ID, but this ratio decreases as IQ decreases (Leonard and Wen 2002). Prevalence estimates are approximately 1%–3% and vary by age, how ID is defined, the methods used to assess individuals, and the population under consideration.

Etiology, Mechanisms, and Risk Factors

Historically, only about 50% of all cases of ID were of known etiology, although studies have suggested that a careful clinical evaluation can now determine etiology in as many as 70% of cases (Croen et al. 2001; Xu and Chen 2003). The most common known causes of ID are described in the section "Congenital Syndromes and Neurobehavioral Phenotypes." Predisposing factors include genetic differences (including inborn errors of metabolism [IEM]), accounting for 40%–50% of cases; environmental influences and exposure to toxins during prenatal development (e.g., fetal alcohol spectrum disorder), which affect 10% of cases; pregnancy and perinatal complications (e.g., trauma, prematurity, hypoxia), affecting 10% of cases; and acquired medical conditions (e.g., lead poisoning), affecting 5% of cases (Srivastava and Schwartz 2014).

Risk factors for ID of unknown etiology continue to be studied. Croen et al. (2001) examined infant and maternal characteristics of more than 11,000 children with ID of unknown cause. Findings showed that low birth weight was the strongest predictor of disability, with systemic inflammation adding considerably to the risk associated with low birth weight (Leviton et al. 2013). Males; children born to black, Asian, and Hispanic women and older women; lower level of maternal education; lower socioeconomic status (SES); multiple births; and second- or later-born children are all risk factors. Both biological and social-environmental factors play a role in the etiology of ID of unknown cause. Moreover, these factors often interact.

Genetic and Molecular Basis of Intellectual Disability

In the last two decades, progress in the field of genetics and genomics has contributed greatly to our understanding of ID. Technological advances and plummeting costs and recognition of the benefits of testing have promoted wider use of aCGH in the clinical context and the application of next-generation sequencing methods such as whole-exome sequencing (WES) and whole-genome sequencing (WGS) to identify rare deleterious variants via research studies. Concomitantly, the proportion of cases of ID that can be positively attributed to a genetic cause has steadily increased.

Historically the focus has been on well-known genetic syndromes ranging from aneuploidies such as DS to copy number variants (CNVs) such as Williams syndrome (WS) to single-gene disorders such as Rett syndrome. In these, a characteristic "behavioral phenotype" for the disorder was fashioned out of patterns of commonly co-occurring cognitive and behavioral features. In combination with defined physiological features these provided the indication for simple first-line genetic testing, although tending to bias diagnosis toward syndromic ID. Targeted single-gene or panel testing was pursued in a minority of cases in which there was strong clinical suspicion. Beginning in the last decade with wider availability of aCGH, a more efficient method of screening, many persons with ID were discovered to have newly identified de novo or inherited CNVs likely accounting for their presentation. In some cases, such as 16p11.2 deletion, these CNVs have proved sufficiently common to become new "syndromes" (Hanson et al. 2015). Pathogenic CNVs may contain many genes, only one or some of which may contribute to the neuropsychiatric phenotype, and are now thought to account for up to an additional 10%–20% of all cases of ID.

Overall, the last two decades of investigation have revealed that the underlying genetic basis of ID encompasses every type of genetic paradigm known in humans, including recessive, dominant, and X-linked inheritance patterns, as well as sporadic de novo occurrences, and multiple types of variation at the single-nucleotide, single-gene, and larger copy number levels. While the standard first-line clinical testing protocol in most centers remains aCGH with fragile X testing, others are now moving rapidly to adopt WES in the clinical context. Of note, while biochemical genetic disorders (IEM) were historically thought to account for 1%–3% of ID, careful specialized testing in this important treatable subgroup may account for more than 10% of cases (Engbers et al. 2008).

These results also considerably strengthen the notion that ID and neurodevelopmental neuropsychiatric disorders in the majority of affected individuals are caused by variations in the genetic control of brain development, maturation, and function from the fetal period through young adulthood, likely by way of alteration to shared signaling and metabolic pathways, cell proliferation and migration, and synaptic function in the brain.

Congenital Syndromes and Neurobehavioral Phenotypes

Within each syndrome much variation in terms of ID severity, attentional and cognitive function, and psychiatric and behavioral patterns exists between individuals. Specific medical, developmental, and psychiatric practice recommendations and interventions are indicated for these and other less common syndromes.

16p11.2 Deletion Syndrome

16p11.2 deletion syndrome (DS) is one of the more common newly defined CNVs, with a likely prevalence of 1:3,000–5,000. It may account for approximately 0.4% of ID cases. Individuals with 16p11.2 DS tend to have mild ID and frequent comorbidity with psychiatric or developmental disorders and lack medical complications other than an association with obesity.

22q11.2 Deletion Syndrome (Velocardiofacial Syndrome)

The constellation of findings grouped historically under a variety of names such as velocardiofacial, DiGeorge, and Shprintzen syndromes were eventually recognized to be the same entity and are now unified under the term *22q11.2 deletion syndrome.* 22q11.2 DS is the most common survivable interstitial deletion in humans—and one of the most common genetic deletion causes of ID—and carries the highest genetic risk for developing schizophrenia. 22q11.2 DS has an estimated prevalence of 1:2,000–4,000, and many individuals with mild symptoms may go undiagnosed. The syndrome is associated with defects in neural crest development, and complications include congenital cardiac anomalies, palatal abnormalities, and T-cell- and thymus-related immune deficiencies. There is a characteristic facial appearance, although this can be quite subtle, particularly in non-Caucasian individuals. Most individuals have developmental delays, and while average IQ is around 70, there is wide variation and often a large split between verbal (higher) and nonverbal IQ. Neurocognitive impairments include difficulties with cognitive control, attention, and social cognition. Speech difficulties are prominent, particularly early in life, and language onset is usually delayed. It is important to specify the etiology of speech deficits, since these may be physiological, and repair of craniofacial defects and medical or surgical interventions for recurrent ear infections optimize development. It is important for child psychiatrists to familiarize themselves with 22q11.2 DS given the known high rates of major psychiatric morbidity, including autism spectrum disorder, attention-deficit/hyperactivity disorder (ADHD), and schizophrenia. Interestingly, studies have demonstrated an association between lower IQ and the presence of psychosis. Anxiety and depression are common.

Angelman Syndrome

Angelman syndrome (AS) is a neurogenetic disorder that occurs at a rate of about 1 per 12,000 to 1 per 20,000 worldwide (Williams 2005). Prevalence in populations with severe ID is 1.4% (King et al. 2005). While severe developmental delays and ID are present from early life, the characteristic neurocognitive profile of severe speech impairment, inattention, gait ataxia and/or tremulous movement of the limbs, inappropriate frequent laughter, happy demeanor, and excitable personality (often with hand flapping) tends to become more prominent in toddlerhood, delaying diagnosis. Hyperactivity and sleep disturbance are common. Generally, language is absent, with few individuals acquiring more than one or two words. Other features include protruding tongue, feeding problems, drooling, sleep disturbance, hypopigmented skin, strabismus, and prognathia (Williams 2005). Delayed head growth usually results in microcephaly by age 2 years. Seizures are common, usually starting before age 3 years. Certain anticonvulsants (vigabatrin and tiagabine) are contraindicated, and carbamazepine is considered less helpful. All three may cause seizure exacerbation. Because of suggested altered dopaminergic metabolism, the use of antipsychotic agents should be approached with caution.

Ciliopathies

The ciliopathies represent a collection or continuum of diseases caused by dysfunction in the primary cilium (PC) that overall affect 1 out of 500 persons. Mutations in individual genes that produce the proteins making up the PC and its basilar transition zone are responsible for the ciliopathies that affect the central nervous system (CNS), namely, Joubert, Bardet-Biedl, and oro-facial-digital syndromes. These syndromes are all associated with varying degrees of ID, and the group as a class is a major cause of ID, affecting collectively some 1 out of 5,000 persons. Individuals with the CNS ciliopathies have malformations of the hindbrain and accordingly may exhibit variable cerebellar signs on neurological examination (ataxia, "cerebellar speech", eye and oral movement control deficits, dysdiadochokinesia, past-pointing, intention tremor) that are useful clues for the psychiatrist as to the etiology of ID. Joubert syndrome is the only genetic cause of ID conclusively associated with specific neuroimaging findings and a molecular mechanism and represents an important exemplar of the future direction of research and clinical practice.

Down Syndrome

DS, or trisomy 21, is found in about 1 in every 1,000 live-born children and is the most common genetic cause of ID. DS is caused by a triplicate state of all or part of the DS critical region (DSCR) on chromosome 21, most often caused by errors in meoisis I of maternal origin increasing with maternal age. The phenotype is characterized by more than 80 features, including cognitive impairments, muscle hypotonia, short stature, malformations of the heart and digestive tract, and a distinctive facial appearance (Aït Yahya-Graison et al. 2007). Physical findings may include a single palmar crease, hyperlax joints, and obesity. Individuals with DS develop the cellular findings associated with Alzheimer's disease at a much earlier age than the general population. Average IQ is 50, although there is variation. Generally, persons with mosaic DS have milder neuropsychiatric phenotypes. A distinct cognitive profile in DS includes relative strengths in visual processing but significant language impairments (King et al. 2005). In adaptive functioning, strengths in social skills relative to communication and other adaptive behavior skill domains have been observed. A generalized deficit in executive function includes problems with attention, impulsivity, hyperactivity, and aggression (King et al. 2005).

Fetal Alcohol Spectrum Disorders

Now understood to be a spectrum disorder, with varying risk according to dose, timing, and pattern of alcohol exposure, fetal alcohol spectrum disorders (FASDs) occur at a rate of about 1% of live births, with the more narrowly defined fetal alcohol syndrome occurring in the United States at a rate of 0.5–2 per 1,000 births (May and Gossage 2001). ID is a hallmark of FASD. Other symptoms include a distinct pattern of facial anomalies (smooth philtrum, thin vermilion border of upper lip, short palpebral fissures), prenatal and/or postnatal growth retardation, and CNS abnormalities. The facial appearance tends to soften with age and may be difficult to identify in older individuals. Cardiovascular, renal, and orthopedic abnormalities may also be present (Manning and Eugene Hoyme 2007). Neuroimaging studies have revealed brain structural defects, such as abnormal brain size and shape, smaller cerebellar and ventricular size, and agenesis of the corpus callosum (Riley and McGee 2005), suggesting that particular brain areas are especially vulnerable. Cognitive and behavioral abnormalities include verbal and nonverbal learning deficits, attention problems, and impairments in executive functioning (Hoyme et al. 2005). Diagnostic criteria for neurobehavioral disorder associated with prenatal alcohol exposure were introduced in DSM-5 as a condition for further study. These criteria highlight impairments in neurocognitive functioning, self-regulation, and adaptive functioning (American Psychiatric Association 2013).

FMR1-Related Disorders (Fragile X Syndrome)

The *FMR1*-related disorders are an interesting example of the "phenotype expansion" that has resulted from modern genetic testing. Complex changes in the X-linked gene *FMR1* (trinucleotide expansion, sometimes with anticipation and methylation) are associated with the disorders. Full or loss-of-function mutations cause fragile X syndrome, whereas premutation status in males (and some females) may cause fragile X–associated tremor/ataxia syndrome (FXTAS) (late-onset progressive cerebellar ataxia and tremor) and in females *FMR1*-related primary ovarian insufficiency.

Fragile X itself is a leading cause of ID, with most males in the moderate range and females in the mild range, although individuals have been reported with normal IQ. The incidence of fragile X syndrome is 1 per 4,000 males and 1 per 8,000 females (Crawford et al. 2001). As many as 25% of individuals with fragile X syndrome also meet the criteria for autism spectrum disorder, but only 2.1% of individuals with autism spectrum disorder have the syndrome. Affected females with average IQ scores show deficits in other areas of cognitive ability, such as executive functioning and social affective abilities. Fragile X syndrome is characterized by a specific neurocognitive profile of strengths and weaknesses and increased risk of psychopathology (for review, see Dykens 2000), but there is significant within-syndrome variability. Behavioral characteristics include hyperarousal, hyperactivity, social anxiety, shyness, and gaze aversion. Individuals with fragile X syndrome are at increased risk for schizotypal disorders, ADHD, and pervasive developmental disorders (King et al. 2005).

Inborn Errors of Metabolism

The IEM or biochemical genetic conditions represent a large class of disorders related to disruptions to genes that make proteins involved in metabolism. Most involve genes that code for enzymes involved in biochemical pathways, including the production and breakdown of neurotransmitters and other molecules crucial to the formation and function of the brain. Generally, the deleterious effects of these disorders result from either the accumulation of substances that prove toxic in excess or the inability to synthesize enough of a required product. Individually, most of these disorders are quite rare. However, collectively, they affect some 1%–1.5% of persons in the population, and many cause neuropsychiatric symptoms and interfere with normal brain development. The IEM are particularly important to consider and diagnose since many have specific treatments to prevent morbidity and mortality and to optimize development, such as supplementation with a deficient enzyme or dietary restriction. Well-known IEM causing ID include phenylketonuria, Lesch-Nyhan syndrome, and the lysosomal and glycogen storage diseases. Specific features in each disorder vary, but the child psychiatrist should consider IEM in the differential diagnosis of every individual with ID, given that these conditions may be responsible for 2%–14% of all cases. In addition, the IEM should be particularly considered when there are associated neuropsychiatric symptoms, such as catatonia, mania, seizures, encephalopathy, and visual hallucinations, and when symptoms are exacerbated by physiological stress and illness or occur with abdominal pain or vomiting or when there is functional regression (Sedel et al. 2007). It is recommended to perform screening laboratory tests during a symptom exacerbation, since assays may be normal during periods of relative metabolic stability. Referral to a specialist biochemical geneticist is recommended for evaluation or management.

MECP2-Related Disorders (Rett Syndrome)

Historically, mutations in the gene *MECP2* were associated solely with Rett syndrome (RS). *MECP2* is located on the X chromosome, and therefore the vast majority of known affected individuals are female, with the mutation in males presumed lethal or causing severe and fatal infant encephalopathy. The population prevalence of RS is approximately 1:8,500, and it is one of the most common causes of severe ID in females. Classic RS is associated with a distinctive "regressive" presentation in which, in girls, there is a period of ostensibly normal development for the first 6–18 months of life, followed by a rapid loss of intellectual functioning and fine and gross motor skills, social withdrawal, the development of stereotypic hand-wringing movements and possible breathing abnormalities, ataxia, and behavioral dysregulation, such as screaming fits and inconsolable crying. The condition then stabilizes, but seizures are present in 90% of cases. Scoliosis, osteopenia, and growth failure are common. More recently, it has been demonstrated that mutations in *MECP2* cause so-called atypical RS with phenotypes resembling AS, ID with spasticity or tremor, more gradual regression ("forme fruste" RS), and even mild learning disability or autism spectrum disorder (Christodoulou and Ho 2001). A new phenotype, called PPM-X syndrome, has been identified in males involving parkinsonism, pyramidal signs, macro-orchidism, and psychosis. Thus, RS has undergone "phenotypic expansion" akin to fragile X, and the continuum has been renamed the *MECP2*-related disorders. Retesting of individuals with suggestive phenotypes but who had previously tested negative may thus be indicated given advances in sequencing of *MECP2*. Diagnosis is important, given the increased incidence of prolonged QTc, T-wave abnormalities, and reduced heart rate variability that may cause sudden death. Patients should receive evaluation from a pediatric cardiologist and the use of psychotropics modified accordingly. Melatonin has been shown to be effective for sleep disturbance and topiramate or the ketogenic diet for seizures.

Prader-Willi Syndrome

Prader-Willi syndrome (PWS) can be caused by either paternal deletion (in about 70% of cases) or maternal uniparental disomy (in about 29% of cases) in the AS/PW region of chromosome 15q11.13. DNA methylation testing of the AS/PW region detects over 99% of cases. PWS is found in 1 per 29,500 births, and there is a distinctive developmental trajectory characterized by hypotonia, global developmental delay, and failure to thrive in infancy giving way to hyperphagia and persistent hunger (even without food stimulus), early obesity, hypogonadism, short stature with small hands and feet, characteristic facies, sleep apnea, and behavioral problems in the older child (Horsthemke and Buiting 2006). All individuals have some degree of cognitive impairment, but the ID is usually mild. Compulsive food-seeking and hoarding behaviors are seen as early as 2 years of age and are lifelong challenges. Other compulsive behaviors are commonly observed, leading to an increased risk of developing obsessive-compulsive disorder. Impulse-control disorders and mood disorders are also often found (King et al. 2005). It has been suggested there is a common behavioral phenotype that includes temper tantrums, stubbornness, and manipulative behaviors. Topiramate has proven effective for self-injurious skin-picking in some studies (Shapira et al. 2004), and selective serotonin reuptake inhibitors (SSRIs) are often used for anxiety and low frustration tolerance, while mood-stabilizing medications appear to be of less benefit (Soni et al. 2007).

Williams Syndrome

WS is caused by a microdeletion on chromosome 7q11.23, has a prevalence of 1:7,500, and is associated with a specific pattern of facial features, including an "elfin" appearance and stellate iris; personality features (excessively friendly, anxious); connective tissue and cardiac abnormalities; hypertension; failure to thrive; and growth deficiency. Many features are likely related to the presence of *ELN*, the gene coding for elastin, in the critical region, and many affected persons have hypertonia, hyperactive reflexes, and cerebellar signs on neurological examination. Individuals with WS most often have mild to moderate IDs and learning disabilities, although in some cases low-average to average intelligence has been reported. WS is also characterized by a distinct personality profile, including social disinhibition and often high levels of indiscriminate social initiation and empathy that may interfere with adaptive social functioning. ADHD behaviors are commonly seen, as well as anxiety disorders (King et al. 2005). Specific phobias (e.g., sounds, bees) are common and may overlap with sensory processing disturbance and sensitivity. Vitamin D should be avoided, and providers should adapt medication strategies where necessary after cardiac consultation for the presence of cardiac abnormalities and monitoring for the emergence of renal stenosis, hypertension, and long QT.

Developmental Course and Prognosis

The developmental course and prognosis for individuals with IDs vary according to the etiology and severity of the disability, underlying genetic syndromes and medical conditions, and environmental and treatment factors. Outcomes range from severe impairment with need for constant supervision to less severe forms of ID. For some, with appropriate treatments and sufficient gains in adaptive functioning, the criteria for a diagnosis of ID may no longer be met.

Sequence and Rate of Development

Some aspects of development in individuals with ID are similar to what we see in typical development, while others vary. In general, the sequence, or ordering, of developmental tasks is the same for all children, with or without a disability. The only exceptions appear to be children with comorbid autism spectrum disorders and some children with uncontrollable seizures (King et al. 2005). The rate of development is generally slowed in individuals with ID, with variation according to age and developmental tasks. For example, in fragile X syndrome, rates of development are steady to 9–10 years of age, after which they slow, while in Down syndrome development slows between 6 and 11 years (King et al. 2005). Children with particular genetic syndromes also show different patterns of development related to skill acquisition and deficits that may be specific to the syndrome or individual and the brain systems affected. Special attention should be paid to diagnosing and treating, where appropriate, functional or physiological barriers to skill acquisition. For example, cleft palate and velopharyngeal insufficiency are common in children with 22q.112DS and may substantially impair speech and language development, although with proper treatment most affected individuals go on to develop a normal cognitive profile. It is also important to diagnose and treat any comorbid ADHD symptoms, which often cause significant barriers to learning and cognitive development.

Evaluation

Clinical History and Physical Examination

The comprehensive clinical evaluation should begin with a prenatal/birth history, family history, and three-generation pedigree (Curry et al. 1997), including medical, psychiatric, and neurological symptoms and diagnoses in the patient and family. A thorough physical and neurological examination is also indicated, given that many genetic syndromes, such as tuberous sclerosis complex, are evidenced through skin changes and/or neuromotor impairments. Photographs and videos can be useful tools in documenting skin conditions, movement disorders, and behavioral characteristics (Battaglia and Carey 2003). Also useful for diagnosis are sequential evaluations of the patient over several years (Curry et al. 1997), as symptoms of many behavioral phenotypes emerge or become more evident over time. In some cases elements such as dysmorphology and motor symptoms become more apparent, and in others, they "soften" over time. Because there is much variability within many of the genetic syndromes, a careful evaluation of attentional and cognitive function as well as psychiatric and behavioral issues should be undertaken.

Cytogenetic Diagnostic Testing

The American College of Medical Genetics (ACMG) provides guidelines for cytogenetic analysis (www.acmg.net) in the evaluation and diagnostic process. The ACMG recommends standard cytogenetic analysis at a minimum of a 550-band level for individuals with ID without a definite diagnosis regardless of whether dysmorphology, a family history, or other clinical features are present. FISH (fluorescence in situ hybridization) analysis or other molecular techniques can be performed on individuals with a provisional diagnosis of microdeletion syndrome concurrent with or before standard testing. Genetic testing technology, practice, and recommendations are evolving rapidly. Many older children, adolescents, and young adults have received testing using technologies or recommendations that are now obsolete. The child psychiatrist should ensure the patient has received testing and a workup conforming to current practice recommendations since these may yield a diagnosis where one was not previously obtainable.

Metabolic Testing

Historically, IEM, also known as the biochemical genetic disorders, were thought to affect a low percentage of individuals with intellectual disabilities. Individually, most IEM are rare, and the ACMG practice guidelines do not recommend routine metabolic testing. However, these diseases may affect 1%–1.5% of the general population. Moreover, IEM are disproportionately represented in persons with ID, and some studies suggest they may account for up to 2.5% of cases after screening by clinicians. More recent studies (Engbers et al. 2008) have shown that even after broad-based metabolic screening, a second line of testing identified metabolic disorders in 14% of patients, many of which were treatable. A careful history should be taken to make sure the patient received usual newborn screening tests and whether this testing followed current recommendations.

Neuroimaging and Electroencephalography

Neuroimaging (see Chapter 6, "Neurological Examination, Electroencephalography, Neuroimaging, and Neuropsychological Testing") has historically most often been performed in patients with micro- or macrocephaly, seizures, neurological signs, and/or loss of psychomotor skills (Curry et al. 1997). Magnetic resonance imaging (MRI) has been useful in elucidating the neurobiology and pathogenesis of intellectual disability. MRI detected frequent cerebral and posterior fossa abnormalities in children with nonspecific intellectual disabilities ranging from mild to severe (Soto-Ares et al. 2003). There have also been published cases of normocephalic patients who were found to have neurological disorders through magnetic resonance spectroscopy, even when results from MRI and cytogenetic and metabolic workups were normal (Battaglia 2003). The diagnostic value of electroencephalographic investigations, such as waking/sleep video-electroencephalographic-polygraphic studies, has also been reported (Battaglia et al. 1999), both in patients with a clinical history of seizures and in those with severe language deficits and/or specific genetic syndromes, such as AS. For an overview of the diagnostic evaluation process and an algorithm to guide decision making regarding the most appropriate tests for the patient with ID, see Battaglia and Carey (2003).

Comorbid Psychopathology

Prevalence

Estimates of the prevalence of psychiatric disorders in children and adolescents with ID range from 30% to 50% (Einfeld et al. 2011), and emotional and behavioral problems are three to seven times higher than in typically developing youth (Dykens 2000). Symptoms of psychiatric disorders are often attributed to the ID rather than recognized as comorbid psychiatric symptomatology. Additionally, some mental health conditions manifest differently in individuals with ID than they do in the general population, and it is important to consider relative developmental stage. For example, individuals with ID may present with apparent psychotic symptoms that in fact represent depression or the extension of the type of magical thinking that is common in younger children. Attentional and executive function deficits are common and may go unrecognized and undertreated. Symptom detection is especially difficult in individuals with severe ID because of their limited cognitive and communication skills. Medical concerns such as urinary tract or ear infections, skin complaints, or constipation should always be considered as underlying causes of behavioral exacerbations in the nonverbal patient. All of the common psychopathologies seen in children without intellectual impairment are also found in youth with ID, but at significantly higher rates. Specific factors that increase risk of comorbid psychiatric disorders include severity of disability, lower adaptive functioning, language impairments, poor socialization, low socioeconomic status, and families with only one biological parent in the home.

Assessment

There are no standardized psychiatric disorder assessment tools specifically for use with youth with ID. Assessment typically involves the child's own report of symptoms and experiences, descriptions from parents and teachers, and observations of behavior. In youth with ID, limited linguistic and communication skills and atypical symptom presentation complicate this process. Therefore, interviews with family, teachers, and other caregivers regarding their observations, as well as assessment of nonverbal aspects of behavior, play a critical role. Additionally, the clinician must be careful to differentiate symptoms of mental illness from symptoms of underlying brain dysfunction. Finally, challenging behaviors (attention seeking, aggression, self-injurious behavior, inappropriate social or sexual behavior), which are common reasons for referral for psychiatric services in youth with disabilities, can be caused or exacerbated by psychiatric disorders but may also be the result of metabolic and/or brain dysfunction. Determining the cause of such behaviors—organic conditions, psychopathology, environment, or a combination—is difficult, yet has important implications for treatment.

Treatment

Prevention

Strategies to prevent intellectual disabilities include prenatal diagnostic testing; prenatal care and education more generally (e.g., regarding exposure to toxins such as alcohol); newborn metabolic screening, which has been highly successful in reducing the incidence and severity of certain syndromes; and folic acid supplementation during prenatal development to reduce neural tube defects and possibly the risk of autism spectrum disorder.

Integrative Treatment

Response to treatment in children and adolescents with ID varies based on level of severity of intellectual impairment, age at which interventions are initiated, family and environmental factors, comorbid psychopathology, and number and severity of problem behaviors being addressed. An integrative approach to treatment—one that considers the youth's developmental level, social and environmental factors, psychological factors influencing capacity to learn problem-solving skills, and biology—is likely to provide the most positive outcome. In addition to direct treatment approaches, there are other avenues for families to explore, such as obtaining guardianship when an adolescent with ID reaches age 18 years.

Behavioral Approaches

Behavioral interventions, including treatments using principles of applied behavior analysis (ABA), have a large evidence base (Beavers et al. 2013). Behavioral approaches begin with an analysis of the cause or function of the behavior (antecedent) and how it is being reinforced. Techniques such as functional communication training (e.g., learning how to request breaks), noncontingent reinforcement (i.e., on a fixed time schedule), and extinction are then used to reduce challenging behaviors (aggression, self-injury, task-avoidant behavior) and promote positive behaviors. Other strategies often employed include breaking tasks down into smaller steps, modifying the teaching approach (more hands on and less verbal instruction), using visual aids, and providing immediate feedback. Behavioral approaches target skills deficits and modifications to the individual's environment and are most effective if applied across multiple settings to promote generalization of skills.

Psychotherapeutic Approaches

Standard psychotherapeutic approaches, such as psychoeducation, behavioral activation, and cognitive-behavioral therapy (CBT) to treat comorbid mental health conditions, are being increasingly studied in populations of individuals with ID. In youth with ID, recent studies with positive results have examined interventions targeting specific skills such as joint engagement in adolescents using reciprocal imitation training (RIT; Ingersoll et al. 2013) as well as parenting programs such as Stepping Stones Triple P to affect child behavior (Roux et al. 2013). A recent meta-analysis showed the most promise for CBT and for individual treatment approaches over group-based interventions; however, there was less benefit overall for children and young people versus adults with ID and mental health problems (Vereenooghe and Langdon 2013). Social skills intervention appears to promise life-enhancing benefits for youth with ID. Successful peer interactions can have significant benefits for youth with ID, affording them the opportunity to learn, practice, and refine social skills; develop friendships; and access support. Increased social competence can also positively affect academic achievement and enhance quality of life (Carter and Hughes 2005). Specific interventions include social interaction skills instruction, peer-delivered training interventions, group training, and peer support (e.g., peer buddy arrangements). Short- to moderate-length effects of such social skills interventions are clear, but long-term effects have been less well evaluated. A recommended approach combines skill-based and support-based strategies (Carter and Hughes 2005).

Pharmacological Treatment

Prevalence of Psychotropic Medication Use

Research finds that more than one-third of persons with ID are receiving at least one psychotropic drug. The general tone of these reports suggests alarm, for example, that the population is "overmedicated" (Holden and Gitlesen 2004) and that drug use is imprecise and appears not to be specific to diagnosis (Shireman et al. 2005). Psychostimulants, antidepressants, antipsychotics, and anticonvulsants account for the vast majority of psychotropic medication prescriptions in ID (Shireman et al. 2005). With respect to the perceived lack of specificity with which psychotropic medications are employed—for example, the off-label use of medications in ID for the treatment of target symptoms such as aggression, hyperarousal, and behavioral disturbance (Haw and Stubbs 2005)—the picture is complicated. Moreover, the atypical antipsychotics risperidone and aripiprazole both have a U.S. Food and Drug Administration (FDA)–approved indication for the treatment of irritability, aggression, and self-injurious behavior in children with autism spectrum disorder.

Review of Drugs by Class

In the use of psychotropic agents in ID, it is worth underscoring that the usual rules generally apply (see Part V of this textbook [Chapters 34–38] for more detailed coverage of psychopharmacology). Although the literature tends to be sparse, perhaps because ID is an exclusionary criterion for most medication efficacy trials, expert consensus is that the starting place for the treatment of psychiatric disorders is the same regardless of the presence of ID. What follows is a brief overview of special considerations, if any, that may be salient to ID.

Antipsychotic Drugs

Antipsychotic agents—increasingly the atypical, or second-generation, agents—are commonly used. Suggested quality assurance includes that the indications for treatment (symptoms and diagnosis) be documented, that the continuing need for the antipsychotic be specifically addressed at least annually for individuals receiving chronic treatment, and that side effects be assessed on a regular basis (Paton et al. 2011). The evidence supporting expanded indications for risperidone, including behavioral disturbances in persons with ID, is greater than that which exists for the other drugs in this class, and it is the most commonly prescribed (Paton et al. 2011). Weight gain and sedation are common side effects. In a 48-week open-label extension study of children who were treated with risperidone for disruptive behavior disorders in the context of borderline to moderate ID, Turgay et al. (2002) reported that average doses of 1.4 mg daily were associated with maintenance of improvement. An average of 4 kg of weight gain was attributed to the drug. Initially elevated prolactin levels retreated into the normal range (albeit significantly higher than at baseline) over the year of treatment.

Open-label studies exist using other atypical antipsychotic agents, and aripiprazole has FDA approval for the treatment of behavioral disturbance in autism spectrum disorder. It is reasonable for a clinician to consider a trial of risperidone for the treatment of extreme irritability, aggression, or self-injury in patients with ID. Other atypical agents could be considered if response was inadequate or use of risperidone is precluded by side effects. Relative doses appear to be much lower when used for this purpose than for the treatment of psychosis, consistent with the general axiom for this population of "start low, go slow." Conversely, when these or other medications are determined not to be helpful, the rate of withdrawal should not be any slower than it would be for a typically developing child who is having a medicine discontinued for lack of efficacy.

Anticonvulsants

Anticonvulsants are also commonly used in persons with ID; prevalence has varied from 23% to 46% across residential settings. A recent population-based study of children with epilepsy in the UK revealed that 40% also had ID. While neurobehavioral disorders were present in the majority of these children, they were often underdiagnosed (Reilly et al. 2014). While in the majority of cases anticonvulsants are prescribed for seizure disorders, as for the general population, this class of medication is also being studied for potential behavioral stabilization.

Antidepressants

Considerable interest exists for understanding the potential utility of SSRIs in children and adolescents, particularly those with repetitive behaviors. Behavioral activation appears to be more common in children and in persons with ID, and recommendations are to begin with extremely low doses.

Adrenergics

Hyperactivity, impulsivity, disinhibition, and behavioral difficulties often pose great problems for parents and teachers of youth with ID. Agarwal et al. (2001) conducted a small randomized, placebo-controlled crossover trial of the α_2 agonist clonidine for symptoms of hyperactivity and impulsivity in children with ID ranging from mild to severe. Ten children were treated with fixed doses of clonidine (4, 6, and 8 μg/day). Clonidine was associated with a significant, dose-related improvement in hyperactivity, impulsivity, and inattention. Half of the children became drowsy, but for most the effect dissipated over time. The investigators concluded that clonidine may have a place in the treatment of impulsive/hyperactive behaviors in youth with ID and that longer-term studies with larger samples are warranted. Handen et al. (2008) evaluated immediate-release guanfacine up to 3 mg daily in a 6-week trial in children with developmental disabilities and symptoms of inattention and hyperactivity. Five of the 11 children in this placebo-controlled crossover trial were deemed responders on the hyperactivity subscale of the Aberrant Behavior Checklist. The use of beta-blocking drugs like propranolol for problem behaviors like aggression has been reported to be helpful in a number of settings, but the evidence base overall is very limited and largely anecdotal (Ward et al. 2013).

Psychostimulants

Stimulant drugs are among the most commonly prescribed psychotropic medications for the treatment of disruptive behavior in children and adolescents with ID (de Bildt et al. 2006). Expert consensus supports the use of methylphenidate and amphetamine formulations as first-line treatments for ADHD symptoms in the setting of ID (Rush and Frances 2000). However, the response rate and effect size are less robust than for the general population with ADHD (Handen et al. 2008; Simonoff et al. 2013). A recent double-blind, placebo-controlled study by Simonoff and colleagues (2013) found that methylphenidate was superior to placebo for ADHD symptoms in the setting of ID but with an effect size of only 0.39 and overall response rate of 40%.

Opioid Antagonists

The opioid antagonist naltrexone has been explicitly studied for the treatment of repetitive self-injurious behavior. The largest controlled trials are negative, and a recent systematic review suggests that available evidence is inconclusive (Gormez et al. 2014). Naltrexone may be an option worthy of consideration in treatment-refractory self-injurious behavior, despite the lack of clear findings in studies and the dearth of recent research.

Other Drugs

Sleep disturbance is a little-studied but often significant problem for some persons with ID. Melatonin has been evaluated for the treatment of insomnia in children with disabilities and, in situations where its administration has led to sleep improvement, behavioral disturbances like self-injury have also been noted to improve (Jan and Freeman 2004). Although these studies support the consideration of melatonin for the treatment of insomnia in children and adolescents with multiple disabilities, the relative numbers of children studied to date remain extremely small, and open trials are problematic.

Educational and Community Services and Supports

Educational programs for youth with ID are often multidisciplinary and include behavior specialists, speech and occupational therapists, special education teachers, and case managers. These professionals collaborate with the individual's family and community to develop individualized treatment plans specific to the child's strengths and needs. Early intervention is essential for optimal development and can be accessed through state-supported programs for children ages birth to 3 years. These programs provide services in multiple settings (home, center) and are designed to target communication, self-help, social, and cognitive development. Developmental preschool programs provided through the public school system serve the same purpose for children ages 3–5.

Once the enters the public school system, an individualized education program (IEP) is developed collaboratively by school staff, social services, and the child's family (see Chapter 48). Specific placement decisions are determined on the basis of level of functioning. Some children with mild impairments can be placed in a regular education classroom, with some time spent during the day in a learning support classroom (or "resource room") to address specific skills deficits. In a resource room, special educators work one-on-one or in small groups with students. Children with greater levels of impairment may be placed in a self-contained special education classroom, where they spend the entire day. Special education and learning support classrooms target academic and independent living skills ("life skills") and also support social skills development and vocational training.

Support services for families of individuals with ID are available through each state's developmental disabilities agency, as well as through organizations such as The Arc and through schools, churches, and other nonprofit groups (Table 7–5). Support services include respite care so that families caring for a child with a high level of need can take short-term breaks to relieve stress, get support, and restore energy; in-home behavioral interventions; and crisis intervention services to help families deal with extreme situations and to ensure the safety of children with ID and their families.

TABLE 7–5. Resources for individuals with intellectual disabilities and their families

Organization or agency	Mission	Contact information
American Association on Intellectual and Developmental Disabilities (AAIDD)	Promotes progressive policies, research, effective practices, and universal human rights for people with ID	501 3rd Street NW, Suite 200, Washington, DC 20001; (202) 387–1968; www.aaidd.org
The Arc of the United States	Advocates for the rights and full participation of all children and adults with intellectual and developmental disabilities; works to improve systems of supports and services, connect families, and influence public policy	1825 K Street NW, Suite 1200, Washington, DC, 20006; (800) 433–5255; e-mail: info@thearc.org; www.thearc.org
Division on Autism and Developmental Disabilities (DADD) of the Council for Exceptional Children	A professional organization of educators, family members, and others working to enhance the competence of those who work with individuals with ID; responding to critical issues in the field; and advocating for individuals with developmental disabilities	Council for Exceptional Children, 2900 Crystal Drive, Suite 1000, Arlington, VA 22202–3557; (888) 232–7733, (866) 915–5000 TTY; e-mail: cec@cec.sped.org; www.cec.sped.org
Wrightslaw Special Education Law and Advocacy	Provides accurate, reliable information about special education law and advocacy for children with disabilities	www.wrightslaw.com

Summary Points

- The term *intellectual disability* (ID) has replaced the term *mental retardation.* There are three diagnostic criteria for a diagnosis of ID: deficits in intellectual function, deficits in adaptive function in one or more areas, and onset during the developmental period.
- About 30%–50% of cases of ID are of unknown etiology, although this number is getting smaller as more sophisticated testing methods are developed and new syndromes are discovered. Current known causes include chromosomal changes and exposure to toxins during prenatal development; heredity, including single-gene abnormalities, chromosomal defects, and inborn errors of metabolism; pregnancy and perinatal complications; acquired medical conditions; and environmental influences.
- Development in children with ID occurs in the same sequence as in children with typical development, but at a different rate, with speeded or slowed development at various ages and/or related to various developmental tasks.
- The clinical evaluation for ID often includes a clinical history and physical exam, cytogenetic diagnostic testing, metabolic testing, and neuroimaging and electroencephalography.
- Youth with ID are at increased risk of developing comorbid psychopathology as compared with youth without ID. Mental health disorders in this population are often unrecognized, undiagnosed, and untreated.
- Treatment for ID should be integrative, taking into account the child's developmental level, social and environmental factors, psychological factors (capacity to learn problem-solving skills), and biology. Behavioral interventions and psychopharmacological approaches currently have the best evidence base.

References

Agarwal V, Sitholey P, Kumar S, et al: Double-blind, placebo-controlled trial of clonidine in hyperactive children with mental retardation. Ment Retard 39(4):259–267, 2001 11448249

Aït Yahya-Graison E, Aubert J, Dauphinot L, et al: Classification of human chromosome 21 gene-expression variations in Down syndrome: impact on disease phenotypes. Am J Hum Genet 81(3):475–491, 2007 17701894

American Association on Intellectual and Developmental Disabilities: Diagnostic and Adaptive Behavior Scale. Washington, DC, American Association on Intellectual and Developmental Disabilities, 2015

American Association on Mental Retardation: Mental Retardation: Definition, Classification and Systems of Supports, 9th Edition. Washington, DC, American Association on Mental Retardation, 1992

American Psychiatric Association: Diagnostic and Statistical Manual of Mental Disorders, 5th Edition. Arlington, VA, American Psychiatric Association, 2013

Battaglia A: Neuroimaging studies in the evaluation of developmental delay/mental retardation. Am J Med Genet C Semin Med Genet 117C(1):25–30, 2003 12561055

Battaglia A, Carey JC: Diagnostic evaluation of developmental delay/mental retardation: an overview. Am J Med Genet C Semin Med Genet 117C(1):3–14, 2003 12561053

Battaglia A, Bianchini E, Carey JC: Diagnostic yield of the comprehensive assessment of developmental delay/mental retardation in an institute of child neuropsychiatry. Am J Med Genet 82(1):60–66, 1999 9916845

Bayley N: Bayley Scales of Infant and Toddler Development, 3rd Edition. San Antonio, TX, Psychological Corporation, 2005

Beavers GA, Iwata BA, Lerman DC: Thirty years of research on the functional analysis of problem behavior. J Appl Behav Anal 46(1):1–21, 2013 24114081

Bracken BA, McCallum RS: Universal Nonverbal Intelligence Test (UNIT). Rolling Meadows, IL, Riverside Publishing, 1998

Bruininks RH, Woodcock RW, Weatherman RF, et al: Scales of Independent Behavior—Revised (SIB-R). Rolling Meadows, IL, Riverside Publishing, 1996

Carter EW, Hughes C: Increasing social interaction among adolescents with intellectual disabilities and their general education peers: effective interventions. Research and Practice for Persons with Severe Disabilities 30:179–193, 2005

Chakrabarti S, Fombonne E: Pervasive developmental disorders in preschool children. JAMA 285(24):3093–3099, 2001 11427137

Christodolou J, Ho G: MECP2-related disorders, in GeneReviews [Internet]. Edited by Pagon RA, Adam MP, Ardinger HH, et al. Seattle, WA, University of Washington, 2001 20301670

Crawford DC, Acuña JM, Sherman SL: FMR1 and the fragile X syndrome: human genome epidemiology review. Genet Med 3(5):359–371, 2001 11545690

Croen LA, Grether JK, Selvin S: The epidemiology of mental retardation of unknown cause. Pediatrics 107(6):E86, 2001 11389284

Curry CJ, Stevenson RE, Aughton D, et al: Evaluation of mental retardation: recommendations of a consensus conference: American College of Medical Genetics. Am J Med Genet 72(4):468–477, 1997 9375733

de Bildt A, Mulder EJ, Scheers T, et al: Pervasive developmental disorder, behavior problems, and psychotropic drug use in children and adolescents with mental retardation. Pediatrics 118:e1860–e1866, 2006

Dykens EM: Psychopathology in children with intellectual disability. J Child Psychol Psychiatry 41(4):407–417, 2000 10836671

Einfeld SL, Ellis LA, Emerson E: Comorbidity of intellectual disability and mental disorder in children and adolescents: a systematic review. J Intellect Dev Disabil 36(2):137–143, 2011 21609299

Elliott CD: Differential Ability Scales, 2nd Edition. San Antonio, TX, Harcourt Assessment, 2006

Engbers HM, Berger R, van Hasselt P, et al: Yield of additional metabolic studies in neurodevelopmental disorders. Ann Neurol 64(2):212–217, 2008 18570304

Gormez A, Rana F, Varghese S: Pharmacological interventions for self-injurious behaviour in adults with intellectual disabilities: abridged republication of a Cochrane systematic review. J Psychopharmacol 28(7):624–632, 2014 24785762

Handen BL, Sahl R, Hardan AY: Guanfacine in children with autism and/or intellectual disabilities. J Dev Behav Pediatr 29(4):303–308, 2008 18552703

Hanson E, Bernier R, Porche K, et al: The cognitive and behavioral phenotype of the 16p11.2 deletion in a clinically ascertained population. Biol Psychiatry 77(9):785–793, 2015 25064419

Harrison P, Oakland T: Adaptive Behavior Assessment Scale, 2nd Edition. San Antonio, TX, Psychological Corporation, 2003

Haw C, Stubbs J: A survey of off-label prescribing for inpatients with mild intellectual disability and mental illness. J Intellect Disabil Res 49(Pt 11):858–864, 2005 16207284

Holden B, Gitlesen JP: Psychotropic medication in adults with mental retardation: prevalence, and prescription practices. Res Dev Disabil 25(6):509–521, 2004 15541629

Horsthemke B, Buiting K: Imprinting defects on human chromosome 15. Cytogenet Genome Res 113(1–4):292–299, 2006 16575192

Hoyme HE, May PA, Kalberg WO, et al: A practical clinical approach to diagnosis of fetal alcohol spectrum disorders: clarification of the 1996 Institute of Medicine criteria. Pediatrics 115(1):39–47, 2005 15629980

Ingersoll B, Walton K, Carlsen D, et al: Social intervention for adolescents with autism and significant intellectual disability: initial efficacy of reciprocal imitation training. Am J Intellect Dev Disabil 118(4):247–261, 2013 23937368

Jan JE, Freeman RD: Melatonin therapy for circadian rhythm sleep disorders in children with multiple disabilities: what have we learned in the last decade? Dev Med Child Neurol 46(11):776–782, 2004 15540640

Kaufman AS, Kaufman NL: Assessment Battery for Children, 2nd Edition (KABC-II). Los Angeles, CA, Western Psychological Services, 2004

King BH, Hodapp RM, Dykens EM: Mental retardation, in Kaplan and Sadock's Comprehensive Textbook of Psychiatry, Vol 2, 8th Edition. Edited by Kaplan HI, Sadock BJ. Baltimore, MD, Lippincott Williams and Wilkins, 2005, pp 3076–3106

Leonard H, Wen X: The epidemiology of mental retardation: challenges and opportunities in the new millennium. Ment Retard Dev Disabil Res Rev 8(3):117–134, 2002 12216056

Leviton A, Fichorova RN, O'Shea TM, et al: Two-hit model of brain damage in the very preterm newborn: small for gestational age and postnatal systemic inflammation. Pediatr Res 73(3):362–370, 2013 23364171

Manning MA, Eugene Hoyme H: Fetal alcohol spectrum disorders: a practical clinical approach to diagnosis. Neurosci Biobehav Rev 31(2):230–238, 2007 16962173

May PA, Gossage JP: Estimating the prevalence of fetal alcohol syndrome. A summary. Alcohol Res Health 25(3):159–167, 2001 11810953

Mullen EM: Mullen Scales of Early Learning. Circle Pines, MN, American Guidance Service, 1995

Newborg J: Battelle Developmental Inventory, 2nd Edition. Rolling Meadows, IL, Riverside Publishing, 2004

Paton C, Flynn A, Shingleton-Smith A, et al: Nature and quality of antipsychotic prescribing practice in UK psychiatry of intellectual disability services. J Intellect Disabil Res 55(7):665–674, 2011 21507097

Reilly C, Atkinson P, Das KB, et al: Neurobehavioral comorbidities in children with active epilepsy: a population-based study. Pediatrics 133(6):e1586–e1593, 2014

Riley EP, McGee CL: Fetal alcohol spectrum disorders: an overview with emphasis on changes in brain and behavior. Exp Biol Med (Maywood) 230(6):357–365, 2005 15956765

Roid GH: Stanford-Binet Intelligence Scales, 5th Edition. Rolling Meadows, IL, Riverside Publishing, 2003

Roid GH, Miller LJ: Leiter International Performance Scale—Revised (Leiter-R). Lutz, FL, Psychological Assessment Resources, 1997

Roux G, Sofronoff K, Sanders M: A randomized controlled trial of group Stepping Stones Triple P: a mixed-disability trial. Fam Process 52(3):411–424, 2013 24033239

Rush AJ, Frances A (eds): Expert consensus guideline series: treatment of psychiatric and behavioral problems in mental retardation (special issue). Am J Ment Retard 105:159–228, 2000

Sedel F, Baumann N, Turpin JC, et al: Psychiatric manifestations revealing inborn errors of metabolism in adolescents and adults. J Inherit Metab Dis 30(5):631–641, 2007 17694356

Shapira NA, Lessig MC, Lewis MH, et al: Effects of topiramate in adults with Prader-Willi syndrome. Am J Ment Retard 109(4):301–309, 2004 15176917

Shireman TI, Reichard A, Rigler SK: Psychotropic medication use among Kansas Medicaid youths with disabilities. J Child Adolesc Psychopharmacol 15(1):107–115, 2005 15741792

Simonoff E, Taylor E, Baird G, et al: Randomized controlled double-blind trial of optimal dose methylphenidate in children and adolescents with severe attention deficit hyperactivity disorder and intellectual disability. J Child Psychol Psychiatry 54(5):527–535, 2013 22676856

Soni S, Whittington J, Holland AJ, et al: The course and outcome of psychiatric illness in people with Prader-Willi syndrome: implications for management and treatment. J Intellect Disabil Res 51(Pt 1):32–42, 2007 17181601

Soto-Ares G, Joyes B, Lemaître MP, et al: MRI in children with mental retardation. Pediatr Radiol 33(5):334–345, 2003 12695867

Sparrow S, Cicchetti D, Balla D: Vineland Adaptive Behavior Scales, 2nd Edition. Circle Pines, MN, American Guidance Service, 2005

Srivastava AK, Schwartz CE: Intellectual disability and autism spectrum disorders: causal genes and molecular mechanisms Neurosci Biobehav Rev 2014 24709068 Epub ahead of print

Turgay A, Binder C, Snyder R, et al: Long-term safety and efficacy of risperidone for the treatment of disruptive behavior disorders in children with subaverage IQs. Pediatrics 110(3):e34, 2002 12205284

Vereenooghe L, Langdon PE: Psychological therapies for people with intellectual disabilities: a systematic review and meta-analysis. Res Dev Disabil 34(11):4085–4102, 2013 24051363

Ward F, Tharian P, Roy M, et al: Efficacy of beta blockers in the management of problem behaviours in people with intellectual disabilities: a systematic review. Res Dev Disabil 34(12):4293–4303, 2013 24171827

Wechsler D: Wechsler Preschool and Primary Scale of Intelligence, 4th Edition. San Antonio, TX, Psychological Corporation, 2012

Wechsler D: Wechsler Intelligence Scale for Children, 5th Edition. San Antonio, TX, Psychological Corporation, 2014

Williams CA: Neurological aspects of the Angelman syndrome. Brain Dev 27(2):88–94, 2005 15668046

Xu J, Chen Z: Advances in molecular cytogenetics for the evaluation of mental retardation. Am J Med Genet C Semin Med Genet 117C(1):15–24, 2003 12561054

CHAPTER 8

Autism Spectrum Disorders

Peter E. Tanguay, M.D.
W. David Lohr, M.D.

In 1943, Leo Kanner, child psychiatrist and author of the first U.S. textbook on child psychiatry, published a paper in which he described 11 children "whose condition differs so markedly and uniquely from anything reported so far, that each case merits—and, I hope will eventually receive—a detailed review of its fascinating peculiarities" (Kanner 1943, p. 217). The following year, Hans Asperger (see Asperger 1991, pp. 37–92), described, in a German publication, a similar disorder. Both reports had the word *autistic* in their title. It was not until DSM-III (American Psychiatric Association 1980) was published that autism became an official and codified diagnosis.

Kanner (1943) believed that "these children have come into the world with innate inability to form the usual, biologically provided affective contact with people" (p. 250). Only when affordable, technically adequate audio and video recording devices were developed in the 1970s was it possible to observe and accurately quantify social responses in infants and children. Since then, many studies have given us a rich understanding of how social interaction develops. The nature and development of human social communication are too complex to be adequately covered in this chapter (for reviews, see Trevarthen and Aitken 2001 and Tuchman 2003), but a brief summary is in order. Children are born with the behavioral propensity to emit social signals. By several months of age they are beginning to engage in a rich experience of communication using eye contact, social smile, social gesture, and body language. By age 15 months they appear to have a rudimentary understanding of "theory of mind" (i.e., that others have minds that differ from their own, and that they can learn from watching the social signals of others). By age 3 or 4 years they begin to engage in to-and-fro conversation and to "mentalize" (i.e., infer others' emotions and intent). In contrast, children who have autism spectrum disorder (ASD) appear to lack the behavioral propensity to interact with their caretakers, or they may begin to do so normally only to lose the ability by 12–15 months of age. They fail to develop joint interaction using eye contact, gesture, prosody, and body language; later they do not develop the capacity to mentalize. Or they may develop some of these skills, but they remain deficient in these skills compared with the general population.

Social communication skills may be continuously distributed in the general population, with people on the autism spectrum being at the most impaired end of the distribution. Constantino et al. (2000) have developed the Social Responsiveness Scale (SRS), comprising 65 items meant to assess a broad spectrum of social communication traits. The scale is capable of distinguishing between children with ASD and children who have other psychiatric disorders. In populations of normally developing school children (Constantino et al. 2000) or neurotypical twins (Constantino and Todd 2003), SRS scores were found to be continuously distributed, with a graph of the distribution resembling a bell-shaped curve. Posserud et al. (2006) have reported a similar continuous distribution of social communication skills in a population of 9,430 children ages 7–9 years, using the parent and teacher versions of the Autism Spectrum Screening Questionnaire. The authors found that 2.7% of children had scores in the extremely abnormal range, with males showing higher scores than females. Hoekstra et al. (2007) found a continuous distribution of Autism Spectrum Quotient scores in a population of 370 18-year-old twins, their 94 siblings, and 128 parents. Males had significantly higher autistic trait scores than females. More recently, Kamio et al. (2013) studied the distribution of SRS (Japanese version) scores of 22,529 children between 6 and 15 years of age. Scaled scores formed a skewed normal distribution with a single factor structure and no significant relation to IQ within the normal intellectual range. There was no evidence of a natural cutoff that could be used to make a specific categorical diagnosis of ASD as opposed to milder forms of the disorder.

Definition, Clinical Description, and Diagnosis

Definition of Autism Spectrum Disorder

The specific criteria for the diagnosis of ASD in DSM-5 are shown in Box 8–1 (American Psychiatric Association 2013). ASD is defined by the presence of persistent deficits in social communication and social interaction across multiple contexts. There must also be symptoms of restrictive and repetitive behaviors and/or stereotyped patterns of interest that are abnormal in their intensity or focus. In the interest of emphasizing that ASD is a continuum, the categories of Asperger's disorder and pervasive developmental disorder not otherwise specified (PDD-NOS), which were listed under the category of pervasive developmental disorder in DSM-IV (American Psychiatric Association 1994), were considered too nonspecific and have been eliminated. Reliability of the discrimination among subtypes was poor, even by experts. In a recent editorial, Ozonoff (2012) reviews the controversy that has been engendered by this change. A study of 4,453 children contrasting the DSM-IV and DSM-5 criteria concluded that most children with a PDD-NOS diagnosis would remain eligible for an ASD diagnosis (Huerta and Lord 2012).

Box 8–1. DSM-5 Diagnostic Criteria for Autism Spectrum Disorder

299.00 (F84.0)

A. Persistent deficits in social communication and social interaction across multiple contexts, as manifested by the following, currently or by history (examples are illustrative, not exhaustive; see text):
   1. Deficits in social-emotional reciprocity, ranging, for example, from abnormal social approach and failure of normal back-and-forth conversation; to reduced sharing of interests, emotions, or affect; to failure to initiate or respond to social interactions.
   2. Deficits in nonverbal communicative behaviors used for social interaction, ranging, for example, from poorly integrated verbal and nonverbal communication; to abnormalities in eye contact and body language or deficits in understanding and use of gestures; to a total lack of facial expressions and nonverbal communication.
   3. Deficits in developing, maintaining, and understanding relationships, ranging, for example, from difficulties adjusting behavior to suit various social contexts; to difficulties in sharing imaginative play or in making friends; to absence of interest in peers.

   Specify current severity:

   Severity is based on social communication impairments and restricted, repetitive patterns of behavior (see Table 2 [DSM-5, p. 52]).

B. Restricted, repetitive patterns of behavior, interests, or activities, as manifested by at least two of the following, currently or by history (examples are illustrative, not exhaustive; see text):
   1. Stereotyped or repetitive motor movements, use of objects, or speech (e.g., simple motor stereotypies, lining up toys or flipping objects, echolalia, idiosyncratic phrases).
   2. Insistence on sameness, inflexible adherence to routines, or ritualized patterns of verbal or nonverbal behavior (e.g., extreme distress at small changes, difficulties with transitions, rigid thinking patterns, greeting rituals, need to take same route or eat same food every day).
   3. Highly restricted, fixated interests that are abnormal in intensity or focus (e.g., strong attachment to or preoccupation with unusual objects, excessively circumscribed or perseverative interests).
   4. Hyper- or hyporeactivity to sensory input or unusual interest in sensory aspects of the environment (e.g., apparent indifference to pain/temperature, adverse response to specific sounds or textures, excessive smelling or touching of objects, visual fascination with lights or movement).

   Specify current severity:

   Severity is based on social communication impairments and restricted, repetitive patterns of behavior (see Table 2 [DSM-5, p. 52]).

C. Symptoms must be present in the early developmental period (but may not become fully manifest until social demands exceed limited capacities, or may be masked by learned strategies in later life).

D. Symptoms cause clinically significant impairment in social, occupational, or other important areas of current functioning.

E. These disturbances are not better explained by intellectual disability (intellectual developmental disorder) or global developmental delay. Intellectual disability and autism spectrum disorder frequently co-occur; to make comorbid diagnoses of autism spectrum disorder and intellectual disability, social communication should be below that expected for general developmental level.

Note: Individuals with a well-established DSM-IV diagnosis of autistic disorder, Asperger's disorder, or pervasive developmental disorder not otherwise specified should be given the diagnosis of autism spectrum disorder. Individuals who have marked deficits in social communication, but whose symptoms do not otherwise meet criteria for autism spectrum disorder, should be evaluated for social (pragmatic) communication disorder.

Specify if:

With or without accompanying intellectual impairment

With or without accompanying language impairment

Associated with a known medical or genetic condition or environmental factor (**Coding note:** Use additional code to identify the associated medical or genetic condition.)

Associated with another neurodevelopmental, mental, or behavioral disorder (**Coding note:** Use additional code[s] to identify the associated neurodevelopmental, mental, or behavioral disorder[s].)

With catatonia (refer to the criteria for catatonia associated with another mental disorder, [DSM-5] pp. 119–120, for definition) (**Coding note:** Use additional code 293.89 [F06.1] catatonia associated with autism spectrum disorder to indicate the presence of the comorbid catatonia.)

Source. Reprinted from the *Diagnostic and Statistical Manual of Mental Disorders*, 5th Edition. Arlington, VA, American Psychiatric Association, 2013. Used with permission.

It should be noted that in DSM-5, there is a new diagnostic category within the chapter "Neurodevelopmental Disorders" called *social (pragmatic) communication disorder* (SPD). It is very similar to ASD, except for the absence of restrictive and repetitive behaviors. SPD is not listed as having a dimensional nature, which is surprising because its social communication symptoms have been well demonstrated to have a dimensional nature. The effect of this becoming a "battle of the diagnoses" is always possible, especially if SPD were deemed to merit less intensive and less costly services.

Clinical Characteristics

Parents are acutely sensitive to delays in certain developmental milestones in their infants and toddlers. A child who is not standing by 15 months, not walking or using words by 20 months, or not using phrases in speech by 30 months will be noticed, leading to efforts to understand and remediate the delay. This is not necessarily so for the more subtle manifestations of the development of social communication, such as use of facial expressions or gestures, the degree of enthusiasm with which the child greets others, the amount of time the child spends in meaningful eye contact, or whether he or she uses gestures to direct another person's attention to things that interest them or that they want. Parents are more likely to notice if their child uses stereotypic hand and finger mannerisms or becomes obsessively preoccupied with certain objects or activities, but not all autistic children behave in this way as infants or toddlers. Therefore, parents might not bring their autistic child for evaluation until age 18 months or later. In addition, children with mild to moderate degrees of ASD may show their least degree of disability when interacting with their mothers, even while interacting less with their siblings, and not at all with persons outside the family. Mothers may report that their child is affectionate with them but entirely aloof from others or that the child will preferentially show a desire to be with them while largely ignoring others.

Certain questions are useful in the specific assessment for social communication disorders: "Does your child talk to you or make sounds to you just to be friendly? Can you have a give-and-take conversation with your child, in which he says something, you reply, he replies in turn, and so on? Can your child choose topics of conversation that take into account your interests rather than just his own interests? Is it difficult to "catch" your child's eye? How has your child responded to others in distress? Does he even notice the distress, and if he notices, does he respond with appropriate empathy and comforting sounds and gestures?" For children ages 3–4 years, play behaviors, both alone and with others, are crucial indicators of social communication deficits. One of the most important functions of play for children is to imitate and master the world in which they live. Even at a very young age, children imitate their parents: pretending to mow the lawn, to cook in the kitchen, to do the things they see their parents do. By age 4 years (or earlier) they play out pretend scenarios of fantastic adventure, but always ones that mirror what they know of the real world. Children who have even mild degrees of social communication deficit do not engage in this *make-believe* play. Their play is obsessive and unimaginative and does not usually involve make-believe imaginary people. They may copy entire stories from television or books, but they play them out without embellishment or change. They do not engage in what is called *symbolic play,* for example, treating a toy car or doll as if it were a real car or a real person. In later years, when they interact with other people, these children are severely handicapped because they are unable to fathom what the other person's intentions are or what his or her interests might be. The child with ASD who has a fascination with and an encyclopedic knowledge of dinosaurs cannot understand why his obsessive dwelling on the topic with other children makes them scorn and reject him.

Beginning with Kanner's original article, it was believed that the social communication symptoms of ASD were present from the first months of life. Several recent studies have suggested that may not be so (Ozonoff et al. 2010, 2014). Two groups of children were studied: 294 at high risk for ASD by virtue of their having a sibling with ASD, and 166 at low risk (with typically developing siblings). Children were evaluated for ASD at ages 6, 12, 18, 24, and 36 months. At 36 months, subjects were classified into three groups: being autistic, having "broad autistic phenotype," or having typical development. At age 6 months the three groups were not distinguishable from one another on measures of social communication. Between ages 6 and 12 months the differences between groups became apparent and continued to broaden over time. Using eye-tracking technology, Jones and Klin (2013) studied high-risk infant siblings of children with ASD. At 2 months infants later diagnosed as having ASD did not differ from those who later were not given an ASD diagnosis. Between 2 and 6 months the former group showed an abrupt decline in attention to eyes as did the latter group, with the decline continuing precipitously. Landa et al. (2013) have shown that at-risk infants may develop symptoms of ASD along different trajectories and that the age at onset of symptoms does not necessarily predict severity of symptoms by toddlerhood.

Many children with ASD have associated deficits in addition to their DSM-IV diagnostic criteria symptoms. Approximately 40% have intellectual deficiency, reflected in IQ scores of less than 70. As a characteristic of ASD, all have deficits in pragmatic communication (i.e., the social aspects of communication), but some persons with ASD have additional deficits in vocabulary and grammar. Some (perhaps 25%) have severe hypersensitivity to sounds, bright lights, touch, or taste. Some have gross and fine motor deficiencies. Such disabilities may emerge before the social handicaps. Only after cataloguing all of the child's problems can the clinician have a sufficient understanding of the child to develop a program of remediation and treatment.

Diagnostic Process

Since there are no biological or laboratory tests to confirm ASD, the diagnosis is based on clinical signs and symptoms. It is possible to suspect ASD at 12 months and to diagnose ASD by 18 months of age. Routine surveillance and screening approaches are recommended. Guevara et al. (2013) studied the degree to which developmental screening tools make a difference in the identification of ASD and other developmental disorders by pediatricians and their staffs. Children from four urban pediatric practices in Philadelphia were enrolled in the study. Each child was randomly assigned to one of three groups. One received evaluations with standard developmental assessment tools filled out by the parents. In the second, parents were given help by the pediatrician's staff in completing the questionnaires. The third group attended a well-baby clinic in which no specific screening tools were used. The results indicated that children with developmental disabilities in the two screening arms were twice as likely to have their developmental disabilities identified and to be referred for services than those who were not. Screening did not over-identify disorders or create false positives, according to the investigators.

The clinical diagnosis of ASD should be made through a multidisciplinary evaluation involving multiple informants and settings and should include parent interview along with direct observation of the child. Further psychological testing is indicated to evaluate cognitive skills, language skills, adaptive function, and academic function (Huerta and Lord 2012; Volkmar et al. 2014).

Evaluation Instruments

Routine early screening of all children for ASD at ages 18 and 24 months is recommended by American Academy of Pediatrics practice guidelines (Johnson et al. 2007). The Checklist for Autism in Toddlers (CHAT) was developed for screening by pediatricians and nurses with children who are ages 18–24 months (Baron-Cohen et al. 1992). It takes less than 10 minutes to administer and uses information from the parent as well as observation of the child. Behaviors that are particularly deficient in toddlers with ASD are proto-declarative pointing (calling the parent's attention to an object of interest), proto-imperative pointing (asking for something), and gaze monitoring. The original CHAT had a high rate of false negatives (failing to identify children who later were diagnosed autistic). A modified version, M-CHAT (Robins et al. 2001), addressed these concerns with improved diagnostic specificity. Recent findings on the use of the M-CHAT support a two-step process in which for children with total scores between 3 and 6 parents are asked in more detail about positive symptoms. Immediate referral is indicated for those with scores of 7 or higher (Chlebowski et al. 2013).

Various instruments exist to guide the clinician in screening and providing diagnostic support. Recent guidelines do not recommend a specific tool but support the use of semistructured interviews and observation as part of a multidisciplinary team evaluation (Falkmer et al. 2013). For children ages 3 years and older, the Autism Diagnostic Interview—Revised (ADI-R; Lord et al. 1994) and the Autism Diagnostic Observation Schedule—Generic (ADOS-G; Lord et al. 2000) are universally recognized as the most comprehensive and valid diagnostic instruments available. The ADI-R is a semistructured interview of the child's primary caretaker that includes many items pertaining to social communication. The diagnosis is reached by means of an algorithm based on scores on clusters of items that correspond to social relationships; verbal and nonverbal communication; and restrictive, repetitive, and stereotypic patterns of behavior. Unfortunately, the ADI takes at least 90 minutes to administer properly, which may diminish its usefulness as a routine instrument in many busy clinics. For this reason the Social Communication Questionnaire (SCQ), a 40-item parent survey derived from the ADI-R, is suggested (Rutter et al. 2003). The ADI-R is the "gold standard" for research. The ADOS-G, designed to be used for both children and adults, consists of a number of age-appropriate social "presses" in which the examiner uses his or her behavior to elicit social responses from the subject. The updated version, Autism Diagnostic Observation Schedule, 2nd Edition (ADOS-2), has a module for toddlers under the age of 3 years. The interview is scored using a template designed to measure social communication domains. Interviewers must be trained, but the interview usually takes 1 hour or less to administer. Neither the ADI nor the ADOS is required for making a clinical diagnosis of ASD.

The Childhood Autism Rating Scale, 2nd Edition (CARS2; Schopler et al. 2010) combines elements of the structured interview with direct observation and may be used for screening and diagnostic supplementation. The Social Responsiveness Scale is a brief but valid quantitative measure that is widely used for screening and measurement of the autistic traits. It has been studied in many different settings and can be easily administered and scored (Constantino 2002; Constantino et al. 2003). For a comprehensive overview of ASD rating instruments, see the article by Falkmer et al. (2013).

Differential Diagnosis: Fragile X Syndrome

The cause of fragile X syndrome is a mutation in the gene *FMR1* (including the occurrence of a greatly expanded trinucleotide repeat) at Xq27.3. The diagnosis is made using Southern blot and polymerase chain reaction testing of persons suspected of having the syndrome. Recent studies indicate that approximately 3%–5% of persons diagnosed with ASD have the *FMR1* mutation (Farzin et al. 2006; Wassink et al. 2001). While small, this prevalence is sufficient to warrant testing of all autistic persons for the mutation, if only because of the implication for family genetic counseling. Study of persons who have fragile X syndrome has revealed social and communication deficits that resemble the symptoms of ASD (Loesch et al. 2007; Rogers et al. 2001). *FMR1* is known to play a role in many neurodevelopmental processes, and some of these may involve systems that are defective in ASD. This suggests that study of the development of these systems might shed light on the pathogenesis of ASD itself.

Epidemiology

In the early 1970s several well-designed epidemiological studies reported that 1 in 2,500 children was autistic. Subsequent epidemiological studies from America, Canada, various European countries, Japan, and China have tracked the steady rise in the prevalence of ASD over at least the past 15 years. Recently, the Centers for Disease Control and Prevention (CDC) reported that 1 in 68 American children was estimated to have ASD (Developmental Disabilities Monitoring Network Surveillance Year 2010 Principal Investigators 2014). What could account for this remarkable increase? No one has been able to answer this satisfactorily. Understanding ASD as a social communication spectrum disorder could account for identifying milder cases, some so mild that one wonders if they deserve a formal diagnosis. The fact that this almost twentyfold increase in the past 30 years has been reported in first, second, and third world countries makes it hard to conceive of an environmental factor that would be common across the globe, although there are enough environmental and food chain toxins that could affect fetal and early child development in first world countries that one could raise numerous scenarios that account for the increase in ASD as well as other developmental disorders. Few of these scenarios have been adequately investigated. Beginning in the late 1990s, vaccination was accused of causing ASD, but numerous studies have since disproven this hypothesis (DeStefano et al. 2013). A workshop convened by the CDC and Autism Speaks in 2011 (Rice et al. 2013) concluded that while documentation of the increase was important, its cause has remained elusive.

Comorbidity

Clinicians who work with persons with ASD have long observed the additional presence of symptoms of other psychiatric disorders. Indeed, Kanner noted in his original paper that anxiety was a prominent feature of the syndrome. In a study of 109 children evaluated with a structured interview, 72% of children with autism had at least one other DSM-IV Axis I diagnosis. More recent studies have corroborated this observation (Leyfer et al. 2006). The most common diagnoses were specific phobia (44%), obsessive-compulsive disorder (OCD) (37%), attention-deficit/hyperactivity disorder (ADHD) (31%), separation anxiety disorder (12%), and major depressive episode (10%). Many children had several comorbid diagnoses. Simonoff et al. (2008) found that 57% of children with autism had one or two additional psychiatric disorders. The most common disorders were social anxiety disorder (29%), ADHD (28%), and oppositional defiant disorder (28%).

Anxiety problems may be more common and severe in ASD than in classical autism. There appears to be a link between anxiety, sensory hypersensitivity, and social impairment (Gadow et al. 2005). As in normally developing youth with anxiety, it appears that specific phobias are more common in younger children with ASD, whereas OCD and social phobia become more common during adolescence. It is difficult to make the diagnosis of anxiety disorders in children with ASD. Symptoms of anxiety may be difficult to pinpoint and may present as nonspecific behaviors or specific increase in repetitive autistic behaviors. Self-report may be difficult in this population because of problems with emotional insight or ability to accurately describe and report one's emotions. Teachers and parents differ in their report of child anxiety (White et al. 2009). For anxiety in ASD to be diagnosed, the signs and symptoms of anxiety must be above and beyond the core symptoms of ASD and should lead to more impaired functioning than can be attributed to the ASD symptoms (Leyfer et al. 2006; Matson and Nebel-Schwalm 2007). It can be very difficult to differentiate OCD from symptoms of ASD. OCD obsessions may be better organized and intrusive than the preoccupations typical of ASD. Also, OCD compulsions may be supported by the presence of pressure or urges to perform a behavior and increased levels of preoccupations (Lubetsky et al. 2011). Validated scales are needed to provide ASD-specific measures of anxiety in a brief clinical format, and a gold standard diagnostic tool for comorbidity in ASD is needed for research on treatment efficacy (Siegel 2012).

The presentation of depression in ASD may also be atypical, and detection may be complicated by the individual's lack of insight into his or her impairment. Persons with better social communication skills may be more likely to have increased self-awareness and thus awareness of their depression. When evaluating an individual with ASD for depression, one should ask about classic DSM diagnostic criteria such as insomnia, anhedonia, self-harm, and motivation and inquire about known predisposing factors to depression, such as family history and recent stresses, and any behavioral changes from the patient's usual state.

ADHD is no longer excluded as a comorbid condition of ASD in DSM-5. Symptoms of inattention and hyperactivity/impulsivity may be common in ASD per se. ADHD should be considered when these symptoms exceed what is typical for the developmental age of the child (American Psychiatric Association 2013). Preoccupation with fixated interests may appear similar to inattention. Overall, up to half of children with ASD may also have symptoms that meet criteria for ADHD. Research supports commonly shared genetic etiological factors (Matson et al. 2013).

Etiology

Genetic Risk Factors

ASD is the most highly heritable of all mental disorders, exceeding the heritability of schizophrenia or bipolar disorder. Twin and family studies have convincingly demonstrated that genetic factors play a role in disorders throughout the autism spectrum (for review see Lauritsen and Ewald 2001). In a recent population-based epidemiological study that included more than two million families, the heritability of ASD and autistic disorder was found to be approximately 50%, with the risk increasing with genetic relatedness (Sandin et al. 2014).

Numerous previous studies have suggested that both maternal and paternal age can influence the likelihood of having a child with ASD (Sandin et al. 2012). This has been confirmed in two large population studies. Idring et al. (2014) examined the Swedish national registry data on more than 400,000 children. ASD was found in 1.1% of the children. Mothers older than 30 years were found to have an increased risk of having a child with ASD, with the likelihood increasing in a linear fashion with advancing age. Fathers older than 32 years also had an increasing risk of having a child with ASD. Frans et al. (2013) estimated that

6% of the risk for ASD was attributable to a paternal age of over 40 years. Even grandfathers' age was important: men who fathered a daughter at greater than 50 years of age were 1.79 times more likely to have a grandchild with ASD. In such a case a de novo mutation was passed from the grandfather through his daughter to his grandchild.

There are no single genes that universally code for ASD. Recent studies have identified numerous gene abnormalities that contribute to ASD, although most play a role in only a small number of cases. Some of the same genes that influence social communication also play a role in other psychiatric and developmental disorders. Copy number variants (CNVs)—submicroscopic chromosome abnormalities involving short microdeletions or duplications of bases within a gene—have been identified in some persons with ASD (Kumar and Christian 2009).

While the identification of gene abnormalities in ASD has led to a plethora of largely uninterpretable findings, it may be time to use different data sources to understand how some of the more frequent findings actually influence brain development at various points from conception onward. A new resource, the BrainSpan atlas, provides investigators with putative three-dimensional maps showing when genes turn on and off in the human brain, from embryo to adult. Using this map, Willsey et al. (2013) have studied the ways in which "high-confidence" gene mutations (those identified in multiple families with ASD) may actually play a role in human brain development. One finding was that such genes play a role in the development of deep cortical layer neurons that send information over long distances. Parikshak et al. (2013) used the atlas to classify ASD-related genes into 12 "families" on the basis of the timing of their expression during brain development, location, and function. In three families, ASD-associated genes whose function it is to establish synaptic functioning during prenatal and early postnatal development were found to be enriched. This type of research, beyond what has been hitherto attempted, has considerable future promise.

Neurobiological Factors

Since the late 1960s investigators have been pursuing neurobiological studies of persons with ASD (for an overview, see DiCicco-Bloom et al. 2006). These "fishing expeditions" have for the most part not been successful. Lately there have been some promising developments in studies based on the normative neurobiology of facial recognition and the circuitry of what has been termed the "social brain network." The relevance of facial recognition as a probe to understand brain function in ASD has been given its impetus by studies of the differences in eye tracking of social scenes by subjects with ASD as compared with control subjects (Klin et al. 2002). While social scenes were being viewed, visual fixations on four regions were coded: mouth, eyes, body, and objects. Significant between-group differences for subjects with ASD and control subjects were obtained for all four regions. The best predictor of ASD was reduced eye region fixation time. Fixation on mouths and objects was significantly correlated with social functioning: increased focus on mouths predicted better social adjustment and less autistic social impairment, whereas more time on objects predicted the opposite relationship. It was concluded that fixation times on mouths and objects, but not on eyes, are strong positive predictors of a lack of social competence.

Previous work in neurotypical subjects demonstrated that facial recognition activates the fusiform gyrus (FG) (more specifically the fusiform face area [FFA]), and it does so in a more pronounced way on the right than on the left side of the brain. This observation has led to a number of studies of FG and FFA activation to facial expression in persons with ASD (Pierce et al. 2001).

In his seminal paper, Kanner (1943) described many persons with ASD as having an increased head circumference (HC). In the past decade studies have shown that growth in HC in persons with ASD accelerates and decelerates over time (Courchesne et al. 2003). Compared with birth HC in healthy infants, birth HC in infants with ASD was significantly smaller ($P<0.001$); after birth, HC increased by 1.67 standard deviations (SDs), and by 6–14 months mean HC was at the 84th percentile. Only 6% of the individual healthy infants in the longitudinal data showed accelerated HC growth trajectories (>2.0 SDs) from birth to 6–14 months; 59% of infants with autistic disorder showed these accelerated growth trajectories. Courchesne and colleagues concluded that the clinical onset of ASD appears to be preceded by two phases of brain growth abnormality: a smaller than typical head size at birth and a sudden and excessive increase in head size at 1–2 months and 6–14 months. However, other studies have shown that HC abnormalities are not characteristic of all children with ASD (Ghaziuddin et al. 1999; Gray et al. 2012).

Psychological Theories

Theory of Mind

The concept of theory of mind originated many years ago in nonhuman primate research with the question "Does one chimpanzee understand that another chimpanzee has a mind different from his own, capable of having different thoughts and intentions?" The answer, for chimps, appears largely to be no. The question was then raised in regard to persons with ASD. Numerous studies using a "false belief" paradigm have reported that many children with ASD may fail the task, but less socially handicapped persons with ASD will not. The latter finding may be due to the tasks being relatively easy to solve. While this concept has been useful in making specific predictions about the impairments in socialization, imagination, and communication shown by people with ASD, it does not provide an explanation of why this might be so.

Folk Psychology Versus Folk Physics

A concept developed by Simon Baron-Cohen et al. (2001) proposes that humans have evolved two neurocognitive adaptations. One is *folk psychology,* for inferring social causality, understanding others' intentions, and predicting their social responses. The other is *folk physics,* for inferring physical causality and for understanding and being fascinated with factual information (e.g., lineages of dinosaurs, the solar system). Baron-Cohen has postulated that each adaptation is under genetic control. It has been amply demonstrated that people with Asperger's disorder can have very good folk physics skills along with very poor folk psychology skills. The concept may be helpful as an organizing principle to understand behaviors seen in verbal persons with ASD who have good intellectual skills. It is possible that genetic and neurobiological research will someday provide a framework for expanding our understanding of these concepts.

Executive Function

Executive function is a term used to describe a set of mental processes that helps us connect past experience with present and future action. Executive function is needed when a person performs such activities as planning, organizing, strategizing, and paying attention to and remembering details. People with executive function problems may also show weakness with "working memory," which is needed to guide one's actions. Many studies have documented that persons with ASD have deficits in the various components of executive functioning (Pennington and Ozonoff 1996). However, such deficits (differing perhaps in degree and profile) have also been reported in many other psychiatric disorders, including schizophrenia. The concept needs to be refined and studied in greater detail in psychiatrically healthy populations before it can be fruitfully applied to understanding the manifestations of various mental illnesses.

Treatment

Behavioral Interventions

Therapeutic interventions can be classified using several parameters. Does the therapist determine what the child should learn (such as a teacher in the classroom who has a specific curriculum), or does the therapist encourage the child to choose the activity and determine how the interaction will proceed? In children with severe ASD, who may not be motivated to attend to others, the therapist has to identify what the child enjoys, join in the activity, and, by varying the parameters of the activity, hope to kindle a nascent relationship with the child. Is the intervention given one-to-one, or is it in a group setting, such as a classroom or a social coaching group? For very handicapped children, a one-to-one engagement, even in the classroom, may be necessary at times. And lastly, are the parents involved, either as co-therapists or as primary therapists in their own right, guided by a consultant on a weekly or biweekly basis? A number of specific therapies are outlined in the following subsections. Many have overlapping approaches, and not all are suitable for all children, given the large variability among persons with ASD in severity of autistic symptoms and differences in intellectual ability and use of language.

Applied Behavior Analysis

Applied behavior analysis (ABA) is one of the oldest of the behavioral therapies, having been developed by Lovaas at UCLA in the 1970s. As its use expanded, it was adapted by many therapists to suit children with different needs. ABA, in a form that came to be called *discrete trial training,* relies on the principles of operant conditioning, in which a stimulus (a question or a command) is presented to evoke a specific response. If necessary, physical prompts are given to encourage the response. Reinforcers (such as small candies or other desired objects) are provided as a reward. In some versions of ABA, incorrect responses might be followed by an aversive stimulus, such as a verbal reprimand. An innovative feature of ABA is that therapists work in the home with the parents as co-therapists. As much as 35 hours a week of ABA therapy has been recommended by some of its proponents. It is essential that therapists be well versed in normal development so that they can choose goals that are within the range of a child's developmental capabilities. ABA is one of the few therapies that has had some empirical validation (McEachin et al. 1993). Studies of Lovaas-based approaches and early intensive behavioral intervention have shown that the interventions result in some improvements in cognitive performance, language skills, and adaptive behavior skills in some children with ASD, although the literature is limited by methodological constraints (Warren et al. 2011). A subsequent ABA approach, *pivotal response training*, was developed by Koegel et al. (2001) with the goal of finding ways to increase the child's motivation, responsiveness to multiple cues, engagement in self-management, and self-initiation of social interactions that were identified as "pivotal" factors in determining the success of behavioral interventions. To increase motivation, the therapist may encourage the child to incorporate self-chosen materials, activities, topics, and toys into the learning situation. Although the clinician follows the child's lead, the therapist assures that the target behaviors are incorporated into the activities, while maintaining the child's attention and decreasing the likelihood that the child will engage in disruptive behavior. Self-management is increased by teaching individuals to discriminate between appropriate and inappropriate behavior. The child is encouraged to actively record how many correct responses he or she makes and to administer self-rewards. Similar approaches are used to help the child learn other pivotal factors, which in turn enhance learning of social skills. Studies of pivotal response training (www.abainternational.org; www.autismprthelp.com) have shown that it can be successful in enhancing adaptive behaviors in persons with ASD.

Treatment and Education of Autistic and Related Communication Handicapped Children

Treatment and Education of Autistic and Related Communication Handicapped Children (TEACCH; www.TEACCH.com), developed by Eric Schopler in the early 1970s, has been expanded into a statewide program in North Carolina that is a model for comprehensive cost-effective intervention in the United States. It focuses on the "culture of autism" and aims to reward and facilitate children's understanding of the structure of events, the communication of visual information, and the acquisition of meaningful knowledge. The program endeavors to develop an individualized person- and family-centered plan for each client or student rather than using a standard curriculum. It summarizes its approach as a family-centered, evidence-based practice for ASD, which is based on a theoretical conceptualization of ASD, supported by empirical research, enriched by extensive clinical expertise, and notable for its flexible and person-centered support of individuals of all ages and skill levels. It sponsors both local and national training programs.

Floor Time

Floor time was developed by Greenspan and Wieder (1998). It has been renamed the Developmental, Individual-Difference, Relationship-Based approach (DIR) (www.icdl.com) to intervention. Like pivotal behavior training, DIR is child-centered. The goal of DIR is to build increasingly larger "circles of interaction" between the therapist and the child in a developmentally appropriate way. Emphasis is on two-way interactions that are gratifying to the child, working up to more sophisticated symbolic interactions. The approach consists of three parts: 1) parents do "floor time" with their child, creating experiences that promote mastery of the milestones in social development; 2) other therapists and educators work with the child, using techniques informed by floor time to deal with the child's specific challenges and to facilitate development; and 3) parents work to improve their own responses and styles of relating with regard to the social milestones to create a family pattern that supports emotional and intellectual growth in all family members. A national network of therapists expert in floor time has been developed to work with parents in implementing DIR. Although the therapy seems reasonable, no empirical studies with control groups have been published. This same criticism could be made for several other behavioral treatments.

Relationship Development Intervention

Relationship Development Intervention (RDI; www.RDIconnect.com) is a parent-based, cognitive-developmental approach, in which primary caregivers are trained to provide daily opportunities for successful functioning in increasingly challenging dynamic systems. It targets behaviors that follow the developmental model of social communication, starting with affective reciprocity and joint attention and culminating in theory of mind and the acquisition of intuitive social knowledge (social mentation). The exercises are designed to catch and hold the child's attention. Parents learn the basics of the treatment at 4-day workshops with Steven Gutstein, the developer of RDI. Regional consultants act as local advisors to the parents. A small outcome study (without control groups but with good diagnostic and measurement instruments) (Gutstein et al. 2007) indicated that the method has promise.

Social Communication, Emotional Regulation and Transactional Support Treatment

Social Communication, Emotional Regulation and Transactional Support Treatment (SCERTS; www.barryprizant.com) was developed by Barry Prizant and Amy Wetherby. It is a child-centered multidisciplinary approach that focuses on the development of the capacity to regulate attention, arousal, and emotional states. Transactional activities are designed and implemented across settings to foster more successful interpersonal interactions and relationships at home, in the school, and in the community. The SCERTS model includes a well-coordinated assessment process that helps a team measure the child's progress and determine the necessary supports to be used by the child's social partners (educators, peers, family members).

Picture Exchange Communication System

Picture Exchange Communication System (PECS; www.pecs.com) is a modified ABA program designed for early nonverbal symbolic communication. It is not designed to teach speech, although speech is indirectly encouraged. Using a trainer and a facilitator (who models the target behaviors for the child), the child is led to understand that requests for objects (using picture cards) can lead to one's receiving the object as a reward. Later iterations of the exercises are designed to teach the child to use cards to express more elaborated requests and to express thanks for the rewards. The program is popular in classrooms for nonverbal autistic children.

Social Stories

Social Stories (www.thegraycenter.org) is a technique developed by Carol Gray, a teacher, in which a Social Story describes a situation, skill, or concept in terms of relevant social cues, perspectives, and common responses in a specifically defined style and format. The goal of a Social Story is to share accurate social information in a patient and reassuring manner that is easily understood by its audience. Half of all Social Stories developed should affirm something that an individual does well. Although the goal of a Social Story should never be solely to change the individual's behavior, that individual's improved understanding of events and expectations may lead to more effective responses. Social Stories may be used with children, adolescents and adults.

Literature Reviews of Behavioral Interventions

Seida et al. (2009) have carried out a comprehensive review of literature reviews of behavioral interventions in ASD. All studies were required to have qualitative or quantitative analysis of their data. Until 1996 there were few studies that met the minimal criteria for inclusion. More than half of the 30 studies that did meet those criteria had been published after 2004. Of these, 83% had major methodological flaws; only three Cochrane review studies did not. The majority of the reviews were of behavioral interventions or communication-focused therapy. The reviews reported positive outcomes, suggesting that some form of treatment is better than no treatment. Among the questions that remain to be addressed are which type of therapy is better for which type of patient, what the effects of any treatment might be over time, and how cost-effective any one therapy might be.

Psychopharmacological Treatment

A substantial body of literature describes trials of psychopharmacological agents in ASD (Kaplan and McCracken 2012). Unfortunately, much of it consists of small open trials, most of which were brief, with little longer-term follow-up (Broadstock et al. 2007). Many studies lacked adequate diagnostic or symptom measurement instruments. No medications have been found to be effective in ameliorating the social, language, or cognitive deficits in ASD. Medications that reduce anxiety may lead to a slight increase in social spontaneity, but this effect is likely to be due to the fact that anxious individuals tend to withdraw from social interaction. There is evidence—some from placebo-controlled studies—that the selective serotonin reuptake inhibitors and the atypical antipsychotics can be effective in reducing aggression, temper outbursts, and self-injurious behavior. They can also reduce stereotyped behaviors. A reduction in these behaviors can allow a person with ASD to participate more fully in treatment, which can lead to better adaptation and learning. To date, the methodologically best investigation has been the Research Units on Pediatric Psychopharmacology (RUPP) study of risperidone treatment of ASD (McDougle et al. 2005). The study consisted of an 8-week double-blind, placebo-controlled trial (N=101) and a 16-week open-label continuation study (N=63) of risperidone for children and adolescents with ASD. Gold-standard instruments were used throughout. Risperidone resulted in significantly greater reductions in scores on the Children's Yale-Brown Obsessive Compulsive Scale and the Maladaptive Behavior domain of the Vineland Adaptive Behavior Scales. This pattern of treatment response was maintained for 6 months. The investigators concluded that risperidone led to significant improvements in the restricted, repetitive, and stereotyped patterns of behavior, interests, and activities of autistic children but did not significantly change their deficits in social interaction and communication. Although in the past, stimulant medications were believed to be contraindicated in persons with ASD, there is some evidence that symptoms of inattention that interfere with learning may be improved with stimulant medication.

On the basis of previous studies that showed that oxytocin (a neuropeptide originally implicated in milk let down and uterine contractions at birth in animals and humans) also plays a role in mediating social behavior in rats, mice, and prairie voles (see Green and Hollander 2010), it has been proposed that oxytocin might be beneficial as a treatment in ASD. Hollander et al. (2007) reported that subjects with ASD who were treated with oxytocin showed a significant improvement on an affective comprehension task and in social memory. Guastella et al. (2008) reported that oxytocin nasal spray increased eye gaze compared with placebo. Other investigators have not found such behavioral improvements (Dadds et al. 2014; Gordon et al. 2013). Despite the mixed findings, oxytocin remains an intriguing therapeutic possibility.

Prognosis

Although ASD has been considered to be a lifetime disability, recent publications have suggested that a small minority of persons with ASD may lose most, if not all, of their symptoms by adulthood. Fein et al. (2013) documented a group of 34 subjects who had initially been judged to meet the criteria for autism but who had lost all symptoms of the disorder by adolescence or young adulthood. As children their social disability had been mild, although of sufficient severity to score within the autistic range on diagnostic instruments. All of these children had verbal and nonverbal IQ scores in the normal range. At the time of follow-up with parental questionnaire and ADOS interview, they were in regular classrooms with no special education services. It was the general impression of the investigators that the subjects' parents were highly involved in the children's treatment programs and in their social lives. It was also their opinion that although such involvement did not guarantee the effectiveness of intervention, it increased the likelihood of such a result.

For most children with ASD, especially those with subnormal intellectual and language skills, such an outcome is infrequent. For many, their lives are socially very constricted, their work opportunities are poor, and they are forced to live with their parents or in special residences (Howlin et al. 2013). There is a severe dearth of school or postsecondary opportunities through which individuals with social impairments can receive social coaching, remedial skill building, and assistance in finding and keeping jobs and in arranging for supervised independent living arrangements. A large national database study of factors associated with employed high school graduates with ASD (Chiang et al. 2013) found that annual household income, parental education, male gender, career counseling in high school, and postsecondary vocational training were important factors associated with participation in employment. A study of participants in the U.S. Rehabilitation Vocational System concluded that persons with ASD were more likely than adults with other impairments to be denied extensive services and were less likely to be competitively employed as adults. In contrast, in England, the supported employment programs not only have led to significant improvement and increase in quality of life but also have been shown to be cost-effective over time as the individuals with ASD gained more independence (Mavranezouli et al. 2013).

In "Sounding a Wake-Up Call," McDougle (2013) proclaims that society (including psychiatrists and psychologists) is not prepared to meet the needs of those with ASD as they become adults. Society is not even aware of what these needs are or what can be done to begin to remedy them. He states that only when we are prepared to meet those needs will "the parents of a newly diagnosed child with autism...have hopes and dreams that may come true" (p. 568). There comes a time, especially in adolescence, when it may be important not to focus solely on what the person cannot do but to focus on the skills at which he or she excels. Examples include persons with Asperger's disorder who were computer experts and were able to find a successfully employed role. One mother reported to this author: "He's a dot-com mathematical guru now, earning a good five-figure salary. He's still autistic, but people don't seem to care about that. He even has a girlfriend."

Summary Points

- Children come into the world with a behavioral propensity to interact socially with others and to learn complex social communication skills even before they learn language. Children with autism spectrum disorder (ASD) may initially have such skills but regress after 6–12 months of age.
- In DSM-5, ASD spectrum disorder is defined as a disorder in which persons have persistent deficits in social communication along with restrictive, repetitive patterns of behavior, interests, and activities. Some may also have impaired language and intellectual abilities, but others can show good language and intellectual abilities.
- Social communication skills are distributed in a continuous pattern in the general population. Persons with ASD lie at the least skillful end of this continuum. No cut-point has been defined for the diagnosis of ASD. Severity is defined in terms of the person's need for treatment.
- Epidemiological studies have indicated that the prevalence of ASD has sharply increased over the past 40 years. According to the Centers for Disease Control and Prevention, as many as 1 in 68 children in America has ASD.
- The most frequent comorbid disorders in ASD are anxiety disorder; attention-deficit/hyperactivity disorder, combined or inattentive type, with or without hyperactivity; and, to a lesser extent, obsessive-compulsive disorder.
- Genetic factors play an important role in ASD, more than in any other psychiatric disorder. The exact nature of the genetic factors is unknown, but they ap-

pear to be numerous and to interact with each other and with as yet unknown environmental factors.

- The diagnosis of ASD is best made through a multidisciplinary process involving multiple informants including parent interviews and direct observations of the child.
- There are many behavioral interventions that have been proposed for the treatment of persons with ASD. There is evidence that such treatment can help, but no single approach has been shown to be superior to others.
- Certain medications, primarily selective serotonin reuptake inhibitors and atypical antipsychotics, have shown promise in alleviating aggressive outbursts, repetitive and stereotyped behaviors, and self-injurious behaviors in persons with ASD. No medication has been shown to be effective in improving the social, language, or cognitive deficits in ASD.
- It is important to focus on what persons with ASD do well, rather than solely on their impairments. Playing to their strengths may enhance the likelihood that they will find some satisfaction in life.

References

American Psychiatric Association: Diagnostic and Statistical Manual of Mental Disorders, 3rd Edition. Washington, DC, American Psychiatric Association, 1980

American Psychiatric Association: Diagnostic and Statistical Manual of Mental Disorders, 4th Edition. Washington, DC, American Psychiatric Association, 1994

American Psychiatric Association: Diagnostic and Statistical Manual of Mental Disorders, 5th Edition. Arlington, VA, American Psychiatric Association, 2013

Asperger H: "Autistic psychopathology" in childhood (1944), in Autism and Asperger Syndrome. Edited by Frith U. Cambridge, UK, Cambridge University Press, 1991, pp 37–92

Baron-Cohen S, Allen J, Gillberg C: Can autism be detected at 18 months? The needle, the haystack, and the CHAT. Br J Psychiatry 161:839–843, 1992 1483172

Baron-Cohen S, Wheelwright S, Spong A, et al: Studies of theory of mind: are intuitive physics and intuitive psychology independent? Journal of Developmental and Learning Disorders 5:47–78, 2001

Broadstock M, Doughty C, Eggleston M: Systematic review of the effectiveness of pharmacological treatments for adolescents and adults with autism spectrum disorder. Autism 11(4):335–348, 2007 17656398

Chiang HM, Cheung YK, Li H, et al: Factors associated with participation in employment for high school leavers with autism. J Autism Dev Disord 43(8):1832–1842, 2013 23224594

Chlebowski C, Robins DL, Barton ML, et al: Large-scale use of the modified checklist for autism in low-risk toddlers. Pediatrics 131(4):e1121–e1127, 2013 23530174

Constantino JN: The Social Responsiveness Scale. Los Angeles, CA, Western Psychological Services, 2002

Constantino JN, Todd RD: Autistic traits in the general population: a twin study. Arch Gen Psychiatry 60(5):524–530, 2003 12742874

Constantino JN, Przybeck T, Friesen D, et al: Reciprocal social behavior in children with and without pervasive developmental disorders. J Dev Behav Pediatr 21(1):2–11, 2000 10706343

Constantino JN, Davis SA, Todd RD, et al: Validation of a brief quantitative measure of autistic traits: comparison of the social responsiveness scale with the autism diagnostic interview-revised. J Autism Dev Disord 33(4):427–433, 2003 12959421

Courchesne E, Carper R, Akshoomoff N: Evidence of brain overgrowth in the first year of life in autism (comment). JAMA 290(3):337–344, 2003 12865374

Dadds MR, MacDonald E, Cauchi A, et al: Nasal oxytocin for social deficits in childhood autism: a randomized controlled trial. J Autism Dev Disord 44(3):521–531, 2014 23888359

DeStefano F, Price CS, Weintraub ES: Increasing exposure to antibody-stimulating proteins and polysaccharides in vaccines is not associated with risk of autism. J Pediatr 163(2):561–567, 2013 23545349

Developmental Disabilities Monitoring Network Surveillance Year 2010 Principal Investigators; Centers for Disease Control and Prevention (CDC): Prevalence of autism spectrum disorder among children aged 8 years—autism and developmental disabilities monitoring network, 11 sites, United States, 2010. MMWR Surveill Summ Mar 28; 63(2):1–21, 2014 24670961

DiCicco-Bloom E, Lord C, Zwaigenbaum L, et al: The developmental neurobiology of autism spectrum disorder. J Neurosci 26(26):6897–6906, 2006 16807320

Falkmer T, Anderson K, Falkmer M, et al: Diagnostic procedures in autism spectrum disorders: a systematic literature review. Eur Child Adolesc Psychiatry 22(6):329–340, 2013 23322184

Farzin F, Perry H, Hessl D, et al: Autism spectrum disorders and attention-deficit/hyperactivity disorder in boys with the fragile X premutation. J Dev Behav Pediatr 27(2 suppl):S137–S144, 2006 16685180

Fein D, Barton M, Eigsti I-M, et al: Optimal outcome in individuals with a history of autism. J Child Psychol Psychiatry 54(2):195–205, 2013 23320807

Frans EM, Sandin S, Reichenberg A, et al: Autism risk across generations: a population-based study of advancing grandpaternal and paternal age. JAMA Psychiatry 70(5):516–521, 2013 23553111

Gadow KD, Devincent CJ, Pomeroy J, et al: Comparison of DSM-IV symptoms in elementary school-age children with PDD versus clinic and community samples. Autism 9(4):392–415, 2005 16155056

Ghaziuddin M, Zaccagnini J, Tsai L, et al: Is megalencephaly specific to autism? J Intellect Disabil Res 43(Pt 4):279–282, 1999 10466865

Gordon I, Vander Wyk BC, Bennett RH, et al: Oxytocin enhances brain function in children with autism. Proc Natl Acad Sci USA 110(52):20953–20958, 2013 24297883

Gray KM, Taffe J, Sweeney DJ, et al: Could head circumference be used to screen for autism in young males with developmental delay? J Paediatr Child Health 48(4):329–334, 2012 22077913

Green JJ, Hollander E: Autism and oxytocin: new developments in translational approaches to therapeutics. Neurotherapeutics 7(3):250–257, 2010 20643377

Greenspan SI, Wieder S: The Child With Special Needs. New York, Pereus Books, 1998

Guastella AJ, Mitchell PB, Dadds MR: Oxytocin increases gaze to the eye region of human faces. Biol Psychiatry 63(1):3–5, 2008 17888410

Guevara JP, Gerdes M, Localio R, et al: Effectiveness of developmental screening in an urban setting. Pediatrics 131(1):30–37, 2013 23248223

Gutstein SE, Burgess AF, Montfort K: Evaluation of the relationship development intervention program. Autism 11(5):397–411, 2007 17942454

Hoekstra RA, Bartels M, Verweij CJ, Boomsma DI: Heritability of autistic traits in the general population. Arch Pediatr Adolesc Med 161(4):372–377, 2007 17404134

Hollander E, Bartz J, Chaplin W, et al: Oxytocin increases retention of social cognition in autism. Biol Psychiatry 61(4):498–503, 2007 16904652

Howlin P, Moss P, Savage S, et al: Social outcomes in mid- to later adulthood among individuals diagnosed with autism and average nonverbal IQ as children. J Am Acad Child Adolesc Psychiatry 52(6):572–581, 2013 23702446

Huerta M, Lord C: Diagnostic evaluation of autism spectrum disorders. Pediatr Clin North Am 59(1):103–111, xi, 2012 22284796

Idring S, Magnusson C, Lundberg M, et al: Parental age and the risk of autism spectrum disorders: findings from a Swedish population-based cohort. Int J Epidemiol 43(1):107–115, 2014 24408971

Johnson CP, Myers SM, American Academy of Pediatrics Council on Children With Disabilities: Identification and evaluation of children with autism spectrum disorders. Pediatrics 120(5):1183–1215, 2007 17967920

Jones W, Klin A: Attention to eyes is present but in decline in 2–6-month-old infants later diagnosed with autism. Nature 504(7480):427–431, 2013

Kanner L: Autistic disturbances of affective contact. Nervous Child 2:217–250, 1943

Kamio Y, Inada N, Moriwaki A, et al: Quantitative autistic traits ascertained in a national survey of 22 529 Japanese schoolchildren. Acta Psychiatr Scand 128(1):45–53, 2013 23171198

Kaplan G, McCracken JT: Psychopharmacology of autism spectrum disorders. Pediatr Clin North Am 59(1):175–187, xii, 2012 22284801

Klin A, Jones W, Schultz R, et al: Visual fixation patterns during viewing of naturalistic social situations as predictors of social competence in individuals with autism. Arch Gen Psychiatry 59(9):809–816, 2002 12215080

Koegel RL, Koegel LK, McNerney EK: Pivotal areas in intervention for autism. J Clin Child Psychol 30(1):19–32, 2001 11294074

Kumar RA, Christian SL: Genetics of autism spectrum disorders. Curr Neurol Neurosci Rep 9(3):188–197, 2009 19348707

Landa RJ, Gross AL, Stuart EA, et al: Developmental trajectories in children with and without autism spectrum disorders: the first 3 years. Child Dev 84(2):429–442, 2013 23110514

Lauritsen M, Ewald H: The genetics of autism. Acta Psychiatr Scand 103(6):411–427, 2001 11401655

Leyfer OT, Folstein SE, Bacalman S, et al: Comorbid psychiatric disorders in children with autism: interview development and rates of disorders. J Autism Dev Disord 36(7):849–861, 2006 16845581

Loesch DZ, Bui QM, Dissanayake C, et al: Molecular and cognitive predictors of the continuum of autistic behaviours in fragile X. Neurosci Biobehav Rev 31(3):315–326, 2007 17097142

Lord C, Risi S, Lambrecht L, et al: The autism diagnostic observation schedule-generic: a standard measure of social and communication deficits associated with the spectrum of autism. J Autism Dev Disord 30(3):205–223, 2000 11055457

Lord C, Rutter M, Le Couteur A: Autism Diagnostic Interview-Revised: a revised version of a diagnostic interview for caregivers of individuals with possible pervasive developmental disorders. J Autism Dev Disord 24(5):659–685, 1994 7814313

Lubetsky MJ, Handen BL, McGonigle JJ: Autism Spectrum Disorder. New York, Oxford University Press, 2011

Matson JL, Nebel-Schwalm MS: Comorbid psychopathology with autism spectrum disorder in children: an overview. Res Dev Disabil 28(4):341–352, 2007 16765022

Matson JL, Rieske RD, Williams LW: The relationship between autism spectrum disorders and attention-deficit/hyperactivity disorder: an overview. Res Dev Disabil 34(9):2475–2484, 2013 23751293

Mavranezouli I, Megnin-Viggars O, Cheema N, et al: The cost-effectiveness of supported employment for adults with autism in the United Kingdom. Autism Int J Res Pract 18(8):975–984, 2013

McDougle CJ: Sounding a wake-up call: improving the lives of adults with autism. J Am Acad Child Adolesc Psychiatry 52(6):566–568, 2013 23702444

McDougle CJ, Scahill L, Aman MG, et al: Risperidone for the core symptom domains of autism: results from the study by the autism network of the research units on pediatric psychopharmacology. Am J Psychiatry 162(6):1142–1148, 2005 15930063

McEachin JJ, Smith T, Lovaas OI: Long-term outcome for children with autism who received early intensive behavioral treatment. Am J Met Retard 97(4):359–391, 1993 8427693

Ozonoff S: Editorial: DSM-5 and autism spectrum disorders—two decades of perspectives from the JCPP. J Child Psychol Psychiatry 53(9):e4–e6, 2012

Ozonoff S, Iosif AM, Baguio F, et al: A prospective study of the emergence of early behavioral signs of autism. J Am Acad Child Adolesc Psychiatry 49(3):256–266, e1–e2, 2010 20410715

Ozonoff S, Young GS, Belding A, et al: The broader autism phenotype in infancy: when does it emerge? J Am Acad Child Adolesc Psychiatry 53(4):398–407, e2, 2014 24655649

Parikshak NN, Luo R, Zhang A, et al: Integrative functional genomic analyses implicate specific molecular pathways and circuits in autism. Cell 155(5):1008–1021, 2013 24267887

Pennington BF, Ozonoff S: Executive functions and developmental psychopathology. J Child Psychol Psychiatry 37(1):51–87, 1996 8655658

Pierce K, Müller RA, Ambrose J, et al: Face processing occurs outside the fusiform 'face area' in autism: evidence from functional MRI. Brain 124(Pt 10):2059–2073, 2001 11571222

Posserud MB, Lundervold AJ, Gillberg C: Autistic features in a total population of 7–9-year-old children assessed by the ASSQ (Autism Spectrum Screening Questionnaire). J Child Psychol Psychiatry 47(2):167–175, 2006 16423148

Rice CE, Rosanoff M, Dawson G, et al: Evaluating changes in the prevalence of the autism spectrum disorders (ASDs). Public Health Rev 34:1–22, 2013

Robins DL, Fein D, Barton ML, et al: The Modified Checklist for Autism in Toddlers: an initial study investigating the early detection of autism and pervasive developmental disorders. J Autism Dev Disord 31(2):131–144, 2001 11450812

Rogers SJ, Wehner DE, Hagerman R: The behavioral phenotype in fragile X: symptoms of autism in very young children with fragile X syndrome, idiopathic autism, and other developmental disorders. J Dev Behav Pediatr 22(6):409–417, 2001 11773805

Rutter M, Bailey A, Lord C: Social Communication Questionnaire (SCQ). Los Angeles, CA, Western Psychological Services, 2003

Sandin S, Hultman CM, Kolevzon A, et al: Advancing maternal age is associated with increasing risk for autism: a review and meta-analysis. J Am Acad Child Adolesc Psychiatry 51(5):477–486, e1, 2012 22525954

Sandin S, Lichtenstein P, Kuja-Halkola R, et al: The familial risk of autism. JAMA 311(17):1770–1777, 2014 24794370

Schopler E, Van Bourgondien ME, Wellman GJ, et al: Childhood Autism Rating Scale, 2nd Edition. Los Angeles, CA, Western Psychological Services, 2010

Seida JK, Ospina MB, Karkhaneh M, et al: Systematic reviews of psychosocial interventions for autism: an umbrella review. Dev Med Child Neurol 51(2):95–104, 2009 19191842

Siegel M: Psychopharmacology of autism spectrum disorder: evidence and practice. Child Adolesc Psychiatr Clin N Am 21(4):957–973, 2012 23040909

Simonoff E, Pickles A, Charman T, et al: Psychiatric disorders in children with autism spectrum disorders: prevalence, comorbidity, and associated factors in a population-derived sample. J Am Acad Child Adolesc Psychiatry 47(8):921–929, 2008 18645422

Trevarthen C, Aitken KJ: Infant intersubjectivity: research, theory, and clinical applications. J Child Psychol Psychiatry 42(1):3–48, 2001 11205623

Tuchman R: Autism. Neurol Clin 21(4):915–932, viii, 2003 14743656

Volkmar F, Siegel M, Woodbury-Smith M, et al: Practice parameter for the assessment and treatment of children and adolescents with autism spectrum disorder. J Am Acad Child Adolesc Psychiatry 53(2):237–257, 2014 24472258

Warren Z, McPheeters ML, Sathe N, et al: A systematic review of early intensive intervention for autism spectrum disorders. Pediatrics 127(5):e1303–e1311, 2011 21464190

Wassink TH, Piven J, Patil SR: Chromosomal abnormalities in a clinic sample of individuals with autistic disorder. Psychiatr Genet 11(2):57–63, 2001 11525418

White SW, Oswald D, Ollendick T: Anxiety in children and adolescents with autism spectrum disorders. Clin Psychol Rev 29(3):216–229, 2009

Willsey AJ, Sanders SJ, Li M, et al: Coexpression networks implicate human midfetal deep cortical projection neurons in the pathogenesis of autism. Cell 155(5):997–1007, 2013 24267886

CHAPTER 9

Neurodevelopmental Disorders: Specific Learning Disorder, Communication Disorders, and Motor Disorders

Karen Pierce, M.D.

Developmental learning, communication, and motor problems affect children throughout development, influencing their lives and personalities. These disorders have long-term implications for children's emotional and regulatory development, affecting their transitions into adulthood. Some of these disorders, when detected and treated early, can be remediated successfully. Others are chronic, and compensatory skills must be taught.

All psychiatric assessments should include the patient's cognitive abilities. All children should be screened and any deficits treated early to prevent long-term sequelae. Many children referred for psychiatric assessment have language impairments, processing deficits, or problems with cognition that remain undetected unless the clinician is thinking about cognition as well as psychiatric symptoms.

In defining learning disorders (LDs) or communication disorders, the various categorical systems often do not agree or even define the same disorder. In DSM-5 (American Psychiatric Association 2013) these disorders are included under the category of *neurodevelopmental disorders.* The federal government's definition used by classroom teachers classifies these disorders somewhat differently. From another perspective, the research criteria proposed by the Insel et al. (2010) include cognitive domains for classifying mental disorders on dimensions of function, including attention, perception, working memory, language behavior, and reception and perception of facial and nonfacial communication.

Processing styles (i.e., strength in either visual or verbal processing) affect behavior and learning, even if deficits do not cross the diagnostic threshold. Clinicians need to define neurodevelopmental disorders according to DSM-5 but must be prepared to adapt their recommendations for educational purposes. Knowledge of both sets of definitions is essential to advocate for and to give comprehensive care to the child patient.

Rarely do learning, communication, and motor disorders occur alone; rather, they typically co-occur with other learning and psychiatric problems. These disorders may or may not be apparent to clinicians when they are evaluating maladaptive behavior and arriving at a psychiatric diagnosis. Since communication is the key to relationships and ultimately to most adaptive functioning, clinicians must be alert to the possibility of deficits in this arena. For example, if a child with an expressive language difficulty answers in one-word sentences or only shakes his head, the clinician might mistake this shyness as mutism or even a thought disorder rather than a communication disorder. If a child routinely loses behavioral or emotional control during the school day, the clinician must determine what class is being taught during that time, since poor frustration tolerance may be related to a learning issue rather than a mood or behavior disorder. A child with poor handwriting secondary to poor fine motor control may become disruptive when writing is required. School subjects that are difficult for the child, such as math or writing, may reveal poor visual processing. Both visuospatial and visual memory deficits can be silent learning issues that may manifest only as behavior problems. The clinician is urged to become familiar with these disorders and their effect on communication and behavior.

Learning Disorders

The specific LD category assumes that LDs are brain-based deficits that interfere with learning. LDs are heterogeneous and persistent. Each individual manifests them differently. Learning disabilities were federally classified as "handicapping conditions" in the United States in the 1960s. Since then, the research into typical learning and treatment of delays has blossomed. More than 8% of youth receive special education, including 60% of the students with either learning issues or communication disorders (U.S. Department of Education Office of Special Education and Rehabilitative Services 2011). The Americans with Disabilities Act Amendments Act of 2008 recognizes reading and communication disorders as meeting the condition of a disability. However, LDs are poorly understood, and the definition is applied differently among schools and states and on the federal level. Because LDs are both an unobservable construct and dimensional, definitions are ambiguous.

Why is an understanding of LD important? As more children receive instruction mainstreamed in regular education classes, the risk of psychiatric symptoms grows as a child faces frustration and limited mastery of academic material. U.S. Department of Education data from 2005–2006 show that students with disabilities who did not complete high school had emotional disturbance (44.9%), speech or language impairments (22.7%), specific learning disabilities (25.1%), intellectual disabilities (22.3%), disabilities (22.3%), and other health impairments (23.4%). Research on adult psychiatric illness demonstrates cognitive impairments in all of the major psychiatric disorders: schizophrenia (Cervellione et al. 2007; Schretlen 2007), bipolar disorder (Dickstein et al. 2007), anxiety disorders (Goldston et al. 2007), and the personality disorder clusters. Cognitive deficits appear to be an important determinant of functional outcomes (Bromley 2007). Cognitive functioning in patients with schizophrenia is associated with community functioning as well as brain imaging studies (Zipursky 2014). Euthymic adult patients with bipolar disorder perform significantly more poorly than control subjects on measures of verbal learning and memory (Martinez-Aran et al. 2004). The link between reading disorder and attention-deficit/hyperactivity disorder (ADHD) is well established (Pennington 2014). White adolescents with reading problems are more likely to have substance use disorders than minority youth (Goldston et al. 2007). Most cognitive impairments appear in childhood and can create subtle issues in personality formation. Not all processing deficits meet the threshold of a diagnosed LD, but they may still affect development.

Children who struggle academically are subject to chronic stress. This chronic stress on the hypothalamic-pituitary-adrenal axis and the autonomic nervous system affects metabolism, cardiovascular, and immune system functioning and even brain development (Noble et al. 2005). Recent meta-analyses of the prevalence of depression in children with learning disabilities show a higher than normal rate of depression (Sideridis 2006). Disruptive and aggressive behavior occurring in school may be the result of poor cognitive skills rather than a psychiatric disorder. Early detection of cognitive disabilities leads to smoother developmental progression and treatment.

Definition

In this section I review the varying definitions of LD, the current federal guidelines, the DSM-5 LD diagnoses, and processing issues in general.

Perhaps the greatest obstacle in discussing LDs is the disparate definitions used by psychiatry, education, advocacy, and law. The lack of clarity has impeded recognition and treatment. Even with special education mandates from the federal government, the threshold for positive identification of LDs and the definition and categories of special education vary from state to state, causing widely discrepant prevalence rates.

In DSM-5 the LD definitions were changed significantly and were placed under neurodevelopmental disorders. There are three specific learning disorders (rated as mild, moderate, or severe), six communication disorders, and two motor disorders.

In 2004, the Office of Special Education and Rehabilitative Services (through the Individuals with Disabilities Education Act) reauthorized the criteria for learning difficulties (for more information, see http://idea.ed.gov). If a child does not achieve adequately or meet state-approved grade-level standards in one or more of the areas listed below, then further intervention is needed. The basic standards are as follows:

- Basic reading skills
- Reading fluency skills
- Reading comprehension
- Mathematics calculation
- Mathematics problem solving
- Written expression
- Oral expression
- Listening comprehension

TABLE 9–1. Comparison of DSM-5 and federal categories of learning disability

DSM-5 diagnosis: specific learning disorder	Federal categories: specific learning disability
With impairment in reading (315.00)	Basic reading skills Reading fluency skills Reading comprehension
With impairment in mathematics (315.1)	Mathematics calculation Mathematics problem solving
With impairment in written expression (315.2) Specify severity: mild, moderate or severe	Written expression

Since these are the categories as defined by federal mandates, they will be given in **bold** as they are discussed in the following subsections. As noted, these are very different definitions of LD from those in DSM-5 (Table 9–1).

Identification of a Learning Disorder

LDs are chronic, heterogeneous disorders that have a negative impact on learning, achievement, and self-esteem. Although there is a strong genetic component, some learning disabilities have environmental causes, such as prenatal exposure to drugs or alcohol, lead toxicity, and brain injury. Whatever the origin, early identification is essential.

Neuropsychological or educational-psychological evaluations provide different and more comprehensive data. It is important to also assess a child's learning strengths, as these will be the resources that the child will use to help him through areas of weakness. Laboratory constructs of learning are not equivalent to cognitive skills and behaviors seen in the clinic.

Astute clinicians can begin to look for possible neuropsychological patterns in the testing data as well as screen for language, visual, and spatial strengths and weaknesses. Often missed are struggling learners who do not meet criteria for an LD or other disabilities.

The current special education law mandates screening all children by measuring the *response to intervention* (RTI; Fuchs et al. 2003). RTI is based on the dual-discrepancy model. The student must both be below the level of same-grade peers and have poor response to carefully planned and precisely delivered instruction. This requires that all classroom teachers develop benchmark- or curriculum-based measures (data norms) for the classroom, grade level, school, and district. This classroom-based evaluation may permit the use of alternative research-based procedures for determining whether a child has a specific LD. If a skill deficit is noted, then an accountability plan is developed to intervene. The plan must describe the intervention, where it is being done, for how long it is being done, the people responsible, and how progress will be measured. These data are compared and shared with the team. Curriculum-based measures determine both the need and the ongoing progress (Fletcher et al. 2007, p. 64).

The goal of any evaluation would be early intervention for those at risk. Requesting an LD evaluation in the schools is no longer the first step; rather, the clinician asks how the child is functioning with relation to his or her peers and the curricula and how he is responding to intervention. As in the DSM-5 system, an LD is diagnosed only when there is both a skill deficit and a resulting functional impairment. The definition of LD automatically excludes children with a visual, hearing, or motor disability; intellectual disability; emotional disturbance; or limited English proficiency; or when cultural factors, environmental factors, or economic disadvantage are involved. The RTI model can make communication with schools harder, since clinicians are taught to make a diagnosis first and then an intervention. Under RTI, intervention starts when a student's performance lags, before a comprehensive assessment is performed.

In general, reading recognition and fluency are easily measured and highly correlated. Reading comprehension and mathematics are a bit more difficult to measure, since there are many brain processes involved. Written expression assessment is difficult, as what defines a disorder is not well established (Fletcher et al. 2007). Speech and language skills assessment is well researched, but higher-level language skills such as pragmatics are just beginning to be studied systematically.

Reading Disorder

In DSM-5 **reading disorder** is defined as impairment of word reading accuracy, reading rate or fluency, or reading comprehension. *Dyslexia* has been suggested as an alternative term. Comments from Colker et al. (2013) show concern with this change, since dyslexia is well described and studied, with clear description of underlying neurobiological and cognitive factors, such as word retrieval difficulties, poor phonemic awareness, and difficulties with word reading and connected text reading. There is appropriate evidence-based treatment for this disorder as well. Dyslexia is the most prevalent LD in children receiving special education services. With more sophisticated testing, boys no longer greatly outnumber girls among those with dyslexia (Rutter et al. 2004). In developmental reading disability, the prevalence ratio of boys to girls is estimated at 1.5–2.1 to 1.

Although the DSM-5 broader label is helpful for psychiatric diagnosis, it lends little specificity and guidance for the school in order to remediate a child's reading skills. For the clinician, knowing the type of weakness in reading can help clinically. Often, children with poor reading fluency show fluency deficits in other areas, such as listening, speaking, and writing, thus giving the clinician a broader understanding of the child's frustrations. The reading processes defined by research and education categories are basic reading skills disability, reading fluency problems, and reading comprehension difficulties.

Basic Reading Skills or Reading Disability

Basic reading skills or reading disability is a common complex condition that is assumed to be based on linguistic or phonological impairment. It is dimensional rather than categorical and is persistent over time (Shaywitz and Shaywitz 2005). Functional brain imaging shows the neurological underpinnings of dyslexia in the areas of the fusiform gyrus, the posterior portion of the middle temporal gyrus, the angular gyrus, and the posterior portion of the superior temporal gyrus.

It is well established in studies using twin, family, and sib-pair designs that dyslexia is a heritable condition (Coch et al. 2007). There have been no specific genes identified, since the complexity and the heterogeneity of this disorder preclude a single genetic deficit. It is also important to recognize that genetic factors do not account for all of the variability; environmental risks also contribute.

All reading skills need the basic building blocks of reading, defined as follows:

- *Phonological awareness* is the metacognitive ability to understand the words we hear and read that have basic structure related to sound. Speech sounds, or phonemes, are patterns that make up words. In spoken language, the listener does not need to decipher each sound. English has 44 phonemes; Spanish has 24. To read, one must break letters into a sound-symbol relationship. How quickly the child does this determines his or her fluency. The best predictor of reading is a child's ability to detect these phonemes. This is true across all languages studied, including Chinese, Greek, Turkish, French, and English (Coch et al. 2007). There is a universal sequence of phonological development from awareness of large units (syllables) to awareness of small units (phonemes).
- *Rapid naming* is the rapid automatized naming of letters and digits. This usually predicts reading skills over time (Schatschneider et al. 2004). Although some authors disagree, most would say the ability to name quickly enhances reading fluency.
- *Phonological memory* is the ability to use working memory to retain sounds and then words. The relationship to poor reading is still not conclusive.
- *Word recognition.* Word-level reading disability or dyslexia is characterized by difficulty in single-word decoding. Without the ability to read a word, fluency and understanding are limited. This is the area where most research has been done. The inability to decode interferes with reading comprehension, word recognition, and fluent reading.
- *Spelling* is the ability to encode words either in isolation or in context and is difficult without word recognition. Some children can spell but not decode. Spelling is a multidimensional skill that is related to both phonological processing and memory.

Since problems can occur in any of these processes, schools need to evaluate each one before intervention is begun. A deficit in any of these processes would manifest as a reading disability. Intervention would vary depending on the deficit. Psychologically, children with reading problems will avoid reading or will procrastinate in this task. Poor reading affects many areas in a child's life, including the ability to read directions, understand signs, or read notes. Even using social networking on the computer or computer games requires reading skills. A clinician can suspect a reading problem if there has been a history of delayed language; problems with the sounds of words, such as rhyming words and pairing sound with symbol; or a family history of reading disorders.

Reading Fluency

Reading speed is the ability to read connected text rapidly, smoothly, and automatically with little attention to decoding (Meyer and Felton 1999). In order to be fluent, a child must recognize words quickly. Children with **reading fluency** problems read more slowly, have a harder time keeping ideas in short-term working memory, and use more energy to read. Most people have a constant reading rate that increases with age. Fluency is easily measured by having a child read a list of words or short passages and dividing the number of words read correctly by the total amount of time reading. Fluency interventions expose children to repeated words and word phrases. The reading material is then scaffolded to the instructional level in reading.

Psychologically, fluency disorders can be very embarrassing when a child is asked to read aloud. Stumbling over words, losing one's place, and having trouble with decoding are easily noticed by peers and can have a profound effect on a child's self-esteem and lead to a child's avoidance of reading aloud. Fluency deficiencies make reading slower, interfering with the efficiency of reading long passages (Paul and Sideridis 2006).

Reading Comprehension

Reading comprehension refers to the ability to understand information in written form. It is a way to connect ideas on the page to what one knows. One needs to be motivated, hold ideas, concentrate, and have good study techniques. There are many places where this process can be derailed, not only with cognitive problems but with behavior, attention, and emotional difficulties. Active readers will monitor how well they understand what they are reading (Swanson 1999). A good assessment requires the reading of a complex text, not usually seen in standard reading tests. A child who reads adequately for a standardized test may fail to read and understand the more complicated ideas in a textbook. Core cognitive processes for comprehension include language skills, listening comprehension, working memory, and the higher-order processing of inference, prior knowledge, comprehension monitoring, and structure sensitivity. A deficit here affects all academic subject areas where reading is required. Reading comprehension is difficult to assess, as there are many aspects of reading for understanding. Reading disorders show high comorbidity with other learning issues. The correlation between ADHD and reading disorders is high, especially if there is slow processing speed.

Intervention is important, since poor reading impairs educational, social, and occupational functioning. Early intervention can protect children at risk from later failure. It is clear that both classroom and small-group tutorial programs are effective, and not all children need individualized one-on-one instruction (Fletcher et al. 2007). Studies of remediation show that there are effective methods of improving word recognition. There are many programs (with a good evidence base) to remediate these disorders. In general, reading programs that are explicit, are oriented to academic content, teach to mastery with scaffolding and emotional support, and monitor progress can be effective (Fletcher et al. 2007). Treatment that includes asking children to ask themselves questions about what they read, predict what will happen next, or retell a story can improve their understanding. Many children can ultimately decode words, but their rate of reading may be slow, making reading less automatic and more effortful. These children should have extended time to decode and read.

Children with reading problems can present to a clinician with avoidance of schoolwork, disruption in class, and oppositional behavior. Children with fluency problems require more mental energy and time to complete tasks and may present with fatigue, poor time management, or slow response to questions. Often, trouble with the basic skills of reading underlies a child's dislike of school. It is important to determine the child's reading skills, as depression or severe anxiety also can impair a child's academic functioning. In a child with low energy, sad mood, and poor concentration, the hallmarks of depression can masquerade as a reading disorder, but a careful history could reveal no earlier problems with reading. Psychiatric disorders often interfere, as a child with depression or poor attention could have trouble reading because of the psychiatric disorder rather than an LD.

Mathematics Disorder

In DSM-5 specific learning disorder in mathematics is divided to include number sense, memorization of arithmetic facts, accurate or fluent calculation, and accurate math reasoning. It is difficult to define a math disability because mathematics is a broad term without consistent standards (Mazzocco and Myers 2003). Research in dyscalculia lags behind that of dyslexia. No core deficits or processes have been identified in the mathematics arena. If a child has trouble in reading, then certain language-based math problems will also be difficult. The prevalence of a math disability is estimated to be 5%–6% (Shalev et al. 2005). Neurobiological studies reveal different neural systems involved with learning mathematics. These systems are best studied in individuals with brain injury, and the correlation with the child with a math LD is not yet available. There is strong evidence for the heritability of math difficulties.

To do math, one must use language, nonverbal problem solving, concept formation, working and long-term memory, processing speed, phonological decoding, attention, and sight word recognition. Research suggests that *number sense,* or the ability to represent and discriminate numbers and to perform arithmetic operations with a limited degree of accuracy, develops early (Feigenson 2005), between ages 2 and 4 years. Clinicians can screen for number sense by asking children to count objects and do simple calculations.

- *Mathematics calculations:* Processes that can be problematic include memory, processing issues in visual memory, and visuospatial problems that make lining up columns and understanding base 10 systems difficult.
- *Mathematics problem solving:* Many areas of brain functioning go into solving a math word problem. Reading, understanding language, finding the salient point, doing multiple steps, and using working memory all are needed to solve a math problem. There are many avenues for a disability to arise in this arena.

Intervention for students with LDs in math includes the need to teach both the foundational skills and higher-order skills in problem solving. No clear research-based interventions have been thoroughly studied, although interventions can be helpful.

Children with math disabilities who have weaknesses in visualization may present to the clinician with socialization problems, such as poor social judgment, poor spatial awareness, and troubles on the playground. Often, children with poor visualization have trouble self-soothing or falling asleep. Children who cannot memorize math facts should be screened for working memory deficits that may impede other areas of learning.

Disorder of Written Expression

Written expression is the last and most complex skill to develop. The DSM-5 definition includes impairment in spelling accuracy, grammar and punctuation, and clarity or organization of written expression. Deficits in this area are not usually noticed until fourth or fifth grade, when the curriculum requires higher-level language and written organization skills. When children present to the clinician in the late fall of fifth grade with sudden onset of behavior issues in school, a query of their writing abilities should be explored. Writing includes the basic skills of spelling, punctuation, and legible writing and more complex skills such as detection of writing errors and planning. Writing requires simultaneous integration of motor skills, memory, language, and organizational strategies. Deficits in fine motor planning affecting legibility, spelling, and spacing can be easily spotted. Messy handwriting is often called *dysgraphia*, defined as a neurological disorder where a person's writing is distorted or incorrect. Often, children with oral language organization difficulties also have trouble with written language.

Remediation strategies include both the mechanics of writing and pencil grip. Occupational therapy can be helpful. Computer keyboarding can help those with illegible writing or poor spacing, but the same skill needed to write with a pencil is required to learn keyboarding. When written organization is a problem, graphic organizers can be helpful, and a variety of types are available. There are computer programs that teach outlining and then turning words into narrative form. Rarely, some children may not be able to master the difficult task of written language and may need oral exams or may need to be permitted to use main ideas rather than a narrative.

Communication Disorders

Communication is a complicated process whose disorders include deficits in language, speech, and communication. For every spoken word, one first must choose and access the semantically correct word and then retrieve the phonological or sound structure of the word. Finally, the word must be encoded in context and planned, produced, and articulated. Then its communication intent must be relayed. This complicated process has a strong neurogenetic basis (Barry et al. 2007). A child with a communication impairment based on speech production skills (articulation) is more likely to be referred for evaluation services than a child with delays in language (vocabulary and syntax) (Tomblin 2006). Clinicians must be alert to language skills, since the clinical interview relies on oral communication as well as nonverbal cues. When assessing speech and language skills, careful consideration must be given to the individual's culture and language context.

Disorders of speech and language are highly comorbid and possibly related to each other. There is growing evidence of the associations between speech-sound disorders and reading disability, as well as specific language impairment and reading disability (Grigorenko 2007). The overall estimated prevalence of speech and language disorders is about 5% of school-age children. This includes voice disorders (3%), stuttering (1%), and developmental disorders (2%–3%). It is widely accepted that all forms of speech and language difficulties occur in families, as seen in studies of first-degree relatives, twins, and adoptees (Grigorenko 2009).

Speech refers to the motor production of speech sounds. Language includes form, function, and the conventional system of symbols. Language is used to communicate information, participate in community, and learn. Communication disorders include both verbal and nonverbal behaviors. In DSM-5, the diagnoses of the communication disorders were changed to the following categories: language disorder, speech sound disorder, childhood-onset fluency disorder (stuttering), social (pragmatic) communication disorder, and unspecified communication disorder.

Speech Disorders

Phonological speech disorders refer to the motor production of speech; *sound skills* refer to the ability to perceive and understand speech sounds that make up words. First one must detect the individual sounds (phonological awareness), then one must retrieve and access the use and name of sounds and then remember the sounds.

DSM-5 speech sound disorder includes difficulties with articulation, such as the inability to use expected speech sounds appropriate for the child's age and dialect, that interfere with communication. Voice pitch, loudness, quality, nasal resonance, and vocal hygiene are important to assess, as they are detected by the listener. The diagnosis of phonological disorder is no longer used, as phonology is typically included as one of the areas of **language,** not of speech.

Childhood-onset fluency disorder (stuttering) is the unexpected disturbance in the normal patterns and flow of speech. The nature and severity of dysfluency may vary at different levels of pragmatic complexity. More typical fluency disorders are hesitations, interjections, phrase revisions, unfinished words, and word repetitions. Less typical fluency problems such as syllable repetitions, sound repetition, prolongations, or blocks usually appear with visible or audible tension. There is some relationship between speech dysfluency and competency in language and phonology.

Language Disorders

Included in DSM-5 are language disorder with receptive and expressive language impairment, unspecified communication disorder (distress or impairment are present, but not all criteria are met), and a new category, social (pragmatic) communication disorder.

Receptive language is the comprehension of single words, language concepts, directions, grammar, concrete/abstract language, auditory memory, inferential reasoning, phonological processing (reading readiness), and combined linguistic skills. *Expressive language* uses vocabulary, word retrieval by context, semantic association skills, grammar, narrative skills, and pragmatic/social language skills (Rhea 2007). The federal guidelines list the disability as problems in **listening comprehension,** though one needs understanding of both the input and the output of language to comprehend the spoken word. *Auditory processing* is a term used to describe what happens when the brain recognizes and interprets sounds (American Speech-Language-Hearing Association 1993). Children with auditory processing disorder often do not recognize subtle differences between sounds in words, even though the sounds themselves are loud and clear. It is not a sensory or hearing impairment. *Auditory processing disorder* is an umbrella term that describes a variety of problems that can interfere with processing auditory information. If a child is having reading difficulty, referral to a speech and language specialist is important.

Oral expression is the ability to convey information and ideas through speech. The child usually understands language better than he or she can communicate. Later this deficit will impact written language. Oral expression requires pragmatic skills.

Social (Pragmatic) Communication Disorder

Pragmatics is the application of language in social or learning situations for problem solving or in expressing affect. Turn taking, language organization, and expression of meaning and content are needed for human interaction. Pragmatic language skills include the following (Bishop 2000):

- Knowing that one has to answer when a question has been asked
- Being able to participate in a conversation by taking turns with the other speaker
- The ability to notice and respond to the nonverbal aspects of language (reacting appropriately to the other person's body language and perceived mood as well as his words)
- Awareness that one has to introduce a topic of conversation in order for the listener to fully understand
- Knowing which words or what sort of sentence type to use when initiating a conversation or responding to something someone has said
- The ability to maintain a topic (or change topic appropriately or interrupt politely)
- The ability to maintain appropriate eye contact (not too much staring and not too much looking away) during a conversation
- The ability to distinguish how to talk and behave toward different communicative partners (formal with some, informal with others)

Pragmatic disorders occur when there are difficulties in using language in a social, situational, or communication context. Children with ADHD have been shown to have a variety of pragmatic deficits (Haynes et al. 2006). Children with thought disorder also have confused language that can be mistaken for a pragmatic deficit, and children with pragmatic deficits can be confused with those who have a thought disorder. In a good screening in a psychiatric interview, the clinician asks a child to tell a story orally and sees how the ideas connect, noting the fluency and organization. Often, clinicians structure an interview by asking a series of questions, which could lead to missing this problem that is so important for the child's friendships and written language.

In DSM-5, this new communication disorder is introduced with little research or definition. When repetitive behavior is present as well as deficits in pragmatic language, autism spectrum disorder is diagnosed (see Chapter 8, "Autism Spectrum Disorders").

Motor Skills Deficits or Developmental Coordination Disorder

Motor disorders and poor coordination are also known as clumsiness or dyspraxia. In DSM-5, the term *developmental coordination disorder* (DCD) is used and includes both fine and gross motor problems that interfere with academic achievement. Not only do gross and fine motor skills require tone, strength, and planning, but movements must also be sequenced and performed at the appropriate speed (Barnhart et al. 2003). There is no consensus if these disorders are developmental or multisensory (Vaivre-Douret 2014). Often, children with motor skills deficits have co-occurring disorders in the area of learning, congenital disorders, or other psychiatric disorders. Few data exist as to the prevalence, severity, or comorbidity of DCD. Martin et al. (2006), reporting the results of a survey of 1,285 twin pairs ages 5–16 years, showed that DCD with fine motor problems and ADHD inattentive subtype were most strongly linked.

Children with movement difficulties may avoid physical activities. This low level of activity puts them at risk for later life problems in motor skills, cardiopulmonary fitness, and weight control. Difficulties with writing and keyboarding prevent a child from demonstrating what he or she learns and interfere with note taking and academic performance.

No universal treatment is recommended for these disorders since they are often heterogeneous. These children can be referred to occupational or physical therapists for further treatment. There are many approaches: cognitive motor intervention with feedback and measurable goals, sensory integration therapy, kinesthetic training, and a variety of others (Wilson 2005).

Clinical Evaluation

Clinicians should pay attention to the learning style in the child whom they are evaluating. A reading disorder may affect only school performance, but if a child's reading weakness includes language deficits or visual processing or fluency deficits, it can have a profound effect on a child's daily functioning. Knowing how a child processes information and his cognitive communication style will make it easier to assess his emotional and behavior styles. Cognitive deficits are not accurately assessed by patient self-report or by the clinical exam. Children with poor oral expression will take longer to interview, and their pauses and word retrieval can be misunderstood as depression or preoccupation. Children with math problem-solving issues may have trouble with visual sequencing and social problem solving, since the parietal lobe is used in social situations and in assessing a problem. Children with fluency issues may be delayed in answering questions, and the interviewer will need to wait for the child both to process the question and to respond fully. Children with expressive language deficits may use physical responses to solve problems, since they do not access their words quickly enough to diffuse the situation. Therapy with a child with poor language skills can be difficult and not helpful. A shy child may have difficulties with language or trouble reading the social situation. An attuned parent often compensates for a child's cognitive weakness, making early identification more difficult. Astute clinicians can begin to look for possible neuropsychological patterns from their clinical exam.

After an evaluation, the clinician may be called on to write a letter and be part of the school's individualized education program process. This communication needs to be clear, accurate, and in the school's language and should indicate why there might be a learning issue in addition to the emotional or behavioral issues.

Summary Points

- Disorders of learning, communication, and motor skills are common and impair behavior.
- Learning disorders (LDs) are common and comorbid, affecting communication and behavior and development of academic skills, social skills, emotional regulation, and problem-solving skills. Cognitive impairment negatively affects activities of daily living, academic competence, prognosis, and adherence to treatment. Being alert to how a child is processing information leads to a better understanding of the child, his or her diagnosis, and the most appropriate treatment plan.
- LDs are neurodevelopmental, with a strong genetic component.
- LD is defined differently by psychiatry, education, advocacy, and law.
- Response to intervention (RTI) is the federal government's model of guidelines for identifying children who need educational intervention on the basis of a dual-discrepancy model of learning as related to same-age peers and poor response to instruction.
- Reading disorder is the most common, best-studied, and most complex learning disorder, with difficulties in word recognition, phonological awareness, rapid naming, phonological memory, fluency, spelling, and comprehension.
- Communication disorders—both articulation difficulties and language problems—are highly correlated with psychiatric disorders.
- Early intervention is imperative and preventive.

References

American Psychiatric Association: Diagnostic and Statistical Manual of Mental Disorders, 5th Edition. Arlington, VA, American Psychiatric Association, 2013

American Speech-Language-Hearing Association: Definitions of communication disorders and variations. Ad Hoc Committee on Service Delivery in the Schools. ASHA Suppl 35(3 suppl 10):40–41, 1993

Barnhart RC, Davenport MJ, Epps SB, et al: Developmental coordination disorder. Phys Ther 83(8):722–731, 2003 12882613

Barry JG, Yasin I, Bishop DV: Heritable risk factors associated with language impairments. Genes Brain Behav 6(1):66–76, 2007 17233642

Bishop DVM: Pragmatic language impairment: a correlate of SLI, a distinct subgroup, or part of the autistic continuum? in Speech and Language Impairments in Children: Causes, Characteristics, Intervention and Outcome. Edited by Bishop DVM, Leonard LB. Hove, UK, Psychology Press, 2000, pp 99–113

Bromley E: Barriers to the appropriate clinical use of medications that improve the cognitive deficits of schizophrenia. Psychiatr Serv 58(4):475–481, 2007 17412848

Cervellione KL, Burdick KE, Cottone JG, et al: Neurocognitive deficits in adolescents with schizophrenia: longitudinal stability and predictive utility for short-term functional outcome. J Am Acad Child Adolesc Psychiatry 46(7):867–878, 2007 17581451

Coch D, Dawson G, Fischer KW: Human Behavior, Learning, and the Developing Brain: Atypical Development. New York, Guilford, 2007

Colker R, Shaywitz S, Shaywitz B, et al: Comments on Proposed DSM-5 Criteria for Specific Learning Disorder from a Legal and Medical/Scientific Perspective. New Haven, CT, Yale Center for Dyslexia and Creativity, 2013. Available at: http://dyslexia.yale.edu/CommentsDSM5ColkerShaywitzSimon.pdf. Accessed April 6, 2015.

Dickstein DP, Nelson EE, McClure EB, et al: Cognitive flexibility in phenotypes of pediatric bipolar disorder. J Am Acad Child Adolesc Psychiatry 46(3):341–355, 2007 17314720

Feigenson L: A double-dissociation in infants' representations of object arrays. Cognition 95(3):B37–B48, 2005 15788156

Fletcher JM, Lyon GR, Fuchs LS, et al: Learning Disabilities: From Intervention to Intervention. New York, Guilford, 2007

Fuchs D, Mock D, Margan PL, et al: Responsiveness-to-intervention: definitions, evidence, and implications for the learning disabilities construct. Learn Disabil Res Pract 18(3):157–171, 2003

Goldston DB, Walsh A, Mayfield Arnold E, et al: Reading problems, psychiatric disorders, and functional impairment from mid- to late adolescence. J Am Acad Child Adolesc Psychiatry 46(1):25–32, 2007 17195726

Grigorenko EL: Rethinking disorders of spoken and written language: generating workable hypotheses. J Dev Behav Pediatr 28(6):478–486, 2007 18091095

Grigorenko EL: Behavior-genetic and molecular studies of disorders of speech and language: an overview, in Handbooks of Genetics. Edited by Kim Y-K. New York, Springer, 2009, pp 300–310

Haynes WO, Pindzola R, Moran M: Communication Disorders in the Classroom: An Introduction for Professionals in School Settings. Boston, MA, Jones and Bartlett, 2006

Insel T, Cuthbert B, Garvey M, et al: Research domain criteria (RDoC): toward a new classification framework for research on mental disorders. Am J Psychiatry 167(7):748–751, 2010 20595427

Martin NC, Piek JP, Hay D: DCD and ADHD: a genetic study of their shared aetiology. Hum Mov Sci 25(1):110–124, 2006 16442650

Martinez-Aran A, Vieta E, Colom F, et al: Cognitive impairment in euthymic bipolar patients: implications for clinical and functional outcomes. Bipolar Disord 6(3):224–232, 2004 15117402

Mazzocco MM, Myers GF: Complexities in identifying and defining mathematics learning disability in the primary school age years. Ann Dyslexia 53(1):218–253, 2003 19750132

Meyer MS, Felton RH: Repeated reading to enhance fluency: old approaches and new directions. Ann Dyslexia 49(1):283–306, 1999

Noble KG, Tottenham N, Casey BJ: Neuroscience perspectives on disparities in school readiness and cognitive achievement. Future Child 15(1):71–89, 2005 16130542

Paul LM, Sideridis GD: Contrasting the effectiveness of fluency interventions for students with or at risk for learning disabilities: a multilevel random coefficient modeling meta-analysis. Learn Disabil Res Pract 21(4):191–210, 2006

Pennington BF: Explaining Abnormal Behavior: A Cognitive Neuroscience Perspective. New York, Guilford, 2014

Rhea P: Language Disorders From Infancy Through Adolescence. St. Louis, MO, Mosby, 2007

Rutter M, Caspi A, Fergusson D, et al: Sex differences in developmental reading disability: new findings from 4 epidemiological studies. JAMA 291(16):2007–2012, 2004 15113820

Schatschneider C, Fletcher JM, Francis DJ, et al: Kindergarten prediction of reading skills: a longitudinal comparative analysis. J Educ Psychol 96(2):265–282, 2004

Schretlen D: The nature and significance of cognitive impairment in schizophrenia. Johns Hopkins Advanced Studies in Medicine 7:72–78, 2007

Shalev RS, Manor O, Gross-Tsur V: Developmental dyscalculia: a prospective six-year follow-up. Dev Med Child Neurol 47(2):121–125, 2005 15707235

Shaywitz SE, Shaywitz BA: Dyslexia (specific reading disability). Biol Psychiatry 57(11):1301–1309, 2005 15950002

Sideridis GD: Understanding low achievement and depression in children with learning disabilities: a goal orientation approach. Int Rev Res Ment Retard 31:163–203, 2006

Swanson HL: Reading comprehension and working memory in learning-disabled readers: Is the phonological loop more important than the executive system? J Exp Child Psychol 72(1):1–31, 1999 9888984

Tomblin JB: A normativist account of language-based learning disabilities. Learn Disabil Res Pract 21(1):8–18, 2006

U.S. Department of Education Office of Special Education and Rehabilitative Services: Trends in High School Dropout and Completion Rates in the United States: 1972–2009. Compendium Report. Washington, DC, U.S. Department of Education, 2011

Vaivre-Douret L: Developmental coordination disorders: state of art. Neurophysiol Clin 44(1):13–23, 2014 24502901

Wilson PH: Practitioner review: approaches to assessment and treatment of children with DCD: an evaluative review. J Child Psychol Psychiatry 46(8):806–823, 2005 16033630

Zipursky RB: Why are the outcomes in patients with schizophrenia so poor? J Clin Psychiatry 75(suppl 2):20–24, 2014 24919167

CHAPTER 10

Attention-Deficit/ Hyperactivity Disorder

Steven R. Pliszka, M.D.

While attention-deficit/hyperactivity disorder (ADHD) is sometimes portrayed as a "modern" condition, George Still (1902) is now credited with the first clinical description of what today would be recognized as ADHD. The first treatment of impulsive, hyperactive, and disruptive behavior with stimulant medication was reported in the 1930s (Bradley 1937). Douglas and Peters (1979) first suggested that *attention deficits* rather than hyperactivity were the core symptoms of the disorder. Since then, the criteria have undergone refinements leading to the current terminology of ADHD in DSM-5 (American Psychiatric Association 2013; see Box 10–1).

Box 10–1. DSM-5 Diagnostic Criteria for Attention-Deficit/Hyperactivity Disorder

A. A persistent pattern of inattention and/or hyperactivity-impulsivity that interferes with functioning or development, as characterized by (1) and/or (2):

1. **Inattention:** Six (or more) of the following symptoms have persisted for at least 6 months to a degree that is inconsistent with developmental level and that negatively impacts directly on social and academic/occupational activities:
   Note: The symptoms are not solely a manifestation of oppositional behavior, defiance, hostility, or failure to understand tasks or instructions. For older adolescents and adults (age 17 and older), at least five symptoms are required.
   a. Often fails to give close attention to details or makes careless mistakes in schoolwork, at work, or during other activities (e.g., overlooks or misses details, work is inaccurate).
   b. Often has difficulty sustaining attention in tasks or play activities (e.g., has difficulty remaining focused during lectures, conversations, or lengthy reading).

c. Often does not seem to listen when spoken to directly (e.g., mind seems elsewhere, even in the absence of any obvious distraction).
d. Often does not follow through on instructions and fails to finish schoolwork, chores, or duties in the workplace (e.g., starts tasks but quickly loses focus and is easily sidetracked).
e. Often has difficulty organizing tasks and activities (e.g., difficulty managing sequential tasks; difficulty keeping materials and belongings in order; messy, disorganized work; has poor time management; fails to meet deadlines).
f. Often avoids, dislikes, or is reluctant to engage in tasks that require sustained mental effort (e.g., schoolwork or homework; for older adolescents and adults, preparing reports, completing forms, reviewing lengthy papers).
g. Often loses things necessary for tasks or activities (e.g., school materials, pencils, books, tools, wallets, keys, paperwork, eyeglasses, mobile telephones).
h. Is often easily distracted by extraneous stimuli (for older adolescents and adults, may include unrelated thoughts).
i. Is often forgetful in daily activities (e.g., doing chores, running errands; for older adolescents and adults, returning calls, paying bills, keeping appointments).

2. **Hyperactivity and impulsivity:** Six (or more) of the following symptoms have persisted for at least 6 months to a degree that is inconsistent with developmental level and that negatively impacts directly on social and academic/occupational activities:
Note: The symptoms are not solely a manifestation of oppositional behavior, defiance, hostility, or a failure to understand tasks or instructions. For older adolescents and adults (age 17 and older), at least five symptoms are required.
a. Often fidgets with or taps hands or feet or squirms in seat.
b. Often leaves seat in situations when remaining seated is expected (e.g., leaves his or her place in the classroom, in the office or other workplace, or in other situations that require remaining in place).
c. Often runs about or climbs in situations where it is inappropriate. (**Note:** In adolescents or adults, may be limited to feeling restless.)
d. Often unable to play or engage in leisure activities quietly.
e. Is often "on the go," acting as if "driven by a motor" (e.g., is unable to be or uncomfortable being still for extended time, as in restaurants, meetings; may be experienced by others as being restless or difficult to keep up with).
f. Often talks excessively.
g. Often blurts out an answer before a question has been completed (e.g., completes people's sentences; cannot wait for turn in conversation).
h. Often has difficulty waiting his or her turn (e.g., while waiting in line).
i. Often interrupts or intrudes on others (e.g., butts into conversations, games, or activities; may start using other people's things without asking or receiving permission; for adolescents and adults, may intrude into or take over what others are doing).

B. Several inattentive or hyperactive-impulsive symptoms were present prior to age 12 years.
C. Several inattentive or hyperactive-impulsive symptoms are present in two or more settings (e.g., at home, school, or work; with friends or relatives; in other activities).
D. There is clear evidence that the symptoms interfere with, or reduce the quality of, social, academic, or occupational functioning.
E. The symptoms do not occur exclusively during the course of schizophrenia or another psychotic disorder and are not better explained by another mental disorder (e.g., mood disorder, anxiety disorder, dissociative disorder, personality disorder, substance intoxication or withdrawal).

Specify whether:

314.01 (F90.2) Combined presentation: If both Criterion A1 (inattention) and Criterion A2 (hyperactivity-impulsivity) are met for the past 6 months.

314.00 (F90.0) Predominantly inattentive presentation: If Criterion A1 (inattention) is met but Criterion A2 (hyperactivity-impulsivity) is not met for the past 6 months.

314.01 (F90.1) Predominantly hyperactive/impulsive presentation: If Criterion A2 (hyperactivity-impulsivity) is met and Criterion A1 (inattention) is not met for the past 6 months.

Specify if:

In partial remission: When full criteria were previously met, fewer than the full criteria have been met for the past 6 months, and the symptoms still result in impairment in social, academic, or occupational functioning.

Specify current severity:

Mild: Few, if any, symptoms in excess of those required to make the diagnosis are present, and symptoms result in no more than minor impairments in social or occupational functioning.

Moderate: Symptoms or functional impairment between "mild" and "severe" are present.

Severe: Many symptoms in excess of those required to make the diagnosis, or several symptoms that are particularly severe, are present, or the symptoms result in marked impairment in social or occupational functioning.

Source. Reprinted from the *Diagnostic and Statistical Manual of Mental Disorders,* 5th Edition. Arlington, VA, American Psychiatric Association, 2013. Used with permission.

Definition, Clinical Description, and Diagnosis

ADHD is a neurodevelopmental disorder in which a child's ability to attend to and control impulses (including inhibiting motor activity when appropriate) 1) is significantly less than that of a typically developing child, 2) causes impairment in the child's academic or social functioning, and 3) is not accounted for by some other medical or psychiatric condition. Box 10–1 presents the specific DSM-5 criteria, including the definition of the three presentations (termed *subtypes* in DSM-IV [American Psychiatric Association 1994]) of ADHD: inattentive, hyperactive-impulsive, and combined. The age of onset is a significant change in the criteria from DSM-IV. In DSM-5 some symptoms are required to be present before age 12 years (formerly age 7 years). The individual symptom descriptions have been broadened to include behaviors typical of an adolescent or adult rather than only young children. Another change is that the diagnosis of ADHD now may be made in the presence of autism spectrum disorder.

Epidemiology

ADHD is among the most common childhood disorders. A review and meta-analysis suggested a worldwide prevalence rate of 5.3% (Polanczyk et al. 2007), but recent data suggest that the rate of diagnosis is on the rise. The 2011 National Survey of Children's Health performed telephone interviews of nearly 100,000 parents of children ages 4–17 years (Visser et al. 2014). Eleven percent of the children had received a diagnosis of ADHD at some point in their lives; 8.8%

were reported as having a current diagnosis of ADHD; and 6.9% were taking medication for ADHD. Parent-reported history of ADHD increased 43% from 2003 to 2011, while medication use increased by 28%. It should be noted that in 2007, less than half of children with ADHD were taking medication. Thus, the increase in medication use reflects growing treatment of the condition.

Comorbidity

As in other psychiatric disorders, comorbidity is common (Barkley 2006; Pliszka 2009). Both oppositional defiant disorder (ODD) and conduct disorder (CD) as well as anxiety disorders are present in 25%–33% of children with ADHD; learning and language disorders afflict another quarter. Many children with ADHD will have two or more comorbid disorders, complicating clinical management. The overlap of ADHD and ODD/CD has been studied best. Compared with children with ADHD alone, those who also have ODD/CD show more severe symptoms of impulsivity, higher rates of aggression, a greater prevalence of learning disorders, and a greater propensity to develop both antisocial personality as adults and substance abuse during their adolescent years (Pliszka 2009). Family studies suggest that ADHD with ODD/CD is a separate genetic subtype from ADHD alone (Biederman et al. 1992).

Compared with those with ADHD alone, those with comorbid anxiety (without ODD/CD) show lower levels of impulsivity on laboratory measures of attention and a greater tendency to respond to psychosocial interventions (Jensen et al. 2001; March et al. 2000; Newcorn et al. 2001). Of interest, it is parent report of anxiety, rather than child report, that predicts such response. ADHD and anxiety appear to arise from independent genetic contributions (Biederman et al. 1992). When children with ADHD have the "double" comorbidity of both anxiety and ODD/CD, they tend to resemble children with ADHD and ODD/CD in their cognitive profile (Newcorn et al. 2001) but show an enhanced response to combined medication and psychosocial intervention (Jensen et al. 2001).

In the Multimodal Treatment Study of Children With ADHD (MTA; Swanson et al. 2008), 11% of children in the sample also met criteria for major depressive disorder (MDD). How depression affects the clinical expression of ADHD has not been explored; family studies suggest that ADHD and MDD might share genetic factors (Biederman et al. 1992). Since treatment of depression rarely leads to remission of ADHD symptoms, it seems unlikely that MDD masquerades as ADHD to any significant degree. If the full DSM-5 criteria for MDD are met in a child with ADHD, this most likely represents the full syndrome of MDD and not a state of demoralization due to the ADHD symptoms (Biederman et al. 1998). The current clinical consensus is that ADHD and MDD represent separate conditions, each requiring its own treatment (Pliszka 2009).

More contentious is the overlap of ADHD and bipolar disorder (BP). Wozniak et al. (1995) found that 16% of a sample of ADHD patients met criteria for mania, while the MTA study (Jensen et al. 2001) did not find it necessary to exclude any child with ADHD because of a diagnosis of BP (although a small subset [n=13] did show signs of "hypomania"). The core of this issue is how to deal with the high rate of emotional dysregulation in children with ADHD. Emotional dysregulation is manifested by chronic irritability, reactive aggressive outbursts, and severe mood lability. It affects 24%–50% of children with ADHD (Shaw et al. 2014). Studies from the National Institute of Mental Health Section on Bipolar Spectrum Disorders suggested that over time, children with emotional dysregulation did *not* develop cycling manic episodes (Stringaris et al. 2009, 2010). In DSM-5, the category *disruptive mood dysregulation disorder* (DMDD) was created, and "the term bipolar disorder is explicitly reserved for episodic presentations of bipolar symptoms" (American Psychiatric Association 2013, p. 257). Following DSM-5 criteria would thus lead to a fairly high rate of comorbidity of ADHD with DMDD but lower rates of co-diagnosis of ADHD and bipolar disorder. See Chapter 13, "Depressive and Disruptive Mood Dysregulation Disorder," and Chapter 14, "Bipolar Disorder," for more discussion of this issue. It is important to note that when dealing with those who meet criteria for *full* cycling bipolar disorder, more than 90% of children and 68% of adolescents will also meet criteria for ADHD (Geller et al. 1998a, 1998b).

Etiology and Risk Factors

Genetics

In twin studies comparing concordance rates for ADHD in monozygotic and dizygotic twins to determine the relative influence of genes and the environment on the variance in symptoms of ADHD, about 71%–90% of the variance in ADHD traits was found to be attributable to genetics (Thapar et al. 2013). Heritability estimates included the effects of gene-environment interaction; thus, the high heritability rates in ADHD do not minimize the effect of environment. Risk alleles of candidate genes mainly involving the dopamine and serotonin systems were associated with ADHD with an odds ratio between 1.11 and 1.68. In contrast, genomewide association studies involving tens of thousands of subjects have *not* revealed any gene variant that passes the very high statistical threshold for genomewide significance (Neale et al. 2010). There is evidence that small deletions or duplications of parts of chromosomes (copy number variants) are found more often in patients with ADHD, particularly those with comorbid developmental disabilities (Williams et al. 2010). The focus in psychiatric genetics is shifting away from genes for individual disorders to genes that underlie variation in traits such as response inhibition or cognitive control.

Environmental Risk Factors

Maternal smoking during pregnancy and prenatal/perinatal adversity have been established as risk factors for ADHD (Mick et al. 2002a, 2002b). Children with ADHD exposed to smoking during pregnancy are at risk for more severe behavioral problems, lower IQ, and poorer neuropsychological test performance than nonexposed children with ADHD (Thakur et al. 2013), even when controlling for income level, ethnicity, and mother's age and alcohol use. In an Australian population-based case control study, more than 12,000 children with ADHD were compared with more than 30,000 control subjects on a wide variety of maternal, pregnancy, and birth data (Silva et al. 2014). Compared with the control group, mothers of children with ADHD were significantly more likely to be younger and single and to have smoked in pregnancy. They also were more likely to have had induced or preterm labor, preeclampsia, or an early term delivery. In contrast, low birth weight, post-term pregnancy, small size for gestational age, fetal distress, and low Apgar scores were not found to be related to ADHD.

Severe head injury can result in ADHD, even when controlling for preinjury ADHD diagnosis (Max et al. 1998, 2002). Lead (Nigg et al. 2010) and polychlorinated biphenyls (PCBs; Sagiv et al. 2010) have been shown to be related to ADHD symptoms, although for PCBs causality has not been established. The interplay between ADHD and family adversity is complex. While children with ADHD are more likely to be exposed to poverty, disruptions in care giving, and harsh discipline, the direction of effect is yet to be worked out (Thapar et al. 2013). These psychosocial correlates may be mediated via genetic effects; that is, parental ADHD results in a father and/or mother who does poorly on the job, smokes, and/or disciplines erratically. Most likely, multiple genes and environmental inputs (as well as epigenetic effects) combine in a complex way to yield ADHD.

The relationship between sleep disorders and ADHD has been controversial. Sleep-disordered breathing (SDB) has a wide range of presentations, from snoring to obstructive sleep apnea; the latter is defined by the number of apneas per hour of sleep. A meta-analysis examined 18 studies involving 1,113 children (874 with SDB who were examined for ADHD symptoms and 239 with ADHD examined for SDB) and 1,405 control subjects (Sedky et al. 2014). SDB was associated with ADHD with a medium effect size (Hedges' g=0.57). In those patients with SDB who underwent adenotonsillectomy, surgery was associated with a decrease in ADHD symptoms (Hedges' g=0.43).

Pathophysiology

Neuropsychology

Recent research has suggested multiple cognitive deficits in children with ADHD (Nigg 2005; Sonuga-Barke et al. 2010). While it is clear that children with ADHD are impulsive behaviorally, it has turned out that inhibitory control as measured in the laboratory does not distinguish those with ADHD from control subjects (Alderson et al. 2007; Lijffijt et al. 2005). In contrast, working memory (WM) deficits robustly delineate ADHD subjects from control subjects, particularly with regard to central executive WM deficits such as updating of WM, manipulating information in WM, and mental manipulation of temporal order (Kasper et al. 2012). Differential response to reward and delay aversion also have been proposed as key deficits in ADHD (Sonuga-Barke et al. 2008, 2010). That is, children with ADHD either cannot tolerate a delay to wait for an anticipated reward or are hyporesponsive to the reward, making their behavior difficult to shape by normal reinforcements and punishments in the environment. More subtle are deficits in temporal processing such as anticipating how much time has gone by, tapping on cue, or discriminating which of two tones has lasted longer (Sonuga-Barke et al. 2010). Children with ADHD are heterogeneous, however, and many show no deficits on either neuropsychological or laboratory testing of cognition.

Neurocircuitry

On the basis of studies of cognitive control in healthy control subjects, a number of brain circuits have been the focus of functional magnetic resonance

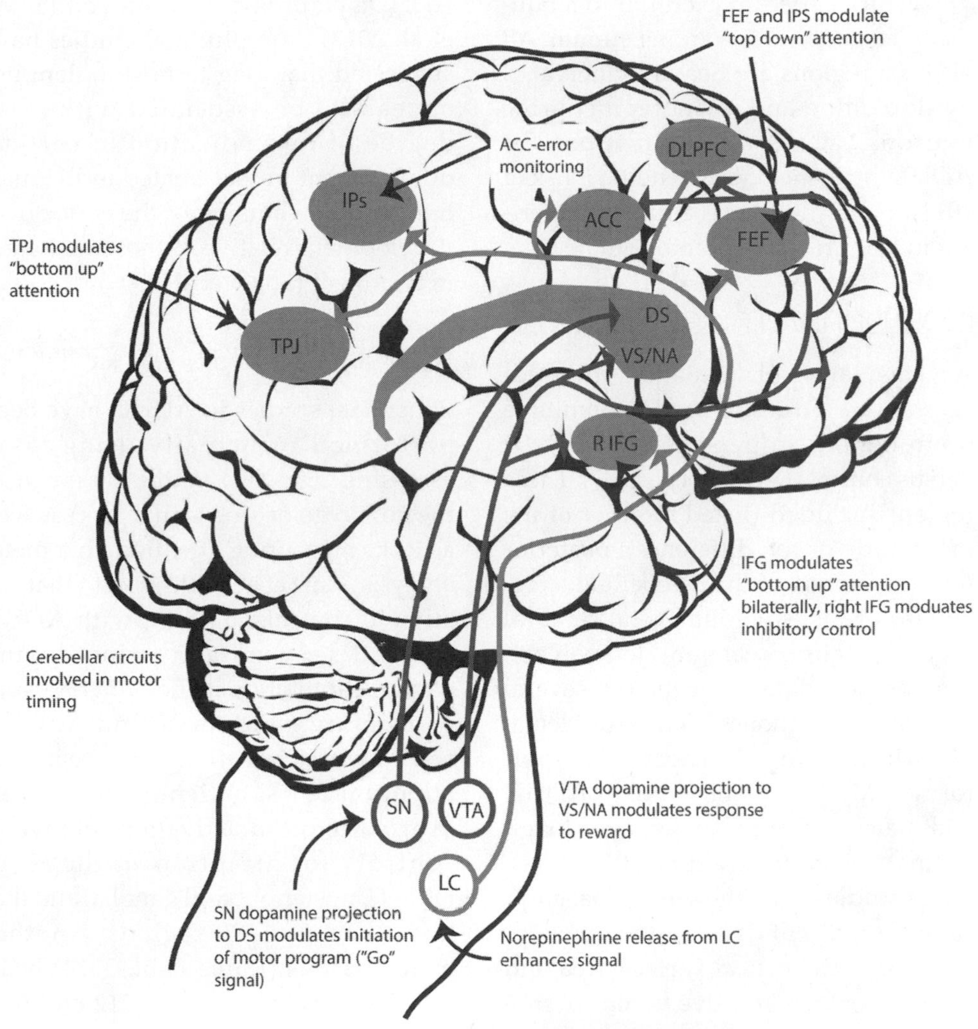

FIGURE 10–1. Brain circuits implicated in the pathophysiology of ADHD.
ACC=anterior cingulate cortex; DLPFC= dorsolateral prefrontal cortex; DS=dorsal striatum; FEF=frontal eye field; IPS=intraparietal sulcus; LC=locus coeruleus; R IFG=right inferior frontal gyrus; SN=substantia nigra; TPJ=temporoparietal junction; VS/NA=ventral striatum/nucleus accumbens; VTA=ventral tegmental area.

imaging (fMRI) studies in ADHD (Posner et al. 2014). These are summarized in Figure 10–1. The frontal eye fields, dorsolateral prefrontal cortex (DLPFC), and intraparietal sulcus are part of the "top-down" system that prepares and applies goal-directed selection for stimuli and responses (Corbetta and Shulman 2002). The temporoparietal junction and inferior frontal cortex (IFC) are specialized for detecting relevant stimuli; this system also responds to novelty. Interestingly, it is right-lateralized, with the right IFC a key region for response inhibition. Effective cognitive control requires a balance in activity between these systems. The anterior cingulate cortex (ACC) is a key region for monitoring ongoing behavior and responding to error; increased activity of the ACC when an error is made leads to improved accuracy on future trials (Carter et al. 1999).

The ventral striatum is critical to modulating response to rewarding stimuli. All of these regions are heavily innervated by dopamine and/or norepinephrine neurons, which all medications for ADHD influence (Arnsten and Pliszka 2011). Finally, the cerebellum is important in tasks requiring motor timing.

Neuroanatomical Findings

A meta-analysis of anatomical MRI studies showed reduced volume of multiple brain regions in persons with ADHD versus controls (Valera et al. 2007). These regions included (listed in order of the magnitude of the difference): posterior inferior vermis of the cerebellum, cerebellar vermis, splenium, total cerebral volume, right cerebellum, left cerebellum, and caudate. Over the last several decades, the National Institute of Mental Health intramural program has performed MRIs on children with ADHD and matched control subjects in a longitudinal design (Shaw et al. 2012, 2013). These studies have shown a global cortical maturational delay in the development of both cortical surface area and cortical thickness relative to control subjects. In control subjects, surface area rises through childhood and peaks around age 12, then declines as pruning progresses. Subjects with ADHD had less cortical surface area than control subjects at entry into the study and delay of about 2 years in reaching peak area, with the effect more pronounced on the right side (Shaw et al. 2012). Cortical thickness followed a similar pattern (peaking in early adolescence, then declining). Subjects with ADHD have a thinner cortex at baseline than control subjects and prune later, but interestingly, decreased pruning (resulting in thickness more similar to that of control subjects) is associated with remission of ADHD symptoms in adulthood (Shaw et al. 2013). Longitudinal studies have suggested that long-term stimulant use appears to be associated with some degree of normalization of cortical development in that treated individuals had reduced thinning of the cortex over development relative to those no longer in treatment (Shaw et al. 2009).

Functional Neuroimaging

Functional studies in ADHD have been performed principally using tasks assessing response inhibition (such as the go/no go or stop signal task) as well as tasks measuring attention. In a meta-analysis, Hart et al. (2013) found that relative to controls, patients with ADHD showed reduced activation during response inhibition in the right IFC, supplementary motor area, and ACC, as well as in striato-thalamic areas. For attention tasks, patients with ADHD showed reduced activation relative to controls for attention in the right DLPFC, posterior basal ganglia, and thalamic and parietal regions. Another meta-analysis (Rubia et al. 2014) of 14 fMRI data sets involving 212 children showed that acute methylphenidate treatment in ADHD consistently enhanced right IFC/insula activation.

Recent fMRI work has shifted from the study of discrete regions activated by tasks to "resting state" networks (Posner et al. 2014). A network is a group of brain regions that operate together. These networks are assessed by having the subject lie in the scanner and not do or think about anything in particular. A key area of study is the default mode network (DMN), consisting of the precuneus/posterior cingulate cortex, medial prefrontal cortex, and lateral/inferior parietal cortex. This circuit is active in task-irrelevant, "daydreaming" activities and is turned off when the attention circuits are activated (see Figure 10–1). Castellanos et al. (2008) first showed that the lack of an anticorrelation (networks were activated or deactivated together rather than having opposite activity levels) between the DMN and these active networks could play a role in ADHD, a result confirmed by four additional studies (Posner et al. 2014). Patients with ADHD may have intrusion of their daydreaming DMN when trying to use cognitive control circuits. A recent large-scale resting state fMRI study compared 481 control subjects with 276 adolescents with ADHD (Sripada et al. 2014). They found ADHD to be associated with a lack of anticorrelation between the DMN and both the ventral attention (bottom-up) and fronto-parietal (top-down) networks. These deficits were found to be right-lateralized.

As noted earlier in the subsection "Neuropsychology," patients with ADHD have difficulty delaying gratification but often seem unresponsive to reward. Plichta and Scheres (2014) reviewed fMRI studies comparing individuals with ADHD to control subjects using reward tasks and found ventral striatal hyporesponsiveness during reward anticipation. In control subjects, anticipation of a reward leads to increased dopamine in the ventral striatum, which is highly reinforcing. This finding suggests that in individuals with ADHD, a lack of ventral striatal activation would mean that normal rewards simply are not as motivating. Such work has shifted ADHD imaging research from the study of "dorsal" cognitive control centers to more limbic areas. As noted earlier in the section "Comorbidity," patients with ADHD have high comorbidity with ODD and mood dysregulation. Relative to control subjects, adolescents with ADHD have greater amygdala activity when looking at subliminal angry faces and greater amygdala-cortical connectivity (Posner et al. 2011). Children with ADHD who have high ratings of emotional lability were found to have greater connectivity between the amygdala and ACC than children with ADHD who were not emotionally labile or control subjects (Hulvershorn et al. 2014). These two studies suggest that patients with ADHD (particularly those with mood dysregulation) have abnormally increased influence of the limbic system on cortical functions.

Course and Prognosis

Barkley and colleagues (Barkley et al. 1990; Fischer et al. 1990) followed up 158 children with ADHD 8–10 years after diagnosis and compared them on a large number of functional measures with a control group of 81 children. Not only did 83% of the children with ADHD still meet criteria for disorder in their late teen years, but they were more likely than control subjects to have had car accidents (Barkley et al. 1993), smoke cigarettes (Barkley et al. 1990), and have failed a grade or been suspended (Fischer et al. 1990). The MTA study found that one-third of the initial sample of 7- to 9-year-old children still met criteria for ADHD 8 years later. These subjects fared poorly on multiple outcome measures, including academic progress, number of psychiatric hospitalizations, and number of police contacts and arrests (Molina et al. 2009). Type of treatment (medication vs. psychosocial therapy) in the first year of the study did not predict outcome. At follow-up, nearly two-thirds of the sample were not on medication for ADHD. Substance abuse also was more common in individuals with ADHD than in control subjects (Molina et al. 2013).

Adults with a childhood history of ADHD have higher than expected rates of antisocial behavior (Barkley et al. 2004), injuries and accidents (Barkley 2004), employment and marital difficulties, health problems, teen pregnancies, and children out of wedlock (Barkley et al. 2006). A 33-year prospective follow-up of 135 boys with ADHD and matched control subjects (Ramos Olazagasti et al. 2013) found 15 deaths in the ADHD group relative to 5 in the control group. Ten of the 15 deaths in the ADHD group were due to suicide, homicide, or accident. Risky sex, driving tickets, and accidents were more prevalent in the ADHD group, with comorbid CD predicting poor outcome.

Clinical Evaluation

The clinician should perform a detailed interview with the parent about each of the 18 ADHD symptoms listed in DSM-5. If a symptom is present, the clinician should inquire about its duration, severity, and frequency. The diagnosis of ADHD requires a chronic course (symptoms do not remit for weeks or months at a time) and onset of symptoms during childhood. After all the symptoms are assessed, the clinician should determine in which settings (school, work, home) impairment occurs. The interview with the parent is most critical, but it is important to also gather data from the child's school, via teacher rating scales (see next paragraph) and/or review of schoolwork. Preschool children or young school-age children (ages 5–8 years) can be interviewed with the parent present, but all children older than age 8 years should be interviewed individually. Observation can yield important information, and the interview, while sometimes not informative with regard to ADHD symptoms, is crucial for differential diagnosis and comorbidity.

A variety of rating scales for quantifying ADHD symptoms are available, including the Conners 3 (Conners 2008), the DuPaul ADHD Rating Scale (DuPaul et al. 1998), and the Vanderbilt ADHD rating scale (Wolraich et al. 2003). While rating scales cannot provide the sole basis for making a diagnosis, they allow the clinician to assess symptoms/impairments in multiple domains (school, home) and establish baseline severity. Follow-up rating scales can then be used to more precisely assess the degree of improvement.

Differential Diagnosis and Comorbidity

The first task is to differentiate children with developmentally appropriate levels of attention, activity, and impulse control from those with ADHD. Lack of any problems in school or symptoms that are not witnessed outside the home are inconsistent with ADHD. On the other hand, lack of evidence of symptoms during the office visit itself should not be used to rule out ADHD. Children with ADHD regularly engage in "fun" activities (video games, sports) without difficulty, so the clinician should inquire about behavior in cognitively demanding situations. Teacher reports of inattention or impulse control problems generally should be accepted unless there is strong evidence to contradict such reports.

The clinician should, in an organized manner, ask the parent about oppositional behavior, conduct and aggression problems, depression, anxiety, and tic disorders. If the child is older than 10 years, queries should be made about tobacco, substance, and alcohol use. The clinician should ask if the child has severe rage outbursts or mood lability. In general, ODD and CD comorbid with ADHD may improve with treatment of the child's ADHD (Newcorn et al. 2005; Spencer et al. 2006). The clinician should determine the presence or absence of depressive symptoms in the child. Intermittent dysphoria over difficulties at home or school is not uncommon in children and adolescents with ADHD, but pervasive depression, neurovegetative signs, or suicidal ideation are strongly suggestive of comorbid MDD. If the attentional symptoms appeared after the depressive symptoms (and full criteria for ADHD are not met), then the clinician should consider whether the depressive symptoms might be causing problems with concentration.

Mania should never be diagnosed on the basis of severe hyperactivity or aggression alone, but the clinician should question the parent regarding periods of intense irritability, rage outbursts, or euphoria. If these periods last for hours a day for several days a week, then a diagnosis of mania should be entertained. However, the clinician should see evidence of associated symptoms, such as decreased need for sleep, grandiosity, hypersexuality, or pathological risk taking (see Chapter 14). If a child has outbursts of verbal or physical aggression in the context of a persistently irritable mood, DMDD should be considered.

Low scores on standardized testing of academic achievement frequently characterize youth with ADHD (Tannock 2002). Academic impairment is commonly due to the ADHD itself. Many months or years of not listening in class, not mastering material in an organized fashion, and not practicing academic skills (e.g., not doing homework) lead to lower achievement than expected for the patient's age and intellectual ability. If the parent and teacher report that the patient performs at (or even above) grade level on subjects when given one-to-one supervision, then a formal learning disorder is less likely. If learning problems are secondary to ADHD, they should begin to resolve within 2–3 months of successful treatment of the ADHD. In other cases, symptoms of comorbid learning/language disorders are present that cannot be accounted for by ADHD. These include deficits in expressive and receptive language, poor phonological processing, poor motor coordination, or difficulty grasping fundamental mathematical concepts (see Chapter 9, "Neurodevelopmental Disorders, Specific Learning Disorders, Communication Disorders, and Motor Disorders").

Clinical Examination and Mental Status Findings

The primary purpose of the interview with the child or adolescent is not to confirm or refute the diagnosis of ADHD. Young children are often unaware of their symptoms of ADHD, and older children and adolescents may be aware of symptoms but will minimize their significance. The interview with the child or adolescent allows the clinician to identify signs or symptoms inconsistent with ADHD or suggestive of comorbid disorders. Careful assessment of mood, anxiety, and symptoms of thought disorder should be performed, as parents may not be aware of such symptoms in their child. In cases of primary ADHD without comorbidity, the mental status examination is generally within normal limits. The child's speech should be assessed for evidence of language delay or articulation problems. Because overt hyperactivity during the one-on-one clinical interview occurs only in the most severe cases, normal attention and activity while alone with the examiner should not be used to rule out ADHD. If the child reports pervasive depression/anxiety, flight of ideas, thought disorder, or suicidal ideation, these are inconsistent with a sole diagnosis of ADHD and may represent either a comorbid disorder or a primary disorder other than ADHD that is impairing attention and impulse control.

Psychological Testing

IQ and achievement testing to rule out learning disorders are not mandatory prior to making a diagnosis of ADHD. Such testing may yield the most valid results after the symptoms of inattention have been controlled. If a child's academic performance does not improve with control of ADHD symptoms or if the developmental history or mental status examination yields evidence of language or motor delays, then IQ and achievement testing and/or speech/language evaluation should be performed, as the child most likely has a comorbid language/learning disorder (see Chapter 9).

Pediatric Evaluation and Laboratory Tests

The child's medical history should be obtained as well as a physical examination within the past year. Patients should be screened for SDB by asking questions about sleep quality, snoring, or abnormal awakenings. If these symptoms are strongly present, and particularly if there are enlarged tonsils, a sleep study (polysomnography) might be considered. A sleep study is not indicated if symptoms of SDB are not present. Children with a history of cardiovascular disease or significant cardiac symptoms (severe palpitations, fainting, exercise intolerance not accounted for by obesity, strong family history of sudden death, unexplained chest pain, family history of arrhythmias, hypertension, syncope) should have consultation with a pediatric cardiologist prior to starting stimulant medication, but there is no need for cardiac screening (i.e., electrocardiogram) in otherwise healthy children and adolescents. Treatment of pediatric ADHD with stimulants has not been associated with cardiac sudden death in the most recent studies (Schelleman et al. 2011).

A neurological examination is not contributory to the diagnosis of ADHD. Children with ADHD may have more nonfocal "soft signs" on a neurological examination than children without ADHD, but such signs are not diagnostic and do not have relevance for selection of treatment (Pine et al. 1993).

Treatment

Pharmacological treatment of ADHD is the best studied intervention in child and adolescent psychiatry. Psychosocial interventions (particularly behavior therapy) also have been extensively studied in the treatment of ADHD (Pelham et al. 1998). Jadad et al. (1999) reviewed six studies that compared pharmacological and nonpharmacological interventions in the treatment of ADHD; superiority of stimulant over nondrug treatment was consistently found. Twenty studies compared combination therapy with a stimulant or psychosocial intervention alone; no evidence of an additive benefit of combination therapy was found.

The MTA study was the most extensive empirical comparison of psychosocial and psychopharmacological intervention (Swanson et al. 2008). Children with ADHD (ages 7–9 years) were randomly assigned to four groups: medication treatment alone, intensive psychosocial treatment alone, a combination of medication management and psychosocial treatment, and community treatment as usual. Medication treatment consisted of monthly supportive appointments in which the dose of medication was carefully titrated according to parent and teacher rating scales. Children in all four treatment groups showed reduced symptoms of ADHD at 14 months relative to baseline. The two groups that received MTA medication management showed a superior outcome with regard to ADHD symptoms compared with those who received intensive behavioral treatment alone or community treatment. Despite the intensity of treatment, those who received behavioral treatment alone were not significantly more improved than those who received community treatment. For the ADHD group *as a whole,* adding psychosocial treatment to medication did not yield a superior outcome to medication alone, but this was not true for all subgroups.

Patients with ADHD *and* comorbid disorders or psychosocial stressors showed greater benefit from a combined pharmacological-psychosocial intervention relative to medication alone. Comorbid anxiety predicted better response to added behavioral treatment; children receiving public assistance and ethnic minorities also showed a better outcome with combined treatment. The most recent follow-up naturalistic findings of the MTA study (Molina et al. 2009) have shown that the four treatment groups continued to converge in outcome, but participation in any treatment for ADHD declined in all four groups. Future studies may need to extend the active study treatment over many years to show a long-term impact. For the present, clinicians should individualize treatment, adding psychosocial treatment when psychopharmacology does not provide optimal control of symptoms.

Pharmacotherapy

Specific information regarding the dosing, titration, and side effects of the agents reviewed in the following subsections can be found in Chapter 35, "Medications Used for Attention-Deficit/Hyperactivity Disorder."

Stimulants

There are voluminous data regarding the efficacy and safety of stimulant treatment for ADHD. Swanson's "review of reviews" (Swanson 1993) reported more than 3,000 citations and 250 reviews of stimulant treatment, principally methylphenidate (MPH). Stimulants are as effective in adolescents (Spencer et al. 2006; Wilens et al. 2006) and preschoolers (Greenhill et al. 2006) as they are in school-age children. Arnold (2000) reviewed studies in which subjects underwent a trial of both amphetamine and MPH. This review suggested that approximately 41% of subjects with ADHD responded equally to MPH and amphetamine, while 44% responded preferentially to one of the classes of stimulants. This suggests that the initial response rate to stimulants may be as high as 85% if both stimulants are tried (in contrast to the finding of a 65%–75% response rate when only one stimulant is tried). At present, however, there is no method to predict which stimulant will produce the best response in a given patient.

Atomoxetine

The nonstimulant agent atomoxetine is a noradrenergic reuptake blocker that has some indirect agonism on dopamine. Numerous studies (Schwartz and Correll 2014) show that it is superior to placebo in the treatment of ADHD in children and adolescents, although in one major study it was less efficacious than long-acting methylphenidate (Newcorn et al. 2008). Its full therapeutic effect may not be seen in some patients until after a month of treatment (Michelson et al. 2002).

The α Agonists

The α_2 receptor agonists clonidine and guanfacine have varied effects on noradrenergic function. In recent years, long-acting versions of both agents have been the focus of studies either as monotherapy or as an add-on to stimulant medication (Hirota et al. 2014). Both α agonists are superior to placebo for treatment of ADHD and ODD symptoms; adding extended-release versions of clonidine or guanfacine to a stimulant significantly improves ADHD symptoms compared with the addition of placebo.

Figure 10–2 shows an algorithm for the pharmacological treatment of ADHD. Stimulants, atomoxetine, or an α agonist can be used as first-line treatment, although stimulants are typically preferred as the initial choice because of larger effect size and rapid onset of action. If one class of stimulant (methylphenidate or amphetamine) does not yield satisfactory results, the other class of stimulant should be used. The α agonists and atomoxetine may be used as monotherapy or may be added to a stimulant for partial responders.

Comorbidity influences the order of agents used for the treatment of ADHD as well as possible supplementary medications (Pliszka et al. 2006). As shown in Figure 10–2, when anxiety is present, atomoxetine may be more likely to treat symptoms of both disorders (Geller et al. 2007). Alternatively, treatment may be initiated with a stimulant for ADHD symptoms, and a selective serotonin reuptake inhibitor may be added in order to address remaining anxiety. When faced with the comorbidity of ADHD and MDD, the clinician should determine which of the two disorders is most severe; the MDD Children's Medication Algorithm Project algorithm (Hughes et al. 2007; also see Chapter 13) should be initiated if the depressive disorder is causing the most impairment. In contrast, if the ADHD is clearly more problematic, pharmacological intervention for it should take precedence. Whichever disorder is treated first, treatment for the comorbid disorder should be added if monotherapy does not lead to remission of both ADHD and depressive symptoms. Finally, the presence of tics is not a contraindication to the use of stimulants for treatment of ADHD (Gadow and Sverd 2006). The clinician should step through the various agents until one is found that reduces ADHD symptoms without worsening tics. Atomoxetine may reduce tics (Allen et al. 2005). In some cases, the ADHD can be controlled only by a stimulant that worsens the child's tics; an α agonist can be added to the stimulant to remedy this situation (Tourette's Syndrome Study Group 2002).

Psychosocial Interventions

A wide range of psychological treatments including behavior therapy have been used in the treatment of ADHD. These techniques are summarized in Chapter 41, "Behavioral Parent Training." A meta-analysis of randomized controlled trials of psychological treatments showed a modest and statistically significant effect of behavioral therapy on parent ratings of ADHD behavior but no effect on the blinded observer ratings (Sonuga-Barke et al. 2013). Daley et al.

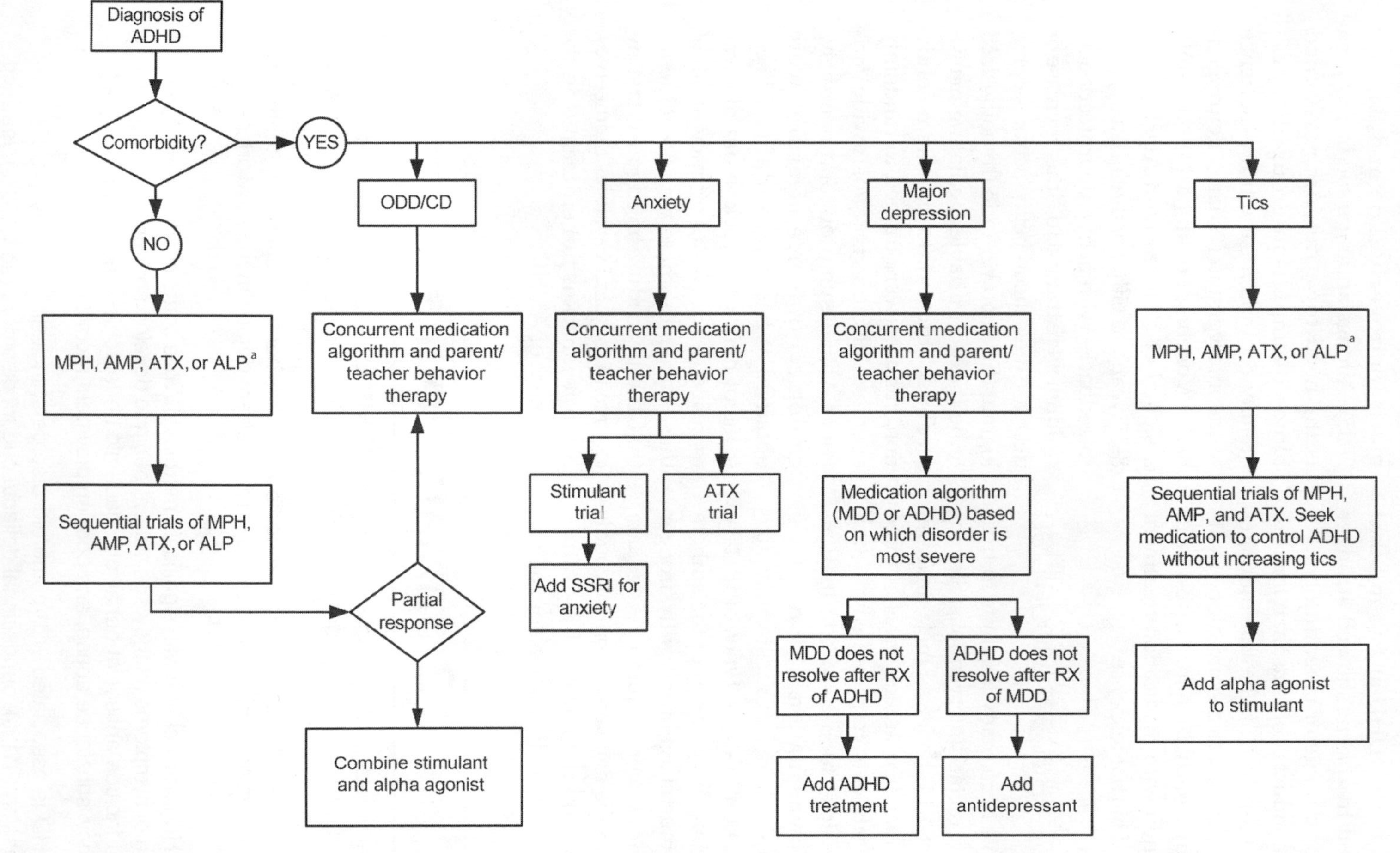

FIGURE 10–2. Algorithm for the treatment of ADHD and its common comorbid disorders.

ALP=α agonist; AMP=amphetamine; ATX=atomoxetine; CD=conduct disorder; MDD=major depressive disorder; MPH=methylphenidate; ODD=oppositional defiant disorder; SSRI=selective serotonin reuptake inhibitor.

[a]Stimulants may be preferred as the initial choice.

(2014) performed an additional meta-analysis of randomized controlled trials in youth with ADHD and found that behavioral treatment showed stronger effects for a range of parenting behaviors and conduct problems than for core ADHD symptoms. Behavior management can be used as a stand-alone treatment (particularly in milder cases) or in combination with medication treatment in cases of partial response.

Other Treatment Modalities

There have been many attempts to treat ADHD via dietary interventions. Stevenson et al. (2014) reviewed meta-analyses of randomized controlled trials of three dietary treatments: restricted elimination diets, artificial food color elimination, and supplementation with free fatty acids. There was a modest effect size (0.17–0.42) for all three types of dietary intervention. The opinion of the authors was that much larger trials with stronger methodology were required. Adequate blinding of the diet versus control conditions was a particular need for future studies. For more than a decade, neurofeedback has been commercially available as a treatment for ADHD, generating much controversy (Loo and Barkley 2005). A longstanding issue in this area is the need for a randomly assigned blinded comparison group that adequately controls for the full experience of the intervention ("sham" neurofeedback). Vollebregt et al. (2014) randomly assigned 41 children with ADHD (ages 8–15 years) to either active or sham neurofeedback. With active neurofeedback, children were trained to either increase or decrease their theta/beta electroencephalogram (EEG) power ratio (hypothesized to be the key variable mediating neurofeedback efficacy). In the sham condition, children were trained to randomly alter their EEG power ratio. A wide variety of ADHD symptom and neuropsychological outcome measures were obtained at baseline and after 30 sessions of neurofeedback. Not only was there a striking lack of efficacy on all of these variables, there was no evidence that the procedure made any lasting change in the EEG variables themselves. Neurofeedback is not efficacious in the treatment of ADHD.

Summary Points

- Attention-deficit/hyperactivity disorder (ADHD) is a neurobiological disorder strongly influenced by genetic factors, occurring in 7%–10% of children and 4% of adults. It most likely involves dysfunction in frontostriatal, cingulate, and cerebellar circuits that underlie inhibitory control, response variability, motor timing, and response to reward. Aberrant default mode network activation is also a likely factor.
- ADHD is associated with significant morbidity. While some children have remission of symptoms as they age, others begin to develop serious adult sequelae that include antisocial behavior, academic underachievement, teenage pregnancy, substance abuse, and poor employment records.
- ADHD is associated with comorbid disorders, including anxiety (~33%), depression (~11%), oppositional defiant/conduct disorders (up to 50%), learning disorders (~20%), and, controversially, bipolar disorder (4%–16%). Comorbid disorders complicate treatment.

- The principal treatment for ADHD is pharmacological, involving stimulants, atomoxetine, and α agonists.
- Psychosocial intervention (primarily behavior therapy) for ADHD should be added when comorbid disorders are present or when response to pharmacological intervention does not result in remission of symptoms.

References

Alderson RM, Rapport MD, Kofler MJ: Attention-deficit/hyperactivity disorder and behavioral inhibition: a meta-analytic review of the stop-signal paradigm. J Abnorm Child Psychol 35(5):745–758, 2007 17668315

Allen AJ, Kurlan RM, Gilbert DL, et al: Atomoxetine treatment in children and adolescents with ADHD and comorbid tic disorders. Neurology 65(12):1941–1949, 2005 16380617

American Psychiatric Association: Diagnostic and Statistical Manual of Mental Disorders, 4th Edition. Washington, DC, American Psychiatric Association, 1994

American Psychiatric Association: Diagnostic and Statistical Manual of Mental Disorders, 5th Edition. Arlington, VA, American Psychiatric Association, 2013

Arnold LE: Methylphenidate vs. amphetamine: comparative review. J Atten Disord 3:200–211, 2000

Arnsten AF, Pliszka SR: Catecholamine influences on prefrontal cortical function: relevance to treatment of attention deficit/hyperactivity disorder and related disorders. Pharmacol Biochem Behav 99(2):211–216, 2011 21295057

Barkley RA: Driving impairments in teens and adults with attention-deficit/hyperactivity disorder. Psychiatr Clin North Am 27(2):233–260, 2004 15063996

Barkley RA: Comorbid disorders, social and family adjustment, and subtyping, in Attention-Deficit Hyperactivity Disorder, 3rd edition. Edited by Barkley RA. New York, Guilford, 2006, pp 184–218

Barkley RA, Fischer M, Edelbrock CS, et al: The adolescent outcome of hyperactive children diagnosed by research criteria: I. An 8-year prospective follow-up study. J Am Acad Child Adolesc Psychiatry 29(4):546–557, 1990 2387789

Barkley RA, Guevremont DC, Anastopoulos AD, et al: Driving-related risks and outcomes of attention deficit hyperactivity disorder in adolescents and young adults: a 3- to 5-year follow-up survey. Pediatrics 92(2):212–218, 1993 8337019

Barkley RA, Fischer M, Smallish L, et al: Young adult follow-up of hyperactive children: antisocial activities and drug use. J Child Psychol Psychiatry 45(2):195–211, 2004 14982236

Barkley RA, Fischer M, Smallish L, et al: Young adult outcome of hyperactive children: adaptive functioning in major life activities. J Am Acad Child Adolesc Psychiatry 45(2):192–202, 2006 16429090

Biederman J, Faraone SV, Keenan K, et al: Further evidence for family genetic risk factors in attention deficit hyperactivity disorder. Patterns of comorbidity in probands and relatives psychiatrically and pediatrically referred samples. Arch Gen Psychiatry 49(9):728–738, 1992 1514878

Biederman J, Mick E, Faraone SV: Depression in attention deficit hyperactivity disorder (ADHD) children: "true" depression or demoralization? J Affect Disord 47(1–3):113–122, 1998 9476751

Bradley C: The behavior of children receiving benzedrine. Am J Psychiatry 94:577–585, 1937

Carter CS, Botvinick MM, Cohen JD: The contribution of the anterior cingulate cortex to executive processes in cognition. Rev Neurosci 10(1):49–57, 1999 10356991

Castellanos FX, Margulies DS, Kelly C, et al: Cingulate-precuneus interactions: a new locus of dysfunction in adult attention-deficit/hyperactivity disorder. Biol Psychiatry 63(3):332–337, 2008 17888409

Conners CK: Conners 3rd Edition. Toronto, ON, Multi-Health Systems, Inc. 2008

Corbetta M, Shulman GL: Control of goal-directed and stimulus-driven attention in the brain. Nat Rev Neurosci 3(3):201–215, 2002 11994752

Daley D, van der Oord S, Ferrin M, et al: Behavioral interventions in attention-deficit/hyperactivity disorder: a meta-analysis of randomized controlled trials across multiple outcome domains. J Am Acad Child Adolesc Psychiatry 53(8):835–847, 2014 25062591

Douglas VI, Peters KG: Toward a clearer definition of the attentional deficit of hyperactive children, in Attention and Cognitive Development. Edited by Hale GA, Lewis M. New York, Plenum, 1979, pp 173–248

DuPaul GJ, Power TJ, Anastopoulos AD, et al: ADHD Rating Scales-IV: Checklists, Norms and Clinical Interpretation. New York, Guilford, 1998

Fischer M, Barkley RA, Edelbrock CS, et al: The adolescent outcome of hyperactive children diagnosed by research criteria: II. Academic, attentional, and neuropsychological status. J Consult Clin Psychol 58(5):580–588, 1990 2254504

Gadow KD, Sverd J: Attention deficit hyperactivity disorder, chronic tic disorder, and methylphenidate. Adv Neurol 99:197–207, 2006 16536367

Geller B, Williams M, Zimerman B, et al: Prepubertal and early adolescent bipolarity differentiate from ADHD by manic symptoms, grandiose delusions, ultra-rapid or ultradian cycling. J Affect Disord 51(2):81–91, 1998a 10743841

Geller B, Warner K, Williams M, et al: Prepubertal and young adolescent bipolarity versus ADHD: assessment and validity using the WASH-U-KSADS, CBCL and TRF. J Affect Disord 51(2):93–100, 1998b 10743842

Geller D, Donnelly C, Lopez F, et al: Atomoxetine treatment for pediatric patients with attention-deficit/hyperactivity disorder with comorbid anxiety disorder. J Am Acad Child Adolesc Psychiatry 46(9):1119–1127, 2007 17712235

Greenhill L, Kollins S, Abikoff H, et al: Efficacy and safety of immediate-release methylphenidate treatment for preschoolers with ADHD. J Am Acad Child Adolesc Psychiatry 45(11):1284–1293, 2006 17023867

Hart H, Radua J, Nakao T, et al: Meta-analysis of functional magnetic resonance imaging studies of inhibition and attention in attention-deficit/hyperactivity disorder: exploring task-specific, stimulant medication, and age effects. JAMA Psychiatry 70(2):185–198, 2013 23247506

Hirota T, Schwartz S, Correll CU: Alpha-2 agonists for attention-deficit/hyperactivity disorder in youth: a systematic review and meta-analysis of monotherapy and add-on trials to stimulant therapy. J Am Acad Child Adolesc Psychiatry 53(2):153–173, 2014 24472251

Hughes CW, Emslie GJ, Crismon ML, et al: Texas Children's Medication Algorithm Project: update from Texas Consensus Conference Panel on medication treatment of childhood major depressive disorder. J Am Acad Child Adolesc Psychiatry 46(6):667–686, 2007 17513980

Hulvershorn LA, Mennes M, Castellanos FX, et al: Abnormal amygdala functional connectivity associated with emotional lability in children with attention-deficit/hyperactivity disorder. J Am Acad Child Adolesc Psychiatry 53(3):351–361, 2014 24565362

Jadad AR, Boyle M, Cunningham C, et al: Treatment of attention-deficit/hyperactivity disorder. Evid Rep Technol Assess (Summ) Nov(11):i–viii, 1–341, 1999 10790990

Jensen PS, Hinshaw SP, Kraemer HC, et al: ADHD comorbidity findings from the MTA study: comparing comorbid subgroups. J Am Acad Child Adolesc Psychiatry 40(2):147–158, 2001 11211363

Kasper LJ, Alderson RM, Hudec KL: Moderators of working memory deficits in children with attention-deficit/hyperactivity disorder (ADHD): a meta-analytic review. Clin Psychol Rev 32(7):605–617, 2012 22917740

Lijffijt M, Kenemans JL, Verbaten MN, et al: A meta-analytic review of stopping performance in attention-deficit/hyperactivity disorder: deficient inhibitory motor control? J Abnorm Psychol 114(2):216–222, 2005 15869352

Loo SK, Barkley RA: Clinical utility of EEG in attention deficit hyperactivity disorder. Appl Neuropsychol 12(2):64–76, 2005 16083395

March JS, Swanson JM, Arnold LE, et al: Anxiety as a predictor and outcome variable in the multimodal treatment study of children with ADHD (MTA). J Abnorm Child Psychol 28(6):527–541, 2000 11104315

Max JE, Arndt S, Castillo CS, et al: Attention-deficit hyperactivity symptomatology after traumatic brain injury: a prospective study. J Am Acad Child Adolesc Psychiatry 37(8):841–847, 1998 9695446

Max JE, Fox PT, Lancaster JL, et al: Putamen lesions and the development of attention-deficit/hyperactivity symptomatology. J Am Acad Child Adolesc Psychiatry 41(5):563–571, 2002 12014789

Michelson D, Allen AJ, Busner J, et al: Once-daily atomoxetine treatment for children and adolescents with attention deficit hyperactivity disorder: a randomized, placebo-controlled study. Am J Psychiatry 159(11):1896–1901, 2002 12411225

Mick E, Biederman J, Faraone SV, et al: Case-control study of attention-deficit hyperactivity disorder and maternal smoking, alcohol use, and drug use during pregnancy. J Am Acad Child Adolesc Psychiatry 41(4):378–385, 2002a 11931593

Mick E, Biederman J, Prince J, et al: Impact of low birth weight on attention-deficit hyperactivity disorder. J Dev Behav Pediatr 23(1):16–22, 2002b 11889347

Molina BS, Hinshaw SP, Swanson JM, et al: The MTA at 8 years: prospective follow-up of children treated for combined-type ADHD in a multisite study. J Am Acad Child Adolesc Psychiatry 48(5):484–500, 2009 19318991

Molina BS, Hinshaw SP, Eugene Arnold L, et al: Adolescent substance use in the multimodal treatment study of attention-deficit/hyperactivity disorder (ADHD) (MTA) as a function of childhood ADHD, random assignment to childhood treatments, and subsequent medication. J Am Acad Child Adolesc Psychiatry 52(3):250–263, 2013 23452682

Neale BM, Medland SE, Ripke S, et al: Meta-analysis of genome-wide association studies of attention-deficit/hyperactivity disorder. J Am Acad Child Adolesc Psychiatry 49(9):884–897, 2010 20732625

Newcorn JH, Halperin JM, Jensen PS, et al: Symptom profiles in children with ADHD: effects of comorbidity and gender. J Am Acad Child Adolesc Psychiatry 40(2):137–146, 2001 11214601

Newcorn JH, Spencer TJ, Biederman J, et al: Atomoxetine treatment in children and adolescents with attention-deficit/hyperactivity disorder and comorbid oppositional defiant disorder. J Am Acad Child Adolesc Psychiatry 44(3):240–248, 2005 15725968

Newcorn JH, Kratochvil CJ, Allen AJ, et al: Atomoxetine and osmotically released methylphenidate for the treatment of attention deficit hyperactivity disorder: acute comparison and differential response. Am J Psychiatry 165(6):721–730, 2008 18281409

Nigg JT: Neuropsychologic theory and findings in attention-deficit/hyperactivity disorder: the state of the field and salient challenges for the coming decade. Biol Psychiatry 57(11):1424–1435, 2005 15950017

Nigg JT, Nikolas M, Mark Knottnerus G, et al: Confirmation and extension of association of blood lead with attention-deficit/hyperactivity disorder (ADHD) and ADHD symptom domains at population-typical exposure levels. J Child Psychol Psychiatry 51(1):58–65, 2010 19941632

Pelham WE Jr, Wheeler T, Chronis A: Empirically supported psychosocial treatments for attention deficit hyperactivity disorder. J Clin Child Psychol 27(2):190–205, 1998 9648036

Pine D, Shaffer D, Schonfeld IS: Persistent emotional disorder in children with neurological soft signs. J Am Acad Child Adolesc Psychiatry 32(6):1229–1236, 1993 8282669

Plichta MM, Scheres A: Ventral-striatal responsiveness during reward anticipation in ADHD and its relation to trait impulsivity in the healthy population: a meta-analytic review of the fMRI literature. Neurosci Biobehav Rev 38:125–134, 2014 23928090

Pliszka SR: Treating ADHD and Comorbid Disorders: Psychosocial and Psychopharmacological Interventions. New York, Guilford, 2009

Pliszka SR, Crismon ML, Hughes CW, et al: The Texas Children's Medication Algorithm Project: revision of the algorithm for pharmacotherapy of attention-deficit/hyperactivity disorder. J Am Acad Child Adolesc Psychiatry 45(6):642–657, 2006 16721314

Polanczyk G, de Lima MS, Horta BL, et al: The worldwide prevalence of ADHD: a systematic review and metaregression analysis. Am J Psychiatry 164(6):942–948, 2007 17541055

Posner J, Nagel BJ, Maia TV, et al: Abnormal amygdalar activation and connectivity in adolescents with attention-deficit/hyperactivity disorder. J Am Acad Child Adolesc Psychiatry 50(8):828–837, e3, 2011 21784302

Posner J, Park C, Wang Z: Connecting the dots: a review of resting connectivity MRI studies in attention-deficit/hyperactivity disorder. Neuropsychol Rev 24(1):3–15, 2014 24496902

Ramos Olazagasti MA, Klein RG, Mannuzza S, et al: Does childhood attention-deficit/hyperactivity disorder predict risk-taking and medical illnesses in adulthood? J Am Acad Child Adolesc Psychiatry 52(2):153–162, 2013 23357442

Rubia K, Alegria AA, Cubillo AI, et al: Effects of stimulants on brain function in attention-deficit/hyperactivity disorder: a systematic review and meta-analysis. Biol Psychiatry 76(8):616–628, 2014 24314347

Sagiv SK, Thurston SW, Bellinger DC, et al: Prenatal organochlorine exposure and behaviors associated with attention deficit hyperactivity disorder in school-aged children. Am J Epidemiol 171(5):593–601, 2010 20106937

Schelleman H, Bilker WB, Strom BL, et al: Cardiovascular events and death in children exposed and unexposed to ADHD agents. Pediatrics 127(6):1102–1110, 2011 21576311

Schwartz S, Correll CU: Efficacy and safety of atomoxetine in children and adolescents with attention-deficit/hyperactivity disorder: results from a comprehensive meta-analysis and metaregression. J Am Acad Child Adolesc Psychiatry 53(2):174–187, 2014 24472252

Sedky K, Bennett DS, Carvalho KS: Attention deficit hyperactivity disorder and sleep disordered breathing in pediatric populations: a meta-analysis. Sleep Med Rev 18(4):349–356, 2014 24581717

Shaw P, Sharp WS, Morrison M, et al: Psychostimulant treatment and the developing cortex in attention deficit hyperactivity disorder. Am J Psychiatry 166(1):58–63, 2009 18794206

Shaw P, Malek M, Watson B, et al: Development of cortical surface area and gyrification in attention-deficit/hyperactivity disorder. Biol Psychiatry 72(3):191–197, 2012 22418014

Shaw P, Malek M, Watson B, et al: Trajectories of cerebral cortical development in childhood and adolescence and adult attention-deficit/hyperactivity disorder. Biol Psychiatry 74(8):599–606, 2013 23726514

Shaw P, Stringaris A, Nigg J, et al: Emotion dysregulation in attention deficit hyperactivity disorder. Am J Psychiatry 171(3):276–293, 2014 24480998

Silva D, Colvin L, Hagemann E, et al: Environmental risk factors by gender associated with attention-deficit/hyperactivity disorder. Pediatrics 133(1):e14–e22, 2014 24298003

Sonuga-Barke EJ, Sergeant JA, Nigg J, et al: Executive dysfunction and delay aversion in attention deficit hyperactivity disorder: nosologic and diagnostic implications. Child Adolesc Psychiatr Clin N Am 17(2):367–384, ix, 2008 18295151

Sonuga-Barke E, Bitsakou P, Thompson M: Beyond the dual pathway model: evidence for the dissociation of timing, inhibitory, and delay-related impairments in attention-deficit/hyperactivity disorder. J Am Acad Child Adolesc Psychiatry 49(4):345–355, 2010 20410727

Sonuga-Barke EJ, Brandeis D, Cortese S, et al: Nonpharmacological interventions for ADHD: systematic review and meta-analyses of randomized controlled trials of dietary and psychological treatments. Am J Psychiatry 170(3):275–289, 2013 23360949

Spencer TJ, Abikoff HB, Connor DF, et al: Efficacy and safety of mixed amphetamine salts extended release (Adderall XR) in the management of oppositional defiant disorder with or without comorbid attention-deficit/hyperactivity disorder in school-aged children and adolescents: A 4-week, multicenter, randomized, double-blind, parallel-group, placebo-controlled, forced-dose-escalation study. Clin Ther 28(3):402–418, 2006 16750455

Sripada C, Kessler D, Fang Y, et al: Disrupted network architecture of the resting brain in attention-deficit/hyperactivity disorder. Hum Brain Mapp 35(9):4693–4705, 2014 24668728

Stevenson J, Buitelaar J, Cortese S, et al: Research review: the role of diet in the treatment of attention-deficit/hyperactivity disorder—an appraisal of the evidence on efficacy and recommendations on the design of future studies. J Child Psychol Psychiatry 55(5):416–427, 2014 24552603

Still GF: Some abnormal psychical conditions in children. Lancet i:1008–1012, 1007–1082, 1163–1168, 1902

Stringaris A, Cohen P, Pine DS, et al: Adult outcomes of youth irritability: a 20-year prospective community-based study. Am J Psychiatry 166(9):1048–1054, 2009 19570932

Stringaris A, Baroni A, Haimm C, et al: Pediatric bipolar disorder versus severe mood dysregulation: risk for manic episodes on follow-up. J Am Acad Child Adolesc Psychiatry 49(4):397–405, 2010 20410732

Swanson JM: Effect of stimulant medication on children with attention deficit disorder: a "review of reviews." Except Child 60(2):154–162, 1993

Swanson J, Arnold LE, Kraemer H, et al: Evidence, interpretation, and qualification from multiple reports of long-term outcomes in the Multimodal Treatment study of Children With ADHD (MTA): part I: executive summary. J Atten Disord 12(1):4–14, 2008 18573923

Tannock R: Cognitive correlates of ADHD, in Attention Deficit Hyperactivity Disorder: State of the Science Best Practices. Edited by Jensen PS, Cooper JR. Kingston, NJ, Civic Research Institute, 2002, pp 8-1–8-27

Thakur GA, Sengupta SM, Grizenko N, et al: Maternal smoking during pregnancy and ADHD: a comprehensive clinical and neurocognitive characterization. Nicotine Tob Res 15(1):149–157, 2013 22529219

Thapar A, Cooper M, Eyre O, et al: What have we learnt about the causes of ADHD? J Child Psychol Psychiatry 54(1):3–16, 2013 22963644

Tourette's Syndrome Study Group: Treatment of ADHD in children with tics: a randomized controlled trial. Neurology 58(4):527–536, 2002 11865128

Valera EM, Faraone SV, Murray KE, et al: Meta-analysis of structural imaging findings in attention-deficit/hyperactivity disorder. Biol Psychiatry 61(12):1361–1369, 2007 16950217

Visser SN, Danielson ML, Bitsko RH, et al: Trends in the parent-report of health care provider-diagnosed and medicated attention-deficit/hyperactivity disorder: United States, 2003–2011. J Am Acad Child Adolesc Psychiatry 53(1):34–46, 2014 24342384

Vollebregt MA, van Dongen-Boomsma M, Buitelaar JK, et al: Does EEG-neurofeedback improve neurocognitive functioning in children with attention-deficit/hyperactivity disorder? A systematic review and a double-blind placebo-controlled study. J Child Psychol Psychiatry 55(5):460–472, 2014 24168522

Wilens TE, McBurnett K, Bukstein O, et al: Multisite controlled study of OROS methylphenidate in the treatment of adolescents with attention-deficit/hyperactivity disorder. Arch Pediatr Adolesc Med 160(1):82–90, 2006 16389216

Williams NM, Zaharieva I, Martin A, et al: Rare chromosomal deletions and duplications in attention-deficit hyperactivity disorder: a genome-wide analysis. Lancet 376(9750):1401–1408, 2010 20888040

Wolraich ML, Lambert W, Doffing MA, et al: Psychometric properties of the Vanderbilt ADHD diagnostic parent rating scale in a referred population. J Pediatr Psychol 28(8):559–567, 2003 14602846

Wozniak J, Biederman J, Kiely K, et al: Mania-like symptoms suggestive of childhood-onset bipolar disorder in clinically referred children. J Am Acad Child Adolesc Psychiatry 34(7):867–876, 1995 7649957

CHAPTER 11

Oppositional Defiant Disorder and Conduct Disorder

Christopher R. Thomas, M.D.

Disruptive and antisocial behavior in youth is the longest and most heavily studied syndrome in child and adolescent mental disorders. This interest is understandable, as externalizing behaviors are often alarming and are easily noticed by caretakers, resulting in disruptive behavior disorders being the most frequent referral problem for youth, accounting for one-third to half of all cases seen in mental health clinics. This focus also reflects the recognition that adult sociopathy is almost always preceded by disruptive behavior in childhood. Our current understanding of the development of antisocial behavior is the most detailed description of the course of any psychopathology over the lifespan. The study of and intervention efforts with antisocial youth had a direct impact on the development of child mental health care in the United States. The founding of juvenile court clinics in 1899 to deal with delinquents directly resulted in the creation of the child guidance movement and the establishment of child and adolescent psychiatry as a subspecialty.

Differences in patterns and outcomes in antisocial youth prompted Jenkins and Hewitt (1944) to propose specific subtypes of disruptive behavior based on the study of clinic-referred youth, including *unsocialized aggressive, socialized delinquent,* and *overinhibited* subtypes. This led to longitudinal studies to determine which features of disruptive children were most predictive of adult outcome, most notably Lee Robins' (1966) *Deviant Children Grown Up.* Environmental factors were the mainstay of scientific inquiry until the groundbreaking studies on temperament by Thomas and Chess in the 1950s (Thomas and Chess 1977). Understanding criminal behavior as a biological or physiological phenomenon has continued with advances in understanding behavior made in the fields of genetics and neuroscience. Current studies are focusing on the complex interaction between constitutional and environmental factors.

The diagnoses of oppositional defiant disorder (ODD) and conduct disorder (CD) are currently included in the chapter on disruptive, impulse-control, and conduct disorders in DSM-5 (American Psychiatric Association 2013).

Oppositional Defiant Disorder

Definition, Clinical Description, and Diagnosis

The behaviors characteristic of ODD can lead to difficulties in all realms of social, academic, and occupational functioning. The central feature is conflict with authority; therefore, problem behaviors are most frequently seen in interactions with authority figures. Requests for or limits on child behavior typically elicit a sharp reaction, and confrontations quickly degenerate into control struggles. The disputes and conflicts may be over seemingly trivial matters, but perceived threats to control and autonomy are critical issues for children with this disorder. Although negative and disobedient behavior can be normative at certain stages of development or in special circumstances, this disorder is characterized by behaviors that are more severe and frequent than normally expected and result in significant functional impairment (Box 11–1).

Box 11–1. DSM-5 Diagnostic Criteria for Oppositional Defiant Disorder

313.81 (F91.3)

A. A pattern of angry/irritable mood, argumentative/defiant behavior, or vindictiveness lasting at least 6 months as evidenced by at least four symptoms from any of the following categories, and exhibited during interaction with at least one individual who is not a sibling.

Angry/Irritable Mood

1. Often loses temper.
2. Is often touchy or easily annoyed.
3. Is often angry and resentful.

Argumentative/Defiant Behavior

4. Often argues with authority figures or, for children and adolescents, with adults.
5. Often actively defies or refuses to comply with requests from authority figures or with rules.
6. Often deliberately annoys others.
7. Often blames others for his or her mistakes or misbehavior.

Vindictiveness

8. Has been spiteful or vindictive at least twice within the past 6 months.

Note: The persistence and frequency of these behaviors should be used to distinguish a behavior that is within normal limits from a behavior that is symptomatic. For children younger than 5 years, the behavior should occur on most days for a period of at least 6 months unless otherwise noted (Criterion A8). For individuals 5 years or older, the behavior should occur at least once per week for at least 6 months, unless otherwise noted (Criterion A8). While these frequency criteria provide guidance on a minimal level of frequency to define symptoms, other factors should also be considered, such as whether the frequency and intensity of the behaviors are outside a range that is normative for the individual's developmental level, gender, and culture.

B. The disturbance in behavior is associated with distress in the individual or others in his or her immediate social context (e.g., family, peer group, work colleagues), or it impacts negatively on social, educational, occupational, or other important areas of functioning.

C. The behaviors do not occur exclusively during the course of a psychotic, substance use, depressive, or bipolar disorder. Also, the criteria are not met for disruptive mood dysregulation disorder.

Specify current severity:

Mild: Symptoms are confined to only one setting (e.g., at home, at school, at work, with peers).

Moderate: Some symptoms are present in at least two settings.

Severe: Some symptoms are present in three or more settings.

Source. Reprinted from the *Diagnostic and Statistical Manual of Mental Disorders,* 5th Edition. Arlington, VA, American Psychiatric Association, 2013. Used with permission. Copyright © American Psychiatric Association.

Epidemiology

Prevalence of ODD in community samples varies among studies, ranging from 1% to 11% and averaging around 3.3% (Canino et al. 2010). The National Comorbidity Survey Replication (NCS-R), a retrospective study of 3,199 adults using DSM-IV criteria, reported a lifetime prevalence of 10.2%: 11.2% for males and 9.2% for females (American Psychiatric Association 1994; Nock et al. 2007). Changes in diagnostic criteria account for some of the variation in reports. Prevalence can also be influenced by social and economic characteristics of the community, as the diagnosis is more often found in children from low socioeconomic status families. Before age 13, ODD is only slightly more common among boys than girls, and there is no apparent gender difference among teenagers (Loeber et al. 2000).

Comorbidity

Attention-deficit/hyperactivity disorder (ADHD) is the most common comorbid condition found with ODD, and, conversely, many children diagnosed with ADHD also have ODD (Lahey et al. 1999). It can be difficult at times to distinguish the behaviors between these two disorders and determine the root cause. Children with ADHD may be described as disobedient when actually their poor compliance is due to inattention and forgetfulness rather than willful defiance. Another important consideration is the possible presence of an anxiety disorder. Separation anxiety disorder and obsessive-compulsive disorder may initially present with complaints of severe tantrums. Children with ODD appear to be at higher risk for developing an anxiety disorder (Rowe et al. 2010b). Similar consideration should be given for the mood disorders, as antagonistic and disobedient behaviors are often associated features for children with mood disorders and studies indicate that children with ODD are at similar increased risk for a comorbid mood disorder (Rowe et al. 2010b).

Etiology, Mechanisms, and Risk Factors

Biological Factors

The frequent clustering of disruptive behaviors in siblings and biological relatives supports the impression that genetic factors may play a role in these disorders, but genetic studies on ODD have reported mixed findings. A twin study suggested genetic vulnerability for comorbid ODD, CD, and ADHD (Nadder et al. 2002). Separate research on 42 candidate genes for ADHD suggested association with ODD (Comings et al. 2000). Other genetic studies have associated ODD with the androgen receptor gene and three dopaminergic genes (*DRD2, DβH, DAT1*), but some of these samples included participants with Tourette's disorder, suggesting that the oppositional defiant behavior is dependent on presence of other concurrent psychopathology.

Most investigations consider the full range of aggressive behaviors rather than ODD alone. Findings must be interpreted carefully, as the samples may include participants with more severe CD or other comorbid conditions, such as ADHD. One study that looked at such distinctions found elevated levels of dehydroepiandrosterone sulfate (DHEAS) in children with ODD in comparison with children with ADHD and control subjects (van Goozen et al. 2000). Elevated DHEAS levels distinguished children with ODD and children with ADHD, while reports from their parents on the Child Behavior Checklist (Achenbach and Rescorla 2000) did not. The study authors speculate that the elevated adrenal androgen functioning in children with ODD indicates a shift in ACTH-β-endorphin functioning in the hypothalamic-pituitary-adrenal axis due to early stress or genetic factors. Another study investigating the role of the norepinephrine transporter gene (*NET1*) found a specific pattern of single nucleotide polymorphisms associated with ADHD comorbid with ODD compared with ADHD alone, especially for measures of argumentative and defiant behaviors (Liu et al. 2014). Further investigation focused on ODD apart from other conditions is needed in order to elucidate any underlying biological features.

Psychological Factors

Temperament is often used to explain difficult behaviors in children, but the evidence of a relationship between temperament and later behavior problems is mixed. Most of the longitudinal studies considering temperament generally support the view that the associated risk for development of later oppositional behaviors depends on the presence of environmental factors. ODD is associated with overreactive response or difficulty calming down. Attachment theory offers a plausible explanation for the development of oppositional behaviors, since they typically involve control struggles with caregivers and issues of autonomy. ODD has been associated with insecure attachment, but only in school-age children, not preschool children. While this might indicate that a secure attachment serves as a protective factor in the face of other risks for the development of the disorder, it may also reflect that early ODD behaviors in children adversely affect child-parent attachment. Research in cognitive processing has focused on how defiant children develop a hostile perspective on the basis of early negative experiences. In comparison with other children, those with ODD are more vigilant for hostile cues from others and twice as likely to generate aggressive responses to problems (Coy et al. 2001). Additional research shows that they have additional deficits in social problem solving, using less pertinent social information and generating fewer alternative reactions. Studies focusing on information processing outside of relationships have found that children with ODD have difficulty with response preservation and motivational inhibition tasks. In one study (van Goozen et al. 2004), the motivational inhibition task correctly discriminated 77% of children as psychiatrically healthy controls or as having ODD. The investigators concluded that when oppositional children are stimulated by possible reward, they are less sensitive to the possibility of punishment.

Sociological Factors

Various environmental factors are correlated with increased risk for ODD. Lower socioeconomic status is associated with risk, but this is probably mediated through family stresses and resulting dysfunction. Many other family attributes are correlated with higher rates of oppositional behaviors, including poor parenting practices; parental discord; domestic violence; low family cohesion; child abuse; and parental mental disorder, especially substance abuse and antisocial personality disorder. Mothers of children at increased risk for oppositional and disruptive behaviors report feeling less competent as parents, have fewer solutions for child behavior problems, and are less assertive in management of child misbehavior (Cunningham and Boyle 2002). Studies also support that harsh or inconsistent limit setting is predictive of later oppositional and antisocial behaviors (Burke et al. 2002). Most developmental theories propose that parental response to normal oppositional behavior in toddlers is central in shaping either adaptive social skills or increased defiance. Patterson's coercion model describes how deviant behavior may be reinforced in parent-child interactions when a parent drops a demand or limit in response to a negative reaction by the child (Patterson et al. 1992). While this dynamic occurs in all families, it becomes critical when it is the predominant parental reaction. It must be remembered that the influences in parent-child interactions go both ways, and extreme negative behaviors of a child can add to family conflict and parental stress.

Prevention

While some prevention efforts focus specifically on ODD behaviors, most also include CD behaviors in the range of disruptive behaviors and long-term outcomes. Prevention efforts for ODD should include for consideration all of the programs that target age groups younger than the usual onset of the disorder: infants, toddlers, and preschoolers. Given the target age group, most of these efforts work on improving parenting skills or the parent-child relationship. Randomized controlled studies of nurse home visitation programs for at-risk mothers have shown outcome differences in lower rates of child abuse and neglect and delinquency (Olds et al. 1998). One of the more extensively studied prevention programs is the Incredible Years series (Webster-Stratton et al. 2008), a parent group training approach that is effective in reducing disruptive behaviors among at-risk children or those with emerging problems. There are now two versions of this program, one for preschool children (ages 2–6 years) and one for school-age children (ages 5–10 years). Both programs train parents in behavioral management techniques and foster better parenting practices and involvement in their child's education and development. Two additional programs with evidence for preventing oppositional behaviors in at-risk children that use parent group training are the Coping Skills Parenting Program (Cunningham et al. 1995) and the DARE to be You program (not associated with the D.A.R.E. program) (Miller-Heyl et al. 1998).

Course and Prognosis

The typical age of onset appears to be around 6 years old, when most children have outgrown earlier normative oppositional behaviors. ODD demonstrates high stability over time, and stability correlates to the severity of the symptoms (Loeber et al. 2000). Longitudinal studies have shown that children diagnosed with the disorder are at significant risk for continued disruptive behavior symptoms. While most children with ODD will not go on to develop CD, they are at greater risk for later development of it, especially childhood-onset CD (Burke et al. 2010). Among boys with ODD, those who developed CD had higher numbers of ODD symptoms than those who did not develop CD. The symptoms of ODD typically persist after the onset of CD. Just as CD is an associated and predictive condition for later development of antisocial personality disorder, so ODD appears to be associated with and predictive of CD. In preschool-age children, the presence of ODD is also predictive of later diagnosis of ADHD (Lavigne et al. 2001).

Evaluation

Interview

Determination of a diagnosis of ODD requires a thorough and complete examination following the general principles of child psychiatric evaluation (see Part I, "Assessment and Diagnosis"). Interviews should be conducted with both the child and the parent or guardian. Information should be collected regarding the presenting problems and any ODD criteria behaviors that are not volunteered by the family. Particular attention should also be given to signs and symptoms of differential diagnoses and comorbid diagnoses. The onset, frequency, and severity of each problem behavior can be helpful in distinguishing ODD from other conditions with defiant behaviors. It is best to conduct separate interviews of the parent and child, as a long litany of parental complaints can be humiliating to the child and potentially can provoke a confrontation during the examination. It can be misleading to take at face value a parent's complaint that a child will not listen or follow directions, since this could reflect a child's inattention, receptive language problems, or hearing impairment rather than defiance. It is better to ask caregivers to describe a recent example or incident. Oppositional youth will typically view their defiance as a justified and appropriate response and will readily tell their side of the story. They are less likely to cooperate if interviewed in a way that implies they are to blame, so it is important to maintain a neutral stance in asking about their behaviors and avoid using pejorative terms. A thorough developmental, family, and social history is critical in distinguishing among ODD, normative behavior, and behaviors due to situational stress. Information should also be collected on parenting practices and expectations, especially response to the oppositional behaviors and previous attempts to deal with them, such as time-outs or star charts. The clinician should be alert to possible physical or sexual abuse and neglect, as these are known risk factors. In addition, disruptive behavior can elicit harsh physical punishment. Collateral information from other sources, such as teachers and other caretakers, is particularly useful in determining if the defiant behavior is seen only in the parent-child relationship or also occurs in other settings.

Rating Scales

A number of rating scales exist that can help in distinguishing deviant oppositional and disruptive behavior from normative development or other conditions. One of the most commonly used is the Child Behavior Checklist (Achenbach and Rescorla 2000) and the related Teacher Report Form, with an aggressive subscale consisting of primarily disruptive and oppositional behaviors. The Eyberg Child Behavior Inventory and Sutter-Eyberg Student Behavior Inventory-Revised are more extensive parent and teacher reports of disruptive behaviors in children and adolescents associated with ODD, CD, and ADHD and are helpful in discriminating among the different disorders and nonclinical conditions (Burns and Patterson 2000). A different approach to assessment of disruptive behaviors is taken by the Home and School Situations Questionnaires (Barkley 1997). These instruments assess the context of the problem behaviors and provide information about potential intervention opportunities based on specific precipitants, settings, or time of day in designing treatment plans and tracking results.

Differential Diagnosis

It is critical to distinguish ODD from developmentally appropriate oppositional behaviors. Studies have shown that the diagnosis can be made reliably in both preschool children and adolescents. Oppositional behaviors that occur as a transient reaction to a specific stressor are more appropriately diagnosed as an adjustment disorder with disturbance of conduct. The presence of more severe antisocial behaviors should indicate the possibility of CD. ODD behaviors do not include physical aggression or violations of the law. As previously noted, many youth with CD will also have symptoms of ODD. The inattentive, impulsive behaviors of ADHD can often appear to be oppositional but are not usually willful defiance. These two diagnoses frequently co-occur, and both diagnoses should be given in those patients meeting criteria for both disorders. Transient oppositional behaviors and irritability can be seen in reaction to stress, such as family move, divorce, physical illness, or sleep deprivation. Because youth with mood and psychotic disorders can exhibit oppositional behavior, ODD should not be diagnosed if the disruptive behaviors are seen only during an episode of a mood or psychotic disorder. Oppositional behaviors can also be seen in children with intellectual disability but should not be diagnosed as ODD unless those behaviors are in excess of what is developmentally appropriate. Failure to follow instructions may also result from impaired hearing or language comprehension problems. While psychotic and autism spectrum disorders can also exhibit hostile and negativistic behaviors, the presence of more bizarre symptoms usually distinguishes these disorders from ODD.

Other Evaluations

A pediatric physical examination can help in screening for illness that might underlie disruptive behaviors as well as signs of abuse or neglect. A hearing examination can also rule out the possibility of hearing impairment or loss. Speech and language evaluation can clarify if there are language processing difficulties. Associated learning impairments can be identified with appropriate intelligence and achievement testing.

Treatment

Pharmacological Treatments

No evidence exists to support an indication for specific medication use in treatment of ODD per se. There are reports of reduction in oppositional behaviors with indicated pharmacological treatment of concurrent disorders such as ADHD. Medications for ADHD, including stimulants, guanfacine, and clonidine, have been noted to reduce comorbid oppositional behaviors along with the primary symptoms of inattention, hyperactivity, and impulsivity (see Chapter 35, "Medications Used for Attention-Deficit/Hyperactivity Disorder"). There are clinical reports that atomoxetine (Bangs et al. 2008) can reduce ODD behaviors in children with comorbid ADHD. Other symptoms of ODD may be reduced with medication treatment of more severe physical aggression (see this chapter on treatment of CD and Chapter 29, "Aggression and Violence"), including the antipsychotic and mood stabilizing agents, but these medications have not been studied in youth with only ODD.

Psychotherapeutic Treatments

Numerous interventions have been developed and tried, usually on the basis of associated parental risk factors and individual social skill deficits that contribute to oppositional and defiant behavior. Reviews and meta-analytic studies have identified several promising, evidence-based treatment approaches. Of these, parent management training and child problem-solving skills training have demonstrated the greatest efficacy with ODD. Parent management training indirectly affects child behavior by improving parent skills in dealing with negative acts and promoting desired behaviors (see Chapter 41, "Behavioral Parent Training"). Child problem-solving skills training derives from cognitive-behavioral therapy techniques in correcting dysfunctional social interactions and focuses on delaying impulsive responses, increasing reflection on alternative solutions, anticipating consequences, and practicing self-assessment of behaviors (Kazdin 2005). Parent management and child problem-solving skills training can be combined, and reports indicate significant additional improvement when they are used together as opposed to using only one approach. As with most conditions, early intervention appears to increase the chances for improvement.

Conduct Disorder

Definition, Clinical Description, and Diagnosis

The central feature of CD is a repetitive pattern of behavior that violates the rights of others or major societal rules. There is no one required or pathognomonic behavior for diagnosis but rather a range of acts that define the condition by their number, severity, and persistence for at least 12 months. Although some of the behaviors may be chargeable offenses and may result in arrest, the diagnosis of CD should not be confused with the legal term of delinquency. The DSM-5 criteria (Box 11–2) have been divided into four clusters: aggression that threatens or harms people or animals, destruction of property, deceitfulness or theft, and serious rule violations. In contrast to the diagnosis of adult antisocial personality disorder, all of the diagnostic criteria for CD are observable, objective behaviors rather than inferred, internal constructs, such as lack of remorse. Repeated studies have found the CD behaviors to be reliable and valid criteria in identifying those youth at greatest risk for continued antisocial behavior (Loeber et al. 2000). DSM-5 and ICD-10 take different approaches to ODD and CD, with the former treating them as related but separate and the latter lumping the two together.

Box 11–2. DSM-5 Diagnostic Criteria for Conduct Disorder

A. A repetitive and persistent pattern of behavior in which the basic rights of others or major age-appropriate societal norms or rules are violated, as manifested by the presence of at least three of the following 15 criteria in the past 12 months from any of the categories below, with at least one criterion present in the past 6 months:

Aggression to People and Animals

1. Often bullies, threatens, or intimidates others.
2. Often initiates physical fights.
3. Has used a weapon that can cause serious physical harm to others (e.g., a bat, brick, broken bottle, knife, gun).
4. Has been physically cruel to people.
5. Has been physically cruel to animals.
6. Has stolen while confronting a victim (e.g., mugging, purse snatching, extortion, armed robbery).
7. Has forced someone into sexual activity.

Destruction of Property

8. Has deliberately engaged in fire setting with the intention of causing serious damage.
9. Has deliberately destroyed others' property (other than by fire setting).

Deceitfulness or Theft

10. Has broken into someone else's house, building, or car.
11. Often lies to obtain goods or favors or to avoid obligations (i.e., "cons" others).
12. Has stolen items of nontrivial value without confronting a victim (e.g., shoplifting, but without breaking and entering; forgery).

Serious Violations of Rules

13. Often stays out at night despite parental prohibitions, beginning before age 13 years.
14. Has run away from home overnight at least twice while living in the parental or parental surrogate home, or once without returning for a lengthy period.
15. Is often truant from school, beginning before age 13 years.

B. The disturbance in behavior causes clinically significant impairment in social, academic, or occupational functioning.

C. If the individual is age 18 years or older, criteria are not met for antisocial personality disorder.

Specify whether:

312.81 (F91.1) Childhood-onset type: Individuals show at least one symptom characteristic of conduct disorder prior to age 10 years.

312.82 (F91.2) Adolescent-onset type: Individuals show no symptom characteristic of conduct disorder prior to age 10 years.

312.89 (F91.9) Unspecified onset: Criteria for a diagnosis of conduct disorder are met, but there is not enough information available to determine whether the onset of the first symptom was before or after age 10 years.

Specify if:

With limited prosocial emotions: To qualify for this specifier, an individual must have displayed at least two of the following characteristics persistently over at least 12 months and in multiple relationships and settings. These characteristics reflect the individual's typical pattern of interpersonal and emotional functioning over this period and not just occasional occurrences in some situations. Thus, to assess the criteria for the specifier, multiple information sources are necessary. In addition to the individual's self-report, it is necessary to consider reports by others who have known the individual for extended periods of time (e.g., parents, teachers, co-workers, extended family members, peers).

Lack of remorse or guilt: Does not feel bad or guilty when he or she does something wrong (exclude remorse when expressed only when caught and/or facing punishment). The individual shows a general lack of concern about the negative consequences of his or her actions. For example, the individual is not remorseful after hurting someone or does not care about the consequences of breaking rules.

Callous—lack of empathy: Disregards and is unconcerned about the feelings of others. The individual is described as cold and uncaring. The person appears more concerned about the effects of his or her actions on himself or herself, rather than their effects on others, even when they result in substantial harm to others.

Unconcerned about performance: Does not show concern about poor/problematic performance at school, at work, or in other important activities. The individual does not put forth the effort necessary to perform well, even when expectations are clear, and typically blames others for his or her poor performance.

Shallow or deficient affect: Does not express feelings or show emotions to others, except in ways that seem shallow, insincere, or superficial (e.g., actions contradict the emotion displayed; can turn emotions "on" or "off" quickly) or when emotional expressions are used for gain (e.g., emotions displayed to manipulate or intimidate others).

Specify current severity:

Mild: Few if any conduct problems in excess of those required to make the diagnosis are present, and conduct problems cause relatively minor harm to others (e.g., lying, truancy, staying out after dark without permission, other rule breaking).

Moderate: The number of conduct problems and the effect on others are intermediate between those specified in "mild" and those in "severe" (e.g., stealing without confronting a victim, vandalism).

Severe: Many conduct problems in excess of those required to make the diagnosis are present, or conduct problems cause considerable harm to others (e.g., forced sex, physical cruelty, use of a weapon, stealing while confronting a victim, breaking and entering).

Source. Reprinted from the *Diagnostic and Statistical Manual of Mental Disorders*, 5th Edition. Arlington, VA, American Psychiatric Association, 2013. Used with permission. Copyright © American Psychiatric Association.

Related to the issue of outcome, various subtypes of CD have been proposed in the past, usually in an attempt to better identify individuals at greatest risk for continuation to antisocial personality disorder. DSM-5 classifies CD into three subtypes on the basis of age of onset: childhood, adolescent, or unspecified. Research indicates that individuals with childhood onset are at greater risk than those with adolescent onset for continued and more severe disruptive and antisocial behaviors (Burke et al. 2010). Childhood onset is defined as the appearance of at least one criterion for CD behavior prior to age 10. Individuals with childhood onset are typically male, exhibit physically aggressive behaviors, previously had ODD, and have concurrent ADHD. Further qualification is given to the subtype classification with description of the symptoms as being mild, moderate, or severe on the basis of the variety and seriousness of the antisocial behaviors, as these features are also predictive of continued disruptive behavior.

Studies have considered the association of interpersonal callousness and CD and compared their ability to predict later psychopathy (Frick et al. 2014), but the relationships are complicated and require further study (Lahey 2014). DSM-5 introduced the limited prosocial specifier for CD for those individuals exhibiting callous and unemotional interactions across multiple settings and relationships. Youth who meet criteria for this specifier tend to have a more severe form of CD (Frick and White 2008) and may not respond to psychotherapy in the same way as others with CD (Hawes and Dadds 2005). Youth with callous-unemotional traits are more likely to exhibit fearless and thrill-seeking behaviors and are less likely to have anxiety or sensitivity to punishment. Callous-unemotional traits are not unique to CD, and only about one-third of youth with these traits meet criteria for diagnosis with CD (Rowe et al. 2010a).

Epidemiology

Prevalence of CD has ranged from 2% to 10% in community studies, with most indicating a rate of about 5% (Costello et al. 2005). As with ODD, prevalence rates for CD vary depending on which DSM edition criteria were used as well as characteristics of the sample. The NCS-R reported a lifetime prevalence of 9.5%: 12% for males and 7.1% for females (Nock et al. 2006). It and some other studies found a slight increase in prevalence with age, while others report no differences in prevalence from childhood to adolescence. The specific CD behaviors show great variation in prevalence by age. For example, the overall prevalence of any physical fighting decreases from childhood to adolescence, but more serious physical assaults tend to increase.

A striking and consistent finding is that CD is more prevalent among boys than girls, with rates three to four times higher (Loeber et al. 2000). This feature has prompted discussion that the diagnostic criteria be modified for girls, since their antisocial behaviors tend to be less aggressive than those of boys. CD is also more common among children and adolescents from low socioeconomic status families and from neighborhoods with high rates of crime and social disorganization (Burke et al. 2002). Although CD is typically perceived as a problem of inner city youth, studies comparing prevalence between urban and rural populations have conflicting results.

Comorbidity

ODD is a frequent precursor of CD, especially among youth with childhood-onset CD (Burke et al. 2010). A major change in DSM-5 is that ODD is diagnosed along with CD if criteria for both are met. The relationship between the two disorders is the focus of extensive research. Some argue it represents a single disorder (Rowe et al. 2005), but other epidemiological studies support the DSM-5 position that they represent two separate but related disorders (Loeber et al. 1998). ADHD is a common current or prior diagnosis in youth with CD, especially those with childhood onset. Longitudinal research on the risk associated with ADHD for later development of CD has been less clear, although retrospective reports in the NCS-R indicated that impulse problems preceded conduct problems (Nock et al. 2006). When CD does appear in children with ADHD, the antisocial behaviors are more severe and appear earlier than in children without ADHD. Substance use is also strongly associated with CD and vice versa. CD typically precedes or coincides with the onset of substance use. Perhaps surprisingly, CD appears to also co-occur with the anxiety disorders.

Studies conflict as to whether the onset of anxiety disorder precedes or follows CD. Symptoms of depression and antisocial behaviors frequently co-occur in adolescence, but studies on the association between major depression and CD have conflicting results. The NCS-R found that CD typically preceded the onset of mood disorders. When they do occur together, resolution of depressive symptoms is correlated with reduction in antisocial behaviors. While bipolar disorder frequently presents with disruptive behaviors, there is little information on its relationship with CD. Among adolescents in their first bipolar episode, if there was a prior childhood psychiatric diagnosis, it was typically a disruptive behavior disorder or ADHD. The risk for development of comorbid disorders is not uniform across all youth with CD (Loeber et al. 2000). Those with childhood-onset CD appear to have a different risk profile than those with adolescent onset, including higher rates of ADHD, low IQ, and other neuropsychiatric disorders. The difference by gender for comorbid disorder is most striking, as girls with CD are at far greater risk for concurrent psychiatric illness, including ADHD, anxiety disorders, mood disorders, and substance use disorders.

Etiology, Mechanisms, and Risk Factors

It is not surprising that no specific etiology has been identified that accounts for all cases of CD, since it is a syndrome defined by a combination of various antisocial acts. Researchers have described an impressive number of factors that increase risk for onset and further development of the condition. Many of these risk factors may be associated with or prove to be causal mechanisms. Several models have been proposed that include many of the factors associated with disruptive behaviors, but there is no agreement on a single etiology, and further research is likely to identify several mechanisms. It is generally agreed that this heterogeneous syndrome is developmental in nature and results from the action of adverse environmental influences on a vulnerable individual at critical stages of growth.

Biological Factors

The occurrence of cases within families and differences in risk by gender support the view of possible genetic influences on CD. Antisocial behavior is likely a polygenetic phenomenon with different genes being expressed at different stages of development, although certain genes may be associated with specific behaviors (Burt and Mikolajewski 2008). Studies report a moderate degree of heritability for aggression, delinquency, and antisocial behavior from childhood to adulthood. Behavioral genetics research also indicates heritability for other factors associated with increased risk of CD, such as impulsivity, temperament, and attention deficits (Niv and Baker 2013). Recent twin studies suggest that the relative importance of genetic and environmental influences may vary for different components of the disorder (Kuny-Slock and Hudziak 2013). Adoption studies demonstrate significant interactions between genetic heritage and adverse environment, although the significance is less than in twin studies. The risk for CD and aggression in the children of biological parents with antisocial behaviors is a function of the relative adverse environment in the adoptive home.

One piece of evidence in support of a genetic contribution to CD is the gender difference in prevalence, but gender differences are also not solely genetic and include social attitudes and conditions. High testosterone levels are associated with aggression and the early onset of aggressive behaviors. Curiously, twin and adoption studies have not revealed any differences by sex in the extent or type of influence for either genetic or environmental influences. The most studied gene associated with antisocial behavior is the gene for monoamine oxidase A (MAOA), an enzyme involved in the metabolism of several neurotransmitters important to behavior and mood regulation. Among abused boys, those with a variant gene for low MAOA activity appear to be twice as likely to develop CD compared with those with normal MAOA activity (Caspi et al. 2002). Environmental influences on this possible genetic vulnerability are critical, as when there is no history of abuse, boys with the low-activity MAOA gene seem to be at no greater risk than other nonabused boys for the later development of antisocial behavior.

Other neurotransmitter differences appear to play a role in antisocial and aggressive behaviors, especially those involved in sympathetic arousal, but the reports are inconsistent. There are contrary findings on activity of both norepinephrine and dopamine metabolites in association with CD, but these inconsistencies may be the result of the differences in age groups sampled or the small numbers of study participants. While low cerebral spinal fluid levels of 5-HIAA, a serotonin metabolite, are found in children with CD, high peripheral blood levels of serotonin are correlated with childhood-onset CD (Unis et al. 1997). The short allele of the serotonin transporter gene promoter region (5HTTLPR) has been associated with aggression in adolescents (Sakai et al. 2006). A related area of research focuses on physiological markers that have associated low sympathetic arousal to CD. Low resting heart rate is predictive of adolescent antisocial behavior and later criminal behavior (Ortiz and Raine 2004). Skin conductance in response to arousing stimuli was found to be inversely correlated in children with CD (Herpertz et al. 2001), but there are conflicting reports. Low-level salivary cortisol is predictive of boys who progress from CD to antisocial personality disorder (Vanyukov et al. 1993). Just as with the genetic studies, many of the physiological differences reported may represent alterations brought about by adverse events or influences at specific stages of development. There is growing evidence from animal and human studies of lasting physical and metabolic changes in the brain as a result of severe stress or insult, which is of particular relevance in our understanding of biological factors affecting antisocial behavior.

Functional neuroimaging studies have found differences in those areas of the brain associated with affect regulation and processing, especially reduced amygdala and ventral prefrontal cortex activation in individuals with CD (Rubia 2011). In particular, those individuals with CD who also have callous and unemotional traits demonstrate the strongest neurophysiological differences (Pope and Blair 2013). While these patterns are not diagnostic, the pathophysiology does appear to be different from that of ADHD.

Development of antisocial behaviors is associated with early toxic exposures, such as lead (Needleman et al. 1996) and opiates and methadone (prenatal) (de Cubas and Field 1993). Maternal smoking during pregnancy also increases risk for CD whether or not there is comorbid ADHD (Wakschlag et al. 2006). Children exposed to prenatal maternal smoking were also more likely to have an earlier onset of delinquent behavior.

Psychological Factors

Several areas of psychological impairment are associated with increased risk for CD. Poor academic achievement is consistently noted, but this association may be reciprocal, with antisocial behaviors disrupting academic performance as well as academic frustration prompting acting-out behaviors. Just as complicated is the association of low IQ and antisocial behaviors. A meta-analytic review of studies conducted by Hogan (1999) found that comorbid ADHD accounted for any relationship between CD and low intelligence, but a more recent study (Simonoff et al. 2004) indicated that low intelligence was significantly correlated with conduct problems. Impaired verbal ability is significantly associated with antisocial behaviors even after controlling for other possible confounds, including race, socioeconomic status, and academic achievement (Moffitt et al. 1993). A key factor in the association between deficits in verbal abilities and antisocial behaviors may be the additional presence of attention problems (Lahey et al. 1995). CD is correlated with other problems in executive functions, including anticipating and planning, inhibition of impulsive behaviors, and abstract reasoning, especially in individuals with comorbid ADHD. Longitudinal studies have found that the presence of these deficits appears to be related to early onset as well as subsequent persistence of antisocial behaviors. As in ODD, CD is associated with deficits in social cognition and essential skills in dealing with confrontations with others. These youth perceive others as hostile, miss important social cues, generate fewer alternative problem-solving responses, and react impulsively in social interactions. Temperament traits of negative emotionality (such as overreactivity) are associated with antisocial behaviors, and there is evidence that fearlessness and stimulation seeking in early childhood are predictive of later aggression. Children with chronic illness or disability are three times more likely to have conduct misbehaviors, and the risk increases to five times more likely if the illness involves the central nervous system (Cadman et al. 1987).

Sociological Factors

Numerous environmental factors are correlated with increased risk of CD, including family and neighborhood characteristics (Burke et al. 2002). Harshly disciplined and physically or sexually abused youth are at greater risk for developing antisocial behaviors. One study reported that sexually abused children were 12 times more likely to develop CD, even when controlling for other factors, although further research in this area is needed (Trickett and Putnam 1998). Physical abuse and neglect are particularly associated with later aggressive and violent behavior. As described previously in the subsection "Biological Factors," physical abuse may be a necessary trigger for aggressive and antisocial behaviors in specifically vulnerable children with low MAOA activity. Parental rejection, neglect, and lack of involvement with their children also contribute to antisocial outcomes (McFadyen-Ketchum et al. 1996). Other family problems associated with increased occurrence of CD include poverty; marital discord; domestic violence; and parental alcohol or substance abuse, criminality, and mental illness. Higher rates of CD are found in disadvantaged neighborhoods characterized by poor housing, crime, substance abuse, and community disorganization. These influences may act by both placing the family under greater stress and presenting negative role models. Exposure to physical violence is consistently found to be a contributing factor in the development of later aggression and other antisocial behaviors, whether it is in the family, in the neighborhood, or through the media. Repeated viewing of violent acts leads to direct imitation and generally increased aggressive behavior. Association with deviant peers is a significant factor in the onset of delinquency and escalation of violence. In addition to serving as role models, peer activities can directly promote antisocial behavior, with two-thirds of all delinquent acts committed by adolescents occurring in groups of two or more (Aultman 1980). The presence of a delinquent adolescent in a peer group can influence the entire group, resulting in delinquent behavior, even if the other adolescents had few prior conduct problems (Patterson et al. 1992). The influence of youth gangs on delinquent and aggressive behavior of members is even greater than associating with antisocial peers (Thomas et al. 2003).

The best theoretical and empirical models propose cumulative risk, with increasing likelihood of CD with each additional negative influence. Longitudinal studies suggest that certain risks exert more or less influence depending on the age of the child, the stage of the disorder, or the presence of some other factor. This might explain contradictory findings of studies focusing on the same risk factor, because their samples differed in key aspects. It is also important to consider that risk factors are not static and can interact with or mediate the influence of other risks, such as marital discord leading to inconsistent discipline. The importance of the various risks is in the accrual and progression of influences over the unfolding development of antisocial behaviors.

Prevention

The emotional and physical costs of this disorder for individuals, their families, and society have prompted numerous attempts at prevention in both the general and at-risk populations (Offord and Bennett 1994). Many prevention efforts are an extension of treatments, such as parent management or individual skills training, in an attempt to improve outcomes by earlier intervention and reduced interference with normal development (Greenberg 2006). Head Start is an example of an enrichment program for academic performance that, as an indirect benefit, reduces adolescent rates of delinquency and antisocial behaviors for high-risk groups of children. Other programs have been developed to target specific early or pathway entry behaviors, such as truancy or bullying (Smith et al. 2003). Preliminary studies indicate that some of the school-based skills programs can lead to reduced rates of disruptive behavior (Mytton et al. 2006).

Protective factors identified as improving resilience (often the converse of specific risk factors) include being female, having a high IQ, or having an easy temperament. Others appear to counterbalance certain risk factors, such as having a positive relationship with at least one parent or adult that can compensate for other negative relationships. Other protective factors include having areas of competence outside of school, good academic skills, and the ability to plan ahead or use other coping strategies. One important area of protection appears to be good interpersonal skills, such as being able to relate to others. Further study is necessary to confirm the exact nature of protective factors within high-risk groups and to determine if they offer new opportunities for prevention programs.

Course and Prognosis

The onset of CD is typically during school age or adolescence, although symptoms may appear as early as the preschool years. Initial symptoms are usually minor behaviors that progress in frequency and intensity and then begin to include more serious and severe acts (Loeber et al. 2009). Individual patterns can vary, and youth with more severe behaviors at an early age tend to have a poorer prognosis. CD is a very stable diagnosis over time, with 45%–90% of individuals still meeting criteria for diagnosis after 3–4 years. About 40% of those diagnosed with CD go on to have antisocial personality disorder. Even among those who do not, most will manifest significant functional impairment in relationships and work. CD has also been linked to other adverse adult outcomes, including substance use and other psychiatric disorders (Nock et al. 2006). Retrospective reports indicate that a history of CD increases the risk for subsequent psychiatric disorder, but remission of CD is associated with significantly lower risk. It remains to be shown whether the adult problems with functioning and mental disorders are a direct result of CD, a consequence of associated conditions and impairments (such as academic failure and incarceration), a result of shared etiological factors, or a combination.

Evaluation

Interview

The examination of complaints of antisocial behaviors should follow the same steps and techniques as described earlier for evaluation of oppositional behaviors. The hostile and often suspicious nature of antisocial youth can present problems in establishing rapport. This is also often true for the parent or guardian, since many of these evaluations have not been initiated by the family but are required by other agencies. It is best to make clear to both the parent and the child the purpose of the evaluation, what will happen during the interview, and with whom the information and conclusions will be shared. It is very important to hear both sides of the story. A matter-of-fact approach that avoids judgmental observations or placing blame is most productive. Research has found self-report of antisocial behavior to be surprisingly accurate, although multiple sources are the most helpful in obtaining a complete picture. It is often mistakenly assumed that antisocial youth will deny or not report their misdeeds. In fact, they usually consider their antisocial behaviors to be justified and appropriate and sometimes are even boastful. Antisocial youth may conceal or lie about their activities if they believe that revealing information will result in consequences or punishment. When confronted with inconsistencies in their explanations for an incident, they will often offer another excuse, without hesitation. Physical agitation and threats should be taken seriously and responded to quickly. The interview should be terminated if there is any question as to the physical safety of persons involved. The onset, frequency, and severity of each antisocial behavior are important in determining the specific subtype and overall severity classification of CD. Presence of risk factors, including history of physical and sexual abuse and family violence and criminality, should be determined. Information about gang membership and peer antisocial behavior, as well as positive peer relationships, is important in determining adverse influences and potential opportunities for change. School information is extremely helpful in assessing academic difficulties and behavior outside the home. Inquiries should be made about any involvement of child protective services and juvenile justice. Legal charges and court history should be ascertained for any delinquency. Frequently associated behaviors and problems, such as substance use and risk-taking behaviors, should be assessed.

Rating Scales

The rating scales described for ODD are useful in assessment of the range and intensity of antisocial behaviors. In addition, there are scales that specifically appraise aggression, delinquency, and sociopathic traits. The Overt Aggression Scale was originally developed to measure verbal and physical aggression among child and adult psychiatric inpatients (Yudofsky et al. 1986). It has proved to be a useful tool in tracking changes in aggressive behaviors in response to treatment. The Children's Aggression Scale is another measure of aggression, specifically developed for children ages 6–11 based on parent or teacher report (Halperin et al. 2002), but there is less information regarding its use. The Antisocial Process Screening Device (Frick and Hare 2001) is a parent and teacher report based on the adult Hare Psychopathy Checklist–Revised that seeks to measure callousness, narcissism, and impulsivity, which are considered features of sociopathy. Callous and unemotional behaviors can be specifically assessed with the Inventory of Callous-Unemotional Traits (Frick and White 2008).

Differential Diagnosis

Antisocial behaviors can be part of many different conditions that merit careful consideration. A single occurrence of deviant behavior or minor incidents of misbehavior may represent isolated antisocial acts or normative risk-taking behaviors. Conduct misbehavior that appears following a significant stressor should merit consideration as an adjustment disorder with disturbance of conduct, but this would not cover preexisting antisocial behaviors exacerbated by stressors. As previously noted, ODD does not include antisocial behaviors, but appearance of antisocial acts that do not yet meet criteria for CD diagnosis may predict the onset of CD. ADHD can be marked by extremely disruptive behaviors that do not conform to rules or expectations but by themselves do not represent a violation of age-appropriate societal norms. When ADHD and CD are found together, both are diagnosed. Conduct problems and irritability are frequently encountered in youth with mood disorders and usually can be distinguished by the occurrence of behavior problems only during episodes of the mood disorder. Psychotic disorders can sometimes mimic the appearance of CD with symptoms of physical aggression or other antisocial acts. Antisocial personality disorder should be considered as the diagnosis for individuals older than age 18 years.

Other Evaluations

A physical examination and medical history are important to assess any concurrent medical problems as well as screen for signs of abuse. Health issues associated with risk-taking behavior should be screened, including head trauma, pregnancy, sexually transmitted diseases, and hepatitis. Serum and urine drug screens can detect and monitor substance abuse. In dealing with academic problems, educational testing is important in screening for and addressing any learning disorders.

Treatment

Many of the difficulties in youth with CD require the involvement of multiple social agencies, including education, mental health, juvenile justice, and child protection. Interventions must deal with various system issues and coordination of care. Comorbid conditions, such as substance use disorders, that confound and interfere with treatment must be addressed. Many treatments have shown efficacy in one demonstration only to have replication efforts fail in a different population. The heterogeneous nature of CD is the greatest challenge in developing treatments, where even specific types of symptoms may have multiple origins that require different intervention approaches. Despite these difficulties, effective and promising treatments for CD do exist. Guidelines have been developed on the basis of these interventions, such as the Treatment of Maladaptive Aggression in Youth (Scotto Rosato et al. 2012) and those by the National Institute for Clinical Excellence (http://pathways.nice.org.uk/pathways/antisocial-behaviour-and-conduct-disorders-in-children-and-young-people).

Pharmacological Treatments

No evidence currently supports the use of medication alone to treat the symptoms of CD. Medications indicated for the treatment of any comorbid disorder should be considered and may result in the reduction of antisocial behaviors as well. Successful treatment of ADHD with stimulants can result in reduction of impulsive, aggressive antisocial behaviors (see Chapter 35). Medications have been reported to be successfully used to treat physical aggression in CD, but most of the reports are uncontrolled studies. Medications that have been shown to reduce aggressive behaviors in youth with CD include lithium, antipsychotics, anticonvulsants, clonidine, and propranolol. Risperidone is one of the most frequently used antipsychotic agents in the treatment of aggression. A meta-analysis of randomized controlled trials found significant improvement in youth (Pappadopulos et al. 2006).

Psychotherapeutic Treatments

Most reported psychotherapies for CD have not been properly studied. A wide variety of treatments have been evaluated, and several meta-analytic studies of those reports have indicated promising interventions demonstrating significant, if modest, effect. Those with the strongest findings include behavioral, skills training, and family-based programs or combinations of these techniques (Woolfenden et al. 2002). Certain treatments, such as shock (i.e., "Scared Straight" programs) or brief, one-time interventions (Lilienfeld 2005), are not only ineffective but may actually exacerbate antisocial behaviors. Two of the most effective treatments for CD are parent management and problem-solving skills training. Parent management training for CD is typically longer in duration than for ODD, ranging from 12 to 25 weeks. It is also modified in some versions to include video modeling to assist in educating parents on problems and techniques. Parent management training is most effective with school-age children or less severe cases, as the results with adolescents are mixed. Problem-solving skills training for CD is similar to that for ODD. Problem-solving skills training appears to be less effective for children with comorbid disorders, intellectual impairments, or extreme family dysfunction.

Functional Family Therapy (FFT) and Multisystemic Therapy (MST) are additional treatments with substantial evidence of efficacy in CD. FFT focuses on understanding and altering problematic interactions and communications between family members that contribute to the family's inability to effectively deal with the child's antisocial behavior (Alexander et al. 1998). All family members attend, and the therapist concentrates on improving family communication patterns. Evaluations of FFT with severe delinquents have demonstrated clear and sustained improvements in behavior compared with traditional interventions. MST, as the name implies, considers antisocial behavior as a result of the various systems with which the adolescent interacts, including peers, school, neighborhood, and family, and seeks to alter the influences of those systems through the family (Henggeler et al. 1998). It requires highly specific training and supervision and is intensive, home based, and typically 3 months in duration. Studies have found it to be superior in outcome and cost-effective in comparison with traditional services and a viable alternative to residential placement.

The longstanding debates on the relationship between CD and antisocial personality disorder and the role of psychopathy in CD have been brought into sharper focus by the introduction of the specifier for limited prosocial emotions in DSM-5, but further research is needed. These debates may seem remote from clinical experience, but they will have profound impact on which children are diagnosed with disruptive behavior disorders and how they will be viewed, as well as the direction of future research into treatment and prevention.

The majority of research on the disruptive behavior disorders has been conducted with boys. The limited research on girls with oppositional and antisocial behaviors indicates there may be key differences between boys and girls. It cannot be assumed that findings with boys can be generalized to girls.

In risk factor research, studies are beginning to bridge from the molecular to the nervous system to the social system by considering the interaction of factors in the progressive stages and pathways of development of oppositional and antisocial behaviors. New techniques in molecular genetics and neuroimaging, coupled with longitudinal prospective studies, will provide a more accurate understanding of the specific mechanisms and psychopathology of these disorders. This knowledge will open new avenues for prevention and treatment.

Summary Points

- Disruptive behavior disorders are the most frequent referral problem for youth, accounting for one-third to half of all cases seen in mental health clinics.
- Multiple risk factors appear to contribute to the onset and influence the course of the disruptive behavior disorders and represent the critical interaction of vulnerable individuals with their surroundings.

- Negative and disobedient behavior can be normal in certain stages of development or in special circumstances, but oppositional defiant disorder differs in that the behaviors are more severe and frequent than normally expected and result in significant functional impairment.
- The central feature of conduct disorder is a repetitive pattern of behavior that violates the rights of others or major societal rules.
- All adults with antisocial personality disorder have a history of conduct disorder, but only about 40% of youth with conduct disorder will become adults with antisocial personality disorder.
- Girls with disruptive behavior disorders have higher rates of comorbid psychiatric disorders than boys with disruptive behavior disorders.
- Careful screening for comorbid disorders is very important, as appropriate treatment of concurrent psychiatric illness may reduce disruptive behaviors as well.
- Effective prevention and treatment programs exist for the disruptive behavior disorders, including parent and child skills training, family therapy, and medication for impulsive aggression.

References

Achenbach TM, Rescorla LA: Manual for the ASEBA School-Age Forms and Profiles. Burlington, Department of Psychiatry, University of Vermont, 2000

Alexander J, Barton C, Gordon D, et al: Functional Family Therapy: Blueprints for Violence Prevention, Book Three. Blueprints for Violence Prevention Series (D.S. Elliott, Series Editor). Boulder, Center for the Study and Prevention of Violence, Institute of Behavioral Science, University of Colorado, 1998

American Psychiatric Association: Diagnostic and Statistical Manual of Mental Disorders, 4th Edition. Washington, DC, American Psychiatric Association, 1994

American Psychiatric Association: Diagnostic and Statistical Manual of Mental Disorders, 5th Edition. Arlington, VA, American Psychiatric Association, 2013

Aultman M: Group involvement in delinquent acts: a study of offense type and male-female participation. Crim Justice Behav 7(2):185–192, 1980

Bangs ME, Hazell P, Danckaerts M, et al: Atomoxetine for the treatment of attention-deficit/hyperactivity disorder and oppositional defiant disorder. Pediatrics 121(2):e314–e320, 2008 18245404

Barkley RA: Defiant Children: A Clinician's Manual for Assessment and Parent Training, 2nd Edition. New York, Guilford, 1997

Burke JD, Loeber R, Birmaher B: Oppositional defiant disorder and conduct disorder: a review of the past 10 years, part II. J Am Acad Child Adolesc Psychiatry 41(11):1275–1293, 2002 12410070

Burke JD, Waldman I, Lahey BB: Predictive validity of childhood oppositional defiant disorder and conduct disorder: implications for the DSM-V. J Abnorm Psychol 119(4):739–751, 2010 20853919

Burns GL, Patterson DR: Factor structure of the Eyberg Child Behavior Inventory: a parent rating scale of oppositional defiant behavior toward adults, inattentive behavior, and conduct problem behavior. J Clin Child Psychol 29(4):569–577, 2000 11126634

Burt SA, Mikolajewski AJ: Preliminary evidence that specific candidate genes are associated with adolescent-onset antisocial behavior. Aggress Behav 34(4):437–445, 2008 18366104

Cadman D, Boyle M, Szatmari P, et al: Chronic illness, disability, and mental and social well-being: findings of the Ontario Child Health Study. Pediatrics 79(5):805–813, 1987 2952939

Canino G, Polanczyk G, Bauermeister JJ, et al: Does the prevalence of CD and ODD vary across cultures? Soc Psychiatry Psychiatr Epidemiol 45(7):695–704, 2010 20532864

Caspi A, McClay J, Moffitt TE, et al: Role of genotype in the cycle of violence in maltreated children. Science 297(5582):851–854, 2002 12161658

Comings DE, Gade-Andavolu R, Gonzalez N, et al: Multivariate analysis of associations of 42 genes in ADHD, ODD and conduct disorder. Clin Genet 58(1):31–40, 2000 10945659

Costello EJ, Egger H, Angold A: 10-year research update review: the epidemiology of child and adolescent psychiatric disorders: I. Methods and public health burden. J Am Acad Child Adolesc Psychiatry 44(10):972–986, 2005 16175102

Coy K, Speltz ML, DeKlyen M, et al: Social-cognitive processes in preschool boys with and without oppositional defiant disorder. J Abnorm Child Psychol 29(2):107–119, 2001 11321626

Cunningham CE, Boyle MH: Preschoolers at risk for attention-deficit hyperactivity disorder and oppositional defiant disorder: family, parenting, and behavioral correlates. J Abnorm Child Psychol 30(6):555–569, 2002 12481971

Cunningham CE, Bremner R, Boyle M: Large group community-based parenting programs for families of preschoolers at risk for disruptive behaviour disorders: utilization, cost effectiveness, and outcome. J Child Psychol Psychiatry 36(7):1141–1159, 1995 8847377

de Cubas MM, Field T: Children of methadone-dependent women: developmental outcomes. Am J Orthopsychiatry 63(2):266–276, 1993 7683453

Frick PJ, Hare RD: Antisocial Process Screening Device (APSD) Technical Manual. North Tonawanda, NY, Multi-Health Systems, Inc, 2001

Frick PJ, White SF: Research review: the importance of callous-unemotional traits for developmental models of aggressive and antisocial behavior. J Child Psychol Psychiatry 49(4):359–375, 2008 18221345

Frick PJ, Ray JV, Thornton LC, et al: Can callous-unemotional traits enhance the understanding, diagnosis, and treatment of serious conduct problems in children and adolescents? A comprehensive review. Psychol Bull 140(1):1–57, 2014 23796269

Greenberg MT: Promoting resilience in children and youth: preventive interventions and their interface with neuroscience. Ann N Y Acad Sci 1094:139–150, 2006 17347347

Halperin JM, McKay KE, Newcorn JH: Development, reliability, and validity of the children's aggression scale-parent version. J Am Acad Child Adolesc Psychiatry 41(3):245–252, 2002 11886018

Hawes DJ, Dadds MR: The treatment of conduct problems in children with callous-unemotional traits. J Consult Clin Psychol 73(4):737–741, 2005 16173862

Henggeler SW, Schoenwald SK, Bordui CM, et al: Multisystemic Treatment of Antisocial Behavior in Children and Adolescents. New York, Guilford, 1998

Herpertz SC, Wenning B, Mueller B, et al: Psychophysiological responses in ADHD boys with and without conduct disorder: implications for adult antisocial behavior. J Am Acad Child Adolesc Psychiatry 40(10):1222–1230, 2001 11589536

Hogan AE: Cognitive functioning in children with oppositional defiant disorder and conduct disorder, in Handbook of Disruptive Behavior Disorders. Edited by Quay HC, Hogan AE. New York, Kluwer Academic/Plenum, 1999, pp 317–335

Jenkins RL, Hewitt LE: Types of personality structure encountered in child guidance clinics. Am J Orthopsychiatry 14:84–94, 1944

Kazdin AE: Parent Management Training: Treatment for Oppositional, Aggressive, and Antisocial Behavior in Children and Adolescents. New York, Oxford University Press, 2005

Kuny-Slock AV, Hudziak JJ: Genetic and environmental influences on aggressive and deviant behavior, in The Origins of Antisocial Behavior: A Developmental Perspective. Edited by Thomas CR, Pope K. New York, Oxford University Press, 2013, pp 39–56

Lahey BB: What we need to know about callous-unemotional traits: comment on Frick, Ray, Thornton, and Kahn (2014). Psychol Bull 140(1):58–63, 2014 24364746

Lahey BB, Loeber R, Hart EL, et al: Four-year longitudinal study of conduct disorder in boys: patterns and predictors of persistence. J Abnorm Psychol 104(1):83–93, 1995 7897057

Lahey BB, Miller TL, Gordon RA, et al: Developmental epidemiology of the disruptive behavior disorders, in Handbook of the Disruptive Behavior Disorders. Edited by Quay HC, Hogan A. New York, Plenum, 1999, pp 23–48

Lavigne JV, Cichetti C, Gibons RD, et al: Oppositional defiant disorder with onset in preschool years: longitudinal stability and pathways to other disorders. J Am Acad Child Adolesc Psyciatry 40(12):1393–1400, 2001 11765284

Lilienfeld SO: Scientifically unsupported and supported interventions for childhood psychopathology: a summary. Pediatrics 115(3):761–764, 2005

Liu L, Cheng J, Li H, et al: The possible involvement of genetic variants of NET1 in the etiology of attention-deficit/hyperactivity disorder comorbid with oppositional defiant disorder. J Child Psychol Psychiatry, 2014 24942521 Epub ahead of print

Loeber R, Burke JD, Lahey BB, et al: Oppositional defiant and conduct disorder: a review of the past 10 years, part I. J Am Acad Child Adolesc Psychiatry 39(12):1468–1484, 2000 11128323

Loeber R, Burke JD, Pardini DA: Development and etiology of disruptive and delinquent behavior. Annu Rev Clin Psychol 5:291–310, 2009 19154139

Loeber R, Keenan K, Russo M, et al: Secondary data analyses for DSM-IV on the symptoms of oppositional defiant disorder and conduct disorder, in DSM-IV-Sourcebook, Vol 4. Edited by Widiger T, Frances A, Pincus H, et al. Arlington, VA, American Psychiatric Association, 1998

McFadyen-Ketchum SA, Bates JE, Dodge KA, et al: Patterns of change in early childhood aggressive-disruptive behavior: gender differences in predictions from early coercive and affectionate mother-child interactions. Child Dev 67(5):2417–2433, 1996 9022248

Miller-Heyl J, MacPhee D, Fritz JJ: DARE to be You: a family support, early prevention program. J Prim Prev 18(3):257–285, 1998

Moffitt TE, Caspi A, Harkness AR, et al: The natural history of change in intellectual performance: who changes? How much? Is it meaningful? J Child Psychol Psychiatry 34(4):455–506, 1993 8509490

Mytton J, DiGuiseppi C, Gough D, et al: School-based secondary prevention programmes for preventing violence. Cochrane Database Syst Rev 3(3):CD004606, 2006 16856051

Nadder TS, Rutter M, Silberg JL, et al: Genetic effects on the variation and covariation of attention deficit-hyperactivity disorder (ADHD) and oppositional-defiant disorder/conduct disorder (Odd/CD) symptomatologies across informant and occasion of measurement. Psychol Med 32(1):39–53, 2002 11883729 (Erratum in Psychol Med 32[2])

Needleman HL, Riess JA, Tobin MJ, et al: Bone lead levels and delinquent behavior. JAMA 275(5):363–369, 1996 8569015

Niv S, Baker LA: Genetic markers for antisocial behavior, in The Origins of Antisocial Behavior: A Developmental Perspective. Edited by Thomas CR, Pope K. New York, Oxford University Press, 2013, pp 3–38

Nock MK, Kazdin AE, Hiripi E, et al: Prevalence, subtypes, and correlates of DSM-IV conduct disorder in the National Comorbidity Survey Replication. Psychol Med 36(5):699–710, 2006 16438742

Nock MK, Kazdin AE, Hiripi E, et al: Lifetime prevalence, correlates, and persistence of oppositional defiant disorder: results from the National Comorbidity Survey Replication. J Child Psychol Psychiatry 48(7):703–713, 2007 17593151

Offord DR, Bennett KJ: Conduct disorder: long-term outcomes and intervention effectiveness. J Am Acad Child Adolesc Psychiatry 33(8):1069–1078, 1994 7982856

Olds D, Henderson CR Jr, Cole R, et al: Long-term effects of nurse home visitation on children's criminal and antisocial behavior: 15-year follow-up of a randomized controlled trial. JAMA 280(14):1238–1244, 1998 9786373

Ortiz J, Raine A: Heart rate level and antisocial behavior in children and adolescents: a meta-analysis. J Am Acad Child Adolesc Psychiatry 43(2):154–162, 2004 14726721

Pappadopulos E, Woolston S, Chait A, et al: Pharmacotherapy of aggression in children and adolescents: efficacy and effect size. J Can Acad Child Adolesc Psychiatry 15(1):27–39, 2006 18392193

Patterson GR, Reid JB, Dishion TJ: A Social Learning Approach, Vol 4: Antisocial Boys. Eugene, OR, Castalia, 1992

Pope K, Blair J: The use of fMRI technology in understanding the neurobiological basis of conduct disorder and psychopathy in children and adolescents, in The Origins of Antisocial Behavior: A Developmental Perspective. Edited by Thomas CR, Pope K. New York, Oxford University Press, 2013, pp 71–85

Robins LN: Deviant Children Grown Up. Baltimore, MD, Williams and Wilkins, 1966

Rowe R, Maughan B, Costello EJ, et al: Defining oppositional defiant disorder. J Child Psychol Psychiatry 46(12):1309–1316, 2005 16313431

Rowe R, Costello EJ, Angold A, et al: Developmental pathways in oppositional defiant disorder and conduct disorder. J Abnorm Psychol 119(4):726–738, 2010a 21090876

Rowe R, Maughan B, Moran P, et al: The role of callous and unemotional traits in the diagnosis of conduct disorder. J Child Psychol Psychiatry 51(6):688–695, 2010b 20039995

Rubia K: "Cool" inferior frontostriatal dysfunction in attention-deficit/hyperactivity disorder versus "hot" ventromedial orbitofrontal-limbic dysfunction in conduct disorder: a review. Biol Psychiatry 69(12):e69–e87, 2011 21094938

Sakai JT, Young SE, Stallings MC, et al: Case-control and within-family tests for an association between conduct disorder and 5HTTLPR. Am J Med Genet B Neuropsychiatr Genet 141B(8):825–832, 2006 16972235

Scotto Rosato N, Correll CU, Pappadopulos E, et al: Treatment of maladaptive aggression in youth: CERT guidelines II. Treatment and ongoing management. Pediatrics 129(6):e1577–e1586, 2012 22641763

Simonoff E, Elander J, Holmshaw J, et al: Predictors of antisocial personality. Continuities from childhood to adult life. Br J Psychiatry 184:118–127, 2004 14754823

Smith PK, Ananiadou K, Cowie H: Interventions to reduce school bullying. Can J Psychiatry 48(9):591–599, 2003 14631879

Thomas A, Chess S: Temperament and Development. New York, Brunner Mazel, 1977

Thomas C, Holzer C, Wall J: Serious delinquency and gang membership. Adolesc Psychiatry 27:61–81, 2003

Trickett PK, Putnam FW: Developmental consequences of child sexual abuse, in Violence Against Children in the Family and the Community. Edited by Trickett PK, Schellenbach CJ. Washington, DC, American Psychological Association, 1998, pp 39–56

Unis AS, Cook EH, Vincent JG, et al: Platelet serotonin measures in adolescents with conduct disorder. Biol Psychiatry 42(7):553–559, 1997 9376451

van Goozen SH, Cohen-Kettenis PT, Snoek H, et al: Executive functioning in children: a comparison of hospitalised ODD and ODD/ADHD children and normal controls. J Child Psychol Psychiatry 45(2):284–292, 2004 14982242

van Goozen SHM, van den Ban E, Matthys W, et al: Increased adrenal androgen functioning in children with oppositional defiant disorder: a comparison with psychiatric and normal controls. J Am Acad Child Adolesc Psychiatry 39(11):1446–1451, 2000 11068901

Vanyukov MM, Moss HB, Plail JA, et al: Antisocial symptoms in preadolescent boys and in their parents: associations with cortisol. Psychiatry Res 46(1):9–17, 1993 8464960

Wakschlag LS, Pickett KE, Kasza KE, et al: Is prenatal smoking associated with a developmental pattern of conduct problems in young boys? J Am Acad Child Adolesc Psychiatry 45(4):461–467, 2006 16601651

Webster-Stratton C, Jamila Reid M, Stoolmiller M: Preventing conduct problems and improving school readiness: evaluation of the Incredible Years Teacher and Child Training Programs in high-risk schools. J Child Psychol Psychiatry 49(5):471–488, 2008 18221346

Woolfenden SR, Williams K, Peat JK: Family and parenting interventions for conduct disorder and delinquency: a meta-analysis of randomised controlled trials. Arch Dis Child 86(4):251–256, 2002 11919097

Yudofsky SC, Silver JM, Jackson W, et al: The Overt Aggression Scale for the objective rating of verbal and physical aggression. Am J Psychiatry 143(1):35–39, 1986 3942284

CHAPTER 12

Substance Use Disorders and Addictions

Oscar G. Bukstein, M.D., M.P.H.

Substance use and abuse by adolescents remain critical problems because of the common use of psychoactive substances by youth, the ensuing consequences, and the persistence into adulthood of pathology related to substance use. Clinicians seeking to understand the risk for substance use and abuse, the acquisition of use behaviors, and their development into substance use disorders (SUDs) should consider neurobiology, all aspects of development, and the characteristics of the individual adolescent. The treatment should focus on specific substance use behaviors as well as risk factors that have a role in the onset and maintenance of SUDs.

Definitions, Clinical Description, and Diagnosis

Substance Use

There is a range of use behaviors and patterns of use. At one end of the use spectrum lies *abstinence*. Substance *use* (often without significant consequences or impairment) applies to the largest group of adolescents. DSM-5 (American Psychiatric Association 2013) presents a significant departure from the DSM-IV (American Psychiatric Association 1994) nomenclature for SUDs. Replacing the two DSM-IV SUD diagnoses of abuse and dependence is a single diagnosis—*substance use disorder,* specified by the type of substance involved (e.g., alcohol use disorder or cannabis use disorder). A DSM-5 SUD diagnosis comprises 11 behavioral and physical signs and symptoms (Criterion A) taken from the criterion list for DSM-IV for both abuse and dependence, with a threshold of 2 symptoms necessary to receive an SUD diagnosis. Severity specifiers—mild, moderate, or severe—are determined by the number of symptoms present. Adolescents' alcohol and drug symptom profiles appear to vary along a severity dimension, rather than fitting into DSM-IV's abuse and dependence categories (Chung and Martin 2005). Many clinicians do not use the DSM criteria, preferring to use single terms such as *addiction* or *chemical dependency* to label substance use pathology. Usually, these terms are not operationally defined (no specific criteria are used).

The diagnosis of an SUD requires evidence of a maladaptive pattern of substance use with clinically significant levels of impairment or distress. Recurrent use in adolescents results in an inability to meet major role obligations, leading to impaired functioning in one or more major areas of their life and an increase in the likelihood of legal problems due to possession, risk-taking behavior, and exposure to hazardous situations. These criteria must be considered within a developmental context. For example, for alcohol use disorders (AUDs), adolescents commonly exhibit tolerance (i.e., requiring increasing amounts of a substance to achieve the same effect) but less frequently show withdrawal or other symptoms of physiological dependence (Chung and Martin 2005). Many adolescents with cannabis and opioid use disorders do manifest withdrawal symptoms (Chung and Martin 2005). Preoccupation with use is often demonstrated by giving up previously important activities, increasing the time spent in activities related to substance use, and using more frequently or for longer amounts of time than planned. The adolescent may use despite the continued existence or worsening of problems caused by substance use. For adolescents, it is important to include criteria such as alcohol-related blackouts, craving, and impulsive sexual behavior when determining if criteria are met. Polysubstance use by adolescents appears to be the rule rather than the exception; therefore, adolescents often present with multiple SUD diagnoses (Chung and Martin 2005).

Gambling and Internet Addiction

Gambling disorder is characterized by recurrent and persistent maladaptive gambling behavior. In DSM-5, pathological gambling was renamed *gambling disorder* and moved to the category for alcohol and drug use disorders. Other changes, based on empirical evidence, include eliminating the "illegal acts" criterion and reducing the threshold for a diagnosis of gambling disorder from five to four symptoms. The specific criteria are similar to those for SUDs, with the addition of typical but specific gambling behavior, such as "chasing" one's losses or relying on others to relieve a desperate financial situation caused by gambling (Leeman and Potenza 2012). A related but unofficial concept is *problem gambling,* which indicates a level of gambling that contributes to financial, social, legal, psychological, school, and vocational consequences (Stinchfield 2010).

In DSM-5, Internet gaming disorder is identified as a condition warranting more clinical research and experience before it might be considered for inclusion in the core manual as a formal disorder. Some individuals develop a preoccupation with certain aspects of the Internet, particularly online games. "Gamers" play compulsively, to the exclusion of other interests, and their persistent and recurrent online activity may result in clinically significant impairment or distress. People with this condition endanger their academic or job functioning because of the amount of time they spend playing. They experience symptoms of withdrawal when prevented from gaming. Preoccupation with the Internet is usually focused on a specific area, not generalized across different activities, and there is evidence that individuals should be classified according to their involvement in specific online activities, such as gambling, shopping, or pornography, which have a more robust basis as "addictions" (Yellowlees and Marks 2007). Individuals with a history of impulse control and other addictive disorders with other SUD risk factors may be at increased risk of using the Internet in a problematic way.

Epidemiology

Data on alcohol and drug use in the United States come from two major sources: 1) the Monitoring the Future (MTF; Johnston et al. 2014) in-school surveys of nationally representative samples of 40,000–50,000 eighth, tenth, and twelfth grade students in more than 400 schools nationwide; and 2) the National Survey on Drug Use and Health (NSDUH; Substance Abuse and Mental Health Services Administration 2013), an annual survey of the noninstitutionalized civilian population of the United States ages 12 years and older. NSDUH rates of youth substance use have been lower than those of MTF, largely because of prevalence rates being reported for the entire 12- to 17-year age group rather than by grade as in the MTF data. Although the two surveys occasionally have shown different trends in youth substance use over a short time period, these two sources of youth behavior have shown very similar long-term trends in prevalence.

Substance Use

A large minority of youth use psychoactive substances. According to the 2013 MTF survey (Johnston et al. 2014), the percentage of U.S. adolescents who use illicit drugs or drink alcohol continued a decade-long drop in 2006, revealing that 15% of eighth graders, less than a third (32%) of tenth graders, and 40% of all twelfth graders had taken an illicit drug (other than alcohol) during their lifetime. According to the NSDUH (Substance Abuse and Mental Health Services Administration 2013), the rate of current illicit drug use among youth ages 12–17 was 11.6% in 2002, 9.9% in 2005, and 9.5% in 2012. In 2012, among youth ages 12–17, 7.2% used marijuana, 2.8% used prescription-type drugs nonmedically, 0.8% used inhalants, 0.6% used hallucinogens, and 0.1% used cocaine (Substance Abuse and Mental Health Services Administration 2013). In 2012, among adults ages 18 years or older, age at first use of marijuana was associated with illicit drug dependence or abuse. Among those who first tried marijuana at age 14 or younger, 13.2% were classified with illicit drug dependence or abuse, which was higher than the 2.2% of adults who had first used marijuana at age 18 or older. In the MTF, when marijuana is removed from the list of illicit drugs, considerably fewer students report use of other illicit drugs. In 2013, 6%, 11%, and 17% of the students in the three grades, respectively, reported using any of these other drugs. Those percentages have dropped gradually since the late 1990s. Both surveys showed decreases between 2002 and 2012 in the percentages of youth who used marijuana, cocaine, 3,4-methylenedioxymethamphetamine (Ecstasy), lysergic acid diethylamide, inhalants, alcohol, and cigarettes in the past month. For current marijuana use, both surveys showed declines from 2002 to 2006 and increases from 2008 to 2011. The legalization of marijuana in Colorado and Washington State has prompted additional concerns about the prospects for future increases in adolescent marijuana use. Already, states with laws permitting medical marijuana may have contributed to increased adolescent access, with 6% of marijuana-using teens in such states reporting having their own marijuana prescription and more than a third reporting getting their marijuana from friends with a prescription. The MTF study has noted increases in perceived risk by all grades, with the prevalence increasing over the past several years, after a decade or more of fairly steady decline.

In the most recent MTF survey, the reported use of synthetic marijuana in the past year dropped sharply—from 11.3% in 2012 to 7.9% in 2013 among twelfth graders, from 8.8% to 7.4% among 10th graders, and from 4.4% to 4.0% among eighth graders. Bath salts, a designer stimulant drug, shows very low annual prevalence rates of 1%, 0.9%, and 0.9% among twelfth, tenth, and eighth graders, respectively. For inhalants, the lifetime prevalence was 10.8%, 8.7%, and 6.9% in the eighth, tenth, and twelfth grades, respectively. The annual prevalence of inhalant use was greatest among eighth graders at 5.2%. Although inhalants briefly showed an increase in use before the mid-1990s, substantial decreases in the prevalence of use have occurred since then.

Alcohol Use

In the MTF survey, the use of alcohol by teens dropped dramatically over roughly the last two decades—particularly among the youngest teens—and continued to drop in 2013. The 30-day prevalence of alcohol use declined in all three grades in 2013, dropping 0.8%, 1.9%, and 2.3% in grades 8, 10, and 12. The prevalence of recent binge drinking (having five or more drinks in a row at least once in the past 2 weeks) was 5.1%, 13.7%, and 22.1% in the three grades. The prevalence of binge drinking was at the lowest point since at least the mid-1990s. In the 2012 NSDUH, the rates of current alcohol use were 2.2% among youth ages 12 and 13, 11.1% of youth ages 14 and 15, 24.8% of 16- and 17-year-olds, and 45.8% of those ages 18–20. Rates of binge alcohol use in 2012 were 0.9% among 12- and 13-year-olds, 5.4% among 14- and 15-year-olds, 15.0% among 16- and 17-year-olds, and 30.5% among persons ages 18–20.

Adults (older than age 21 years) who had first used alcohol before age 21 were more likely than adults who had their first drink at or after age 21 to be classified with alcohol dependence or abuse. Adults ages 21 or older who had first used alcohol at age 14 or younger were more than seven times as likely to be classified with alcohol dependence or abuse than adults who had their first drink at or after age 21 (15.2% vs. 2.1%).

Tobacco Use

In the 2013 MTF survey, the percentage of students reporting any cigarette smoking in the prior 30 days (30-day prevalence) continued a decrease from the last several decades (4.5% among eighth graders, 9.1% among tenth graders, and 16.3% among twelfth graders. Since smoking by youth reached a peak in the late 1990s, the rates of current (past 30-day) smoking have fallen by nearly 80% among eighth graders, 70% among tenth graders, and more than 50% among twelfth graders, with even greater decreases in daily smoking. In 2013, 1.8% of eighth graders, 4.4% of tenth graders, and 8.5% of twelfth graders reported daily cigarette use. Only 3.4% of twelfth graders reported smoking half a pack or more of cigarettes per day. Similarly, in the NSDUH, the rate of past month tobacco use among 12- to 17-

year-olds declined from 15.2% in 2002 to 8.6% in 2012.

One important cause of these declines in current smoking among youth is the marked decrease in the number of youth who have ever started to smoke. In 1996, 49% of eighth graders said they had tried cigarettes, but by 2013 only 15% had tried cigarettes—a drop of 70% in smoking initiation since the mid to late 1990s (Johnston et al. 2014).

In the 2013 MTF survey, 30-day prevalence rates for smokeless tobacco use were 2.8%, 6.4%, and 8.1% among eighth, tenth, and twelfth graders, respectively. From the mid-1990s to the early 2000s, there was a substantial decline in the use of smokeless tobacco among teens, plateauing briefly from the mid-2000s through 2010 but showing declines from 2010 through 2012.

Substance Use Disorders

The prevalence of SUDs increases with age through young adulthood. Current statistics are limited to studies examining DSM-IV prevalence rates, with no major studies examining rates of DSM-5 SUDs. In the NSDUH, the rate of illicit drug dependence or abuse among youth ages 12–17 was 4.0% in 2012, which was lower than the rates in 2010 (4.7%) and 2002 (5.6%). The rate of alcohol dependence or abuse among youth ages 12–17 was 3.4% in 2012 but declined from 4.6% in 2010 and from 5.9% in 2002. Results from the National Comorbidity Survey–Adolescent Supplement found an overall lifetime SUD prevalence of 11.4%–8.9% of adolescents with drug abuse/dependence and 6.4% with alcohol abuse/dependence. The prevalence of DSM-IV SUDs for illicit drugs was 3.4% in youth ages 13–14 years and 16.5% in the 17- to 18-year age group (Swendsen et al. 2012). The median age of onset for illicit drug use was 13 years, the median age for drug abuse with dependence was 14 years, and the median age for drug abuse without dependence was 15 years. For AUDs, 5.2% of all adolescents met criteria for alcohol abuse without dependence and 1.3% met criteria for abuse with dependence. The rate for abuse with or without dependence was 1.3% for adolescents ages 13–14 and 15.1% for adolescents ages 17–18. Median age of onset for first alcohol use was 13 years, and median age for regular use or abuse (with or without dependence) was 14 years. SUDs were somewhat more frequent in males, and a fivefold to elevenfold increase in prevalence was observed across increasing age groups. Although male and female adolescents had equivalent rates of use, there were modestly higher rates of regular use and abuse by males because of greater rates in older males (17–18 years). For illicit drugs, the gender findings are similar to those for alcohol. For both alcohol and illicit drugs, white and Hispanic adolescents showed higher rates of use and abuse than African American youth.

Gambling

Between 60% and 80% of adolescents reported having engaged in some form of gambling during the past year (Derevensky 2007), with most described as social, recreational, and occasional gamblers, although 3%–8% of adolescents may have a very serious gambling problem, with another 10%–15% at risk for the development of a gambling problem. A survey of youth found the prevalence of youth problem gambling to be 2.1%. In the past year, 68% of the youth had gambled; 11% had gambled more often than twice a week. Males had much higher gambling involvement (23% were frequent gamblers, and 14%

were at-risk or problem gamblers) than females (Welte et al. 2008).

Internet Addiction

Although using nonstandardized criteria, the prevalence of Internet addiction or problem Internet use has ranged from 1%–2% to 11%–13% (Kuss et al. 2013). Using a modified version of the Minnesota Impulsive Disorders Inventory, 4% of U.S. high school students were identified as addicted to using the Internet (Liu et al. 2011). Higher rates have been described in Asian countries (e.g., Taiwan, Singapore, South Korea, China) (Kuss et al. 2013).

Comorbidity

In both community surveys of adolescents with SUD and samples of adolescents in addiction treatment, the majority have a co-occurring non-substance-related mental disorder (Hser et al. 2001). More than half of those adolescents in addiction treatment who have a co-occurring mental illness have three or more co-occurring psychiatric disorders (Chan et al. 2008). The most commonly comorbid psychiatric disorders among youth in addiction treatment include conduct problems, attention-deficit/hyperactivity disorder (ADHD), mood disorders (e.g., depression), and trauma-related symptoms (Grella et al. 2001).

Comorbid psychopathology may precede, exacerbate, or follow the onset of heavy substance use. A review of adolescent community surveys found that childhood mental illness generally predicted earlier initiation of substance use and SUD onset, particularly in relation to conduct disorder (Armstrong and Costello 2002). The early symptoms of most psychiatric disorders, excluding depression, typically emerged prior to the onset of substance use; full criteria for a nonsubstance psychiatric disorder were typically met prior to SUD onset in adolescence (Kaminer and Bukstein 2008). Among treated adolescents, comorbid psychopathology, particularly conduct problems (Chan et al. 2008) and major depression (Cornelius et al. 2004), predicted early return to substance use. Co-occurring psychopathology also predicted a more persistent course of substance involvement over 1-year follow-up (Grella et al. 2001). Comorbidity of SUDs with disruptive behavior disorders (DBDs) is high, with a median prevalence of 46% in community samples compared with between 7% and 8% for those without DBDs and a fourfold increase of risk for DBD in youth using or abusing substances (Armstrong and Costello 2002). Conduct disorder confers increased risk for substance use initiation across all substance classes at age 15 years, with greater relative risk for illicit substances compared with licit substances (e.g., alcohol). This effect continues until age 18 years, with the weakest effect for alcohol (Hopfer et al. 2013).

ADHD is an independent risk factor for developing SUDs and nicotine dependence (Charach et al. 2011; Lee et al. 2011). Conduct disorder during childhood increases the risk and remains the strongest predictor of SUD severity (Lee et al. 2011). The prevalence of SUDs is high among adolescents with ADHD, and adolescents with SUDs have higher rates of comorbid ADHD than those without SUDs.

Cannabis use is associated with an approximate doubling of the risk of anxiety disorder (Degenhardt et al. 2013). Evidence indicates that the use of cannabis is also associated with an increased risk of major depression. Increasing frequency of cannabis use has been found to be associated with increasing depressive symptoms (Chen et al. 2002). Comorbidity of SUD and other psychiatric disorders increases the risk of suicidal behavior and the severity of the psychiatric disorders, especially mood disorders (Pompili et al. 2012). Prospective data suggest that bipolar disorder during adolescence is a risk factor for the subsequent development of substance use (Goldstein and Bukstein 2010) and that adolescents with comorbid bipolar and substance use disorders have significant functional impairment and high suicide risk (Goldstein and Bukstein 2010). Epidemiological research has provided extensive evidence of associations between cannabis use and psychosis (Compton et al. 2009). Cannabis use has been associated with both subclinical psychotic experiences and clinical psychotic disorders.

In general, the presence of psychiatric disorders–SUD comorbidity predicts lower age of onset of use and SUD, more rapid progression of use to SUD, greater SUD severity, and more persistent SUD (Kaminer and Bukstein 2008).

Etiology, Mechanisms, and Risk Factors

First experiences with substance use most often take place in a social context with the use of "gateway" substances, such as alcohol and cigarettes, which are legal for adults and readily available to minors (Kandel and Yamaguchi 2002). The wide availability of marijuana prompts consideration of this as a gateway substance as well. Initial use may occur because of adolescent curiosity or the availability of a substance. Progressively fewer adolescents advance to later and more serious levels of substance use, with the risk for and rate of progression to SUD being the same whether consumption begins with a legal or illegal drug (Tarter et al. 2006). The early onset of substance use and a more rapid progression through the stages of substance use are among the risk factors for the development of SUDs (Behrendt et al. 2009). The literature on the development of substance use and SUDs in adolescents has identified an assortment of individual, peer, family, and community risk factors. Both temperament and social interactions (e.g., family and peer relations) have a critical role in adolescent SUD outcomes. Many family factors have been implicated in increasing SUD risk in children and adolescents. The most widely recognized factors involve affectional bonding, parental supervision, discipline style, and adherence to religious practices (Clark et al. 1998). Affiliation with socially deviant peers has been shown in many studies to promote substance use (Kosterman et al. 2000). Affiliation with older peers may be especially hazardous because of premature exposure to risky situations, including drugs, sex, automobile travel, and social settings without adult supervision.

Although adoption, twin, and extended-family designs have established that there is a strong heritable (genetic) component to liability to nicotine, alcohol, and illicit drug dependence, shared environmental influences are relatively stronger at earlier stages of substance involvement (e.g., initiation, use) (Kendler et al. 2003; Lynskey et al. 2010). There is considerable overlap in the genetic influences associated with SUDs across drug classes, and shared genetic influences contribute to the commonly observed associations between substance use disorders and externalizing disorders (Lynskey et al. 2010). This research supports an etiologic model of individual differences in substance use, in which initiation and early patterns of use are strongly influenced by social and familial environmental factors, while later levels of use are strongly influenced by genetic factors.

Understanding the risk for the development of SUDs can be noted in the emerging view of adolescence as characterized by an imbalance between early emerging subcortical "bottom-up" systems (i.e., more primitive and earlier developing parts of the brain) that may express reactivity to motivational stimuli and later developing "top-down" cognitive control regions, which include executive functions (Casey and Jones 2010). Studies show curvilinear development of the subcortical brain regions, with a peak from 13 to 17 years. In contrast, prefrontal regions, the top-down cortical regions, show a linear pattern of development into young adulthood that parallels that seen in behavioral studies of impulsivity. The imbalance between these developing systems during adolescence may lead to cognitive control processes being more vulnerable to incentive-based (reward) modulation and increased susceptibility to the motivational properties of alcohol and other drugs (Casey and Jones 2010). Psychopathology that further compromises reward mechanisms and increases impulsivity (e.g., ADHD) further increases the risk for SUDs (Bukstein 2011).

Prevention

Most prevention interventions are based on social learning models, including educational approaches, family-based interventions, and community-based projects. Empirically based prevention efforts primarily involve strengthening resilience factors and reducing risk factors for the development of SUDs (National Institute on Drug Abuse 2003) (see Table 12–1). School-based and some community-based prevention methods can be effective in reducing substance use.

Course

In examining the clinical course of AUDs in community samples, among adolescents with an AUD, 55% had an AUD at young adult follow-up (Rohde et al. 2001), suggesting some remission with maturation, as well as a more chronic course of adolescent-onset AUD for certain individuals. Although the majority of treated adolescents return to some substance use following treatment, treated adolescents generally show reductions in substance use and problems over both short- and longer-term follow-up.

Changes in different domains of psychosocial functioning occurred at different rates: school functioning generally improved within the first year of follow-up, but improvements in family functioning emerged only after 2 years (Chung and Martin 2011). Despite significant reductions in substance involvement and improvements in school performance, interpersonal relations, and other areas, treated adolescents continued to show greater problem severity across multiple domains compared with a community sample (Chung and Martin 2011). Thus, adolescent-onset SUD, likely in combination with co-occurring psychopathology and other risk factors (e.g., negative environmental influences), interferes with the achievement of normative adolescent developmental tasks.

TABLE 12–1. Principles for effective prevention programs

Principle 1: Prevention programs should enhance protective factors and reverse or reduce risk factors.

Principle 2: Prevention programs should address all forms of drug abuse, alone or in combination, including the underage use of legal drugs (e.g., tobacco, alcohol); the use of illegal drugs (e.g., marijuana, heroin); and the inappropriate use of legally obtained substances (e.g., inhalants), prescription medications, or over-the-counter drugs.

Principle 3: Prevention programs should address the type of drug abuse problem in the local community, target modifiable risk factors, and strengthen identified protective factors.

Principle 4: Prevention programs should be tailored to address risks specific to population or audience characteristics, such as age, gender, and ethnicity, to improve program effectiveness.

Principle 5: Family-based prevention programs should enhance family bonding and relationships and include parenting skills; practice in developing, discussing, and enforcing family policies on substance abuse; and training in drug education and information.

Principle 6: Prevention programs can be designed to intervene as early as preschool to address risk factors for drug abuse, such as aggressive behavior, poor social skills, and academic difficulties.

Principle 7: Prevention programs for elementary school children should target improving academic and social-emotional learning to address risk factors for drug abuse, such as early aggression, academic failure, and school dropout. Education should focus on the following skills:

- Self-control
- Emotional awareness
- Communication
- Social problem-solving
- Academic support, especially in reading

Principle 8: Prevention programs for middle or junior high and high school students should increase academic and social competence with the following skills:

- Study habits and academic support
- Communication
- Peer relationships
- Self-efficacy and assertiveness
- Drug-resistance skills
- Reinforcement of antidrug attitudes
- Strengthening of personal commitments against drug abuse

Principle 9: Prevention programs aimed at general populations at key transition points, such as the transition to middle school, can produce beneficial effects even among high-risk families and children. Such interventions do not single out risk populations and, therefore, reduce labeling and promote bonding to school and community.

Principle 10: Community prevention programs that combine two or more effective programs, such as family- and school-based programs, can be more effective than a single program.

Principle 11: Community prevention programs reaching populations in multiple settings (e.g., schools, clubs, faith-based organizations, the media) are most effective when they present consistent communitywide messages in each setting.

Principle 12: When communities adapt programs to match their needs, community norms, or differing cultural requirements, they should retain core elements of the original research-based intervention that include the following:

- Structure (how the program is organized and constructed)
- Content (what the information, skills, and strategies of the program are)
- Delivery (how the program is adapted, implemented, and evaluated)

TABLE 12–1. Principles for effective prevention programs *(continued)*

Principle 13: Prevention programs should be long term, with repeated interventions (i.e., booster programs) to reinforce the original prevention goals. Research shows that the benefits from middle school prevention programs diminish without follow-up programs in high school.
Principle 14: Prevention programs should include teacher training on good classroom management practices, such as rewarding appropriate student behavior. Such techniques help to foster students' positive behavior, achievement, academic motivation, and school bonding.
Principle 15: Prevention programs are most effective when they employ interactive techniques, such as peer discussion groups and parent role-playing, that allow for active involvement in learning about drug abuse and reinforcing skills.
Principle 16: Research-based prevention programs can be cost-effective.

Source. Adapted from National Institute on Drug Abuse 2003.

Evaluation

Perhaps the most critical skill for clinicians is evaluation, which includes screening, baseline assessment, and ongoing assessment of progress. For more detailed guidelines to both evaluation and treatment, the reader is referred to the article by Bukstein et al. (2005).

Validity of Adolescent Report

Although the clinician should always question whether any self-report about substance use is truthful, the majority of adolescents in drug clinics or schools give temporally consistent reports of substance use (Winters et al. 1990–1991). Most youth in drug treatment settings admit to use of substances; few treatment-seeking adolescents endorse questions that indicate blatant faking of responses (e.g., admitting to the use of a fictitious drug). Specific populations, especially extremely antisocial youth, have much higher responses of "faking good" than clinical samples (Winters et al. 1990–1991).

Both clinicians and investigators have noted an "intake-discharge effect" in which level of use reported at discharge and problems as well as SUDs are higher than those endorsed at admission to a treatment program (Stinchfield 1997). The possible causes of the intake-discharge effect include factors at intake such as denial, reluctance to self-disclose due to embarrassment, and wish to avoid sanctions for use, as well as ability of the adolescent in treatment to more carefully examine the extent of substance use.

The use of structured interviews or standardized questionnaires may also serve to support or validate the self-report. The adolescent may feel less threatened by self-report questionnaires, many of which have questions to ascertain response bias. The use of toxicological methods such as urine drug screens can validate self-report by testing for the use of a specific agent. Finally, the attitude and skill of the interviewer are often the best promoters of the validity of self-report, as engagement with the adolescent predicts more valid responses.

Levels of Assessment

There are two levels of assessment: screening and comprehensive assessment. Screening is a process by which adolescents are identified according to characteristics that indicate that they possibly have a problem with substance use.

Screening does not inform the clinician of the severity of the adolescent's substance use or the presence of SUDs. Screening identifies the need for a comprehensive assessment and is not a substitute for an assessment. The comprehensive assessment is a thorough process that includes variables or factors contributing to and maintaining substance abuse, the severity of the problems, and the variety of consequences associated with the adolescent's substance use. Screening is appropriate for nonclinical settings (such as schools), primary medical care settings, and nonspecialized mental health settings (those not specifically treating SUD-related problems).

Screening

Screening instruments are required in order to screen large numbers of youth. Youth selected for screening may be at high risk for having or developing an SUD (e.g., those with other psychiatric diagnoses or having parents with SUDs). The two alternative approaches to screening involve 1) specific screening only for substance use and related behaviors or 2) screening for SUDs as part of a multidomain screen that includes mental health problems and high-risk behaviors.

Screening, Brief Intervention, and Referral to Treatment (SBIRT) is a comprehensive integrated approach to the screening and identification of individuals engaged in alcohol and drug use and the delivery of early brief interventions to these people in order to reduce risky use (Mitchell et al. 2013). The limited evidence suggests that brief interventions (described below) may be effective with adolescents.

Primary health care physicians and nurses typically use a brief series of questions to screen for substance use problems (e.g., the CRAFFT screening tool) (Knight et al. 2002), while mental health professionals use one of a variety of available screening instruments. In a primary care setting, questions for all youth about substance use follow a general inquiry about health behaviors and should include questions about cigarette, alcohol, and other substance use. In settings such as child welfare, mental health, or juvenile justice, the high-risk status is sufficient to require screening of each adolescent. Although specific interview questions with established validity such as the CRAFFT tool are often sufficient, many clinicians use specific screening instruments (for representative screening and assessment instruments, see Bukstein et al. 2005; Winters and Kaminer 2008).

Professionals need to decide what screening threshold will trigger a comprehensive assessment. Generally, adolescent report of regular substance use (e.g., greater than two times a month for several consecutive months) and/or consequences of use is sufficient for referral for a comprehensive assessment. Other factors, such as past history of substance use, high-risk behaviors, or moderate to severe high-risk status, may prompt such a referral even in the absence of an adolescent report of regular use or consequences.

Comprehensive Assessment

The assessment process is used to identify those individuals who have an SUD and whether they meet criteria for a DSM-5 SUD diagnosis. Substance use behaviors, the pattern of use, and any consequences of use are also discussed. The results of the comprehensive assessment will usually identify which individuals require treatment, what level of treatment is needed, and other problems as well as strengths of the adolescent that may be helpful.

A comprehensive evaluation requires assessment of many domains of functioning in the adolescent's life. These domains include substance use behaviors, psychiatric and behavioral problems, school and occupational functioning, family functioning, social competency and peer relations, and leisure/recreation.

Interview

A comprehensive substance use history includes age at onset; duration; frequency; and route of ingestion for each individual drug, including alcohol, tobacco, illicit drugs, inhalants, over-the-counter medications, and prescription drugs such as benzodiazepines, opiates, and stimulants. Additional inquiry should cover negative consequences as well as attempts and motivation to control use or quit. Areas covered by questions detailing the context of use include the setting of use (time and place), whether the adolescent uses alone or with peers, and the attitudes of those peers about substance use. Variability in quantity and frequency of adolescent substance use is often great. The adolescent may report periods of abstinence as well as periods of rapid acceleration of use and heavy use of particular agents. A timeline chart or calendar is often useful to allow the adolescent to report quantity, frequency, and variability data across time, with important dates, holidays, and other time cues as a guide. Additional substance use–related information includes attitudes and/or expectancies of use and motivation(s) to use or perceived benefits of use. Assessment of substance use behavior may follow a functional analysis of use to determine usual antecedents to use and consequences of use. Such an analysis may allow a more specific targeting of relevant antecedents during treatment. Along with specific attitudes and beliefs about substance use, the clinician should also inquire about the adolescent's values and attitudes in general.

Although substance use may be the target domain for the assessment, the other domains are also very important. In choosing the level of inquiry into psychopathology, the clinician is guided by the setting and the purpose of the assessment. Screening questions about depression, suicidality, aggression, psychosis, and treatment history may be sufficient to augment other information in determining when an adolescent should be referred for a more detailed, comprehensive psychiatric evaluation. The medical history and possible physical examination search for symptoms and illnesses that may be related to SUDs and behaviors, including trauma, pregnancy, HIV/AIDS, other sexually transmitted diseases, infections or wounds, and possible liver disease. School/vocational, peer, and family domains emphasize family and peer substance use and attitudes toward use, parental monitoring and supervision, family history of SUDs and psychiatric disorders, and the effect of substance use on academic and/or vocational functioning. Inquiry into recreational or prosocial activities such as sports, interests, and hobbies will provide the clinician with information about the adolescent's social repertoire and whether this will have to be targeted for change.

Confidentiality

Both the Health Insurance Portability and Accountability Act and state law (in most states) protect confidential information that an adolescent may provide during assessment and/or treatment. Adolescents are more likely to provide truthful information if they believe that their information (at least the details) will not be shared. Prior to the interview, the clinician should review with the adolescent exactly what information the clinician is obliged to share and with whom. Typically, a clinician should inform the adolescent that a threat of danger to self or others or information about physical or sexual abuse will force the clinician to reveal otherwise confidential information. The clinician should be knowledgeable about state and federal laws that limit what information may be released from drug and alcohol treatment programs. Confidentiality statutes include information about illegal behavior such as selling drugs, who sells the adolescent drugs, and peer behaviors. In order for the assessment team to speak with the adolescent's family, school, or legal staff members, the adolescent must sign a consent form. In some states, parents must also sign a consent form. The clinician should encourage and support the adolescent's revealing to parents the extent of substance use and other problems. The clinician should discuss what information the adolescent will allow the clinician to reveal, such as a general recommendation for treatment or impressions rather than a detailed report of specific behaviors.

Toxicology

Toxicological tests—of bodily fluids (usually urine but also saliva) and of hair samples—to detect the presence of specific substances (Table 12–2) should be part of the formal evaluation and the ongoing assessment of substance use (Levy et al. 2014), especially in SUD treatment settings. The optimal use of urine screening requires proper collection techniques, including monitoring of obtaining the sample, evaluation of positive results, and specific plan(s) of action should the specimen be positive or negative for the presence of substance(s). Prior to testing, the clinician should establish rules regarding the confidentiality of the results. Because of the limited time a drug will remain in the urine and possible adulteration, a negative urine screen does not indicate that the youth does not use drugs. A positive specimen indicates only the presence of specific drug(s) and not necessarily the presence of an SUD or a specific pattern of use.

Outcome Assessment

Ongoing evaluation of the effects of treatment on relevant variables is critical to planning treatment and determining whether existing treatment is working. Ongoing assessment generally consists of toxicology in addition to questioning the adolescent about the extent of his or her recent or interim substance use (usually the number of days of use or abstinence in the past week or month). In addition to substance use, clinicians should monitor the effects of treatment on other domains of functioning.

Treatment

Reviews of studies of adolescent treatment outcome have concluded that treatment for adolescent SUDs is better than no treatment (Tanner-Smith et al. 2013; Williams et al. 2000). In the year following treatment, adolescents report decreased heavy drinking, marijuana and other illicit drug use, and criminal involvement, as well as improved psychological adjustment and school performance (Grella et al. 2001; Hser et al. 2001). Longer duration of treatment is associated with more favorable outcomes (Hser et al. 2001; Tanner-Smith et al. 2013). Some reviews have identified such variables as co-occurring psychopathology, nonwhite race, higher severity of substance use, criminality, and lower educational status as predicting poorer

TABLE 12–2. Urine toxicology

Substance	Half-life, hours	Detection after last use, days
Amphetamines	10–15	1–2
Barbiturates	20–96	3–21
Benzodiazepines	20–90	2–42
Cocaine	0.8–6.0	0.2–10 (metabolites)
Methaqualone	20–60	7–24
Opiates	2–4	1–2
Phencyclidine	7–16	2–8
Cannabinoids	10–40	2–8 (acute), 14–60 (chronic)
Alcohol		Up to 12 hours
Heroin	2–3	1–3
Methadone	15–60	7–10
Hydromorphone	2.6	1–2

Note. Drugs not usually tested: lysergic acid diethylamide (LSD); psilocybin; methylenedioxymethamphetamine (MDMA); 3,4-methylenedioxyamphetamine (MDA); and other designer drugs. These drugs may be tested by chromatography methods.

adolescent SUD outcomes (Bukstein 1995). These reviews have also identified the provision of comprehensive services such as housing, academic assistance, and recreation and posttreatment association with nonusing peers and involvement in leisure time activities, work, and school as predicting more positive outcomes. Other studies reported treatment completion, low pretreatment use, and peer and parent social support and nonuse of substances to be most consistently related to positive outcomes for adolescents receiving SUD treatment (Grella et al. 2001). A more recent meta-analysis did not find that any of these variables predicted improved treatment outcomes (Tanner-Smith et al. 2013).

Table 12–3 lists principles of treatment for adolescents with SUDs (National Institute on Drug Abuse 2014). The primary goal for the treatment of adolescents with SUDs is achieving and maintaining abstinence from substance use. While abstinence should remain the explicit long-term goal for treatment, a realistic view recognizes both the chronicity of SUDs in some populations of adolescents and the self-limited nature of substance use and substance use–related problems in others. Taken from a comprehensive review of the treatment literature, the average rate of sustained abstinence is 38% at 6 months (ranging from 30% to 55%) and 32% at 12 months (ranging from 14% to 47%) (Williams et al. 2000). Given these considerations, harm reduction may be an interim implicit acceptable outcome, if not the goal, of treatment. Included in the concept of harm reduction is a reduction in the use and negative consequences of substances, a reduction in the severity and frequency of relapses, and an improvement in one or more domains of the adolescent's functioning (e.g., academic performance, family functioning). While adolescents in treatment may not initially be motivated to stop substance use, the attainment of skills to deal with substance use may provide the adolescent with greater self-efficacy to not only reduce use but also ultimately to move toward the future goal of abstinence.

TABLE 12–3. Principles of adolescent substance use disorder treatment

1. Adolescent substance use needs to be identified and addressed as soon as possible.
2. Adolescents can benefit from a drug abuse intervention even if they are not addicted to a drug.
3. Routine annual medical visits are an opportunity to ask adolescents about drug use.
4. Legal interventions and sanctions or family pressure may play an important role in getting adolescents to enter, stay in, and complete treatment.
5. Substance use disorder treatment should be tailored to the unique needs of the adolescent.
6. Treatment should address the needs of the whole person, rather than just focusing on his or her drug use.
7. Behavioral therapies are effective in addressing adolescent drug use.
8. Families and the community are important aspects of treatment.
9. Effectively treating substance use disorders in adolescents requires also identifying and treating any other mental health conditions they may have.
10. Sensitive issues such as violence and child abuse or risk of suicide should be identified and addressed.
11. It is important to monitor drug use during treatment.
12. Staying in treatment for an adequate period of time and continuity of care afterward are important.
13. Testing adolescents for sexually transmitted diseases like HIV, as well as hepatitis B and C, is an important part of drug treatment.

"Controlled use" of any nonprescribed substance of abuse should never be an explicit goal in the treatment of adolescents. In addition, control of substance use should not be the only goal of treatment. A broad concept of rehabilitation involves targeting associated problems and domains of functioning for treatment. Integrated interventions that concurrently deal with coexisting psychiatric and behavioral problems, family functioning, peer and interpersonal relationships, and academic or vocational functioning not only will produce general improvements in psychosocial functioning but most likely will yield improved outcomes in the primary treatment goal of achieving and maintaining abstinence.

On the basis of the combination of empirical research and current clinical consensus, the clinician dealing with adolescents with SUDs should develop a treatment plan that uses modalities that target a number of salient areas (see Table 12–3). Only a small percentage of adolescents with SUDs actually receive any treatment. The rate and number of youth ages 12–17 years who needed treatment for an illicit drug or alcohol use problem in 2012 (6.3% and 1.6 million) were lower than in 2011 (7.0% and 1.7 million), 2010 (7.5% and 1.8 million), and 2002 (9.1% and 2.3 million). Of the 1.6 million youth who needed treatment in 2012, 157,000 received treatment at a specialty facility (about 10% of the youth who needed treatment), leaving about 1.4 million who needed treatment for a substance use problem but did not receive it (Substance Abuse and Mental Health Services Administration 2013).

Pharmacological Treatments

The majority of the research in pharmacotherapy of adolescents with SUD relates to the treatment of comorbid psychiatric disorders, such as depression and ADHD. Strategies in pharmacological interventions for SUDs include substitution therapies, detoxification, blocking therapies, craving reduction, and aversion therapies (Bukstein and Horner 2010).

Substitution therapies, which are used to prevent withdrawal, eliminate drug craving, and block the euphoric effects of illicit opioid use, use an agonist (e.g., nicotine replacement therapy [NRT] for nicotine dependence, methadone maintenance for opioid dependence) or a partial agonist (e.g., buprenorphine for opioid dependence) that acts on the same receptors that mediate the psychotropic effects of a substance.

Detoxification strategies generally use agonists or medications that provide symptomatic relief (e.g., clonidine for opioid withdrawal, benzodiazepines for alcohol withdrawal). In the absence of specific research, it is reasonable to use for adolescent pharmacotherapy protocols similar to those used in adults, when needed. Aversive interventions, such as disulfiram (Antabuse), blocking strategies (e.g., naltrexone for opioid dependence), and anticraving medications (naltrexone, acamprosate, and ondansetron for alcohol; bupropion for nicotine; buprenorphine for opioids), require medication adherence and are likely most effective among patients with high motivation (Bukstein and Horner 2010). With the possible exception of bupropion and buprenorphine, there is very modest evidence supporting their use in adolescents. These agents should be prescribed to youth only after a thorough consideration of previous treatment attempts.

In an 8-week double-blind randomized placebo-controlled trial of *N*-acetylcysteine (NAC), an agent presumed to affect glutamate modulation, treatment-seeking cannabis-dependent adolescents who took NAC had more than twice the odds, compared with those receiving placebo, of having negative urine cannabinoid test results during treatment (Gray et al. 2012a). Exploratory secondary abstinence outcomes favored NAC but were not statistically significant. NAC was well tolerated, with minimal adverse events.

Tobacco use or nicotine dependence is commonly present in adolescents with SUDs and/or psychiatric disorders, but few of them are diagnosed with nicotine dependence and offered smoking cessation treatment (Upadhyaya et al. 2005). NRTs (transdermal patch, gum, inhaler, lozenge), varenicline, and bupropion sustained-release (SR) are currently approved by the U.S. Food and Drug Administration for smoking cessation in adults. NRTs and bupropion SR are the agents most studied for adolescent smokers, with most studies of NRTs using the transdermal nicotine patch. The efficacy of the transdermal nicotine patch and gum has been modest among adolescents, with resulting abstinence rates ranging from 5% to 18% (Moolchan et al. 2005). Nicotine withdrawal symptoms may be a significant problem in situations where adolescents with nicotine dependence cannot smoke, such as psychiatric hospitals, and NRT may need to be provided to counter nicotine withdrawal symptoms, even to nontreatment-seeking adolescent smokers (Upadhyaya et al. 2005). Bupropion has also shown promise in the treatment of adolescent smokers in an open study (Upadhyaya et al. 2005) and a randomized controlled trial (RCT; Gray et al. 2011). In a randomized, blinded comparison of bupropion XL with varenicline, both agents improved nicotine abstinence, although no difference between the agents was reported (Gray et al. 2012b).

Buprenorphine is a partial agonist. It is difficult to overdose on buprenorphine, and its combination with naloxone (opiate antagonist) makes it difficult to abuse intravenously. Naloxone is not absorbed orally and hence is not active if the combination is taken sublingually (buprenorphine alone is taken sublingually). If the combination medication is injected, naloxone blocks the opiate receptors and any euphoric effects of buprenorphine. Two double-blind placebo-controlled trials have demonstrated the efficacy of buprenorphine in retention in treatment and reducing the number of positive urine tests for opioids compared with clonidine (Marsch et al. 2005), and there are fewer dropouts from maintenance treatment (Woody et al. 2008). Current evidence does not support use of pharmacotherapy for any other SUDs or other drug use (e.g., cocaine, stimulants, sedative/hypnotics, club drugs) in adolescents.

Comorbid Psychiatric Disorders

Recent emerging research and experience suggest that pharmacotherapy can be used safely and effectively in adolescents with SUDs (Bukstein and Horner 2010). While most evidence points to improvement in the comorbid disorder (e.g., depression, bipolar disorder—one RCT each—and ADHD—three RCTs, one each with fluoxetine, lithium, and stimulants), there are several studies showing no effect.

Overall, these results suggest that pharmacological treatment in comorbid adolescents (e.g., with SUDs and MDD, bipolar disorder, or ADHD) may result in improvements in the psychiatric target but will have little, if any, effect on the substance use, especially without concurrent and specific therapy for the SUD. However, there appears to be little medical risk or increase in adverse effects with treatment, and no evidence of abuse or diversion.

Some commonly used pharmacological agents, such as psychostimulants and benzodiazepines, have inherent abuse potential. The risk of diversion or misuse of a therapeutic agent by the adolescent, his or her peer group, or family members should prompt a thorough assessment of the risk of this outcome (e.g., history of abuse of the specific or other potentially abusable agents, family/parental history of substance abuse or antisocial behavior). Often, parental or adult supervision of medication administration can alleviate concerns about potential abuse. The clinician should also consider alternative agents to psychostimulants, such as atomoxetine, α agonists, or bupropion, which do not have abuse potential. The long-acting stimulant preparations may offer less potential for abuse or diversion because of their form of administration, reduced level of reinforcement due to more gradual and longer time to maximum plasma concentration, and ability to more easily monitor and supervise once-a-day dosing. In particular, because of their formulations (see Chapter 35, "Medications Used for Attention-Deficit/Hyperactivity Disorder") both osmotic-release oral system methylphenidate and lisdexamfetamine have minimal, if any, effects if snorted or injected. Many anxiety symptoms or disorders in adolescents can be treated successfully with psychosocial methods such as behavior therapy. If pharmacotherapy is required, the use of selective serotonin reuptake inhibitors or buspirone is preferred over benzodiazepines.

Psychotherapeutic Treatments

A meta-analysis conducted by Waldron and Turner (2008) reviewed findings from 17 randomized clinical trials and the 46 treatment conditions embedded within them. Their results showed generally beneficial treatment effects that were especially positive for multidimensional family therapy (MDFT), Functional Family Therapy, and cognitive-behavioral therapy (CBT). Other family models, including Multisystemic Therapy (MST), Brief Strategic Family Therapy (BSFT), and Behavioral Family Therapy (BFT), are probably efficacious; Adolescent Community Reinforcement Approach (A-CRA) and other individual CBT approaches appear promising, but additional research is needed. Evidence-based therapies are listed in Table 12–4.

Family therapy approaches have the most empirical support (Tanner-Smith et al. 2013; Waldron and Turner 2008; Williams et al. 2000). Family interventions for substance abuse treatment have common goals: providing psychoeducation about SUDs, which decreases familial resistance to treatment and increases motivation and engagement; assisting parents and family to initiate and maintain efforts to get the adolescent into appropriate treatment and achieve abstinence; assisting parents and family to establish or reestablish structure with consistent limit setting and careful monitoring of the adolescent's activities and behavior; improving communication among family members; and getting other family members into treatment and/or support programs. Specific engagement procedures have been incorporated as part of many family-based interventions. Other family-based treatments such as MDFT (Liddle et al. 2009) and MST (Henggeler et al. 1999) also have strong engagement goals and components.

Although not ideal, treatment can be effective without participation of the adolescent (Waldron et al. 2001). Similarly, interventions with the adolescent alone or in groups of teenagers (e.g., CBT or CBT plus motivational enhancement therapy) are also effective and are likely the most cost-effective (French et al. 2008). Individual approaches such as CBT, with or without motivational enhancement, have been shown to be efficacious (Azrin et al. 2001; Waldron et al. 2001). Contingency management (CM) approaches using contingency contracting and vouchers also appear to be promising (Stanger and Budney 2010). Evidence is accumulating to support the efficacy of brief interventions, especially as part of SBIRT, for the treatment of substance-using adolescents and those with SUDs. These are generally one to four sessions in duration and are usually based on motivational interviewing (MI) principles (Mitchell et al. 2013) (see Chapter 45, "Motivational Interviewing").

MI is a client-centered counseling style directed at exploring and resolving ambivalence about changing personal behaviors and has been used to target both substance use and pathological use (Naar-King and Suarez 2011; Sussman et al. 2012). A majority of the MI-based interventions tested have resulted in significant improvements in substance use outcomes. Practical application of brief interventions in such venues as primary care (Yuma-Guerrero et al. 2012), emergency departments, and schools potentially extends access to intervention to a large proportion of adolescents. MI-based interventions are also commonly combined with other interventions such as CBT and/or CM (Stanger and Budney 2010).

Twelve-step approaches, using Alcoholics Anonymous (AA) and Narcotics Anonymous (NA) as a basis for treatment, are perhaps the most common approaches for treatment in the United

TABLE 12–4. Evidence-based interventions for adolescents with substance use disorders

Intervention	Type	Population	Reference
Adolescent Community Reinforcement Approach (A-CRA)	Family	Youth ages 13–17 Girls/boys Outpatient/home	Godley et al. 2007
Brief Strategic Family Therapy (BSFT)	Family	Youth ages 13–17 Girls/boys Outpatient/home	Santisteban et al. 1996
Family behavior therapy	Family	Youth ages 13–17 Girls/boys Outpatient/home	Donohue and Azrin 2012
Family support network	Family	Youth ages 13–17 Girls/boys Outpatient/home	Dennis et al. 2004
Functional Family Therapy (FFT)	Family	Youth ages 13–17 Girls/boys Outpatient/home	Waldron et al. 2001
Motivational enhancement therapy (MET)/ Cognitive-behavioral therapy (CBT) 5 or 12	Individual/group	Youth ages 13–17 Girls/boys Outpatient/home	Dennis et al. 2004
MET and motivational interviewing	Individual/group	Youth ages 13–17	
Multidimensional family therapy (MDFT)	Family	Youth ages 13–17 Girls/boys Outpatient/home	Liddle et al. 2009
Multidimensional Treatment Foster Care (MTFC)	Individual/group family	Youth ages 13–17 MTFC foster home	Chamberlain and Reid 1998
Multisystemic Therapy (MST)	Brief Individual	Youth ages 13–17 Home, school, or community	Henggeler et al. 1999

TABLE 12–4. Evidence-based interventions for adolescents with substance use disorders *(continued)*

Intervention	Type	Population	Reference
Teen Intervene	Individual	Youth ages 12–19 Outpatient, school, or juvenile detention setting	Winters et al. 2012
The Seven Challenges Program	Individual	Youth ages 13–17 Outpatient	Stevens et al. 2007
Seeking Safety	Group or individual	Youth ages 13–17 Outpatient, inpatient, residential	Najavits et al. 2006
Parenting with Love and Limits (PLL)	Family	Youth ages 13–17	Smith et al. 2006
Chestnut Health Systems-Bloomington Adolescent Outpatient (OP) and Intensive Outpatient (IOP) Treatment Model	Individual/group	Youth ages 12–18	Godley et al. 2010

States. Naturalistic studies of adolescent SUD treatment find that attendance in aftercare treatment or self-support groups (e.g., AA, NA) is related to positive outcomes (Kelly and Myers 2007) and higher rates of abstinence and other measures of improved outcome when compared with adolescents not participating in such groups following treatment (Kelly et al. 2000).

SUDs are often chronic disorders requiring ongoing intervention. Participation in aftercare services following treatment in a program is related to improved outcomes (Williams et al. 2000). Adolescents attending more intensive aftercare programs involving case management and community reinforcement were more likely than those who did not receive these services to be abstinent from marijuana and to reduce their alcohol use at 3 months postdischarge (Godley et al. 2002). Empirical studies have found aftercare interventions for adolescents with SUDs to be efficacious (Godley et al. 2007). After acute treatment for substance use, ongoing attention should be paid to comorbid psychopathology and other comprehensive needs of the adolescent and his or her family.

Although not specifically an intervention, juvenile drug courts offer an option for youth adjudicated for drug-related offenses to receive SUD treatment rather than juvenile justice placements. Recent research suggests that adolescents in juvenile drug courts received significantly more substance abuse treatment, family-based services, probation supervision, and drug testing than those in outpatient treatment and were significantly more satisfied with treatment (Ives et al. 2010). At follow-up, juvenile drug court participants showed significantly greater reductions in days of substance abuse problems and emotional problems. Much of the ultimate success of drug courts may depend on their ability to identify and refer to high-quality programs using evidence-based interventions (Henggeler et al. 2006).

Treatment of Gambling and Internet Addiction

There are few controlled studies to guide treatment planning for gambling and Internet addiction. On the basis of the parallels between these problems and SUDs, similar approaches appear reasonable pending future studies. Some investigators have proposed modified CBT for adolescent gambling (Derevensky 2007) and for Internet addiction (King et al. 2012). As motivation to desist may be an issue, motivational interviewing or enhancement may be useful as a lead-in or adjunct to specific treatment for these problems. Although the intervention approaches may be similar, such youth should not be treated in SUD programs if they do not have SUDs.

Summary Points

- Clinicians should distinguish among substance use, misuse, abuse, dependence, and diversion.
- Some illicit substance use is normative for many adolescents; however, preoccupation, compulsive use, and/or negative consequences of use indicate potential pathology.

- Risk factors for the development of substance use disorders (SUDs) include individual, peer, and family factors; risk factors are likely not specific for a particular substance but are common across substances.
- While most adolescents start with gateway drugs that are legal for older individuals (e.g., tobacco, alcohol), they may start with other drugs such as marijuana and bypass gateway drugs.
- Comorbidity with other psychiatric disorders is the rule rather than the exception in adolescents with SUDs.
- Comorbid psychiatric disorders should be treated concurrently with SUDs.
- Evidence-based practices for SUDs include specific family therapies, CBT, and motivational interviewing/enhancement.
- Aftercare and involvement in prosocial activities with nondeviant peers are critical following an acute treatment episode.
- Empirically based prevention interventions primarily involve strengthening resilience factors and reducing risk factors for the development of SUDs.

References

American Psychiatric Association: Diagnostic and Statistical Manual of Mental Disorders, 4th Edition. Washington, DC, American Psychiatric Association, 1994

American Psychiatric Association: Diagnostic and Statistical Manual of Mental Disorders, 5th Edition. Arlington, VA, American Psychiatric Association, 2013

Armstrong TD, Costello EJ: Community studies on adolescent substance use, abuse, or dependence and psychiatric comorbidity. J Consult Clin Psychol 70(6):1224–1239, 2002 12472299

Azrin NH, Donohue B, Teichner GA, et al: A controlled evaluation and description of individual-cognitive problem solving and family behavior therapies in dually diagnosed conduct-disordered and substance-dependent youth. J Child Adolesc Subst Abuse 11(1):1–43, 2001

Behrendt S, Wittchen HU, Höfler M, et al: Transitions from first substance use to substance use disorders in adolescence: is early onset associated with a rapid escalation? Drug Alcohol Depend 99(1–3):68–78, 2009 18768267

Bukstein OG: Adolescent Substance Abuse: Assessment, Treatment and Prevention Perspectives. New York, Wiley, 1995

Bukstein OG: Attention deficit hyperactivity disorder and substance use disorders, in Behavioral Neuroscience of Attention Deficit Hyperactivity Disorder and Its Treatment (Current Topics in Behavioral Neurosciences). Edited by Stanford C, Tannock R. Berlin, Springer-Verlag, 2011, pp 146–172

Bukstein OG, Horner MS: Management of the adolescent with substance use disorders and comorbid psychopathology. Child Adolesc Psychiatr Clin N Am 19(3):609–623, 2010 20682224

Bukstein OG, Bernet W, Arnold V, et al: Practice parameter for the assessment and treatment of children and adolescents with substance use disorders. J Am Acad Child Adolesc Psychiatry 44(6):609–621, 2005 15908844

Casey BJ, Jones RM: Neurobiology of the adolescent brain and behavior: implications for substance use disorders. J Am Acad Child Adolesc Psychiatry 49(12):1189–1201, quiz 1285, 2010 21093769

Chamberlain P, Reid JB: Comparison of two community alternatives to incarceration for chronic juvenile offenders. Child J Consult Clin Psychol 66(4):624–633, 1998 9735578

Chan YF, Dennis ML, Funk RR: Prevalence and comorbidity of major internalizing and externalizing problems among adolescents and adults presenting to substance abuse treatment. J Subst Abuse Treat 34(1):14–24, 2008 17574804

Charach A, Yeung E, Climans T, et al: Childhood attention-deficit/hyperactivity disorder and future substance use disorders: comparative meta-analyses. J Am Acad Child Adolesc Psychiatry 50(1):9–21, 2011 21156266

Chen CY, Wagner FA, Anthony JC: Marijuana use and the risk of major depressive episode: epidemiological evidence from the United States National Comorbidity Survey. Soc Psychiatry Psychiatr Epidemiol 37(5):199–206, 2002 12107710

Chung T, Martin CS: Classification and short-term course of DSM-IV cannabis, hallucinogen, cocaine, and opioid disorders in treated adolescents. J Consult Clin Psychol 73(6):995–1004, 2005 16392973

Chung T, Martin CS: Adolescent substance use and substance use disorders: prevalence and clinical course, in Clinical Manual of Adolescent Substance Abuse Treatment. Edited by Kaminer Y, Winters KC. Arlington, VA, American Psychiatric Publishing, 2011, pp 1–23

Clark DB, Neighbors BD, Lesnick LA, et al: Family functioning and adolescent alcohol use disorders. J Fam Psychol 12(1):81–92, 1998

Compton MT, Kelley ME, Ramsay CE, et al: Association of pre-onset cannabis, alcohol, and tobacco use with age at onset of prodrome and age at onset of psychosis in first-episode patients. Am J Psychiatry 166(11):1251–1257, 2009 19797432

Cornelius JR, Maisto SA, Martin CS, et al: Major depression associated with earlier alcohol relapse in treated teens with AUD. Addict Behav 29(5):1035–1038, 2004 15219354

Degenhardt L, Coffey C, Romaniuk H, et al: The persistence of the association between adolescent cannabis use and common mental disorders into young adulthood. Addiction 108(1):124–133, 2013 15501373

Dennis M, Godley SH, Diamond G, et al: The Cannabis Youth Treatment (CYT) Study: main findings from two randomized trials. J Subst Abuse Treat 27(3):197–213, 2004

Derevensky JL: Gambling behaviors, in Adolescent Substance Abuse: Psychiatric Comorbidity and High Risk Behaviors. Edited by Kaminer Y, Bukstein OG. New York, Haworth Press, 2007, pp 403–433

Donohue B, Azrin NH: Treating Adolescent Substance Abuse Using Family Behavior Therapy: A Step-by-Step Approach. Hoboken, NJ, Wiley, 2012

French MT, Zavala SK, McCollister KE, et al: Cost-effectiveness analysis of four interventions for adolescents with a substance use disorder. J Subst Abuse Treat 34(3):272–281, 2008 17600651

Godley MD, Godley SH, Dennis ML, et al: Preliminary outcomes from the assertive continuing care experiment for adolescents discharged from residential treatment. J Subst Abuse Treat 23(1):21–32, 2002 12127465

Godley MD, Godley SH, Dennis ML: The effect of assertive continuing care on continuing care linkage, adherence and abstinence following residential treatment for adolescents with substance use disorders. Addiction 102(1):81–93, 2007 17207126

Godley SH, Garner BR, Passetti LL, et al: Adolescent outpatient treatment and continuing care: main findings from a randomized clinical trial. Drug Alcohol Depend 110(1–2):44–54, 2010 20219293

Goldstein BI, Bukstein OG: Comorbid substance use disorders among youth with bipolar disorder: opportunities for early identification and prevention. J Clin Psychiatry 71(3):348–358, 2010 19961811

Gray KM, Carpenter MJ, Baker NL, et al: Bupropion SR and contingency management for adolescent smoking cessation. J Subst Abuse Treat 40(1):77–86, 2011 20934835

Gray KM, Carpenter MJ, Baker NL, et al: A double-blind randomized controlled trial of N-acetylcysteine in cannabis-dependent adolescents. Am J Psychiatry 169(8):805–812, 2012a 22706327

Gray KM, Carpenter MJ, Lewis AL, et al: Varenicline versus bupropion XL for smoking cessation in older adolescents: a randomized, double-blind pilot trial. Nicotine Tob Res 14:234–239, 2012b

Grella CE, Hser YI, Joshi V, et al: Drug treatment outcomes for adolescents with comorbid mental and substance use disorders. J Nerv Ment Dis 189(6):384–392, 2001 11434639

Henggeler SW, Pickrel SG, Brondino MJ: Multisystemic treatment of substance-abusing and dependent delinquents:

outcomes, treatment fidelity, and transportability. Ment Health Serv Res 1(3):171–184, 1999 11258740

Henggeler SW, Halliday-Boykins CA, Cunningham PB, et al: Juvenile drug court: enhancing outcomes by integrating evidence-based treatments. J Consult Clin Psychol 74(1):42–54, 2006 16551442

Hopfer C, Salomonsen-Sautel S, Mikulich-Gilbertson S, et al: Conduct disorder and initiation of substance use: a prospective longitudinal study. J Am Acad Child Adolesc Psychiatry 52(5):511–518, e4, 2013 23622852

Hser YI, Grella CE, Hubbard RL, et al: An evaluation of drug treatments for adolescents in 4 US cities. Arch Gen Psychiatry 58(7):689–695, 2001 11448377

Ives ML, Chan Y-F, Modisette KC, et al: Characteristics, needs, services, and outcomes of youths in juvenile treatment drug courts as compared to adolescent outpatient treatment. Drug Court Review 7:10–56, 2010

Johnston LD, O'Malley PM, Bachman JG, et al: Monitoring Future National Survey Results On Drug Use, 1975–2013, Vol 1: Secondary School Students. Ann Arbor, Institute for Social Research, University of Michigan, 2014. Available at: http://monitoringthefuture.org//pubs/monographs/mtf-vol1_2013.pdf. Accessed July 3, 2014.

Kaminer Y, Bukstein OG: Adolescent Substance Abuse: Psychiatric Comorbidity and High Risk Behaviors. New York, Routledge Mental Health, 2008

Kandel D, Yamaguchi K: Stages of drug involvement in the U.S. population, in Stages and Pathways of Drug Involvement: Examining the Gateway Hypothesis. Edited by Kandel D. New York, Cambridge University Press, 2002, pp 65–89

Kelly JF, Myers MG: Adolescents' participation in Alcoholic Anonymous and Narcotics Anonymous: Review, implications and future directions. J Psychoactive Drugs 39(3):259–269, 2007 18159779

Kelly JF, Myers MG, Brown SA: A multivariate process model of adolescent 12-step attendance and substance use outcome following inpatient treatment. Psychol Addict Behav 14(4):376–389, 2000 11130156

Kendler KS, Jacobson KC, Prescott CA, et al: Specificity of genetic and environmental risk factors for use and abuse/dependence of cannabis, cocaine, hallucinogens, sedatives, stimulants, and opiates in male twins. Am J Psychiatry 160(4):687–695, 2003 12668357

King DL, Delfabbro PH, Griffiths MD, et al: Cognitive-behavioral approaches to outpatient treatment of Internet addiction in children and adolescents. J Clin Psychol 68(11):1185–1195, 2012 22976240

Knight JR, Sherritt L, Shrier LA, et al: Validity of the CRAFFT substance abuse screening test among adolescent clinic patients. Arch Pediatr Adolesc Med 156(6):607–614, 2002 12038895

Kosterman R, Hawkins JD, Guo J, et al: The dynamics of alcohol and marijuana initiation: patterns and predictors of first use in adolescence. Am J Public Health 90(3):360–366, 2000 10705852

Kuss DJ, Van Rooij AJ, Shorter GW, et al: Internet addiction in adolescents: prevalence and risk factors. Comput Human Behav 29(5):1987–1996, 2013

Lee SS, Humphreys KL, Flory K, et al: Prospective association of childhood attention-deficit/hyperactivity disorder (ADHD) and substance use and abuse/dependence: a meta-analytic review. Clin Psychol Rev 31(3):328–341, 2011 21382538

Leeman RF, Potenza MN: Similarities and differences between pathological gambling and substance use disorders: a focus on impulsivity and compulsivity. Psychopharmacology (Berl) 219(2):469–490, 2012 22057662

Levy S, Siqueira LM, Committee on Substance Abuse, et al: Testing for drugs of abuse in children and adolescents. Pediatrics 133:e1798–e1807, 2014

Liddle HA, Rowe CL, Dakof GA, et al: Multidimensional family therapy for young adolescent substance abuse: twelve-month outcomes of a randomized controlled trial. J Consult Clin Psychol 77(1):12–25, 2009 19170450

Liu TC, Desai RA, Krishnan-Sarin S, et al: Problematic Internet use and health in adolescents: data from a high school survey in Connecticut. J Clin Psychiatry 72(6):836–845, 2011 21536002

Lynskey MT, Agrawal A, Heath AC: Genetically informative research on adolescent substance use: methods, findings, and challenges. J Am Acad Child Adolesc Psychiatry 49(12):1202–1214, 2010 21093770

Marsch LA, Bickel WK, Badger GJ, et al: Comparison of pharmacological treatments for opioid-dependent adolescents: a randomized controlled trial. Arch Gen Psychiatry 62(10):1157–1164, 2005 16203961

Mitchell SG, Gryczynski J, O'Grady KE, et al: SBIRT for adolescent drug and alcohol use: current status and future directions. J Subst Abuse Treat 44(5):463–472, 2013 23352110

Moolchan ET, Robinson ML, Ernst M, et al: Safety and efficacy of the nicotine patch and gum for the treatment of adolescent tobacco addiction. Pediatrics 115(4):e407–e414, 2005 15805342

Naar-King S, Suarez M: Motivational Interviewing With Adolescents and Young Adults. New York, Guilford, 2011

Najavits LM, Gallop RJ, Weiss RD: Seeking safety therapy for adolescent girls with PTSD and substance use disorder: a randomized controlled trial. J Behav Health Serv Res 33(4):453–463, 2006 16858633

National Institute on Drug Abuse: Preventing Drug Use Among Children and Adolescents: A Research-Based Guide for Parents, Educators, and Community Leaders, 2nd Edition. Rockville, MD, National Institute on Drug Abuse/National Institutes of Health, 2003

National Institute on Drug Abuse: Principles of Adolescent Substance Use Disorder Treatment: A Research-Based Guide. Bethesda, MD, National Institute on Drug Abuse, 2014. Available at: http://www.drugabuse.gov/sites/default/files/podata_1_17_14.pdf. Accessed July 7, 2014.

Pompili M, Serafini G, Innamorati M, et al: Substance abuse and suicide risk among adolescents. Eur Arch Psychiatry Clin Neurosci 262(6):469–485, 2012 23304731

Rohde P, Lewinsohn PM, Kahler CW, et al: Natural course of alcohol use disorders from adolescence to young adulthood. J Am Acad Child Adolesc Psychiatry 40(1):83–90, 2001 11195569

Santisteban DA, Szapocznik J, Perez-Vidal A: Efficacy of intervention for engaging youth and families into treatment and some variables that may contribute to differential effectiveness. J Fam Psychol 10:35–944 1996

Smith TE, Sells SP, Rodman J, et al: Reducing adolescent substance abuse and delinquency: pilot research of a family oriented psycho-education curriculum. J Child Adolesc Subst Abuse 15(4):105–115, 2006

Stanger C, Budney AJ: Contingency management approaches for adolescent substance use disorders. Child Adolesc Psychiatr Clin N Am 19(3):547–562, 2010 19951806

Stevens SJ, Schwebel R, Ruiz B: The Seven Challenges: an effective treatment for adolescents with co-occurring substance abuse and mental health problems. J Soc Work Pract Addict 7(3):29–49, 2007

Stinchfield R: Reliability of adolescent self-reported pretreatment alcohol and other drug use. Subst Use Misuse 32(4):425–434, 1997 9090804

Stinchfield R: A critical review of adolescent problem gambling assessment instruments. Int J Adolesc Med Health 22(1):77–93, 2010 20491419

Substance Abuse and Mental Health Services Administration: Results from the 2012 National Household Survey on Drug Use and Health: National Findings. Rockville, MD, Office of Applied Studies, 2013. Available at: http://archive.samhsa.gov/data/NSDUH/2012SummNatFindDetTables/NationalFindings/NSDUHresults2012.htm. Accessed July 3, 2014.

Sussman S, Sun P, Rohrbac LA, et al: One-year outcomes of a drug abuse prevention program for older teams and emerging adults: evaluating a motivational interviewing booster. Health Psychol 31(4):476–485, 2012 21988096

Swendsen J, Burstein M, Case B, et al: Use and abuse of alcohol and illicit drugs in US adolescents: results of the National Comorbidity Survey–Adolescent Supplement. Arch Gen Psychiatry 69(4):390–398, 2012 22474107

Tanner-Smith EE, Wilson SJ, Lipsey MW: The comparative effectiveness of outpatient treatment for adolescent substance abuse: a meta-analysis. J Subst Abuse Treat 44(2):145–158, 2013 22763198

Tarter RE, Vanyukov M, Kirisci L, et al: Predictors of marijuana use in adolescents before and after licit drug use: examination of the gateway hypothesis. Am J Psychiatry 163(12):2134–2140, 2006 17151165

Upadhyaya H, Deas D, Brady K: A practical clinical approach to the treatment of nicotine dependence in adolescents. J Am Acad Child Adolesc Psychiatry 44(9):942–946, 2005 16113623

Waldron HB, Turner CW: Evidence-based psychosocial treatments for adolescent substance abuse. J Clin Child Adolesc Psychol 37(1):238–261, 2008 18444060

Waldron HB, Slesnick N, Brody JL, et al: Treatment outcomes for adolescent substance abuse at 4- and 7-month assessments. J Consult Clin Psychol 69(5):802–813, 2001 11680557

Welte JW, Barnes GM, Tidwell MC, et al: The prevalence of problem gambling among U.S. adolescents and young adults: results from a national survey. J Gambl Stud 24(2):119–133, 2008

Williams RJ, Chang SY, Addiction Centre Adolescent Research Group: A comprehensive and comparative review of adolescent substance abuse treatment outcome. Clinical Psychology: Science & Practice 7:138–166, 2000

Winters KC, Kaminer Y: Screening and assessing adolescent substance use disorders in clinical populations. J Am Acad Child Adolesc Psychiatry 47(7):740–744, 2008 18574399

Winters KC, Stinchfield RD, Henly GA, et al: Validity of adolescent self-report of alcohol and other drug involvement. Int J Addict 25(11A):1379–1395, 1990–1991 2132719

Winters KC, Fahnhorst T, Botzet A, et al: Brief intervention for drug-abusing adolescents in a school setting: outcomes and mediating factors. J Subst Abuse Treat 42(3):279–288, 2012 22000326

Woody GE, Poole SA, Subramaniam G, et al: Extended vs short-term buprenorphine-naloxone for treatment of opioid-addicted youth: a randomized trial. JAMA 300(17):2003–2011, 2008 18984887

Yellowlees PM, Marks S: Problematic Internet use or Internet addiction? Comput Human Behav 23(3):1447–1450, 2007

Yuma-Guerrero PJ, Lawson KA, Velasquez MM, et al: Screening, brief intervention, and referral for alcohol use in adolescents: a systematic review. Pediatrics 130(1):115–122, 2012 22665407

CHAPTER 13

Depressive and Disruptive Mood Dysregulation Disorders

Boris Birmaher, M.D.
David A. Brent, M.D.

Definition, Clinical Description, and Diagnosis

Depressive disorders are familial recurrent illnesses associated with significant morbidity and mortality. Early identification and effective treatment may reduce the impact of depression on the child's normal development and psychosocial functioning and reduce the risk for suicide and other conditions such as substance abuse.

The criteria for *major depressive disorder* (MDD) used in this chapter are consistent with DSM-5 (American Psychiatric Association 2013). However, it is important to note that all existing research is based on prior versions of DSM. What was referred to as *dysthymic disorder* (DD) in DSM-IV (American Psychiatric Association 1994) now falls under the category of *persistent depressive disorder,* which includes both chronic MDD and the previous DD. Unless specified, in this chapter the term *depression* encompasses MDD and persistent depressive disorder. However, since there are few clinical studies for the treatment of persistent depressive disorders and dysthymic disorder in youths, the information included in this chapter, particularly regarding treatment, pertains mainly to MDD. DSM-5 also includes a new disorder in the depressive disorders section: *disruptive mood dysregulation disorder* (DMDD), which is discussed at the end of this chapter.

Unless specified, the term *youth* refers to both children and adolescents.

Depressive Disorders

Epidemiology

The prevalence of MDD is approximately 2% in children and 4%–8% in adolescents, with a male-female ratio of 1:1 during childhood and 1:2 during adolescence (Birmaher et al. 1996). The risk for depression increases by a factor of two to four after puberty, particularly in females, and the cumulative prevalence by age 18 is approximately 20% in community samples. Approximately 5%–10% of children and adolescents have subsyndromal symptoms of MDD. These youth have considerable psychosocial impairment and high family loading for depression. They are at increased risk for suicide and developing full symptoms of depression (Birmaher et al. 1996).

There are no studies of persistent depressive disorder. The few epidemiological studies that include DD report a prevalence of 0.6%–1.7% in children and 1.6%–8.0% in adolescents (Birmaher et al. 1996).

Clinical Description

Currently, the diagnosis of MDD in youth is made according to the DSM-5 criteria (Box 13–1) or the ICD-10 (World Health Organization 1992). The DSM-5 criteria for MDD are similar to the DSM-IV criteria with the exception that bereavement is no longer an exclusion criterion because the risk factors, phenomenology, and course of depression are similar in depressions associated with bereavement and those that are not (Hamdan et al. 2012). Thus, bereavement is now considered a severe stressor that can precipitate a major depressive episode.

Box 13–1. DSM-5 Diagnostic Criteria for Major Depressive Disorder

A. Five (or more) of the following symptoms have been present during the same 2-week period and represent a change from previous functioning; at least one of the symptoms is either (1) depressed mood or (2) loss of interest or pleasure.

Note: Do not include symptoms that are clearly attributable to another medical condition.

1. Depressed mood most of the day, nearly every day, as indicated by either subjective report (e.g., feels sad, empty, hopeless) or observation made by others (e.g., appears tearful). (**Note:** In children and adolescents, can be irritable mood.)
2. Markedly diminished interest or pleasure in all, or almost all, activities most of the day, nearly every day (as indicated by either subjective account or observation).
3. Significant weight loss when not dieting or weight gain (e.g., a change of more than 5% of body weight in a month), or decrease or increase in appetite nearly every day. (**Note:** In children, consider failure to make expected weight gain.)
4. Insomnia or hypersomnia nearly every day.
5. Psychomotor agitation or retardation nearly every day (observable by others, not merely subjective feelings of restlessness or being slowed down).
6. Fatigue or loss of energy nearly every day.
7. Feelings of worthlessness or excessive or inappropriate guilt (which may be delusional) nearly every day (not merely self-reproach or guilt about being sick).
8. Diminished ability to think or concentrate, or indecisiveness, nearly every day (either by subjective account or as observed by others).
9. Recurrent thoughts of death (not just fear of dying), recurrent suicidal ideation without a specific plan, or a suicide attempt or a specific plan for committing suicide.

B. The symptoms cause clinically significant distress or impairment in social, occupational, or other important areas of functioning.
C. The episode is not attributable to the physiological effects of a substance or to another medical condition.

Note: Criteria A–C represent a major depressive episode.

Note: Responses to a significant loss (e.g., bereavement, financial ruin, losses from a natural disaster, a serious medical illness or disability) may include the feelings of intense sadness, rumination about the loss, insomnia, poor appetite, and weight loss noted in Criterion A, which may resemble a depressive episode. Although such symptoms may be understandable or considered appropriate to the loss, the presence of a major depressive episode in addition to the normal response to a significant loss should also be carefully considered. This decision inevitably requires the exercise of clinical judgment based on the individual's history and the cultural norms for the expression of distress in the context of loss.[1]

D. The occurrence of the major depressive episode is not better explained by schizoaffective disorder, schizophrenia, schizophreniform disorder, delusional disorder, or other specified and unspecified schizophrenia spectrum and other psychotic disorders.
E. There has never been a manic episode or a hypomanic episode.

   Note: This exclusion does not apply if all of the manic-like or hypomanic-like episodes are substance-induced or are attributable to the physiological effects of another medical condition.

Coding and Recording Procedures

The diagnostic code for major depressive disorder is based on whether this is a single or recurrent episode, current severity, presence of psychotic features, and remission status. Current severity and psychotic features are only indicated if full criteria are currently met for a major depressive episode. Remission specifiers are only indicated if the full criteria are not currently met for a major depressive episode. Codes are as follows:

Severity/course specifier	Single episode	Recurrent episode*
Mild ([DSM-5] p. 188)	296.21 (F32.0)	296.31 (F33.0)
Moderate ([DSM-5] p. 188)	296.22 (F32.1)	296.32 (F33.1)
Severe ([DSM-5] p. 188)	296.23 (F32.2)	296.33 (F33.2)
With psychotic features** ([DSM-5] p. 186)	296.24 (F32.3)	296.34 (F33.3)

[1] In distinguishing grief from a major depressive episode (MDE), it is useful to consider that in grief the predominant affect is feelings of emptiness and loss, while in MDE it is persistent depressed mood and the inability to anticipate happiness or pleasure. The dysphoria in grief is likely to decrease in intensity over days to weeks and occurs in waves, the so-called pangs of grief. These waves tend to be associated with thoughts or reminders of the deceased. The depressed mood of MDE is more persistent and not tied to specific thoughts or preoccupations. The pain of grief may be accompanied by positive emotions and humor that are uncharacteristic of the pervasive unhappiness and misery characteristic of MDE. The thought content associated with grief generally features a preoccupation with thoughts and memories of the deceased, rather than the self-critical or pessimistic ruminations seen in MDE. In grief, self-esteem is generally preserved, whereas in MDE feelings of worthlessness and self-loathing are common. If self-derogatory ideation is present in grief, it typically involves perceived failings vis-à-vis the deceased (e.g., not visiting frequently enough, not telling the deceased how much he or she was loved). If a bereaved individual thinks about death and dying, such thoughts are generally focused on the deceased and possibly about "joining" the deceased, whereas in MDE such thoughts are focused on ending one's own life because of feeling worthless, undeserving of life, or unable to cope with the pain of depression.

Severity/course specifier	Single episode	Recurrent episode*
In partial remission ([DSM-5] p. 188)	296.25 (F32.4)	296.35 (F33.41)
In full remission ([DSM-5] p. 188)	296.26 (F32.5)	296.36 (F33.42)
Unspecified	296.20 (F32.9)	296.30 (F33.9)

*For an episode to be considered recurrent, there must be an interval of at least 2 consecutive months between separate episodes in which criteria are not met for a major depressive episode. The definitions of specifiers are found on the indicated pages.
**If psychotic features are present, code the "with psychotic features" specifier irrespective of episode severity

In recording the name of a diagnosis, terms should be listed in the following order: major depressive disorder, single or recurrent episode, severity/psychotic/remission specifiers, followed by as many of the following specifiers without codes that apply to the current episode.

Specify:

With anxious distress ([DSM-5] p. 184)
With mixed features ([DSM-5] pp. 184–185)
With melancholic features ([DSM-5] p. 185)
With atypical features ([DSM-5] pp. 185–186)
With mood-congruent psychotic features ([DSM-5] p. 186)
With mood-incongruent psychotic features ([DSM-5] p. 186)
With catatonia ([DSM-5] p. 186). **Coding note:** Use additional code 293.89 (F06.1).
With peripartum onset ([DSM-5] pp. 186–187)
With seasonal pattern (recurrent episode only) ([DSM-5] pp. 187–188)

Source. Reprinted from the *Diagnostic and Statistical Manual of Mental Disorders*, 5th Edition. Arlington, VA, American Psychiatric Association, 2013. Used with permission.

Overall, the clinical picture of MDD in children and adolescents is similar to that in adults, but there are some differences that can be attributed to the child's psychosocial developmental stage (Birmaher et al. 1996; Lewinsohn et al. 2003b; Luby et al. 2004; Yorbik et al. 2004). For example, children, when compared with adolescents, tend to be more irritable and present with low frustration tolerance, temper tantrums, somatic complaints, hallucinations, and/or social withdrawal instead of verbalizing feelings of depression. Adolescents may also show the above symptoms, but they usually have more melancholic symptoms and suicide attempts.

Subtypes of MDD have prognostic and treatment implications (Birmaher et al. 1996; Hughes et al. 2007). DSM-5 added a new specifier *with mixed features* to denote the presence of at least three manic symptoms that are insufficient to satisfy criteria for a manic or hypomanic episode. Youth with mixed features respond less to treatment for depression and may be at risk of developing bipolar disorder. Also, to emphasize the presence of anxiety and because comorbidity with anxiety predicts better response to the combination of cognitive-behavioral therapy (CBT) plus medication versus medication alone (Asarnow et al. 2009), a *with anxious distress* specifier was added. *Psychotic depression* has been associated with family history of bipolar disorder and psychotic depression, more severe depression, greater long-term morbidity, resistance to antidepressant monotherapy, and, most notably, increased risk of bipolar disorder. MDD can be manifested with *atypical symptoms* such as increased reactivity to rejection, lethargy (leaden paralysis), increased appetite, craving for carbohydrates, and hypersomnia. Youth with *seasonal affective disorder* have symptoms of depression mainly during the season with less daylight. However, seasonal affective disorder should be differentiated from depression triggered by school stress because both usually coincide with the school calendar.

The DSM-5 criteria for persistent depressive disorder are enumerated in Box 13–2. This disorder now includes DD and consists of a long-term change in mood that generally is less intense but more chronic than in MDD. It is often overlooked or misdiagnosed. Prior studies showed that although the symptoms of DD are not as severe as in MDD, DD is associated with more psychosocial impairment than MDD (Kovacs et al. 1994; Masi et al. 2001).

Box 13–2. DSM-5 Diagnostic Criteria for Persistent Depressive Disorder (Dysthymia)

300.4 (F34.1)

This disorder represents a consolidation of DSM-IV-defined chronic major depressive disorder and dysthymic disorder.

A. Depressed mood for most of the day, for more days than not, as indicated by either subjective account or observation by others, for at least 2 years.

   Note: In children and adolescents, mood can be irritable and duration must be at least 1 year.

B. Presence, while depressed, of two (or more) of the following:

   1. Poor appetite or overeating.
   2. Insomnia or hypersomnia.
   3. Low energy or fatigue.
   4. Low self-esteem.
   5. Poor concentration or difficulty making decisions.
   6. Feelings of hopelessness.

C. During the 2-year period (1 year for children or adolescents) of the disturbance, the individual has never been without the symptoms in Criteria A and B for more than 2 months at a time.

D. Criteria for a major depressive disorder may be continuously present for 2 years.

E. There has never been a manic episode or a hypomanic episode, and criteria have never been met for cyclothymic disorder.

F. The disturbance is not better explained by a persistent schizoaffective disorder, schizophrenia, delusional disorder, or other specified or unspecified schizophrenia spectrum and other psychotic disorder.

G. The symptoms are not attributable to the physiological effects of a substance (e.g., a drug of abuse, a medication) or another medical condition (e.g. hypothyroidism).

H. The symptoms cause clinically significant distress or impairment in social, occupational, or other important areas of functioning.

Note: Because the criteria for a major depressive episode include four symptoms that are absent from the symptom list for persistent depressive disorder (dysthymia), a very limited number of individuals will have depressive symptoms that have persisted longer than 2 years but will not meet criteria for persistent depressive disorder. If full criteria for a major depressive episode have been met at some point during the current episode of illness, they should be given a diagnosis of major depressive disorder. Otherwise, a diagnosis of other specified depressive disorder or unspecified depressive disorder is warranted.

Specify if:

With anxious distress ([DSM-5] p. 184)
With mixed features ([DSM-5] pp. 184–185)
With melancholic features ([DSM-5] p. 185)
With atypical features ([DSM-5] pp. 185–186)
With mood-congruent psychotic features ([DSM-5] p. 186)
With mood-incongruent psychotic features ([DSM-5] p. 186)
With peripartum onset ([DSM-5] pp. 186–187)

Specify if:

In partial remission ([DSM-5] p. 188)
In full remission ([DSM-5] p. 188)

Specify if:

Early onset: If onset is before age 21 years.
Late onset: If onset is at age 21 years or older.

Specify if (for most recent 2 years of persistent depressive disorder):

With pure dysthymic syndrome: Full criteria for a major depressive episode have not been met in at least the preceding 2 years.

With persistent major depressive episode: Full criteria for a major depressive episode have been met throughout the preceding 2-year period.

With intermittent major depressive episodes, with current episode: Full criteria for a major depressive episode are currently met, but there have been periods of at least 8 weeks in at least the preceding 2 years with symptoms below the threshold for a full major depressive episode.

With intermittent major depressive episodes, without current episode: Full criteria for a major depressive episode are not currently met, but there has been one or more major depressive episodes in at least the preceding 2 years.

Specify current severity:

Mild ([DSM-5] p. 188)
Moderate ([DSM-5] p. 188)
Severe ([DSM-5] p. 188)

Source. Reprinted from the *Diagnostic and Statistical Manual of Mental Disorders*, 5th Edition. Arlington, VA, American Psychiatric Association, 2013. Used with permission.

Comorbidity

Depending on the setting, source of referral, and methodology used to ascertain comorbid disorders, 40%–90% of youth with depressive disorders also have other psychiatric disorders, with up to 50% having two or more comorbid diagnoses. The most frequent comorbid diagnoses are anxiety disorders, followed by disruptive disorders, attention-deficit/hyperactivity disorder (ADHD), and, in adolescents, substance use disorders. Depressive disorders usually manifest after the onset of other psychiatric disorders (e.g., anxiety), but depression also increases the risk for the development of nonmood psychiatric problems such as conduct and substance abuse disorders (Angold et al. 1999; Birmaher et al. 1996; Fombonne et al. 2001; Lewinsohn et al. 2003b). MDD and DD may occur together (the so-called "double depression"), and either disorder can be accompanied by medical or neurological illness.

Etiology, Mechanisms, and Risk Factors

As evidenced by high-risk, bottom-up (families of depressed youth), adoption, and twin studies, MDD runs in families (Birmaher et al. 1996; Caspi et al. 2003; Kendler et al. 2005; Pilowsky et al. 2006; Weissman et al. 2006a). In fact, the single most predictive factor associated with the risk of developing MDD is high family loading for this disorder (Birmaher et al. 1996). The heritability of MDD is about 40%–60% (Craddock et al. 2005), with evidence that vulnerability to depression interacts with stressful life events to result in depressive symptoms. In some reports, people who are homozygous or heterozygous for the less functional allele for the neuronal serotonin presynaptic reuptake site are most likely to develop MDD when they are also exposed to recurrent negative life events (Caspi et al. 2003; Kendler et al. 2005). Thus, the onset and/or recurrences of major depression may be precipitated by the presence of stressors such as losses, physical or sexual abuse, neglect, ongoing conflicts, exposure to violence, and frustrations. The effects of these stressors also depend on the child's cognitive and coping styles with stress, IQ, socioeconomic status, family and social support, and perhaps other genetic factors. For example, subjects who have negative cognitive styles and a tendency toward rumination and hopelessness are at high risk to become depressed when exposed to negative life events (the cognitive vulnerability-transactional stress model) (Alloy and Abramson 2007).

Parental history of other disorders such as anxiety and substance abuse and the youth's characteristics such as prior history of depression, subsyndromal depressive symptoms, presence of other psychiatric disorders (e.g., anxiety, substance abuse, ADHD, eating disorders), medical illness (e.g., diabetes), medications (e.g., corticosteroids), and sociocultural factors have also been related to the development and maintenance of depressive symptomatology (Alloy and Abramson 2007; Birmaher et al. 1996; Caspi et al. 2003; Costello et al. 2002; Kendler et al. 2005; Pine et al. 1998; Reinherz et al. 2003; Weissman et al. 2006a, 2006b).

Neurochemical, inflammation, neuroimaging, and to a lesser extent genetic studies are promising but not yet relevant to clinical practice (Hulvershorn et al. 2011; Zalsman et al. 2006). For example, neuroimaging studies have shown that depressed youth have disturbances in the circuits associated with cognitive and emotional regulation of mood.

Prevention

Strategies for the prevention of onset or recurrence of depression include the amelioration of risk factors such as subsyndromal symptoms of depression, underlying psychiatric disorders (e.g., anxiety disorders), ongoing stressful situations, and parental psychopathology (Birmaher et al. 1996; Horowitz and Garber 2006). The relationship between stress or conflict and depression is often bidirectional. Depression can make a person more irritable, which then increases interpersonal tension, causing others to distance themselves from the depressed person, which then leads the patient to experience loneliness and lack of support. Involvement in deviant peer groups may lead to antisocial behavior, generating more stressful life events and increasing the likelihood of depression (Fergusson et al. 2003). Thus, for those with recurrent depression, a proactive plan to avoid and/or cope with ongoing or anticipated difficulties may be helpful to diminish or prevent the risk for relapse and recurrence. Also, early identification of signs and symptoms of depression may help to abort relapses or new episodes of depression.

Successful treatment of mothers with depression was associated with significantly fewer new psychiatric diagnoses and higher remission rates of existing disorders in their children (Pilowsky et al. 2008; Weissman et al. 2006b). Maternal depression has also been associated with less response in youth to CBT for depression (Brent et al. 1998). These findings support the importance of early identification of depressed mothers in primary care or psychiatric clinics and vigorous treatment (Gunlicks and Weissman 2008).

Meta-analysis evaluated 30 studies of psychoeducation; cognitive, coping, and social skills; and family therapy to assess efficacy of the prevention of new onset or worsening of depressive symptomatology in general populations (universal studies) or youth at high risk of developing MDD because of parental depression or subsyndromal depression (Horowitz and Garber 2006). Programs for populations at risk were more effective than those targeting general populations, particularly for females and older subjects. However, the effects of these treatments were small to modest, both immediately postintervention and at an average follow-up of 6 months.

Early-onset dysthymia is associated with an increased risk of MDD (Kovacs et al. 1994), indicating the need for early treatment. Also, there is evidence that anxiety disorder is a precursor of depression (Birmaher et al. 1996; Pine et al. 1998; Weissman et al. 2006a), and treatment of anxiety may reduce the onset and recurrences of depression (Dadds et al. 1999; Hayward et al. 2000). Since selective serotonin reuptake inhibitors (SSRIs) appear to have much greater efficacy for anxiety than for depression, vigorous detection and treatment of anxiety disorders may reduce the risk for subsequent depression.

Finally, although less well studied, prevention may include lifestyle modifications—regular and adequate sleep, exercise, a coping plan for stress (e.g., meditation, yoga, exercise, social activities), pursuit of enjoyable and meaningful activities, and avoidance of situations that are predictably stressful and nonproductive.

Clinical Course and Outcome

The median duration of a major depressive episode in clinically referred youth is about 8 months and in community samples about 1–2 months. Although most children and adolescents recover from their first depressive episode, longitudinal studies of both clinical and community samples of depressed youth have shown that the probability of recurrence reaches 20%–60% by 1–2 years after remission and climbs to 70% after 5 years (Birmaher et al. 2002; Costello et al. 2002). Recurrences can persist throughout life, and a substantial proportion of children and adolescents with MDD will continue to have MDD episodes as adults. For the most part, the predictors of recovery, relapse, and recurrence overlap. In general, greater severity, chronicity or multiple recurrent episodes, comorbidity, hopelessness, presence of residual subsyndromal symptoms, presence of manic/hypomanic symptoms, negative cognitive style, family problems, low socioeconomic status, and exposure to ongoing negative events (e.g., abuse, family conflict) are associated with poor outcome (Birmaher et al. 2002, 2007).

Childhood depression, compared with adolescent-onset depression, appears to be more heterogeneous. Some children have a strong family history of mood disorders and high risk for recurrences, whereas others are more likely to develop behavior problems and substance abuse than depression (Birmaher et al. 2002). About 20%–40% of depressed youth develop bipolar disorder. Those with high risk of developing bipolar disorder seem to have more psychotic depression, family history of depression, and pharmacologically induced mania or hypomania (Birmaher et al. 2002; see Chapter 14, "Bipolar Disorder").

Childhood DD (persistent depressive disorder) has a protracted course, with a mean episode length of approximately 3–4 years for clinical and community samples, and is associated with an increased risk for subsequent MDD and substance use disorders (Birmaher et al. 2002; Kovacs et al. 1994).

If untreated, depressive disorders affect the development of a child's emotional, cognitive, and social skills and interfere considerably with family relationships (Birmaher et al. 1996, 2002; Lewinsohn et al. 2003a). Suicide attempts and completion are among the most significant and devastating sequelae of MDD, with approximately 60% reporting having thought about suicide and 30% actually attempting suicide (Brent et al. 1999; see Chapter 27, "Youth Suicide"). The risk for suicidal behavior increases if there is a history of suicide attempts, comorbid psychiatric disorders (e.g., disruptive disorders, substance abuse), impulsivity and aggression, availability of lethal agents (e.g., firearms), exposure to negative events (e.g., physical or sexual abuse, violence), or family history of suicidal behavior.

Youth with depressive disorders are also at high risk for substance abuse (including nicotine dependence); legal problems; exposure to negative life events; physical illness; early pregnancy; and poor work, academic, and psychosocial functioning. After an acute episode of depression, a slow and gradual improvement in psychosocial functioning may occur unless there are relapses or recurrences. However, psychosocial difficulties and subsyndromal depressive symptoms frequently persist after the remission of the depressive episode, underscoring the need for continuing treatment for the depression as well as treatment that addresses associated psychosocial and contextual issues (Fergusson and Woodward 2002; Fergusson et al. 2005; Hammen et al. 2004; Lewinsohn et al. 2003a).

Evaluation

General Considerations

The most useful tool for diagnosing depressive disorders is a comprehensive psychiatric diagnostic evaluation that is sensitive to the child's developmental stage, sex, race, environmental conditions, and cultural and religious background. No biological or imaging tests are clinically validated for the diagnosis of depression.

The evaluation should ascertain information from both the child and the parents regarding DSM-5 or ICD-10 (World Health Organization 1992) symptoms and subtypes of depressive disorders (e.g., seasonal, psychotic), bipolar depression, other psychiatric and medical disorders, current and past treatments (types, dose, response, side effects), the child's current and past psychosocial functioning (e.g., school, family, social), the child's and family's strengths, exposure to acute and ongoing stressful life events (e.g., conflicts, abuse, exposure to violence), and family psychiatric and medical history (See Part I, "Assessment and Diagnosis," in this book).

In the first episode of depression, it is difficult to differentiate unipolar major depression from the depressive phase of bipolar disorder. Certain indicators such as high family loading for bipolar disorder, psychosis, subclinical symptoms of mania/hypomania, and history of pharmacologically induced mania or hypomania may herald the development of bipolar disorder (Birmaher et al. 1996). It is important to evaluate carefully for the presence of subtle or short-duration hypomanic symptoms because these symptoms often are overlooked, and these children and adolescents may be more likely to become manic when treated with antidepressant medications (Martin et al. 2004). However, it is also important to note that 5%–10% of children who receive an antidepressant may become "disinhibited." Not all of these children will develop bipolar disorder (Wilens et al. 1998).

Depressive disorders need to be differentiated from other psychiatric (e.g., anxiety, ADHD, oppositional defiant disorder, autism spectrum disorder, substance use disorder, premenstrual dysphoric disorder) and medical (e.g., hypothyroidism, mononucleosis, anemia, certain cancers, autoimmune diseases, chronic fatigue syndrome) disorders, as well as conditions such as depressive reactions to stressors (adjustment disorder). However, stressors may trigger an episode of MDD. Finally, there are chronic medical conditions that appear to have higher rates of depression, such as those involving the central nervous system (e.g., migraine, epilepsy) and those with prominent inflammatory components (e.g., asthma, inflammatory bowel disease). Also, the above conditions may mimic or induce symptoms of depression such as poor self-esteem, demoralization, tiredness, sleep disturbances, and poor concentration. Medications (e.g., stimulants, corticosteroids, contraceptives) can also induce depression-like symptomatology. A depressive disorder is not diagnosed unless the youth meets the criteria.

Suicidal ideation and behaviors are very common in youth with depressive disorders. Thus, it is crucial to evaluate their presence before, during, and after treatment as well as the risks (e.g., age, sex, stressors, comorbid conditions, hopelessness, impulsivity) and protective factors (e.g., religious belief, concern not to hurt family) that might influence the desire to attempt suicide (see Chapter 27). The presence of guns or other potential suicidal (or homicidal) methods in the home should be ascertained, and the clinician should recommend that the parents secure or remove them (Brent et al. 1993b). Clinicians should also differentiate suicidal behavior from other types of self-harm behaviors, the goal of which is to relieve negative affect. Nonsuicidal self-injury most commonly involves repetitive self-cutting, with clear motivation to relieve anger, sadness, or loneliness rather than to end one's life.

Homicidal ideation and behaviors may occur in youth with depressive symptoms and co-occur with suicidal ideation in the same individuals. About one-third of adolescent suicide victims in one study had homicidal ideation in the week before their suicide (Brent et al.

1993a). Thus, clinicians must conduct an assessment similar to that described for suicidal ideation with regard to what factors are influencing, either positively or negatively, the degree of likelihood the patient will carry out a homicidal act.

Finally, the clinician, together with the child and parents, should evaluate the appropriate intensity and restrictiveness of care (e.g., hospitalization). The decision for the level of care will depend primarily on levels of function and safety to self and others, which in turn are determined by the severity of depression, presence of suicidal and/or homicidal symptoms, psychosis, substance dependence, agitation, child's and parents' adherence to treatment, parental psychopathology, and family environment.

Instruments

Standardized structured and semistructured interviews such as the Diagnostic Interview Schedule for Children (DISC; Shaffer et al. 2000), the Schedule for Affective Disorders and Schizophrenia (KSADS; Kaufman et al. 1997), and the Anxiety Disorders Interview Schedule (ADIS; Silverman and Albano 1996) are available for the evaluation of psychiatric symptoms in children older than 7 years and more recently in younger children. The interviews are typically too long to be carried out in nonresearch settings and require special training.

In the assessment of the onset and course of mood disorders, it is helpful to use a mood diary and a mood timeline that use school years, birthdays, holidays, and significant events as anchors. Mood is rated from very happy to very sad and/or as very irritable to nonirritable. Normative and non-normative stressors as well as treatments are noted. The mood timeline can help children and their parents to visualize the course of their mood and comorbid conditions, identify events that may have triggered the depression, and examine the relationship between treatment and response.

Clinician-based scales such as the Children's Depression Rating Scale, Revised (CDRS-R; Poznanski and Mokros 1995), the Hamilton Depression Rating Scale (HDRS; Hamilton 1960), and parent and child self-report instruments such as the Mood and Feelings Questionnaire (Daviss et al. 2006), the Children's Depression Inventory (CDI; Kovacs 1985), and the Beck Depression Inventory (Beck et al. 1961) may be useful to assess the severity of the depressive symptoms before, during, and after treatment. Also, there are several mobile applications that can be used to track mood symptomatology.

Clinician-based and self-report scales to evaluate for the presence of comorbid disorders (e.g., anxiety, ADHD, substance abuse) are also indicated (see other chapters in Part II, "Neurodevelopmental and Other Psychiatric Disorders").

Treatment

The treatment of depression is usually divided into three phases: acute, continuation, and maintenance (Birmaher et al. 2007). The main goal of the acute phase is to achieve response and ultimately *full* symptomatic remission. (For definitions of outcome, see Table 13–1.) Continuation treatment is required for all depressed youth to consolidate the response to treatment and avoid relapses. Finally, maintenance treatment is used to avoid recurrences or new episodes (Emslie et al. 2008; Kennard et al. 2008).

The choice of treatment at each phase should be governed by factors such as age and cognitive development; severity and subtype of depression; chronicity;

TABLE 13–1. Definitions of outcome

	Definition
Response	No symptoms or a significant reduction in depressive symptoms for at least 2 weeks
Remission	A period of at least 2 weeks and less than 2 months with no or very few depressive symptoms
Recovery	Absence of significant symptoms of depression (e.g., no more than one to two symptoms) for 2 months
Relapse	A DSM episode of depression during the period of remission
Recurrence	Emergence of symptoms of depression during the period of recovery (a new episode)

comorbid conditions; family psychiatric history; family and social environment; family and patient treatment preference and expectations; ethnic, cultural, and religious issues; and availability of expertise in pharmacotherapy and/or psychotherapy. During all treatment phases, clinicians should arrange frequent follow-up contacts that allow sufficient time to monitor the subject's clinical status (e.g., symptoms of depression, development of mania or hypomania, comorbid disorders, functioning) and environmental conditions.

Treatment response is usually defined as the absence of MDD criteria (e.g., no more than one DSM symptom) or a significant reduction (e.g., 50%) in symptom severity. However, using the latter criterion, patients deemed "responders" may still have considerable residual symptoms. Therefore, an absolute final score on the CDRS-R (Poznanski and Mokros 1995) of 28 or lower, together with persistent improvement in the patient's functioning for at least 2 weeks or longer, may better reflect a satisfactory response. Overall improvement has also been measured using the Clinical Global Impression Scale, Improvement subscale (Guy 1976).

Since the goal is to restore function and not just reduce symptoms, a lack of progress in functional status is an important clue that the depression is incompletely treated or that impaired functional status is due to a comorbid psychiatric or medical disorder or environmental factors. Functional improvement can be tracked using a score of 70 or greater on the Global Assessment of Functioning (GAF; American Psychiatric Association 2013) or the Children's Global Assessment Scale (Shaffer et al. 1983).

If a patient is being treated with medication, it is important to evaluate adherence to medication treatment, presence of side effects, and youth and parent beliefs about the medication's benefits and its side effects that may contribute to poor adherence or premature discontinuation of treatment. History of suicidality, homicidal ideation, or somatic symptoms should be evaluated before starting the pharmacological treatment, to assist in differentiating from symptoms of mood and other psychiatric or medical conditions or medication side effects during treatment.

Psychoeducation and Supportive Management

Each phase of treatment should include psychoeducation, supportive management for the family and patient, and school involvement (Birmaher et al. 2007; see also Chapter 40, "Parent Counseling, Psychoeducation, and Parent Support Groups"). Parents and patient (and sometimes teachers) should be enlisted as collaborators in the diagnosis and treatment plan. Family members, the patient, and, if appropriate, school personnel should be educated about the causes, symptoms, course, and treatments of depression and the risks associated with these treatments as well as the risks of no treatment. Also, written material and reliable Web sites about depression and its treatment can be provided. Psychoeducation improves adherence to treatment and reduces the symptoms of depression (Ackerson et al. 1998; Brent et al. 1993c; Goodyer et al. 2007; Renaud et al. 1998; Sanford et al. 2006). For families with depressed parents, psychoeducation with or without further interventions improves the ability of families to solve problems around parental illness and children's behavior and attitudes.

The clinician and the family may need to advocate for school accommodations (e.g., schedule, workload) until recovery has been achieved. However, if after recovery the child continues to have academic difficulties, then the clinician should suspect the presence of subclinical symptoms of depression or comorbid conditions (e.g., developmental learning disorders, ADHD, anxiety, substance abuse, bipolar disorder) or environmental factors that might explain the child's persistent difficulties. Students with a depressive disorder may qualify for the emotional disturbance disability categorization under the Individuals With Disabilities Education Act and therefore be eligible to receive school-based services (e.g., counseling) and accommodations that enable them to continue to learn (see Chapter 48, "School-Based Interventions").

It is crucial to involve the family to ascertain symptoms, assure that the youth is safe and adherent to treatment, and monitor progress and possible pharmacological side effects. Interventions with the family must take into account the family's cultural and religious background and focus on strengthening the relationship between the identified patient and caregiver(s), provide parenting guidance (e.g., management of conflicts), reduce family dysfunction, and facilitate treatment referral for caregivers or siblings with psychiatric disorders and for marital conflict (Birmaher et al. 2000; Garber et al. 2002; Hammen et al. 2004; Nomura et al. 2002).

Evidence that supportive management may help comes from pharmacotherapy and psychotherapy randomized controlled trials (RCTs), which have shown that up to an average of 50%–60% of children and adolescents with MDD respond to placebo (Bridge et al. 2007). Moreover, 15%–30% respond to very brief nonspecific treatments (Goodyer et al. 2007; Renaud et al. 1998). Thus, it is reasonable, for a patient with a mild or brief depression, mild psychosocial impairment, and the absence of clinically significant suicidality or psychosis, to begin treatment with education, support, and case management related to environmental stressors in the family and school. Response is expected after 4–6 weeks of supportive therapy. However, when patients do not respond to supportive management; are more severely depressed; and have significant melancholic symptoms, hopelessness, or suicidal ideation/behaviors, supportive treatment is insufficient (Barbe et al. 2004b; March et al. 2004; Mufson et al. 1999; Renaud et al. 1998), and these youth need a trial of specific psychotherapy and/or antidepressants.

Acute Treatment

Although it is still not clear which treatment is best for a particular youth with acute MDD, the choice of treatment may be dictated by availability, patient and family preference, or clinical presentation (e.g., a very irritable or a psychotic or agitated depressed child will not be able to engage in psychotherapy).

Psychotherapy

Several types of psychotherapy are being used for the treatment of youth with depression. However, only CBT and interpersonal psychotherapy (IPT) have evidence of efficacy from RCTs, particularly for depressed adolescents (Weisz et al. 2006; see also Chapter 43, "Interpersonal Psychotherapy for Depressed Adolescents," and Chapter 44, "Cognitive-Behavioral Treatment for Anxiety and Depression"). Psychodynamic therapy is widely used in clinical practice despite lack of evidence for efficacy. Because family interaction is related to the onset and course of adolescent depression (Birmaher et al. 2000; Nomura et al. 2002; Pilowsky et al. 2006), the improvement of family interactions is a logical treatment target in adolescent depression. While one RCT examined the impact of family therapy and found that CBT was superior to systemic behavioral family therapy in the short-term reduction of adolescent depression (Brent et al. 1997), more recently, attachment-based family therapy was shown to be superior to supportive clinical management for depressed youth (Diamond et al. 2010). Also, IPT is emerging as another efficacious psychotherapy for adolescent depression, especially in patients who are moderately or severely depressed and in older teens (Mufson et al. 2004; see also Chapter 43). While IPT as formulated by Mufson and colleagues is an individual treatment, it has a strong dyadic (parent-child) component focusing on parent-child discord. IPT has been shown to be more efficacious than CBT in one study and less efficacious than CBT in another in study by the same research group (Rosselló et al. 2008). IPT appears to be easy to disseminate, insofar as therapists in school-based health clinics with brief training and supervision were able to improve depression using IPT compared with treatment as usual (Mufson et al. 2004).

In general, the overall effects of specific psychotherapy for the acute treatment of depressed youth, when compared with a control psychosocial treatment of comparable intensity, are modest (d=0.35) (Weisz et al. 2006). The few psychotherapy studies that included follow-up after acute treatment showed that the beneficial effects of psychotherapy appear durable for the initial months, but results of different types of interventions tend to converge over time, in part because of the effects of open treatment provided in these studies. Use of CBT during the continuation phase to prevent relapse appears to be promising as an intervention (Kennard et al. 2008). Thus, more studies are needed to evaluate the effects of "boosters" and continuation therapy. Also, few studies have assessed suicidality as an outcome. On average, these studies showed a small reduction in suicidality without clear specific treatment effects, emphasizing the need for more targeted techniques to address this worrisome symptom (Stanley et al. 2009; Weisz et al. 2006). Finally, the effects of the psychotherapy for depressed youth also improved anxiety but not externalizing symptoms, indicating the need for modified psychotherapy techniques to manage comorbid disruptive disorders.

The most widely studied type of psychotherapy for the treatment of youth with MDD is CBT. This psychotherapy is effective and appears to be more efficacious even in the face of comorbidity, suicidal ideation, and hopelessness. However, when there is a history of sexual abuse or when one of the parents is depressed, CBT does not appear to perform as well (Asarnow et al. 2009; Barbe et al. 2004a). Clinical trials also suggest that CBT can be delivered effectively in primary care settings to depressed children and adolescents and results in better outcomes than treatment as usual (Asarnow et al. 2005; Weersing et al. 2006).

In contrast with most CBT studies, a large RCT (Treatment for Adolescents With Depression Study [TADS]) did not find differences between CBT and placebo for adolescents with MDD after 12 weeks of treatment (March et al. 2004), although CBT was superior to placebo when assessed 18 weeks post-initiation of treatment (March et al. 2007). Moreover, while the combination of CBT and fluoxetine showed a more rapid decline in depressive symptoms and better baseline-adjusted endpoint outcomes, rates of clinical improvement were not different among groups (Kennard et al. 2006; Kratochvil et al. 2006). Also, the combined treatment was better than fluoxetine alone mainly for mild to moderate depression and for depression with high levels of cognitive distortion but not for severe depression (Curry et al. 2006). The combination treatment did result in a greater rate of remission than in any of the other treatments, but the effects were modest (remission rate 37% in combined treatment) (Kennard et al. 2006). It is unclear why CBT did not differ from placebo in this study with regard to acute treatment. Possible explanations include that the adolescents were not blind to medication assignment in the two CBT cells and that treatment delivered a "low dose" of a large number of skills and techniques, whereas some of the more successful treatment studies with CBT used a flexible protocol that focused mainly on cognitive restructuring and behavior activation (Weisz et al. 2006). Other RCTs examining the effects of combined treatment versus medication alone have also been disappointing. Goodyer et al. (2007) found that in moderately to severely depressed adolescents who did not respond to a brief psychosocial treatment, the combination of CBT plus an SSRI was no better than the SSRI alone in relief of depressive symptoms or improvement in overall outcome. Melvin et al. (2006) were unable to demonstrate the superiority of combined sertraline and CBT over either treatment alone for adolescents with mild to moderate depression, although this study was underpowered to detect differences among active treatments. After acute treatment, CBT was found to be superior to sertraline alone, which may suggest an advantage to CBT but might also be explained by the relatively low sertraline dose. Clarke et al. (2005) compared the addition of CBT to SSRI management in primary care and found some modest improvement on quality of life but not on the primary outcome. Moreover, an unexpected result of the combined treatment was that those patients were more likely to discontinue their SSRIs. Finally, recent meta-analyses showed that for adolescents with MDD, combination treatment was better than antidepressant monotherapy for functional outcome but not for suicidality or depression (Dubicka et al. 2010).

Most of the above-noted clinical trials were carried out with adolescents rather than younger children. However, randomized CBT trials for symptomatic volunteers have suggested that this therapy may be useful for younger children (Weisz et al. 2006). Most clinicians recommend the adaptation of cognitive, interpersonal, and psychodynamic techniques for younger children. In addition, because of the prominent role of family issues in early onset depression and the greater dependency of the child on parents, some form of family intervention is recommended. However, no RCTs of psychotherapy have been conducted in clinically referred depressed children.

Pharmacotherapy

Efficacy

A meta-analysis of all published and unpublished pharmacological RCTs for MDD in youth showed an average response rate of 61% (95% confidence interval [CI], 58%–63%) for the SSRI antidepressants and 50% (95% CI, 47%–53%) for placebo, yielding a risk difference of 11% (95% CI, 7%–15%) (Bridge et al. 2007). Using these data, the number needed to treat to yield one response attributable to active treatment was 10 overall (95% CI, 7%–15%). Several studies showed small or no differences between the SSRI and placebo, in part because the rates of placebo response were high. This was more obvious in depressed children than adolescents. Thus, it is possible that depressive symptoms in youth may be highly responsive to supportive management; these studies included subjects with mild depression; or other methodological issues, such as low medication doses, are responsible for the lack of difference between medication and placebo. Interestingly, the difference between the responses to SSRIs and placebo was inversely related to the number of sites involved in the study (Bridge et al. 2007).

Fluoxetine showed a larger difference between medication and placebo than other antidepressants and is the only agent that also shows superiority to placebo in prepubertal depressed youth. This may be due to actual differences in the effect of the fluoxetine or other related properties of this medication (e.g., long half-life may lessen the effect of poor adherence to treatment) or because the studies involving fluoxetine were better designed and conducted or included more severely depressed patients.

The rate of remission, usually defined as a CDRS-R score of 28, ranged between 30% and 40% (Bridge et al. 2005). Possible explanations for this low rate are that it may take longer to observe higher rates of remission after response, optimal pharmacological treatment may involve a higher dose or longer duration of treatment, the lack of treatment of comorbid conditions might affect depressive symptoms, and/or some children and adolescents need to receive a combination of pharmacological and psychosocial interventions.

Few trials have evaluated the effects of other classes of antidepressants for the treatment of depressed youth (Hughes et al. 2007). RCTs have shown no differences between venlafaxine or mirtazapine and placebo (Bridge et al. 2007). Secondary analysis of the venlafaxine trials showed an age effect, with drug being better than placebo for depressed adolescents but not depressed children. However, children were treated with low doses (Emslie et al. 2007). One study showed better response in most measurements between nefazodone and placebo for adolescents with MDD, but a second study including depressed children and adolescents was negative. Finally, RCTs as well as a meta-analysis have shown that tricyclic antidepressants (TCAs) are no more efficacious than placebo for the treatment of child and adolescent depression (Hazell et al. 2002). For this reason, as well as side effect profile and fatality after an overdose, TCAs should be far down the list of choices for treatment of youth depression.

Side Effects

The side effects of antidepressants are described in Chapter 36, "Antidepressants." Of these side effects, in addition to the rare risk of triggering hypomania in certain children, the most serious side effect of the antidepressants is the small but statistically significant risk of onset or worsening of suicidal ideation and, more rarely, suicide attempts. A meta-analysis that reanalyzed the U.S. Food and Drug Administration (FDA) analyses (Hammad et al. 2006), including more published and unpublished antidepressant RCTs and using more appropriate statistical analyses (Bridge et al. 2007), found that for MDD, obsessive-compulsive disorder (OCD), and non-OCD anxiety disorders, the pooled risk difference for new or increased *spontaneously reported* suicidal ideation or suicidal behaviors for all antidepressants (SSRIs, venlafaxine, and bupropion) to be 0.7% (95% CI, 0.1%–1.3%). This and other studies have suggested that 1–3 in 100 youth exposed to antidepressants had a new or worsening spontaneously reported suicidal ideation or behavior. There were very few suicide attempts and *no completed suicides*. Interestingly, when the analyses were done for each disorder separately, there were no significant differences between the antidepressants and placebo. For example, for MDD the rates of suicidal ideation/attempts were 3% (95% CI, 2%–4%) for those taking the antidepressants and 2% (95% CI, 1%–2%) for those receiving placebo, yielding a risk difference of 1% (95% CI, –0.1%–2%). Using these data, the number of depressed subjects needed to treat to observe one adverse event (number needed to "harm") that can be attributed to the active treatment for antidepressants was 112 (Bridge et al. 2007).

In contrast to the analyses of *spontaneously* suicidal reported adverse events, evaluation of suicidal ideation and attempts ascertained through rating scales in 17 studies did not show significant onset or worsening of suicidality (risk ratios approximately 0.90) (Hammad et al. 2006). Most recently, a large pharmacoepidemiological naturalistic study found that youth ages 24 years and younger who were started at above the modal dose for an antidepressant (e.g., 40 mg of fluoxetine) were more likely to engage in deliberate self-harm than those started at the usual dose (Miller et al. 2014). However, it is possible that more severe cases received higher doses of antidepressants. In any case, it is good practice to begin antidepressant treatment at the equivalent of 10 mg of fluoxetine, then increase to 20 mg for the next 3 weeks and reevaluate to see if the patient responds or might benefit from further dose increases (Birmaher et al. 2007).

As stated by the FDA (Hammad et al. 2006), the implications and clinical significance regarding the findings noted earlier are uncertain, since coincident with the increase in use of SSRIs there had been a dramatic decline in adolescent suicide (Olfson et al. 2003). In contrast, after the black box warning for all antidepressants was imposed by the FDA, the prescription of antidepressants diminished (Libby et al. 2007), and although not proven to be due to the reduction of antidepressant use, the rates of suicide increased (Hamilton et al. 2007). Pharmacoepidemiological studies, while correlative rather than causal, support a positive relationship between SSRI use and the reduction in the adolescent and young adult suicide rate (Gibbons et al. 2006; Valuck et al. 2004). Also, a study showed increased suicide attempts only immediately before the SSRIs were administered (Simon and Savarino 2007) and, as in TADS, a decreased rate of attempts after treatment was initiated. However, as noted previously, higher dosages of antidepressants were found to be associated with increased risk for self-harm (Miller et al. 2014).

In summary, in acute RCTs, the SSRIs and venlafaxine minimally but statistically significantly increase *spontaneously* reported suicidal ideation and, to a lesser extent, suicide attempts. Nevertheless, given the greater number of patients who benefit from SSRIs than those who experience these side effects, the lack of any completed suicides in the RCTs, and the decline in overall suicidality seen on rating scales, the risk-benefit ratio for carefully monitored SSRI use in pediatric depression appears to be favorable.

Continuation Treatment

The few continuation pharmacotherapy and psychotherapy studies suggest that the relapse rate is higher in youth who do not continue treatment, particularly in those with residual symptoms (Brent et al. 2001; Emslie et al. 2008). Given these data, together with the fact that the rate of relapse is very high even after successful acute treatment, it is recommended that after acute response every child and adolescent should continue treatment for at least 6–12 months (Birmaher et al. 2007). There is also evidence that a wellness-oriented CBT delivered during continuation medication treatment adds further protection against relapse (Kennard et al. 2008).

When indicated, discontinuation can be tried during the summer so that a relapse would be less disruptive to school function. However, it is important to note that the treatment for depression can also be helping other disorders (e.g., anxiety) and that medication discontinuation may accelerate the symptoms of these other conditions. During the continuation phase, patients typically are seen at least monthly, depending on clinical status, functioning, support systems, environmental stressors, motivation for treatment, and presence of comorbid psychiatric or medical disorders. In this phase, psychotherapy consolidates the skills learned during the acute phase and helps patients cope with the psychosocial sequelae of the depression and also addresses the antecedents, contextual factors, environmental stressors, and internal as well as external conflicts that may contribute to a relapse. Moreover, if the patient is taking antidepressants, follow-up sessions should continue to foster medication adherence, optimize the dose, and evaluate for the presence of side effects.

Maintenance Treatment

Although there are no maintenance studies in youth with depression, once a youth has been asymptomatic for approximately 6–12 months, the clinician must decide whether maintenance therapy is indicated, which therapy, and for how long (Birmaher et al. 2007). Extrapolation from adult studies would suggest that youth with more than two episodes of depression or severe or chronic depression should have maintenance treatment for 1 year or longer. Also, youth with double depression (major depressive disorder comorbid with persistent depressive disorder or DD), subsyndromal symptoms of depression, other psychiatric or medical conditions, psychosis, suicidality, past or ongoing stressors (e.g., abuse, divorce, conflicts), family psychopathology, or lack of community support may also need maintenance treatment. During the maintenance phase, visits may be monthly to quarterly or more frequent, depending on the patient's clinical status, functioning, support systems, environmental stressors, motivation for treatment, existence of comorbid psychiatric/medical disorders, and availability of the clinician.

Use of Antidepressants

The general use of antidepressants is described in Chapter 36; in this subsection we briefly focus on the use of antidepressants for youth with MDD. Overall, it appears that the doses of antidepressants in children and adolescents are similar to those used for adult patients. However, the half-lives of sertraline, citalopram, paroxetine, and sustained-release bupropion are shorter than reported in adults (Axelson et al. 2002; Findling et al. 2006). Therefore, clinicians should be alert to the possibility of daily withdrawal side effects when these medications are prescribed once a day. Also, to avoid side effects and improve adherence to treatment, it is recommended to start with a low dose and increase it slowly until an appropriate dose is reached. Clinical response should be assessed at 4- to 6-week intervals, and if the child has tolerated the antidepressant, the dose may be increased if a complete response has not been obtained (Hughes et al. 2007). At each step, adequate time should be allowed for clinical response, and frequent early dose adjustments should be avoided. By about 12 weeks of treatment, the goal should be remission of symptoms, and in youth who are not remitted by that time, alternative treatment options may be warranted (Birmaher et al. 2007). Although some studies have shown no relationship between drug concentration and clinical response, others have shown that, for citalopram and fluoxetine, higher concentration may increase the probability of response (Sakolsky et al. 2011).

All patients receiving antidepressants should be monitored for the minimal but plausible possibility of worsening or de novo suicidal thoughts and behavior, as well as other side effects. The FDA recommends that depressed youth should be seen every week for the first 4 weeks and biweekly thereafter. However, it is not always possible to schedule weekly face-to-face appointments. In this case, evaluations should be carried out briefly by telephone. It is important to emphasize that there are no data to suggest that either the monitoring schedule proposed by the FDA or telephone calls have any impact on the risk of suicide. Monitoring is important for all patients, but patients at increased risk for suicide (e.g., those with current or prior suicidality, impulsivity, substance abuse, history of sexual abuse, family history of suicide) should be followed particularly closely (Birmaher et al. 2007). Those with a family history of bipolar disorder should be carefully monitored for onset of mania or mixed state. After the continuation and maintenance phases are over, or when the antidepressants need to be discontinued, all antidepressants, except for fluoxetine, should be discontinued slowly. Abrupt discontinuation of antidepressants may induce withdrawal symptoms, some of which may mimic a relapse or recurrence of a depressive episode (e.g., tiredness, irritability, and severe somatic symptoms). Sometimes withdrawal symptoms can be accompanied by worsening or emergent suicidal symptoms. The withdrawal symptoms can appear after as few as 6–8 weeks on an antidepressant and within 24–48 hours of discontinuation.

Careful attention to possible medication interactions is recommended because most antidepressants are metabolized by hepatic cytochrome P450 isoenzymes. In addition, interactions of antidepressants with other serotonergic and/or noradrenergic medications, in particular monoamine oxidase inhibitors, may induce serotonin syndrome, marked by agitation, confusion, and hyperthermia

Treatment of Subtypes of Depression

Psychotic Depression

Extrapolating from adult studies suggests the atypical antipsychotic medications combined with SSRIs as the treatment of choice for depressed youth who are psychotic (Hughes et al. 2007). Vague or mild psychotic symptoms in a depressed youth may respond to antidepressants alone. How long the antipsychotic should be continued after the psychotic symptoms have improved is unclear, but the recommendation is to slowly taper these medications, with the eventual goal of keeping the youth on monotherapy with an antidepressant. If the youth is going to be maintained for long periods of time on both medications, side effects associated with the use of atypical antipsychotics and possible interactions with the antidepressants need to be monitored. Noncontrolled reports suggest that electroconvulsive therapy (ECT) may be useful for depressed psychotic adolescents.

Seasonal Affective Disorder

A small RCT showed that bright light therapy is efficacious for youth with seasonal affective disorder (Swedo et al. 1997). Morning sessions are recommended, but morning hours may be difficult on school days and for youth who refuse to wake up early in the morning. Bright light therapy has been associated with some side effects, such as headaches and eye strain. Some authors have recommended an ophthalmological evaluation before initiating light therapy, but the need for this practice is not established unless the patient has a history of eye illness. Treatment with light may induce episodes of hypomania or mania in vulnerable patients.

Bipolar Depression

Early in the course of illness, it is difficult to determine whether a patient has unipolar or bipolar depression. If a depressed youth has indicators of risk for bipolar disorder such as psychosis or family history of bipolar disorder, the clinician should discuss with the patient and family the pros and cons of initiating mood stabilizers. For mild to moderate unipolar depression in patients with a bipolar diathesis, it may be best to start with psychotherapy because the risk for manic conversion with the use of antidepressants is substantial (Martin et al. 2004). (For further discussion, see Chapter 14.)

Treatment-Resistant Depression

Each of the strategies noted in the previous section requires implementation in a systematic fashion, education of the patient and family, and support and education to reduce the potential for the patient to become hopeless.

Many factors can account for a depressed youth's failure to respond to treatment, including misdiagnosis, unrecognized or untreated comorbid psychiatric or medical disorders (e.g., anxiety, dysthymia, eating disorders, substance use, personality disorders, hypothyroidism), undetected bipolar disorder, inappropriate pharmacotherapy or psychotherapy, inadequate length of treatment or dose, lack of adherence to treatment, medication side effects, exposure to chronic or severe life events (such as sexual abuse or ongoing family conflicts), personal identity issues (such as concern about same-sex attraction), cultural/ethnic factors, and inadequate fit with or skill level of the psychotherapist (Birmaher et al. 1996, 2007; Hughes et al. 2007).

In a National Institute of Mental Health (NIMH) multicenter study, the Treatment of Resistant Depression in Adolescents (TORDIA; Brent et al. 2008), depressed adolescents who failed to respond to an adequate trial with an SSRI were randomly assigned to one of four interventions using a balanced, two-by-two design: switch to another SSRI, switch to venlafaxine, switch to another SSRI plus addition of CBT, or switch to venlafaxine plus CBT. There were no differences in outcome between switching to another SSRI or venlafaxine, although there were more side effects in youth treated with venlafaxine. However, the combination of CBT plus medication was superior to medication alone. This study also identified significant predictors of treatment response, such as drug concentration, adherence, and presence of subsyndromal manic symptoms, and moderators of treatment response, namely, comorbidity, which favored the combination treatment, and a history of abuse, which was associated with a better response to medication monotherapy. On the basis of this study, in depressed youth who do not respond to an adequate trial with an SSRI, the best next step is to switch to another SSRI and to add CBT. This study is one of the few head-to-head comparisons of different antidepressants. Venlafaxine, fluoxetine, and citalopram all had similar response rates.

Several psychopharmacological strategies that have been recommended for adults with resistant depression may be applicable to youth: optimization (extending the initial medication trial and/or adjusting the dose; adding CBT or IPT), switching to another agent in the same or a different class of medications, or a combination (e.g., adding lithium or triiodothyronine) (Hughes et al. 2007). Optimization and augmentation strategies are usually used when patients have shown a partial response to the current regimen, and switching is usually used when patients have not responded to or cannot tolerate the medications, but no studies have validated these practices in children.

Finally, the use of somatic therapies that have not been well studied in children, such as transcranial magnetic stimulation, or more intensive somatic therapies for depressed teens, such as ECT, may be considered.

Management of Comorbid Conditions

There are very few studies to guide the clinician in how to sequence the treatment of depression and comorbid disorders (Hughes et al. 2007). Usually, clinicians make a determination of which condition is causing the greatest distress and functional impairment and begin treatment of that disorder. Also, if recovery from depression is unlikely until a comorbid condition is addressed (e.g., severe malnutrition in anorexia or severe substance dependence, such as cocaine or intravenous drug dependence), then the comorbid condition must be addressed first.

Several psychosocial and pharmacological treatments used to treat depression may also be useful for the treatment of comorbid conditions (e.g., anxiety, substance use disorders, ADHD; see respective chapters in this book). For depressed youth with comorbid substance abuse, it is important to treat both disorders because depressive symptomatology increases the risk of persistent substance abuse and vice versa: substance abuse worsens the prognosis of the depression, and depression comorbid with substance abuse is a potent risk factor for completed suicide. One RCT suggested that 16 weeks of CBT plus fluoxetine was better than CBT plus placebo for the treatment of MDD symptoms in adolescents with substance abuse and conduct disorders (Riggs et al. 2007). Further studies regarding the use of psychosocial and pharmacological treatments for depressed youth with comorbid substance abuse are necessary. Finally, a recent study showed that successful treatment of depression with either a combination of fluoxetine and CBT or fluoxetine monotherapy was accompanied by improvement in anxiety, ADHD, and behavior symptoms (Hilton et al. 2013).

There are few published studies examining the efficacy of psychopharmacological or psychotherapeutic treatments for depression in medically ill children and adolescents. Brief CBT and supportive therapy were equally efficacious for youth with depression comorbid with inflammatory bowel disorder (Szigethy et al. 2010). Studies are necessary, however, because diagnosable depression may occur frequently in children and adolescents with medical diseases, and medical illness and its treatment may change the natural course of depression (Lewinsohn et al. 1996). Furthermore, the pharmacokinetics, pharmacodynamics, and side effects of antidepressants may be affected by both the medical illnesses and the medications used to treat these illnesses. Psychotherapy is useful not only for treating depression in these children but for helping these patients and their families cope with the medical illness (Kovacs et al. 1996; Szigethy et al. 2010).

Disruptive Mood Dysregulation Disorder (DMDD)

DSM-5 includes a new disorder in the category of the depressive disorders, *disruptive mood dysregulation disorder* (DMDD). This disorder is characterized by frequent, severe, recurrent temper outbursts and chronically irritable and/or angry mood, both of which must be present for at least a year and cannot be accounted for by other mood disorders (Box 13–3). DMDD shares many characteristics of ODD, including irritable mood and temper outbursts but not the oppositional component.

Box 13–3. DSM-5 Diagnostic Criteria for Disruptive Mood Dysregulation Disorder

296.99 (F34.8)

A. Severe recurrent temper outbursts manifested verbally (e.g., verbal rages) and/or behaviorally (e.g., physical aggression toward people or property) that are grossly out of proportion in intensity or duration to the situation or provocation.
B. The temper outbursts are inconsistent with developmental level.
C. The temper outbursts occur, on average, three or more times per week.
D. The mood between temper outbursts is persistently irritable or angry most of the day, nearly every day, and is observable by others (e.g., parents, teachers, peers).
E. Criteria A–D have been present for 12 or more months. Throughout that time, the individual has not had a period lasting 3 or more consecutive months without all of the symptoms in Criteria A–D.
F. Criteria A and D are present in at least two of three settings (i.e., at home, at school, with peers) and are severe in at least one of these.

G. The diagnosis should not be made for the first time before age 6 years or after age 18 years.
H. By history or observation, the age at onset of Criteria A–E is before 10 years.
I. There has never been a distinct period lasting more than 1 day during which the full symptom criteria, except duration, for a manic or hypomanic episode have been met.
   Note: Developmentally appropriate mood elevation, such as occurs in the context of a highly positive event or its anticipation, should not be considered as a symptom of mania or hypomania.
J. The behaviors do not occur exclusively during an episode of major depressive disorder and are not better explained by another mental disorder (e.g., autism spectrum disorder, posttraumatic stress disorder, separation anxiety disorder, persistent depressive disorder [dysthymia]).
   Note: This diagnosis cannot coexist with oppositional defiant disorder, intermittent explosive disorder, or bipolar disorder, though it can coexist with others, including major depressive disorder, attention-deficit/hyperactivity disorder, conduct disorder, and substance use disorders. Individuals whose symptoms meet criteria for both disruptive mood dysregulation disorder and oppositional defiant disorder should only be given the diagnosis of disruptive mood dysregulation disorder. If an individual has ever experienced a manic or hypomanic episode, the diagnosis of disruptive mood dysregulation disorder should not be assigned.
K. The symptoms are not attributable to the physiological effects of a substance or to another medical or neurological condition.

Source. Reprinted from the *Diagnostic and Statistical Manual of Mental Disorders*, 5th Edition. Arlington, VA, American Psychiatric Association, 2013. Used with permission.

DMDD was included in DSM-5 primarily to reduce the misdiagnosis of bipolar disorder in children with chronic irritability and temper outbursts but without the episodicity that characterizes bipolar disorder (Axelson 2013). However, the high degree of overlap with symptoms of depression and oppositional defiant disorder has raised questions as to whether DMDD represents a distinct disorder or simply a more severe form of the above-noted existing conditions.

To construct DMDD, the DSM-5 work group used part of the criteria created for severe mood dysregulation (SMD; Leibenluft 2011). SMD also is manifested by chronic irritability, but in contrast to DMDD, it includes some symptoms of ADHD, mania, and depression such as distractibility, insomnia, agitation, racing thoughts, flight of ideas, pressured speech, intrusiveness, and sadness. Youth with SMD are predominantly male (66%), and all have comorbid ADHD and/or ODD. In addition, they tend to have anxiety disorders (58%) and major depressive disorder (16%). When compared with youth with bipolar disorder, youth with SMD did not show mood episodes and had lower familial rates of bipolar disorder, very low rates of manic and hypomanic episodes over follow-up, and a variety of differences in neurocognitive and neuroimaging tests (Leibenluft 2011).

Using a retrospective proxy diagnosis of SMD, a secondary analysis of the Great Smoky Mountains Study showed a prevalence of 1.8% in community youth ages 9–13 years. Youth with SMD had similar demographic and clinical characteristics to those in the NIMH studies but, as expected for a community sample, lower rates of comorbid disorders. Longitudinal follow-up of these youth showed low stability of the diagnosis of SMD and increased risk of developing depressive and anxiety disorders (Leibenluft 2011). Interestingly, similar to the SMD studies, longitudinal follow-up studies of youth with ODD who have high levels of irritability also showed increased risk for depression and anxiety disorders (Rowe et al. 2010; Stringaris et al. 2009).

Using criteria for DMDD retrospectively, analysis of the Duke Preschool Anxiety (ages 2–5), the Great Smoky Mountains (ages 9–13), and the Caring for Children in the Community (ages 9–17) epidemiological studies showed a prevalence of DMDD of 3.3%, 1.1%, and 0.8%, respectively (Copeland et al. 2013). DMDD co-occurred with other disorders in 62%–92% of the cases, particularly with ODD and depressive disorders. Of note, the prevalence of DMDD in children ages 2–5 was higher than in older children, questioning the DSM-5 decision to exclude these children from the diagnosis of DMDD. In a prospective study of the Great Smoky Mountains sample, young adults with a history of a retrospective diagnosis of childhood DMDD showed elevated rates of anxiety and depression and more general psychopathology, health problems, and poor functioning than subjects with no history of childhood psychiatric disorders or subjects meeting criteria for psychiatric disorders other than DMDD in childhood or adolescence (Copeland et al. 2014).

Recently, in a large sample of outpatient youth included in the Longitudinal Assessment of Manic Symptoms study, the prevalence, stability over 2 years, and family history of a retrospective constructed DMDD diagnosis were examined (Axelson et al. 2012). As anticipated, severe recurrent temper outbursts and chronic irritability were common symptoms across all psychiatric disorders. DMDD was highly comorbid with disruptive behavior disorders to the point that it could not be clearly differentiated from oppositional defiant and conduct disorders. DMDD was also present in 40%–50% of youth diagnosed with anxiety, depressive, and bipolar spectrum disorders. DMDD did not show longitudinal stability, and it was not specifically associated with a parental history of ADHD or mood, anxiety, conduct, or substance use disorders. Finally, in this study DMDD at intake did not specifically predict future onset of mood or anxiety disorders over follow-up.

In summary, the scarce literature and the facts that irritable mood and temper outbursts are ubiquitous across psychiatric disorders in youth, DMDD is highly comorbid with other disorders, DSM-5 field studies showed that DMDD had very low reliability (Regier et al. 2013), and the diagnosis of DMDD does not appear to diminish the rate of diagnosis of bipolar disorder (Margulies et al. 2012) raise questions about whether it was premature to include DMDD in DSM-5. Moreover, although the diagnosis of DMDD was established to help clinicians discriminate these phenomena from pediatric bipolar disorder, in fact, the offspring of bipolar parents have increased rates of DMDD relative to the offspring of parents with other psychiatric disorders and healthy control subjects (Sparks et al. 2014). In any case, the controversy about DMDD (and SMD) brought attention to an important subgroup of children with severe mood dysregulation, fostering phenomenology, family, biological, longitudinal, and treatment studies that will shed light on whether this is a real disorder or a phenotype shared by several psychiatric disorders. In the meantime, clinicians should be careful when assessing youth with chronic irritability and temper tantrums, and instead of hastening to diagnose DMDD, they should search for the presence of underlying disorders for which there are known treatments. There are currently no studied treatments for DMDD.

Summary Points

- Depressive disorders are familial recurrent illnesses associated with significant psychosocial morbidity and mortality.
- Depressive disorders have onset during childhood and equally affect males and females. Their prevalence increases after puberty, affecting twice as many females as males.
- There are age differences in the clinical expression of the depressive disorders.
- Although most depressions remit, a substantial proportion of youth experience depressive recurrences.
- The etiology of depressive disorders seems to be determined by the interaction of certain genes with the environment and support systems and the youth's cognitive and coping style.
- There are no biological tests that guide the diagnosis and treatment of depressed youth. The diagnosis is based on a comprehensive evaluation with a youth and other informants, such as parents and teachers.
- The goal of treatment is to achieve remission and good psychosocial functioning and to prevent recurrences.
- During all phases of treatment, depressed youth and their families should be offered education and support. Some mildly depressed youth may respond well to a short course of management with education and support.
- There is evidence that CBT, IPT, and the SSRI antidepressants (in particular, fluoxetine) are efficacious for the treatment of depressed youth. The combination of therapy plus antidepressants seems to be more efficacious for some depressed youth.
- Antidepressants may induce side effects (e.g., agitation, disinhibition, gastrointestinal symptoms, and, in predisposed individuals, mania), and about 1–3 in 100 children and adolescents treated with these medications may show onset or worsening of suicidal ideation and, more rarely, suicide attempts.
- Depending on the severity and chronicity of the depression and other factors (e.g., environment, child and parental motivation, IQ), treatment during the acute phase should include antidepressants and/or psychotherapy. Moderate depression may respond to CBT or IPT alone. More severe depressive episodes will generally require treatment with antidepressants. Treatment with antidepressants may be administered alone until the child is amenable to psychotherapy, or, if appropriate, it can be combined with psychotherapy from the beginning of treatment.

- After successful acute treatment, all youth should be offered continuation treatment with SSRIs and/or psychotherapy for at least 6–12 months to prevent relapses.
- Depressed youth who do not respond to prior monotherapy, either psychotherapy or an antidepressant, require a combination of these two treatment modalities.
- After the continuation phase, some depressed youth, especially those with severe depression or frequent recurrences, should have maintenance treatment with SSRIs and/or psychotherapy for at least 1 year or more to prevent recurrences.
- Management of resistant depression should consider factors associated with poor response to treatment such as poor adherence to treatment, misdiagnoses, ongoing negative life events, and presence of comorbid disorders. In patients who do not respond to an initial trial with an SSRI antidepressant, the recommended next step is to switch to another SSRI and add CBT. Although not well studied, sometimes the combination of medications (e.g., adding bupropion or lithium to the SSRI) or, rarely, ECT may be indicated. Treatment of subtypes of depression, including seasonal, psychotic, and bipolar depression, may require special treatments such as light therapy, antipsychotics, and mood stabilizers, respectively.
- Management of comorbid disorders, ongoing conflicts, and family psychopathology is necessary to achieve remission.
- Studies are needed to evaluate whether DMDD is a distinct condition or simply a more extreme phenotype of depression and/or ODD or a phenotype ubiquitous among several psychiatric disorders. Regardless, management of irritability symptoms and a better understanding of the determinants, course, and treatment are crucial for the well-being of the child and the family.

References

Ackerson J, Scogin F, McKendree-Smith N, et al: Cognitive bibliotherapy for mild and moderate adolescent depressive symptomatology. J Consult Clin Psychol 66(4):685–690, 1998 9735587

Alloy LB, Abramson LY: The adolescent surge of depression and emergence of gender differences: a biocognitive vulnerability-stress model in developmental context, in Adolescent Psychopathology and Developing Brain. Edited by Romer D, Walker EF. New York, Oxford University Press, 2007

American Psychiatric Association: Diagnostic and Statistical Manual of Mental Disorders, 4th Edition. Washington, DC, American Psychiatric Association, 1994

American Psychiatric Association: Diagnostic and Statistical Manual of Mental Disorders, 5th Edition. Arlington, VA, American Psychiatric Association, 2013

Angold A, Costello EJ, Erkanli A: Comorbidity. J Child Psychol Psychiatry 40(1):57–87, 1999 10102726

Asarnow JR, Jaycox LH, Duan N, et al: Effectiveness of a quality improvement intervention for adolescent depression in primary care clinics: a randomized controlled trial. JAMA 293(3):311–319, 2005 15657324

Asarnow JR, Emslie G, Clarke G, et al: Treatment of selective serotonin reuptake inhibitor-resistant depression in adolescents: predictors and moderators of treatment response. J Am Acad Child Adolesc Psychiatry 48(3):330–339, 2009 19182688

Axelson D: Taking disruptive mood dysregulation disorder out for a test drive. Am J Psychiatry 170(2):136–139, 2013 23377631

Axelson DA, Perel JM, Birmaher B, et al: Sertraline pharmacokinetics and dynamics in adolescents. J Am Acad Child Adolesc Psychiatry 41(9):1037–1044, 2002 12218424

Axelson D, Findling RL, Fristad MA, et al: Examining the proposed disruptive mood dysregulation disorder diagnosis in children in the Longitudinal Assessment of Manic Symptoms study. J Clin Psychiatry 73(10):1342–1350, 2012 23140653

Barbe RP, Bridge JA, Birmaher B, et al: Lifetime history of sexual abuse, clinical presentation, and outcome in a clinical trial for adolescent depression. J Clin Psychiatry 65(1):77–83, 2004a 14744173

Barbe RP, Bridge J, Birmaher B, et al: Suicidality and its relationship to treatment outcome in depressed adolescents. Suicide Life Threat Behav 34(1):44–55, 2004b 15106887

Beck AT, Ward CH, Mendelson M, et al: An inventory for measuring depression. Arch Gen Psychiatry 4:561–571, 1961 13688369

Birmaher B, Arbelaez C, Brent D: Course and outcome of child and adolescent major depressive disorder. Child Adolesc Psychiatr Clin N Am 11(3):619–637, x, 2002 12222086

Birmaher B, Ryan ND, Williamson DE, et al: Childhood and adolescent depression: a review of the past 10 years. Part I. J Am Acad Child Adolesc Psychiatry 35(11):1427–1439, 1996 8936909

Birmaher B, Brent DA, Kolko D, et al: Clinical outcome after short-term psychotherapy for adolescents with major depressive disorder. Arch Gen Psychiatry 57(1):29–36, 2000 10632230

Birmaher B, Brent D, Bernet W, et al: Practice parameter for the assessment and treatment of children and adolescents with depressive disorders. J Am Acad Child Adolesc Psychiatry 46(11):1503–1526, 2007 18049300

Brent DA, Perper JA, Moritz G, et al: Firearms and adolescent suicide. A community case-control study. Am J Dis Child 147(10):1066–1071, 1993a 8213677

Brent DA, Johnson B, Bartle S, et al: Personality disorder, tendency to impulsive violence, and suicidal behavior in adolescents. J Am Acad Child Adolesc Psychiatry 32(1):69–75, 1993b 8428886

Brent DA, Poling K, McKain B, et al: A psychoeducational program for families of affectively ill children and adolescents. J Am Acad Child Adolesc Psychiatry 32(4):770–774, 1993c 8340297

Brent DA, Holder D, Kolko D, et al: A clinical psychotherapy trial for adolescent depression comparing cognitive, family, and supportive therapy. Arch Gen Psychiatry 54(9):877–885, 1997 9294380

Brent DA, Kolko DJ, Birmaher B, et al: Predictors of treatment efficacy in a clinical trial of three psychosocial treatments for adolescent depression. J Am Acad Child Adolesc Psychiatry 37(9):906–914, 1998 9735610

Brent DA, Baugher M, Bridge J, et al: Age- and sex-related risk factors for adolescent suicide. J Am Acad Child Adolesc Psychiatry 38(12):1497–1505, 1999 10596249

Brent DA, Birmaher B, Kolko D, et al: Subsyndromal depression in adolescents after a brief psychotherapy trial: course and outcome. J Affect Disord 63(1–3):51–58, 2001 11246080

Brent D, Emslie G, Clarke G, et al: Switching to another SSRI or to venlafaxine with or without cognitive behavioral therapy for adolescents with SSRI-resistant depression: the TORDIA randomized controlled trial. JAMA 299(8):901–913, 2008 18314433

Bridge JA, Salary CB, Birmaher B, et al: The risks and benefits of antidepressant treatment for youth depression. Ann Med 37(6):404–412, 2005 16203613

Bridge JA, Iyengar S, Salary CB, et al: Clinical response and risk for reported suicidal ideation and suicide attempts in pediatric antidepressant treatment: a meta-analysis of randomized controlled trials. JAMA 297(15):1683–1696, 2007 17440145

Caspi A, Sugden K, Moffitt TE, et al: Influence of life stress on depression: moderation by a polymorphism in the 5-HTT gene. Science 301(5631):386–389, 2003 12869766

Clarke G, Debar L, Lynch F, et al: A randomized effectiveness trial of brief cognitive-behavioral therapy for depressed adolescents receiving antidepressant medication. J Am Acad Child Adolesc Psychiatry 44(9):888–898, 2005 16113617

Copeland WE, Angold A, Costello EJ, et al: Prevalence, comorbidity, and correlates of DSM-5 proposed disruptive mood dysregulation disorder. Am J Psychiatry 170(2):173–179, 2013 23377638

Copeland WE, Shanahan L, Egger H, et al: Adult diagnostic and functional outcomes of DSM-5 disruptive mood dysregulation disorder. Am J Psychiatry 171(6):668–674, 2014 24781389

Costello EJ, Pine DS, Hammen C, et al: Development and natural history of mood disorders. Biol Psychiatry 52(6):529–542, 2002 12361667

Craddock N, O'Donovan MC, Owen MJ: The genetics of schizophrenia and bipolar disorder: dissecting psychosis. J Med Genet 42(3):193–204, 2005 15744031

Curry J, Rohde P, Simons A, et al: Predictors and moderators of acute outcome in the Treatment for Adolescents with Depression Study (TADS). J Am Acad Child Adolesc Psychiatry 45(12):1427–1439, 2006 17135988

Dadds MR, Holland DE, Laurens KR, et al: Early intervention and prevention of anxiety disorders in children: results at 2-year follow-up. J Consult Clin Psychol 67(1):145–150, 1999 10028219

Daviss WB, Birmaher B, Melhem NA, et al: Criterion validity of the Mood and Feelings Questionnaire for depressive episodes in clinic and non-clinic subjects. J Child Psychol Psychiatry 47(9):927–934, 2006 16930387

Diamond GS, Wintersteen MB, Brown GK, et al: Attachment-based family therapy for adolescents with suicidal ideation: a randomized controlled trial. J Am Acad Child Adolesc Psychiatry 49(2):122–131, 2010 20215934

Dubicka B, Elvins R, Roberts C, et al: Combined treatment with cognitive-behavioural therapy in adolescent depression: meta-analysis. Br J Psychiatry 197(6):433–440, 2010 21119148

Emslie GJ, Findling RL, Yeung PP, et al: Venlafaxine ER for the treatment of pediatric subjects with depression: results of two placebo-controlled trials. J Am Acad Child Adolesc Psychiatry 46(4):479–488, 2007 17420682

Emslie GJ, Kennard BD, Mayes TL, et al: Fluoxetine versus placebo in preventing relapse of major depression in children and adolescents. Am J Psychiatry 165(4):459–467, 2008 18281410

Fergusson DM, Woodward LJ: Mental health, educational, and social role outcomes of adolescents with depression. Arch Gen Psychiatry 59(3):225–231, 2002 11879160

Fergusson DM, Wanner B, Vitaro F, et al: Deviant peer affiliations and depression: confounding or causation? J Abnorm Child Psychol 31(6):605–618, 2003 14658741

Fergusson DM, Horwood LJ, Ridder EM, et al: Subthreshold depression in adolescence and mental health outcomes in adulthood. Arch Gen Psychiatry 62(1):66–72, 2005 15630074

Findling RL, McNamara NK, Stansbrey RJ, et al: The relevance of pharmacokinetic studies in designing efficacy trials in juvenile major depression. J Child Adolesc Psychopharmacol 16(1–2):131–145, 2006 16553534

Fombonne E, Wostear G, Cooper V, et al: The Maudsley long-term follow-up of child and adolescent depression. 1. Psychiatric outcomes in adulthood. Br J Psychiatry 179:210–217, 2001 11532797

Garber J, Keiley MK, Martin C: Developmental trajectories of adolescents' depressive symptoms: predictors of change. J Consult Clin Psychol 70(1):79–95, 2002 11860059

Gibbons RD, Hur K, Bhaumik DK, et al: The relationship between antidepressant prescription rates and rate of early adolescent suicide. Am J Psychiatry 163(11):1898–1904, 2006 17074941

Goodyer I, Dubicka B, Wilkinson P, et al: Selective serotonin reuptake inhibitors (SSRIs) and routine specialist care with and without cognitive behaviour therapy in adolescents with major depression: randomised controlled trial. BMJ 335(7611):142–146, 2007 17556431

Gunlicks ML, Weissman MM: Change in child psychopathology with improvement in parental depression: a systematic review. J Am Acad Child Adolesc Psychiatry 47(4):379–389, 2008 18388766

Guy W: ECDEU Assessment Manual of Psychopharmacology. U.S. Department of Health, Education, and Welfare Publication (ADM). Rockville, MD, National Institute of Mental Health, Psychopharmacology Research Branch, 1976

Hamdan S, Melhem NM, Porta G, et al: The phenomenology and course of depression in parentally bereaved and non-bereaved youth. J Am Acad Child Adolesc Psychiatry 51(5):528–536, 2012 22525959

Hamilton BE, Miniño AM, Martin JA, et al: Annual summary of vital statistics: 2005. Pediatrics 119(2):345–360, 2007 17272625

Hamilton M: A rating scale for depression. J Neurol Neurosurg Psychiatry 23:56–62, 1960 14399272

Hammad TA, Laughren T, Racoosin J: Suicidality in pediatric patients treated with antidepressant drugs. Arch Gen Psychiatry 63(3):332–339, 2006 16520440

Hammen C, Brennan PA, Shih JH: Family discord and stress predictors of depression and other disorders in adolescent children of depressed and nondepressed women. J Am Acad Child Adolesc Psychiatry 43(8):994–1002, 2004 15266194

Hayward C, Varady S, Albano AM, et al: Cognitive-behavioral group therapy for social phobia in female adolescents: results of a pilot study. J Am Acad Child Adolesc Psychiatry 39(6):721–726, 2000 10846306

Hazell P, O'Connell D, Heathcote D, et al: Tricyclic drugs for depression in children and adolescents. Cochrane Database Syst Rev (2):CD002317, 2002 DOI: 10.1002/14651858.CD002317 12076448

Hilton RC, Rengasamy M, Mansoor B, et al: Impact of treatments for depression on comorbid anxiety, attentional, and behavioral symptoms in adolescents with selective serotonin reuptake inhibitor-resistant depression. J Am Acad Child Adolesc Psychiatry 52(5):482–492, 2013 23622849

Horowitz JL, Garber J: The prevention of depressive symptoms in children and adolescents: a meta-analytic review. J Consult Clin Psychol 74(3):401–415, 2006 16822098

Hughes CW, Emslie GJ, Crismon ML, et al: Texas Children's Medication Algorithm Project: update from Texas Consensus Conference Panel on Medication Treatment of Childhood Major Depressive Disorder. J Am Acad Child Adolesc Psychiatry 46(6):667–686, 2007 17513980

Hulvershorn LA, Cullen K, Anand A: Toward dysfunctional connectivity: a review of neuroimaging findings in pediatric major depressive disorder. Brain Imaging Behav 5(4):307–328, 2011 21901425

Kaufman J, Birmaher B, Brent D, et al: Schedule for Affective Disorders and Schizophrenia for School-Age Children-Present and Lifetime Version (K-SADS-PL): initial reliability and validity data. J Am Acad Child Adolesc Psychiatry 36(7):980–988, 1997 9204677

Kendler KS, Kuhn JW, Vittum J, et al: The interaction of stressful life events and a serotonin transporter polymorphism in the prediction of episodes of major depression: a replication. Arch Gen Psychiatry 62(5):529–535, 2005 15867106

Kennard B, Silva S, Vitiello B, et al: Remission and residual symptoms after short-term treatment in the Treatment of Adolescents with Depression Study (TADS). J Am Acad Child Adolesc Psychiatry 45(12):1404–1411, 2006 17135985

Kennard BD, Emslie GJ, Mayes TL, et al: Cognitive-behavioral therapy to prevent relapse in pediatric responders to pharmacotherapy for major depressive disorder. J Am Acad Child Adolesc Psychiatry 47(12):1395–1404, 2008 18978634

Kovacs M: The Children's Depression Inventory (CDI). Psychopharmacol Bull 21(4):995–998, 1985 4089116

Kovacs M, Akiskal HS, Gatsonis C, et al: Childhood-onset dysthymic disorder. Clinical features and prospective naturalistic outcome. Arch Gen Psychiatry 51(5):365–374, 1994 8179460

Kovacs M, Mukerji P, Iyengar S, et al: Psychiatric disorder and metabolic control among youths with IDDM. A longitudinal study. Diabetes Care 19(4):318–323, 1996 8729153

Kratochvil C, Emslie G, Silva S, et al: Acute time to response in the Treatment for Adolescents with Depression Study (TADS). J Am Acad Child Adolesc Psychiatry 45(12):1412–1418, 2006 17135986

Leibenluft E: Severe mood dysregulation, irritability, and the diagnostic boundaries of bipolar disorder in youths. Am J Psychiatry 168(2):129–142, 2011 21123313

Lewinsohn PM, Seeley JR, Hibbard J, et al: Cross-sectional and prospective relationships between physical morbidity and depression in older adolescents. J Am Acad Child Adolesc Psychiatry 35(9):1120–1129, 1996 8824055

Lewinsohn PM, Rohde P, Seeley JR, et al: Psychosocial functioning of young adults who have experienced and recovered from major depressive disorder during adolescence. J Abnorm Psychol 112(3):353–363, 2003a 12943014

Lewinsohn PM, Pettit JW, Joiner TE Jr, et al: The symptomatic expression of major depressive disorder in adolescents and young adults. J Abnorm Psychol 112(2):244–252, 2003b 12784834

Libby AM, Brent DA, Morrato EH, et al: Decline in treatment of pediatric depression after FDA advisory on risk of suicidality with SSRIs. Am J Psychiatry 164(6):884–891, 2007 17541047

Luby JL, Mrakotsky C, Heffelfinger A, et al: Characteristics of depressed preschoolers with and without anhedonia: evidence for a melancholic depressive subtype in young children. Am J Psychiatry 161(11):1998–2004, 2004 15514399

March J, Silva S, Petrycki S, et al: Fluoxetine, cognitive-behavioral therapy, and their combination for adolescents with depression: Treatment for Adolescents With Depression Study (TADS) randomized controlled trial. JAMA 292(7):807–820, 2004 15315995

March JS, Silva S, Petrycki S, et al: The Treatment for Adolescents With Depression Study (TADS): long-term effectiveness and safety outcomes. Arch Gen Psychiatry 64(10):1132–1143, 2007 17909125

Margulies DM, Weintraub S, Basile J, et al: Will disruptive mood dysregulation disorder reduce false diagnosis of bipolar disorder in children? Bipolar Disord 14(5):488–496, 2012 22713098

Martin A, Young C, Leckman JF, et al: Age effects on antidepressant-induced manic conversion. Arch Pediatr Adolesc Med 158(8):773–780, 2004 15289250

Masi G, Favilla L, Mucci M, et al: Depressive symptoms in children and adolescents with dysthymic disorder. Psychopathology 34(1):29–35, 2001 11150928

Melvin GA, Tonge BJ, King NJ, et al: A comparison of cognitive-behavioral therapy, sertraline, and their combination for adolescent depression. J Am Acad Child Adolesc Psychiatry 45(10):1151–1161, 2006 17003660

Miller M, Swanson SA, Azrael D, et al: Antidepressant dose, age, and the risk of deliberate self-harm. JAMA Intern Med 174(6):899–909, 2014 24782035

Mufson L, Weissman MM, Moreau D, et al: Efficacy of interpersonal psychotherapy for depressed adolescents. Arch Gen Psychiatry 56(6):573–579, 1999 10359475

Mufson L, Dorta KP, Wickramaratne P, et al: A randomized effectiveness trial of interpersonal psychotherapy for depressed adolescents. Arch Gen Psychiatry 61(6):577–584, 2004 15184237

Nomura Y, Wickramaratne PJ, Warner V, et al: Family discord, parental depression, and psychopathology in offspring: ten-year follow-up. J Am Acad Child Adolesc Psychiatry 41(4):402–409, 2002 11931596

Olfson M, Shaffer D, Marcus SC, et al: Relationship between antidepressant medication treatment and suicide in adolescents. Arch Gen Psychiatry 60(10):978–982, 2003 14557142

Pilowsky DJ, Wickramaratne P, Nomura Y, et al: Family discord, parental depression, and psychopathology in offspring: 20-year follow-up. J Am Acad Child Adolesc Psychiatry 45(4):452–460, 2006 16601650

Pilowsky DJ, Wickramaratne P, Talati A, et al: Children of depressed mothers 1 year after the initiation of maternal treatment: findings from the STAR*D-Child Study. Am J Psychiatry 165(9):1136–1147, 2008 18558646

Pine DS, Cohen P, Gurley D, et al: The risk for early adulthood anxiety and depressive disorders in adolescents with anxiety and depressive disorders. Arch Gen Psychiatry 55(1):56–64, 1998 9435761

Poznanski EO, Mokros HB: Children's Depression Rating Scale, Revised (CDRS-R) Manual. Los Angeles, CA, Western Psychological Services, 1995

Regier DA, Kuhl EA, Kupfer DJ: The DSM-5: Classification and criteria changes. World Psychiatry 12(2):92–98, 2013 23737408

Reinherz HZ, Paradis AD, Giaconia RM, et al: Childhood and adolescent predictors of major depression in the transition to adulthood. Am J Psychiatry 160(12):2141–2147, 2003 14638584

Renaud J, Brent DA, Baugher M, et al: Rapid response to psychosocial treatment for adolescent depression: a two-year follow-up. J Am Acad Child Adolesc Psychiatry 37(11):1184–1190, 1998 9808930

Riggs PD, Mikulich-Gilbertson SK, Davies RD, et al: A randomized controlled trial of fluoxetine and cognitive behavioral therapy in adolescents with major depression, behavior problems, and substance use disorders. Arch Pediatr Adolesc Med 161(11):1026–1034, 2007 17984403

Rosselló J, Bernal G, Rivera-Medina C: Individual and group CBT and IPT for Puerto Rican adolescents with depressive symptoms. Cultur Divers Ethnic Minor Psychol 14(3):234–245, 2008 18624588

Rowe R, Costello EJ, Angold A, et al: Developmental pathways in oppositional defiant disorder and conduct disorder. J Abnorm Psychol 119(4):726–738, 2010 21090876

Sakolsky DJ, Perel JM, Emslie GJ, et al: Antidepressant exposure as a predictor of clinical outcomes in the Treatment of Resistant Depression in Adolescents (TORDIA) study. J Clin Psychopharmacol 31(1):92–97, 2011 21192150

Sanford M, Boyle M, McCleary L, et al: A pilot study of adjunctive family psychoeducation in adolescent major depression: feasibility and treatment effect. J Am Acad Child Adolesc Psychiatry 45(4):386–495, 2006 16601642

Shaffer D, Gould MS, Brasic J, et al: A children's global assessment scale (CGAS). Arch Gen Psychiatry 40(11):1228–1231, 1983 6639293

Shaffer D, Fisher P, Lucas CP, et al: NIMH Diagnostic Interview Schedule for Children Version IV (NIMH DISC-IV): description, differences from previous versions, and reliability of some common diagnoses. J Am Acad Child Adolesc Psychiatry 39(1):28–38, 2000 10638065

Silverman W, Albano A: The Anxiety Disorders Interview Schedule for Children–IV (Child and Parent Versions). San Antonio, TX, Psychological Corporation, 1996

Simon GE, Savarino J: Suicide attempts among patients starting depression treatment with medications or psychotherapy. Am J Psychiatry 164(7):1029–1034, 2007 17606654

Sparks GM, Axelson DA, Yu H, et al: Disruptive mood dysregulation disorder and chronic irritability in youth at familial risk for bipolar disorder. J Am Acad Child Adolesc Psychiatry 53(4):408–416, 2014 24655650

Stanley B, Brown G, Brent DA, et al: Cognitive-behavioral therapy for suicide prevention (CBT-SP): treatment model, feasibility, and acceptability. J Am Acad Child Adolesc Psychiatry 48(10):1005–1013, 2009 19730273

Stringaris A, Cohen P, Pine DS, et al: Adult outcomes of youth irritability: a 20-year prospective community-based study. Am J Psychiatry 166(9):1048–1054, 2009 19570932

Swedo SE, Allen AJ, Glod CA, et al: A controlled trial of light therapy for the treatment of pediatric seasonal affective disorder. J Am Acad Child Adolesc Psychiatry 36(6):816–821, 1997 9183137

Szigethy E, McLafferty L, Goyal A: Inflammatory bowel disease. Child Adolesc Psychiatr Clin N Am 19(2):301–318, ix, 2010 20478501

Valuck RJ, Libby AM, Sills MR, et al: Antidepressant treatment and risk of suicide attempt by adolescents with major depressive disorder: a propensity-adjusted retrospective cohort study. CNS Drugs 18(15):1119–1132, 2004 15581382

Weersing VR, Iyengar S, Kolko DJ, et al: Effectiveness of cognitive-behavioral therapy for adolescent depression: a benchmarking investigation. Behav Ther 37(1):36–48, 2006 16942959

Weissman MM, Wickramaratne P, Nomura Y, et al: Offspring of depressed parents: 20 years later. Am J Psychiatry 163(6):1001–1008, 2006a 16741200

Weissman MM, Pilowsky DJ, Wickramaratne PJ, et al: Remissions in maternal depression and child psychopathology: a STAR*D-child report. JAMA 295(12):1389–1398, 2006b 16551710

Weisz JR, McCarty CA, Valeri SM: Effects of psychotherapy for depression in children and adolescents: a meta-analysis. Psychol Bull 132(1):132–149, 2006 16435960

Wilens TE, Wyatt D, Spencer TJ: Disentangling disinhibition. J Am Acad Child Adolesc Psychiatry 37(11):1225–1227, 1998 9808935

World Health Organization: International Classification of Diseases, 10th Revision (ICD-10). Geneva, Switzerland, World Health Organization, 1992

Yorbik O, Birmaher B, Axelson D, et al: Clinical characteristics of depressive symptoms in children and adolescents with major depressive disorder. J Clin Psychiatry 65(12):1654–1659, quiz 1760–1761, 2004 15641870

Zalsman G, Oquendo MA, Greenhill L, et al: Neurobiology of depression in children and adolescents. Child Adolesc Psychiatr Clin N Am 15(4):843–868, vii–viii, 2006 16952764

CHAPTER 14

Bipolar Disorder

Gabrielle A. Carlson, M.D.
Caroly Pataki, M.D.
Stephanie E. Meyer, Ph.D.

Bipolar disorder (BP) clearly exists in children and adolescents (Pavuluri et al. 2005). The relevant issues concern its prevalence, continuity between the various conceptualizations of BP in youth and BP in adults, and the treatment and research implications of missing the diagnosis of BP versus misdiagnosis of another condition as BP.

Definition

Bipolar I disorder (BP-I) is defined by episodes of mania. Bipolar II disorder (BP-II) is characterized by hypomania—briefer duration of manic symptoms with less impairment. In DSM-5 (American Psychiatric Association 2013) other specified or unspecified bipolar and related disorder, manic symptoms are of insufficient number and/or duration to meet mania or hypomania criteria. Depressive episodes, at all levels of severity and duration, need not occur in BP-I but usually do. In BP-II, full major depression occurs with hypomania. Cyclothymic disorder refers to cycles of subsyndromal mania and depression.

Changes in mania criteria in DSM-5 (Box 14–1 and Box 14–2) include the following: 1) "abnormally and persistently increased goal-directed activity or energy" has been added to the "A" criterion of "abnormally and persistently elevated, expansive, or irritable mood." 2) These symptoms should be present "most of the day, nearly every day." 3) Added to the "B" criteria (i.e., other symptoms of mania) is the statement that these symptoms must be present to a significant degree *and represent a noticeable change from usual behavior.* 4) A full manic or hypomanic episode that occurs during antidepressant treatment and continues at a fully syndromic level *beyond* (emphasis ours) the physiological effect of that treatment is sufficient evidence for a manic episode and, therefore, a diagnosis of bipolar I disorder. As with other

DSM-5 conditions, qualifiers of *mild, moderate,* and *severe* have been added and there are new specifiers, including *with anxious distress* and *with catatonia.*

Box 14–1. DSM-5 Diagnostic Criteria for Bipolar I Disorder

For a diagnosis of bipolar I disorder, it is necessary to meet the following criteria for a manic episode. The manic episode may have been preceded by and may be followed by hypomanic or major depressive episodes.

Manic Episode

A. A distinct period of abnormally and persistently elevated, expansive, or irritable mood and abnormally and persistently increased goal-directed activity or energy, lasting at least 1 week and present most of the day, nearly every day (or any duration if hospitalization is necessary).

B. During the period of mood disturbance and increased energy or activity, three (or more) of the following symptoms (four if the mood is only irritable) are present to a significant degree and represent a noticeable change from usual behavior:

   1. Inflated self-esteem or grandiosity.
   2. Decreased need for sleep (e.g., feels rested after only 3 hours of sleep).
   3. More talkative than usual or pressure to keep talking.
   4. Flight of ideas or subjective experience that thoughts are racing.
   5. Distractibility (i.e., attention too easily drawn to unimportant or irrelevant external stimuli), as reported or observed.
   6. Increase in goal-directed activity (either socially, at work or school, or sexually) or psychomotor agitation (i.e., purposeless non-goal-directed activity).
   7. Excessive involvement in activities that have a high potential for painful consequences (e.g., engaging in unrestrained buying sprees, sexual indiscretions, or foolish business investments).

C. The mood disturbance is sufficiently severe to cause marked impairment in social or occupational functioning or to necessitate hospitalization to prevent harm to self or others, or there are psychotic features.

D. The episode is not attributable to the physiological effects of a substance (e.g., a drug of abuse, a medication, other treatment) or to another medical condition.

   Note: A full manic episode that emerges during antidepressant treatment (e.g., medication, electroconvulsive therapy) but persists at a fully syndromal level beyond the physiological effect of that treatment is sufficient evidence for a manic episode and, therefore, a bipolar I diagnosis.

Note: Criteria A–D constitute a manic episode. At least one lifetime manic episode is required for the diagnosis of bipolar I disorder.

Hypomanic Episode

A. A distinct period of abnormally and persistently elevated, expansive, or irritable mood and abnormally and persistently increased activity or energy, lasting at least 4 consecutive days and present most of the day, nearly every day.

B. During the period of mood disturbance and increased energy and activity, three (or more) of the following symptoms (four if the mood is only irritable) have persisted, represent a noticeable change from usual behavior, and have been present to a significant degree:

   1. Inflated self-esteem or grandiosity.
   2. Decreased need for sleep (e.g., feels rested after only 3 hours of sleep).
   3. More talkative than usual or pressure to keep talking.

4. Flight of ideas or subjective experience that thoughts are racing.
5. Distractibility (i.e., attention too easily drawn to unimportant or irrelevant external stimuli), as reported or observed.
6. Increase in goal-directed activity (either socially, at work or school, or sexually) or psychomotor agitation.
7. Excessive involvement in activities that have a high potential for painful consequences (e.g., engaging in unrestrained buying sprees, sexual indiscretions, or foolish business investments).

C. The episode is associated with an unequivocal change in functioning that is uncharacteristic of the individual when not symptomatic.

D. The disturbance in mood and the change in functioning are observable by others.

E. The episode is not severe enough to cause marked impairment in social or occupational functioning or to necessitate hospitalization. If there are psychotic features, the episode is, by definition, manic.

F. The episode is not attributable to the physiological effects of a substance (e.g., a drug of abuse, a medication, other treatment).

   Note: A full hypomanic episode that emerges during antidepressant treatment (e.g., medication, electroconvulsive therapy) but persists at a fully syndromal level beyond the physiological effect of that treatment is sufficient evidence for a hypomanic episode diagnosis. However, caution is indicated so that one or two symptoms (particularly increased irritability, edginess, or agitation following antidepressant use) are not taken as sufficient for diagnosis of a hypomanic episode, nor necessarily indicative of a bipolar diathesis.

Note: Criteria A–F constitute a hypomanic episode. Hypomanic episodes are common in bipolar I disorder but are not required for the diagnosis of bipolar I disorder.

Major Depressive Episode

A. Five (or more) of the following symptoms have been present during the same 2-week period and represent a change from previous functioning; at least one of the symptoms is either (1) depressed mood or (2) loss of interest or pleasure.

   Note: Do not include symptoms that are clearly attributable to another medical condition.

   1. Depressed mood most of the day, nearly every day, as indicated by either subjective report (e.g., feels sad, empty, or hopeless) or observation made by others (e.g., appears tearful). (**Note:** In children and adolescents, can be irritable mood.)
   2. Markedly diminished interest or pleasure in all, or almost all, activities most of the day, nearly every day (as indicated by either subjective account or observation).
   3. Significant weight loss when not dieting or weight gain (e.g., a change of more than 5% of body weight in a month), or decrease or increase in appetite nearly every day. (**Note:** In children, consider failure to make expected weight gain.)
   4. Insomnia or hypersomnia nearly every day.
   5. Psychomotor agitation or retardation nearly every day (observable by others; not merely subjective feelings of restlessness or being slowed down).
   6. Fatigue or loss of energy nearly every day.
   7. Feelings of worthlessness or excessive or inappropriate guilt (which may be delusional) nearly every day (not merely self-reproach or guilt about being sick).
   8. Diminished ability to think or concentrate, or indecisiveness, nearly every day (either by subjective account or as observed by others).
   9. Recurrent thoughts of death (not just fear of dying), recurrent suicidal ideation without a specific plan, or a suicide attempt or a specific plan for committing suicide.

B. The symptoms cause clinically significant distress or impairment in social, occupational, or other important areas of functioning.

C. The episode is not attributable to the physiological effects of a substance or another medical condition.

Note: Criteria A–C constitute a major depressive episode. Major depressive episodes are common in bipolar I disorder but are not required for the diagnosis of bipolar I disorder.

Note: Responses to a significant loss (e.g., bereavement, financial ruin, losses from a natural disaster, a serious medical illness or disability) may include the feelings of intense sadness, rumination about the loss, insomnia, poor appetite, and weight loss noted in Criterion A, which may resemble a depressive episode. Although such symptoms may be understandable or considered appropriate to the loss, the presence of a major depressive episode in addition to the normal response to a significant loss should also be carefully considered. This decision inevitably requires the exercise of clinical judgment based on the individual's history and the cultural norms for the expression of distress in the context of loss.[1]

Bipolar I Disorder

A. Criteria have been met for at least one manic episode (Criteria A–D under "Manic Episode" above).

B. The occurrence of the manic and major depressive episode(s) is not better explained by schizoaffective disorder, schizophrenia, schizophreniform disorder, delusional disorder, or other specified or unspecified schizophrenia spectrum and other psychotic disorder.

Coding and Recording Procedures

The diagnostic code for bipolar I disorder is based on type of current or most recent episode and its status with respect to current severity, presence of psychotic features, and remission status. Current severity and psychotic features are only indicated if full criteria are currently met for a manic or major depressive episode. Remission specifiers are only indicated if the full criteria are not currently met for a manic, hypomanic, or major depressive episode. Codes are as follows:

Bipolar I disorder	Current or most recent episode manic	Current or most recent episode hypomanic*	Current or most recent episode depressed	Current or most recent episode unspecified**
Mild ([DSM-5] p. 154)	296.41 (F31.11)	NA	296.51 (F31.31)	NA
Moderate ([DSM-5] p. 154)	296.42 (F31.12)	NA	296.52 (F31.32)	NA

[1] In distinguishing grief from a major depressive episode (MDE), it is useful to consider that in grief the predominant affect is feelings of emptiness and loss, while in MDE it is persistent depressed mood and the inability to anticipate happiness or pleasure. The dysphoria in grief is likely to decrease in intensity over days to weeks and occurs in waves, the so-called pangs of grief. These waves tend to be associated with thoughts or reminders of the deceased. The depressed mood of a MDE is more persistent and not tied to specific thoughts or preoccupations. The pain of grief may be accompanied by positive emotions and humor that are uncharacteristic of the pervasive unhappiness and misery characteristic of a major depressive episode. The thought content associated with grief generally features a preoccupation with thoughts and memories of the deceased, rather than the self-critical or pessimistic ruminations seen in a MDE. In grief, self-esteem is generally preserved, whereas in a MDE, feelings of worthlessness and self-loathing are common. If self-derogatory ideation is present in grief, it typically involves perceived failings vis-à-vis the deceased (e.g., not visiting frequently enough, not telling the deceased how much he or she was loved). If a bereaved individual thinks about death and dying, such thoughts are generally focused on the deceased and possibly about "joining" the deceased, whereas in a major depressive episode such thoughts are focused on ending one's own life because of feeling worthless, undeserving of life, or unable to cope with the pain of depression.

Bipolar I disorder	Current or most recent episode manic	Current or most recent episode hypomanic*	Current or most recent episode depressed	Current or most recent episode unspecified**
Severe ([DSM-5] p. 154)	296.43 (F31.13)	NA	296.53 (F31.4)	NA
With psychotic features*** ([DSM-5] p. 152)	296.44 (F31.2)	NA	296.54 (F31.5)	NA
In partial remission ([DSM-5] p. 154)	296.45 (F31.73)	296.45 (F31.71)	296.55 (F31.75)	NA
In full remission ([DSM-5] p. 154)	296.46 (F31.74)	296.46 (F31.72)	296.56 (F31.76)	NA
Unspecified	296.40 (F31.9)	296.40 (F31.9)	296.50 (F31.9)	NA

*Severity and psychotic specifiers do not apply; code 296.40 (F31.0) for cases not in remission.
**Severity, psychotic, and remission specifiers do not apply. Code 296.7 (F31.9).
***If psychotic features are present, code the "with psychotic features" specifier irrespective of episode severity.

In recording the name of a diagnosis, terms should be listed in the following order: bipolar I disorder, type of current or most recent episode, severity/psychotic/remission specifiers, followed by as many specifiers without codes as apply to the current or most recent episode.

Specify:

With anxious distress ([DSM-5] p. 149)
With mixed features ([DSM-5] pp. 149–150)
With rapid cycling ([DSM-5] pp. 150–151)
With melancholic features ([DSM-5] p. 151)
With atypical features ([DSM-5] pp. 151–152)
With mood-congruent psychotic features ([DSM-5] p. 152)
With mood-incongruent psychotic features ([DSM-5] p. 152)
With catatonia ([DSM-5] p. 152). **Coding note:** Use additional code 293.89 (F06.1).
With peripartum onset ([DSM-5] pp. 152–153)
With seasonal pattern ([DSM-5] pp. 153–154)

Source. Reprinted from the *Diagnostic and Statistical Manual of Mental Disorders*, 5th Edition. Arlington, VA, American Psychiatric Association, 2013. Used with permission.

Box 14–2. DSM-5 Diagnostic Criteria for Bipolar II Disorder

296.89 (F31.81)

For a diagnosis of bipolar II disorder, it is necessary to meet the following criteria for a current or past hypomanic episode *and* the following criteria for a current or past major depressive episode:

Hypomanic Episode

A. A distinct period of abnormally and persistently elevated, expansive, or irritable mood and abnormally and persistently increased activity or energy, lasting at least 4 consecutive days and present most of the day, nearly every day.

B. During the period of mood disturbance and increased energy and activity, three (or more) of the following symptoms have persisted (four if the mood is only irritable), represent a noticeable change from usual behavior, and have been present to a significant degree:

1. Inflated self-esteem or grandiosity.
2. Decreased need for sleep (e.g., feels rested after only 3 hours of sleep).
3. More talkative than usual or pressure to keep talking.
4. Flight of ideas or subjective experience that thoughts are racing.
5. Distractibility (i.e., attention too easily drawn to unimportant or irrelevant external stimuli), as reported or observed.
6. Increase in goal-directed activity (either socially, at work or school, or sexually) or psychomotor agitation.
7. Excessive involvement in activities that have a high potential for painful consequences (e.g., engaging in unrestrained buying sprees, sexual indiscretions, or foolish business investments).

C. The episode is associated with an unequivocal change in functioning that is uncharacteristic of the individual when not symptomatic.

D. The disturbance in mood and the change in functioning are observable by others.

E. The episode is not severe enough to cause marked impairment in social or occupational functioning or to necessitate hospitalization. If there are psychotic features, the episode is, by definition, manic.

F. The episode is not attributable to the physiological effects of a substance (e.g., a drug of abuse, a medication or other treatment).

   Note: A full hypomanic episode that emerges during antidepressant treatment (e.g., medication, electroconvulsive therapy) but persists at a fully syndromal level beyond the physiological effect of that treatment is sufficient evidence for a hypomanic episode diagnosis. However, caution is indicated so that one or two symptoms (particularly increased irritability, edginess, or agitation following antidepressant use) are not taken as sufficient for diagnosis of a hypomanic episode, nor necessarily indicative of a bipolar diathesis.

Major Depressive Episode

A. Five (or more) of the following symptoms have been present during the same 2-week period and represent a change from previous functioning; at least one of the symptoms is either (1) depressed mood or (2) loss of interest or pleasure.

   Note: Do not include symptoms that are clearly attributable to a medical condition.

1. Depressed mood most of the day, nearly every day, as indicated by either subjective report (e.g., feels sad, empty, or hopeless) or observation made by others (e.g., appears tearful). (**Note:** In children and adolescents, can be irritable mood.)
2. Markedly diminished interest or pleasure in all, or almost all, activities most of the day, nearly every day (as indicated by either subjective account or observation).
3. Significant weight loss when not dieting or weight gain (e.g., a change of more than 5% of body weight in a month), or decrease or increase in appetite nearly every day. (**Note:** In children, consider failure to make expected weight gain.)
4. Insomnia or hypersomnia nearly every day.
5. Psychomotor agitation or retardation nearly every day (observable by others; not merely subjective feelings of restlessness or being slowed down).
6. Fatigue or loss of energy nearly every day.
7. Feelings of worthlessness or excessive or inappropriate guilt (which may be delusional) nearly every day (not merely self-reproach or guilt about being sick).
8. Diminished ability to think or concentrate, or indecisiveness, nearly every day (either by subjective account or as observed by others).
9. Recurrent thoughts of death (not just fear of dying), recurrent suicidal ideation without a specific plan, a suicide attempt, or a specific plan for committing suicide.

B. The symptoms cause clinically significant distress or impairment in social, occupational, or other important areas of functioning.
C. The episode is not attributable to the physiological effects of a substance or another medical condition.

Note: Criteria A–C above constitute a major depressive episode.

Note: Responses to a significant loss (e.g., bereavement, financial ruin, losses from a natural disaster, a serious medical illness or disability) may include the feelings of intense sadness, rumination about the loss, insomnia, poor appetite, and weight loss noted in Criterion A, which may resemble a depressive episode. Although such symptoms may be understandable or considered appropriate to the loss, the presence of a major depressive episode in addition to the normal response to a significant loss should be carefully considered. This decision inevitably requires the exercise of clinical judgment based on the individual's history and the cultural norms for the expression of distress in the context of loss.[2]

Bipolar II Disorder

A. Criteria have been met for at least one hypomanic episode (Criteria A–F under "Hypomanic Episode" above) and at least one major depressive episode (Criteria A–C under "Major Depressive Episode" above).
B. There has never been a manic episode.
C. The occurrence of the hypomanic episode(s) and major depressive episode(s) is not better explained by schizoaffective disorder, schizophrenia, schizophreniform disorder, delusional disorder, or other specified or unspecified schizophrenia spectrum and other psychotic disorder.
D. The symptoms of depression or the unpredictability caused by frequent alternation between periods of depression and hypomania causes clinically significant distress or impairment in social, occupational, or other important areas of functioning.

Coding and Recording Procedures

Bipolar II disorder has one diagnostic code: 296.89 (F31.81). Its status with respect to current severity, presence of psychotic features, course, and other specifiers cannot be coded but should be indicated in writing (e.g., 296.89 [F31.81] bipolar II disorder, current episode depressed, moderate severity, with mixed features; 296.89 [F31.81] bipolar II disorder, most recent episode depressed, in partial remission).

---

[2] In distinguishing grief from a major depressive episode (MDE), it is useful to consider that in grief the predominant affect is feelings of emptiness and loss, while in a MDE it is persistent depressed mood and the inability to anticipate happiness or pleasure. The dysphoria in grief is likely to decrease in intensity over days to weeks and occurs in waves, the so-called pangs of grief. These waves tend to be associated with thoughts or reminders of the deceased. The depressed mood of a MDE is more persistent and not tied to specific thoughts or preoccupations. The pain of grief may be accompanied by positive emotions and humor that are uncharacteristic of the pervasive unhappiness and misery characteristic of a MDE. The thought content associated with grief generally features a preoccupation with thoughts and memories of the deceased, rather than the self-critical or pessimistic ruminations seen in a MDE. In grief, self-esteem is generally preserved, whereas in a MDE feelings of worthlessness and self-loathing are common. If self-derogatory ideation is present in grief, it typically involves perceived failings vis-à-vis the deceased (e.g., not visiting frequently enough, not telling the deceased how much he or she was loved). If a bereaved individual thinks about death and dying, such thoughts are generally focused on the deceased and possibly about "joining" the deceased, whereas in a MDE such thoughts are focused on ending one's own life because of feeling worthless, undeserving of life, or unable to cope with the pain of depression.

Specify current or most recent episode:

Hypomanic

Depressed

Specify if:

With anxious distress ([DSM-5] p. 149)

With mixed features ([DSM-5] pp. 149–150)

With rapid cycling ([DSM-5] pp. 150–151)

With melancholic features ([DSM-5] p. 151)

With atypical features ([DSM-5] pp. 151–152)

With mood-congruent psychotic features ([DSM-5] p. 152)

With mood-incongruent psychotic features ([DSM-5] p. 152)

With catatonia ([DSM-5] p. 152). **Coding note:** Use additional code 293.89 (F06.1).

With peripartum onset ([DSM-5] pp. 152–153)

With seasonal pattern ([DSM-5] pp. 153–154): Applies only to the pattern of major depressive episodes.

Specify course if full criteria for a mood episode are not currently met:

In partial remission ([DSM-5] p. 154)

In full remission ([DSM-5] p. 154)

Specify severity if full criteria for a mood episode are currently met:

Mild ([DSM-5] p. 154)

Moderate ([DSM-5] p. 154)

Severe ([DSM-5] p. 154)

Source. Reprinted from the *Diagnostic and Statistical Manual of Mental Disorders*, 5th Edition. Arlington, VA, American Psychiatric Association, 2013. Used with permission.

BP is further classified by the temporal relationship of episodes and symptoms. When episodes of mania and depression follow each other without a euthymic interval, the type is said to be *circular.* The presence of four or more episodes per year defines *rapid cycling*. The specifier *mixed features* has replaced *mixed episode.* Mixed features indicates that in the presence of an episode of either hypomania/mania or depression, at least several symptoms of the other mood are manifest, but full criteria for the opposite mood state are not met.

Finally, there is a severity spectrum. At the less severe end are mood-congruent psychotic symptoms (those consistent with an elevated or depressed mood). More severe are mood-incongruent symptoms (most often paranoia and other delusions and hallucinations less related to a mood state) and then schizoaffective mania, where more prominent symptoms typical of schizophrenia occur. Schizoaffective disorder, depressive type, may be closer to schizophrenia than to a mood disorder.

Controversy remains in the child and adolescent BP literature as to whether the condition should be defined more narrowly/conservatively or more broadly/liberally. This disparity emerged inadvertently as a result of differing interpretations by clinicians and researchers of the ambiguities in the transition from DSM-III (American Psychiatric Association 1980) to DSM-IV-TR (American Psychiatric Association 2000) literature (Carlson and Klein 2014).

Clinical Description

According to Goodwin and Jamison (2007), conservatively defined mania has an acute onset and lasts several months, during which a person experiences a roller coaster of feelings. Among youth, prodromal symptoms may last longer than in adults. Even in predominantly euphoric mania, the mood is labile with highs and lows, irritability, and anxiety. Simultaneously, energy, activity level, speech, and flow of ideas are on "overdrive." Patience is short and anger can intrude quickly. Sleep is unnecessary and time is filled with extravagant plans. Delusional thinking and sometimes hallucinations are present about half of the time, although psychosis is not usually sustained. Patients may cycle out gradually or quickly and return to a euthymic state or plunge immediately into a depressive episode, which is as bleak, despairing, and enervating as mania is ebullient, optimistic, and activated. Depressive episodes are longer than manic episodes, taking up to a year to remit.

Case Example 1: Child With Early Onset BP (Conservatively/Narrowly Defined)

Nicola, a girl age 12 years and 9 months who was previously shy, helpful, and academically normal, presented with a sudden onset of behavior change over 2–3 weeks consisting of a change in dress to very revealing clothes, uninhibited talking to strangers by telephone and Internet, increased energy around the clock, and extreme mood changes from laughing hysterically one minute to swearing and smashing things the next to crying uncontrollably, all without much provocation.

Nicola's only prior mental health problem had been an apparent depression at age 10 following the death of her grandmother. She recovered with brief psychotherapy. She had menarche at age 12 and started middle school the same year.

Nicola could be heard in the waiting room talking with everyone loudly and rapidly, bragging about waiting for a cell phone call from a famous actor. She frantically tried to organize playroom toys, becoming furious when another parent told her to calm down. She was suspicious about letting her parents be interviewed alone and furious when asked about drug and alcohol use (which she denied).

Nicola's father was a Wall Street broker who had become depressed with stock reversals in the past. He also drank heavily. Her mother had suffered from a postpartum depression.

Case Example 2: Possible Liberally/Broadly Defined BP

Lynda, an 11-year-old girl, had been hyperactive, disinhibited, and impulsive since preschool. Increasing problems academically and with peers prompted medication treatment. Stimulant treatments since age 8 resulted in only partially controlled symptoms. She did not have a learning disorder. At school she could not sit still and talked too much, often about topics unrelated to the task. Social skills were poor because she was bossy and intrusive. She was oppositional, sometimes insubordinate, but basically manageable in class.

Over the year prior to referral, Lynda had become increasingly angry, irritable, provocative, destructive, and capricious. She bullied smaller children and expressed interest in lewd material on the Internet. She was often a show-off, and when lots of people were around, she would act silly and repeat jokes long past the time they were funny. In spite of poor grades, she told her family that she planned to be a doctor, a record producer, a professional wrestler, or an acrobat. Her rages when she did not get her way, or when a demand was made on her, were severe and could last for several hours. She would scream, curse, throw dishware, and occasionally threaten with a knife. As a result of this behavior, she was sent to a psychiatric emergency room for an overnight stay.

On interview, Lynda was calm but disrespectful to her parents and tried to be a "femme fatale" with the young male resident who was interviewing her. She could focus on what she wanted but would ask irrelevant questions trying to control the direction of conversation.

Alone, Lynda admitted to being distractible, forgetful, and restless. She often felt sad, was suicidal when angry, and admitted to flying off the handle easily. She had many complaints about her parents and unfair treatment by the girls in school. She denied euphoria but said her speech was rapid, although emergency room staff did not observe this. She complained of insomnia (i.e., not getting to sleep until 1:00 A.M. but sleeping until 3:00 P.M. the following afternoon). She was starting to smoke and experiment with marijuana and sex. In terms of the future, she thought she could go to law school if she brought up her grades.

There is a history in first-degree relatives of depression, hypomania, and attention-deficit/hyperactivity disorder (ADHD).

The two cases just described, annotated for each criterion of mania, were rated by child psychiatrists in the United States and United Kingdom (Dubicka et al. 2008). In Case Example 1, the patient was diagnosed with mania by 96% of the U.S. clinicians and 92% of the U.K. clinicians. For Case Example 2, however, 75% of U.S. child psychiatrists diagnosed mania, usually with comorbid ADHD, versus 33% of U.K. child psychiatrists ($P<0.001$). The remainder of U.K. clinicians conceptualized Lynda as exhibiting ADHD and/or a behavior disorder only. The cases serve to illustrate that despite 40 years of work since DSM-III to operationalize criteria and assessments, persisting ambiguities in the criteria and their interpretation have produced inconsistencies in differentiating children and adolescents with ADHD and emotion regulation problems from those with mania/bipolar I disorder. The criteria changes in DSM-5 are an attempt to correct these ambiguities. However, continued controversy regarding applying a narrow or broad definition of mania in children complicates the research on BP (Carlson and Klein 2014; Pataki and Carlson 2013).

Epidemiology

Among adults in the United States, rates of lifetime BP-I disorder vary between 0.8% and 1.6%, while the rate of lifetime BP-II is about 1.1%; the lifetime rate of subthreshold manic symptoms ranges from 2.4% to about 6%. In teens, rates of diagnosis and of comorbidities depend on who is interviewed, how information is combined, what interview is used, and whether the shared symptoms of ADHD and BP are simply counted toward each condition or must intensify during the episode (Carlson and Klein 2014; Galanter et al. 2012). Thus, rates of lifetime mania vary from 0.1% (Lewinsohn et al. 1995; Stringaris et al. 2010) to 1.7% (Merikangas et al. 2012). Rates of bipolar spectrum disorder are as high as 6.7% (Van Meter et al. 2011), with high rates of conversion from bipolar disorder not otherwise specified (BP-NOS) to BP-I over 4 years (Axelson et al. 2011) as opposed to negligible rates over 30 years (Shankman et al. 2009). Children younger than age 9 have not been studied in community samples. In the Great Smoky Mountains epidemiological study of children ages 9–13 years no children were found to have had a manic episode (Costello et al. 1996), using a 3-month current window (not lifetime).

Between the 1990s and the twenty-first century, for many reasons there has been a significant increase in the diagnoses of BP in youth in the United States but not in the United Kingdom. In the United States the estimated annual number of office-based visits of youth with a diagnosis of bipolar disorder increased from 25 in 100,000 in 1994–1995 to 1,003 in 100,000 in 2002–2003 (Moreno et al. 2007). Hospital discharge diagnoses using the National Hospital Discharge Survey jumped from 1.4 in 10,000 to 7.3 in 10,000 in 9- to 13-year-olds and from 5.1 in 10,000 to 20.4 in 10,000 in 14- to 19-year-olds (Blader and Carlson 2007). This was not found in U.K. hospital discharges (James et al. 2014). This change in diagnostic practice in the United States, associated with the increased use of atypical antipsychotic agents, was sufficiently concerning that the DSM-5 committee tightened the mania criteria and used data on severe mood dysregulation (Leibenluft et al. 2003) to create a new condition, disruptive mood dysregulation disorder (see Chapter 13, "Depressive and Disruptive Mood Dysregulation Disorder").

Comorbidity

Children who meet criteria for mania almost invariably qualify for at least one other disorder. The most common simultaneous comorbidities (ADHD, oppositional defiant disorder [ODD], conduct disorder [CD], anxiety) occur during mania, and it may be difficult to distinguish these comorbidities from mania without a careful and detailed history. The comorbid symptoms may represent a halo effect of a manic or depressive episode, subsiding when the mood disorder is treated. The comorbid disorder often has its own comorbidities. Thus, ADHD is often comorbid with ODD and CD, anxiety, and specific learning disorders. Multiple anxiety disorders often occur together.

ADHD, which begins prior to BP, may be found in up to 90% of prepubertal children and about half of adolescents with BP (Faraone et al. 1997; Tillman et al. 2003). The Longitudinal Assessment of Manic Symptoms (LAMS) study (Arnold et al. 2011) found that among children with BP, 69% met the criteria for ADHD. The authors concluded that comorbid ADHD and BP are better accounted for as independent concurrent disorders, rather than ADHD posing a risk factor for BP.

CD may precede or co-occur with BP. The combination of externalizing disorders and BP may represent a phenotype specific to prepubertal children (Biederman et al. 2000). Adults with BP-I and co-occurring substance abuse have significantly higher rates of adolescent CD compared with those without substance abuse. Substance abuse or dependence in adolescents is also a significant comorbidity, one that often perpetuates mood cycles.

Anxiety disorders occur with surprising frequency, although rates vary widely depending on whether the disorder is diagnosed when the patient is euthymic (Dickstein et al. 2005).

BP in children with autism spectrum disorder (ASD) is less well studied (for review, see Gutkovich and Carlson 2008). About 20% of children diagnosed with mania also had comorbid ASD, but up to 60% of patients with mood disorders obtained parent ratings of autism spectrum behaviors in the "likely ASD" range.

Substance and alcohol abuse are common comorbidities in adolescents with BP. ADHD and CD, which may be comorbid in early onset BP, are both risk factors for the development of substance and alcohol abuse. However, early onset BP itself appears to increase rates of substance abuse over and above other externalizing disorders. Cannabis abuse increases rates of psychosis in general. Substance and alcohol abuse also complicate BP by increasing both the severity and number of episodes. Finally, DSM-5 recognizes that mania or depression frequently occurs secondary to substance abuse and that the episode may remit when the drugs of abuse are discontinued. Disentangling these entities is next to impossible while drug and alcohol abuse continue.

Etiology, Mechanisms, and Risk Factors

Genetic Factors

Twin studies of adults suggest that genetic influences explain approximately 60%–93% of the variance in BP, while shared and unique environmental factors account for 30%–40% and 10%–21%, respectively (Althoff et al. 2005). Findings from "top-down" studies over the past 30 years depend both on how conservatively bipolar disorder is diagnosed and on study setting (i.e., community, response to advertisements, tertiary care clinics). Rates of mania in high-risk offspring who have been followed into adulthood vary from 2% to 7%; rates of bipolar spectrum disorder are as high as 20%. Rates of depression and other psychopathology are even higher, however (for a review, see Carlson and Klein 2014). High-risk offspring also exhibit more anxiety, behavioral disturbance, and mood dysregulation (Birmaher et al. 2013) than healthy comparison samples. Since these high-risk samples are compared with healthy control subjects, it is not clear if these figures represent specific bipolar harbingers, the impact of having a mentally ill parent, or both.

In "bottom-up" studies, one-third to almost half of the first-degree relatives of bipolar spectrum probands have a bipolar spectrum disorder (including recurrent depression). Rates are much lower in the comparison groups (Brotman et al. 2007; Geller et al. 2006; Rende et al. 2007).

Environmental risk factors like physical and sexual abuse (Leverich et al. 2002), irritable and negative parenting styles (Geller et al. 2004; Meyer et al. 2006), poor social support, and prenatal alcohol exposure (O'Connor et al. 2002) may interact with genetic vulnerability to enhance early age at onset of BP, as well as a variety of negative course indicators, including rapid cycling, substance use, elevated risk of suicidal behavior, and high comorbidity rates (Alloy et al. 2005).

Brain Structure and Function

There is a convergence of data to suggest key roles for the amygdala, anterior paralimbic cortices, and connections among these structures in the emotional dysregulation of bipolar disorder (Strakowski et al. 2012; Terry et al. 2009; Wang et al. 2012). The functions subserved by their more widely distributed connection sites suggest that broader system dysfunction could account for the range of functions—from neurovegetative to cognitive—disrupted in the disorder. Some of these abnormalities are apparent by adolescence, while others, such as those in rostral prefrontal regions, appear to progress over adolescence and young adulthood, suggesting a neurodevelopmental model of the disorder (Schneider et al. 2012). Early onset pediatric/adolescent BD may signify a more malignant course of illness in which extensive executive neurocognitive deficits are found early and may persist, with some potential for improvement during remission and perhaps with treatment (Garrett et al. 2012; Whitney et al. 2012). However, some findings conflict, which may reflect the small sample sizes and methodological differences among studies. Furthermore, the clinical heterogeneity that confounds the diagnostic, genetic, and treatment studies of bipolar disorder complicates interpretation of imaging studies as well (Strakowski et al. 2012).

Age at Onset, Course, and Prognosis

Age at onset varies by whether it is dated from emergence of a full mood episode or from displays of symptoms believed to be harbingers of BP. BP often begins with depression or dysthymia, followed by mania occurring in adolescence and young adulthood. On the other hand, if broad phenotype BP is included in age of onset data, it is possible that onset could be dated to the preschool years.

Over a 2- to 4-year follow-up in U.S. samples, early onset BP (both broad and narrow phenotypes) is characterized by slow response to treatment, persistent mood fluctuations, elevated risk for suicide attempts, and severe psychosocial impairment. Although rates of remission are variable over the short term, if cases are followed long enough, almost everyone remits. However, rates of recurrence, albeit varying with time to follow-up, are as high as 70%.

In spite of what appears to be a rather pessimistic picture, a latent class analysis of the Course of Bipolar Youth (COBY) sample over 8 years revealed that 24% of young patients with bipolar disorder (BP-I, BP-II, and BP-NOS) were euthymic on average for 84.4% of the follow-up period (Birmaher et al. 2014), another 19.1% remained ill early in follow-up but started to improve greatly at around 3 years, 34.6% were moderately euthymic (about 47.3% of the time), and 22.3% were persistently mood disordered. The "predominantly euthymic" group, compared with the more chronic group, was older at first symptoms and first episode and less likely to have experienced associated depressive behaviors such as self-injurious and suicidal behavior. Their condition overall was less complicated, with lower rates of comorbid ADHD and anxiety. Rates of psychiatric disorders (bipolar disorder, ADHD, and other disorders) in their parents were lower, socioeconomic status was higher, families were more often intact, and rates of prior physical and sexual abuse were lower. Half of the "predominantly euthymic" group had no additional mood episodes over the follow-up period compared with the more chronic group (49.9% vs. 8.5%) and appeared to have had fewer episodes prior to the study.

Follow-up studies report that impairment is most profound among the youngest patients with bipolar disorder. Fewer than half of child samples experienced remission at 6- and 12-month follow-up, and subthreshold symptoms of mania and depression and comorbid conditions often persist between episodes (Birmaher et al. 2006; Strober et al. 1995).

Nonadherence with pharmacological treatment, low socioeconomic status, low maternal warmth, psychosis, comorbid anxiety, and rapid cycling are poor prognostic indicators (Birmaher et al. 2006; DelBello et al. 2007; Geller et al. 2004).

Children with BP-NOS, now identified in DSM-5 as *other specified bipolar and related disorder*, suffer from a more chronic course than youth with BP-I or BP-II, with persistent subthreshold symptoms and slower response to acute treatment. Within 4 years of follow-up, 40% of individuals in the COBY sample initially diagnosed with BP-NOS converted to BP-I or BP-II (Axelson et al. 2011). However, in other studies with different definitions of subsyndromal bipolar disorder, rates of conversion from subsyndromal mania to BP-I were negligible (Brotman et al. 2006; Findling et al. 2013d).

Evaluation

Evaluation of a serious childhood psychiatric disorder includes screening, an interview with parents and child, and other diagnostic information as needed. This is difficult to accomplish in less than 2 hours, even with articulate parents.

Screening

Standardized rating scales that address mood symptoms and other psychiatric behaviors and disorders are important to obtain. The Child Behavior Checklist (CBCL) has been studied most and detects high rates of internalizing and externalizing disorder comorbidity. Elevated anxiety/depression, aggression, and attention subscale scores on the CBCL (T scores ≥67) have been called the CBCL-dysregulated phenotype. While the CBCL is not diagnostic for bipolar disorder, acutely manic youth may present with those subscale elevations.

Screening instruments directed more specifically at mania/hypomania include parent-completed versions of the General Behavior Inventory (P-GBI), Child Mania Rating Scale (P-CMRS), and Young Mania Rating Scale (P-YMRS; Youngstrom et al. 2006). As with most other conditions in child psychiatry, cross-informant agreement is low.

Parent Interview

Parents are the most useful source of information, and they should be interviewed first, regardless of the patient's age. After the clinician elicits parent concerns and a general psychiatric history, details about the child's mood and activity level should be elicited. Antecedents to "mood swings" or aggressive, agitated, explosive behavior (rages) and how or if they differ from the child's "usual self" must be established. Fatigue, hunger, and sedating medications may increase such behaviors. This information is necessary for planning interventions.

Family History

Family history of mood disorders (bipolar and unipolar) and other psychiatric disorders must be elicited. It is difficult to confirm an accurate diagnosis of BP disorder in a relative reported to have predominantly depressive symptoms or significant comorbidity, even with a stated history of lithium response. Adults are sometimes incorrectly given a BP diagnosis in lieu of more pessimistic or stigmatizing diagnoses (e.g., schizophrenia, substance use disorder, personality disorder).

Child Interview

Besides ascertaining the presence of manic and depressive symptoms germane to the diagnosis of BP, it is necessary to directly assess the child's language; presence of thought disorder, psychosis, anxiety, suicidal behavior, physical/sexual abuse, and illicit substance use; and evidence of racing thoughts and flight of ideas.

It is important to reconcile parent and child information. If child information does not agree with parent information, the child should be told what his or her parent has said and asked for clarification. Parents sometimes misinterpret; children sometimes deny.

Other Evaluations

Teacher information is important to establish the pervasiveness of mania or depression. A child with rages at home who is completely asymptomatic at school is likely to have a different condition from one who is similarly symptomatic in both places. For a child having scholastic difficulties, a psychoeducational evaluation (IQ and achievement tests) is needed. For children with communication problems, a language evaluation with a speech sample is needed. In addition to a good medical history (or information from the primary care physician), polysomnography (for possible sleep apnea), a thorough neurological assessment, or laboratory tests may be needed. The complex nature of early onset BP requires an assessment beyond ascertainment of mania and depression criteria alone.

Systematic Interviews

Semistructured and structured interviews, such as the Schedule for Affective Disorders and Schizophrenia for School-Age Children (K-SADS) and the National Institute of Mental Health Diagnostic Interview Schedule for Children, Version IV (DISC-IV; Shaffer et al. 2000), are the cornerstones of most clinical research. In clinical settings, these may be used to confirm diagnosis after the clinician himself or herself has obtained a good history or enough information to know that the diagnoses of interest are covered by the systematic interview.

Interview Rating Scales

Rating scales may guide treatment response and track mania (including mood lability), depression, anxiety, ADHD, aggression, and psychosis. The Young Mania Rating Scale (YMRS) (Young et al. 1978) has been used in drug studies to assess significant severity (a cutoff score of 20). Ironically, the YMRS does not assess all the symptoms of mania. The Children's Depression Rating Scale—Revised (Poznanski and Mokros 1996) was developed for children and is used to rate the severity of depression. Scores over 40 are indicative of moderately severe depression. Neither instrument replaces a history.

Differential Diagnosis

In preadolescents, ADHD and bipolar disorder are the conditions that appear to be most often confused. This is in part because some children with ADHD have severe outbursts, and one school of thought believes that these outbursts are pathognomonic for bipolar disorder. However, severe outbursts occur in youth with ADHD and ODD/CD or ASD, in children exposed to severe abuse or domestic violence, and in children with panic attacks who respond to the fear stimulus with "fight" rather than "flight or freeze." The new DSM-5 condition called disruptive mood dysregulation disorder (see Chapter 13) is characterized by such outbursts in the context of chronic irritability. The clinical relevance is whether one treats the mood dysregulation first, as a form of mania, or treats the other disorder first because it is considered to be the reason for the mood dysregulation (Carlson 2012; Kowatch et al. 2005).

Clearly defined mood episodes with duration longer than a week that are clearly distinguishable from the premorbid state are more easily diagnosed. Depression is often the reason for which children and teens seek treatment. It is important to look for hints of mania or hypomania in their past, recognizing there may be none. It may take a number of years for a manic episode to occur (as seen in Case Example 1). Postpubertal mania and depression can include very severe psychosis, which brings schizophrenia and substance-induced psychosis into the differential diagnosis.

The following are areas in which careful history and symptom ascertainment are necessary to make distinctions (for a review, see Carlson and Meyer 2006).

Symptoms

- The silly, disinhibited behavior of a child with ADHD trying to be funny and not knowing when to quit versus someone with an elated mood
- Impulsivity versus pleasure seeking without heeding consequences
- A child's resistance to bedtime versus a reduced need for sleep

Onset of Illness

- The exacerbation of subthreshold ADHD symptoms because of increased late elementary or middle school demands versus the start of a mood disorder
- The progression of ADHD symptoms to include more oppositional/explosive/conduct disordered behavior in the context of family, school, and/or peer difficulties

Mental Status

- The pragmatic, distracted, or odd language seen in children who have language disorders as part of ADHD or an autism spectrum disorder versus the flight of ideas and thought disorder of mania
- The "hallucinations" seen in a very anxious child versus mood-incongruent symptoms of a mood disorder
- The mood-incongruent psychotic symptoms of mania or depression versus symptoms of early schizophrenia

Finally, teens who are abusing marijuana, alcohol, or other drugs may have psychosis and/or mood symptoms. While a positive toxicology screen helps document the ingestion of drugs, negative drug screens do not rule out substance abuse, and symptoms of mania may continue for a number of weeks even if the patient is drug-free.

Treatment

Although medication treatment of BP is vital, adequate preparation for treatment is more likely to ensure its success.

Psychoeducation and Psychosocial Management

1. Educate patient and family members about BP (including any comorbidities).

2. Include in the treatment recommendations the advantages, limitations, and risks of medication use, as well as consequences of no use.
3. Remind parents to keep medications secure and to administer them reliably.
4. Try to obtain baseline laboratory test results: complete blood count, platelets, fasting blood sugar, liver and renal functioning, cholesterol, lipids, and thyroid-stimulating hormone (TSH).
5. To separate psychiatric adverse events from baseline disorder and to evaluate medication benefit, obtain baseline ratings for the major symptom areas being addressed (e.g., aggression/irritability, psychosis, hyperactivity, inattention, anxiety, depression, episode shifts). For children with rages or outbursts, establish their frequency, intensity, number, and duration.
6. Discuss medication risks. If side effects are minimal and treatment efficacy is clear, continue treatment. If adverse events appear to be worse than the condition being treated, change treatment. If there is no improvement after several months, there is no reason to continue that treatment. It is necessary to establish a clear baseline of symptoms and functional impairment in order to assess treatment efficacy. The decision to try another (similar or different) medication or that same medication at a different dose must be made on a case-by-case basis.
7. Prepare patient and family for the fact that different strategies may be needed and tell parents to give each dose adequate time to work.
8. Address educational aspects of the disorder with necessary teacher rating scales, psychoeducational testing, classroom observation, and development of an individualized education program.
9. If the child has comorbid ADHD, ASD, anxiety, or ODD/CD, address these conditions.
10. Recommend treatment for parents so that they can effectively manage their child. The family impact of BP is profound and reciprocal, and rates of family mental illness are quite high.

Specific Psychosocial Interventions

There are six empirically supported psychosocial interventions for early onset bipolar spectrum disorders. These include child- and family-focused cognitive-behavioral therapy, multi/individual family psychoeducation, family-focused treatment for adolescents, dialectical behavioral therapy for adolescents, interpersonal and social rhythm therapy for adolescents, and cognitive-behavioral therapy for bipolar disorders in adolescents (for a review, see Weinstein et al. 2013).

Pharmacological Treatment

Medication remains the major treatment for BP; however, the medication choice should be based on evidence of effectiveness, phase of illness, subtype of disorder (psychosis, mixed episode, rapid cycling), comorbidities, the side effect profile with respect to the particular patient, the patient's history of medication response, and possibly a family member's history of medication response. This is a rapidly changing area, so clinicians must keep abreast of the evidence and the literature (see also Chapter 37, "Mood Stabilizers," and Chapter 38, "Antipsychotic Medications").

As of 2014, 10 medications (lithium, chlorpromazine, divalproex, extended-release carbamazepine, olanzapine, quetiapine, risperidone, aripiprazole, ziprasidone, asenapine) have U.S. Food and Drug Administration (FDA) approval in *adults* for the treatment of acute mania, 6 of them for mixed episodes. Lithium and olanzapine have FDA indications for adolescent mania, along with risperidone and aripiprazole for children ages 10–17 years. There has been a positive trial of ziprasidone in youth but as yet not an FDA-approved indication prior to age 18 years. Asenapine was recently granted FDA approval for youth ages 10–17 years.

Mania medication trials last 3–8 weeks depending on the medication. Efficacy has been measured in three ways: 1) change from baseline on the YMRS (Young et al. 1978) score; 2) response, which is usually a 50% reduction in YMRS entry score (which averages about 30); and 3) remission, which is variously defined as a YMRS score less than 12, a Clinical Global Improvement score on manic symptoms rating the child as improved or very much improved, or both. Completion rates for studies conducted with children and adolescents have been 60%–80%.

The results from placebo-controlled trials of atypical antipsychotics for mania/mixed mania show a larger effect size (ES) than mood stabilizers (ES 0.65, confidence interval [CI] 0.53–0.78 compared with ES 0.20, CI 0.02–0.39) (Correll et al. 2010). Using response as measured by a 50% reduction in YMRS entry score, 50%–70% of subjects improved on active atypical antipsychotic medication versus 20%–37% on placebo. The number needed to treat in successful trials where drug was better than placebo varied from 3.8 to 5.3. Atypical antipsychotics with FDA-approved indications for acute/mixed mania include olanzapine for adolescents and risperidone, aripiprazole, and quetiapine for youth ages 10–17 years. Ziprasidone has also been studied but does not presently have this FDA indication. See Table 14–1.

Although divalproex has an FDA treatment indication for mania in adults, its efficacy in bipolar youth is less robust. It was better than placebo in one unpublished 8-week study, but divalproex ER was not better than placebo in a 4-week industry-sponsored study (Wagner et al. 2009). Other anticonvulsants—topiramate and oxcarbazepine—have not been found to be significantly better than placebo (DelBello et al. 2005; Wagner et al. 2006).

There have been three randomized (but not placebo-controlled) studies comparing divalproex (DVP) or divalproex extended release (DVP-ER) and lithium to an atypical antipsychotic, either quetiapine or risperidone. In the three studies, response rate to the atypical antipsychotic was 68.5% (Geller et al. 2012), 72% (DelBello et al. 2006), and 78.1% (Pavuluri et al. 2010), while the comparable response rate for DVP was 24%, 40%, and 45.5%. Where it was measured, the time to response for atypicals was shorter than for divalproex. Importantly, the less robust response of DVP in the Treatment of Early Age Mania (TEAM) study (Geller et al. 2012; Stringaris 2012) was not due to inadequate blood levels. It most likely had do to with the >90% rate of comorbid ADHD plus ODD, whereas rates of ADHD plus ODD in the other studies were about 30%. ADHD implications are discussed in the following subsection.

Lithium has been used in children for more than 70 years. However, until recently there have been no large placebo-controlled studies examining efficacy in children with mania. In the TEAM study (Geller et al. 2012), patients were

TABLE 14–1. Treatment studies in youth and adults with bipolar disorder

	Studies in bipolar youth		FDA-approved treatments for bipolar disorder in adults			
	FDA approved	Trial status	Mania	Mixed	Depression	Maintenance
Apripiprazole (Findling et al. 2009, 2012, 2013a)	Mania (ages 10–17)		×	×		×
Asenapine		Positive mania	×	×		
Carbamazepine (Kowatch et al. 2000) Extended release (Wagner et al. 2006)		Negative mania	×	×		
Chlorpromazine			×			
Lamotrigine		In process				×
Lithium (Geller et al. 2012)	Mania (ages 12–17)		×			×
Lurasidone					×	
Olanzapine (Tohen et al. 2007)	Mania (ages 13–17)		×	×		×
Olanzapine/fluoxetine combination (OFC)		Positive depression			×	
Quetiapine (DelBello et al. 2002; Findling et al. 2013c; Pathak et al. 2013)	Mania (ages 10–17)	Negative depression	×		×	
Risperidone (Haas et al. 2009; Geller et al. 2012; Pavuluri et al. 2010)	Mania		×	×		
Valproate (DelBello et al. 2006; Geller et al. 2012) Divalproex extended release (Wagner et al. 2009)		Negative mania	×			
Ziprasidone (Findling et al. 2013b)		Positive mania	×	×		

randomly assigned to risperidone, lithium, or divalproex. In this study, the lithium response rate was 35.6%. Keeping in mind that the placebo response rate in industry-sponsored trials in mania is consistently between 25% and 30%, lithium would not have beaten placebo in that study. It did not appear that lithium protected against mania relapse after hospital discharge (for a review, see Kowatch et al. 2005). However, the Collaborative Lithium Trials (CoLT) investigators recently presented findings showing a 4.5 point difference on the YMRS scale at week 8, with lithium-treated participants showing more improvement than placebo-treated youth ($p=0.031$). Rates of response (≥50% drop in YMRS) did not differ significantly between lithium and placebo groups (37.7% vs. 28.6%, respectively) (Robb et al. 2014). Regarding relapse prevention (at least for mania), there are suggestions that aripiprazole in one study (Findling et al. 2013a) and lamotrigine in another (Findling et al. 2014) increases the time to relapse for mania.

Published treatment algorithms for mania emphasize the presence or absence of psychotic symptoms. If psychosis is absent, the first-line treatment may include a single antimanic drug, including lithium, valproate, carbamazepine, or any of the atypical or even typical antipsychotic medications. If psychosis is present or mania is severe, from the outset lithium or one of the aforementioned anticonvulsants is combined with an antipsychotic medication. If response is poor, combinations other than the one that has not worked are used. Electroconvulsive therapy or clozapine is reserved for the most treatment-resistant cases.

Given the level of severity and impairment with which most children and teens begin a bipolar treatment study, the improvement, when it occurs, is noteworthy but often is not sufficient. Few data are available to predict treatment response. Using more than one medication has increasingly become acceptable for treating mania or BP in both adults and young people. In youth, there are three types of studies: 1) comparing two medications to one, such as combined divalproex and quetiapine versus quetiapine alone (DelBello et al. 2002); 2) adding one medication to another if the first drug does not work, for example, adding risperidone to lithium or divalproex (Pavuluri et al. 2004); and 3) starting two medications together, for instance, lithium and divalproex, and discontinuing one (Findling et al. 2006). This last study was designed as a maintenance treatment study and suggested that a child stabilized on two medications needs to be maintained on both since the relapse rate on one drug alone was high. These data suggest that at least these medication combinations are additive, both in effectiveness and in side effects.

Mania and/or ADHD

There are increasing data that comorbid externalizing disorders (including ADHD) are important in determining treatment response and type of intervention. It remains unclear whether mania plus ADHD represents a subtype of bipolar disorder or an emotionally dysregulated subtype of ADHD. Either way, response to both ADHD treatments and mood-stabilizing treatments is often less robust than in the uncomplicated versions of either condition. Atypical antipsychotics alone appear to be more effective than mood stabilizers alone.

In the case of clear acute mania, consensus documents recommend stabilizing the mood disorder symptoms first and then treating the comorbid disorder (Kowatch et al. 2005; McClellan et al.

2007). ADHD is the only comorbid condition that has been systematically studied in children with mania or BP-NOS. Although there have been concerns about treating ADHD in children with definite or possible mania, an increasing number of studies are substantiating the utility of doing so either with or without prior mood stabilization (Miller et al. 2013).

In cases where clinicians cannot distinguish between possible mania and ADHD, recommendations include discussing with parents the risks and benefits of using atypical antipsychotics or mood stabilizers first versus ADHD treatment first. If the child becomes more irritable or aggressive with ADHD treatment, it makes most sense to begin an atypical antipsychotic or a mood stabilizer, perhaps followed by retrying the ADHD treatment. There are no diagnostic implications of poor stimulant response or stimulant rebound.

Bipolar Depression

Three medications (olanzapine and fluoxetine combined [OFC], quetiapine, and lurasidone) have FDA-approved indications for bipolar depression in adults. Lithium may be helpful, but it has an indication only for prevention of mania or depression. In young people, there has been a positive trial for OFC but negative small studies for lithium and quetiapine. As of this writing, the only studies of lamotrigine have been open trials, although an industry-sponsored discontinuation trial is being completed. The use of antidepressants alone or in combination with lithium/divalproex appears to be less useful than in adults. Moreover, the risk of "switching" or developing mood elevation as a result of medications used to improve mood is a contentious topic. Extrapolating from information about activation in studies of selective serotonin reuptake inhibitors, rates are higher in children than in adolescents and adults and may average about 10%–20% (Perlis et al. 2010; Safer and Zito 2006).

Of particular relevance to youth is a first episode of depression in a patient with a family history of bipolar disorder. Here, the risks of precipitating a manic/hypomanic/bipolar course with an antidepressant must be weighed against treating with medications for which there are either minimal or no data regarding effectiveness in children or adolescents. Any history suggestive of a bipolar diathesis (including clear bipolar history in first-degree relatives), the reliability of parent observation and child adherence to treatment, and family preference should be carefully considered in the decision-making process.

Maintenance

In adults, two medications have FDA-approved indications for maintenance treatment in BP: lithium for prevention of mania and lamotrigine for bipolar depression. Young people with BP have higher relapse rates than adults. Lithium alone has not been successful as a maintenance medication in this age group. Six-month extension data from recent studies of atypical antipsychotics are not yet available. However, both the available data and clinical experience suggest that if remission is achieved on a particular regimen, it should be continued as long as possible, at least until the child or adolescent has navigated his or her most important developmental, academic, and social milestones.

Prevention

Although it is well known that offspring of parents with bipolar I disorder are at elevated risk for developing psychopathology in general and bipolar spectrum symptoms in particular, there are not yet

TABLE 14–2. Treatments for mania and conditions confused with mania

Treatment type	Mania/BP	MDD	PDD	Abuse	Aggression	ADHD
Lithium	×				×	
Divalproex	×		×		×	
Antipsychotics	×		×		×	
Antidepressants		×	×		×	
ADHD medications			×		×	×
Specific IEP			×			
Language therapy			×			
Psychotherapy	Family-focused therapy, cognitive-behavioral strategies, BP psychoeducation	CBT	Social skills, social stories; collaborative problem solving	CBT, other therapy	Behavior modification	Behavior modification, ADHD, psychoeducation
Child Protective Services				×		

Note. ADHD=attention-deficit/hyperactivity disorder; BP=bipolar disorder; CBT=cognitive-behavioral therapy; IEP=individualized education program; MDD=major depressive disorder; PDD=pervasive developmental disorder.

any proven methods of prevention. Several small trials using lithium, divalproex, risperidone, and quetiapine as well as one study of family-focused treatment in high-risk youth with BP-NOS have been undertaken. Insofar as quetiapine reduced symptoms in these children, it was felt to be an effective prevention. In the other interventions, both the treatment and comparison groups improved at the same rate. Prevention of psychosis or symptom attenuation, not actual mania prevention, were the goals (McNamara et al. 2012).

Treatment Implications for Broad and Narrow Phenotypes

At this time, no definitive recommendations can be made regarding the relative efficacy of treatment response in youth with narrow versus broad phenotype/disruptive mood dysregulation disorder. Atypical antipsychotics appear to have considerable effectiveness. The data are mixed for divalproex and lithium. If youth with severe mood dysregulation/broad phenotype have a condition that is continuous with mixed, rapid cycling, then strategies aimed at these subtypes are warranted. Insofar as rapid cycles are often between bipolar depression and hypomania and depressive symptoms are prominent in mixed episodes, medications aimed at bipolar depression are recommended in adults. Unfortunately, there are no data in children or adolescents on rapid cycling bipolar disorder.

Nicola, described in Case Example 1, responded well to lithium, although she developed a sufficiently severe postmanic depression that she needed to be placed in a special education program for the following year. Lynda was in and out of hospitals and tried various medications, responding well while hospitalized and relapsing when she returned home. She was sent to live with a relative out of state and appeared most stable on mixed amphetamine salts and a low-dose atypical antipsychotic.

BP in children and young adolescents is an important condition to recognize and treat. However, it is also important not to overlook other conditions in which mood dysregulation can figure prominently because the treatment implications can be quite different. Table 14–2 outlines some of the differences in treatment that should be considered.

Summary Points

- Bipolar disorder (BP) and mania in youth are defined with a range of narrow to broad application of DSM criteria by different investigators and clinicians. The degree to which these variations in definition identify the same children and predict a course consistent with the diagnosis of BP in adults is the subject of ongoing study.
- Simultaneous comorbidity of mania and externalizing disorders is higher in prepubertal children than in adolescents. Anxiety and developmental disorders are other important comorbidities. Substance abuse is both a complication and comorbidity of BP in teens.
- Neurobiological validators are being sought through the use of neuroimaging studies. There is some consistency to the finding of decreased amygdala volume and abnormalities in the prefrontal cortex.

- BP in youth is a largely heritable condition with environmental contributions. Complex comorbidity in parents may confer higher rates of psychopathology on offspring. Candidate genes are being sought.
- Age at onset varies by definition (first behavior disorder symptoms, first mood episode, first manic episode). Early onset episodes appear to have worse outcome, in both episode recurrence and functional impairment.
- Evaluation requires interview of parent and child and, if possible, confirmatory information from another source. Comorbidities need to be assessed.
- The differential diagnosis of BP includes ADHD, anxiety disorders, schizophrenia, substance use disorder, and conditions characterized by poor emotion regulation. There are no easy strategies for establishing the diagnosis definitively.
- Treatment modalities for early onset mania are evolving. Currently, there is more evidence for the efficacy of atypical antipsychotics than for lithium or anticonvulsants. There are no placebo-controlled studies of treatment for bipolar depression in youth. Maintenance and prophylactic studies are also needed.

References

Alloy LB, Abramson LY, Urosevic S, et al: The psychosocial context of bipolar disorder: environmental, cognitive, and developmental risk factors. Clin Psychol Rev 25(8):1043–1075, 2005 16140445

Althoff RR, Faraone SV, Rettew DC, et al: Family, twin, adoption, and molecular genetic studies of juvenile bipolar disorder. Bipolar Disord 7(6):598–609, 2005 16403185

American Psychiatric Association: Diagnostic and Statistical Manual of Mental Disorders, 3rd Edition, Washington, DC, American Psychiatric Association, 1980

American Psychiatric Association: Diagnostic and Statistical Manual of Mental Disorders, 4th Edition, Text Revision. Washington, DC, American Psychiatric Association, 2000

American Psychiatric Association: Diagnostic and Statistical Manual of Mental Disorders, 5th Edition. Arlington, VA, American Psychiatric Association, 2013

Arnold LE, Demeter C, Mount K, et al: Pediatric bipolar spectrum disorder and ADHD: comparison and comorbidity in the LAMS clinical sample. Bipolar Disord 13(5–6):509–521, 2011 22017220

Axelson DA, Birmaher B, Strober MA, et al: Course of subthreshold bipolar disorder in youth: diagnostic progression from bipolar disorder not otherwise specified. J Am Acad Child Adolesc Psychiatry 50(10):1001–1016, e3, 2011 21961775

Biederman J, Mick E, Faraone SV, et al: Pediatric mania: a developmental subtype of bipolar disorder? Biol Psychiatry 48(6):458–466, 2000 11018219

Birmaher B, Axelson D, Strober M, et al: Clinical course of children and adolescents with bipolar spectrum disorders. Arch Gen Psychiatry 63(2):175–183, 2006 16461861

Birmaher B, Goldstein BI, Axelson DA, et al: Mood lability among offspring of parents with bipolar disorder and community controls. Bipolar Disord 15(3):253–263, 2013 23551755

Birmaher B, Gill MK, Axelson DA, et al: Longitudinal trajectories and associated baseline predictors in youths with bipolar spectrum disorders. Am J Psychiatry 171(9):990–999, 2014

Blader JC, Carlson GA: Increased rates of bipolar disorder diagnoses among U.S. child, adolescent, and adult inpatients, 1996–2004. Biol Psychiatry 62(2):107–114, 2007 17306773

Brotman MA, Schmajuk M, Rich BA, et al: Prevalence, clinical correlates, and longitudinal course of severe mood dysregulation in children. Biol Psychiatry 60(9):991–997, 2006 17056393

Brotman MA, Kassem L, Reising MM, et al: Parental diagnoses in youth with narrow phenotype bipolar disorder or severe mood dysregulation. Am J Psychiatry 164(8):1238–1241, 2007 17671287

Carlson GA: Differential diagnosis of bipolar disorder in children and adolescents. World Psychiatry 11(3):146–152, 2012 23024665

Carlson GA, Klein DN: How to understand divergent views on bipolar disorder in youth. Annu Rev Clin Psychol 10:529–551, 2014 24387237

Carlson GA, Meyer SE: Phenomenology and diagnosis of bipolar disorder in children, adolescents, and adults: complexities and developmental issues. Dev Psychopathol 18(4):939–969, 2006 17064424

Correll CU, Sheridan EM, DelBello MP: Antipsychotic and mood stabilizer efficacy and tolerability in pediatric and adult patients with bipolar I mania: a comparative analysis of acute, randomized, placebo-controlled trials. Bipolar Disord 12(2):116–141, 2010 20402706

Costello EJ, Angold A, Burns BJ, et al: The Great Smoky Mountains Study of Youth. Goals, design, methods, and the prevalence of DSM-III-R disorders. Arch Gen Psychiatry 53(12):1129–1136, 1996 8956679

DelBello MP, Schwiers ML, Rosenberg HL, et al: A double-blind, randomized, placebo-controlled study of quetiapine as adjunctive treatment for adolescent mania. J Am Acad Child Adolesc Psychiatry 41(10):1216–1223, 2002 12364843

DelBello MP, Findling RL, Kushner S, et al: A pilot controlled trial of topiramate for mania in children and adolescents with bipolar disorder. J Am Acad Child Adolesc Psychiatry 44(6):539–547, 2005 15908836

DelBello MP, Kowatch RA, Adler CM, et al: A double-blind randomized pilot study comparing quetiapine and divalproex for adolescent mania. J Am Acad Child Adolesc Psychiatry 45(3):305–313, 2006 16540815

DelBello MP, Hanseman D, Adler CM, et al: Twelve-month outcome of adolescents with bipolar disorder following first hospitalization for a manic or mixed episode. Am J Psychiatry 164(4):582–590, 2007 17403971

Dickstein DP, Rich BA, Binstock AB, et al: Comorbid anxiety in phenotypes of pediatric bipolar disorder. J Child Adolesc Psychopharmacol 15(4):534–548, 2005 16190786

Dubicka B, Carlson GA, Vail A, et al: Prepubertal mania: diagnostic differences between US and UK clinicians. Eur Child Adolesc Psychiatry 17(3 suppl):153–161, 2008 17876503

Faraone SV, Biederman J, Wozniak J, et al: Is comorbidity with ADHD a marker for juvenile-onset mania? J Am Acad Child Adolesc Psychiatry 36(8):1046–1055, 1997 9256584

Findling RL, McNamara NK, Stansbrey R, et al: Combination lithium and divalproex sodium in pediatric bipolar symptom re-stabilization. J Am Acad Child Adolesc Psychiatry 45(2):142–148, 2006 16429084

Findling RL, Nyilas M, Forbes RA, et al: Acute treatment of pediatric bipolar I disorder, manic or mixed episode, with aripiprazole: a randomized, double-blind, placebo-controlled study. J Clin Psychiatry 70(10):1441–1451, 2009 19906348

Findling RL, Youngstrom EA, McNamara NK et al: Double-blind, randomized, placebo-controlled long-term maintenance study of aripiprazole in children with bipolar disorder. J Clin Psychiatry 73:57–63, 2012

Findling RL, Correll CU, Nyilas M, et al: Aripiprazole for the treatment of pediatric bipolar I disorder: a 30-week, randomized, placebo-controlled study. Bipolar Disord 15(2):138–149, 2013a 23437959

Findling RL, Cavuş I, Pappadopulos E, et al: Efficacy, long-term safety, and tolerability of ziprasidone in children and adolescents with bipolar disorder. J Child Adolesc Psychopharmacol 23:545–557, 2013b

Findling RL, Pathak S, Earley WR, et al: Safety, tolerability, and efficacy of quetiapine in youth with schizophrenia or bipolar I disorder: a 26-week, open-label, continuation study. J Child Adolesc Psychopharmacol 23(7):490–501, 2013c 24024534

Findling RL, Jo B, Frazier TW, et al: The 24-month course of manic symptoms in children. Bipolar Disord 15(6):669–679, 2013d 23799945

Findling RL, Chang KD, Robb A, et al: Double-blind, placebo-controlled, 36 week maintenance study of lamotrigine in youth with bipolar I disorder. Presented at the American Academy of Child and Adolescent Psychiatry Annual Meeting, San Diego, CA, October 21–25, 2014

Galanter CA, Hundt SR, Goyal P, et al: Variability among research diagnostic interview instruments in the application of DSM-IV-TR criteria for pediatric bipolar disorder. J Am Acad Child Adolesc Psychiatry 51(6):605–621, 2012 22632620

Garrett AS, Reiss AL, Howe ME, et al: Abnormal amygdala and prefrontal cortex activation to facial expressions in pediatric bipolar disorder. J Am Acad Child Adolesc Psychiatry 51(8):821–831, 2012 22840553

Geller B, Tillman R, Bolhofner K, et al: Controlled, blindly rated, direct-interview family study of a prepubertal and early adolescent bipolar I disorder phenotype: morbid risk, age at onset, and comorbidity. Arch Gen Psychiatry 63(10):1130–1138, 2006 17015815

Geller B, Tillman R, Craney JL, et al: Four-year prospective outcome and natural history of mania in children with a prepubertal and early adolescent bipolar disorder phenotype. Arch Gen Psychiatry 61(5):459–467, 2004 15123490

Geller B, Luby JL, Joshi P, et al: A randomized controlled trial of risperidone, lithium, or divalproex sodium for initial treatment of bipolar I disorder, manic or mixed phase, in children and adolescents. Arch Gen Psychiatry 69(5):515–528, 2012 22213771

Goodwin FK, Jamison KR: Manic-Depressive Illness: Bipolar Disorders and Recurrent Depression. New York, Oxford University Press, 2007

Gutkovich ZA, Carlson GA: Medication treatment of bipolar disorder in developmentally disabled children and adolescents. Minerva Pediatr 60(1):69–85, 2008 18277367

Haas M, DelBello MP, Pandina G, et al: Risperidone for the treatment of acute mania in children and adolescents with bipolar disorder: a randomized, double-blind, placebo-controlled study. Bipolar Disord 11(7):687–700, 2009 19839994

James A, Hoang U, Seagroatt V, et al: A comparison of American and English hospital discharge rates for pediatric bipolar disorder, 2000 to 2010. J Am Acad Child Adolesc Psychiatry 53(6):614–624, 2014 24839880

Kowatch RA, Suppes T, Carmody TJ, et al: Effect size of lithium, divalproex sodium, and carbamazepine in children and adolescents with bipolar disorder. J Am Acad Child Adolesc Psychiatry 39(6):713–720, 2000 10846305

Kowatch RA, Fristad M, Birmaher B, et al: Treatment guidelines for children and adolescents with bipolar disorder. J Am Acad Child Adolesc Psychiatry 44(3):213–235, 2005 15725966

Leibenluft E, Charney DS, Towbin KE, et al: Defining clinical phenotypes of juvenile mania. Am J Psychiatry 160(3):430–437, 2003 12611821

Leverich GS, McElroy SL, Suppes T, et al: Early physical and sexual abuse associated with an adverse course of bipolar illness. Biol Psychiatry 51(4):288–297, 2002 11958779

Lewinsohn PM, Klein DN, Seeley JR: Bipolar disorders in a community sample of older adolescents: prevalence, phenomenology, comorbidity, and course. J Am Acad Child Adolesc Psychiatry 34(4):454–463, 2995 7751259

McClellan J, Kowatch R, Findling RL, Work Group on Quality Issues: Practice parameter for the assessment and treatment of children and adolescents with bipolar disorder. J Am Acad Child Adolesc Psychiatry 46(1):107–125, 2007 17195735

McNamara RK, Strawn JR, Chang KD, et al: Interventions for youth at high risk for bipolar disorder and schizophrenia. Child Adolesc Psychiatr Clin N Am 21(4):739–751, 2012 23040899

Merikangas KR, Cui L, Kattan G, et al: Mania with and without depression in a community sample of US adolescents. Arch Gen Psychiatry 69(9):943–951, 2012 22566563

Meyer SE, Carlson GA, Wiggs EA, et al: A prospective high-risk study of the association among maternal negativity, apparent frontal lobe dysfunction, and the development of bipolar disorder. Dev Psychopathol 18(2):573–589, 2006 16600068

Miller S, Chang KD, Ketter TA: Bipolar disorder and attention-deficit/hyperactivity disorder comorbidity in children and adolescents: evidence-based approach to diagnosis and treatment. J Clin Psychiatry 74(6):628–629, 2013 23842014

Moreno C, Laje G, Blanco C, et al: National trends in the outpatient diagnosis and treatment of bipolar disorder in youth. Arch Gen Psychiatry 64(9):1032–1039, 2007 17768268

O'Connor MJ, Shah B, Whaley S, et al: Psychiatric illness in a clinical sample of children with prenatal alcohol exposure. Am J Drug Alcohol Abuse 28(4):743–754, 2002 12492268

Pataki C, Carlson GA: The comorbidity of ADHD and bipolar disorder: any less confusion? Curr Psychiatry Rep 15(7):372, 2013 23712723

Pathak S, Findling RL, Earley WR, et al: Efficacy and safety of quetiapine in children and adolescents with mania associated with bipolar I disorder: a 3-week, double-blind, placebo-controlled trial. J Clin Psychiatry 74(1):e100–e109, 2013 23419231

Pavuluri MN, Henry DB, Carbray JA, et al: Open-label prospective trial of risperidone in combination with lithium or divalproex sodium in pediatric mania. J Affect Disord 82(suppl 1):S103–S111, 2004 15571784

Pavuluri MN, Birmaher B, Naylor MW: Pediatric bipolar disorder: a review of the past 10 years. J Am Acad Child Adolesc Psychiatry 44(9):846–871, 2005 16113615

Pavuluri MN, Henry DB, Findling RL, et al: Double-blind randomized trial of risperidone versus divalproex in pediatric bipolar disorder. Bipolar Disord 12(6):593–605, 2010 20868458

Perlis RH, Ostacher MJ, Goldberg JF, et al: Transition to mania during treatment of bipolar depression. Neuropsychopharmacology 35(13):2545–2552, 2010 20827274

Poznanski E, Mokros H: Children's Depression Rating Scale–Revised (CDRS-R). Los Angeles, CA, WPS, 1996

Rende R, Birmaher B, Axelson D, et al: Childhood-onset bipolar disorder: Evidence for increased familial loading of psychiatric illness. J Am Acad Child Adolesc Psychiatry 46(2):197–204, 2007 17242623

Robb AS, Findling RL, McNamara NK: Lithium in the acute treatment of a manic or mixed episode in pediatric bipolar I disorder: a randomized, double-blind, placebo-controlled study. Presented at the American Academy of Child and Adolescent Psychiatry Annual Meeting, San Diego, CA, October 22–25, 2014

Safer DJ, Zito JM: Treatment-emergent adverse events from selective serotonin reuptake inhibitors by age group: children versus adolescents. J Child Adolesc Psychopharmacol 16(1–2):159–169, 2006 16553536

Schneider MR, DelBello MP, McNamara RK, et al: Neuroprogression in bipolar disorder. Bipolar Disord 14(4):356–374, 2012 22631620

Shaffer D, Fisher P, Lucas CP, et al: NIMH Diagnostic Interview Schedule for Children Version IV (NIMH DISC-IV): description, differences from previous versions, and reliability of some common diagnoses. J Am Acad Child Adolesc Psychiatry 39(1):28–38, 2000 10638065

Shankman SA, Lewinsohn PM, Klein DN, et al: Subthreshold conditions as precursors for full syndrome disorders: a 15-year longitudinal study of multiple diagnostic classes. J Child Psychol Psychiatry 50(12):1485–1494, 2009 19573034

Strakowski SM, Adler CM, Almeida J, et al: The functional neuroanatomy of bipolar disorder: a consensus model. Bipolar Disord 14(4):313–325, 2012 22631617

Stringaris A: What we can all learn from the Treatment of Early Age Mania (TEAM) trial. J Am Acad Child Adolesc Psychiatry 51(9):861–863, 2012 22917198

Stringaris A, Santosh P, Leibenluft E, et al: Youth meeting symptom and impairment criteria for mania-like episodes lasting less than four days: an epidemiological enquiry. J Child Psychol Psychiatry 51(1):31–38, 2010 19686330

Strober M, Schmidt-Lackner S, Freeman R, et al: Recovery and relapse in adolescents with bipolar affective illness: a five-year naturalistic, prospective follow-up. J Am Acad Child Adolesc Psychiatry 34(6):724–731, 1995 7608045

Terry J, Lopez-Larson M, Frazier JA: Magnetic resonance imaging studies in early onset bipolar disorder: an updated review.

Child Adolesc Psychiatr Clin N Am 18(2):421–439, ix–x, 2009 19264271

Tillman R, Geller B, Bolhofner K, et al: Ages of onset and rates of syndromal and subsyndromal comorbid DSM-IV diagnoses in a prepubertal and early adolescent bipolar disorder phenotype. J Am Acad Child Adolesc Psychiatry 42(12):1486–1493, 2003 14627884

Tohen M, Kryzhanovskaya L, Carlson G, et al: Olanzapine versus placebo in the treatment of adolescents with bipolar mania. Am J Psychiatry 164(10):1547–1556, 2007 17898346

Van Meter AR, Moreira AL, Youngstrom EA: Meta-analysis of epidemiologic studies of pediatric bipolar disorder. J Clin Psychiatry 72(9):1250–1256, 2011 21672501

Wagner KD, Kowatch RA, Emslie GJ, et al: A double-blind, randomized, placebo-controlled trial of oxcarbazepine in the treatment of bipolar disorder in children and adolescents. Am J Psychiatry 163(7):1179–1186, 2006 16816222

Wagner KD, Redden L, Kowatch RA, et al: A double-blind, randomized, placebo-controlled trial of divalproex extended-release in the treatment of bipolar disorder in children and adolescents. J Am Acad Child Adolesc Psychiatry 48(5):519–532, 2009 19325497

Wang F, Bobrow L, Liu J, et al: Corticolimbic functional connectivity in adolescents with bipolar disorder. PLoS ONE 7(11):e50177, 2012 23185566

Weinstein SM, West AE, Pavuluri M: Psychosocial intervention for pediatric bipolar disorder: current and future directions. Expert Rev Neurother 13(7):843–850, 2013 23898854

Whitney J, Joormann J, Gotlib IH, et al: Information processing in adolescents with bipolar I disorder. J Child Psychol Psychiatry 53(9):937–945, 2012 22390273

Young RC, Biggs JT, Ziegler VE, et al: A rating scale for mania: reliability, validity and sensitivity. Br J Psychiatry 133:429–435, 1978 728692

Youngstrom E, Meyers O, Youngstrom JK, et al: Diagnostic and measurement issues in the assessment of pediatric bipolar disorder: implications for understanding mood disorder across the life cycle. Dev Psychopathol 18(4):989–1021, 2006 17064426

CHAPTER 15

Anxiety Disorders

Sucheta D. Connolly, M.D.
Liza M. Suárez, Ph.D.
Andrea M. Victor, Ph.D.
Alexandra D. Zagoloff, Ph.D.
Gail A. Bernstein, M.D.

When providing care to anxious youth, clinicians must distinguish normal, transient, developmentally appropriate worries and fears, as well as responses to the stressors of daily life, from anxiety disorders. Worries and fears are distinct concepts: *worry* involves anxious apprehension and thoughts focused on the possibility of negative future events, while *fear* is related to the response to threat or danger that is perceived as actual or impending. Occasional worry is normative in children. The fears reported by children tend to decline with increasing age and change over time from immediate and tangible concerns to anticipatory and less tangible ones, whereas the content and complexity of worries increase with age and cognitive ability.

Common fears among infants include loud noises, being startled or dropped, and later normal separation anxiety. Toddlers typically experience fears of imaginary creatures or monsters and darkness. These normative fears diminish after age 6. From ages 5 to 6, worries about physical well-being (e.g., injury, kidnapping) emerge, and later fears of natural events (storms) develop. The most commonly reported fears in children ages 8–13 include concerns about the dark, spiders, and thunderstorms. From age 8, worries about school performance, behavioral competence, rejection by peers, and health and illness emerge, and by age 12 and into adolescence, worries about social competence, social evaluation, and psychological well-being become prominent.

In this chapter we address the diagnosis, epidemiology, assessment, and treatment of seven childhood anxiety disorders: generalized anxiety disorder (GAD), separation anxiety disorder (SAD), social anxiety disorder (SOC), selective mutism (SM), specific phobia, panic disorder, and agoraphobia as well as the symptom of school refusal, which is related to several diagnoses. In DSM-5 (American Psychiatric Association 2013), SAD and SM were moved to the anxiety disorders section.

Diagnostic Criteria and Additional Features

In order for patients to receive an anxiety disorder diagnosis, in addition to presence of the symptom criteria, there must be significant interference in functioning or marked distress for the child. Also, the symptoms cannot be attributable to substance abuse, medication, or other medical condition or better explained by another mental disorder. In order to reduce the overdiagnosis of transient fears or worry in children and adolescents as anxiety disorders, DSM-5 requires that symptoms be present for at least 6 months for specific phobia, social anxiety disorder, and agoraphobia. In this section we summarize the DSM-5 diagnostic criteria and highlight changes from DSM-IV-TR (American Psychiatric Association 2000). We also provide additional clinical features to aid clinicians in diagnosis of these anxiety disorders.

Generalized Anxiety Disorder

GAD is characterized by excessive and uncontrollable anxiety and worry (apprehensive expectation) regarding numerous situations or activities, occurring most days for at least 6 months. The anxiety and worry are associated with at least three of the following six symptoms in adults and at least one in children: 1) restlessness or feeling on edge, 2) fatigue, 3) decreased concentration or mind going blank, 4) irritability, 5) muscle tension, or 6) difficulty sleeping.

Additional Features

- Anxiety and worry occur in a number of areas (school, interpersonal relationships, health/safety of self, health/safety of others, family, natural disasters, future events), and the types of worries exhibited by children with GAD are more typical of adults.
- Excessive self-consciousness; frequent reassurance-seeking from parents, peers, and teachers; cognitive distortions; and persistent worry about negative consequences are characteristic.
- Youth with GAD are perfectionistic, display unreasonable expectations regarding their own performance, and are excessively critical of themselves when they cannot meet these expectations; worries persist in the absence of realistic concerns.
- Somatic complaints are common, including gastrointestinal distress, headaches, frequent urination, sweating, and tremor.
- Prior to DSM-IV (American Psychiatric Association 1994), children with excessive worry were diagnosed with overanxious disorder.

Specific Phobia

Specific phobia is characterized by marked fear or anxiety about a specific object or situation (e.g., flying, heights, animals, receiving an injection, seeing blood). The object or situation almost always provokes immediate intense fear or anxiety and is actively avoided or endured with intense fear or anxiety.

Additional Features

- Specific phobia typically develops following a traumatic event (e.g., being attacked by an animal or stuck in an elevator), observation of others going through a traumatic event (e.g., watching someone drown), an unexpected panic attack in the to-be-feared situation (e.g., while on the subway), or informational transmission (e.g., intensive media coverage of a plane crash).

- It is common for individuals to have multiple phobias.
- In children, the anxiety may be expressed by crying, tantrums, freezing, or clinging rather than a recognizable anxiety response.
- The fear or anxiety may take the form of a full or limited symptom panic attack (*expected panic attack*).
- The fear or anxiety response is out of proportion to the actual danger posed by the specific object or situation and the sociocultural context.
- Individuals with situational, natural environment, and animal specific phobias are likely to show increased sympathetic nervous system arousal. Individuals with *injection-injury specific phobia* often demonstrate a vasovagal fainting or near fainting response that is marked by initial brief acceleration of heart rate and elevation of blood pressure followed by a deceleration of heart rate and drop in blood pressure.
- Young children have a hard time understanding the concept of *avoidance,* and thus it is important to gather additional information from those who know the child well.
- Transient fears are common in young children. It is important to consider the degree of impairment; duration of the fear, anxiety, and/or avoidance; and whether the fear is typical of the child's developmental stage to determine if diagnosis of specific phobia is appropriate.

Separation Anxiety Disorder

SAD is a developmentally appropriate response in young children on separation from their primary caregivers. This is normal for infants from ages 6 to 30 months and usually intensifies between ages 13 and 18 months. Separation anxiety typically declines between ages 3 and 5 years as a result of the child's cognitive maturation that allows the child to comprehend that separation from a caregiver is temporary. SAD is diagnosed when the child demonstrates developmentally inappropriate distress associated with separation from a primary caregiver (American Psychiatric Association 2013). The separation anxiety must occur for at least 4 weeks and cause significant impairment in the child's daily functioning related to home, school, and social settings. Three or more of the following must occur to meet diagnostic criteria for SAD:

- Recurrent and excessive distress in anticipation of or when separation occurs from home or primary attachment figures
- Persistent, excessive anxiety about losing primary attachment figures or something bad happening to primary attachment figures
- Significant anxiety that an event will occur that would lead to prolonged separation (e.g., getting lost, being kidnapped)
- Reluctance or refusal to go places (e.g., school, friend's house) due to fear of separation
- Fear of being or reluctance to be home alone or in other settings without primary attachment figures
- Reluctance or refusal to sleep away from home or fall asleep away from primary attachment figures

- Recurring nightmares regarding separation
- Complaints of physical symptoms (e.g., headaches, stomachaches, nausea, vomiting) when separation is anticipated or occurs

Panic Disorder

Panic disorder is characterized by recurrent unexpected panic attacks. A panic attack is an abrupt surge of intense fear or discomfort that reaches a peak within minutes, during which time four or more of the following physical and cognitive symptoms occur: (1) palpitations, pounding heart, or accelerated heart rate; (2) sweating; (3) trembling or shaking; (4) sensations of shortness of breath or smothering; (5) feeling of choking; (6) chest pain or discomfort; (7) nausea or abdominal distress; (8) feeling dizzy, unsteady, light-headed, or faint; (9) chills or heat sensations; (10) paresthesias; (11) derealization (feelings of unreality) or depersonalization (being detached from oneself); (12) fear of losing control or going crazy; or (13) fear of dying. An unexpected panic attack occurs with no obvious cue or trigger, happening "out of the blue." Worries about having a panic attack are usually associated with physical concerns, such as worry that panic attacks are indicative of life-threatening illnesses (e.g., heart disease, seizure disorder); social concerns, such as embarrassment or fear of being judged negatively by others because of visible panic symptoms; and concerns about mental functioning, such as "going crazy" or losing control.

Additional Features

- A panic attack per se is not a DSM diagnosis. Panic attacks can occur in the context of any anxiety disorder as well as other mental disorders and some medical conditions. When panic attacks happen in the context of other disorders, *panic attack* should be noted as a specifier.
- Panic disorder is rare in childhood, but adults with panic disorder often report that the first occurrence of "fearful spells" was in childhood. Symptoms in adolescents with panic disorder are similar to those in adults, but adolescents tend to worry less about future panic attacks than young adults do.
- Panic disorder is less common in younger children, and the presentation is slightly different. For example, panic attacks experienced by younger children are usually cued or triggered by a specific event or stressor, and the experience of out-of-the-blue panic attacks is rare.
- Adolescents may be less willing than adults to openly discuss panic attacks. Therefore, clinicians need to be attuned to this possibility when encountering adolescents with episodes of intense fear or distress or paroxysmal physical symptoms.

Agoraphobia

Agoraphobia involves marked fear or anxiety about two (or more) of the following situations: (1) using public transportation (e.g., automobiles, buses, trains, ships, planes); (2) being in open spaces (e.g., parking lots, market places, bridges); (3) being in enclosed places (e.g., shops, theaters, cinemas); (4) standing in line or being in a crowd; or (5) being outside of the home alone. Situations are avoided because of thoughts that escape might be difficult or help might not be available in the event of developing panic-like symptoms or other incapacitating or embarrassing symptoms (e.g., fear of falling, fear of incontinence).

Additional Features

- In DSM-5 agoraphobia is classified as a separate diagnosis and is no longer linked to the presence or absence of panic disorder.
- The percentage of individuals with agoraphobia reporting panic attacks or panic disorder is high (30% in community samples and more than 50% in clinic samples) (American Psychiatric Association 2013). The majority of individuals with panic disorder show signs of anxiety and agoraphobia before the onset of panic disorder.
- Among children with agoraphobia, being outside of the home alone is the most frequent situation feared, and cognitions most commonly pertain to becoming lost.
- When criteria for panic disorder are met, agoraphobia should not be diagnosed unless the criterion for avoidance of two or more agoraphobic situations is met.

Social Anxiety Disorder

SOC is characterized by a marked, intense, and consistent fear or anxiety that occurs in one or more social situations in which the individual may be scrutinized by others.

- The individual worries that he or she will act in a way or have anxiety symptoms (e.g., blushing, trembling, sweating, difficulty speaking, staring) that will be negatively evaluated by others (i.e., will lead to humiliation, embarrassment, or rejection or offend others).
- The social situations almost always produce fear or anxiety, but the severity and type of fear or anxiety can vary (e.g., anticipatory anxiety, panic attack). The anticipatory anxiety can begin long before the feared situation.
- The social situations that provoke fear are avoided or if endured result in intense anxiety.
- In children, the anxiety must also occur with peers and not only with adults. Also, the fear may be displayed as crying, tantrums, freezing, clinging, shrinking, or refusal to speak in social situations.
- The fear is excessive and is not consistent with the threat posed by the social situation (e.g., being bullied or tormented by others) or the sociocultural context.
- The fear or avoidance usually has been experienced for 6 months or more.
- Specify *performance only* if the fear or avoidance is restricted to public speaking or performance. These individuals do not have anxiety in nonperformance social situations. In contrast, DSM-IV-TR specified *generalized* SOC if the individual was anxious in most social situations.

Additional Features

- Commonly feared social situations in children include giving public performances (reading aloud in front of the class, music or athletic performances), being in ordinary social situations (starting conversations, joining in on conversations, speaking to adults), ordering food in a restaurant, attending dances or parties, taking tests, working or playing with other children, and asking the teacher for help.
- Individuals with SOC are often shy or withdrawn, share little about themselves, often lack assertiveness, and are too submissive but, less commonly, may be highly controlling of the conversation. They may have rigid posture and limited eye contact or speak softly (American Psychiatric Association 2013).

- Characteristics in children include restricted social skills, longer speech latencies, few or no friends, limited involvement in extracurricular or peer activities, and school refusal.

Selective Mutism

Children with SM are consistently unable to speak in certain social situations (e.g., at school) despite an established capacity to speak in other situations (e.g., at home). The duration of the mutism is at least 1 month and is not limited to the first month of school. The mutism is not due to a lack of knowledge or comfort with the language required. The mutism is not better explained by a communication disorder and does not occur exclusively during the course of autism spectrum disorder, schizophrenia or another psychotic disorder, or severe intellectual disability. If these disorders are present, SM should be diagnosed only when there is an ability to speak in some social situations.

Additional Features

- Transient mutism may occur during transitional periods or in response to stressors, such as the first month of school or a move to a new home. Also, children may initially refuse to speak after they have immigrated to a new country because of lack of knowledge of the new language. However, if refusal to speak persists after comprehension of the new language is established, selective mutism needs to be considered.
- Associated features may include "excessive shyness, fear of social embarrassment, social isolation and withdrawal, clinging, compulsive traits, negativism, temper tantrums, or mild oppositional behavior" (American Psychiatric Association 2013, p. 195).
- SM commonly co-occurs with other anxiety disorders. Research increasingly supports the relationship of SM to SOC (Vecchio and Kearney 2005). If the social anxiety and avoidance in SOC is associated with SM, then both diagnoses may be given. Children with SM usually have normal language development but may have an associated communication disorder that, unlike the SM, is not restricted to a specific social situation.

School Refusal

Unlike SAD, school refusal is not a DSM diagnosis; it is a symptom associated with several diagnoses, including SAD, GAD, SOC, major depression, and ODD. School refusal is often defined as difficulty attending school associated with emotional distress, especially anxiety and depression (King and Bernstein 2001). Terms such as *separation anxiety* and *school phobia* have been used synonymously with school refusal. However, the term *school refusal* is favored because it is descriptive and inclusive and does not imply etiology (King and Bernstein 2001). School refusal does not typically include youth who are not attending school because of truancy or conduct disorder.

School refusal covers a spectrum of avoidance, including complete absence from school, initial attendance at school but leaving during the school day, going to school after intense behavioral resistance (e.g., tantrums), or extreme distress while at school and pleading with parents to allow staying home in the future (Kearney and Albano 2007). School refusers are a heterogeneous group of youth with various associated psychopathology (Suveg et al. 2005). Although the clinical picture can vary greatly, commonly seen features are pleas to parents to be allowed to stay home from school, distress when going to school, somatic complaints, and associated peer and family relationship difficulties.

Kearney and Albano (2007) classify school refusal behavior as serving a function of negative reinforcement (i.e., to avoid unpleasant stimuli or social/evaluative situations at school) or positive reinforcement (i.e., to pursue pleasant situations outside of school). For example, children may refuse school to avoid one or more of the following: riding the school bus, going to gym class, using the school bathroom, encountering bullies, giving a speech or reading aloud, or interacting with teachers. In such cases, the school refusal behavior is negatively reinforced because staying home from school reduces anxiety. On the other hand, if the child is allowed to engage in pleasurable activities such as playing computer games or spending special time with a parent when refusing school, the behavior is positively reinforced by pleasurable emotional experiences.

Epidemiology and Comorbidity

Prevalence, Course, and Prognosis

Large community studies in the United States and other countries have shown that anxiety disorders are among the most common psychiatric disorders in children and adolescents. Lifetime prevalence of "any anxiety disorder" in children and adolescents is between 15% and 32%, and the period prevalence (1 year or 6 months) for any anxiety disorder ranges from 3.1% to 18% (see review by Essau and Gabbidon 2013). Specific prevalence rates are lower in studies where impairment criteria are applied. Table 15–1 summarizes research findings on prevalence, course, and prognosis. Anxiety disorders are common in preschool children, and they follow similar patterns as in older children (Egger and Angold 2006).

Prospective longitudinal data from the Great Smoky Mountains Study showed that anxiety disorders in childhood are predictors of a range of psychiatric disorders in adolescence (Bittner et al. 2007). More specifically, SAD in childhood predicted SAD in adolescence; overanxious disorder (OAD) was associated with later OAD, panic attacks, depression, and conduct disorder; childhood SOC was associated with adolescent OAD, SOC, and attention-deficit/hyperactivity disorder (ADHD); and GAD was related only to conduct disorder.

Anxiety disorders in childhood often precede the onset of other disorders such as disruptive behavior disorders (emerging in mid childhood) and depression (emerging in late childhood). Children with anxiety disorders are at greater risk of developing substance abuse and conduct problems and have increased use of long-term psychiatric and medical services and greater overall functional impairment (Marquenie et al. 2007). A childhood diagnosis of anxiety disorder is associated with high severity and impairment, familial risk, and greater risk of developing a range of disorders across the life span (Egger and Angold 2006).

Comorbidity

Anxiety disorders are highly comorbid with other anxiety disorders (Verduin and Kendall 2003) and with other psychiatric disorders, including depression (Lewinsohn et al. 1997) and ADHD (Kendall et al. 2001). Approximately one-

TABLE 15–1. Prevalence, course, and prognosis of specific anxiety disorders in childhood and adolescence

Prevalence	Course and prognosis
Generalized anxiety disorder (GAD)	
Community samples of children and adolescents	
Prevalence increases with age Lifetime prevalence 0.4%–2.2% Period prevalence (1 year or 6 months) 0.2%–3.6% More equal gender ratio in youth than adults (females 2:1) (Essau and Gabbidon 2013)	Chronic condition with rates of full remission very low Waxing and waning course Individuals with GAD early in life have more comorbidities and greater impairment (American Psychiatric Association 2013)
Separation anxiety disorder (SAD)	
Childhood prevalence 3%–5% (Shear et al. 2006) More common in children than adolescents Higher occurrence in females compared with males (American Psychiatric Association 2013)	Early predictors of SAD: parental depression, parental panic disorder, strong stranger anxiety during infancy (Lavallee et al. 2011) Predictors of persistent SAD: comorbid diagnosis of ODD, ADHD symptoms, reported maternal marital dissatisfaction (Foley et al. 2004) May be related to the later development of panic disorder and depressive disorder (Lewinsohn et al. 2008) Adults with SAD typically have a history of SAD during childhood (Silove et al. 2010)
Specific phobias	
Prevalence 5% in children and 16% in 13- to 17-year-olds Twice as common in females; animal, natural environment, and situational specific phobias are predominantly experienced by females, whereas blood-injection-injury phobia has similar rates across genders (American Psychiatric Association 2013) Typically develops in early childhood; majority of cases prior to age 10 Median age of onset is 7–11 years (mean=10) Situational phobias have later age of onset compared with other types	Specific phobias that develop in childhood and adolescence tend to wax and wane, but phobias that persist into adulthood are unlikely to remit (American Psychiatric Association 2013) Youth with natural environment-type phobias have poorer outcomes and are less responsive to treatment (Ollendick et al. 2010b)

TABLE 15–1. Prevalence, course, and prognosis of specific anxiety disorders in childhood and adolescence *(continued)*

Prevalence	Course and prognosis
Panic disorder	
Community samples	
Panic attacks: 16%–63% of adolescents; panic disorder: 0.6%–5% of adolescents Prevalence <4% before age 14 Rate of onset gradually increases during adolescence, particularly for females, peaking in adulthood (American Psychiatric Association 2013)	Typical age at onset is late adolescence and early adulthood Less common in younger children Usual course if untreated is chronic but waxing and waning Some individuals have episodic outbreaks with years of remission in between; others have continuous severe symptoms (American Psychiatric Association 2013)
Agoraphobia	
Yearly estimated prevalence of 1.7% for adolescents and adults combined May occur in childhood, but incidence peaks in late adolescence and early adulthood Onset in childhood is rare; overall mean age at onset is 17 years, but without preceding panic attacks of panic disorder age of onset is 25–29 years (American Psychiatric Association 2013)	Course is persistent and chronic Complete remission is rare unless treated (American Psychiatric Association 2013)
Social Anxiety Disorder (SOC)	
Community samples in children and adolescents	*Children and adults*
Lifetime prevalence rates 1.6%–9.1% Period prevalence rates 0.27%–6.3% Lower prevalence in countries outside the United States (Essau and Gabbidon 2013) Rates higher for females, especially in adolescents and young adults (American Psychiatric Association 2013)	Relatively stable problem, likely to persist over time if left untreated Median age of onset is 13 years, and 75% have onset between 8 and 15 years Adolescents endorse a broader pattern of fear and avoidance compared with younger children (American Psychiatric Association 2013) Generalized subtype shows earlier age at onset, greater functional impairment, and association with higher risk for comorbid conditions relative to the nongeneralized subtype (Velting and Albano 2001)
Clinical samples	
Youth and adults have reported equal or higher prevalence rates in males than females (American Psychiatric Association 2013) Generalized subtype predominates	

TABLE 15–1. Prevalence, course, and prognosis of specific anxiety disorders in childhood and adolescence *(continued)*

Prevalence	Course and prognosis
Selective mutism (SM)	
Point prevalence ranges from 0.03% to 1% depending on the setting (clinic, school, community) and ages of the individuals in the sample Prevalence does not seem to vary by gender, race, or ethnicity More likely to manifest in young children than adolescents or adults (American Psychiatric Association 2013)	Onset between 3 and 5 years of age Course tends to be chronic; children who do not improve prior to adolescence may have a more persistent form (see review by Cohan et al. 2006) Although some individuals outgrow SM, in many cases social anxiety persists even when SM is resolved
School refusal	
Prevalence about 1% of school-age children (Heyne et al. 2001) Prevalence about 5% in clinic-referred children (Heyne et al. 2001) Five to twenty-eight percent of youth refuse school at some point during their education (Kearney and Bensaheb 2006) Equally common in boys and girls; may be equal across school years or may increase at transitions (e.g., school entry, change in schools) Not linked with learning disabilities, intelligence, socioeconomic status, or single-parent families	Contributes to poorer educational development and may contribute to employment difficulties in adulthood (Heyne et al. 2001) Leads to impaired peer and romantic social development; may contribute to agoraphobia in adulthood Dysthymia, SOC, and learning difficulties predict poorer functional outcomes (McShane et al. 2004)

Note. ADHD=attention-deficit/hyperactivity disorder; ODD=oppositional defiant disorder third of children in the Multimodal Treatment Study of Children with ADHD had co-occurring anxiety disorders (Jensen et al. 2001). Other conditions that frequently co-occur with anxiety include oppositional defiant disorder (ODD), learning disorders, and language disorders (Manassis and Monga 2001). The co-occurrence of anxiety and depression increases with age and is associated with greater impairment and severity (Bernstein 1991). Accurate diagnosis is made difficult by the frequency of overlapping symptoms between anxiety disorders and comorbid conditions (Connolly et al. 2007). Symptoms of inattention, for example, may be indicative of anxiety, ADHD, depression, learning disorders, and substance abuse. Childhood anxiety disorders, particularly SOC, increase the risk of later developing alcohol abuse (Marquenie et al. 2007).

The high degree of comorbidity may have implications for level of functional impairment and treatment outcomes. Several studies have demonstrated, for example, a greater severity of internalizing symptoms among highly comorbid children (Nottelmann and Jensen 1995). In studies of children with SM, nearly all children also met criteria for SOC (Vecchio and Kearney 2005). Developmental disorders/delay, communication disorders, and elimination disorders were also common in some studies of SM (Kristensen 2000).

Verduin and Kendall (2003) compared comorbidity rates in 199 children (8–13 years) with a primary diagnosis of GAD, SAD, or SOC. Children with SAD had a higher mean number of comorbid diagnoses compared with children with GAD or SOC. Furthermore, children with SAD were the least likely to have a comorbid mood disorder and most likely to be diagnosed with sleep terror disorder. Children with SAD had a higher rate of specific phobia compared with children with SOC and a similar rate as children with GAD. ODD was determined to occur relatively evenly among the three anxiety disorders (12% in SAD, 10% in GAD, 5% in SOC).

In clinical samples of school refusers (Kearney and Albano 2004; McShane et al. 2001), more youth met criteria for a psychiatric diagnosis compared with a community sample. Greater than 50% of the participants from each sample had at least one psychiatric diagnosis. The primary categories of diagnoses were anxiety, mood, and disruptive behavior disorders. The two studies showed similar patterns of diagnoses among the participants with school refusal. The most prominent anxiety disorder among the school refusers was SAD (22%, Kearney and Albano 2004; 20%, McShane et al. 2001). Other common anxiety disorders included GAD, SOC, specific phobia, and panic disorder. Major depressive disorder was the most prominent mood disorder (5%, Kearney and Albano 2004; 30%, McShane et al. 2001). The most prominent disruptive behavior disorder was ODD (8.4%, Kearney and Albano 2004; 24%, McShane et al. 2001).

Anxious children are also more likely to have health problems, including asthma, gastrointestinal disorders, and allergies.

Etiology, Mechanisms, and Risk Factors

Genetic predisposition can lead to the development of specific anxiety disorders as a result of the interplay with environmental influences (Gar et al. 2005). Table 15–2 summarizes common biological and environmental influences on the development of childhood anxiety.

TABLE 15–2. Common biological and environmental influences on the development of childhood anxiety

Biological influences

Heredity

Strong familial aggregation and high heritability are found among anxiety disorders (Bolton et al. 2006).

Trait anxiety (a more stable personality characteristic guiding responses to anxiety-provoking situations) is more genetically determined than is state anxiety (a transitory pattern of anxiety symptoms in response to stressors) (Lau et al. 2006).

Temperament

Behavioral inhibition in young children (e.g., tendency toward being shy, timid, quiet, and initially avoidant of novel and uncertain stimuli) is associated with the development of anxiety (for a review, see Degnan et al. 2010).

Autonomic reactivity

Children with anxiety disorders show greater autonomic reactivity in response to stress and have different patterns of cortisol dysregulation than healthy children (Feder et al. 2004).

Children at risk for anxiety disorders have gastrointestinal distress in response to stressors (Campo et al. 2003) and are more likely to have irregularities in sleeping and eating patterns (Ong et al. 2006).

Anxiety sensitivity

Anxiety sensitivity, a tendency to ascribe negative consequences to physiological responses typically associated with anxiety (e.g., shortness of breath, increased heart rate, trembling), is common among children at risk for anxiety disorders.

Longitudinal studies show a specific link between anxiety sensitivity and the development of panic disorder (e.g., Weems et al. 2002).

Environmental influences

Attachment styles

Parents of anxious children are likely to display insecure attachment styles (Shamir-Essakow et al. 2005).

Early insecure attachment styles in children have been associated with subsequent development of anxiety disorders.

Parenting behaviors (for a review, see Suárez et al. 2008)

Control: High levels of parental control (overprotective/overcontrolling parenting) are thought to encourage children's dependence on parents and lower their sense of mastery and control in difficult situations, thus contributing to higher levels of anxiety.

Acceptance: Low levels of parental warmth and sensitivity and higher levels of parental rejection and criticism are thought to influence children's ability to regulate their own emotions and tolerate negative affect, including their experiences of anxiety.

Anxious parenting: By modeling anxious responses to potentially threatening situations, parents may reinforce the child's own anxious coping responses, reducing the likelihood of learning effective strategies to reduce anxiety.

Overinvolved parenting when the child is young increases the risk of the child showing signs of behavioral inhibition, which may then lead to anxiety problems later in childhood.

Peer/social problems (for a review, see Kingery et al., 2010)

Early peer victimization experiences (bullying)

Rejection and neglect by peers

Social skills deficits and a greater tendency toward negative self-evaluations in social situations

TABLE 15–2. Common biological and environmental influences on the development of childhood anxiety *(continued)*

Negative/stressful life events
Negative life events (losing a family member, experiencing parental separation, moving to another school, experiencing a natural disaster)
Exposure to community violence
Childhood adversity (parental mental illness, physical abuse) was related to childhood anxiety among Mexican youth (Benjet et al. 2010).
Antenatal maternal stress has also been linked to increased risk for anxiety in children, and these findings are clinically significant even when considered independently from the effects on childhood outcomes associated with parental postnatal depression and anxiety (Talge et al. 2007).

As described in Table 15–2, several characteristics within the family and specific parenting behaviors have been identified as playing a key role in childhood anxiety. However, it is important to consider the interaction between parent and child variables. For example, Whaley et al. (1999) examined parent-child communication among mothers with and without anxiety. Clinically anxious mothers show higher levels of criticism and tendency to catastrophize compared with mothers with normal anxiety levels, and these behaviors, in turn, predict childhood anxiety. Mothers of anxious children show less warmth and less granting of autonomy than mothers of comparison children (Moore et al. 2004). This relationship is likely to be circular, with parenting behaviors intensifying in reaction to the characteristics of the child. Behavioral inhibition, insecure attachment, and detached and overprotective parenting have additive effects on child anxiety symptoms (van Brakel et al. 2006).

Two parenting dimensions can facilitate or inhibit a sense of control in children: 1) warmth, consistency, and contingency and 2) encouragement of autonomy (Barlow 2002). A sense of uncontrollability and inability to cope lies at the core of the experience of anxious individuals when faced with challenging situations and unpredictable events, leading to more negative emotional responses (Suárez et al. 2008). A diminished sense of personal control (external locus of control) mediates the relationship between environmental family characteristics and the development of anxiety.

Some evidence suggests that parenting by fathers also influences child outcomes (for a review, see Bögels and Phares 2008). Elevated child anxiety has been associated with paternal control, lack of affection, anxious rearing, and paternal anxiety. Also, fathers of anxious children tend to be more (physically) controlling, tend to provide less guidance, and are more rigid. They report having more marital problems. Paternal behaviors that are most likely to be associated with child anxiety include not setting limits on or ignoring their child's avoidant behaviors, less involvement with the child, and lack of encouragement of the child's autonomy. Anxious children are three times more likely to have fathers with an anxiety disorder. The father's responses (e.g., avoidance) in the face of possible threat have a greater influence on children than do the mother's responses, and this can increase the development of child anxiety in the future.

Gunnar et al. (2006) summarized social influences on the regulation of cortisol levels early in human development. High cortisol responsivity, associated with higher levels of anxiety, diminishes with responsive caregiving. Children learn that they can count on their parents for support when in distress and therefore respond more confidently in the face of threat. This is particularly true in children who are anxious and fearful or easily angered and frustrated. This review links early parenting behaviors (overcontrolling and lack of warmth) with impaired child coping responses and the expression of neurobiological processes associated with anxiety.

Evidence for the interaction between biological and environmental influences can also be found in school experiences. Anxious solitude (tendency for children to be shy and socially anxious and to prefer to play alone) assessed at preschool predicted peer rejection and victimization in first grade, while classroom climate (teacher and peer interactions that contribute to positive and negative experiences) was associated with subsequent emotional adjustment (Gazelle 2006).

Barlow (2002) described an interacting set of three vulnerabilities or diatheses leading to the development of anxiety disorders and related conditions. These include 1) a generalized (heritable) biological vulnerability contributing to the development of anxiety and negative affect; 2) a generalized psychological vulnerability related to early developmental experiences that leads to a diminished sense of control (e.g., low levels of parental warmth, consistency, and contingency; lack of encouragement of autonomy); and 3) specific psychological vulnerabilities relating to early learning experiences that focus anxiety on specific life circumstances, leading to the development of specific anxiety disorders. For example, a child with a biological predisposition for anxiety (as indicated by a family history of anxiety disorders) who is also reared by overcontrolling parents is likely to develop anxiety symptoms. The specific type of anxiety disorder that this child develops, however, may be determined by learning experiences, such as being in a dangerous or threatening situation (e.g., a dog attack leading to specific phobia of dogs) or experiencing a false alarm within a specific context (e.g., a panic attack during a speech could mark the beginning of SOC), or vicarious conditioning such as by observing or being told that a situation is dangerous (e.g., observing parents become alarmed by their own physiological responses to fear could lead to the development of panic disorder) (Suárez et al. 2008).

Mineka and Zinbarg (2006) apply a contemporary learning theory perspective to the etiology of childhood anxiety, which considers the interaction between existing vulnerabilities (e.g., genetics/temperament, prior conditioning, perceptions of controllability) and stress (perception of controllability and predictability of stressful events, direct/vicarious traumatic conditioning experience, properties of the conditioned stimulus such as fear relevance, interoceptive versus exteroceptive experiences, temporal proximity to stressful events). These, in turn, influence the quality (e.g., anxiety vs. panic) and intensity of the conditioned association, which then influence the quality and intensity of the expression of conditioned panic and/or anxiety. In the context of existing child vulnerabilities and stressors, child rearing that focuses on facilitating the development of a strong sense of mastery, as well as extensive exposure to nonanxious ways to respond, should lead to more positive outcomes.

Screening and Assessment

Anxiety disorders in children and adolescents remain underrecognized and undertreated. Recommendations to increase the likelihood of identification and early and appropriate treatment (Connolly et al. 2007) include the following:

- Routine screening for anxiety symptoms should be done during the initial mental health assessment.
- If the screening indicates significant anxiety, further evaluation should follow to determine which anxiety disorders are present, along with the severity of the anxiety symptoms and functional impairment.
- The psychiatric assessment should include differential diagnosis of physical conditions and other psychiatric disorders that may mimic anxiety symptoms.
- Comorbid conditions should be assessed.

Screening and Clinical Interview

Obtaining information about anxiety symptoms from multiple informants, including the child, parents, teacher, and other care providers, is important because of variable agreement between informants (Choudhury et al. 2003). Young children may lack the understanding and vocabulary needed to communicate anxiety symptoms or related distress directly, and parental report is essential. Also, children with SAD may not experience as much distress or frustration as their caregivers, who cannot leave the house or even go to another part of the house without their child accompanying them. Alternatively, the child's anxiety may cause significant internal distress but be behaviorally less evident to others (e.g., GAD). Teachers may be more readily aware of anxiety symptoms that affect a child's academic or social functioning relative to same-age peers (e.g., SOC). An anxious child's desire to please adults and concerns about performance during the assessment can also affect the child's report. The clinician needs to be sensitive to the severity of the child's anxiety and monitor the child's physical and emotional cues from the beginning of the evaluation process. In their efforts to please the clinician and their parents, some children with anxiety may attempt to do what is asked of them despite experiencing internal distress or feeling overwhelmed and then acutely shut down. Even discussing anxiety symptoms during the evaluation may be too much for some children, and they may want parents to give details initially.

Various rating scales have been developed to use in conjunction with a clinical interview. Broadband measures, such as the Behavior Assessment System for Children, Second Edition (BASC-2; Reynolds and Kamphaus 2004), offer multiple perspectives of the child's functioning. The Multidimensional Anxiety Scale for Children-2 (MASC-2; March et al. 1997), the Screen for Child Anxiety Related Emotional Disorders (SCARED; Birmaher et al. 1999), and the Spence Children's Anxiety Scale (SCAS; Spence 1998) are self-report measures that focus on symptoms commonly associated with anxiety disorders in children, are specific and sensitive to assessing clinical levels of anxiety in youth, are sensitive to change, and are clinically useful. Screening tools for detection of anxiety disorders in young children are being studied and focus on parent report measures. The Preschool Anxiety Scale is a parent report adapted from the SCAS that was developed for this purpose. The SCARED (ages 8–17), SCAS (ages 7–14), and Preschool Anxiety Scale (ages 2.5–6.5) are free and accessible online (www.wpic.pitt.edu/research; www.scaswebsite.com).

Measures are available for assessment and follow-up of specific anxiety disorders in youth, including specific phobias, SOC, and SM. The Fear Survey Schedule for Children–Revised (FSSC-R; Ollendick 1983) is a self-report screening instrument for specific phobias. The Social Anxiety Scale for Children–Revised (SASC-R; La Greca 1999) and the Social Anxiety Scale for Adolescents–Revised (SAS-A; La Greca 1999) have both parent report and self-report for social anxiety disorder symptoms, and the Social Phobia Anxiety Index–Child Version (SPAI-C; Beidel et al. 1995) is self-report. The Selective Mutism Questionnaire has parent and teacher report forms that can assist with baseline assessment and clinical monitoring of SM (Bergman et al. 2008).

Early detection of anxiety disorders is critical for effective intervention, and the primary care setting plays a key role. Pediatricians and family practitioners can consider the Pediatric Symptom Checklist (PSC), which has a parent report that can be used for ages 4–16 and youth self-report (Y-PSC) for ages 11 and older, with both versions free and accessible online. The Social Anxiety Scale, the Social Worries Questionnaire, and the social phobia subscale of the SCARED are brief screening measures for SOC that are useful in a pediatric primary care (Bailey et al. 2006). Differentiating and diagnosing the specific anxiety disorders can be challenging. Structured interviews lead to more reliable anxiety diagnoses than unstructured interviews (Silverman and Ollendick 2005). The Anxiety Disorders Interview Schedule for DSM-IV: Child Version (ADIS-IV-C; Silverman and Albano 1996), Child and Parent Interview Schedules, is well studied and the most commonly used semistructured interview for anxiety disorders in youth ages 6–17 years. An updated version for DSM-5 is being developed. It is also sensitive to treatment effects and outcome (Silverman and Ollendick 2005). The ADIS-IV-C may be used in its entirety, or sections corresponding to specific disorders may be used to supplement the clinical interview, confirm an anxiety diagnosis, or assist in discriminating among childhood anxiety disorders. It uses language and situations that are developmentally appropriate for children and adolescents and evaluates the presence and severity of anxiety disorders along with comorbid depressive disorders and externalizing disorders. Children with anxiety symptoms who do not meet full DSM criteria for anxiety disorders may still have significant functional impairment and distress and be at risk for development of anxiety disorders in the future. The ADIS-IV-C has a Feelings Thermometer (ratings from 0 to 8) that allows the child and parents to quantify the severity of anxiety symptoms and interference with the child's functioning. The ratings can be used to assist in diagnosis, structure self-monitoring and parent monitoring of anxiety, and assess treatment progress over time. Younger children may prefer visual tools for rating, such as smiley faces and upset faces.

Family assessment can determine possible environmental reinforcements for anxious and avoidant behaviors in children. Clinical observations of parenting styles (controlling, critical, overprotective) and family responses to a child's anxiety symptoms and assessment of parental expectations and coping approaches modeled by parents are helpful. The presence of an anxiety disorder in a parent should be considered during treatment planning.

Often, children with SAD, SOC, or SM are not able to separate from parents to meet alone with the clinician, so the interview needs to be conducted with the parent and child together. It is helpful if the other parent, a sibling, or another familiar person is present at the evaluation to stay with the child so that the clinician can meet with a parent alone to discuss the child's symptoms. This is also necessary when even discussing the anxiety symptoms is too overwhelming for the child. It is also helpful to contact teachers, other school personnel, or day care providers to gather additional information regarding the child's functioning in settings outside the home and away from parents.

There are no consensus guidelines for the assessment of school refusal. Since school refusal is often associated with anxiety, guidelines developed for childhood anxiety disorders (Connolly et al. 2007) are helpful. Youth with school refusal vary in their clinical presentation; therefore, it is most beneficial to use a multimodal assessment with multiple informants (e.g., youth, parents, school personnel) (King and Bernstein 2001). On the basis of the vulnerabilities and symptoms associated with school refusal, a comprehensive evaluation may include several of the following components: clinical interview, semistructured diagnostic interview, examination of factors contributing to the school refusal, self-ratings and parent and teacher ratings of symptoms of anxiety and depression, evaluation of family functioning, and review of school attendance. It may also be helpful to complete psychoeducational and language evaluations to assess for learning and language deficits that could be contributing to school refusal.

The School Refusal Assessment Scale—Revised (SRAS-R; parent and child versions) was developed to assess the primary function of school refusal behavior (Kearney 2002). The SRAS-R assesses the strength of four functional conditions that often maintain school refusal behavior: avoidance of school-related stimuli that trigger negative affect, escape from negative social and/or evaluative situations, getting attention from others, and/or receipt of tangible reinforcements when not in school. One study found that school refusal among children with separation anxiety was most associated with attention-seeking, while children with ODD or conduct disorder were reinforced by tangible rewards (Kearney and Albano 2004). This assessment tool may be helpful in planning effective treatment.

Physical Examination, Mental Status Findings, and Laboratory Tests

It is common for children with anxiety disorders to present with physical symptoms such as muscle tension, headaches, abdominal complaints, restlessness, and difficulty sleeping, which they may not relate to anxiety symptoms. It is important to inquire about and document somatic symptoms during the evaluation to help the child and parents understand these symptoms and their relation to the anxiety disorder.

There are no standard laboratory tests for children or adolescents with anxiety disorders. The clinician needs to consider family history of medical illness and physical symptoms in each child that may warrant further work-up. However, a thyroid panel (thyroid-stimulating hormone, T_3, T_4) should be considered, especially if there is a family history of thyroid disease or comorbid depressive symptoms.

Developmental Considerations

The evaluation should include differentiating anxiety disorders from developmentally appropriate worries or fears and normal responses to stressors. Significant psychosocial stressors or traumas should be carefully considered to determine how they may be contributing to the development or maintenance of anxiety symptoms. Anxiety disorders in children may manifest with behavioral symptoms such as crying, irritability, angry outbursts or tantrums, and argumentativeness. These behaviors may be misunderstood by adults as oppositionality or disobedience, when in fact they could represent the child's expression of overwhelming fear or effort to avoid the anxiety-provoking object or situation. Children with anxiety disorders may not recognize their fears or worry as unreasonable or excessive, even when it is evident to others that their anxiety and avoidance are far out of proportion to actual danger and impair their functioning and judgment.

Differential Diagnosis

Assessment of anxiety disorders in youth should include a differential diagnosis of psychiatric conditions and physical conditions that may mimic anxiety symptoms (Table 15–3). When distinguishing SAD from other anxiety disorders, it is important to understand what the child fears will happen when he or she is separated from a primary caregiver. Children with SAD fear that something bad will happen to them or their primary caretaker that will result in permanent separation. Children and adolescents diagnosed with other anxiety disorders (e.g., GAD, SOC, panic disorder) may also worry about being separated from their primary caretaker; however, the reason for their fear is different. Children with SOC may be concerned about being away from their parents because of the anxiety they experience in social and evaluative situations. Children with panic disorder may be resistant to being separated from their parents because they are fearful they may need their parents' help if a panic attack occurs. Children with GAD endorse multiple worries, which may include worry about the health and safety of themselves and family members, but these worries do not impair their ability to separate from their parents. Another distinguishing factor is that children with SAD exhibit minimal anxiety when with their primary caretaker, whereas children with other anxiety disorders often continue to worry even in the presence of their primary caretaker.

Treatment

Treatment Planning

Treatment planning for childhood anxiety disorders should consider both severity and impairment. For children with anxiety disorders of mild severity that are associated with minimal impairment, it is recommended that treatment begin with evidence-based psychotherapy (Connolly et al. 2007). However, combination treatment with medication and psychotherapy may be necessary for acute symptom reduction in a severely anxious child, concurrent treatment of a comorbid disorder, or partial response to psychotherapy. Residual symptoms of an anxiety disorder can increase the risk for persistence or relapse of the same or another anxiety disorder (Birmaher et al. 2003). Functional impairment, not just reduction of

TABLE 15–3. Differential diagnosis of psychiatric and physical conditions with symptoms similar to those of anxiety disorders

Condition	Symptoms or medications
Psychiatric disorders	
Attention-deficit/hyperactivity disorder	Motor restlessness, fidgeting, inattention
Depression	Poor concentration, insomnia, somatic complaints
Autism spectrum disorder	Social awkwardness, withdrawal, social skills deficits, communication deficits, repetitive behaviors, adherence to routines
Learning disorders	Persistent worries focused on school performance; school refusal
Bipolar disorder	Restlessness, irritability, insomnia
Psychotic disorders	Restlessness, agitation, social withdrawal
Physical conditions	
More common conditions	Hyperthyroidism, caffeinism (including carbonated beverages, energy drinks), migraine, asthma, seizure disorder, lead intoxication
Less common conditions	Hypoglycemic episodes, pheochromocytoma, central nervous system disorders (e.g., delirium, brain tumors), cardiac arrhythmias, allergic rhinitis, chronic pain/illness (e.g., Crohn's disease), diabetes, dysmenorrhea
Medication side effects	
Prescription medications	Antiasthmatics, sympathomimetics, steroids, selective serotonin reuptake inhibitors, antipsychotics (akathisia), haloperidol, pimozide (neuroleptic-induced separation anxiety disorder), and atypical antipsychotics
Nonprescription medications	Diet pills, antihistamines, cold medicines

Source. Connolly et al. 2007.

anxiety symptoms, needs to be monitored during the treatment process.

Effective treatment of children with anxiety disorders often includes child and parent psychoeducation, school consultation, cognitive-behavioral therapy (CBT), and a selective serotonin reuptake inhibitor (SSRI). Similar to youth with anxiety disorders, youth with school refusal benefit most from a multimodal treatment approach. The function of the school refusal behavior should be considered in developing an effective individualized treatment protocol (Kearney and Albano 2004).

Psychotherapeutic Treatments

Among the psychotherapies, exposure-based CBT has received the most empirical support from randomized controlled studies for the treatment of anxiety disorders in children and adolescents and is currently the psychotherapy of choice for this population (see reviews by Compton et al. 2004; In-Albon and Schneider 2007). CBT has been shown to reduce anxiety symptoms and is superior to wait list control; however, relative efficacy and effectiveness compared with other psychotherapeutic interventions (except as described in the following subsections) have not been investigated.

Cognitive-Behavioral Therapy

CBT is a diverse group of interventions that are administered by trained clinicians in a flexible manner for the patient presenting with one disorder or comorbid disorders (Compton et al. 2004). Behavioral therapies are grounded in conditioning and social learning models and have guided interventions used to treat specific phobias and SOC. CBT for childhood anxiety disorders consists of several components: psychoeducation, somatic management, cognitive restructuring, problem solving, exposure, and relapse prevention. (For more detail see Chapter 44, "Cognitive-Behavioral Treatment for Anxiety and Depression.")

Psychoeducation about anxiety disorders showed efficacy comparable to CBT in youth with anxiety disorders in two studies (Last et al. 1998; Silverman et al. 1999). In these studies, psychoeducation and supportive therapy alone may have led to self-directed exposure that in turn reduced anxiety. The current evidence base supports the short-term efficacy and long-term effectiveness (Nevo and Manassis 2009) of child-focused, individual, and group CBT for youth with anxiety disorders. However, these studies indicate that 20%–50% of children may continue to meet criteria for an anxiety disorder after treatment with child-focused CBT. Additional psychosocial interventions and multimodal treatments need to be flexibly considered when needed.

Identifying and treating childhood anxiety disorders at an early age may improve child and parent anxiety management skills, prevent impairment in the child's self-concept, and improve socialization and learning over time (Hirshfeld-Becker et al. 2010). Empirically supported modifications to CBT for younger children (ages 4–7 years) include age-appropriate self-instruction to manage their anxiety, exposure exercises that incorporate games and immediate and frequent positive reinforcement, increased parental participation in modeling, and parental reinforcement of coping strategies. In addition, teaching parental anxiety management strategies and parental skills training is helpful (Hirshfeld-Becker et al. 2010).

Emerging adulthood is a term applied to individuals ages 18–25 years who are navigating issues such as career goals, financial independence, and sexual identity. Treatment approaches are being designed to help those for whom anxiety is interfering with this transition. The Launching Emerging Adults Program (LEAP; Albano 2014) addresses the needs of the young adult with an anxiety or mood disorder as well as the parental behavior that maintains the difficulties. Consistent with the cognitive-behavioral model, the program includes psychoeducation (especially related to areas of transition), treatment hierarchies and exposure (e.g., anxiety related to getting a job), evaluation of negative predictions, and assertiveness training. The treatment formally addresses parental anxiety regarding watching the young adult learn from mistakes.

Parent-Child and Family Interventions

Parents and families have an important role in the development and maintenance of childhood anxiety disorders. Child-focused interventions may not address risk factors such as parental anxiety, insecure attachment, and parenting styles. Interventions that improve parent-child relationships, strengthen family problem-solving and communication skills, reduce parental anxiety, and foster parenting skills that reinforce healthy coping and autonomy in the child are often integrated into treatment with anxious children in clinical settings (Connolly et al. 2007).

The benefits of adding a parental component to established child-focused CBT for childhood anxiety, in addition to standard psychoeducation and coaching, need further study. Parental involvement has been shown to be most critical when the parent is anxious (Cobham et al. 1998). Parental overinvolvement, criticism, and control are some of the variables felt to contribute to development and maintenance of childhood anxiety. Integrative models for family treatment of anxious children have been proposed that consider the interaction between attachment, parent-child learning processes, and behavioral and temperamental characteristics of both the child and parent, but they still need further evaluation.

Although most family studies on etiology and treatment for anxiety include mothers, research suggests that fathers play an important role different from that of mothers (Bögels and Phares 2008). The authors suggest that paternal factors that could be the target of treatment include paternal involvement, warmth, encouragement of autonomy, and addressing the father's own anxiety.

Other Psychotherapeutic Treatments

Psychodynamic psychotherapy has been used in the clinical treatment of anxiety disorders in children and adolescents, but empirical evidence regarding efficacy or effectiveness is very limited (In-Albon and Schneider 2007).

Applications of CBT and Other Interventions for Specific Anxiety Disorders and School Refusal

Generalized Anxiety Disorder

Children with GAD may benefit from modifications to standard CBT to target core symptoms of uncontrollable worry and physical signs of anxiety (Keeton et al. 2009). Relaxation skills such as diaphragmatic breathing and progressive muscle relaxation techniques can be introduced early and practiced often to target physical symptoms. Cognitive restructuring is a vital component in treatment of GAD to identify and challenge persistent worries and negative thought patterns in a range of situations. On the basis of the abstract nature of some of their worries (e.g., health-related issues, death), children with GAD can benefit from imaginal exposures to visualize and face the feared situation and practice coping strategies and self-talk. Problem solving is a useful technique to generate possible solutions and then prospectively develop a realistic action plan to respond to various challenging situations.

Specific Phobias

Systematic desensitization procedures have substantial research support and usually involve three components: 1) induction of muscle relaxation; 2) development of a fear-producing stimulus hierarchy; and 3) systematic, graduated pairing of items in the hierarchy with relaxation. Developmentally appropriate adaptations of systematic desensitization procedures for children with specific phobias may include use of real life desensitization programs (in vivo), emotive imagery (narrative stories), live modeling (demonstration of nonphobic response), participant modeling (physical contact with the model-therapist and the phobic object), and contingency management (shaping, positive reinforcement, extinction) (King et al. 2005). Different types of specific phobias may warrant specific treatment modifications. For example, patients with blood-injection-injury phobias should use applied tension strategies to prevent fainting.

Intensive, one-session treatment for specific phobias that combine gradual in vivo exposure, participant modeling, reinforcement, psychoeducation, cognitive challenges, and skills training have shown positive results not only on the primary phobia but also on secondary phobias and other comorbid anxiety disorders (Ollendick et al. 2010a).

Panic Disorder

CBT strategies employed to treat panic disorder include psychoeducation about physiological processes that lead to physical sensations, progressive muscle relaxation, breathing retraining, cue-controlled relaxation, cognitive coping, and gradual exposure to agoraphobic situations (Barlow and Craske 2007). Additionally, interoceptive exposure (gradual exposure to somatic sensations such as dizziness, shortness of breath, and sweating by using exercise that induces these sensations) has been used effectively to manage worry about future panic attacks (Barlow and Craske 2007). Developmental adaptations from adult models of panic control treatment have been developed specifically for adolescents (Hoffman and Mattis 2000). Modifications include 1) the use of clear, simple language with verbal and visual examples; 2) parental participation; and 3) reframing exposures as "hypothesis testing" activities.

An evaluation of Panic Control Treatment for Adolescents demonstrated significant and stable treatment gains (Pincus et al. 2010). The 12-session manualized intervention includes psychoeducation and exposure exercises, guidelines for delivering an intensive (8-day) adaptation of the panic control treatment, and recommendations for tailoring the intervention to youth of various ages (Pincus et al. 2008a, 2008b).

Social Anxiety Disorder

Programs for SOC have included exposure-based CBT with an emphasis on social skills training. In a preliminary study, Cognitive Behavioral Group Treatment for Adolescents, which included skills training and exposure-based CBT with a parent component, showed significant improvement in self-report measures of anxiety and depression throughout treatment and at 1-year follow-up (Albano et al. 1995). Social Effectiveness Therapy for Children (SET-C) includes a peer generalization component in which children join a group of nonanxious peers in a group activity. Children treated with SET-C showed maintenance of a majority of posttreatment gains at 3-year follow-up, with 72% of treated children free of SOC diagnosis (Beidel et al. 2005).

Selective Mutism

There is good evidence to support behavioral interventions for SM (Cohan et al. 2006). However, most behavioral interventions evaluated have not targeted communication deficits, developmental delays, or second-language acquisition, and addressing these comorbidities may be promising. A small randomized controlled pilot study that combined clinic-based sessions and phone communication with teachers suggested efficacy of exposure-based behavior therapy for SM (Bergman et al. 2013). A home- and school-based CBT intervention for SM showed efficacy in a recent randomized controlled treatment study (Oerbeck et al. 2014).

A multimodal psychosocial treatment approach has been proposed for SM with comorbid SOC and mutism at school (Cohan et al. 2006). Psychotherapy focused on verbal and nonverbal communication skills and anxiety management is combined with a behavioral program in the school to shape appropriate communication. Social interactions and communication in all settings are rewarded along a hierarchy of feared speaking situations. Adults, siblings, and classmates are encouraged not to speak for the child. Efforts at nonverbal communication (pointing and participating in activities) are reinforced, and over time verbal behaviors (mouthing words, whispering, speaking in a soft voice) are rewarded as the child learns to manage anxiety through standard CBT strategies. Stimulus fading (gradual removal of people or objects that increase the child's comfort level) can be used initially to develop comfort with the therapist and later to develop comfort with individuals and areas in the school setting in order to generalize speech. This may involve inviting peers to settings where the child is comfortable (home) and then moving play dates to the child's classroom. In the classroom, teachers or classmates can be faded in and out systematically from the periphery of the classroom while a comfortable person such as a parent is present. When comfort develops, the parent can be faded out.

Separation Anxiety Disorder

CBT is the best proven psychotherapeutic treatment for youth with SAD (Eisen and Schaefer 2005). Initial psychoeducation provides information to the parent and youth regarding behaviors that sustain SAD (e.g., avoidance of anxiety-provoking situations) and treatment approaches (e.g., thought identification, cognitive modification, behavioral exposures) that are effective in alleviating anxiety.

Children with SAD often report fearful thoughts related to anxiety-provoking situations (e.g., going to school, being away from the parent, attending sleepovers). Common anxious thoughts include "Mom will forget to pick me up from school"; "Mom will die when we are not together and I will never see her again"; and "I will get lost and never be able to see Mom again." Cognitive modification teaches youth to recognize their anxiety-provoking thoughts and to challenge these maladaptive thoughts with more realistic and rational thoughts.

As a result of anxious thoughts about separation, children change their behavior to prevent separation from their parents (e.g., school refusal, unwillingness to leave parents to go to a friend's house). Since youth with SAD believe that these dangerous and feared outcomes have a high likelihood of occurring, it is crucial to challenge these thoughts and predictions with behavioral exposure exercises. Parents, who may also suffer from anxiety, may need support to withstand the child's distress and implement the exposure long enough for anxiety reduction to occur.

Limited intervention research has been conducted with children younger than 7 years of age who are diagnosed with SAD. Parent-Child Interaction Therapy (PCIT) is empirically supported as a treatment for children with disruptive behavior disorders and has been adapted to be used in the treatment of young children with SAD (Pincus et al. 2005). PCIT uses play to teach parents specific skills to help develop and strengthen a nurturing and secure relationship between the parent and child. During play-based interactions, parents learn to encourage prosocial behaviors and discourage negative behaviors, which often results in an improvement in attachment and warmth between parent and child. It is expected that this may ultimately help the child separate from the parent by strengthening the child's feeling of security. PCIT also incorporates parenting skills that are important in decreasing child anxiety (e.g., parental attention toward child, differential reinforcement, behavioral modification, clear commands).

School Refusal

Psychotherapeutic treatments aimed at school refusal are primarily cognitive-behavioral combined with a family systems approach that incorporates relaxation training, cognitive modification, social skills training, exposure-based activities, and contracting and contingency management (Kearney and Albano 2007). Therapist and parent books have been written to guide treatment (Kearney and Albano 2007). Relaxation training, cognitive modification, and social skills training are typically completed prior to engaging in exposure-based activities to prepare the youth for school reentry. Prior to school reentry, a plan must be developed with the youth and parent that includes a hierarchy of steps toward full-day entry. Youth with mild or acute school refusal are more likely to start with immediate full-day return to school. School reentry is often a difficult process for youth with chronic school refusal; therefore, return should be phased (King et al. 2001), and contingency contracts are helpful to motivate the youth to begin and continue the reentry process. Using homebound services or changing schools is generally not recommended.

In addition to using CBT techniques with the youth, it is crucial to work with parents and school personnel, who often need to play active roles in helping the child return to school. Parents learn to set appropriate limits that do not reinforce the child's school refusal behaviors (e.g., escort child to school, limit access to attention and pleasurable activities when at home). School personnel are essential to ensure that the youth remains at school for the planned amount of time. Teachers can help integrate the child back into the classroom, and counselors can help manage anxiety if necessary. School personnel perceive different categories of absent students (e.g., legitimately versus illegitimately ill), and their perceptions influence their responses to students (Torrens Armstrong et al. 2011). "Frequent fliers" is a label applied to students who visit the nurse frequently. Providers were found to distinguish between those students believed to have legitimate illnesses (e.g., asthma) and those who do not have demonstrable medical illness or may attempt to use their illness to manipulate the system. School personnel identified the following types of absent students: defiant, adult, failing, bored, invisible, physically refusing, socially uncomfortable, sick, and victim. These types differed with respect to their perceptions of parental control, parental awareness, student locus of control, placement of blame for absenteeism, and victim status. Related to these constructs, school staff were more or less likely to emphasize support or discipline as a strategy for intervention. Youth, parents, school personnel, and outside providers (psychologists, psychiatrists) must work as a team to ensure successful school reentry.

CBT is an efficacious treatment for youth with school refusal; however, additional research needs to be conducted for it to gain well-established empirical status. King and colleagues (1998, 1999) have published results from two studies of CBT for school refusal. In both studies, children who received CBT significantly improved their school attendance and demonstrated improvements on self-report measures of emotional distress and coping. Sixteen of the children who received CBT completed a 3- to 5-year follow-up assessment (King et al. 2001). Thirteen of the 16 children had a normal school attendance at follow-up and did not endorse any new psychological problems.

Kearney and Bensaheb (2006) summarized suggestions for school-based interventions. Support groups have been created to address triggers for absenteeism, including bullying, safety for gay and lesbian students, and teen pregnancy. For children with separation anxiety, the morning transition can be especially challenging. Once the child has entered the building, it is recommended that the child initially be allowed to spend the whole day in one place (e.g., the lobby) rather than return home. Such an approach provides the child with exposure to the school setting and does not reinforce avoidance behavior. When children seek excessive reassurance, adults are encouraged to answer the question the first time so that the child receives accurate information and then politely ignore future repetitive questions. Allowing a child to call his or her parent later in the day can be used as a reward for engaging in school-based activities. When children present to the nurse's office, they should be kept in school whenever possible. Brief anxiety-management breaks in the nurse's office can be formally incorporated into a 504 plan when necessary. A two-pronged approach is useful for addressing somatic complaints (headaches, stomachaches). First, students should gradually increase their school participation (e.g., adding an hour per day) and can spend other times in the library. Second, the student should learn and implement anxiety-management strategies (relaxation, breathing) whenever possible. When students attend class despite symptoms of anxiety, prompt rewards are encouraged.

Other Treatment Modalities

Classroom-based accommodations may be part of the treatment plan for anxious children. It is often beneficial to educate the teacher and other school personnel regarding the child's anxiety and effective strategies to help the child cope in the classroom. It is helpful to identify an adult other than the teacher (e.g., school nurse, school social worker) to assist the child with problem-solving or anxiety management strategies. If performance or test anxiety is present, then testing in a quiet, private environment and increased time allowed for testing may reduce excess anxiety. For speeches or performances, the child may practice in a stepwise fashion using a recording device, then in the classroom without others present, and gradually with familiar students and finally including the teacher. Specific recommendations for the anxiety disorder can be written into the student's 504 plan or individualized education program.

Pharmacological Treatments

Selective Serotonin Reuptake Inhibitors

Medications are considered when the severity of anxiety symptoms or related impairment makes participation in psychotherapy difficult or treatment with psychotherapy alone results in a partial response. In addition, medication is considered as a part of a multimodal treatment plan when anxiety symptoms are moderate to severe and associated with substantial impairment. The age of the child is a factor. Older children are more likely to be prescribed medications compared with younger children. The SSRIs are the first-line pharmacological treatment for pediatric anxiety disorders (Connolly et al. 2007; Kodish et al. 2011; Strawn et al. 2012). These medications are covered in Chapter 36, "Antidepressants."

A number of randomized placebo-controlled trials have established the short-term efficacy and safety of SSRIs (primarily fluoxetine and sertraline) for the treatment of childhood anxiety disorders (Table 15–4). SAD, GAD, and SOC often occur together and are treated with similar pharmacological strategies. They have been often been studied together in medication trials (Birmaher et al. 2003; The Research Unit on Pediatric Psychopharmacology Anxiety Study Group 2001; Walkup et al. 2008). Specific anxiety disorders with controlled SSRI trials include SM with SOC (Black and Uhde 1994), SOC (Beidel et al. 2007; Wagner et al. 2004), and GAD (Rynn et al. 2001).

A study of paroxetine in SOC showed significant adverse effects in the treatment group, such as vomiting, decreased appetite, and insomnia, and there were concerns about elevated rate of suicidal ideation and behavior (Wagner et al. 2004). The use of paroxetine declined dramatically between 2005 and 2009, related to U.S. Food and Drug Administration (FDA) warnings and studies showing lack of efficacy in trials for pediatric depression and the risk of side effects (Lam et al. 2013).

A multisite study compared the relative efficacy of fluoxetine, pill placebo, and SET-C in the treatment of 122 children and adolescents with SOC (Beidel et al. 2007). Both fluoxetine and SET-C were shown to be efficacious for SOC and superior to placebo in reducing social distress and avoidance and improving general functioning. However, SET-C was superior to fluoxetine in all these areas, and SET-C alone was superior to placebo in improving social skills and enhancing social competence. This study did not examine combined treatments.

There are no randomized controlled trials of escitalopram for pediatric anxiety disorders, although an open-label trial (ages 10–17) with dosing 2–20 mg/day (Isolan et al. 2007) and a retrospective chart review in preschool children with dosing 2–10 mg/day (Coşun et al. 2012) suggested positive effects.

TABLE 15–4. Randomized placebo-controlled pharmacological treatment studies[a]

	Treatment	Demographics	Diagnoses	Results
Selective serotonin reuptake inhibitors				
Black and Uhde 1994	Fluoxetine (12–27 mg/day), 12 weeks	*N*=15, ages 6–11	SM plus SOC or AD	Fluoxetine>Pbo
The Research Unit on Pediatric Psychopharmacology Anxiety Study Group 2001	Fluvoxamine (50–250 mg/day child, 50–300 mg/day adolescent), 8 weeks	*N*=128, ages 6–17	SOC, SAD, GAD	Fluvoxamine>Pbo
Rynn et al. 2001	Sertraline (50 mg/day), 9 weeks	*N*=22, ages 5–17	GAD	Sertraline>Pbo
Birmaher et al. 2003	Fluoxetine (20 mg/day), 12 weeks	*N*=74, ages 7–17	SOC, SAD, GAD	GAD or SOC: Fluoxetine>Pbo SAD: Fluoxetine=Pbo
Wagner et al. 2004	Paroxetine (10–50 mg/day), 16 weeks	*N*=322, ages 8–17	SOC	Paroxetine>Pbo
Beidel et al. 2007	Fluoxetine (10–40 mg/day), 12 weeks	*N*=65, ages 7–17	SOC	Fluoxetine>Pbo
Walkup et al. 2008	Sertraline (25–200 mg/day), 12 weeks	*N*=209, ages 7–17	SOC, SAD, GAD	Sertraline>Pbo
Serotonin norepinephrine reuptake inhibitors				
March et al. 2007	Venlafaxine ER (37.5–225 mg/day), 16 weeks	*N*=293, ages 8–17	SOC	Venlafaxine ER>Pbo
Rynn et al. 2007	Venlafaxine ER (37.5–225 mg/day), 8 weeks	*N*=320, ages 6–17 (two studies combined)	GAD	Venlafaxine ER>Pbo (study 1) Venlafaxine ER=Pbo (study 2)
Strawn et al. 2015	Duloxetine (30–120 mg/day), 10 weeks	*N*=272, ages 7–17	GAD	Duloxetine>Pbo
Selective norepinephrine reuptake inhibitors				
Geller et al. 2007	Atomoxetine (mean final dose of 1.3 mg/kg/day), 12 weeks	*N*=176, ages 8–17	ADHD plus SOC, SAD, GAD	Atomoxetine>Pbo for anxiety and ADHD symptoms

Note. AD=avoidant disorder; ADHD=attention-deficit/hyperactivity disorder; ER=extended release; GAD=generalized anxiety disorder; Pbo=placebo; SAD=separation anxiety disorder; SM=selective mutism; SOC=social anxiety disorder.

[a]Data reported in this table reflect medication arm of multimodal study only.

There are no controlled studies in youth of medication treatment for panic disorder. Clinically, SSRIs are considered the first-line treatment in youth with panic disorder and may be combined with benzodiazepines (clonazepam or lorazepam) when severe panic disorder is present (Reinblatt and Riddle 2007).

The first-choice medication for children and adolescents with school refusal is an SSRI, on the basis of evidence supporting the efficacy of SSRIs for treating youth with anxiety disorders. School refusal associated with depression may also be addressed with an SSRI (Cheung et al. 2005).

Children with anxiety disorders generally tolerate SSRIs. Side effects are covered in Chapter 36. Acute changes in level of active defiance, "mouthiness," or heightened emotional reactivity that can be part of disinhibition need to be distinguished from improvement in spontaneity and assertiveness that are positive effects of SSRIs in anxious children. In a retrospective chart review of escitalopram used for anxiety disorders in preschoolers, the most common side effect was behavioral disinhibition, often requiring discontinuation of the medication (Coşun et al. 2012).

Other Medications

Alternative medications that have been used to treat pediatric anxiety disorders include serotonin norepinephrine reuptake inhibitors (SNRIs), tricyclic antidepressants (TCAs), benzodiazepines, atomoxetine, and buspirone (for reviews, see Kodish et al. 2011; Strawn et al. 2012).

Serotonin Norepinephrine Reuptake Inhibitors

One large study evaluated venlafaxine ER for the treatment of GAD in children and adolescents (Rynn et al. 2007), and another large study evaluated venlafaxine ER for SOC in youth (March et al. 2007). In the study of youth with GAD, venlafaxine ER was significantly more effective than placebo, with a response rate of 69% in the venlafaxine group and 48% in the placebo group (Rynn et al. 2007). In the study of SOC, venlafaxine ER was significantly better than placebo, with response rates of 56% in the medication group compared with 37% in the placebo group (March et al. 2007). Side effects included anorexia, weight loss, and sedation. Suicidal ideation was reported in 2% of participants on active medication compared with 0% on placebo (March et al. 2007). These two studies provide some support for the use of venlafaxine in treating youth with GAD and/or SOC.

Another SNRI, duloxetine, was evaluated for the treatment of children and adolescents with GAD (Strawn et al. 2015). The response rate for duloxetine (59%) was significantly greater than placebo (42%), and the remission rate for duloxetine (50%) was significantly greater than placebo (34%). Duloxetine was recently approved by the FDA for the treatment of GAD in youth ages 7–17 years. Significant side effects include nausea, vomiting, decreased appetite, dizziness, cough, oropharyngeal pain, and palpitations.

Tricyclic Antidepressants

TCAs have more side effects than SSRIs, especially cardiovascular effects, and are dangerous in overdose. Furthermore, the use of TCAs requires monitoring of electrocardiograms and blood levels. Results of randomized controlled trials are conflicting regarding the efficacy of TCAs for anxiety-based school refusal and SAD (Strawn et al. 2012). The lack of agreement is explained by small sample sizes, differing drug dosages, lack of control of adjunctive therapies, and different comorbidity patterns. In any case, inconsistent findings regarding efficacy and the side effect profile move TCAs far down the line of treatment options.

Benzodiazepines

Benzodiazepines have not shown efficacy in controlled trials of childhood anxiety disorders, despite established efficacy in adult trials. Clinically, they can be used as an adjunctive short-term treatment to achieve acute reduction in severe anxiety symptoms while an SSRI is titrated up. They may reduce anxiety symptoms enough to permit initiation of the exposure phase of CBT for school refusal, panic disorder, or specific phobias. Benzodiazepines should be used cautiously in youth because of the possibility of developing physical and psychological dependence (Reinblatt and Riddle 2007). They are contraindicated in youth with a history of substance abuse. Possible side effects include sedation, disinhibition (aggression, irritability), behavioral dyscontrol, and cognitive impairment that can impede learning. Withdrawal symptoms may be severe, especially if the medication is stopped abruptly, and may include insomnia, anxiety, gastrointestinal upset, and seizures. A gradual taper down of the benzodiazepine is needed to reduce the likelihood of withdrawal symptoms. Because of potential harm to the fetus and nursing infant, benzodiazepines are not recommended in girls who are pregnant or breastfeeding.

Atomoxetine

Atomoxetine, a selective norepinephrine reuptake inhibitor, was studied in children and adolescents with ADHD and comorbid anxiety disorder (i.e., SAD, GAD, and/or SOC) (Geller et al. 2007). Subjects were randomly assigned to 12 weeks of atomoxetine (n=87) versus placebo (n=89). Using last observation carried forward, the atomoxetine group was significantly improved on both anxiety and ADHD symptoms compared with the placebo group. These findings are encouraging because approximately one-fourth of children with ADHD have comorbid anxiety disorders.

Buspirone

Two randomized placebo-controlled studies (N=559) examined the efficacy and tolerability of buspirone (15–60 mg/day) for GAD in children and adolescents (Bristol-Meyers Squibb Company 2010). Despite good evidence in adults with GAD, there were no significant differences between buspirone and placebo in reducing GAD symptoms in children and adolescents.

Clinical Approach to Pharmacological Treatment of Pediatric Anxiety Disorders

There is no evidence that a particular SSRI is more effective than another for the treatment of childhood anxiety disorders. The clinician can consider side effect profile, drug-drug interactions, duration of action and patient compliance, and positive response to one of the SSRIs in a first-degree relative with anxiety. Anxious children and parents are very sensitive to any worsening of somatic symptoms or the development of even mild or transient side effects. Therefore, careful assessment of somatic symptoms at baseline prior to starting medication trials is important. The clinician should also routinely screen for symptoms of bipolar disorder and family history of bipolar disorder prior to initiating an SSRI or other antidepressant because mania and hypomania can be side effects of SSRIs. In addition, it is important to evaluate psychosocial factors that may predispose a patient to risk for aggression or suicidal behavior (Seidel and Walkup 2006).

Although the FDA issued a black box warning in 2004 for use of any antidepressant medication in the pediatric population, the risk for suicidality does not seem to be elevated in pediatric anxiety trials. This, along with the larger effect size of SSRIs for childhood anxiety disorders compared with depression, suggests that the risk-benefit ratio is more favorable for anxiety disorders than that for depression (Seidel and Walkup 2006). (See Chapter 36 for more detail.)

Currently, there are no specific dosing guidelines for use of SSRIs in youth with anxiety disorder. Clinicians should start at low doses, monitor side effects closely, and increase the dose slowly on the basis of treatment response and tolerability. Especially for young children, using the liquid form of SSRI medications allows for starting at very low doses, which may reduce the likelihood of side effects. Clinicians should consider increasing the SSRI dose by the fourth week of treatment if significant improvement in anxiety symptoms or impairment is not achieved by then. Also, because improvement on SSRI medication does not result in full resolution of symptoms in about half of anxious children (Walkup et al. 2008), it is suggested that higher doses of medication or multimodal treatments be considered in some cases, especially if baseline anxiety symptoms are severe. Pine (2002) recommended that clinicians consider a medication-free trial for children who achieve marked improvement in anxiety or depressive symptoms and associated impairment. The medication-free trial can occur during the first low-stress period (such as vacations) after 1 year of remission of anxiety symptoms with SSRI treatment. Children who exhibit signs of relapse during the taper down or discontinuation of medication should be promptly restarted on the SSRI.

There are limited data to guide combinations of medications when a single medication is ineffective or there is a partial response. It is important to make sure that the diagnosis is accurate, the medication trial is of adequate length, and the dose is optimized (Reinblatt and Riddle 2007; Seidel and Walkup 2006). Switching SSRIs in a child with treatment-resistant anxiety has been shown to be a useful treatment strategy (Walkup et al. 2002). Comorbid diagnoses are strongly considered in selection of medication (Connolly et al. 2007; Reinblatt and Riddle 2007).

Pharmacological Treatment of Young Children with Anxiety Disorders

The American Academy of Child and Adolescent Psychiatry Preschool Psychopharmacology Working Group developed recommendations for psychopharmacological treatment in young children (Gleason et al. 2007). The algorithm for anxiety disorders included SAD, GAD, SM, and specific phobia. Initially, psychotherapy for a minimum of 12 weeks is recommended. If psychotherapy alone is not effective, fluoxetine is the first-choice medication, in liquid form, starting at very low doses (1 mg) and monitored closely. The medication is increased slowly in small increments to minimize side effects. Dosages as low as 5–8 mg/day of fluoxetine may be effective. If an adequate trial of fluoxetine is not successful, switching to another SSRI is recommended. Paroxetine, α-agonists, and TCAs were not recommended. Benzodiazepines were listed under "not-endorsed practices" for preschoolers, except for extreme anxiety for medical or dental procedures.

Multimodal Treatment

The Child-Adolescent Anxiety Multimodal Study (CAMS) compared the effectiveness of 12 weeks of sertraline, CBT, sertraline plus CBT, and placebo in the treatment of 488 children and adolescents with moderate to severe SAD, GAD, and/or SOC (Walkup et al. 2008). At posttreatment, 55% of those who received sertraline, 60% of those who received CBT, 81% of those who received combination treatment, and 24% of those who received placebo were rated as very much or much improved on the CGI scale. Combination treatment was significantly superior to each of the monotherapies. Sertraline and CBT were equivalent. All active treatments were significantly more effective than placebo. Greater severity of anxiety at baseline, greater caregiver strain, and a primary diagnosis of SOC predicted poorer outcome in all groups (Compton et al. 2014). This study demonstrated that an SSRI plus CBT results in the most positive outcome for youth with SAD, GAD, and/or SOC. However, any of the three active treatments (SSRI, CBT, combination) may be recommended, on the basis of the availability of specific interventions, cost, time constraints, and patient and family preference (Walkup et al. 2008).

The 24- and 36-week follow-ups in CAMS examined response and remission rates over time and revealed that more than 80% of acute responders maintained their positive response at both 24 and 36 weeks (Piacentini et al. 2014). During the follow-up period, participants who had been treated with sertraline were maintained on medication, while participants who had received CBT participated in six monthly booster sessions. Those who received combination treatment continued on medication and received boosters. On dimensional outcomes (e.g., Children's Global Assessment Scale), the combination group maintained superiority over the two monotherapies at both follow-up points. On most categorical outcomes (e.g., remission of diagnosis) the three treatment groups did not differ over the follow-up period. The sertraline group was more likely to receive nonstudy concomitant psychosocial treatments compared with the combination and CBT groups. In the naturalistic 6-year follow-up of youth from CAMS, close to half were in remission a mean of 6 years after being randomly assigned to treatment (Ginsburg et al. 2014). Remission was defined as absence of all entry anxiety diagnoses. The participants who were responders to the acute treatment were more likely to be in remission at 6 years posttreatment. Nearly half of the acute responders relapsed during the follow-up period. The authors argue that acute CBT and SSRI treatments lead to durable gains if maintenance treatment is provided, as a substantial number of children and adolescents with anxiety disorders need more intensive or extended treatment.

In a study of multimodal treatment for 63 school-refusing adolescents with anxiety and major depressive disorders, subjects were randomly assigned to 8 weeks of imipramine plus CBT or 8 weeks of placebo plus CBT (Bernstein et al. 2000). Over the course of the study, school attendance significantly improved in the imipramine group but not in the placebo group. Fifty-four percent of the imipramine group and 17% of the placebo group achieved remission (school attendance greater than 75%) at 8 weeks. The low remission rate in the placebo group reflected the severe symptoms of participants and supports the need for multimodal intervention in treating severe school refusal in teenagers.

Early Intervention, Prevention, and Dissemination

Early intervention can alleviate some of the difficulties experienced by youth with anxiety. Severity and impairment increase with age (Hirshfeld-Becker and Biederman 2002). Effective prevention efforts should target known risk factors that can be treated with evidence-based interventions. Efforts should include screening and early assessments, interventions in community settings, psychoeducation, and parent skills training (Connolly et al. 2007).

Although anxiety disorders are common in children, only a small proportion of those affected receive care. Prevention efforts targeting youth at risk, and even universal interventions in schools, should be considered (Farrell and Barrett 2007). The FRIENDS program (Barrett 2004) is a CBT approach for children that has been proven effective in clinical samples, among youth identified at risk, and in settings where the program was delivered to entire classrooms of youth not identified with anxiety disorders. The FRIENDS program teaches youth skills to manage stress, anxiety, and depression and has been found to reduce symptoms of anxiety (Farrell and Barrett 2007).

It is important to target both parents and youth in the prevention of childhood anxiety disorders. Parent skills training programs can improve parent-child relationships, parenting style, family functioning, and anxiety management (Hirshfeld-Becker and Biederman 2002). In addition, school-based early intervention programs have been shown to be effective in treating children with mild to moderate anxiety disorders (e.g., Bernstein et al. 2005).

Promotion of healthy family relationships, encouragement of independent behavior in children, and support of children's involvement in school and extracurricular activities may reduce school refusal. Proactive problem solving about stressors in the school environment (e.g., bullies) will also be beneficial. At the earliest signs of school refusal, parents and school officials should promote a swift return to the classroom with support in place for the anxious child, as treatment resistance increases with chronicity.

Adaptation and transportability of evidence-informed interventions for childhood anxiety disorders to community practice were recently reviewed (Connolly et al. 2011). Intervention studies have been conducted primarily with white, middle to upper class youth in academic settings, and generalization of these findings to children in community settings and from diverse backgrounds is being explored. In addition, culturally sensitive adaptations of CBT are being developed for school psychologists to address the growing needs of Mexican American students in U.S. public schools. Many anxious youth cannot access or use treatment with CBT because of limited availability of trained CBT providers, cost of treatment, and time required to complete CBT programs. Bibliotherapy (step-by-step written guide for parents without therapist contact), while not as efficacious as standard group CBT, has yielded positive results. Adding contact with a therapist by phone or Internet to a bibliotherapy program may extend the reach of effective treatment. A CBT stepped care model has been proposed that begins with minimal therapist involvement and increases the intensity of interventions in a stepwise fashion up to full therapist-directed treatment, based on the individual needs of the child and family (for a review, see Connolly et al. 2011). The feasibility of guided CBT self-help in primary care for childhood anxiety disorders has recently been evaluated as an alternative to standard CBT treatment (Creswell et al. 2010). Short-term CBT self-help with bibliotherapy via a parent in conjunction with guidance from existing primary mental health workers in the community yielded promising results in increasing access. The role of the primary mental health worker was to encourage the parent(s) to move through the book and rehearse key skills and to advise the parent(s) when challenges arose.

Much attention is being paid to interventions that can be delivered electronically, given the significant discrepancy between the need for mental health care and the availability of practitioners trained in evidence-based treatments (Khanna 2014). Such treatments can address barriers in geography, affordability, consistency, and anonymity. Computer-based cognitive behavioral treatments include BRAVE, BRAVE-ONLINE, and Camp Cope-A-Lot (for a review, see Khanna 2014). Videoteleconferencing involves a clinician providing services via the Internet; data support this modality for youth with Tourette's disorder and family-based therapy for youth with obsessive-compulsive disorder (see Chapter 33, "Telemental Health"). Two promising avenues for parents to receive training are www.anxietybc.com and www.copingcatparents.com. In addition to educational material, parents will find resources to help manage their child's anxiety. Finally, smartphone applications afford youth and their parents greater access to tools taught in CBT sessions (e.g., the Mayo Clinic Anxiety Coach app). Many of these resources have demonstrated superior outcomes in comparison with wait list control and have been considered acceptable by families.

Summary Points

- Anxiety disorders are common, and routine screening is recommended.
- ADHD and depression are common comorbid disorders.
- School refusal is not a DSM-5 diagnosis; it is a symptom that is commonly associated with anxiety or depressive disorders in youth.
- To understand the etiology of anxiety disorders, it is important to consider the interplay between key biological (e.g., heredity, behavioral inhibition) and environmental (e.g., parenting styles, negative life experiences, peer/social problems) risk factors.
- Assessment and treatment planning should consider severity of the anxiety disorder, functional impairment, comorbid conditions, and information from several sources/informants.
- The presence of parental anxiety disorders needs to be considered in the treatment process.

- Exposure-based CBT and medication with SSRIs are evidence-based treatments for childhood anxiety disorders and school refusal.
- A multimodal treatment plan is beneficial for success in treating anxiety disorders and school refusal.
- School refusal behavior is often maintained through positive reinforcement (i.e., engagement in pleasant activities) and/or negative reinforcement (i.e., avoidance of unpleasant situations).
- Prevention and early intervention efforts have been successful in clinical and school settings.

References

Albano AM: A developmental approach to treating anxiety and depression in the transitional years (18–25). Workshop presented at the annual conference of the Anxiety and Depression Association of America, Chicago, IL, March, 2014

Albano AM, Marten PA, Holt CS, et al: Cognitive-behavioral group treatment for social phobia in adolescents. A preliminary study. J Nerv Ment Dis 183(10):649–656, 1995 7561811

American Psychiatric Association: Diagnostic and Statistical Manual of Mental Disorders, 4th Edition. Washington, DC, American Psychiatric Association, 1994

American Psychiatric Association: Diagnostic and Statistical Manual of Mental Disorders, 4th Edition, Text Revision. Washington, DC, American Psychiatric Association, 2000

American Psychiatric Association: Diagnostic and Statistical Manual of Mental Disorders, 5th Edition. Arlington, VA, American Psychiatric Association, 2013

Bailey KA, Chavira DA, Stein MT, et al: Brief measures to screen for social phobia in primary care pediatrics. J Pediatr Psychol 31(5):512–521, 2006 16034004

Barlow DH: The origins of anxious apprehension, anxiety disorders, and related emotional disorders: triple vulnerabilities, in Anxiety and Its Disorders: The Nature and Treatment of Anxiety and Panic, 2nd Edition. Edited by Barlow DH. New York, Guilford, 2002, pp 252–291

Barlow DH, Craske MG: Mastery of Your Anxiety and Panic: Therapist Guide. New York, Oxford University Press, 2007

Barrett PM: Friends for Life! For Children. Participant Workbook and Leader's Manual. Brisbane, Australia, Australian Academic Press, 2004

Beidel DC, Turner SM, Morris TL, et al: A new inventory to assess childhood social anxiety and phobia: the Social Phobia and Anxiety Inventory for Children. Psychol Assess 7(1):73–79, 1995

Beidel DC, Turner SM, Young B, et al: Social effectiveness therapy for children: three-year follow-up. J Consult Clin Psychol 73(4):721–725, 2005 16173859

Beidel DC, Turner SM, Sallee FR, et al: SET-C versus fluoxetine in the treatment of childhood social phobia. J Am Acad Child Adolesc Psychiatry 46(12):1622–1632, 2007 18030084

Benjet C, Borges G, Medina-Mora ME: Chronic childhood adversity and onset of psychopathology during three life stages: childhood, adolescence and adulthood. J Psychiatr Res 44(11):732–740, 2010 20144464

Bergman RL, Keller ML, Piacentini J, et al: The development and psychometric properties of the selective mutism questionnaire. J Clin Child Adolesc Psychol 37(2):456–464, 2008 18470781

Bergman RL, Gonzalez A, Piacentini J, et al: Integrated behavior therapy for selective mutism: a randomized controlled pilot study. Behav Res Ther 51(10):680–689, 2013 23933108

Bernstein GA: Comorbidity and severity of anxiety and depressive disorders in a clinic sample. J Am Acad Child Adolesc Psychiatry 30(1):43–50, 1991 2005063

Bernstein GA, Borchardt CM, Perwien AR, et al: Imipramine plus cognitive-behavioral therapy in the treatment of school refusal.

J Am Acad Child Adolesc Psychiatry 39(3):276–283, 2000 10714046

Bernstein GA, Layne AE, Egan EA, et al: School-based interventions for anxious children. J Am Acad Child Adolesc Psychiatry 44(11):1118–1127, 2005 16239860

Birmaher B, Brent DA, Chiappetta L, et al: Psychometric properties of the Screen for Child Anxiety Related Emotional Disorders (SCARED): a replication study. J Am Acad Child Adolesc Psychiatry 38(10):1230–1236, 1999 10517055

Birmaher B, Axelson DA, Monk K, et al: Fluoxetine for the treatment of childhood anxiety disorders. J Am Acad Child Adolesc Psychiatry 42(4):415–423, 2003 12649628

Bittner A, Egger HL, Erkanli A, et al: What do childhood anxiety disorders predict? J Child Psychol Psychiatry 48(12):1174–1183, 2007 18093022

Black B, Uhde TW: Treatment of elective mutism with fluoxetine: a double-blind, placebo-controlled study. J Am Acad Child Adolesc Psychiatry 33(7):1000–1006, 1994 7961338

Bögels S, Phares V: Fathers' role in the etiology, prevention and treatment of child anxiety: a review and new model. Clin Psychol Rev 28(4):539–558, 2008 17854963

Bolton D, Eley TC, O'Connor TG, et al: Prevalence and genetic and environmental influences on anxiety disorders in 6-year-old twins. Psychol Med 36(3):335–344, 2006 16288680

Bristol-Meyers Squibb Company: Buspirone (package insert). Princeton, NJ, Bristol-Meyers Squibb Company, 2010

Campo JV, Dahl RE, Williamson DE, et al: Gastrointestinal distress to serotonergic challenge: a risk marker for emotional disorder? J Am Acad Child Adolesc Psychiatry 42(10):1221–1226, 2003 14560172

Cheung AH, Emslie GJ, Mayes TL: Review of the efficacy and safety of antidepressants in youth depression. J Child Psychol Psychiatry 46(7):735–754, 2005 15972068

Choudhury MS, Pimentel SS, Kendall PC: Childhood anxiety disorders: parent-child (dis)agreement using a structured interview for the DSM-IV. J Am Acad Child Adolesc Psychiatry 42(8):957–964, 2003 12874498

Cobham VE, Dadds MR, Spence SH: The role of parental anxiety in the treatment of childhood anxiety. J Consult Clin Psychol 66(6):893–905, 1998 9874902

Cohan SL, Chavira DA, Stein MB: Practitioner review: Psychosocial interventions for children with selective mutism: a critical evaluation of the literature from 1990–2005. J Child Psychol Psychiatry 47(11):1085–1097, 2006 17076747

Compton SN, March JS, Brent D, et al: Cognitive-behavioral psychotherapy for anxiety and depressive disorders in children and adolescents: an evidence-based medicine review. J Am Acad Child Adolesc Psychiatry 43(8):930–959, 2004 15266189

Compton SN, Peris TS, Almirall D, et al: Predictors and moderators of treatment response in childhood anxiety disorders: results from the CAMS trial. J Consult Clin Psychol 82(2):212–224, 2014 24417601

Connolly SD, Bernstein GA, Work Group on Quality Issues: Practice parameter for the assessment and treatment of children and adolescents with anxiety disorders. J Am Acad Child Adolesc Psychiatry 46(2):267–283, 2007 17242630

Connolly SD, Suarez L, Sylvester C: Assessment and treatment of anxiety disorders in children and adolescents. Curr Psychiatry Rep 13(2):99–110, 2011 21225481

Coşun M, Öztürk M, Zoroğlu S: Escitalopram treatment in preschool children with anxiety disorders: a case series. Bull Clin Psychopharmacol 22(3):262–267, 2012

Creswell C, Hentges F, Parkinson M, et al: Feasibility of guided cognitive behaviour therapy (CBT) self-help for childhood anxiety disorders in primary care. Ment Health Fam Med 7(1):49–57, 2010 22477922

Degnan KA, Almas AN, Fox NA: Temperament and the environment in the etiology of childhood anxiety. J Child Psychol Psychiatry 51(4):497–517, 2010 20158575

Egger HL, Angold A: Common emotional and behavioral disorders in preschool children: presentation, nosology, and epidemiology. J Child Psychol Psychiatry 47(3–4):313–337, 2006 16492262

Eisen AR, Schaefer CE: Separation Anxiety in Children and Adolescents: An Individualized Approach to Assessment and Treatment. New York, Guilford, 2005

Essau CA, Gabbidon J: Epidemiology comorbidity and mental health service utilization, in The Wiley-Blackwell Handbook of Treatment of Childhood and Adolescent Anxiety, 1st Edition. Edited by Essau CA, Ollendick TH. Chichester, UK, Wiley-Blackwell, 2013, pp 23–42

Farrell LJ, Barrett PM: Prevention of childhood emotional disorders: reducing the burden of suffering associated with anxiety and depression. Child Adolesc Ment Health 12(2):58–65, 2007

Feder A, Coplan JD, Goetz RR, et al: Twenty-four-hour cortisol secretion patterns in prepubertal children with anxiety or depressive disorders. Biol Psychiatry 56(3):198–204, 2004 15271589

Foley DL, Pickles A, Maes HM, et al: Course and short-term outcomes of separation anxiety disorder in a community sample of twins. J Am Acad Child Adolesc Psychiatry 43(9):1107–1114, 2004 15322414

Gar NS, Hudson JL, Rapee RN: Family factors and the development of anxiety disorders, in Psychopathology and the Family. Edited by Hudson JL, Rapee RM. Oxford, UK, Elsevier, 2005

Gazelle H: Class climate moderates peer relations and emotional adjustment in children with an early history of anxious solitude: a Child X Environment model. Dev Psychol 42(6):1179–1192, 2006 17087551

Geller D, Donnelly C, Lopez F, et al: Atomoxetine treatment for pediatric patients with attention-deficit/hyperactivity disorder with comorbid anxiety disorder. J Am Acad Child Adolesc Psychiatry 46(9):1119–1127, 2007 17712235

Ginsburg GS, Becker EM, Keeton CP, et al: Naturalistic follow-up of youths treated for pediatric anxiety disorders. JAMA Psychiatry 71(3):310–318, 2014 24477837

Gleason MM, Egger HL, Emslie GJ, et al: Psychopharmacological treatment for very young children: contexts and guidelines. J Am Acad Child Adolesc Psychiatry 46(12):1532–1572, 2007 18030077

Gunnar MR, Fisher PA, Early Experience, Stress, and Prevention Network: Bringing basic research on early experience and stress neurobiology to bear on preventive interventions for neglected and maltreated children. Dev Psychopathol 18(3):651–677, 2006 17152395

Heyne D, King NJ, Tonge BJ, et al: School refusal: epidemiology and management. Paediatr Drugs 3(10):719–732, 2001 11706923

Hirshfeld-Becker DR, Biederman J: Rationale and principles for early intervention with young children at risk for anxiety disorders. Clin Child Fam Psychol Rev 5(3):161–172, 2002 12240705

Hirshfeld-Becker DR, Masek B, Henin A, et al: Cognitive behavioral therapy for 4- to 7-year-old children with anxiety disorders: a randomized clinical trial. J Consult Clin Psychol 78(4):498–510, 2010 20658807

Hoffman EC, Mattis SG: A developmental adaptation of panic control treatment for panic disorder in adolescence. Cognit Behav Pract 7(3):253–261, 2000

In-Albon T, Schneider S: Psychotherapy of childhood anxiety disorders: a meta-analysis. Psychother Psychosom 76(1):15–24, 2007 17170560

Isolan L, Pheula G, Salum GA Jr, et al: An open-label trial of escitalopram in children and adolescents with social anxiety disorder. J Child Adolesc Psychopharmacol 17(6):751–760, 2007 18315447

Jensen PS, Hinshaw SP, Kraemer HC, et al: ADHD comorbidity findings from the MTA study: comparing comorbid subgroups. J Am Acad Child Adolesc Psychiatry 40(2):147–158, 2001 11211363

Kearney CA: Identifying the function of school refusal behavior: a revision of the School Refusal Assessment Scale. J Psychopathol Behav Assess 24(4):235–245, 2002

Kearney CA, Albano AM: The functional profiles of school refusal behavior: diagnostic aspects. Behav Modif 28:147–161, 2004

Kearney CA, Albano AM: When Children Refuse School: A Cognitive-Behavioral Therapy Approach, 2nd Edition. New York, Oxford University Press, 2007

Kearney CA, Bensaheb A: School absenteeism and school refusal behavior: a review and suggestions for school-based health professionals. J Sch Health 76(1):3–7, 2006 16457678

Keeton CP, Kolos AC, Walkup JT: Pediatric generalized anxiety disorder: epidemiology, diagnosis, and management. Paediatr Drugs 11(3):171–183, 2009 19445546

Kendall PC, Brady EU, Verduin TL: Comorbidity in childhood anxiety disorders and treatment outcome. J Am Acad Child Adolesc Psychiatry 40(7):787–794, 2001 11437017

Khanna MS: A primer on internet interventions for child anxiety. The Behavior Therapist 37(5):122–125, 2014

King NJ, Bernstein GA: School refusal in children and adolescents: a review of the past 10 years. J Am Acad Child Adolesc Psychiatry 40(2):197–205, 2001 11211368

King NJ, Tonge BJ, Heyne D, et al: Cognitive-behavioral treatment of school-refusing children: a controlled evaluation. J Am Acad Child Adolesc Psychiatry 37(4):395–403, 1998 9549960

King NJ, Tonge BJ, Tuner S, et al: Brief cognitive-behavioural treatment for anxiety-disordered children exhibiting school refusal. Clin Psychol Psychother 6(1):39–45, 1999

King NJ, Tonge BJ, Heyne D, et al: Cognitive-behavioural treatment of school-refusing children: maintenance of improvement at 3- to 5-year follow-up. Scandinavian Journal of Behaviour Therapy 30:85–89, 2001

King NJ, Muris P, Ollendick TH: Childhood fears and phobias: assessment and treatment. Child Adolesc Mental Health 10(2):50–56, 2005

Kingery JN, Erdley CA, Marshall KC, et al: Peer experiences of anxious and socially withdrawn youth: an integrative review of the developmental and clinical literature. Clin Child Fam Psychol Rev 13(1):91–128, 2010 20069362

Kodish I, Rockhill C, Ryan S, et al: Pharmacotherapy for anxiety disorders in children and adolescents. Pediatr Clin North Am 58(1):55–72, x, 2011 21281848

Kristensen H: Selective mutism and comorbidity with developmental disorder/delay, anxiety disorder, and elimination disorder. J Am Acad Child Adolesc Psychiatry 39(2):249–256, 2000 10673837

La Greca AM: Manual and Instructions for the SASC, SASC-R, SAS-A, and Parent Versions of the Scales. Coral Gables, FL, University of Miami, 1999

Lam D, Gorman DA, Patten S, et al: The pharmacoepidemiology of selective serotonin reuptake inhibitors for children and adolescents in Canada from 2005 to 2009: a database analysis. Paediatr Drugs 15(4):319–327, 2013 23529865

Last CG, Hansen C, Franco N: Cognitive-behavioral treatment of school phobia. J Am Acad Child Adolesc Psychiatry 37(4):404–411, 1998 9549961

Lau JY, Eley TC, Stevenson J: Examining the state-trait anxiety relationship: a behavioural genetic approach. J Abnorm Child Psychol 34(1):19–27, 2006 16557359

Lavallee K, Herren C, Blatter-Meunier J, et al: Early predictors of separation anxiety disorder: early stranger anxiety, parental pathology and prenatal factors. Psychopathology 44(6):354–361, 2011 21847002

Lewinsohn PM, Zinbarg R, Seeley JR, et al: Lifetime comorbidity among anxiety disorders and between anxiety disorders and other mental disorders in adolescents. J Anxiety Disord 11(4):377–394, 1997 9276783

Lewinsohn PM, Holm-Denoma JM, Small JW, et al: Separation anxiety disorder in childhood as a risk factor for future mental illness. J Am Acad Child Adolesc Psychiatry 47(5):548–555, 2008 18356763

Manassis K, Monga S: A therapeutic approach to children and adolescents with anxiety disorders and associated comorbid conditions. J Am Acad Child Adolesc Psychiatry 40(1):115–117, 2001 11195553

March JS, Parker JDA, Sullivan K, et al: The Multidimensional Anxiety Scale for Children (MASC): factor structure, reliability, and validity. J Am Acad Child Adolesc Psychiatry 36(4):554–565, 1997 9100431

March JS, Entusah AR, Rynn M, et al: A randomized controlled trial of venlafaxine ER versus placebo in pediatric social anxiety disorder. Biol Psychiatry 62(10):1149–1154, 2007 17553467

Marquenie LA, Schadé A, van Balkom AJ, et al: Origin of the comorbidity of anxiety disorders and alcohol dependence: findings of a general population study. Eur Addict Res 13(1):39–49, 2007 17172778

McShane G, Walter G, Rey JM: Characteristics of adolescents with school refusal. Aust N Z J Psychiatry 35(6):822–826, 2001 11990893

McShane G, Walter G, Rey JM: Functional outcome of adolescents with 'school refusal.' Clin Child Psychol Psychiatry 9(1):53–60, 2004

Mineka S, Zinbarg R: A contemporary learning theory perspective on the etiology of anxiety disorders: it's not what you thought it was. Am Psychol 61(1):10–26, 2006 16435973

Moore PS, Whaley SE, Sigman M: Interactions between mothers and children: impacts of maternal and child anxiety. J Abnorm Psychol 113(3):471–476, 2004 15311992

Nevo GA, Manassis K: Outcomes for treated anxious children: a critical review of long-term follow-up studies. Depress Anxiety 26(7):650–660, 2009 19496175

Nottelmann ED, Jensen PS: Comorbidity of disorders in children and adolescents: developmental perspectives. Advances in Clinical Child Psychology 17:109–155, 1995

Oerbeck B, Stein MB, Wentzel-Larsen T, et al: A randomized controlled trial of a home and school-based intervention for selective mutism-defocused communication and behavioural techniques. Child Adolesc Ment Health 19:192–198, 2014

Ollendick TH: Reliability and validity of the Revised Fear Surgery Schedule for Children (FSSC-R). Behav Res Ther 21(6):685–692, 1983 6661153

Ollendick TH, Öst LG, Reuterskiöld L, et al: Comorbidity in youth with specific phobias: impact of comorbidity on treatment outcome and the impact of treatment on comorbid disorders. Behav Res Ther 48(9):827–831, 2010a 20573338

Ollendick TH, Raishevich N, Davis TE 3rd, et al: Specific phobia in youth: phenomenology and psychological characteristics. Behav Ther 41(1):133–141, 2010b 20171334

Ong SH, Wickramaratne P, Tang M, et al: Early childhood sleep and eating problems as predictors of adolescent and adult mood and anxiety disorders. J Affect Disord 96(1–2):1–8, 2006 16844230

Piacentini J, Bennett S, Compton SN, et al: 24- and 36-week outcomes for the Child/Adolescent Anxiety Multimodal Study (CAMS). J Am Acad Child Adolesc Psychiatry 53(3):297–310, 2014 24565357

Pincus D, Eyberg S, Choate M: Adapting parent-child interaction therapy for young children with separation anxiety disorder. Education and Treatment of Children 28(2):163–181, 2005

Pincus DB, Ehrenreich J, Mattis S: Mastery of Anxiety and Panic for Adolescents. New York, Oxford University Press, 2008a

Pincus DB, Ehrenreich J, Spiegel D: Riding the Wave Workbook. New York, Oxford University Press, 2008b

Pincus DB, Ehrenreich MJ, Whitton SW, et al: Cognitive-behavioral treatment of panic disorder in adolescence. J Clin Child Adolesc Psychopharmacology 39:638–649, 2010

Pine DS: Treating children and adolescents with selective serotonin reuptake inhibitors: how long is appropriate? J Child Adolesc Psychopharmacol 12(3):189–203, 2002 12427293

Reinblatt SP, Riddle MA: The pharmacological management of childhood anxiety disorders: a review. Psychopharmacology (Berl) 191(1):67–86, 2007 17205317

The Research Unit on Pediatric Psychopharmacology Anxiety Study Group: Fluvoxamine for the treatment of anxiety disorders in children and adolescents. N Engl J Med 344(17):1279–1285, 2001 11323729

Reynolds CR, Kamphaus RW: Behavior Assessment System for Children, 2nd Edition. Circle Pines, MN, American Guidance Service, 2004

Rynn MA, Siqueland L, Rickels K: Placebo-controlled trial of sertraline in the treatment of children with generalized anxiety disorder. Am J Psychiatry 158(12):2008–2014, 2001 11729017

Rynn MA, Riddle MA, Yeung PP, et al: Efficacy and safety of extended-release venlafaxine in the treatment of generalized anxiety disorder in children and adolescents: two placebo-controlled trials. Am J Psychiatry 164(2):290–300, 2007 17267793

Seidel L, Walkup JT: Selective serotonin reuptake inhibitor use in the treatment of the pediatric non-obsessive-compulsive disorder anxiety disorders. J Child Adolesc Psychopharmacol 16(1–2):171–179, 2006 16553537

Shamir-Essakow G, Ungerer JA, Rapee RM: Attachment, behavioral inhibition, and anxiety in preschool children. J Abnorm Child Psychol 33(2):131–143, 2005 15839492

Shear K, Jin R, Ruscio AM, et al: Prevalence and correlates of estimated DSM-IV child and adult separation anxiety disorder in the National Comorbidity Survey Replication. Am J Psychiatry 163(6):1074–1083, 2006 16741209

Silove DM, Marnane CL, Wagner R, et al: The prevalence and correlates of adult separation anxiety disorder in an anxiety clinic. BMC Psychiatry 10:21–27, 2010 20219138

Silverman WK, Albano AM: Anxiety Disorders Interview Schedule for DSM-IV: Child Version, Child and Parent Interview Schedules. San Antonio, TX, Psychological Corporation, 1996

Silverman WK, Ollendick TH: Evidence-based assessment of anxiety and its disorders in children and adolescents. J Clin Child Adolesc Psychol 34(3):380–411, 2005 16026211

Silverman WK, Kurtines WM, Ginsburg GS, et al: Contingency management, self-control, and education support in the treatment of childhood phobic disorders: a randomized clinical trial. J Consult Clin Psychol 67(5):675–687, 1999 10535234

Spence SH: A measure of anxiety symptoms among children. Behav Res Ther 36(5):545–566, 1998 9648330

Strawn JR, Sakolsky DJ, Rynn MA: Psychopharmacologic treatment of children and adolescents with anxiety disorders, in Anxiety Disorders. Edited by Rynn MA, Vidair HB, Blackford JR. Philadelphia, PA, WB Saunders, 2012

Strawn JR, Prakash A, Zhang Q, et al: Contingency management, self-control, and education support in the treatment of childhood phobic disorders: a randomized clinical trial. J Am Acad Child Adolesc Psychiatry 54(4):283–293, 2015 25791145

Suárez L, Barlow D, Bennett S, et al: Understanding anxiety disorders from a "triple vulnerabilities" framework, in Handbook of Anxiety and the Anxiety Disorders. Edited by Anthony M, Stein M. New York, Oxford University Press, 2008

Suveg C, Aschenbrand SG, Kendall PC: Separation anxiety disorder, panic disorder, and school refusal. Child Adolesc Psychiatr Clin N Am 14(4):773–795, ix, 2005 16171702

Talge NM, Neal C, Glover V, et al: Antenatal maternal stress and long-term effects on child neurodevelopment: how and why? J Child Psychol Psychiatry 48(3–4):245–261, 2007 17355398

Torrens Armstrong AM, McCormack Brown KR, Brindley R, et al: Frequent fliers, school phobias, and the sick student: school health personnel's perceptions of students who refuse school. J Sch Health 81(9):552–559, 2011 21831068

van Brakel AML, Muris P, Bögels SM, et al: A multifactorial model for the etiology of anxiety in nonclinical adolescents: main and interactive effects of behavioral inhibition, attachment and parental rearing. J Child Fam Stud 15(5):569–579, 2006

Vecchio JL, Kearney CA: Selective mutism in children: comparison to youths with and without anxiety disorders. J Psychopathol Behav Assess 27(1):31–37, 2005

Velting ON, Albano AM: Current trends in the understanding and treatment of social phobia in youth. J Child Psychol Psychiatry 42(1):127–140, 2001 11205621

Verduin TL, Kendall PC: Differential occurrence of comorbidity within childhood anxiety disorders. J Clin Child Adolesc Psychol 32(2):290–295, 2003 12679288

Wagner KD, Berard R, Stein MB, et al: A multicenter, randomized, double-blind, placebo-controlled trial of paroxetine in children and adolescents with social anxiety disorder. Arch Gen Psychiatry 61(11):1153–1162, 2004 15520363

Walkup J, Labellarte M, Riddle MA, et al: Treatment of pediatric anxiety disorders: an open-label extension of the research units on pediatric psychopharmacology anxiety study. J Child Adolesc Psychopharmacol 12(3):175–188, 2002 12427292

Walkup JT, Albano AM, Piacentini J, et al: Cognitive behavioral therapy, sertraline, or a combination in childhood anxiety. N Engl J Med 359(26):2753–2766, 2008 18974308

Weems CF, Hayward C, Killen J, et al: A longitudinal investigation of anxiety sensitivity in adolescence. J Abnorm Psychol 111(3):471–477, 2002 12150423

Whaley SE, Pinto A, Sigman M: Characterizing interactions between anxious mothers and their children. J Consult Clin Psychol 67(6):826–836, 1999 10596505

CHAPTER 16

Posttraumatic Stress Disorder and Persistent Complex Bereavement Disorder

Judith A. Cohen, M.D.
Anthony P. Mannarino, Ph.D.

Posttraumatic stress disorder (PTSD) was first introduced in DSM in 1980 (American Psychiatric Association 1980), making it one of the more recently accepted psychiatric disorders. PTSD develops in response to one or more traumatic life events (Box 16–1; American Psychiatric Association 2013). Since the introduction of PTSD into the psychiatric lexicon, the disorder has been documented in children exposed to a wide variety of traumas, including child abuse, domestic violence, natural disasters, medical trauma, war, terrorism, community violence, and multiple and complex trauma experiences. Substantial progress has been made in understanding the developmental manifestations of PTSD, the complexities of evaluating PTSD in children, and how to effectively treat this disorder in children and adolescents, but much remains to be learned. When parents or other important attachment figures die, most children have normal or typical grief. However, some children may develop maladaptive grief responses. When these responses persist and interfere with the child's functioning, they may meet criteria for a psychiatric disorder. Children's maladaptive grief responses have variously been referred to as *childhood traumatic grief* or *complicated bereavement.* In DSM-5 the criteria for this condition have been incorporated into a new disorder, *persistent complex bereavement disorder,* which is included in the DSM-5 section "Conditions for Further Study" (Box 16–2; American Psychiatric Association 2013).

Box 16–1. DSM-5 Diagnostic Criteria for Posttraumatic Stress Disorder

309.81 (F43.10)

Posttraumatic Stress Disorder

Note: The following criteria apply to adults, adolescents, and children older than 6 years. For children 6 years and younger, see corresponding criteria below.

A. Exposure to actual or threatened death, serious injury, or sexual violence in one (or more) of the following ways:

1. Directly experiencing the traumatic event(s).
2. Witnessing, in person, the event(s) as it occurred to others.
3. Learning that the traumatic event(s) occurred to a close family member or close friend. In cases of actual or threatened death of a family member or friend, the event(s) must have been violent or accidental.
4. Experiencing repeated or extreme exposure to aversive details of the traumatic event(s) (e.g., first responders collecting human remains; police officers repeatedly exposed to details of child abuse).

   Note: Criterion A4 does not apply to exposure through electronic media, television, movies, or pictures, unless this exposure is work related.

B. Presence of one (or more) of the following intrusion symptoms associated with the traumatic event(s), beginning after the traumatic event(s) occurred:

1. Recurrent, involuntary, and intrusive distressing memories of the traumatic event(s).

   Note: In children older than 6 years, repetitive play may occur in which themes or aspects of the traumatic event(s) are expressed.

2. Recurrent distressing dreams in which the content and/or affect of the dream are related to the traumatic event(s).

   Note: In children, there may be frightening dreams without recognizable content.

3. Dissociative reactions (e.g., flashbacks) in which the individual feels or acts as if the traumatic event(s) were recurring. (Such reactions may occur on a continuum, with the most extreme expression being a complete loss of awareness of present surroundings.)

   Note: In children, trauma-specific reenactment may occur in play.

4. Intense or prolonged psychological distress at exposure to internal or external cues that symbolize or resemble an aspect of the traumatic event(s).
5. Marked physiological reactions to internal or external cues that symbolize or resemble an aspect of the traumatic event(s).

C. Persistent avoidance of stimuli associated with the traumatic event(s), beginning after the traumatic event(s) occurred, as evidenced by one or both of the following:

1. Avoidance of or efforts to avoid distressing memories, thoughts, or feelings about or closely associated with the traumatic event(s).
2. Avoidance of or efforts to avoid external reminders (people, places, conversations, activities, objects, situations) that arouse distressing memories, thoughts, or feelings about or closely associated with the traumatic event(s).

D. Negative alterations in cognitions and mood associated with the traumatic event(s), beginning or worsening after the traumatic event(s) occurred, as evidenced by two (or more) of the following:

1. Inability to remember an important aspect of the traumatic event(s) (typically due to dissociative amnesia and not to other factors such as head injury, alcohol, or drugs).
2. Persistent and exaggerated negative beliefs or expectations about oneself, others, or the world (e.g., "I am bad," "No one can be trusted," "The world is completely dangerous," "My whole nervous system is permanently ruined").
3. Persistent, distorted cognitions about the cause or consequences of the traumatic event(s) that lead the individual to blame himself/herself or others.
4. Persistent negative emotional state (e.g., fear, horror, anger, guilt, or shame).
5. Markedly diminished interest or participation in significant activities.
6. Feelings of detachment or estrangement from others.
7. Persistent inability to experience positive emotions (e.g., inability to experience happiness, satisfaction, or loving feelings).

E. Marked alterations in arousal and reactivity associated with the traumatic event(s), beginning or worsening after the traumatic event(s) occurred, as evidenced by two (or more) of the following:
   1. Irritable behavior and angry outbursts (with little or no provocation) typically expressed as verbal or physical aggression toward people or objects.
   2. Reckless or self-destructive behavior.
   3. Hypervigilance.
   4. Exaggerated startle response.
   5. Problems with concentration.
   6. Sleep disturbance (e.g., difficulty falling or staying asleep or restless sleep).

F. Duration of the disturbance (Criteria B, C, D, and E) is more than 1 month.

G. The disturbance causes clinically significant distress or impairment in social, occupational, or other important areas of functioning.

H. The disturbance is not attributable to the physiological effects of a substance (e.g., medication, alcohol) or another medical condition.

Specify whether:

With dissociative symptoms: The individual's symptoms meet the criteria for posttraumatic stress disorder, and in addition, in response to the stressor, the individual experiences persistent or recurrent symptoms of either of the following:

1. **Depersonalization:** Persistent or recurrent experiences of feeling detached from, and as if one were an outside observer of, one's mental processes or body (e.g., feeling as though one were in a dream; feeling a sense of unreality of self or body or of time moving slowly).
2. **Derealization:** Persistent or recurrent experiences of unreality of surroundings (e.g., the world around the individual is experienced as unreal, dreamlike, distant, or distorted).

Note: To use this subtype, the dissociative symptoms must not be attributable to the physiological effects of a substance (e.g., blackouts, behavior during alcohol intoxication) or another medical condition (e.g., complex partial seizures).

Specify if:

With delayed expression: If the full diagnostic criteria are not met until at least 6 months after the event (although the onset and expression of some symptoms may be immediate).

Posttraumatic Stress Disorder for Children 6 Years and Younger

A. In children 6 years and younger, exposure to actual or threatened death, serious injury, or sexual violence in one (or more) of the following ways:

1. Directly experiencing the traumatic event(s).
2. Witnessing, in person, the event(s) as it occurred to others, especially primary caregivers.

   Note: Witnessing does not include events that are witnessed only in electronic media, television, movies, or pictures.
3. Learning that the traumatic event(s) occurred to a parent or caregiving figure.

B. Presence of one (or more) of the following intrusion symptoms associated with the traumatic event(s), beginning after the traumatic event(s) occurred:

1. Recurrent, involuntary, and intrusive distressing memories of the traumatic event(s).

   Note: Spontaneous and intrusive memories may not necessarily appear distressing and may be expressed as play reenactment.
2. Recurrent distressing dreams in which the content and/or affect of the dream are related to the traumatic event(s).

   Note: It may not be possible to ascertain that the frightening content is related to the traumatic event.
3. Dissociative reactions (e.g., flashbacks) in which the child feels or acts as if the traumatic event(s) were recurring. (Such reactions may occur on a continuum, with the most extreme expression being a complete loss of awareness of present surroundings.) Such trauma-specific reenactment may occur in play.
4. Intense or prolonged psychological distress at exposure to internal or external cues that symbolize or resemble an aspect of the traumatic event(s).
5. Marked physiological reactions to reminders of the traumatic event(s).

C. One (or more) of the following symptoms, representing either persistent avoidance of stimuli associated with the traumatic event(s) or negative alterations in cognitions and mood associated with the traumatic event(s), must be present, beginning after the event(s) or worsening after the event(s):

Persistent Avoidance of Stimuli

1. Avoidance of or efforts to avoid activities, places, or physical reminders that arouse recollections of the traumatic event(s).
2. Avoidance of or efforts to avoid people, conversations, or interpersonal situations that arouse recollections of the traumatic event(s).

Negative Alterations in Cognitions

3. Substantially increased frequency of negative emotional states (e.g., fear, guilt, sadness, shame, confusion).
4. Markedly diminished interest or participation in significant activities, including constriction of play.
5. Socially withdrawn behavior.
6. Persistent reduction in expression of positive emotions.

D. Alterations in arousal and reactivity associated with the traumatic event(s), beginning or worsening after the traumatic event(s) occurred, as evidenced by two (or more) of the following:

1. Irritable behavior and angry outbursts (with little or no provocation) typically expressed as verbal or physical aggression toward people or objects (including extreme temper tantrums).
2. Hypervigilance.
3. Exaggerated startle response.

4. Problems with concentration.
5. Sleep disturbance (e.g., difficulty falling or staying asleep or restless sleep).

E. The duration of the disturbance is more than 1 month.
F. The disturbance causes clinically significant distress or impairment in relationships with parents, siblings, peers, or other caregivers or with school behavior.
G. The disturbance is not attributable to the physiological effects of a substance (e.g., medication or alcohol) or another medical condition.

Specify whether:

With dissociative symptoms: The individual's symptoms meet the criteria for posttraumatic stress disorder, and the individual experiences persistent or recurrent symptoms of either of the following:

1. **Depersonalization:** Persistent or recurrent experiences of feeling detached from, and as if one were an outside observer of, one's mental processes or body (e.g., feeling as though one were in a dream; feeling a sense of unreality of self or body or of time moving slowly).
2. **Derealization:** Persistent or recurrent experiences of unreality of surroundings (e.g., the world around the individual is experienced as unreal, dreamlike, distant, or distorted).

Note: To use this subtype, the dissociative symptoms must not be attributable to the physiological effects of a substance (e.g., blackouts) or another medical condition (e.g., complex partial seizures).

Specify if:

With delayed expression: If the full diagnostic criteria are not met until at least 6 months after the event (although the onset and expression of some symptoms may be immediate).

Source. Reprinted from the *Diagnostic and Statistical Manual of Mental Disorders*, 5th Edition. Arlington, VA, American Psychiatric Association, 2013. Used with permission.

Box 16–2. DSM-5 Proposed Criteria for Persistent Complex Bereavement Disorder

---

A. The individual experienced the death of someone with whom he or she had a close relationship.
B. Since the death, at least one of the following symptoms is experienced on more days than not and to a clinically significant degree and has persisted for at least 12 months after the death in the case of bereaved adults and 6 months for bereaved children:

1. Persistent yearning/longing for the deceased. In young children, yearning may be expressed in play and behavior, including behaviors that reflect being separated from, and also reuniting with, a caregiver or other attachment figure.
2. Intense sorrow and emotional pain in response to the death.
3. Preoccupation with the deceased.
4. Preoccupation with the circumstances of the death. In children, this preoccupation with the deceased may be expressed through the themes of play and behavior and may extend to preoccupation with possible death of others close to them.

C. Since the death, at least six of the following symptoms are experienced on more days than not and to a clinically significant degree, and have persisted for at least 12 months after the death in the case of bereaved adults and 6 months for bereaved children:

Reactive distress to the death

1. Marked difficulty accepting the death. In children, this is dependent on the child's capacity to comprehend the meaning and permanence of death.
2. Experiencing disbelief or emotional numbness over the loss.
3. Difficulty with positive reminiscing about the deceased.
4. Bitterness or anger related to the loss.
5. Maladaptive appraisals about oneself in relation to the deceased or the death (e.g., self-blame).
6. Excessive avoidance of reminders of the loss (e.g., avoidance of individuals, places, or situations associated with the deceased; in children, this may include avoidance of thoughts and feelings regarding the deceased).

Social/identity disruption

7. A desire to die in order to be with the deceased.
8. Difficulty trusting other individuals since the death.
9. Feeling alone or detached from other individuals since the death.
10. Feeling that life is meaningless or empty without the deceased, or the belief that one cannot function without the deceased.
11. Confusion about one's role in life, or a diminished sense of one's identity (e.g., feeling that a part of oneself died with the deceased).
12. Difficulty or reluctance to pursue interests since the loss or to plan for the future (e.g., friendships, activities).

D. The disturbance causes clinically significant distress or impairment in social, occupational, or other important areas of functioning.

E. The bereavement reaction is out of proportion to or inconsistent with cultural, religious, or age-appropriate norms.

Specify if:

With traumatic bereavement: Bereavement due to homicide or suicide with persistent distressing preoccupations regarding the traumatic nature of the death (often in response to loss reminders), including the deceased's last moments, degree of suffering and mutilating injury, or the malicious or intentional nature of the death.

Source. Reprinted from the *Diagnostic and Statistical Manual of Mental Disorders,* 5th Edition. Arlington, VA, American Psychiatric Association, 2013. Used with permission. Copyright © American Psychiatric Association.

Definition, Clinical Description, and Diagnosis

In DSM-5 (American Psychiatric Association 2013), PTSD is no longer classified with the anxiety disorders. It is one of several disorders that are newly categorized as *trauma- and stressor-related disorders,* in which exposure to a traumatic or stressful event is explicitly listed as a diagnostic criterion. The disorder has also been revised to account for the diversity of individual responses to traumatic experiences. Although many responses can be understood within the context of fear or anxiety conditioning, for others the most prominent characteristics are dysphoric, angry, or dissociative symptoms or a combination of these symptoms. As a result, DSM-5 PTSD criteria no longer require that children respond to the traumatic event with intense fear, helplessness, or horror (or, in young children, with disorganized or agitated behavior). With the addition of a new symptom cluster (Cluster D), the revised DSM-5 criteria acknowledge the centrality of cognitive and mood changes in PTSD (American Psychiatric Association 2013, pp. 271–272). DSM-5 also recognizes the importance of developmental factors in the manifestation of clinical symptoms by including empirically validated alternative criteria for diagnosing PTSD in children 6 years old and younger as described in Box 16–1.

When a parent or other important person dies, most children have normal or typical grief responses. Tasks of normal child bereavement include accepting the reality of the death, fully experiencing the pain of the death, adjusting to an environment and self-identity without the deceased, converting the relationship with the deceased from one of interaction to one of memory, finding meaning in the death, and experiencing continuing supportive relationships with adults. Children who develop maladaptive grief responses struggle to negotiate these tasks (Kaplow et al. 2012). A new condition, persistent complex bereavement disorder, has been proposed in DSM-5 under "Conditions for Further Study" to describe maladaptive grief responses (American Psychiatric Association 2013, p. 789). This condition has already been subject to significant debate. The diagnostic criteria for this condition will likely be revised on the basis of additional research that elucidates how maladaptive grief is manifested across the developmental spectrum.

The current version of persistent complex bereavement disorder (Box 16–2) requires the child to have at least one symptom of death preoccupation and six symptoms related to reactive distress or social/identity disruption for at least 6 months after the death of someone close. Reactive distress symptoms largely overlap with PTSD symptoms as seen in Box 16–2. The child is considered to have *traumatic bereavement* (or *traumatic grief*) if the death resulted from homicide or suicide and was followed by persistent preoccupation related to the traumatic nature of the death. These criteria for traumatic bereavement overlap very closely with those previously described for childhood traumatic grief (Cohen and Mannarino 2004; Kaplow et al. 2012). As noted previously, controversy is ongoing about persistent complex bereavement disorder, and it is likely that the diagnostic criteria for this condition will change substantially in new iterations of DSM as new data become available.

Epidemiology and Risk Factors

PTSD is more common among girls than boys. Certain genotypes may be protective or increase risk of PTSD after trauma exposure. Greater trauma exposure is a risk factor for developing PTSD, as is perceived life threat, personal injury, and interpersonal violence (particularly trauma perpetrated by a caregiver such as child abuse or domestic violence). Other risk factors associated with developing PTSD after disasters include increased media viewing after a disaster, experiencing peritraumatic panic symptoms, delayed evacuation after a disaster, and the presence of a predisaster anxiety disorder (Thienkrua et al. 2006). Negative appraisals, negative coping strategies, and lack of social support are also risk factors for developing PTSD.

Risk factors for developing persistent complex bereavement disorder have not been firmly established because of the preliminary nature of this diagnosis. Data suggest that disturbances in caregiver emotional support or being female may be risk factors for developing this disorder (American Psychiatric Association 2013).

Comorbidity

Comorbidity is common in children with PTSD, including depressive, anxiety, and/or behavioral problems. Some child samples have shown comorbidity of up to 60% with depressive disorders; this is consistent with adult PTSD cohorts. Externalizing symptoms are common as well. Comorbid conditions may include attention-deficit/hyperactivity disorder (ADHD) or oppositional defiant or conduct disorders. Older children and adolescents may engage in substance use or abuse, which may represent attempts to avoid trauma reminders or may be signs of an independent substance use disorder that may predate the trauma. After early ongoing trauma that involves attachment disruption (e.g., child abuse, domestic violence), children may develop complex PTSD, which is often misdiagnosed as a variety of other conditions (Briere and Spinazzola 2005). It is possible that the revisions to the DSM-5 diagnostic criteria will result in improved recognition of youth with complex trauma.

Common comorbidities with persistent complex bereavement disorder are PTSD, depression, and substance use disorders (American Psychiatric Association 2013). PTSD is particularly common when the death occurred under traumatic circumstances (Cohen et al. 2004b, 2006; Melhem et al. 2007).

Etiology

As noted earlier in the chapter, experiencing or learning about a serious traumatic event is a required etiological factor for developing PTSD. Fear conditioning and failure of inhibitory learning have been hypothesized as underlying mechanisms for the development of PTSD following exposure to a potentially traumatic event. It is proposed that fear and danger experienced during the traumatic event are reinforced when the child is exposed to trauma reminders, that is, to innocuous circumstances or situations that are associated with the trauma. These reminders lead to overgeneralized intrusion, avoidance, and negative cognitions/mood changes and arousal (typical PTSD symptoms) in response to trauma reminders. Inhibitory learning (Craske et al. 2008) may mitigate this process if the child is exposed to experiences that challenge or contradict the fear/danger paradigm, that is, that enable the child to learn that the innocuous circumstances or situations are not dangerous and do not have to be feared or avoided. However, as noted earlier in the chapter, not all individuals with PTSD have a preponderance of fear or anxiety symptoms. It is important to take into account developmental and cognitive factors when considering the nature of traumatic stressors. In addition to the requirement of a trauma, there is growing evidence of a genetic predisposition related to the development of PTSD (Stein et al. 2002).

Other than the death of an important attachment figure, the etiology of persistent complex bereavement disorder is not clear.

Prevention

Early identification of at-risk children may be possible through early screening of children exposed to trauma. This is particularly crucial after community-level traumas such as natural disasters, in which large numbers of children may be affected. School- or community-based screening and treatment may be the most efficient way to serve many of these children, who would not otherwise receive such interventions. Screening instruments such as the UCLA PTSD Reaction Index for DSM-5 (R.S. Pynoos and A. Steinberg, unpublished instrument, 2013) or the Child PTSD Symptom Scale (CPSS; Foa et al. 2001) may be used in this regard.

Widespread screening following a large-scale disaster may require triage by nonprofessional mental health workers. PsySTART is a 13-question instrument that can be used for rapid triage; it was used after the 2004 Asian tsunami to inquire about experiences rather than symptoms. The PsySTART triage screen successfully predicted risk factors for developing PTSD and depression 9 months posttsunami in 7- to 14-year-old children (Thienkrua et al. 2006).

A secondary prevention program has been successful in preventing the development of chronic PTSD in children and adolescents. The Child and Family Traumatic Stress Intervention (CFTSI; Berkowitz et al. 2011) is a brief (four session) intervention that is initiated with children and parents within the first 30 days after exposure to a potentially traumatic event. The intervention includes psychoeducation for parent and child about trauma responses and symptoms, provision of relaxation and other coping skills that are targeted to the child's specific trauma symptoms (on the basis of assessment instruments that the child completes serially during the treatment process), and ongoing parent-child communication and enhanced support about the child's symptoms. Final assessment, feedback, and disposition are included during the final session. Compared with a supportive comparison condition, at 3 month follow-up children in the CFTSI group demonstrated significantly fewer partial and full PTSD diagnoses than those in the comparison group (Berkowitz et al. 2011).

No preventive interventions are currently available for persistent complex bereavement disorder.

Course and Prognosis

There is some evidence that "natural recovery" from PTSD occurs in children—that is, that the overall percentage of children qualifying for a PTSD diagnosis decreases over time (La Greca et al. 1998)—although other studies have not found a natural decrease over time (Scheeringa et al. 2005). Researchers agree that for a core group of children, PTSD symptoms persist, and for these children the prognosis is grim without effective intervention. PTSD is a significant risk factor for increased suicide attempts, major depression, dissociation, and impaired global emotional functioning.

Persistent complex bereavement disorder can occur at any age. Symptoms usually begin soon after the death, although there can be a delay of months, or even years, before the syndrome appears. Although grief responses typically appear immediately after a death, this condition is not diagnosed in children until the symptoms have persisted for 6 months. The course of the disorder may change during development, with young children showing more developmental regression, protest and anxiety at separation and reunion, and separation distress. Older children may develop clearer PTSD symptoms and risk for comorbid depression and substance abuse.

Clinical Evaluation

The following information pertains to clinical rather than forensic evaluations. PTSD is one of the most challenging disorders to accurately diagnose in children and adolescents. Clinicians face the paradox of needing children to describe experiences that the very essence of this disorder makes them avoid thinking and talking about. Many PTSD diagnostic criteria are not even comprehensible to young children, who are not developmentally capable of describing complex internal experiences or emotional states. Clinicians assessing these children should be familiar with the diagnostic criteria for young children and how to conduct a clinical interview with parents to elicit these children's PTSD symptoms.

The evaluation of persistent complex bereavement disorder is challenging because of the lack of a consensus-validated child and adolescent assessment instrument.

Multiple Informants

As with any child psychiatric evaluation, assessing children for possible PTSD requires information from multiple sources. This should always include information from the child and parent or caretaker, although for very young children, information from the child will be primarily observational and subjective, with the parent completing validated instruments. Because of privacy concerns, the family may not want the school to know the child is receiving an evaluation, and they will need to be assured about confidentiality, if this is appropriate. In some cases it may be necessary or possible to complete the evaluation without receiving teacher reports. In many instances, the evaluation of a child for PTSD will also include obtaining records and possibly additional information from a pediatrician, forensic evaluator, police investigator, or child protection worker (e.g., if there was alleged child abuse prior to the evaluation). Agencies such as crime victims' assistance programs, domestic violence shelters, child advocacy centers, and/or other therapists or agencies that provide services to the child and family might serve as useful supplemental sources of information.

Multiple informants may also be helpful in evaluating persistent complex bereavement disorder. For example, in addition to obtaining information from the child's parent or caregiver, obtaining information from the child's school may elucidate information about maladaptive grief symptoms the child is exhibiting only in that setting (Cohen and Mannarino 2011).

Rating Scales and Standardized Interviews

Evaluators should include the use of parent and/or child rating scales for assessing PTSD. Several validated self- and parent-report instruments are available for this purpose, including the UCLA PTSD Reaction Index for DSM-5, the CPSS, and others. Some children are more comfortable acknowledging symptoms on a paper-and-pencil instrument than in a face-to-face interview, or vice versa. Providing both options may optimize the evaluator's opportunity to learn about the child's symptoms. Semistructured interviews for PTSD (see review by Cohen et al. 2010) are also available but are too time-consuming to be feasible for most clinical settings.

There is currently no standardized rating scale or interview to assess persistent complex bereavement disorder in children and adolescents. Collaborations are under way to develop such an instrument (Kaplow et al. 2012).

Differential Diagnosis

Other psychiatric conditions may manifest with symptoms similar to those seen in PTSD. Children with PTSD may appear to have ADHD because of poor attention, restlessness, hyperactivity, and disorganized and/or agitated play. Arousal symptoms such as difficulty sleeping and poor concentration may also mimic ADHD. Unless clinicians obtain a careful history regarding the timing of onset or worsening of these symptoms in relation to trauma exposure, it may be impossible to distinguish these conditions. PTSD may also mimic oppositional defiant disorder because of arousal symptoms presenting as angry outbursts or irritability. These symptoms may be particularly prominent if the child is exposed to modeling of anger as a successful strategy for controlling one's environment (e.g., living with a perpetrator of domestic violence or in a context of ongoing bullying).

PTSD may present as panic disorder or social anxiety disorder if the child exhibits striking anxiety and distress on exposure to reminders of the trauma and avoidance of talking about the traumatic event. PTSD may be difficult to distinguish from other anxiety disorders if children develop phobias, fears, or avoidance of cues associated with their traumatic experiences. PTSD may also mimic major depressive disorder because of the presence of self-injury as a means of avoidant coping, sleep problems, social withdrawal, and/or affective numbing. PTSD may also be misdiagnosed as a primary substance use disorder since drugs and/or alcohol may be used to numb and avoid trauma reminders. Conversely, it is important to keep in mind that youth with a trauma history may have a primary substance use disorder with few trauma symptoms; such youth will likely benefit more from receiving interventions for substance use disorder rather than PTSD.

PTSD may be misdiagnosed as bipolar disorder. Some children with PTSD, particularly those who have been abused or exposed to ongoing domestic violence, may present with severe affective, behavioral, and/or cognitive dysregulation. These problems may be due to experiencing physiological changes as well as having been forced to tolerate ongoing abuse without protest. Such children may display extreme outbursts of anger, silliness, confusion, sexualized behavior, aggression, self-injury, and other symptoms suggestive of bipolar disorder. It is also possible for PTSD and bipolar disorder to coexist. Obtaining a history of trauma exposure and how it may be influencing symptoms is critically important in accurately diagnosing these children.

PTSD should be distinguished from psychotic disorders, which PTSD may mimic because of the presence of flashbacks, hypervigilance, sleep disturbance, numbing, and/or social withdrawal. PTSD should also be differentiated from milder adjustment disorders. PTSD can mimic physical conditions including migraine, asthma, caffeinism, seizure disorder, hyperthyroidism, or side effects from a variety of prescription medications and nonprescription drugs. PTSD is often associated with somatic symptoms such as headaches and abdominal pain. Children presenting with significant medical symptoms of unknown origin with a history of trauma should be considered for a mental health evaluation, which should include a complete assessment for PTSD symptoms.

Persistent complex bereavement disorder should be distinguished from normal grief by the presence of severe grief reactions that persist for 6 months after the death. Persistent complex bereavement disorder shares sadness, crying, and suicidal ideation with major depression and dysthymia (DSM-5 persistent depressive disorder) but is distinguished from these disorders in that it is characterized by a focus on the loss. Persistent complex bereavement disorder should be distinguished from separation anxiety disorder. While the former involves distress about separation from a deceased person, the latter involves distress about separation from current living attachment figures.

Persistent complex bereavement disorder should also be distinguished from PTSD. Although children can develop both disorders concurrently, children who have the former have a preoccupation with the loss and yearning for the deceased, which is absent in PTSD.

Clinical Examination and Mental Status Findings

Evaluators may have particular difficulty distinguishing oppositional behavior from avoidance ("I don't want to talk about it") or appropriate resolution of a troubling experience ("I'm over it, and I'm tired of everyone asking me about that stuff"). One way to assess this is to ask the child to describe the experience "so I can reassure your parent who is concerned about you that everything is really okay." Another is to evaluate the child's adaptive functioning: if the child is doing well in most domains (school, friends, family, self-image, neurovegetative functioning) and has no apparent dysfunctional thoughts about the traumatic experience, PTSD symptoms, or other psychiatric symptoms, the clinician may judge this avoidance to be adaptive. Avoidant symptoms may alternate with intrusion symptoms; at times children may exhibit a predominance of one or the other. Finally, as always, the clinician should discuss these findings with the parent, as the parent's reason for coming for the evaluation and other information may be pertinent in coming to a conclusion.

Treatment

Among the available treatments for childhood PTSD, there is more evidence for trauma-focused psychotherapy (i.e., therapies that specifically address and focus on children's traumatic experiences) than for pharmacotherapies. Therefore, in most cases, clinicians should provide children with evidence-based psychotherapy prior to starting medication unless there is a compelling reason to do otherwise. In some cases, there may be justification for starting medication immediately; for example, there may be a comorbid condition for which there is a proven pharmacological treatment, the child may be so dysregulated or dangerous to self or others that a medication is required for immediate safety, or the child is unable to function without the immediate addition of medication for another reason (e.g., sleep is severely impaired and the condition has not responded to reasonable psychosocial interventions). Since psychotherapeutic treatments are preferred as a first-line intervention in most cases, these are described first.

Many child PTSD treatments have been applied for children who have maladaptive grief responses, particularly for those children who experienced traumatic bereavement. Since persistent complex bereavement disorder is a newly introduced condition, no data are available in regard to treating children with this specific condition. Information about effective treatments for earlier descriptions of this condition (e.g., childhood traumatic grief) is provided where applicable in the following treatment subsections.

Psychotherapeutic Treatments

Several evidence-based treatment models are currently available for children with PTSD or symptoms of persistent complex bereavement disorder. These models have a number of common principles, concepts, and components that have guided their development and cut across their differences in orientation, style, format, and specific content. The National Child Traumatic Stress Network (NCTSN; www.nctsn.org) provides information sheets that describe core components of evidence-based treatments for child PTSD, including cultural competency. Underlying tenets of effective treatments for children with PTSD and persistent complex bereavement disorder include the following:

1. Demonstrate developmental sensitivity
2. Be informed by the neurobiological impact of trauma or traumatic bereavement on children
3. Include parents/caretakers/families (i.e., show an awareness of the centrality of the family constellation in children's lives)
4. Demonstrate cultural sensitivity in the broadest sense of "culture"
5. Reestablish safety/trust
6. Address trauma, loss, and change reminders
7. Address significant areas of dysfunction (e.g., cognitive distortions regarding the trauma and/or death, negative child-parent interactions, school problems) in order to regain optimal developmental trajectory and momentum

In matching evidence-based or evidence-informed treatments to specific children with PTSD, posttrauma symptoms, and/or persistent complex bereavement disorder, clinicians should consider each child's developmental level; the setting in which it is either most efficient to provide services or most likely that the child/family will accept them; acceptability of different treatments in terms of duration, cost, privacy, and cultural match for a given family; comorbid conditions; type of trauma; and perhaps other individual factors. These factors are addressed in the following descriptions of the well-established evidence-based models for childhood PTSD and, where appropriate, their application for children with persistent complex bereavement disorder.

Trauma-Focused Cognitive-Behavioral Therapy

Trauma-focused cognitive-behavioral therapy (TF-CBT) has the strongest evidence base for effectively treating children who have PTSD. The core components of TF-CBT are summarized by the acronym PRACTICE: psychoeducation, parenting skills, relaxation, affective modulation, cognitive processing, trauma narrative and processing, in vivo mastery of trauma reminders, conjoint child-parent sessions, and enhancing safety (Cohen and Mannarino, in press). There are currently 15 published TF-CBT randomized controlled trials (RCTs) that include more than 700 children ages 3–18 years who experienced diverse traumas, including multiple and complex traumas across different cultures. These trials have demonstrated the superiority of TF-CBT over comparison treatments or a wait list condition in improving child and adolescent PTSD as well as depressive, anxiety, behavioral, cognitive, and other problems (e.g., Cohen et al. 2004a, 2011; Deblinger et al. 1996; Jensen et al. 2014; O'Callaghan et al. 2013). Several TF-CBT studies also documented differential improvement in the personal symptoms and parenting skills for those parents who participated in TF-CBT treatment.

TF-CBT has also been tested in effectiveness trials for children with traumatic bereavement. In these trials, the following grief-related components were added to the TF-CBT PRACTICE components: grief psychoeducation, grieving the loss and resolving ambivalent feelings about the deceased, preserving positive memories, redefining the relationship from one of interaction to one of memory, and treatment closure issues. In two open effectiveness trials (Cohen et al. 2004b, 2006), children receiving this version of TF-CBT experienced significant improvement in traumatic bereavement, PTSD, anxiety, depression, and behavior problems.

Cognitive-Behavioral Interventions for Trauma in Schools

A parallel treatment model to TF-CBT, cognitive-behavioral intervention for trauma in schools (CBITS) provides similar PRACTICE components described in TF-CBT, with the exception that CBITS is provided in group therapy, which is conducted during the school day at the child's school, and therefore parental involvement typically does not occur. In the CBITS model, the trauma narrative occurs in individual breakout sessions with the group therapist. Advantages of school-based treatments like CBITS include that they may greatly improve accessibility and acceptability of treatment for families who cannot or will not seek clinic-based services. Additionally, children may experience a decreased sense of stigmatization and improvement of other symptoms specifically through participating in group treatment. CBITS has been compared with a wait list condition in one RCT and one quasi-RCT for children exposed to community violence, including primarily Latino immigrant children (Kataoka et al. 2003; Stein et al. 2003). It has also been used for children exposed to disasters.

Child-Parent Psychotherapy

For very young traumatized children, child-parent psychotherapy (CPP) is a relationship-based model delivered in joint child-parent treatment sessions focusing on improving interactions between the young child and his or her parent. Often the parent or caregiver has experienced trauma as well, so this treatment allows both child and parent to learn improved ways of interacting, as well as correcting dysfunctional thoughts and developing a joint trauma narrative. In one RCT, young children (ages 3–7 years) who participated in CPP with their domestic violence–exposed mothers experienced significantly greater improvement in PTSD and behavioral symptoms than those who received case management and individual psychotherapy (Lieberman et al. 2005). CPP has also been successfully applied for young children experiencing traumatic bereavement (Lieberman et al. 2003).

Narrative Exposure Therapy for Children

Narrative Exposure Therapy for Children (KidNET) is a structured cognitive-behavioral child treatment for children and adolescents exposed to war and refugee experiences. KidNET was adapted from a parallel evidence-based treatment for adults with PTSD, Narrative Exposure Therapy. KidNET was provided to refugee children exposed to war and was found to be superior to a wait list control condition in improving PTSD symptoms and diagnosis (Ruf et al. 2010).

Trauma Grief Component Therapy for Adolescents

Trauma Grief Component Therapy for Adolescents (TGCT-A; formerly UCLA Trauma/Grief Program for Adolescents) is a cognitive-behaviorally based group treatment model that includes five modules sequentially addressing trauma- and grief-related issues: traumatic experiences, trauma and loss reminders, posttraumatic stress and adversities, bereavement and the interplay of trauma and grief, and resumption of developmental progression It is typically provided in school settings. It has been used in quasi-randomized and open studies internationally and in the United States for youth exposed to disasters, terrorism, war, and community violence (CATS Consortium 2010; Layne et al. 2001; Saltzman et al. 2001) and in one non-blinded randomized controlled trial in Bosnia (Layne et al. 2008) that compared this program to classroom-based psychoeducation and skills intervention alone. In this trial TGCT-A was superior to the comparison condition in improving PTSD and depression.

Trauma Systems Therapy

Trauma systems therapy (TST) combines an individual intervention such as TF-CBT with a more systematic approach for children with complex needs. For example, TST includes acute stabilization up to and including inpatient hospitalization; psychotropic medication management; intensive home-based behavioral- or family-based interventions; and liaison with multiple other systems including medical, justice, child welfare, child protection, educational, and law enforcement. TST was associated with improvement in children's PTSD symptoms in one open trial (Saxe et al. 2005).

Other Psychosocial Treatments

Treatments are being developed and tested for children with complex trauma and a variety of comorbid conditions. For example, Trauma Affect Regulation: Guidelines for Education and Therapy (TARGET; Ford et al. 2012), a treatment for youth with complex trauma, has been tested with juvenile justice–involved teen girls in outpatient and residential treatment settings with promising results. Seeking Safety, a treatment originally developed for adults with comorbid PTSD and substance use disorders, has been adapted for adolescents and tested in a small pilot study with positive outcomes for PTSD symptoms (Najavits et al. 2006).

Interest has grown regarding optimal strategies for disseminating and implementing evidence-based treatments for traumatized children. One approach uses a Web-based curriculum (http://tfcbt.musc.edu) to train large numbers of clinicians in the TF-CBT model. More than 200,000 learners from more than 120 countries have registered for this online course since its introduction in 2005. Surveys show that completers gained significant knowledge about TF-CBT and had high levels of satisfaction in using the course. The NCTSN is also using innovative dissemination strategies, including adaptation of the Institute for Healthcare Improvement's (www.ihi.org) learning collaborative model to spread innovative evidence-based treatments community-wide. TF-CBT, CPP, and TST learning collaboratives have been sponsored by the NCTSN, individual states, and other organizations within the United States and internationally. Data suggest that these programs are successfully disseminating evidence-based treatments to participant agencies and communities.

Pharmacological Treatments

A number of neurotransmitter systems have been studied in connection with the development and maintenance of PTSD symptoms. This has led to the use of medications such as anti-adrenergic agents, anticonvulsants, antidepressants, morphine, and antipsychotics. Despite the failure of several randomized controlled treatment trials to document that pharmacological agents effectively treat PTSD in the pediatric age group, many medications are prescribed for children with PTSD symptoms (for an excellent review of this topic, see Wilkinson and Carrion 2012).

Small open trials have suggested the potential benefit of selective serotonin reuptake inhibitors (e.g., Seedat et al. 2002), propranolol (Famularo et al. 1988), and clonidine (Harmon and Riggs 1996; Perry 1994) for treating childhood PTSD. A case report suggested the potential benefit for prazosin for improving reexperiencing and hyperarousal symptoms (Strawn et al. 2009). Open trials have been conducted with two additional medications, neither of which would typically be routinely prescribed for traumatized children in outpatient settings. Saxe et al. (2001) conducted a naturalistic study examining morphine doses for acutely burned children who required hospitalization. These researchers documented a linear association between mean morphine dosage (mg/kg/day) and 6-month reduction in PTSD symptoms, after controlling for subjective experience of pain. Morphine would likely be considered a first-line treatment for PTSD only among acutely injured or possibly other acutely traumatized children seen in hospital settings. An open trial using risperidone demonstrated remission from severe PTSD symptoms in 13 of 18 boys (Horrigan and Barnhill 1999). This cohort had high rates of serious comorbid conditions (e.g., bipolar disorder, ADHD, aggression); such factors would need to be weighed carefully when considering potential risks versus potential benefits of using atypical antipsychotic medications in children.

Because of the strong placebo effect in children, it is important not to assume that because a child's PTSD symptoms improve after taking a prescribed medication the improvement was due to the medication. Once the child seems to respond, the temptation is to leave the child on the medication, even if the symptoms then return. It is essential to carefully balance the potential risks and benefits in such situations, particularly since there is no empirical evidence to back up such prescribing practices. An alternative approach if symptoms recur would be to decrease or discontinue the medication, rather than increasing the dose, under an alternative assumption that the response was not due to medication in the first place but was rather a placebo response or was due to supportive evaluation and psychoeducation. This has the advantages of not continuing children on ineffective medications, avoiding unnecessary and possibly detrimental polypharmacy, and using a rational pharmacology approach to prescribing. Current recommendations are to provide children who have PTSD with trauma-focused psychotherapy as a first-line treatment, prior to starting medication, unless there is a clear indication that medication is warranted (Cohen et al. 2010).

Other Treatments for PTSD

Eye movement desensitization and reprocessing (EMDR) has been adapted for children and tested in one well-controlled trial, which showed that children receiving EMDR demonstrated more improvement in intrusion symptoms—but not in avoidance or hyperarousal symptoms—than a wait list control group (Ahmad and Sundelin-Wahlsten 2008). A recent well-controlled study comparing EMDR with TF-CBT showed these treatments to be equally effective and efficient in treating children's PTSD symptoms, with TF-CBT showing superiority to EMDR in treating co-occurring problems such as depression and behavior problems (Diehle et al. 2015). Debate is ongoing regarding the mechanism of efficacy for EMDR; deconstructive studies have documented that EMDR is equally effective with or without bilateral eye movements, and Ahmad and Sundelin-Wahlsten (2008, p. 131) noted that their adaptation was effective for children because of its similarity to cognitive therapy.

Unproven techniques, such as severely restricting movement through binding, restricting nutritional intake, or using "rebirthing" techniques, are sometimes used for traumatized children. These interventions have led to serious complications, including death. Professional organizations, including the American Academy of Child and Adolescent Psychiatry (www.aacap.org) and the American Professional Society on the Abuse of Children (www.apsac.org), recommend that these interventions not be used.

Summary Points

- Posttraumatic stress disorder (PTSD) is a difficult condition to accurately diagnose in children. Many children have experienced multiple traumas, making it challenging to anchor PTSD symptoms to specific traumatic experiences. Clinicians must ask about symptoms in developmentally appropriate ways, obtain information from parents or other caretakers as well as from the children, and realize that avoidance leads to underreporting in many cases.
- Although natural recovery can occur, many children do not spontaneously recover from PTSD. Children with subsyndromal PTSD symptoms often experience the same functional impairments as those meeting full diagnostic criteria. When the clinician is in doubt, treatment should be provided.
- Effective treatments are available for childhood PTSD throughout the developmental spectrum, from infants through adolescents.
- In general, treatment should start with psychotherapy, not pharmacotherapy, unless there is a clear reason to give medication (e.g., a comorbid diagnosis for which there is an effective pharmacotherapy, clear dangerousness requiring immediate medication, symptoms so severe that psychotherapy is deemed unable to provide relief).

- Parents should be included in trauma-focused therapy whenever feasible; however, therapy should not be denied to children if parents are not available. School-based treatments can provide access to treatment for children who might not otherwise receive it.
- Following the death of an important person, some children will develop persistent complex bereavement disorder, which is currently included in DSM-5 as a condition for further study.
- Individual and group treatment models for PTSD are being applied for children with persistent complex bereavement disorder, particularly when the person died under traumatic circumstances.
- Preliminary evidence suggests that integrating trauma- and grief-focused components is effective in reducing persistent complex bereavement disorder and related difficulties for children and adolescents.
- More research is needed to further validate child assessment instruments and treatments for persistent complex bereavement disorder.
- Resources for clinicians, parents, and teachers are available at www.nctsn.org.

References

Ahmad A, Sundelin-Wahlsten V: Applying EMDR on children with PTSD. Eur Child Adolesc Psychiatry 17(3):127–132, 2008 17846813

American Psychiatric Association: Diagnostic and Statistical Manual of Mental Disorders, 3rd Edition. Washington, DC, American Psychiatric Association, 1980

American Psychiatric Association: Diagnostic and Statistical Manual of Mental Disorders, 5th Edition, Arlington, VA, American Psychiatric Association, 2013

Berkowitz SJ, Stover CS, Marans SR: The Child and Family Traumatic Stress Intervention: secondary prevention for youth at risk of developing PTSD. J Child Psychol Psychiatry 52(6):676–685, 2011 20868370

Briere J, Spinazzola J: Phenomenology and psychological assessment of complex posttraumatic states. J Trauma Stress 18(5):401–412, 2005 16281238

CATS Consortium: Implementation of CBT for youth affected by the World Trade Center disaster: matching need to treatment intensity and reducing trauma symptoms. J Trauma Stress 23(6):699–707, 2010 21171130

Cohen JA, Mannarino AP: Treatment of childhood traumatic grief. J Clin Child Adolesc Psychol 33(4):819–831, 2004 15498749

Cohen JA, Mannarino AP: Supporting children with traumatic grief: what educators need to know. Sch Psychol Int 32:117–131, 2011

Cohen JA, Mannarino AP: Trauma-focused cognitive behavioral therapy for traumatized children and families. Child Adolesc Psychiatr Clin N Am (in press)

Cohen JA, Deblinger E, Mannarino AP, et al: A multisite, randomized controlled trial for children with sexual abuse-related PTSD symptoms. J Am Acad Child Adolesc Psychiatry 43(4):393–402, 2004a 15187799

Cohen JA, Mannarino AP, Knudsen K: Treating childhood traumatic grief: a pilot study. J Am Acad Child Adolesc Psychiatry 43(10):1225–1233, 2004b 15381889

Cohen JA, Mannarino AP, Staron V: A pilot study of modified cognitive-behavioral therapy for childhood traumatic grief (CBT-CTG). J Am Acad Child Adolesc Psychiatry 45(12):1465–1473, 2006 17135992

Cohen JA, Bukstein O, Walter W, et al: Practice parameter for the assessment and treatment of children and adolescents with posttraumatic stress disorder. J Am Acad Child Adolesc Psychiatry 49(4):414–430, 2010 20410735

Cohen JA, Mannarino AP, Iyengar S: Community treatment of PTSD for children exposed to intimate partner violence: a randomized controlled trial. Arch Pediatr Adolesc Med 165(1):16–21, 2011

Craske MG, Kircanski K, Zelikowsky M, et al: Optimizing inhibitory learning during exposure therapy. Behav Res Ther 46(1):5–27, 2008 18005936

Deblinger E, Lippmann J, Steer R: Sexually abused children suffering posttraumatic stress symptoms: initial treatment outcome findings. Child Maltreat 1:310–321, 1996

Diehle J, Opmeer BC, Boer F, et al: Trauma-focused cognitive behavioral therapy or eye movement desensitization and reprocessing: what works in children with posttraumatic symptoms? A randomized controlled trial. Eur Child Adolesc Psychiatry 24(2):227–236, 2015 24965797

Famularo R, Kinscherff R, Fenton T: Propranolol treatment for childhood posttraumatic stress disorder, acute type. A pilot study. Am J Dis Child 142(11):1244–1247, 1988 3177336

Foa EB, Johnson KM, Feeny NC, et al: The child PTSD Symptom Scale: a preliminary examination of its psychometric properties. J Clin Child Psychol 30(3):376–384, 2001 11501254

Ford JD, Steinberg KL, Hawke J, et al: Randomized trial comparison of emotion regulation and relational psychotherapies for PTSD with girls involved in delinquency. J Clin Child Adolesc Psychol 41(1):27–37, 2012 22233243

Harmon RJ, Riggs PD: Clonidine for posttraumatic stress disorder in preschool children. J Am Acad Child Adolesc Psychiatry 35(9):1247–1249, 1996 8824068

Horrigan JP, Barnhill LJ: Risperidone and PTSD in boys. J Neuropsychiatry Clin Neurosci 11:126–127, 1999

Jensen T, Holt T, Ormhaug S, et al: A randomized effectiveness study comparing trauma-focused cognitive behavioral therapy with therapy as usual for youth. J Clin Child Adolesc Psychol 43(3):356–369, 2014 23931093

Kaplow JB, Layne CM, Pynoos RS, et al: DSM-V diagnostic criteria for bereavement-related disorders in children and adolescents: developmental considerations. Psychiatry 75(3):243–266, 2012 22913501

Kataoka SH, Stein BD, Jaycox LH, et al: A school-based mental health program for traumatized Latino immigrant children. J Am Acad Child Adolesc Psychiatry 42(3):311–318, 2003 12595784

La Greca AM, Silverman WK, Wasserstein SB: Children's predisaster functioning as a predictor of posttraumatic stress following Hurricane Andrew. J Consult Clin Psychol 66(6):883–892, 1998 9874901

Layne CM, Pynoos RS, Saltzman WR, et al: Trauma/grief-focused group psychotherapy: school-based postwar intervention with traumatized Bosnian adolescents. Group Dyn 5(4):277–290, 2001

Layne CM, Saltzman WR, Poppleton L, et al: Effectiveness of a school-based group psychotherapy program for war-exposed adolescents: a randomized controlled trial. J Am Acad Child Adolesc Psychiatry 47(9):1048–1062, 2008 18664995

Lieberman AF, Compton NC, Van Horn P, et al: Losing a Parent to Death in the Early Years: Guidelines for the Treatment of Traumatic Bereavement in Infancy and Early Childhood. Washington, DC, Zero to Three Press, 2003

Lieberman AF, Van Horn P, Ippen CG: Toward evidence-based treatment: child-parent psychotherapy with preschoolers exposed to marital violence. J Am Acad Child Adolesc Psychiatry 44(12):1241–1248, 2005 16292115

Melhem NM, Moritz G, Walker M, et al: Phenomenology and correlates of complicated grief in children and adolescents. J Am Acad Child Adolesc Psychiatry 46(4):493–499, 2007 17420684

Najavits LM, Gallop RJ, Weiss RD: Seeking safety therapy for adolescent girls with PTSD and substance use disorder: a randomized controlled trial. J Behav Health Serv Res 33(4):453–463, 2006 16858633

O'Callaghan P, McMullen J, Shannon C, et al: A randomized controlled trial of trauma-focused cognitive behavioral therapy for sexually exploited, war-affected Congolese girls. J Am Acad Child Adolesc Psychiatry 52(4):359–369, 2013 23582867

Perry BD: Neurobiological sequelae of childhood trauma: PTSD in children, in Catecholamine Function in Posttraumatic Stress Disorder: Emerging Concepts. Edited by Murburg MM. Washington,

DC, American Psychiatric Press, 1994, pp 223–255

Ruf M, Schauer M, Neuner F, et al: Narrative exposure therapy for 7- to 16-year-olds: a randomized controlled trial with traumatized refugee children. J Trauma Stress 23(4):437–445, 2010 20684019

Saltzman WR, Pynoos RS, Layne CM, et al: Trauma- and grief-focused intervention for adolescents exposed to community violence: results of a school-based screening and group treatment protocol. Group Dyn 5(4):291–303, 2001

Saxe G, Stoddard F, Courtney D, et al: Relationship between acute morphine and the course of PTSD in children with burns. J Am Acad Child Adolesc Psychiatry 40(8):915–921, 2001 11501691

Saxe G, Ellis BH, Fogler J, et al: Comprehensive care for traumatized children: an open trial examines treatment using trauma systems therapy. Psychiatr Ann 35(5):443–448, 2005

Scheeringa MS, Zeanah CH, Myers L, et al: Predictive validity in a prospective follow-up of PTSD in preschool children. J Am Acad Child Adolesc Psychiatry 44(9):899–906, 2005 16113618

Seedat S, Stein DJ, Ziervogel C, et al: Comparison of response to selective serotonin reuptake inhibitor in children, adolescents, and adults with posttraumatic stress disorder. J Child Adolesc Psychopharmacol 12(1):37–46, 2002 12014594

Stein M, Jang KL, Taylor S, et al: Genetic and environmental influences on trauma exposure and posttraumatic stress disorder symptoms: a twin study. Am J Psychiatry 159(10):1675–1681, 2002 12359672

Stein BD, Jaycox LH, Kataoka SH, et al: A mental health intervention for schoolchildren exposed to violence: a randomized controlled trial. JAMA 290(5):603–611, 2003 12902363

Strawn JR, Delbello MP, Geracioti TD: Prazosin treatment of an adolescent with posttraumatic stress disorder. J Child Adolesc Psychopharmacol 19(5):599–600, 2009 19877989

Thienkrua W, Cardozo BL, Chakkraband ML, et al: Symptoms of posttraumatic stress disorder and depression among children in tsunami-affected areas in southern Thailand. JAMA 296(5):549–559, 2006 16882961

Wilkinson JM, Carrion VG: Pharmacotherapy in pediatric PTSD: a developmentally focused review of the evidence. Curr Psychopharmacol 1(3):252–270, 2012

CHAPTER 17

Obsessive-Compulsive Disorder

Daniel A. Geller, M.B.B.S., FRACP
Kyle Williams, M.D.

Definition, Clinical Description, and Diagnosis

Obsessive-compulsive disorder (OCD) is defined by the presence of *either* obsessions (*worries* is a more user-friendly term for children) *or* compulsions (*rituals* is a more user-friendly term for children), although both may be present. Although OCD was categorized among the anxiety disorders in DSM-IV (American Psychiatric Association 1994, 2000), a variety of hidden or poorly articulated affects may drive the symptoms. In DSM-5 (American Psychiatric Association 2013), OCD was removed from the anxiety disorders section, and instead a new category was created for obsessive-compulsive (OC) "spectrum" disorders. These related disorders include body dysmorphic disorder, hoarding disorder, trichotillomania (hair-pulling disorder), and excoriation (skin-picking) disorder. Box 17–1 shows the DSM-5 criteria for OCD. The specifier *with poor insight* may be especially relevant to the diagnosis in youth since children's ability to explain their obsessions and the fears driving their compulsions may be quite limited. There is also a new *tic-related* specifier, reflecting the high prevalence of tic disorder comorbidity in individuals with OCD.

This chapter is dedicated to the memory of Henrietta Leonard, M.D., esteemed clinician, researcher, teacher, mentor, and colleague.

Box 17–1. DSM-5 Diagnostic Criteria for Obsessive-Compulsive Disorder

300.3 (F42)

A. Presence of obsessions, compulsions, or both:

Obsessions are defined by (1) and (2):

1. Recurrent and persistent thoughts, urges, or images that are experienced, at some time during the disturbance, as intrusive and unwanted, and that in most individuals cause marked anxiety or distress.
2. The individual attempts to ignore or suppress such thoughts, urges, or images, or to neutralize them with some other thought or action (i.e., by performing a compulsion).

Compulsions are defined by (1) and (2):

1. Repetitive behaviors (e.g., hand washing, ordering, checking) or mental acts (e.g., praying, counting, repeating words silently) that the individual feels driven to perform in response to an obsession or according to rules that must be applied rigidly.
2. The behaviors or mental acts are aimed at preventing or reducing anxiety or distress, or preventing some dreaded event or situation; however, these behaviors or mental acts are not connected in a realistic way with what they are designed to neutralize or prevent, or are clearly excessive.

Note: Young children may not be able to articulate the aims of these behaviors or mental acts.

B. The obsessions or compulsions are time-consuming (e.g., take more than 1 hour per day) or cause clinically significant distress or impairment in social, occupational, or other important areas of functioning.

C. The obsessive-compulsive symptoms are not attributable to the physiological effects of a substance (e.g., a drug of abuse, a medication) or another medical condition.

D. The disturbance is not better explained by the symptoms of another mental disorder (e.g., excessive worries, as in generalized anxiety disorder; preoccupation with appearance, as in body dysmorphic disorder; difficulty discarding or parting with possessions, as in hoarding disorder; hair pulling, as in trichotillomania [hair-pulling disorder]; skin picking, as in excoriation [skin-picking] disorder; stereotypies, as in stereotypic movement disorder; ritualized eating behavior, as in eating disorders; preoccupation with substances or gambling, as in substance-related and addictive disorders; preoccupation with having an illness, as in illness anxiety disorder; sexual urges or fantasies, as in paraphilic disorders; impulses, as in disruptive, impulse-control, and conduct disorders; guilty ruminations, as in major depressive disorder; thought insertion or delusional preoccupations, as in schizophrenia spectrum and other psychotic disorders; or repetitive patterns of behavior, as in autism spectrum disorder).

Specify if:

With good or fair insight: The individual recognizes that obsessive-compulsive disorder beliefs are definitely or probably not true or that they may or may not be true.

With poor insight: The individual thinks obsessive-compulsive disorder beliefs are probably true.

With absent insight/delusional beliefs: The individual is completely convinced that obsessive-compulsive disorder beliefs are true.

Specify if:

Tic-related: The individual has a current or past history of a tic disorder.

Clinical Features

OCD in childhood is distinct in important ways from the disorder in adults. Pediatric OCD generally has a prepubertal age of onset, is male predominant, and is characterized by a distinct pattern of OC symptoms and psychiatric comorbidity. Relative to OCD beginning in adulthood, pediatric OCD may in some cases be etiologically related to immune-mediated pathology (e.g., pediatric autoimmune neuropsychiatric disorders associated with streptococcal infection [PANDAS]). Additionally, pediatric OCD is more highly familial and generally has a better prognosis. The secretive nature of OCD symptoms and the isolated and idiosyncratic functional deficits, which may be severe but domain-specific and variable, contribute to OCD being underrecognized and underdiagnosed in youth.

Despite overlap between children and adults in phenotypic presentation, issues such as limited insight and the evolution of symptom profiles that follow developmental themes over time differentiate children and adults with OCD. In addition, children with OCD frequently perform rituals without well-developed obsessions (e.g., feeling bad or uneasy rather than specific cognitions) (Rettew et al. 1992), making these symptoms harder to target using cognitive-behavioral therapy (CBT). The majority of children with OCD exhibit multiple obsessions as well as compulsions. Neither gender nor age at onset determine the number or severity of OCD symptoms. Boys are more likely to report sexual obsessions (including unwanted anxiety-provoking thoughts about being gay), and girls are more likely to report hoarding symptoms (Mataix-Cols et al. 2008). Often, children's obsessions center on fear of a catastrophic family event (e.g., death of a parent), leading to checking and other behaviors resembling separation anxiety disorder but with no premorbid history of this disorder and a later age of onset. Contamination, sexual or somatic obsessions, and scruples (overly moralistic thoughts) are the most commonly reported obsessions. Washing, repeating, checking, and ordering are the most commonly reported compulsions (Geller et al. 2001a). While OCD symptoms tend to wax and wane, they persist in the majority of patients but change over time, so the initially presenting symptom constellation is not maintained (Rettew et al. 1992). Frequently, parents are intimately involved in their child's rituals, especially in reassurance seeking, a form of "verbal checking." Geller et al. (2001a) found that religious and sexual obsessions were overrepresented in adolescents compared with children and adults. Hoarding compulsions, when seen in isolation, lead to a hoarding disorder diagnosis, yet when seen along with other more typical OC symptoms, hoarding compulsions are then included in the OCD diagnosis. Factor analytic methods identify consistent symptom "dimensions" of OCD that may be more informative for understanding its causes. One four-factor solution explaining 60% of symptom variance is characterized by 1) symmetry/ordering/repeating/checking, 2) contamination/cleaning/aggressive behavior/somatic symptoms, 3) hoarding, and 4) sexual/religious symptoms (Stewart et al. 2007). This dimensional approach to phenotyping OCD may yield important biological signals in genetic, translational, and treatment studies, whereas more traditional categorical approaches do not.

Pediatric OCD is characterized by male preponderance (3:2 male to female). Boys may have an earlier age at onset than girls. Adult gender patterns (slight female preponderance) appear in late adolescence. The mean age at onset of OCD is 9–10 years, with the majority of childhood onset falling between ages 6 and 12.5 years. On average, age at clinical presentation is 2 or more years after age at onset (Geller et al. 2001a). Interest in the neuropsychological "endophenotype" of children with OCD grows out of clinical experience that many children have academic difficulties that are not wholly explained by their primary disorder. Given the potential involvement of frontal-striatal systems in OCD, several aspects of neuropsychological performance have been especially relevant to its study, especially measures of visuospatial integration, short-term memory, attention, and executive functions. Early studies of children with OCD yielded inconsistent results regarding significant neuropsychological deficits (for a review, see Abramovitch et al. 2012). While academic dysfunction is common, the demonstrated reduced processing speed and reduced performance on visuospatial and working memory tasks in children with OCD may be related to the primary symptoms.

Epidemiology

Prevalence rates of pediatric OCD are around 1%–2% in the United States and elsewhere (Apter et al. 1996; Flament et al. 1988). In the first epidemiological study of pediatric OCD (Flament et al. 1988), most subjects identified through screening who were later diagnosed with OCD had been previously undiagnosed. In the British Child Mental Health Survey of more than 10,000 children and adolescents ages 5–15 years, the point prevalence was 0.25%. Almost 90% of cases identified had been undetected and untreated. In this study, lower socioeconomic status and lower intelligence quotient were associated with OCD in youth (Heyman et al. 2001). There are two peaks of incidence for OCD across the life span, one occurring in preadolescent children and a later peak in early adult life (mean age of 21 years) (Geller et al. 2001a). Childhood onset occurs in at least 30%–50% of cases (Pauls et al. 1995).

Comorbidity

OCD in youth is usually accompanied by other psychopathology. Epidemiological studies find comorbid psychiatric diagnoses in more than 50% of children with OCD (Flament et al. 1988), and rates are higher in clinically referred samples (Geller et al. 2001a). This comorbid psychopathology often shows a distinct chronology, so assessment and treatment approaches must evolve with time. Rates of comorbidity vary widely, but samples of youth with OCD consistently have high rates of not only tic disorders but also mood, anxiety, disruptive behavior, and specific developmental disorders, attention-deficit/hyperactivity disorder (ADHD), and enuresis (Figure 17–1).

Regardless of age at ascertainment, an earlier age at onset for OCD predicts increased risk for ADHD and anxiety disorders. In contrast, mood and psychotic disorders are associated with older age and are more prevalent in adolescent subjects with OCD. Tourette's disorder is associated with both age at onset (earlier onset is more likely to be associated with comorbid Tourette's disorder) and chronological age (adolescents usually show remission of tics).

An important issue is whether comorbid disorders modify the expression of OCD. There is some evidence that this is true in the case of Tourette's disorder,

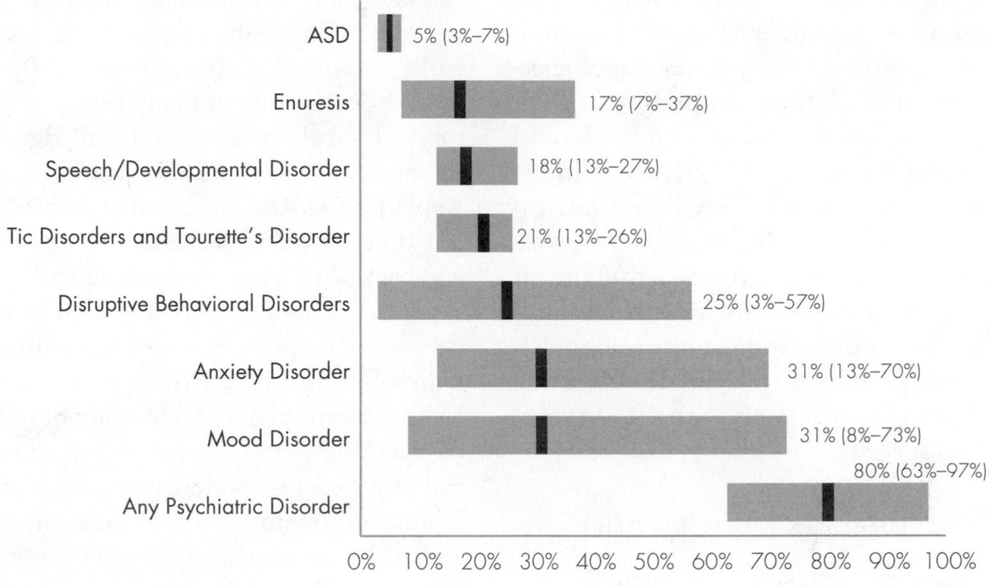

FIGURE 17–1. Comorbid disorders in pediatric obsessive-compulsive disorder: review of clinical studies.

Note. ASD=autism spectrum disorder.
Source. Adapted from Geller et al. 1998.

where specific symptoms (touching, tapping, repeating) appear to be more common than in patients without tic disorders (Leckman et al. 2003). By contrast, the OCD phenotype appears to be independent of the presence or absence of ADHD in symptoms, patterns of comorbid disorders, or OCD-specific functional impairment (Geller et al. 2003c). In any case, the presence (or absence) of comorbid psychopathology is important for clinicians to identify and address. Comorbidities are associated with a greater rate of relapse following treatment (Geller et al. 2003a).

Pathophysiology, Mechanisms, and Risk Factors

Several frontal cortico-striatal-thalamic circuits have been implicated in the pathophysiology of OCD, and several neurotransmitter systems modulate this feedback loop, including the excitatory amine glutamate and dopamine- and serotonin-containing neurons (Pauls et al. 2014). The frontostriatal model of OCD hypothesizes that increased glutamate can result from both the internal globus pallidus–substantia nigra pars reticulata interaction with the thalamus and the interactions between the striatum and external globus pallidus (Kalra and Swedo 2009). Major brain structures central to OCD include the orbitofrontal cortex, anterior cingulate cortex, caudate, and thalamus (Pauls et al. 2014). Pediatric imaging studies appear similar to those in adults, detecting structural abnormalities in the cingulate cortex, basal ganglia, and thalami of pediatric OCD patients (Abramovitch et al. 2012). A handful of functional imaging studies conducted with children at rest and following treatment have yielded results compatible with those in adults. Fitzgerald et al. (2000) used multislice proton magnetic resonance spectroscopic imaging in pediatric OCD patients and matched controls and found a significant reduction in *N*-acetylaspartate (NAA)/choline and NAA/creatine/phosphocreatine levels bilaterally in the medial thalami of affected children compared with control subjects. Furthermore, reductions in left medial thalamic NAA levels were inversely correlated with OCD symptom severity.

PANDAS and Pediatric Acute Neuropsychiatric Syndrome

Perhaps no issue in OCD remains as controversial as the debate around PANDAS, originally described by Swedo et al. (1997) (Leckman et al. 2011). The central hypothesis of PANDAS derives from observations of neurobehavioral disturbance accompanying Sydenham chorea, a sequel of rheumatic fever. An immune response to group A β-hemolytic streptococcus (GABHS) infections leads to cross-reactivity with and inflammation of basal ganglia with a distinct neurobehavioral syndrome that includes OCD and tics. Diagnostic criteria laid out by Swedo et al. (1997) (Table 17–1) have been used in a variety of studies of antibiotic prophylaxis (Garvey et al. 1999; Snider et al. 2005) and immune-modulating therapies (such as plasmapheresis). Some research has found significant associations between GABHS infections and OCD/Tourette's disorder diagnoses (e.g., Mell et al. 2005), as well as structural brain differences between PANDAS patients and healthy controls. For example, a magnetic resonance imaging analysis by Giedd et al. (2000) found increased caudate, pallidal, and putaminal volume in PANDAS patients compared with controls. However, detractors argue that GABHS is but one of many nonspecific physiological stressors that can trigger an increase in tics or OCD (Kurlan and Kaplan 2004). The weight of evidence at this time supports the belief that among a subset of children with OCD and/or Tourette's disorder, both onset and clinical exacerbations are linked to GABHS (Kurlan et al. 2008). However, data are lacking as to which children are at risk (PANDAS-affected children are reported to have an unexpectedly high rate of familial autoimmune illness [Murphy et al. 2010]) and what are the most effective treatments. Recently, the notion of a postinfectious autoimmune neuropsychiatric disorder has been decoupled from a specific pathogen (e.g., GABHS) to a broader, more inclusive category of dramatic-onset OCD or severe food restriction, captured by the term *pediatric acute onset neuropsychiatric syndrome* (Murphy et al. 2014), although the clinical features and diagnostic boundaries are challenging to define. The discovery of autoimmune encephalitis induced by anti-*N*-methyl-D-aspartate (NMDA) receptor antibodies (Dalmau et al. 2008) has rekindled interest in postinfectious autoimmune mediated etiology in early onset OCD.

Genetics

The contribution of genetic factors to the development of OCD has been explored in twin, family genetic, and segregation analysis studies (Nestadt et al. 2000; Pauls et al. 1995). The concordance rates for monozygotic twins are significantly higher than for dizygotic twins (van Grootheest et al. 2005), and heritability rates for early onset OCD range from 0.45 to 0.65 (Pauls et al. 2014). While family studies consistently demonstrate that

TABLE 17–1. Diagnostic criteria for PANDAS

1. Obsessive-compulsive disorder and/or a tic disorder
2. Prepubertal onset between 3 and 12 years of age, or Tanner I or II
3. Episodic course (abrupt onset and/or exacerbations)
4. Symptom onset/exacerbations temporally related to documented GABHS infections on two occasions
5. Association with neurological abnormalities

Note. GABHS=group A β-hemolytic streptococcus; PANDAS=pediatric autoimmune neuropsychiatric disorders associated with streptococcal infection.

Source. Swedo et al. 1997.

OCD is familial (Pauls et al. 1995, 2014), the risk of OCD in first-degree relatives appears to be greater for index cases with a childhood onset. For example, in their multisite family study of OCD, Nestadt et al. (2000) found a risk for OCD of around 12% in first-degree relatives, while relatives of pediatric OCD probands have shown age-corrected morbid risks of 24%–26% (do Rosario-Campos et al. 2005). These findings suggest greater genetic loading in pediatric-onset OCD. Further, a substantial proportion of relatives (5%–15%) is affected with subthreshold OC symptoms that may be genetic (Nestadt et al. 2000) and may also be relevant to family functioning. Segregation analyses suggest that familial patterns of OCD are consistent with genetic models that include genes of major effect (Nestadt et al. 2000), with possible sex effects. It is highly likely that there are many genes of small but cumulative effect that are important for the expression of this complex disorder. A genomewide linkage scan for OCD showed evidence for susceptibility loci on chromosomes 3q, 7p, 1q, 15q, and 6q (Shugart et al. 2006). The glutamate transporter gene *SLC1A1* on 9p24 has also been identified as a positive candidate gene (Walitza et al. 2010), and a genome-wide association study of OCD found a trend of associations for genes such as *NEUROD6*, *SV2A*, and *PTPRD* (Mattheisen et al. 2014). A genomewide meta-analysis (Stewart et al. 2013) suggests that OCD gene discovery will approximate that of schizophrenia and bipolar disorder, requiring very large sample sizes to identify multiple genes of small effect (Ruderfer et al. 2014).

Environmental Factors

While the aforementioned studies emphasize genetic factors, they also point clearly to major effects of *nongenetic* influences in the expression of OCD. For example, twin studies show that even among monozygotic twins, OCD is *not* fully concordant. In a cross-cultural sample of 4,246 twin pairs (Hudziak et al. 2004), genetic (45%–58%) and unique environmental (42%–55%) factors were almost equally important. In a population sample of 527 female twin pairs (Jonnal et al. 2000), heritability was 33% for obsessions and 26% for compulsions. Furthermore, a study of 4,662 pediatric twin pairs found a moderate correlation (r=0.40) between "normative" ritualistic behaviors in childhood and the subsequent onset of OCD, suggesting not only a potential risk factor for OCD onset but also that nonshared environmental factors can trigger the disorder (Pauls et al. 2014). Clearly, nonheritable etiological factors contribute to the risk of developing OCD as much as, if not more than, genetic factors. In fact, many to most cases of OCD arise *without* a positive family history of the disorder. However, these occurrences, known as sporadic cases, do not rule out a genetic etiology (for example, due to spontaneous mutations). Consequently, both familial and sporadic "subtypes" of OCD have repeatedly been identified (Nestadt et al. 2000; Pauls et al. 1995), leading to speculation about the differing impact of environmental and genetic factors on familial and nonfamilial forms of the disorder. Information regarding environmental triggers of the disorder may be especially relevant for the sporadic form, since the presence of OCD cannot be explained by the presence of an affected relative.

Perinatal Factors in Pediatric OCD

Lensi et al. (1996) found a higher rate of perinatal trauma (defined by dystocic delivery, use of forceps, breech presentation, or prolonged hypoxia) in males with an earlier onset of OCD. Geller et al. (2008) found that children with OCD had mothers with significantly higher rates of illness requiring medical care during pregnancy, as well as more birth difficulties (e.g., induced labor, forceps delivery, nuchal cord, prolonged labor). Among the OCD-affected children, there were significant associations between adverse perinatal experiences and earlier age at onset, increased OCD severity, and increased risk for comorbid ADHD, chronic tic disorder, anxiety disorder, and major depressive disorder.

Role of the Family in Pediatric OCD

Parents are often intimately involved in their children's OC symptoms and may unwittingly reinforce compulsive behaviors by providing verbal reassurance or other "assistance" to their children (e.g., handling objects that their children avoid, such as opening doors; laundering "contaminated" clothes and linens excessively; even wiping children on the toilet who will not do it themselves). Because OCD, and an anxiety diathesis in general, is highly familial, disentangling parental psychopathology from disturbed family functioning resulting from the child's OCD is critical, especially in younger patients. Increasingly, the central role of family members for children affected with OCD (both for maintenance of pathology as well as proxy therapy agents) has been recognized and is reflected both in a broader assessment that evaluates family function (e.g., Family Accommodation Scale for OCD–Interviewer Rated [FAS-IR; Calvocoressi et al. 1999]) and in newer models of treatment intervention (e.g., the Pediatric Obsessive Compulsive Treatment Study for Young Children [POTS Jr.; Freeman et al. 2014]) (see the section "Treatment" later in this chapter).

Course and Prognosis

Precipitating psychosocial events such as physical or sexual assault, being home alone during a forced breaking and entering, or witnessing serious or fatal domestic violence, are occasionally associated with the onset of OCD, sometimes dramatically (Lafleur et al. 2011). However, the majority of pediatric OCD cases have a gradual onset without a history of precipitating stressors. Sixteen samples reported in 22 studies with a total of 521 children with OCD and follow-up periods ranging from 1 to 15.6 years (mean 5.7 years) showed pooled mean persistence rates of 41% for *full* OCD and 60%

for *full* or *subthreshold* OCD (Stewart et al. 2004). Earlier age at onset, longer duration of OCD, and inpatient treatment predicted persistence. Comorbid psychiatric illness and poor initial treatment response were also poor prognostic factors. One pediatric OCD study found a significant relationship between OCD and PTSD, suggesting that psychological trauma may predict the onset of OCD (Lafleur et al. 2011). The occurrence of pediatric OCD is also commonly associated with compromised long-term psychosocial functioning, including a lower likelihood of cohabitation and marriage and a higher likelihood of living with parents as adults and/or hiding symptoms from family members. These studies also report high levels of social/peer problems (55%–100%), isolation, and unemployment (45%). The average educational level of those experiencing pediatric OCD did not differ from control subjects, with 30%–70% having attended college.

The long-term prognosis for pediatric OCD is better than originally thought (Stewart et al. 2004) and is better than in individuals with adult-onset OCD (Pauls et al. 2014). Many children will remit partially or entirely. Adverse prognostic factors include very early age at onset, concurrent psychiatric diagnoses, poor initial treatment response, long duration of illness, and a positive first-degree family history of OCD.

Evaluation

Making the Diagnosis

The simplest probes derive from the DSM-5 diagnostic criteria of the American Psychiatric Association (2013): "Do you ever have unwanted thoughts that upset you and that you cannot suppress?" "Do you ever have ideas, images or urges that make you anxious?" For younger children the question might be phrased, "Do you have worries that just won't go away?" It is reasonable to offer some examples at this time such as "worries about things not being clean" or "worrying that something bad might happen to yourself or a loved one." For compulsions a similar probe might be, "Do you ever have to do rituals over and over even though you know they don't make sense?" "Do you do things or have habits that you don't want because you feel anxious or worried about something?" For younger children the question might be phrased, "Do you have habits that you can't stop?" Examples such as washing, checking, repeating, ordering, and counting can be offered.

Sometimes adults must infer obsessions from observing a child's behavior when the obsessions are not articulated or even acknowledged by the child. Examples include avoidance behaviors such as not entering a room or handling an object. If screening questions suggest that OC symptoms are present, clinicians should follow with more in-depth assessment using the DSM-5 criteria of 1) time occupied by OC symptoms, 2) level of subjective distress, and 3) functional impairment, as well as a standardized inventory of symptoms and scalar assessment of severity, subjective distress, impairment, resistance, control, and insight, such as the Children's Yale-Brown Obsessive Compulsive Scale (CY-BOCS; Scahill et al. 1997).

The CY-BOCS is a 10-item anchored ordinal scale (0–4) that rates the clinical severity of the disorder by scoring the time occupied (0=no time, 4=more than 8 hours per day), degree of life interference (0=none, 4=extreme), subjective distress (0=none, 4=extreme), internal resistance (0=always, 4=none), and degree of control (0=excellent, 4=none) for both obsessions and compulsions. The CY-BOCS also includes a checklist of more than 60 obsessions and compulsions categorized by the predominant theme involved, such as contamination, hoarding, washing, checking, and so forth. Scores of 8–15 are considered to represent mild illness, 16–23 moderate illness, and ≥24 severe illness. Equally important are quantitative measures of avoidance, insight, indecisiveness, pathological responsibility and doubt, and slowness. The CY-BOCS is a clinician-administered instrument that is most informative when given to both children and their parents, and a "worst report" algorithm that combines the two reports is likely to be most accurate.

While the CY-BOCS is the current standard assessment tool for pediatric OCD, there are several important limitations to this scale. The first is that the avoidance rating is not included in the quantitative score of the scale (although later it is assigned an ordinal score from 0 to 4) and thus may underestimate severity when avoidance is a large part of the presenting behavior. Second, the scale is not linear, which makes it difficult to use to monitor treatment progress. Marked reductions in time occupied by obsessions or compulsions are not reflected in a proportional drop in scale scores. It is for this reason that a 25%–40% reduction in CY-BOCS scores is considered a clinically significant response.

Families may become deeply involved in their children's OCD. Parental efforts to relieve a child's anxiety may inadvertently lead to accommodation and reinforcement of OC behaviors. The very high intensity of affect and irritability displayed by some children may make it difficult for parents to react with the supportive yet detached responses needed for effective behavioral treatment. The familial nature of anxiety disorders and OCD are added factors in families' responses to a child with OCD. The role of individual family members in maintenance and management of OC symptoms is important to assess and can be done with the FAS-IR (Calvocoressi et al. 1999). Detailed and specific questions about activities of daily living may be needed to understand the cycle of OC behaviors at home.

Differential Diagnosis

Typical toddlers and preschoolers frequently engage in ritualistic behavior, such as mealtime or bedtime routines. As a rule, these routines do not cause impairment in family functioning, and interruption of these rituals does not create severe distress in the child. For some children, however, excessive rituals early in life may be a marker for later onset of OCD (Leonard et al. 1990). Perhaps the most difficult differential diagnosis occurs in the context of autism spectrum disorder. Core symptoms of this syndrome include stereotypic, repetitive behaviors and a restricted and narrow range of interests and activities that may easily be confused with OCD, especially in young children. A small number of children with OCD (5%–7%) may also meet criteria for DSM-IV Asperger's syndrome or pervasive developmental disorder (PDD; Geller et al. 2001a). In OCD, symptoms are ego-dystonic and are associated with anxiety-driven obsessional fears. Children with PDD engage in repetitive behaviors with apparent gratification and will become upset only when their preferred activities are interrupted. Left to their rituals, they do not display anxiety or discomfort. While younger children with OCD may not be able to articulate their concerns, evidence of anxiety is usually discernible. If symptoms are typical of OCD (such as washing, cleaning, or checking), one can infer obsessional concern.

Another diagnostic dilemma occurs in the context of poor insight into obsessional ideas that merges into overvalued ideation and even delusional thinking, suggesting psychosis. In children with OCD, insight is not static but rather varies with anxiety level and is best assessed when anxiety is at a minimum. While OC symptoms may herald a psychotic or schizophreniform disorder in youth, especially adolescents, other positive or negative symptoms of psychosis will usually be present or emerge to assist in differential diagnosis. The nature of obsessional ideation in patients with psychosis is often atypical (e.g., a fear that he will turn into another person or that her parent has been replaced by an alien).

Clinical Examination

Best-estimate diagnostic formulations should include information from *all* available sources, including the child, parents and other caregivers, teachers, and other clinicians involved. School and educational history provides an ecologically important and valid measure of function and illness severity. OC symptoms that spill into the school setting imply more anxiety, stronger compulsions, less insight, and less resistance and control. Therefore, educational impairment denoted by falling grades or the need for extra help or special class placement indicates more urgency for treatment and could justify more aggressive interventions, including medications. Neuropsychological assessment should be considered in children with OCD who are struggling at school.

Attention to GABHS infection as a potential precipitant for PANDAS-associated OCD is indicated in acute and dramatic onsets or exacerbations in preadolescent patients or when a child in remission suddenly relapses. Neurological signs such as Sydenham chorea should prompt a search for prior GABHS infection and other evidence of rheumatic fever but may not occur for many months after infection. Softer neurological signs such as tremor, coordination difficulties, and soft motor abnormalities contribute to one criterion for the PANDAS diagnosis (Swedo et al. 1997). Since the immunology of streptococcus and its role in infection-triggered neuropsychiatric symptoms is poorly understood, recommendations regarding antibody assay are uncertain. In acute and abrupt onset cases, antistreptolysin O and anti-DNase B titers may be helpful. A 0.2 log rise in either antibody or absolute levels more than twice the upper limit of the normal range suggest a recent GABHS infection. Intercurrent titers are also helpful as a baseline if there are subsequent exacerbations that may be associated with sudden increase in antibody levels. Titers at intervals of less than 3 months are not likely to be helpful (Kurlan et al. 2008).

Treatment

Overview

CBT is the first-line treatment for mild to moderate cases of OCD in children. Since the publication of a CBT treatment manual that operationalized and systematized this method (March and Mulle 1998), numerous studies have shown its acceptability and efficacy (March et al. 2001; Piacentini et al. 2003). Severe OCD, concurrent psychopathology (e.g., comorbid anxiety or major depressive or disruptive behavior disorders), lack of family cohesion, poor insight, and lack of skilled CBT practitioners are factors to consider in deciding when to use medication. Scores >23 on the CY-BOCS or Clinical Global Impressions—Severity scale (CGI-S) scores of "marked" to "severe" impairment provide a threshold for consideration of drug intervention. In addition, any situation that could impede the successful delivery of CBT should be cause for earlier consideration of medication treatment. For instance, poor insight into the irrational nature of the obsessions and associated compulsions can lead to resistance to CBT. Chaotic or nonintact family situations will make close family involvement in implementation of CBT more difficult. Finally, there is a dire shortage of skilled CBT practitioners. Site-specific differences in CBT outcomes in the National Institute of Mental Health (NIMH)–funded Pediatric OCD Treatment Study (POTS; March et al. 2004) suggest that expert delivery will improve response rates to CBT. In the POTS study, CBT alone did not differ from sertraline alone, and both were better than placebo.

Concurrent psychopathology may reduce the patient's acceptance of or compliance with CBT and may require medication itself. For example, a depressed adolescent with a mood-congruent anhedonic view of the future may see little point in making the effort to tolerate exposure and response prevention. Similarly, comorbid diagnoses have been shown to reduce the success of pharmacological treatment. In one study examining treatment with paroxetine, patients with comorbid ADHD, tic disorder, or oppositional defiant disorder demonstrated significantly lower response rates (56%, 53%, and 39%, respectively) than patients with OCD only (75%), despite strong overall treatment response among children and adolescents (71%; Geller et al. 2003a). Furthermore, comorbidity was associated with a greater rate of relapse (46% for ≥1 comorbid disorder [P=0.04] and 56% for ≥2 comorbid disorders [P<0.05] vs. 32% for no comorbidity). More recent analysis of data from the POTS comparative treatment trial (March et al. 2004) looked at symptom reduction on the CY-BOCS after 12 weeks of treatment. Those children with a comorbid tic disorder failed to respond to sertraline and did not separate statistically from placebo-treated patients, while response in youth with OCD without tics replicated previously published intent-to-treat outcomes. In children with tics, sertraline was helpful only when combined with CBT, while CBT alone was effective. Moreover, the presence of disruptive behavior disorders may represent a therapeutic challenge for clinicians, especially cognitive-behavioral clinicians. Storch et al. (2008) found that among children treated with CBT, those with OCD and one or more comorbid diagnoses had lower response and remission rates relative to those without a comorbid diagnosis. The number of comorbid conditions was negatively related to outcome.

Pharmacological Treatments

The past decade has seen rapid advances in our knowledge of the pharmacotherapy of OCD. Clomipramine, approved in 1989, was the first agent widely used in pediatric OCD populations. Subsequent multisite randomized controlled trials (RCTs), many of which were industry sponsored, have demonstrated significant efficacy of the selective serotonin reuptake inhibitors (SSRIs) compared with placebo, including sertraline (March et al. 1998), fluvoxamine (Riddle et al. 2001), fluoxetine (Geller et al.

2001b), and paroxetine (Geller et al. 2002). No comparative treatment studies have yet been performed, and there is little to guide clinicians in the choice of therapeutic agents. Clomipramine and three SSRIs (fluoxetine, fluvoxamine, and sertraline) have U.S. Food and Drug Administration (FDA)–approved pediatric indications, but paroxetine and citalopram are also used. Expert consensus guidelines for pediatric OCD (American Academy of Child and Adolescent Psychiatry 2012) suggest starting medication at the lowest dose and titrating slowly (for example, three weekly increments) to a target dose (see Table 17–2), with close monitoring for response and adverse effects over the first 6–8 weeks. The FDA recommends weekly review over the first 4 weeks, then every other week for 4 weeks, and then at week 12 following initiation of SSRIs in children, despite a lack of evidence that such a schedule alters outcome. Visits at 2- to 3-week intervals are more typical in practice. Most importantly, clinicians should be readily available for urgent communications during this period, and parents and youth should be encouraged to contact their physician or therapist with any concerns.

The cumulative data accrued from RCTs of pediatric OCD are now sufficient to examine the overall effect of medication treatment. One meta-analysis of all published RCTs (12) in children and adolescents with OCD (N=1,044) assessed evidence for differential efficacy based on type of drug, study design, and outcome measure (Geller et al. 2003b). There were four SSRIs (paroxetine, fluoxetine, fluvoxamine, sertraline) plus clomipramine, four study designs (parallel, withdrawal, substitution, crossover), four dependent outcome measures (CY-BOCS, NIMH Global Obsessive Compulsive Scale, CGI-S, Leyton Obsessional Inventory—Child Version), and two types of outcome scores (change and posttreatment). The effect size, expressed as a pooled standardized mean difference for results of all studies, was 0.46 (95% confidence interval [CI], 0.37–0.55) and showed a highly significant difference between drug and placebo treatment (z=9.87, P<0.001) (see Table 17–3).

Multivariate regression of drug effect, while controlling for other variables, showed that clomipramine was significantly superior to each of the SSRIs but that the other SSRIs were comparably effective. Clinically speaking, overall effect sizes of medication treatment were modest, with CY-BOCS scores for active medication improving about 6 points more than with placebo. Since then, the POTS (March et al. 2004) confirmed these findings with an effect size of 0.66 (95% CI, 0.12–1.2) for sertraline. A recent meta-analysis of 10 RCTs (Watson and Rees 2008) showed an overall drug effect size of 0.48 (95% CI, 0.36–0.61) and a clomipramine effect size of 0.85 (95% CI, 0.32–1.39). One limitation in interpreting published reports of medication trials is the numerous exclusion criteria used to select samples (Geller et al. 2003a). Because many comorbid conditions were excluded, the drug effect in clinical settings may be lower than meta-analyses suggest. Long-term studies suggest that there is a cumulative benefit over longer periods of drug exposure with gradually declining scalar scores and increasing remission rates for sertraline (Wagner et al. 2003) and paroxetine (Hollander et al. 2003) for up to 1 year.

Beyond these commonly used first-line pharmacological agents, there has been recent interest in agents targeting glutamatergic transmission (Chakrabarty et al. 2005), particularly NMDA receptors. NMDA receptors have a well-established role in the induction of long-term potenti-

TABLE 17–2. Dose range for serotonin reuptake inhibitors in children with obsessive-compulsive disorder

Drug	Starting dose, mg		Typical dose range, mg (mean dose)[a]
	Preadolescent	Adolescent	
Clomipramine[b,c]	6.25–25	25	50–200
Fluoxetine[c,d]	2.5–10	10–20	10–80 (25)
Sertraline[c,d]	12.5–25	25–50	50–200 (178)
Fluvoxamine[b,c]	12.5–25	25–50	50–300 (165)
Paroxetine[e]	2.5–10	10	10–60 (32)
Citalopram[d]	2.5–10	10–20	10–60

Note. [a]Mean daily doses used in controlled trials.
[b]Doses <25 mg/day may be administered by compounding 25 mg into 5 mL suspension.
[c]Approved by the U.S. Food and Drug Administration for obsessive-compulsive disorder in children and adolescents.
[d]Oral concentrate commercially available.
[e]Oral suspension commercially available.

TABLE 17–3. Effect size by drug in meta-analysis of pediatric obsessive-compulsive disorder trials

Drug	Standardized mean difference	95% confidence interval
Paroxetine	0.405	0.204–0.606
Fluoxetine	0.546	0.353–0.738
Fluvoxamine	0.375	0.167–0.584
Sertraline	0.327	0.160–0.493
Clomipramine	0.693	0.475–0.910

Source. Adapted from Geller et al. 2003b.

ation and have been implicated in the acquisition and retention of fear extinction (Morishita et al. 2001; Song and Huganir 2002). Because of the critical involvement of learning and memory mechanisms in OCD, additional research on such pharmacological agents is necessary in order to fully understand their possible utility (Davis and Myers 2002).

Riluzole, an anti-glutamatergic agent, is one such pharmacological intervention that has had success in reducing anxiety symptoms among adults with various anxiety disorders (Zarate and Manji 2008). Studies in child populations have had mixed results: a 12-week open-label study found substantial OCD symptom reduction in four out of six participants (ages 8–16; Grant et al. 2007), while a 12-week RCT of youth with treatment-resistant OCD (ages 7–17 years) failed to find a significant difference between riluzole and placebo (Grant et al. 2014). However, this finding may be a result of methodological limitations (e.g., sample characteristics, high rates of concomitant medications), so future studies should continue to explore the potential benefits of riluzole in child populations.

Comorbidities may influence the type of pharmacological treatment recommended. For OCD with Tourette's disorder, augmentation of SSRIs with clomipramine is an effective strategy, and often SSRIs or clomipramine are combined with either a typical or atypical antipsychotic agent (in all cases, QTc levels should be monitored) or with an α_2 agonist. Comorbid bipolar disorder, occurring in 5%–10% of OCD cases, is difficult to treat with medications, as SSRIs can exacerbate mood and behavioral changes associated with hypomania. It is recommended that clinicians focus pharmacological treatments toward mood episodes before OCD. Mood stabilizers or atypical antipsychotic agents may be effective at counteracting the activating effects of SSRIs. Furthermore, psychotic symptoms, which were found to occur in a small sample of OCD patients (Eisen and Rasmussen 1993), should be evaluated during treatment, as they can predict a poor response to medication. Finally, for patients exhibiting both OCD and ADHD, it is recommended that clinicians focus on the OCD treatment first, as stimulants can increase OCD symptoms and anxiety. Medications like clomipramine, atomoxetine, and bupropion should be considered. α-Agonist agents such as clonidine or guanfacine may be especially beneficial for treating hyperactivity and impulsivity symptoms in patients with comorbid ADHD.

Psychotherapeutic Treatments

Cognitive-Behavioral Therapy

The protocol used in the POTS (March et al. 2004) consists of 14 visits over 12 weeks spread across five phases: 1) psychoeducation, 2) cognitive training, 3) mapping OCD, 4) exposure and response prevention, and 5) relapse prevention and generalization training. Except for weeks 1 and 2, when patients come twice weekly, all visits are 1 hour per week. There is one between-visit, 10-minute telephone contact scheduled during each of weeks 3 through 12. Each session includes a statement of goals, review of the preceding week, provision of new information, therapist-assisted practice, homework for the coming week, and monitoring procedures.

The principle of *exposure and response prevention* (ERP), as illustrated in Figure 17–2, relies on the fact that anxiety usually attenuates after sufficient duration of contact with a feared stimulus. Repeated exposure is associated with decreased anxiety across exposure trials, with anxiety reduction largely specific to the domain of exposure, until the child no longer fears contact with specifically targeted phobic stimuli. Adequate exposure depends on blocking the negative reinforcement effect of rituals or avoidance behavior, a process termed *response prevention.* ERP is typically implemented gradually (sometimes termed *graded exposure*), with exposure targets under the patient's or, less desirably, the therapist's control (March et al. 2001).

In a recent meta-analysis of five RCTs of CBT in children (N=161) with OCD, Watson and Rees (2008) found a large mean pooled effect size of 1.45 (95% CI, 0.68–2.22). CBT studies have greater heterogeneity than pharmacotherapy trials. Although both treatments are significantly superior to control, CBT yields a larger treatment effect, consistent with treatment outcomes in adult OCD populations. These findings support the recommendations of the American Academy of Child and Adolescent Psychiatry (2012) practice parameters guidelines that CBT should be the first-line treatment for mild to moderate pediatric OCD, followed by pharmacotherapy.

Several variations in delivering CBT have been studied and reported, includ-

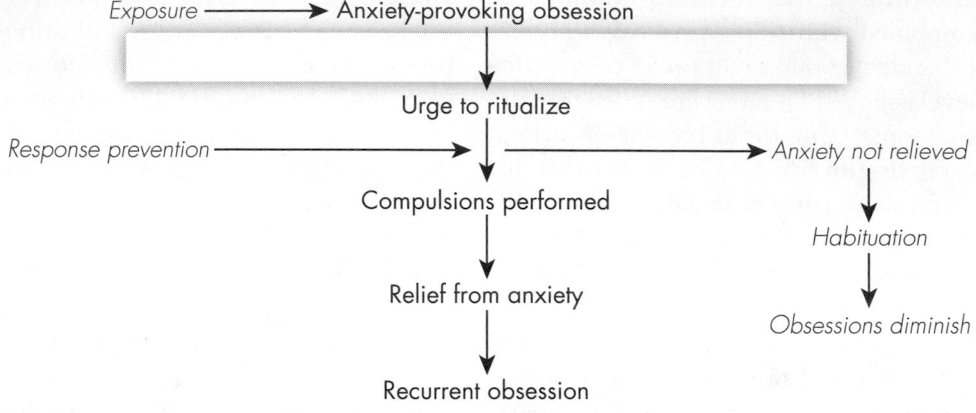

FIGURE 17–2. Theoretical basis of cognitive-behavioral treatment (exposure and response prevention).

ing those that use family-based approaches (Barrett et al. 2004; Storch et al. 2008), particularly with very young children whose parents still control most of the contingencies for their child's behavior. A recent multisite randomized controlled trial, POTS Jr. (Freeman et al. 2014), found family-based CBT superior to a control intervention (family-based relaxation treatment) in 127 children ages 5–8 years. Another variation that may be helpful is CBT delivered through group settings, where positive elements of both group therapy and CBT are combined (Thienemann et al. 2001). Intensive CBT approaches work well for children who subscribe in advance to this approach (Storch et al. 2007). Intensive approaches may be especially useful for treatment-resistant OCD or for patients who desire a very rapid response. Such treatment can now be found in several specialized intensive outpatient or residential treatment centers in the United States.

Recent research has explored two additional nonpharmacological methods of treatment for children with OCD. Acceptance and commitment therapy (ACT), like CBT, focuses on cognitive processes, but while CBT seeks to alter the content of maladaptive thoughts, ACT is concerned with the process and function of thoughts in specific contexts (Park and Geller 2014). Patients are encouraged to accept their thoughts as simply thoughts, rather than reality or truth, while avoiding specific experiences that run counter to this acceptance (Coyne et al. 2011). ACT has demonstrated empirical efficacy in adult trials (Forman et al. 2007), but there is some concern that the method is too complex and abstract for children and adolescents. A limited number of reports and case studies with various clinical pediatric populations have noted the successful application of ACT (Metzler et al. 2000), as well as other mindfulness-based therapies (Burke 2010), but there is a dearth of empirical research specifically examining ACT for pediatric OCD.

Another nonpharmacological treatment alternative is attention bias modification (ABM). Studies suggest that attention biases toward threat-related stimuli may contribute to the etiology and maintenance of anxiety disorders (Bar-Haim et al. 2011). Therefore, ABM aims to retrain these attention biases away from threat, thus potentially reducing the anxiety associated with those stimuli. ABM typically employs a computer-based dot probe task, in which a visual probe is repeatedly presented over neutral stimuli to implicitly retrain attention away from threatening stimuli (Pine 2007). ABM has demonstrated success in reducing the symptoms of children with various anxiety disorders (Bar-Haim et al. 2011; Eldar et al. 2012) and has also been an effective adjunct to CBT in adolescent populations (Shechner et al. 2014). No studies have specifically examined the application of ABM for pediatric OCD, but its success with other anxiety-related disorders has positive implications for its use with this population, particularly for youth who may be averse to standard CBT.

Combined Treatment

For greatest efficacy, the combination of CBT with medication is the treatment of choice. Recommendations from the POTS (March et al. 2004) were to start treatment with either CBT alone or CBT plus medication. The combined treatment showed the greatest decrease in symptom scores and the greatest remission rate, with an effect size that approximated the arithmetic sum of the component treatments (effect size combined=1.4, CBT=0.97, and sertraline=0.67). Fifty-four percent of children receiving combined treatment achieved a remission. This result was supported by a follow-up study (POTS II; Franklin et al. 2011). In this latter study, medication plus CBT "instruction" delivered as part of pharmacotherapy visits was not superior to medication alone, while protocol-driven systematic CBT plus medication improved outcome significantly. This supports the notion that rigorous expert CBT is the method of choice for nonpharmacological intervention. It is possible that medication enhances the effect of CBT by decreasing anxiety and improving a child's ability to tolerate ERP. Although sertraline was the medication used in the POTS, other investigators have reported similar combination treatment approaches with different drugs, including clomipramine (Foa et al. 2005) and fluvoxamine (Neziroglu et al. 2000), so it is reasonable to extrapolate the POTS findings to other medications that have independently shown efficacy for OCD in children. A meta-analysis of 18 studies found that combined treatment was the most efficacious in reducing OCD symptoms, reporting an effect size of 1.7 (Sánchez-Meca et al. 2014).

Augmentation Strategies

Medication augmentation strategies are reserved for treatment-resistant cases. By expert consensus, the term *treatment resistant* applied to children with OCD indicates a child who has *persistent* and *substantial* OCD symptoms in the face of *adequate* treatment known to be effective in childhood OCD. Persistent symptoms of at least moderate severity (e.g., CY-BOCS ≥16 or CGI-S of marked or severe impairment) are useful guidelines. At least two serotonin reuptake inhibitor trials are necessary to declare adequate medication therapy. Therefore, failure of adequate trials of at least two SSRIs, or one SSRI and one clomipramine trial, as well as a failure of adequately delivered CBT, would constitute treatment resistance. Children should have a minimum of 10 weeks of each SSRI or clomipramine at maximum recommended (or tolerated) doses, with no change in dose for the preceding 3 weeks. In terms of adequate CBT dose, if a child has not shown *any* improvement after 8–10 total sessions (or 5–6 sessions of exposure) or has substantial residual OC psychopathology after completing standard CBT treatment, the child may be considered a

CBT nonresponder. To summarize, failure of at least two monotherapies as well as combined treatment is required prior to considering the OCD to be treatment-resistant.

Adding clomipramine to an SSRI may be helpful. The rationale is to combine the serotonergic effects of each while minimizing adverse events across differing drug classes. Even low-dosage augmentation (25–75 mg/day) may be useful; however, electrocardiogram indices must be monitored when combining clomipramine with CYP450 2D6 (primary), or 3 A4 inhibitors such as fluoxetine, paroxetine, or fluvoxamine, as potentially toxic increases in clomipramine levels may occur. Clonazepam has also been used in combination with SSRIs in several small adult trials (e.g., Crockett et al. 2004). By far, the most common drug augmentation strategies have employed atypical antipsychotic agents. High-quality RCTs employing atypical antipsychotics have been done in adults with OCD (summarized by Bloch et al. [2006] in a comprehensive meta-analysis), but only case reports and open trials exist for children. However, expert consensus suggests that many children with treatment-resistant OCD will benefit from judicious augmentation with an atypical antipsychotic, particularly children with tic disorders, autism spectrum disorder symptoms, or mood instability. One open label augmentation trial for pediatric tic-related OCD found that risperidone and aripiprazole were effective augmentation strategies for children who did not respond to SSRI monotherapy (Masi et al. 2013). Augmentation with venlafaxine or duloxetine has also been found to be efficacious in adults (Dell'Osso et al. 2006). Finally, there are numerous novel augmentation strategies being tested, including stimulants, α agonists, and glutamatergic drugs like riluzole (Grant et al. 2014). None of these novel augmentation strategies yet meet minimal standards that permit recommendation for routine use, but they provide directions for future research.

In addition to purely pharmacological augmentation strategies, recent studies have focused on the augmentation of CBT, in particular ERP, with D-cycloserine (DCS). DCS, a partial glutamate agonist, has been found to enhance NMDA neurotransmission within the brain structures involved in fear extinction and learning. In adult trials, DCS has been found to improve the effects of treatment (Otto et al. 2010), as well as the overall speed of treatment effects. A pilot study investigating the augmentation of CBT for pediatric OCD with DCS found moderate to small effect sizes on the CY-BOCS (d=0.67 for the main effect for the group, d=0.31 for the group by time interaction) and a moderate effect size on the CGI-S (d=0.47) for patients treated with DCS compared with placebo. The average CY-BOCS reduction for the CBT plus DCS arm was 72% versus 58% for the CBT plus placebo arm, providing preliminary evidence that DCS may be an effective augmentation strategy for CBT in pediatric OCD (Storch et al. 2010). A NIMH-funded multisite study is currently being conducted to further explore the augmenting effects of DCS with ERP in 7- to 17-year-old children with OCD (E.A. Storch and D.A. Geller, principal investigators). DCS is a well-tolerated agent with few related adverse events, and its potential for providing rapid treatment gains warrants further research.

Putative PANDAS cases of OCD have also attracted novel and experimental treatment interventions. Antibiotic prophylaxis with penicillin failed to prevent streptococcal infections in one study

(Garvey et al. 1999) but was effective in a subsequent study: results showed a reduction in both infections and OCD symptoms in the year of prophylaxis compared with the previous baseline year (Snider et al. 2005). Data are not sufficient to meet minimal standards to recommend antibiotic prophylaxis for children with OCD, even when PANDAS is suspected. Instead, standard treatments for both OCD and streptococcal infections are recommended. Plasmapharesis and other immune-modulating therapies such as intravenous immunoglobulin (IVIG) remain experimental. A recently completed NIMH intramural trial of IVIG for children with putative PANDAS-associated OCD failed to show efficacy above sham IVIG (K. Williams, personal communication, March 2015).

Other Treatment Modalities

Insight-oriented psychotherapy has proven disappointing in children and adolescents with OCD. Nevertheless, sequelae of OC symptoms should be considered for further treatment, especially when OCD has been longstanding. Children with OCD who have experienced the following may benefit from supportive individual or family psychotherapy: 1) decreased function in some important domain of life (e.g., in school grades, ability to maintain friendships) and 2) loss of self-esteem or marked conflict at home that has disrupted primary relationships.

Non-CBT psychotherapeutic intervention may also be effective for comorbid psychopathology. Particular attention to social function is recommended because of the long-term outcome data suggesting that this domain is often compromised, even when affected children have successful educational outcomes. Collaborative engagement with clinicians such as CBT therapists, educational psychologists, and school personnel, as well as immediate, and at times extended, family, is essential for best outcomes.

Furthermore, there is preliminary evidence in adults for the efficacy of interventional psychiatric treatments, including deep brain stimulation (DBS; Rauch et al. 2006) and repetitive transcranial magnetic stimulation (Mantovani et al. 2006). For example, Greenberg et al. (2006) found significant long-term improvement in Y-BOCS scores for adults with OCD after DBS. More research is necessary for these treatment modalities, especially with regard to pediatric applications, prior to their recommended or widespread use.

Summary Points

- Obsessive-compulsive disorder (OCD) affects 1%–2% of children and adolescents and is frequently underdiagnosed and undertreated because of the hidden nature of its symptoms.
- Families often become entangled in their children's rituals.
- Most often, OCD in children is accompanied by comorbid psychopathology that has a significant impact on functioning and treatment outcome.
- Simple probes for the presence of anxiety, "worries," and rituals will identify most children with OCD.

- Gathering information from both parents and children is essential.
- Assessment should include a standardized quantitative or scalar measure of symptoms along with an inventory of "target" symptoms.
- CBT is the treatment of choice for mild to moderate childhood cases.
- Medications are reserved for cases of OCD that are more severe, have multiple comorbid conditions, are accompanied by poor insight, or are CBT resistant; medications are also recommended in situations where adequate CBT resources cannot be found.
- SSRIs are the first recommended medicines for OCD at any age.

References

Abramovitch A, Mittelman A, Henin A, et al: Neuroimaging and neuropsychological findings in pediatric obsessive-compulsive disorder: A review and developmental considerations. Neuropsychiatry 2(4):313–329, 2012

American Academy of Child and Adolescent Psychiatry: Practice parameter for the assessment and treatment of children and adolescents with obsessive-compulsive disorder. J Am Acad Child Adolesc Psychiatry 51(1):98–113, 2012 22176943

American Psychiatric Association: Diagnostic and Statistical Manual of Mental Disorders, 4th Edition. Washington, DC, American Psychiatric Association, 1994

American Psychiatric Association: Diagnostic and Statistical Manual of Mental Disorders, 4th Edition, Text Revision. Washington, DC, American Psychiatric Association, 2000

American Psychiatric Association: Diagnostic and Statistical Manual of Mental Disorders, 5th Edition. Arlington, VA, American Psychiatric Association, 2013

Apter A, Fallon TJ Jr, King RA, et al: Obsessive-compulsive characteristics: from symptoms to syndrome. J Am Acad Child Adolesc Psychiatry 35(7):907–912, 1996 8768350

Bar-Haim Y, Morag I, Glickman S: Training anxious children to disengage attention from threat: a randomized controlled trial. J Child Psychol Psychiatry 52(8):861–869, 2011 21250993

Barrett P, Healy Farrell L, March JS: Cognitive-behavioral family treatment of childhood obsessive-compulsive disorder: a controlled trial. J Am Acad Child Adolesc Psychiatry 43(1):46–62, 2004 14691360

Bloch MH, Peterson BS, Scahill L, et al: Adulthood outcome of tic and obsessive-compulsive symptom severity in children with Tourette syndrome. Arch Pediatr Adolesc Med 160(1):65–69, 2006 16389213

Burke CA: Mindfulness-based approaches with children and adolescents: a preliminary review of current research in an emergent field. J Child Fam Stud 19(2):133–144, 2010

Calvocoressi L, Mazure CM, Kasl SV, et al: Family accommodation of obsessive-compulsive symptoms: instrument development and assessment of family behavior. J Nerv Ment Dis 187(10):636–642, 1999 10535658

Chakrabarty K, Bhattacharyya S, Christopher R, et al: Glutamatergic dysfunction in OCD. Neuropsychopharmacology 30(9):1735–1740, 2005 15841109

Coyne LW, McHugh L, Martinez ER: Acceptance and commitment therapy (ACT): advances and applications with children, adolescents, and families. Child Adolesc Psychiatr Clin N Am 20(2):379–399, 2011 21440862

Crockett BA, Churchill E, Davidson JRT: A double-blind combination study of clonazepam with sertraline in obsessive-compulsive disorder. Ann Clin Psychiatry 16(3):127–132, 2004 15517844

Dalmau J, Gleichman AJ, Hughes EG, et al: Anti-NMDA-receptor encephalitis: case series and analysis of the effects of antibodies. Lancet Neurol 7(12):1091–1098, 2008 18851928

Davis M, Myers KM: The role of glutamate and gamma-aminobutyric acid in fear extinction: clinical implications for exposure therapy. Biol Psychiatry 52(10):998–1007, 2002 12437940

Dell'Osso B, Nestadt G, Allen A, et al: Serotonin-norepinephrine reuptake inhibitors in the treatment of obsessive-compulsive disorder: A critical review. J Clin Psychiatry 67(4):600–610, 2006 16669725

do Rosario-Campos MC, Leckman JF, Curi M, et al: A family study of early onset obsessive-compulsive disorder. Am J Med Genet B Neuropsychiatr Genet 136B(1):92–97, 2005 15892140

Eisen JL, Rasmussen SA: Obsessive compulsive disorder with psychotic features. J Clin Psychiatry 54(10):373–379, 1993 8262879

Eldar S, Apter A, Lotan D, et al: Attention bias modification treatment for pediatric anxiety disorders: a randomized controlled trial. Am J Psychiatry 169(2):213–220, 2012 22423353

Fitzgerald KD, Moore GJ, Paulson LA, et al: Proton spectroscopic imaging of the thalamus in treatment-naive pediatric obsessive-compulsive disorder. Biol Psychiatry 47(3):174–182, 2000 10682215

Flament MF, Whitaker A, Rapoport JL, et al: Obsessive compulsive disorder in adolescence: an epidemiological study. J Am Acad Child Adolesc Psychiatry 27(6):764–771, 1988 3264280

Foa EB, Liebowitz MR, Kozak MJ, et al: Randomized, placebo-controlled trial of exposure and ritual prevention, clomipramine, and their combination in the treatment of obsessive-compulsive disorder. Am J Psychiatry 162(1):151–161, 2005 15625214

Forman EM, Herbert JD, Moitra E, et al: A randomized controlled effectiveness trial of acceptance and commitment therapy and cognitive therapy for anxiety and depression. Behav Modif 31(6):772–799, 2007 17932235

Franklin ME, Sapyta J, Freeman JB, et al: Cognitive behavior therapy augmentation of pharmacotherapy in pediatric obsessive-compulsive disorder: the Pediatric OCD Treatment Study II (POTS II) randomized controlled trial. JAMA 306(11):1224–1232, 2011 21934055

Freeman J, Sapyta J, Garcia A, et al: Family based treatment of early childhood obsessive-compulsive disorder: the Pediatric Obsessive-Compulsive Disorder Treatment Study for Young Children (POTS Jr)—a randomized clinical trial. JAMA Psychiatry 71(6):689–698, 2014 24759852

Garvey MA, Perlmutter SJ, Allen AJ, et al: A pilot study of penicillin prophylaxis for neuropsychiatric exacerbations triggered by streptococcal infections. Biol Psychiatry 45(12):1564–1571, 1999 10376116

Geller DA, Biederman J, Jones J, et al: Is juvenile obsessive-compulsive disorder a developmental subtype of the disorder? A review of the pediatric literature? J Am Child Adolesc Psychiatry 37(4):420–427, 1998 9549963

Geller DA, Biederman J, Faraone S, et al: Developmental aspects of obsessive compulsive disorder: findings in children, adolescents, and adults. J Nerv Ment Dis 189(7):471–477, 2001a 11504325

Geller DA, Hoog SL, Heiligenstein JH, et al: Fluoxetine treatment for obsessive-compulsive disorder in children and adolescents: a placebo-controlled clinical trial. J Am Acad Child Adolesc Psychiatry 40(7):773–779, 2001b 11437015

Geller DA, Wagner KD, Emslie GJ, et al: Efficacy of paroxetine in pediatric OCD: results of a multi-center study. Poster presented at the New Clinical Drug Evaluation Unit Annual Meeting, Boca Raton, FL, June 2002

Geller DA, Biederman J, Stewart SE, et al: Impact of comorbidity on treatment response to paroxetine in pediatric obsessive-compulsive disorder: is the use of exclusion criteria empirically supported in randomized clinical trials? J Child Adolesc Psychopharmacol 13 (suppl 1):S19–S29, 2003a 12880497

Geller DA, Biederman J, Stewart SE, et al: Which SSRI? A meta-analysis of pharmacotherapy trials in pediatric obsessive-compulsive disorder. Am J Psychiatry 160(11):1919–1928, 2003b 14594734

Geller DA, Coffey B, Faraone S, et al: Does comorbid attention-deficit/hyperactivity disorder impact the clinical expression of pediatric obsessive-compulsive disorder? CNS Spectr 8(4):259–264, 2003c 12679741

Geller DA, Wieland N, Carey K, et al: Perinatal factors affecting expression of obsessive compulsive disorder in children and adolescents. J Child Adolesc Psychopharmacol 18(4):373–379, 2008 18759647

Giedd JN, Rapoport JL, Garvey MA, et al: MRI assessment of children with obsessive-compulsive disorder or tics associated with streptococcal infection. Am J Psychiatry 157(2):281–283, 2000 10671403

Grant P, Lougee L, Hirschtritt M, et al: An open-label trial of riluzole, a glutamate antagonist, in children with treatment-resistant obsessive-compulsive disorder. J Child Adolesc Psychopharmacol 17(6):761–767, 2007 18315448

Grant PJ, Joseph LA, Farmer CA, et al: 12-week, placebo-controlled trial of add-on riluzole in the treatment of childhood-onset obsessive-compulsive disorder. Neuropsychopharmacology 39(6):1453–1459, 2014 24356715

Greenberg BD, Malone DA, Friehs GM, et al: Three-year outcomes in deep brain stimulation for highly resistant obsessive-compulsive disorder. Neuropsychopharmacology 31(11):2384–2393, 2006 16855529

Heyman I, Fombonne E, Simmons H, et al: Prevalence of obsessive-compulsive disorder in the British nationwide survey of child mental health. Br J Psychiatry 179:324–329, 2001 11581112

Hollander E, Allen A, Steiner M, et al: Acute and long-term treatment and prevention of relapse of obsessive-compulsive disorder with paroxetine. J Clin Psychiatry 64(9):1113–1121, 2003 14628989

Hudziak JJ, Van Beijsterveldt CE, Althoff RR, et al: Genetic and environmental contributions to the Child Behavior Checklist Obsessive-Compulsive Scale: a cross-cultural twin study. Arch Gen Psychiatry 61(6):608–616, 2004 15184240

Jonnal AH, Gardner CO, Prescott CA, et al: Obsessive and compulsive symptoms in a general population sample of female twins. Am J Med Genet 96(6):791–796, 2000 11121183

Kalra SK, Swedo SE: Children with obsessive-compulsive disorder: are they just "little adults"? J Clin Invest 119(4):737–746, 2009 19339765

Kurlan R, Kaplan EL: The pediatric autoimmune neuropsychiatric disorders associated with streptococcal infection (PANDAS) etiology for tics and obsessive-compulsive symptoms: hypothesis or entity? Practical considerations for the clinician. Pediatrics 113(4):883–886, 2004 15060240

Kurlan R, Johnson D, Kaplan EL, et al: Streptococcal infection and exacerbations of childhood tics and obsessive-compulsive symptoms: a prospective blinded cohort study. Pediatrics 121(6):1188–1197, 2008 18519489

Lafleur DL, Petty C, Mancuso E, et al: Traumatic events and obsessive compulsive disorder in children and adolescents: is there a link? J Anxiety Disord 25(4):513–519, 2011 21295942

Leckman JF, Pauls DL, Zhang H, et al: Obsessive-compulsive symptom dimensions in affected sibling pairs diagnosed with Gilles de la Tourette syndrome. Am J Med Genet B Neuropsychiatr Genet 116B(1):60–68, 2003 12497616

Leckman J, King R, Gilbert D, et al: Streptococcal upper respiratory tract infections and exacerbations of tic and obsessive-compulsive symptoms: a prospective longitudinal study. J Am Acad Child Adolesc Psychiatry 50(2):108–118, 2011 21241948

Lensi P, Cassano GB, Correddu G, et al: Obsessive-compulsive disorder. Familial-developmental history, symptomatology, comorbidity and course with special reference to gender-related differences. Br J Psychiatry 169(1):101–107, 1996 8818377

Leonard HL, Goldberger EL, Rapoport JL, et al: Childhood rituals: normal development or obsessive-compulsive symptoms? J Am Acad Child Adolesc Psychiatry 29(1):17–23, 1990 2295573

Mantovani A, Lisanby SH, Pieraccini F, et al: Repetitive transcranial magnetic stimulation (rTMS) in the treatment of obsessive-compulsive disorder (OCD) and Tourette's syndrome (TS). Int J Neuropsychopharmacol 9(1):95–100, 2006 15982444

March JS, Mulle K: OCD in Children and Adolescents: A Cognitive-Behavioral Treatment Manual. New York, Guilford, 1998

March JS, Biederman J, Wolkow R, et al: Sertraline in children and adolescents with obsessive-compulsive disorder: a multicenter randomized controlled trial. JAMA 280(20):1752–1756, 1998 9842950

March JS, Franklin M, Nelson A, et al: Cognitive-behavioral psychotherapy for pediatric obsessive-compulsive disorder. J Clin Child Psychol 30(1):8–18, 2001 11294080

March JS, Foa EB, Gammon P, et al: Cognitive-behavior therapy, sertraline, and their combination for children and adolescents with obsessive-compulsive disorder: the Pediatric OCD Treatment Study (POTS) randomized controlled trial. JAMA 292(16):1969–1976, 2004 15507582

Masi G, Pfanner C, Brovedani P: Antipsychotic augmentation of selective serotonin reuptake inhibitors in resistant tic-related obsessive-compulsive disorder in children and adolescents: a naturalistic comparative study. J Psychiatr Res 47(8):1007–1012, 2013 23664673

Mataix-Cols D, Nakatani E, Micali N, et al: Structure of obsessive-compulsive symptoms in pediatric OCD. J Am Acad Child Adolesc Psychiatry 47(7):773–778, 2008 18344900

Mattheisen M, Samuels JF, Wang Y, et al: Genome-wide association study in obsessive-compulsive disorder: results from the OCGAS. Mol Psychiatry 13(May):1–8, 2014 24821223

Mell LK, Davis RL, Owens D: Association between streptococcal infection and obsessive-compulsive disorder, Tourette's syndrome, and tic disorder. Pediatrics 116(1):56–60, 2005 15995031

Metzler CW, Biglan A, Noell J, et al: A randomized controlled trial of a behavioral intervention to reduce high-risk sexual behavior among adolescents in STD clinics. Behav Ther 31(1):27–54, 2000

Morishita W, Connor JH, Xia H, et al: Regulation of synaptic strength by protein phosphatase 1. Neuron 32(6):1133–1148, 2001 11754843

Murphy TK, Storch EA, Turner A, et al: Maternal history of autoimmune disease in children presenting with tics and/or obsessive-compulsive disorder. J Neuroimmunol 229(1–2):243–247, 2010 20864184

Murphy TK, Patel PD, McGuire JF, et al: Characterization of the Pediatric Acute-Onset Neuropsychiatric Syndrome phenotype. J Child Adolesc Psychopharmacol 2014 Epub ahead of print

Nestadt G, Samuels J, Riddle M, et al: A family study of obsessive-compulsive disorder. Arch Gen Psychiatry 57(4):358–363, 2000 10768697

Neziroglu F, Yaryura-Tobias JA, Walz J, et al: The effect of fluvoxamine and behavior therapy on children and adolescents with obsessive-compulsive disorder. J Child Adolesc Psychopharmacol 10(4):295–306, 2000 11191690

Otto MW, Tolin DF, Simon NM, et al: Efficacy of d-cycloserine for enhancing response to cognitive-behavior therapy for panic disorder. Biol Psychiatry 67(4):365–370, 2010 19811776

Park JM, Geller DA: Novel approaches in treatment of pediatric anxiety. F1000Prime Rep 6:30, 2014 24860652

Pauls DL, Alsobrook JP 2nd, Goodman W, et al: A family study of obsessive-compulsive disorder. Am J Psychiatry 152(1):76–84, 1995 7802125

Pauls DL, Abramovitch A, Rauch SL, et al: Obsessive-compulsive disorder: an integrative genetic and neurobiological perspective. Nat Rev Neurosci 15(6):410–424, 2014 24840803

Piacentini J, Bergman RL, Keller M, et al: Functional impairment in children and adolescents with obsessive-compulsive disorder. J Child Adolesc Psychopharmacol 13(suppl 1):S61–S69, 2003 12880501

Pine DS: Research review: a neuroscience framework for pediatric anxiety disorders. J Child Psychol Psychiatry 48(7):631–648, 2007 17593144

Rauch SL, Dougherty DD, Malone D, et al: A functional neuroimaging investigation of deep brain stimulation in patients with obsessive-compulsive disorder. J Neurosurg 104(4):558–565, 2006 16619660

Rettew DC, Swedo SE, Leonard HL, et al: Obsessions and compulsions across time in 79 children and adolescents with obsessive-compulsive disorder. J Am Acad Child Adolesc Psychiatry 31(6):1050–1056, 1992 1429404

Riddle MA, Reeve EA, Yaryura-Tobias JA, et al: Fluvoxamine for children and adolescents with obsessive-compulsive disorder: a randomized, controlled, multicenter trial. J Am Acad Child Adolesc Psychiatry 40(2):222–229, 2001 11211371

Ruderfer DM, Fanous AH, Ripke S, et al: Polygenic dissection of diagnosis and clinical dimensions of bipolar disorder and schizophrenia. Mol Psychiatry 19(9):1017–1024, 2014 24280982

Sánchez-Meca J, Rosa-Alcázar AI, Iniesta-Sepúlveda M, et al: Differential efficacy of cognitive-behavioral therapy and pharmacological treatments for pediatric obsessive-compulsive disorder: a meta-analysis. J Anxiety Disord 28(1):31–44, 2014 24334214

Scahill L, Riddle MA, McSwiggin-Hardin M, et al: Children's Yale-Brown Obsessive Compulsive Scale: reliability and validity. J Am Acad Child Adolesc Psychiatry 36(6):844–852, 1997 9183141

Shechner T, Rimon-Chakir A, Britton JC, et al: Attention bias modification treatment augmenting effects on cognitive behavioral therapy in children with anxiety: randomized controlled trial. J Am Acad Child Adolesc Psychiatry 53(1):61–71, 2014 24342386

Shugart YY, Samuels J, Willour VL, et al: Genomewide linkage scan for obsessive-compulsive disorder: evidence for susceptibility loci on chromosomes 3q, 7p, 1q, 15q, and 6q. Mol Psychiatry 11(8):763–770, 2006 16755275

Snider LA, Lougee L, Slattery M, et al: Antibiotic prophylaxis with azithromycin or penicillin for childhood-onset neuropsychiatric disorders. Biol Psychiatry 57(7):788–792, 2005 15820236

Song I, Huganir RL: Regulation of AMPA receptors during synaptic plasticity. Trends Neurosci 25(11):578–588, 2002 12392933

Stewart SE, Geller DA, Jenike M, et al: Long-term outcome of pediatric obsessive-compulsive disorder: a meta-analysis and qualitative review of the literature. Acta Psychiatr Scand 110(1):4–13, 2004 15180774

Stewart SE, Rosario MC, Brown TA, et al: Principal components analysis of obsessive-compulsive disorder symptoms in children and adolescents. Biol Psychiatry 61(3):285–291, 2007 17161383

Stewart SE, Yu D, Scharf JM, et al: Genome-wide association study of obsessive-compulsive disorder. Mol Psychiatry 18(7):788–798, 2013 22889921

Storch EA, Geffken GR, Merlo LJ, et al: Family based cognitive-behavioral therapy for pediatric obsessive-compulsive disorder: comparison of intensive and weekly approaches. J Am Acad Child Adolesc Psychiatry 46(4):469–478, 2007 17420681

Storch EA, Merlo LJ, Larson MJ, et al: Clinical features associated with treatment-resistant pediatric obsessive-compulsive disorder. Compr Psychiatry 49(1):35–42, 2008 18063039

Storch EA, Murphy TK, Goodman WK, et al: A preliminary study of d-cycloserine augmentation of cognitive-behavioral therapy in pediatric obsessive-compulsive disorder. Biol Psychiatry 68(11):1073–1076, 2010 20817153

Swedo SE, Leonard HL, Mittleman BB, et al: Identification of children with pediatric autoimmune neuropsychiatric disorders associated with streptococcal infections by a marker associated with rheumatic fever. Am J Psychiatry 154(1):110–112, 1997 8988969

Thienemann M, Martin J, Cregger B, et al: Manual-driven group cognitive-behavioral therapy for adolescents with obsessive-compulsive disorder: a pilot study. J Am Acad Child Adolesc Psychiatry 40(11):1254–1260, 2001 11699798

van Grootheest DS, Cath DC, Beekman AT, et al: Twin studies on obsessive-compulsive disorder: a review. Twin Res Hum Genet 8(5):450–458, 2005 16212834

Wagner KD, Cook EH, Chung H, et al: Remission status after long-term sertraline treatment of pediatric obsessive-compulsive disorder. J Child Adolesc Psychopharmacol 13(suppl 1):S53–S60, 2003 12880500

Walitza S, Wendland JR, Gruenblatt E, et al: Genetics of early onset obsessive-compulsive disorder. Eur Child Adolesc Psychiatry 19(3):227–235, 2010 20213231

Watson HJ, Rees CS: Meta-analysis of randomized, controlled treatment trials for pediatric obsessive-compulsive disorder. J Child Psychol Psychiatry 49(5):489–498, 2008 18400058

Zarate CA, Manji HK: Riluzole in psychiatry: a systematic review of the literature. Expert Opin Drug Metab Toxicol 4(9):1223–1234, 2008 18721116

CHAPTER 18

Early Onset Schizophrenia

Ian Kodish, M.D., Ph.D.
Jon M. McClellan, M.D.

Schizophrenia, a neurodevelopmental disorder that most often manifests in late adolescence or early adulthood, causes significant disturbances in perception, emotion, executive cognitive function, and social relatedness. Early onset schizophrenia (EOS) is a less common form of the illness, defined as onset prior to age 18 years. Childhood-onset schizophrenia (COS) refers to the rare occurrences of onset before age 13 years. EOS is considered to be continuous with adult-onset schizophrenia (AOS), as both exhibit related clinical features and neurobiological abnormalities, yet youth incidence is further impacted by unique developmental and social challenges. In this chapter we provide a description of schizophrenia in children and adolescents, including its history, etiology, genetic contributions, and clinical presentation. Special emphasis will be placed on EOS and the neurodevelopmental impact of illness across the lifespan. Current research highlighting effective psychosocial and pharmacological interventions will then be reviewed, including clinical recommendations to help guide effective and comprehensive care for youth with schizophrenia and related disorders.

History

Accounts of psychotic symptoms and madness date back to antiquity. In the early 1900s, Emil Kraepelin described a form of psychotic illness in young adults as *dementia praecox* (dementia of the young), a neurodegenerative condition separate in character from episodic mania and from dementias observed in old age. Eugene Bleuler later coined the term *schizophrenia* to mean a splitting of psychic functioning, resulting in a loosening of associations, disturbances of affectivity, ambivalence, and autism. The clinical description also came to characterize psychotic symptoms most often seen in adulthood, while schizophrenia was rarely found in children.

Later, Bender, Kanner, and others focused on the neurodevelopmental context of EOS by highlighting developmental deficits across language, perception, and movement (Fish 1977). During this era, developmental lags characterized within the broader rubric of childhood schizophrenia included conditions now considered autism spectrum disorders (ASDs). In the 1970s, seminal research differentiated the developmental features of schizophrenia from those of autism (Kolvin 1971; Rutter 1972). Since that time, autism and schizophrenia have been classified as distinct entities. Research continues to support this distinction, as well as supporting the use of the same diagnostic criteria for schizophrenia in youth and adults, given similarities in symptoms, course of illness, neurobiological features, and outcome.

Epidemiology

In the general population, the estimated lifetime prevalence of schizophrenia ranges from approximately 0.3% to 0.7% (American Psychiatric Association 2013). Onset prior to age 13 is rare and then increases sharply during adolescence, with the peak onset between ages 15 and 25 years for men and ages 20 and 30 years for women. EOS tends to be diagnosed more often in males (McClellan et al. 2013). Population-based registries in Denmark suggest that the diagnosed incidence of EOS has increased over the last four decades, from 1.80 per 100,000 for youth during the period 1971–1993 to 5.15 per 100,000 for youth during the period 1994–2010 (Okkels et al. 2013). Over this time, the relative proportion of females diagnosed with EOS has also increased. It is not clear whether the increased rates are due to differences in diagnostic criteria, community practices, or true changes in the incidence of the disorder. The National Institute of Mental Health (NIMH) Childhood-onset Schizophrenia Study suggests that the incidence of COS is less than 0.04% (Driver et al. 2013). Although there are reported cases of schizophrenia in youth younger than 6 years of age, the diagnostic validity of the illness in preschoolers has not been established.

Neurodevelopment and Etiology

Schizophrenia appears to be characterized by extreme etiologic heterogeneity. Current evidence suggests that the development of schizophrenia is best explained by a neurodevelopmental model, whereby the illness stems from a multitude of genetic and environmental exposures that disrupt critical elements of brain development (Rapoport et al. 2012).

Genetic Factors

Family, twin, and adoption studies reveal a strong genetic component for schizophrenia. The lifetime risk of developing the illness is 5–20 times higher in first-degree relatives of affected probands compared with the general population. The rate of concordance among monozygotic twins is 40%–60%, whereas the rate of concordance in dizygotic twins and other siblings ranges from 5% to 15% (Cardno and Gottesman 2000).

The genetic architecture underlying schizophrenia remains mostly unknown. Much of the research examining genetic contributions to schizophrenia is based on the hypothesis that the illness stems from the collective effects of different genetic risk variants, each contributing only a small degree of risk. This *common-disease, common-variant* model posits that some combination of common risk variants and/or exposures to environmental risk factors ultimately leads to the illness. Some postulate that thousands of risk alleles, each conferring very small risk, are responsible for a substantial portion of the illness (International Schizophrenia Consortium et al. 2009).

Research based on the common-disease, common-variant model has identified scores of candidate genomic loci and candidate genes. Genomewide association studies, using large collaborative international cohorts, have published findings implicating different genomic regions and genes, including the major histocompatibility complex (6p21.1), the microRNA 137 (*MIR137*), and different genes involved with calcium signaling (Giusti-Rodríguez and Sullivan 2013). However, the search for common risk alleles in schizophrenia has been hampered by small and diminishing effect sizes, variable findings, lack of replication, and the difficulty in establishing definitive causality for any given candidate gene or haplotype (McClellan and King 2010). A targeted study of the 14 most promising candidate genes in 1,870 individuals with schizophrenia and 2,002 control subjects found no evidence of association for any of the previously reported risk alleles (Sanders et al. 2008). More generally, across all of medicine, putative common risk variants do not explain the vast majority of genetic liability for complex disease (Manolio et al. 2009).

There is now strong evidence supporting the role of rare deleterious genetic mutations, many de novo or recent in origin, for complex human diseases, including neuropsychiatric conditions such as schizophrenia (McClellan and King 2010). Persons with schizophrenia are significantly more likely than unaffected persons to harbor rare gene-disrupting genomic duplications and deletions, known as copy number variants (CNVs; Rapoport et al. 2012; Walsh et al. 2008). Individuals with EOS, particularly those with COS, appear to have an even greater risk of harboring one or more large deleterious CNVs. Genes affected by rare damaging CNVs in persons with schizophrenia function disproportionately in cellular signaling and neurodevelopmental processes, including neuregulin and glutamate pathways (Walsh et al. 2008). Most rare deleterious copy number mutations detected in affected persons are unique; others recur independently at genomic hotspots, including chromosomes 1q21.1, 3q29, 15q11.2, 15q13.3, 16p11.2, 16p12.1, 16p13.11, 17p12, and 22q11.2 (McClellan and King 2010). Persons with autism and intellectual disability are also more likely to have rare damaging CNVs, including many of the same recurrent hotspot mutations (McClellan and King 2010).

Given advanced sequencing technologies, it is now possible to efficiently detect smaller mutations genomewide. Recent findings demonstrate the importance of rare damaging point mutations and small insertions and deletions, either de novo or inherited, in schizophrenia (Fromer et al. 2014; Gulsuner et al. 2013; Purcell et al. 2014; Xu et al. 2011). Affected individuals harbor more damaging de novo mutations than their healthy siblings (Gulsuner et al. 2013). The genes disrupted by these events are highly co-expressed in fetal prefrontal cortex and operate in pathways critical to brain development, including neuronal migration and synaptic integrity. In a large case-control exome sequencing study (Purcell et al. 2014), persons with schizophrenia were more likely than control subjects to harbor a rare damaging mutation in genes regulating activity-dependent cytoskeleton-associated scaffolding and *N*-methyl-D-aspartate receptor postsynaptic signaling complexes in genes that are targets of the FMR1 protein and in genes previously implicated in studies of schizophrenia and autism. The same neurobiological processes were implicated in a related study of de novo mutations in schizophrenia (Fromer et al. 2014).

The importance of rare deleterious mutations for human disease reflects evolutionary forces that shape the human genome (Manolio et al. 2009). All humans carry dozens of de novo point mutations, small insertions and deletions, and larger CNVs. The rate of de novo mutations increases with paternal age (Kong et al. 2012), which helps explain the increased risk of schizophrenia and ASD with advancing age of fathers. The steady influx of new mutations can account for the persistence of complex neuropsychiatric disorders, despite their significant impact on reproductive fitness (McClellan and King 2010).

Schizophrenia appears to be characterized by vast genetic heterogeneity. To date, no single gene or genomic locus explains more than approximately 1% of schizophrenia. Instead, the illness appears to be caused by multiple different mutations in multiple different genes and genomic loci. Additionally, the same mutation (or different mutations in the same gene) may lead to different neuropsychiatric phenotypes in different individuals, including ASD, bipolar disorder, or intellectual disability. Potential contributions from somatic mutations, epigenetic mechanisms, gene-by-gene and/or gene-by-environment interactions, and environmental exposures further add to causal complexity. Given the vast number of genes and genomic regulatory mechanisms related to brain development, and the number of mutational mechanisms that can disrupt these processes, it is possible that most affected people have a unique genetic cause (McClellan and King 2010).

Environmental Factors

Numerous environmental exposures have been associated with increased incidence of schizophrenia (Brown 2011). Environmental exposures may mediate disease risk via a number of different mechanisms, including direct neurological damage, gene-environment interactions, epigenetic effects, and de novo mutations. Risk factors most commonly linked with schizophrenia include in utero exposure to famine, advanced paternal age, prenatal infection, obstetric complications, and marijuana use. The effects of these exposures on illness incidence may be impacted by prior susceptibility, including potentially heralding onset at an earlier age. Other social factors such as urban living, ethnic minority status, cultural migration, and lack of social support further increase the risk of schizophrenia and may operate through shared mechanisms that foster maladaptive reorganization of regulatory circuits (Meyer-Lindenberg and Tost 2012).

Neuroanatomical Abnormalities

Multiple neuroanatomical abnormalities have been reported in studies of adults with schizophrenia, including decreased total brain volumes and losses of gray matter in the anterior cingulate, frontal and temporal lobes, hippocampus, amygdala, thalamus, and insula (Shepherd et al. 2012). A key feature of schizophrenia appears to be brain dysconnectivity, that is, aberrant connections with and between different brain regions (Fitzsimmons et al. 2013). Although volumetric reductions are subtle and often vary across studies, alterations tend to be present by time of first diagnosis, regardless of age (Ganzola et al. 2014; Rapoport et al. 2012). Cortical thickness differences in prefrontal, temporal, and parietal regions further reveal gray matter loss in schizophrenia and related disorders (Narr et al. 2005), thought to be driven by dendritic reductions in synaptic connectivity (Glausier and Lewis 2013) with sparing of neuronal cell bodies (Selemon and Goldman-Rakic 1999).

Earlier onset of illness may be associated with greater neuroanatomical aberrations. The NIMH study measured volumetric changes across illness progression in youth with COS. Illness was associated with significant gray matter volumetric reductions and a more rapid progressive loss of gray matter over time, revealing a much greater rate of synaptic elimination across adolescence compared with controls (Rapoport et al. 2012). Synaptic density normally increases through early childhood until neurodevelopmental refinements begin to sculpt over-elaborated networks to allow for specialization and efficiency, resulting in synaptic elimination. Synaptic refinements proceed with regional and temporal specificity, generally in a caudal to frontal pattern, with increasing complexity to support increasingly integrative demands. The heightened rate of synaptic elimination in COS progresses in a similar orientation toward frontal regions (Gogtay et al. 2004b; Toga et al. 2006).

Adolescence is a critical period for sculpting neuronal networks to drive specialization of integrative networks that support higher cognitive functions and decision-making skills. In EOS, disruptions evident during this period of development may herald impairments in abstract thinking, working memory, emotion regulation, or empathic responses. The accelerated reduction in cortical gray matter was observed in medication-naive patients and appears to be specific to COS, as the findings were not noted in adolescents with transient psychosis (Gogtay et al. 2004a) or in studies of adults (Greenstein et al. 2006; Narr et al. 2005). Interestingly, localized increases in cortical thickness in COS patients were associated with symptom remission following hospitalization and antipsychotic treatment (Greenstein et al. 2008; Mattai et al. 2010).

There is some variation in findings across studies. Other COS cohorts exhibit volumetric reductions in anterior cingulate (Marquardt et al. 2005), hippocampus (Mattai et al. 2011), and fornix (Kendi et al. 2008). Yet COS was also correlated with volumetric increases in the superior temporal gyrus (Taylor et al. 2005), a language processing center, as well as increased caudate volume (Juuhl-Langseth et al. 2012), suggesting that neuronal changes in COS may be neither uniformly atrophic nor limited to cortical regions. In adults, volumetric reductions have been associated with either more severe (Gur et al. 2000) or less severe (Gur et al. 1998; Vidal et al. 2006) symptoms. Further, some unaffected siblings show similar brain alterations, and increased rates of frontal cortical thinning were not found to be associated with cognitive impairments (Gochman et al. 2005). Cumulative antipsychotic treatment may also play a role in cortical reduction (Fusar-Poli et al. 2013).

Follow-up studies show that the accelerated rate of cortical thinning in COS appears to plateau in early adulthood, with findings more consistent with those reported in adult-onset patients (Greenstein et al. 2006). A study of youth with EOS revealed a plateau effect of illness across adolescence, as cortical thickness did not exhibit the neurodevelopmental refinements of healthy teenagers (Thormodsen et al. 2013). The normative trajectory of early synaptic overproduction and subsequent elimination is thus altered in schizophrenia, suggesting that developmental impairments in anatomical plasticity and specialization likely contribute to clinical onset.

In addition to synaptic abnormalities, white matter impairments have also been implicated in schizophrenia, suggesting deficits in multiple domains of network connectivity (see Fitzsimmons et al. 2013). A longitudinal study of COS revealed progression of white matter deficits in a rostro-caudal pattern, again paralleling the growth trajectory of maturation in healthy adolescents (Gogtay et al. 2008). Alterations found in EOS impact the neurodevelopmental regulation of multiple aspects of anatomic plasticity, including synaptic elaboration and network connectivity, likely contributing to impairments during critical stages of cognitive maturation.

Clinical Presentation

Patients with schizophrenia face tremendous challenges, including shorter lifespan and reduced access to appropriate health care. Accurate diagnosis and early effective intervention are imperative (McClellan et al. 2013). EOS is diagnosed using the same criteria as for adults (Box 18–1). Misdiagnosis in youth is common, particularly at initial onset. Psychotic symptoms are the hallmark feature of schizophrenia, characterized by severe disruption in thought and reality testing, and are generally divided into two broad clusters. Positive symptoms include hallucinations, delusions, and disorganized thought. Negative symptoms include affective flattening, alogia, avolition, and anhedonia. Among youth with a variety of psychotic illnesses, negative symptoms appear to be the most specifically associated with EOS. Hallucinations, disordered thought, and affective flattening are also common in EOS, whereas complex delusions and catatonia occur less frequently. Evaluation of disordered thinking in EOS further demands an appreciation of developmental context and contributing language or communication deficits but is generally characterized by loose associations and illogical thinking (Caplan et al. 1989).

Box 18–1. DSM-5 Diagnostic Criteria for Schizophrenia

295.90 (F20.9)

A. Two (or more) of the following, each present for a significant portion of time during a 1-month period (or less if successfully treated). At least one of these must be (1), (2), or (3):
   1. Delusions.
   2. Hallucinations.
   3. Disorganized speech (e.g., frequent derailment or incoherence).
   4. Grossly disorganized or catatonic behavior.
   5. Negative symptoms (i.e., diminished emotional expression or avolition).

B. For a significant portion of the time since the onset of the disturbance, level of functioning in one or more major areas, such as work, interpersonal relations, or self-care, is markedly below the level achieved prior to the onset (or when the onset is in childhood or adolescence, there is failure to achieve expected level of interpersonal, academic, or occupational functioning).

C. Continuous signs of the disturbance persist for at least 6 months. This 6-month period must include at least 1 month of symptoms (or less if successfully treated) that meet Criterion A (i.e., active-phase symptoms) and may include periods of prodromal or residual symptoms. During these prodromal or residual periods, the signs of the disturbance may be manifested by only negative symptoms or by two or more symptoms listed in Criterion A present in an attenuated form (e.g., odd beliefs, unusual perceptual experiences).

D. Schizoaffective disorder and depressive or bipolar disorder with psychotic features have been ruled out because either 1) no major depressive or manic episodes have occurred concurrently with the active-phase symptoms, or 2) if mood episodes have occurred during active-phase symptoms, they have been present for a minority of the total duration of the active and residual periods of the illness.

E. The disturbance is not attributable to the physiological effects of a substance (e.g., a drug of abuse, a medication) or another medical condition.

F. If there is a history of autism spectrum disorder or a communication disorder of childhood onset, the additional diagnosis of schizophrenia is made only if prominent delusions or hallucinations, in addition to the other required symptoms of schizophrenia, are also present for at least 1 month (or less if successfully treated).

Specify if:

The following course specifiers are only to be used after a 1-year duration of the disorder and if they are not in contradiction to the diagnostic course criteria.

First episode, currently in acute episode: First manifestation of the disorder meeting the defining diagnostic symptom and time criteria. An *acute episode* is a time period in which the symptom criteria are fulfilled.

First episode, currently in partial remission: *Partial remission* is a period of time during which an improvement after a previous episode is maintained and in which the defining criteria of the disorder are only partially fulfilled.

First episode, currently in full remission: *Full remission* is a period of time after a previous episode during which no disorder-specific symptoms are present.

Multiple episodes, currently in acute episode: Multiple episodes may be determined after a minimum of two episodes (i.e., after a first episode, a remission and a minimum of one relapse).

Multiple episodes, currently in partial remission

Multiple episodes, currently in full remission

Continuous: Symptoms fulfilling the diagnostic symptom criteria of the disorder are remaining for the majority of the illness course, with subthreshold symptom periods being very brief relative to the overall course.

Unspecified

Specify if:

With catatonia (refer to the criteria for catatonia associated with another mental disorder, [DSM-5] pp. 119–120, for definition).

Coding note: Use additional code 293.89 (F06.1) catatonia associated with schizophrenia to indicate the presence of the comorbid catatonia.

Specify current severity:

Severity is rated by a quantitative assessment of the primary symptoms of psychosis, including delusions, hallucinations, disorganized speech, abnormal psychomotor behavior, and negative symptoms. Each of these symptoms may be rated for its current severity (most severe in the last 7 days) on a 5-point scale ranging from 0 (not present) to 4 (present and severe). (See Clinician-Rated Dimensions of Psychosis Symptom Severity in the chapter "Assessment Measures.")

Note: Diagnosis of schizophrenia can be made without using this severity specifier.

Source. Reprinted from the *Diagnostic and Statistical Manual of Mental Disorders,* 5th Edition. Arlington, VA, American Psychiatric Association, 2013. Used with permission.

Clinical expertise, comprehensive assessment, and rigorous application of diagnostic criteria improve accuracy of diagnosis (McClellan et al. 2013). In DSM-5 (American Psychiatric Association 2013), the diagnosis of schizophrenia requires that one of three cardinal psychotic symptoms—hallucinations, delusions, or disorganized speech—be present. In DSM-5, the subtypes of schizophrenia were eliminated because of their lack of predictive stability and clinical utility (American Psychiatric Association 1994; Tandon et al. 2013). Instead, specifiers are used to describe impairments that further characterize illness severity and course when lasting for longer than a year.

In both youth and adults, schizophrenia is characterized by four phases: prodromal, acute, recovery, and residual (McClellan et al. 2013). Patients typically progress through the last three phases once the illness is established. Individuals are often first assessed during an active acute phase of disease, which is commonly characterized by significant positive symptoms. During this phase, patients may be grossly disorganized, confused, and potentially dangerous to themselves or others. Recovery from the active phase marks a shift to a predominance of negative symptoms. The time to recovery generally takes 1–6 months or longer, depending on response to treatment. In youth, recovery is often incomplete. Longer duration of untreated psychosis and greater severity of negative symptoms at the time of diagnosis predict greater functional impairment over time (Clarke et al. 2006). Individuals who recover from an acute phase generally have persistent functional deficits, residual disordered thinking, and negative symptoms. Most youth with EOS demonstrate some degree of chronic impairment.

Prior to the onset of positive symptoms, individuals generally experience a decline in function that presages the illness. Abnormalities during this prodromal period include social isolation, academic difficulties, odd or idiosyncratic preoccupations, and mood symptoms. This phase can last from days to weeks or follow a more chronic course of years. COS tends to have a more chronic onset with signs in early childhood, while the presentation in adolescence can have either an acute or a more insidious onset (McClellan et al. 2013).

In addition, the majority of youth with EOS have histories of premorbid problems, including cognitive delays, learning problems, behavioral difficulties or oddities, and social withdrawal (McClellan et al. 2013). Approximately 10%–20% of individuals with EOS have intellectual deficits, with impairments ranging from mild to severe. Commonly co-occurring and/or premorbid psychiatric disorders include attention-deficit/hyperactivity disorder, disruptive behavior disorders, and anxiety and mood disorders, in addition to substance use disorders in adolescents (Frazier et al. 2007). Although effective treatment for psychosis may lead to improvement in these domains, treatment planning needs to account for these conditions.

Suicide is a major cause of death among individuals with schizophrenia. At least 5%–13% of affected individuals complete suicide (Pompili et al. 2007). Risk factors include male gender, history of prior suicide attempts, depression, substance abuse, hopelessness, social isolation, and concurrent stressors. Regular assessment and monitoring for suicidal ideation and for associated risk factors are important elements of clinical care.

Differential Diagnosis: Other Psychotic Syndromes

Given the symptomatic heterogeneity of schizophrenia and complexities in accurately diagnosing youth, it is important to recognize other conditions that manifest with overlapping presentations (McClellan et al. 2013). Table 18–1 lists the differential diagnoses of EOS that should be considered when evaluating possible psychosis, some of which require urgent management. Appropriate diagnostic evaluation (Table 18–2) requires strategies to evaluate for comorbid and confounding medical and psychiatric disorders, including detailed symptom phenomenology, prodromal symptoms, family history, and social stressors.

Medical Conditions

Numerous medical conditions can result in symptoms of psychosis. Recognition and correction of these conditions can often result in the remission of psychotic symptoms and may prevent life-threatening illness (see Table 18–1). Psychosis caused by an underlying medical condition is often associated with delirium, characterized by intermittent disturbances in consciousness and autonomic regulation, resulting in significantly increased morbidity and mortality. Delirium may result from numerous medical etiologies. Treatment calls for urgent medical and neurological evaluation to determine underlying causes, especially in cases with acute onset or rapid progression of symptoms. Delirium also shares many features of neuroleptic malignant syndrome and malignant catatonia, also concerns in EOS populations, but each calls for different management. Agitation or cognitive abnormalities from delirium may call for judicious psychopharmacological treatment with antipsychotic medication until the underlying cause can be addressed and should include frequent assessments given the waxing and waning nature of the disease process (DeMaso et al. 2009).

TABLE 18–1. Differential diagnosis of early onset schizophrenia

Psychiatric disorder
Psychotic disorder due to another medical condition
Bipolar disorder
Unipolar major depression with psychotic features
Schizoaffective disorder
Posttraumatic stress disorder
Obsessive-compulsive disorder
Autism spectrum disorder
Nonpsychotic emotional and behavioral disorders
Psychosocial factors
Abuse or neglect
Traumatic stress
Secondary gain for symptom reporting
Medical condition
Substance intoxication, overdose
Delirium
Brain neoplasm
Autoimmune encephalitis
Head injury
Seizure disorder
Meningitis
Porphyria
Wilson's disease
Cerebrovascular accident
AIDS
Electrolyte or fluid abnormalities
Blood glucose abnormalities
Endocrine abnormalities

TABLE 18–2. Components of a diagnostic evaluation for patients with psychotic symptoms

A comprehensive psychiatric history focusing on the longitudinal characterization of the patient's current and past symptoms; information from multiple sources is helpful to improve accuracy
A comprehensive psychosocial history including academic and interpersonal functioning, in utero exposures, familial psychiatric history, past exposure to trauma or neglect, and current familial strengths
A comprehensive physical examination to rule out nonpsychiatric medical conditions as a cause of psychotic symptoms
Laboratory evaluations and neuroimaging as clinically indicated
Standardized rating scales and, if warranted, neuropsychological testing to assess for learning and developmental disability and offer insights into academic supports

Intoxication

Psychosis can result from a wide range of intoxicants, in addition to several prescription agents. These include corticosteroids, anesthetics and inhalants, anticholinergics, antihistamines, amphetamines, and dextromethorphan. Patients should be warned of potential risks and encouraged to seek care for identification and elimination of the offending agent. Poison control should be contacted in cases of greater concern such as overdose or severe symptoms. Symptomatic management may also include temporary use of psychopharmacological approaches, with heightened concern for potential toxicity.

Experimentation with mind-altering substances can be particularly risky in youth. Drugs of abuse that frequently result in psychosis include dextromethorphan, lysergic acid diethylamide (LSD), mushrooms, psilocybin, peyote, cannabis, stimulants, salvia, and inhalants. Newer synthetic agents have also been recognized to cause brief psychotic states, and individuals may respond to similar agents in idiosyncratic ways. Some intoxicants cannot be detected by current blood assays or can be quickly metabolized, making detection difficult.

More concerning clinically, drugs such as methamphetamine, methylenedioxyamphetamine (MDA), and dextromethorphan may result in lasting neurocognitive impairment. Chronic psychotic states produced by these substances can be similar in character to schizophrenia, with persistent severe impairments in functioning, and may respond to similar treatment approaches. It is unclear whether these prolonged episodes represent independent drug effects or an environmental stimulus for the expression of schizophrenia in a vulnerable individual.

Schizoaffective Disorder

Although schizoaffective disorder is defined in youth by the same criteria as in adults, early onset schizoaffective disorder has not been well characterized, and the reliability of diagnosis in clinical settings is poor. Diagnosis requires the presence of psychotic symptoms in addition to prominent mood episodes meeting full criteria for mania or depression. DSM-5 diagnosis further requires that these episodes be present for the majority of the total duration of the active and residual portions of the illness. On the basis of previous diagnostic criteria, youth with schizoaffective disorder exhibited similar severe impairments to those with schizophrenia in addition to concurrent severe mood disturbances (Frazier et al. 2007).

Affective Psychosis

Psychotic episodes caused by mood disorders (especially bipolar disorders; see Chapter 14, "Bipolar Disorder") can manifest with a variety of affective and psychotic symptoms. In children and adolescents with schizophrenia, negative symptoms may be mistaken for depression, especially since it is common for patients to experience dysphoria with their illness. Alternatively, mania in teenagers often manifests with florid psychosis, including hallucinations, delusions, and thought disorder. Psychotic depression may manifest with mood congruent or incongruent psychotic features, including hallucinations or delusions, and represents a severe form of illness. The overlap in symptoms increases the likelihood of misdiagnosis at the time of schizophrenia onset. Longitudinal reassessment is needed to ensure accuracy of diagnosis. Family psychiatric history may also be a helpful differentiating factor.

Differentiating True Psychotic Symptoms From Other Phenomena

Many children may report symptoms of hallucinations and delusions, yet most children reporting such symptoms do not have a true psychotic disorder (Garralda 1984; Hlastala and McClellan 2005). The assessment of psychosis in youth requires an appreciation of their developmental context, including cognitive and affective functioning. Active imaginations are often healthy and important in early development, particularly in preadolescent children or individuals with developmental delay. Gauging whether hallucinations or unrealistic beliefs represent true psychotic phenomena can be difficult. The accuracy of diagnosis is enhanced when mental status evaluations and historical patterns of symptom presentation are incorporated into the diagnostic formulation (e.g., direct observations of disorganized thought and bizarre behavior).

Experiential effects of trauma, neglect, or externalizing behavior also contribute to reporting experiences of psychotic-like phenomena. Youth with conduct disorder or emotional disorders, including posttraumatic stress disorder (PTSD), reported more of these atypical psychotic symptoms (Hlastala and McClellan 2005). Instead of thought disorder, symptoms may represent hypervigilance or styles of cognitive coping that often affect perceptual fidelity, particularly during times of heightened emotional demands. This is reflected in refinements to the diagnosis of PTSD in DSM-5, which now incorporates hallucinations into reexperiencing symptoms of PTSD without the need for additional classification as a psychotic disorder.

Behaviorally, children with PTSD are found to exhibit more restricted or repetitive play, while youth with obsessive-compulsive disorder may exhibit private, and sometimes bizarre, compulsive behaviors as a result of anxious distress. Alternatively, the report of psychotic-like symptoms can be behaviorally reinforced, as it often elicits increased emotional support, so a functional appreciation of familial response to symptoms is also important.

Clinically, differentiation is best determined by the presence or absence of disorganized thought and behavior, the qualitative nature of the symptom report, the context within which symptoms are reported, the association with sleep phase transitions, and the pattern of symptom progression (Hlastala and McClellan 2005).

Autism Spectrum Disorders

ASDs can be distinguished from EOS by the absence or transitory nature of psychotic symptoms and by the characteristic predominance of abnormal communication and social relatedness with repetitive behavioral repertoires. An earlier age at onset is also typical of ASD. Premorbid abnormalities in individuals with EOS tend to be less pervasive and less severe than in those with autism. DSM-5 refinements to ASD diagnosis highlight its dimensional nature, clustering former classifications of pervasive developmental disorder and Asperger's disorder into a broader framework of ASD with an emphasis on degree of impairment. Higher-functioning children with ASD may lack the marked language disturbances seen in other forms of ASD but present with deficits in contextual communication (particularly social cues) and a restricted (and often unusual) range of interests. Similarly, youth with schizophrenia also often have premorbid histories characterized by social oddities and aloofness, some of whom initially receive a diagnosis of ASD. This may reflect common neurodevelopmental processes (de Lacy and King 2013). The lack of overt hallucinations and delusions distinguishes ASD from schizophrenia. Transient symptoms of psychosis in patients with ASD (lasting less than a month) do not meet criteria for schizophrenia, although such symptoms do warrant ongoing monitoring.

Psychosocial Factors

Psychological or social factors, by themselves, do not appear to cause schizophrenia. However, psychosocial factors are thought to interact with neurobiological factors to mediate the timing of onset, course, and severity of the disorder. Parenting factors and other relationships have been shown to influence the course of illness, both positively and negatively. Unfortunately, in the past, families of individuals with schizophrenia were unfairly blamed for causing psychosis in their children. Family support is essential for nurturing the development of effective communication and emotion regulation in all youth, particularly those at risk for EOS.

Family Influence

Family interaction styles can influence the course and morbidity of schizophrenia and are also potentially amenable to treatment (Pharoah et al. 2010). Criticism, emotional overinvolvement, and hostility in families (known as high expressed emotion) have been associated with worse outcomes in adults with schizophrenia and are strong predictors of future symptom severity (Butzlaff and Hooley 1998). In contrast, positive remarks from caregivers are associated with decreased negative symptoms and improved social functioning in adolescents and young adults (O'Brien et al. 2006). Higher adult scores on warmth scales are also associated with decreased relapse and improved social functioning (Breitborde et al. 2007).

Rather than simply being a causal factor, high expressed emotion may partially be a response of caregivers to a family member severely affected by emotional and behavioral difficulties. Culture also appears to mediate the effect of high expressed emotion; in African American families, high expressed emotion was not found to be a predictor of relapse. Instead, high levels of critical and intrusive family behavior were associated with improved outcome in adults with schizophrenia over a 2-year follow-up period (Rosenfarb et al. 2006).

Interestingly, a study of Mexican American families found a curvilinear association between emotional overinvolvement and relapse (Breitborde et al. 2007). In this study, midlevel emotional overinvolvement and high-level warmth were associated with improved outcome, possibly reflective of the importance of family involvement tempered with a respect for independence. Although these associations may not be present in all families with schizophrenia, focusing on the familial environment may enhance insight into ways to foster healthy individuation in at-risk youth while also nurturing meaningful interpersonal connections (López et al. 2004).

Peer Relationships

During childhood and adolescence, success in relationships with peers of similar age is a core developmental goal. During normal development, children transition from more family-centered to peer-centered relationships. However, youth with schizophrenia are especially vulnerable to difficulties managing interpersonal relationships. In assessing recent onset schizophrenia, functional deficits are associated with experiential deprivation and lack of empowerment (Horan et al. 2005). Even prior to the onset of the illness, most affected youth experience a prodromal period characterized by relationship difficulties and withdrawal (Cannon et al. 2001). Greater deficits in peer relations and social relatedness predict a poorer outcome, highlighting the importance of early intervention strategies aimed at social functioning. Families should be encouraged to foster supportive opportunities for consistent and meaningful relationships, emphasizing structured activities within a network of family, peers, and the wider community. Conversely, problems such as escalating peer conflicts, disinterest in socialization, neglect of hygiene, or strong preference for fantasy over interpersonal relatedness may be signs of emerging psychosis and should lower the threshold for seeking clinical intervention.

Cultural and Diversity Issues

Cultural factors can greatly influence the assessment and treatment of psychiatric symptoms. Prevalence rates of schizophrenia are relatively similar across cultures when using narrow definitions of the disorder but vary more widely with broad definitions (Brown 2011). This may relate either to different environmental influences on symptom presentation or to differences across cultures in how potential symptoms are characterized. One environmental factor that does appear to influence the prevalence of schizophrenia is migration status. First- and second-generation immigrants show an increased risk of schizophrenia (Cantor-Graae and Selten 2005). Living in urban settings is also associated with increased risk for schizophrenia (Brown 2011).

Societal beliefs must also be considered in the interpretation of psychotic symptoms. Even within cultures, norms may vary considerably, as social and religious values highly influence the way events are interpreted and experiences are reported. Differentiating a psychotic thought process from a culturally or religiously reinforced belief can be a challenge, and symptoms should also be examined more broadly by evaluating multiple domains of functioning. Psychosis is characterized by dramatic shifts in thought processes and behavior. Clinical judgment is required to distinguish delusional thinking from unusual strongly held personal beliefs. In some situations, a cultural consultation may be helpful toward better understanding the context of unfamiliar belief systems.

In addition, cultural factors often highly influence attitudes toward treatment, creating significant treatment challenges. Many cultures have negative views of mental illness that contribute to denial of symptoms, reluctance to seek treatment, and nonadherence with recommended care. Maintaining cultural sensitivity and destigmatizing mental illness can be essential components for engaging patients and their families in effective treatments.

Treatment

Treatment of EOS requires a comprehensive and integrated approach, combining medication with psychosocial interventions. Developmentally appropriate interventions that focus on cognitive, behavioral, and social functioning to reduce symptomatic impairments and improve quality of life are needed. The management of EOS mirrors that of affected adults, with special emphasis on developmental concerns and familial factors.

Controlled trials have established the short-term effectiveness of antipsychotics for the treatment of adults with schizophrenia, with improvements in overall functioning, psychotic symptoms, and likelihood for relapse (Lehman et al. 2004). Despite widespread assumptions to the contrary, comparative trials have indicated that the newer atypical (second-generation) agents do not appear to be superior to traditional neuroleptics (first-generation agents) in regard to long-term response or side effect profiles in either adults or youth with EOS (Jones et al. 2006; Lieberman et al. 2005, Sikich et al. 2008). Furthermore, many affected individuals are unable to continue with the same agent for the long term, highlighting the impact of side effects and noncompliance, as well as the clinical importance of longitudinal assessment and adjusting treatment strategies.

Medication treatment guidelines for EOS are increasingly supported by randomized placebo-controlled trials. However, trials comparing the efficacy and safety of different agents are limited, and clinical practice is often guided by findings from adult populations. Short-term controlled trials in EOS support the efficacy of traditional agents (e.g., haloperidol, loxapine, thioridazine, thiothixene), as well as several second-generation antipsychotics (for a review, see McClellan et al. 2013). Risperidone, olanzapine, paliperidone, quetiapine, and aripiprazole are currently approved by the U.S. Food and Drug Administration (FDA) for the treatment of adolescents 13 years and older with schizophrenia. To be most clinically effective, these agents should be used in conjunction with psychotherapeutic interventions.

Comparative studies are also limited but have revealed mild differences in the efficacy and safety profile of various antipsychotic agents. The largest comparative randomized controlled trial of EOS spectrum disorders compared olanzapine, risperidone, and molindone over 8 weeks and found no significant differences between groups in response rate or degree of symptom improvement

(Sikich et al. 2008). For more detail on antipsychotic agents, see Chapter 38, "Antipsychotic Medications."

Clinical determination of which agent to choose is based on FDA approval status, side effect profile, patient and family preferences, past treatment responses, compliance concerns, and cost. Procedures for the use and monitoring of medications in EOS are available to help guide clinical practice (McClellan et al. 2013). Individual responses vary among agents. If a treatment response is insufficient after approximately 4–6 weeks at an adequate dosage, use of an alternative antipsychotic agent is indicated. Risks of weight gain and metabolic effects with olanzapine raise caution regarding its use as a first-line agent in youth. Clozapine is the only antipsychotic agent with established superiority for schizophrenia, in both EOS and AOS populations, and should be considered for refractory cases. Given the significant risk profile of clozapine, intensive monitoring protocols are required.

Antipsychotic treatment of youth with EOS requires medical monitoring and careful assessment of potential side effects. Extrapyramidal symptoms, including dystonia, akathisia, tardive dyskinesia, and neuroleptic malignant syndrome, may occur with traditional or atypical agents and require periodic assessment throughout treatment. It is also important to regularly monitor weight gain and metabolic functions. Youth appear to be particularly prone to the metabolic side effects of atypical antipsychotics, contributing to long-term risks of hyperlipidemia and diabetes (Correll et al. 2009). Patients and their families should therefore be advised of the importance of a healthy lifestyle, including sleep hygiene, healthy diet, and routine exercise. If weight increases significantly or signs of metabolic syndrome are emerging (obesity, hypertension, dyslipidemia, insulin resistance), a different antipsychotic agent with lower metabolic risk may be tried, or, alternatively, an agent that targets metabolic derangements (e.g., metformin) may be added.

Clinical consensus further suggests that children and adolescents will most likely benefit from comprehensive intervention strategies that focus on behavioral and family functioning in addition to efforts at enhancing medication and treatment compliance. Evidence supporting psychosocial interventions for the treatment of schizophrenia is primarily based on adult studies, which show benefits from psychoeducational strategies, family interventions, skills training, and relapse prevention (Patterson and Leeuwenkamp 2008). Cognitive-behavioral interventions focusing on identifying and addressing deficits in thought processes have shown lasting effects in symptom management, in addition to medication compliance (Pilling et al. 2002). Assertive community intervention strategies show improvement in rates of hospitalization, housing stability, and relapse (Lehman 1998). Skills training has been associated with improved role functioning, self-efficacy, and patient satisfaction (Bellack et al. 2005). Family and environmentally based therapies have been shown to improve compliance, decrease relapse, and lower hospital admissions in adults (Pilling et al. 2002). Behavioral, psychoeducational, and supportive family intervention strategies also appear to provide enduring positive effects (Pharoah et al. 2010).

In youth with EOS, comprehensive treatment strategies that promote stable nurturing environments are essential to illness management and require significant family education and support. Parental burden is high with schizophrenia, given the effects of the illness on family functioning, the potential grief at witnessing a highly impaired child, the frustration inherent in dealing with complex and often confusing mental health care systems, and the financial burdens of caring for a child with significant health needs. Efforts to provide support, decrease isolation, validate frustrations, and empower families can enhance quality of lives and improve outcomes by fostering the family's ability to care for their child.

There are few psychosocial treatment studies that specifically address EOS. For young patients, clinical consensus suggests that skills training designed to target social deficits can aid in skill acquisition and alleviate distress in social situations. A small study of patients with EOS found that family psychoeducation seminars, problem-solving sessions, hospital milieu therapy, and reintegration into community and school networks were associated with decrease in relapse rate and global improvement of functioning (Rund 1994). Youth with greater premorbid functional deficits demonstrated more significant benefits, highlighting the importance of comprehensive care in severe cases.

Cognitive remediation has also been shown to be beneficial in EOS. When receiving cognitive remediation combined with psychoeducation, youth exhibited sustained improvements in visual information processing (Ueland and Rund 2005), and when they received cognitive remediation combined with standard therapy, youth demonstrated improved planning ability and cognitive flexibility (Wykes et al. 2007). Interventions should focus on remedying functional impairments and should be tailored to the interpersonal skill and developmental level of the patient.

Summary Points

- Early onset schizophrenia may represent a more severe variant of the adult-onset form.
- Childhood schizophrenia is rare and is associated with significant cognitive and developmental impairments.
- Most children reporting psychotic-like symptoms do not have a psychotic illness. The diagnosis is made on the basis of characteristic patterns of symptoms, course of illness, and mental status examination.
- Premorbid signs and symptoms may occur early in childhood and warrant close attention to optimize supports.
- Severity of negative symptoms and duration of untreated psychosis are associated with poor quality of life and long-term functioning.
- Individuals with schizophrenia are at significant risk for suicide.
- Schizophrenia appears to be characterized by marked genetic heterogeneity.
- Genetic vulnerability and environmental exposures interact across neurodevelopment to influence the onset and progression of schizophrenia.
- Several neurodevelopmental and neuroanatomical abnormalities are associated with schizophrenia, with many present at disease onset.

- Effective treatment requires a comprehensive approach combining psychopharmacology with psychotherapeutic and environmental interventions.
- Comorbid illnesses are common and should be an additional focus of treatment.

References

American Psychiatric Association: Diagnostic and Statistical Manual of Mental Disorders, 4th Edition. Washington, DC, American Psychiatric Association, 1994

American Psychiatric Association: Diagnostic and Statistical Manual of Mental Disorders, 5th Edition. Arlington, VA, American Psychiatric Association, 2013

Bellack AS, Dickinson D, Morris SE, et al: The development of a computer-assisted cognitive remediation program for patients with schizophrenia. Isr J Psychiatry Relat Sci 42(1):5–14, 2005 16134402

Breitborde NJ, López SR, Wickens TD, et al: Toward specifying the nature of the relationship between expressed emotion and schizophrenic relapse: the utility of curvilinear models. Int J Methods Psychiatr Res 16(1):1–10, 2007 17425243

Brown AS: The environment and susceptibility to schizophrenia. Prog Neurobiol 93(1):23–58, 2011 20955757

Butzlaff RL, Hooley JM: Expressed emotion and psychiatric relapse: a meta-analysis. Arch Gen Psychiatry 55(6):547–552, 1998 9633674

Cannon M, Walsh E, Hollis C, et al: Predictors of later schizophrenia and affective psychosis among attendees at a child psychiatry department. Br J Psychiatry 178:420–426, 2001 11331557

Cantor-Graae E, Selten JP: Schizophrenia and migration: a meta-analysis and review. Am J Psychiatry 162(1):12–24, 2005 15625195

Caplan R, Guthrie D, Fish B, et al: The Kiddie Formal Thought Disorder Rating Scale: clinical assessment, reliability, and validity. J Am Acad Child Adolesc Psychiatry 28(3):408–416, 1989 2738008

Cardno AG, Gottesman II: Twin studies of schizophrenia: from bow-and-arrow concordances to star wars Mx and functional genomics. Am J Med Genet 97(1):12–17, 2000 10813800

Clarke M, Whitty P, Browne S, et al: Untreated illness and outcome of psychosis. Br J Psychiatry 189:235–240, 2006 16946358

Correll CU, Manu P, Olshanskiy V, et al: Cardiometabolic risk of second-generation antipsychotic medications during first-time use in children and adolescents. JAMA 302(16):1765–1773, 2009 19861668

de Lacy N, King BH: Revisiting the relationship between autism and schizophrenia: toward an integrated neurobiology. Annu Rev Clin Psychol 9:555–587, 2013 23537488

DeMaso DR, Martini DR, Cahen LA, et al: Practice parameter for the psychiatric assessment and management of physically ill children and adolescents. J Am Acad Child Adolesc Psychiatry 48(2):213–233, 2009 20040826

Driver DI, Gogtay N, Rapoport JL: Childhood onset schizophrenia and early onset schizophrenia spectrum disorders. Child Adolesc Psychiatr Clin N Am 22(4):539–555, 2013 24012072

Fish B: Neurobiologic antecedents of schizophrenia in children. Evidence for an inherited, congenital neurointegrative defect. Arch Gen Psychiatry 34(11):1297–1313, 1977 263819

Fitzsimmons J, Kubicki M, Shenton ME: Review of functional and anatomical brain connectivity findings in schizophrenia. Curr Opin Psychiatry 26(2):172–187, 2013 23324948

Frazier JA, McClellan J, Findling RL, et al: Treatment of early onset schizophrenia spectrum disorders (TEOSS): demographic and clinical characteristics. J Am Acad Child Adolesc Psychiatry 46(8):979–988, 2007 17667477

Fromer M, Pocklington AJ, Kavanagh DH, et al: De novo mutations in schizophrenia implicate synaptic networks. Nature 506(7487):179–184, 2014 24463507

Fusar-Poli P, Smieskova R, Kempton MJ, et al: Progressive brain changes in schizophrenia related to antipsychotic treatment? A meta-analysis of longitudinal MRI studies. Neurosci Biobehav Rev 37(8):1680–1691, 2013 23769814

Ganzola R, Maziade M, Duchesne S: Hippocampus and amygdala volumes in children and young adults at high-risk of schizophrenia: research synthesis. Schizophr Res 156(1):76–86, 2014 24794883

Garralda ME: Hallucinations in children with conduct and emotional disorders: II. The follow-up study. Psychol Med 14(3):597–604, 1984 6494368

Giusti-Rodríguez P, Sullivan PF: The genomics of schizophrenia: update and implications. J Clin Invest 123(11):4557–4563, 2013 24177465

Glausier JR, Lewis DA: Dendritic spine pathology in schizophrenia. Neuroscience 251:90–207, 2013 22546337

Gochman PA, Greenstein D, Sporn A, et al: IQ stabilization in childhood-onset schizophrenia. Schizophr Res 77(2–3):271–277, 2005 15913958

Gogtay N, Sporn A, Clasen LS, et al: Comparison of progressive cortical gray matter loss in childhood-onset schizophrenia with that in childhood-onset atypical psychoses. Arch Gen Psychiatry 61(1):17–22, 2004a 14706940

Gogtay N, Giedd JN, Lusk L, et al: Dynamic mapping of human cortical development during childhood through early adulthood. Proc Natl Acad Sci USA 101(21):8174–8179, 2004b 15148381

Gogtay N, Lu A, Leow AD, et al: Three-dimensional brain growth abnormalities in childhood-onset schizophrenia visualized by using tensor-based morphometry. Proc Natl Acad Sci USA 105(41):15979–15984, 2008 18852461

Greenstein D, Lerch J, Shaw P, et al: Childhood onset schizophrenia: cortical brain abnormalities as young adults. J Child Psychol Psychiatry 47(10):1003–1012, 2006 17073979

Greenstein DK, Wolfe S, Gochman P, et al: Remission status and cortical thickness in childhood-onset schizophrenia. J Am Acad Child Adolesc Psychiatry 47(10):1133–1140, 2008 18724254

Gulsuner S, Walsh T, Watts AC, et al: Spatial and temporal mapping of de novo mutations in schizophrenia to a fetal prefrontal cortical network. Cell 154(3):518–529, 2013 23911319

Gur RE, Cowell P, Turetsky BI, et al: A follow-up magnetic resonance imaging study of schizophrenia. Relationship of neuroanatomical changes to clinical and neurobehavioral measures. Arch Gen Psychiatry 55(2):145–152, 1998 9477928

Gur RE, Cowell PE, Latshaw A, et al: Reduced dorsal and orbital prefrontal gray matter volumes in schizophrenia. Arch Gen Psychiatry 57(8):761–768, 2000 10920464

Hlastala SA, McClellan J: Phenomenology and diagnostic stability of youths with atypical psychotic symptoms. J Child Adolesc Psychopharmacol 15(3):497–509, 2005 16092913

Horan WP, Ventura J, Nuechterlein KH, et al: Stressful life events in recent-onset schizophrenia: reduced frequencies and altered subjective appraisals. Schizophr Res 75(2–3):363–374, 2005 15885527

International Schizophrenia Consortium, Purcell SM, Wray NR, et al: Common polygenic variation contributes to risk of schizophrenia and bipolar disorder. Nature 460(7256):748–752, 2009 19571811

Jones PB, Barnes TR, Davies L, et al: Randomized controlled trial of the effect on quality of life of second- vs first-generation antipsychotic drugs in schizophrenia: Cost Utility of the Latest Antipsychotic Drugs in Schizophrenia Study (CUtLASS 1). Arch Gen Psychiatry 63(10):1079–1087, 2006 17015810

Juuhl-Langseth M, Rimol LM, Rasmussen IA Jr, et al: Comprehensive segmentation of subcortical brain volumes in early onset schizophrenia reveals limited structural abnormalities. Psychiatry Res 203(1):14–23, 2012 22917502

Kendi M, Kendi AT, Lehericy S, et al: Structural and diffusion tensor imaging of the fornix in childhood- and adolescent-onset schizophrenia. J Am Acad Child Adolesc Psychiatry 47(7):826–832, 2008 18520955

Kolvin I: Studies in the childhood psychoses, I: diagnostic criteria and classification. Br J Psychiatry 118(545):381–384, 1971 5576635

Kong A, Frigge ML, Masson G, et al: Rate of de novo mutations and the importance of father's age to disease risk. Nature 488(7412):471–475, 2012 22914163

Lehman AF: Public health policy, community services, and outcomes for patients with schizophrenia. Psychiatr Clin North Am 21(1):221–231, 1998 9551498

Lehman AF, Lieberman JA, Dixon LB, et al: Practice guideline for the treatment of patients with schizophrenia, second edition. Am J Psychiatry 161(2 suppl):1–56, 2004

Lieberman JA, Stroup TS, McEvoy JP, et al: Effectiveness of antipsychotic drugs in patients with chronic schizophrenia. N Engl J Med 353(12):1209–1223, 2005 16172203

López SR, Nelson Hipke K, Polo AJ, et al: Ethnicity, expressed emotion, attributions, and course of schizophrenia: family warmth matters. J Abnorm Psychol 113(3):428–439, 2004 15311988

Manolio TA, Collins FS, Cox NJ, et al: Finding the missing heritability of complex diseases. Nature 461(7265):747–753, 2009 19812666

Marquardt RK, Levitt JG, Blanton RE, et al: Abnormal development of the anterior cingulate in childhood-onset schizophrenia: a preliminary quantitative MRI study. Psychiatry Res 138(3):221–233, 2005 15854790

Mattai A, Chavez A, Greenstein D, et al: Effects of clozapine and olanzapine on cortical thickness in childhood-onset schizophrenia. Schizophr Res 116(1):44–48, 2010 19913390

Mattai A, Hosanagar A, Weisinger B, et al: Hippocampal volume development in healthy siblings of childhood-onset schizophrenia patients. Am J Psychiatry 168(4):427–435, 2011 21245087

McClellan J, King MC: Genetic heterogeneity in human disease. Cell 141(2):210–217, 2010 20403315

McClellan J, Stock S, American Academy of Child and Adolescent Psychiatry (AACAP) Committee on Quality Issues (CQI): Practice parameter for the assessment and treatment of children and adolescents with schizophrenia. J Am Acad Child Adolesc Psychiatry 52(9):976–990, 2013 23972700

Meyer-Lindenberg A, Tost H: Neural mechanisms of social risk for psychiatric disorders. Nat Neurosci 15(5):663–668, 2012 22504349

Narr KL, Bilder RM, Toga AW, et al: Mapping cortical thickness and gray matter concentration in first episode schizophrenia. Cereb Cortex 15(6):708–719, 2005 15371291

O'Brien MP, Gordon JL, Bearden CE, et al: Positive family environment predicts improvement in symptoms and social functioning among adolescents at imminent risk for onset of psychosis. Schizophr Res 81(2–3):269–275, 2006 16309893

Okkels N, Vernal DL, Jensen SO, et al: Changes in the diagnosed incidence of early onset schizophrenia over four decades. Acta Psychiatr Scand 127(1):62–68, 2013 22906158

Patterson TL, Leeuwenkamp OR: Adjunctive psychosocial therapies for the treatment of schizophrenia. Schizophr Res 100(1–3):108–119, 2008 18226500

Pharoah F, Mari J, Rathbone J, et al: Family intervention for schizophrenia. Cochrane Database Syst Rev 12(12):CD000088, 2010 21154340

Pilling S, Bebbington P, Kuipers E, et al: Psychological treatments in schizophrenia: I. Meta-analysis of family intervention and cognitive behaviour therapy. Psychol Med 32(5):763–782, 2002 12171372

Pompili M, Amador XF, Girardi P, et al: Suicide risk in schizophrenia: learning from the past to change the future. Ann Gen Psychiatry 6:10, 2007 17367524

Purcell SM, Moran JL, Fromer M, et al: A polygenic burden of rare disruptive mutations in schizophrenia. Nature 506(7487):185–190, 2014 24463508

Rapoport JL, Giedd JN, Gogtay N: Neurodevelopmental model of schizophrenia: update 2012. Mol Psychiatry 17(12):1228–1238, 2012 22488257

Rosenfarb IS, Bellack AS, Aziz N: Family interactions and the course of schizophrenia in African American and White patients. J Abnorm Psychol 115(1):112–120, 2006 16492102

Rund BR: Cognitive dysfunctions and psychosocial treatment of schizophrenics: research of the past and perspectives on the future. Acta Psychiatr Scand Suppl 384:9–16, 1994 7879650

Rutter M: Childhood schizophrenia reconsidered. J Autism Child Schizophr 2(4):315–337, 1972 4581613

Sanders AR, Duan J, Levinson DF, et al: No significant association of 14 candidate genes with schizophrenia in a large European ancestry sample: implications for psychiatric genetics. Am J Psychiatry 165(4):497–506, 2008 18198266

Selemon LD, Goldman-Rakic PS: The reduced neuropil hypothesis: a circuit based model of schizophrenia. Biol Psychiatry 45(1):17–25, 1999 9894571

Shepherd AM, Laurens KR, Matheson SL, et al: Systematic meta-review and quality assessment of the structural brain alterations in schizophrenia. Neurosci Biobehav Rev 36(4):1342–1356, 2012 22244985

Sikich L, Frazier JA, McClellan J, et al: Double-blind comparison of first- and second-generation antipsychotics in early onset schizophrenia and schizo-affective disorder: findings from the treatment of early onset schizophrenia spectrum disorders (TEOSS) study. Am J Psychiatry 165(11):1420–1431, 2008 18794207

Tandon R, Gaebel W, Barch DM, et al: Definition and description of schizophrenia in the DSM-5. Schizophr Res 150(1):3–10, 2013 23800613

Taylor JL, Blanton RE, Levitt JG, et al: Superior temporal gyrus differences in childhood-onset schizophrenia. Schizophr Res 73(2–3):235–241, 2005 15653266

Thormodsen R, Rimol LM, Tamnes CK, et al: Age-related cortical thickness differences in adolescents with early onset schizophrenia compared with healthy adolescents. Psychiatry Res 214(3):190–196, 2013 24144503

Toga AW, Thompson PM, Sowell ER: Mapping brain maturation. Trends Neurosci 29(3):148–159, 2006 16472876

Ueland T, Rund BR: Cognitive remediation for adolescents with early onset psychosis: a 1-year follow-up study. Acta Psychiatr Scand 111(3):193–201, 2005 15701103

Vidal CN, Rapoport JL, Hayashi KM, et al: Dynamically spreading frontal and cingulate deficits mapped in adolescents with schizophrenia. Arch Gen Psychiatry 63(1):25–34, 2006 16389194

Walsh T, McClellan JM, McCarthy SE, et al: Rare structural variants disrupt multiple genes in neurodevelopmental pathways in schizophrenia. Science 320(5875):539–543, 2008 18369103

Wykes T, Newton E, Landau S, et al: Cognitive remediation therapy (CRT) for young early onset patients with schizophrenia: an exploratory randomized controlled trial. Schizophr Res 94(1–3):221–230, 2007 17524620

Xu B, Roos JL, Dexheimer P, et al: Exome sequencing supports a de novo mutational paradigm for schizophrenia. Nat Genet 43(9):864–868, 2011 21822266

PART III

Disorders Affecting Somatic Function

CHAPTER 19

Psychiatric Aspects of Chronic Physical Disorders

D. Richard Martini, M.D.
Kelly Walker Lowry, Ph.D.
John V. Lavigne, Ph.D., ABPP

Approximately 10–20 million children in the United States experience a medical condition that requires periodic intervention (Wallander et al. 2003). For most of these children, the condition is mild, but approximately 10% of these children and adolescents have conditions that affect them nearly every day (Wallander et al. 2003). Advances in medicine have improved survival to such an extent that nearly 90% of children whose conditions were at one time considered terminal are now living into adulthood (Thompson and Gustafson 1996). While some of these individuals will experience a full recovery, the number of people who must live with a chronic condition will continue to increase.

Psychological Adjustment

While most children with chronic physical illnesses are not affected emotionally, behaviorally, or developmentally by their condition (American Academy of Pediatrics Committee on Children With Disabilities and Committee on Psychosocial Aspects of Child and Family Health 1993), there is evidence that children and adolescents with chronic illnesses are at increased risk for emotional or behavioral problems (Pinquart and Shen 2011; Wallander et al. 2003). In general, specific disease-related factors seem to play a smaller part in affecting the child's psychological adjustment than psychosocial factors do; thus, family factors and parental mental health are more strongly associated with child adjustment problems than is illness severity (Lavigne and Faier-Routman 1993).

One disease-related factor associated with psychological problems of physical disorders in children and adolescents is the degree to which the central nervous system (CNS) is involved in the disease process. Disorders affecting CNS functioning (e.g., epilepsy, cerebral palsy, hydrocephalus) show higher rates of psychological problems than other disorders (DeMaso et al. 1990; Lavigne and Faier-Routman 1992; Noeker et al. 2005). Numerous studies have found little relationship between disease severity and psychosocial adjustment (Campis et al. 1995; DeMaso et al. 1991, 1995; Shaw and DeMaso 2006) among conditions not involving the brain (e.g., cystic fibrosis, diabetes mellitus, asthma). Exceptions include children and adolescents with multiple chronic physical conditions (Newacheck et al. 1991) or long-term physical disability (Holmbeck et al. 2003).

Models of Adaptation and Coping

The biopsychosocial factors associated with psychological adjustment of children with chronic physical disorders are complex. Over the years, a variety of models of the effects of chronic illness on adjustment have been proposed. Early models tended to emphasize one or two core psychological factors as critical factors associated with the child or adolescent's psychological adjustment. One of the earliest models was proposed by Beatrice Wright (1960), who posited a central role for the effects of chronic illness on the self-system, including body image. Wright argued that the impact of a chronic physical condition would be greater if it impacted something central or peripheral to self-concept (e.g., ability to excel in athletics for some individuals) or body image (e.g., facial appearance). Subsequently, Pless and Pinkerton (1975) integrated her insights on self-concept with early work by coping researchers and advanced a model indicating that both the self-system and coping processes were central to the adjustment of children and adolescents to chronic illness. These models served a heuristic function but generated little research.

More recently, better articulated and integrative models of adaptation to pediatric illnesses (Thompson 1985; Thompson and Gustafson 1996; Wallander and Varni 1992) have been developed that emphasize the interplay between child and parent adaptation in adjustment. Successful adaptation to the chronic illness by the patient and family is dependent on an interaction between the disease and a variety of biomedical, developmental, and psychosocial factors (Wallander et al. 2003). The transactional model emphasizes the interplay between chronic illness and exposure to negative life events in the etiology of adjustment disorders.

Factors Affecting Adaptation to Illness

Coping Style

An individual's approach to illness is affected by the cognitive, emotional, and behavioral responses that characterize coping style. For example, a coping method that directly handles the stressor and the subsequent emotional response is considered to be *approach-oriented.* An *avoidance-oriented* style seeks to control upset by evading the stressor (Hubert et al. 1988). Some patients and families may also deal with distress by taking a practical approach and focusing primarily on the problems at hand. Others struggle to maintain emotional control and cope by regulating their emotional responses (Folkman and Lazarus 1988).

The child with an acute or chronic medical illness should be encouraged to take advantage of the coping style that he or she identifies as most comfortable (Shaw and DeMaso 2006). There is no single preferred method, although some evidence suggests that a problem-focused coping style may be more effective in cases of chronic pediatric illness (Band and Weisz 1988).

Developmental Factors

Adaptation to physical illness and the ability to garner the necessary coping resources depend on a variety of developmental factors. The understanding and use of medical information, the sense of illness causality and personal responsibility, and the need for adherence to treatment are all addressed in the context of the child's developmental level (Shaw and DeMaso 2006; Thompson and Gustafson 1996). Preschool children typically cannot understand the complexities of medical diagnosis and treatment, so their adjustment is affected by fear of the unknown and unexpected (Melamed et al. 1982; Simeonsson et al. 1979). School-age children can recall and comprehend information about medical diagnosis and treatment. They worry over loss of control and an inability to protect themselves from harm. Adolescents may experience physical illness as an assault on their quest for autonomy and a sense of identity. When the illness is chronic, the age and developmental level of patients do not have a significant effect on the development of psychological problems (Wallander et al. 2003).

History of Illness and Medical Experience

Children may be traumatized by difficult and painful medical procedures, some of which recur as part of a treatment regimen and others that are repeated when clinicians are unsuccessful in their initial attempts. The patient anxiously anticipates similar experiences during subsequent hospital or clinic visits (Dahlquist et al. 1986). As a result, both child and family may begin to avoid contact with medical professionals for fear of reexperiencing these situations and the emotional aftermath. Medical care suffers because the patient does not receive routine services, increasing the likelihood of unforeseen medical complications that require aggressive attention and possibly invasive procedures.

Temperament

A child's temperament can influence the choices he or she makes in response to acute and chronic medical illness (Rudolph et al. 1995). Anxious children avoid medical interventions and in the process become more noncompliant. Children who are less affected by the illness are more likely to participate actively in treatment and inquire about their care and prognosis. Young patients with certain temperamental styles, such as slow-to-warm-up children or children with difficult temperaments, are more likely to suffer long-term behavioral and emotional complications (Wallander et al. 2003).

Parent and Family Factors

Anxious parents are more likely to be distressed by procedures and the uncertainty that frequently accompanies medical diagnoses. Unfortunately, their personal preoccupations leave them less available to address their children's emotional needs. They cannot, for example, help their children generate appropriate coping strategies and deal with the immediate and long-term effects of the illness (Melamed 1993; Shaw and DeMaso 2006). Studies of parental psychopathology find that maternal depression and anxiety play an important role in long-term emotional adjustment of the child (DeMaso et al. 1991, 1995, 2004; Wallander et al. 2003).

Families adapt to physical illness in three distinct phases: crisis, chronic, and terminal (Rolland and Walsh 2006). The crisis or acute phase occurs immediately before and after the diagnosis of an illness, when most energy is spent to understand and manage the symptoms while coping with the grief that accompanies the loss of a healthy child. Medical disorders may be stable, progressive, or episodic in nature. The family adjusts to these characteristics during the chronic phase, with an emphasis on maintaining family stability, minimizing the impact of the illness, and providing appropriate medical care. The terminal phase both anticipates and follows the death of the child and involves managing and processing the feelings and preparing the young patient and the family for the end of life.

Comorbidity of Medical and Psychiatric Conditions: Somatopsychic and Psychosomatic Relationships

There is a constant interplay between organic and functional factors in an illness, and it is often difficult, therefore, to describe a child's disorder as simply either medical or psychiatric. Patients' symptoms evolve over time in a relationship that is clearly bidirectional. The inability to recognize psychiatric disorder in a physically ill child may prolong and unnecessarily complicate the treatment course. Psychiatric disorders in physically ill children include those conditions that existed prior to or following the onset of the medical illness and those that develop as a direct consequence of the disease. The former can be classified as coincidental comorbidity and the latter as causal comorbidity. An example of coincidental comorbidity is the care of a patient with preexisting attention-deficit/hyperactivity disorder who is diagnosed with diabetes. An example of causal comorbidity is the development of depression in patients with Addison disease, because a deficiency in cortisol can lead to symptoms of mood disorder. Recurrent physical complaints that do not correlate with the medical findings are characteristic of mood, anxiety, and psychosomatic disorders. A good example is the patient with functional abdominal pain who also presents with panic disorder (Shaw and DeMaso 2006).

Psychiatric disorder not only affects the child's medical adherence, lifestyle, and adjustment to the illness, but there is also a direct impact on physiology and the disease process. For example, children with diabetes are at greater risk for depressive disorders (Kovacs et al. 1997). Young diabetics with comorbid depression who do not follow the treatment regimen are hospitalized more frequently and experience more disease-related complications (Freeman and Freeman 2006; Kovacs et al. 1995). Young asthmatics frequently suffer from depressive symptoms, and for inner-city children, mood disorder is associated with a worse prognosis (Waxmonsky et al. 2006). Dysfunctional and chaotic families exacerbate the child's depression and increase asthma symptom severity (Wood et al. 2006).

Categorical and Noncategorical Approaches

Psychological adjustment to illness is typically considered in the context of either a categorical (diagnosis-specific) experience or a broader noncategorical experience (Knapp and Harris 1998; Lavigne and Faier-Routman 1993; Thompson and Gustafson 1996; Wallander et al. 2003). Within a categorical approach, each illness is thought to differ from others in important ways psychologically. For example, asthma, diabetes, and recurrent abdominal pain are identified as medical diagnoses with characteristic patterns of behavior and reasonably well-understood interactions between the psychological and physiological aspects of illness. Therefore, from a categorical viewpoint, it is important to take a diagnosis-specific approach and consider these factors when planning treatment for certain aspects of these disorders (Campo et al. 2004; Hocking and Lochman 2005; Wamboldt et al. 1998).

A noncategorical approach identifies common aspects of the illness experience (e.g., visible/invisible, fatal/nonfatal, stable/unpredictable) when evaluating the child's response to a disease (Knapp and Harris 1998; Shaw and DeMaso 2006). For example, posttraumatic stress symptoms may appear following a number of medical interventions in both diagnostic and treatment settings (Stuber and Shemesh 2006). Developmentally, young patients who are paraplegic as a result of traumatic injury or congenital malformation frequently experience symptoms of anxiety and depression when faced with the expectations of self-sufficiency during adolescence and young adulthood. The family dimensions of cohesion, flexibility, affection, and expressiveness are important factors in determining patient outcome regardless of medical illness (Fisher and Weihs 2000; Lewis and Vitulano 2003; Vitulano 2003). The general illness models discussed in the subsection "Models of Adaptation and Coping" are applicable across disease groups and tend to be noncategorical in their approach. The models recognize that individual differences might affect outcomes—for example, children with certain temperamental styles may do better than others in dealing with an illness, and presumably that would be true across types of illness. The general models posit, however, that key aspects of adjusting to a chronic illness are the same across disorders and that it is not necessary to conceptualize the psychological aspects of each disorder differently.

Impact of Chronic Illness on the Family

Most families with a medically ill child are well adjusted and productive. Individual members, however, are more likely than the general population to experience symptoms of irritability, anxiety, depression, and somatic complaints (Jacobs 2000). Shaw and DeMaso (2006) suggest that the amount of disability, predictability of the disease course and prognosis, any stigma associated with the disorder, and how much monitoring is required may affect the family's experience of, and adjustment to, the disorder. Parental behavior must also be understood in the context of family beliefs and prior experience with illness and death (Shaw and DeMaso 2006).

Along with providing the instrumental care and emotional support their child needs, parents must also deal with their own feelings about being unable to protect their child from disease and their loss of control over their child's life. Forced to rely on professional help, parents are obliged to surrender certain degrees of control and may need to forsake their traditional roles. While successful coping may require parents to develop a good understanding of their child's illness, parents can become overly concerned with medical information and neglect both their child's and family's psychosocial needs.

The demands of caring for an ill child may affect the parents' marital relationship (Kazak et al. 2003). Parents may be highly supportive of each other and even be drawn closer to each other, but there is a risk that the marital relationship may be weakened, particularly if marital problems existed before the child's illness developed. When genetic factors are known contributors to the illness, a parent blaming himself or the other parent is not uncommon.

Parental response to illness can have both a beneficial and deleterious effect on the behavior of the physically ill child (for review, see Shaw and DeMaso 2006). In addition, family factors play a larger role in the child's adjustment to illness than do illness-related factors (Lavigne and Faier-Routman 1993). Both inappropriate responses (e.g., threats, punishment, relinquishing control to the child) and over-responding to the child (via excessive parental attention, reassurance, empathy, and apologies) can interfere with the child's ability to cope with his or her illness (Frank et al. 1995; Logan and Scharff 2005). Generally, a calm supportive response, the continuation of familiar "family rules," and appropriate limit setting are important for helping the child adjust to his or her illness (Pederson and Harbaugh 1995).

Siblings

Siblings of chronically ill children also show increased levels of emotional and behavioral difficulties, including increased shyness or anxiety when compared with control subjects (Kazak et al. 2003; Siemon 1984; Shaw and DeMaso 2006).

Depending on the illness severity, siblings may be partially "frozen out" of families preoccupied with meeting the demands imposed by the child's illness, occasionally becoming emotionally disengaged from busy parents, less able to engage in activities with the affected child, and jealous of the attention directed toward the ill child and feeling guilt about not being affected. Roles can change if a sibling's achievements surpass those of the child who is now limited by the physical illness. At times, siblings take on a parental role for the other siblings and do more caretaking for the ill child.

General Considerations in Psychiatric Management

Psychopharmacology

Psychotropic medications may be effective in the management of emotional and behavioral problems that accompany medical illness. Frequently, psychopharmacological interventions are instituted when the medical team believes that the psychiatric symptoms in the child are affecting the patient's care. The diagnosis of a psychiatric disorder is rarely made in these situations, and the treatment targets specific symptoms rather than syndromes (Shaw and DeMaso 2006).

Before starting the patient on a medication, the clinician should be aware of possible interactions between the illness and the treatment as a way to minimize adverse effects. Patients and caregivers should provide information on any alternative treatments or over-the-counter preparations taken by the patient as well as current medication regimens. Psychotropic drugs may have a variety of effects on the pharmacokinetic and pharmacodynamic properties of other medications, and these factors should be considered in treatment planning. Clinicians should proactively monitor for side effects and drug interactions, whether through physical examination or laboratory studies.

Young patients may be affected by illnesses that impair organ systems and change drug metabolism—particularly patients with hepatic, gastrointestinal, renal, and cardiac diseases. Therefore, it is wise to follow the axiom "start low, go slow" when initiating medication. Drug levels for psychotropic medications are not reliable indicators of efficacy or toxicity. In medically ill children, it is best to use one medication at a time and choose a drug with a short half-life that can be administered in single doses and that quickly reaches a therapeutic level. The medically ill child and caregiver are already overwhelmed with complicated therapeutic regimens. Simple and direct psychopharmacological recommendations will improve adherence.

Pharmacokinetics

Pharmacokinetics involves the absorption, distribution, and metabolism of medications (Robinson and Owen 2005). Medical illness, particularly as it affects organ systems, alters pharmacokinetics. Most psychotropic medications, with the exception of lithium, venlafaxine, divalproex sodium, methylphenidate, gabapentin, and topiramate, are bound to protein at a rate of 80%–90%. The unbound drug is considered "active." Patients with chronic diseases of the liver and kidney lose protein and as a result are likely to have more unbound active drug. Most psychotropic medications are absorbed in the gastrointestinal tract, metabolized in the liver and gastrointestinal tract, and excreted through the kidneys. Diseases of these organ systems require dose reductions in order to prevent toxicity. In addition, any medication or illnesses that reduce hepatic metabolism, renal excretion, or blood flow to the liver or kidneys should be considered when choosing a drug or medication dose (Shaw and DeMaso 2006).

Pharmacodynamics

Pharmacodynamics involves changes in the drug's effectiveness as a consequence of drug-drug interactions or modifications in drug receptor site binding. For example, the hepatic cytochrome P450 (CYP450) system is responsible for most drug metabolism and interactions. Clinicians should be aware of medications that either potentiate or inhibit the CYP450, particularly in medically ill patients on multiple drug regimens. In these situations, drug metabolism is altered and drug-drug interactions are more likely (Shaw and DeMaso 2006).

Medication Use in Specific Illnesses

Hepatic Disease

Hepatic disease lowers the first-pass extraction and biotransformation of medications. In the presence of liver failure, there is a greater risk for medication side effects, particularly after oral administration and with drugs that have a narrow therapeutic index (like tricyclic antidepressants). Liver disease affects the ability of medications to bind to proteins and affects the metabolism of most antidepressants, benzodiazepines like diazepam, and neuroleptics, including haloperidol. With chronic liver failure, there should be a 25%–50% reduction in dose because medications that are not bound to protein are more active. In cases of acute hepatic disease, alterations in drug dose are not necessary. Among antidepressant medications, nefazodone, phenelzine, imipramine, amitriptyline, duloxetine, trazodone, and bupropion have the greatest risk for hepatotoxicity. Citalopram, escitalopram, paroxetine, and fluvoxamine are the least hepatotoxic (Voican et al. 2014). Clinicians should also avoid carbamazepine, valproate, and the phenothiazines because of hepatotoxicity. Patients with impaired hepatic function are more likely to develop orthostatic hypotension as a side effect of antipsychotic medications. Intravenous drug administration avoids first-pass metabolism by the CYP450 system and may allow medication doses more typical for patients with normal hepatic function (Beliles 2000; Shaw and DeMaso 2006).

Gastrointestinal Disease

Drug absorption is affected by gastrointestinal mucosal integrity and motility, particularly when medications are given orally. Motility is altered by medications, including psychotropic agents (particularly those with anticholinergic side effects), and a variety of medical conditions, including colitis and diabetes. Delays in gastric emptying or diseases of the small bowel (e.g., Crohn's disease) that affect the integrity of the intestine lead to poor absorption. This may also inhibit protein binding, leading to uneven drug distribution. Extended-release preparations generally produce less gastrointestinal upset because of the gradual exposure to the medication and the slower increase in plasma levels (Beliles 2000).

Renal Disease

Renal disease does not generally affect the metabolism of psychotropic medications because these drugs are typically fat soluble, easily pass through the blood-brain barrier, are not dialyzable, and are metabolized by the liver and excreted in bile. The exceptions are lithium, gabapentin, methylphenidate, venlafaxine, divalproex sodium, and topiramate. Lithium is excreted unchanged in the urine, and toxicity in the presence of renal disease is associated with a decrease in renal concentration ability. Occasionally, patients have nephrogenic diabetes insipidus with lithium toxicity. These problems are typically reversible with the use of thiazides or amiloride but can become permanent if uncorrected (Freeman and Freeman 2006). Decreases in psychotropic medication doses in the presence of renal disease are usually a consequence of common problems that accompany the disorders, including protein deficiency and fluid and electrolyte shifts. A good general rule is to decrease the dose by one-third in patients with renal disease. Hemodialysis initially lowers the plasma blood concentrations, followed by a rebound when the drug moves from the periphery to the circulation. Protein-bound medications are not typically cleared by hemodialysis.

Cardiac Disease

Cardiovascular disease affects perfusion of the liver and kidneys and the volume of distribution for medication. This is particularly true with congestive heart failure and the associated fluid retention. Psychotropic medications may have direct effects on the cardiovascular system. Tricyclic antidepressants cause both blood pressure and heart rate increases and are class I antiarrhythmics with quinidine-like properties that are potentially fatal in overdose. These medications are contraindicated in patients with heart disease and in patients with a history of suicidal behavior. Selective serotonin reuptake inhibitors (SSRIs) are associated with a moderate slowing of the heart rate but are not contraindicated in patients with heart disease. Bupropion increases blood pressure in adults, but similar changes are not documented in children. Lithium occasionally causes sinus node dysfunction and arrhythmias, including bradycardia and atrioventricular block (Freeman and Freeman 2006). Episodes of syncope with T wave flattening and inversion (typically benign) are also possible. Clonidine decreases systolic blood pressure and decreases cardiac output and heart rate, although the medication does not generally cause clinically significant hypotension when used for psychiatric indications. Low-potency antipsychotics (e.g., chlorpromazine, thioridazine) with anticholinergic, antihistaminic, and α-adrenergic blocking effects may cause hypotension. In addition, both typical and atypical antipsychotics have quinidine-like effects on conduction with QT prolongation that are most often associated with chronic use. Haloperidol, administered parenterally in high doses, is associated with lengthening of the QT interval, torsades de pointes, and multifocal ventricular tachycardia. Clozapine treatment is associated with myocarditis and cardiomyopathy in a small number of adult and pediatric patients (Chow et al. 2014; Mackin 2008). Stimulant medication is used with caution in patients with preexisting heart disease, including postoperative tetralogy of Fallot, coronary artery abnormalities, subaortic stenosis, or hypertrophic cardiomyopathy (Pliszka and American Academy of Child and Adolescent Psychiatry Work Group on Quality Issues 2007). Patients with a history of syncope, dizziness, chest pain, and palpitations are considered at risk for sudden cardiac death, particularly with a positive family history, and should receive a thorough physical examination including a cardiac evaluation before beginning treatment (Pliszka and American Academy of Child and Adolescent Psychiatry Work Group on Quality Issues 2007; Shaw and DeMaso 2006). Screening electrocardiograms for cardiac disease rarely lead to changes in the management of stimulant medication.

Pulmonary Disease

Hypoxia and hypercarbia can affect pharmacokinetics of psychoactive medications by changing pH and affecting drug absorption and distribution. Patients in respiratory distress may experience symptoms of anxiety and panic in a direct response to increasing levels of carbon dioxide. Use of anxiolytics, particularly benzodiazepines, requires great caution if used in patients with respiratory disease because of their tendency to decrease respiratory drive. Should benzodiazepines be required, as in cases when it is necessary to alleviate anxiety in a patient in critical care as he or she is being weaned from a ventilator, doses must be titrated carefully. SSRIs can effectively treat anxiety in patients with comorbid respiratory disease. Buspirone is also considered an anxiolytic that is not associated with respiratory depression and may have mild respiratory stimulant effects.

Epilepsy

Psychotropic medications should be used with caution in patients with epilepsy, primarily because of a lowering of the seizure threshold. First- and second-generation antipsychotics can be used judiciously, with the exception of chlorpromazine and clozapine. Haloperidol has a relatively low seizure risk. SSRIs generally do not present a significant risk; neither does trazodone or the α-agonists. Tricyclic antidepressants present a greater epileptogenic risk than SSRIs (Haddad and Dursun 2008). Bupropion is contraindicated because it lowers the seizure threshold. Lithium is considered a proconvulsant but can be used with care in appropriate cases. Although antidepressant medications can improve outcome, no specific antidepressant medications are recommended for the treatment of comorbid depression and epilepsy (Mehndiratta and Sajatovic 2008). The U.S. Food and Drug Administration (FDA) states that stimulants are contraindicated in patients with comorbid seizure disorders, but data suggest that the medications can be used safely, particularly when the seizures are well controlled (Gucuyener et al. 2003; Hemmer et al. 2001). Benzodiazepines are administered as anticonvulsants but can cause seizures if withdrawn too quickly.

Psychosocial Interventions

Individual Psychotherapy

Psychotherapy provides the child with an opportunity to discuss his or her concerns and feelings about dealing with the illness or disability (Shaw and DeMaso 2006). While Wright (1960) emphasized the role of the self-system and altering inappropriate values in counseling with individuals with chronic illness, more recently a bereavement model has been found to be useful in conceptualizing the process of adaptation to a physical illness as well as guiding treatment (Shaw and DeMaso 2006). The child's emotional responses to a physical illness or disability may be viewed as a process beginning with shock and denial and moving toward an assimilation of illness information and adjustment (Shaw and DeMaso 2006). There are several models of individual psychotherapies used with physically ill children.

In supportive treatment, the therapist seeks to provide a climate of understanding and acceptance through which the child can relate his or her experiences, begin to manage the strong feelings he or she feels, and get help improving the coping mechanisms needed to deal with the chronic illness experience (Green 2000).

In applying principles of psychodynamic psychotherapy, the therapist seeks to help the individual understand the emotional conflicts that contribute to the problem behaviors while adjusting to the chronic illness or disability. As Shaw and DeMaso (2006) note, the usefulness of this type of therapy is often limited by patients' diminished cognitive skills due to the illness itself and the brief time often available for therapy in the pediatric setting.

Narrative therapy allows children and their families the opportunity to share, organize, and validate their experiences and physical condition. Studies have shown significant benefits to patients given the opportunity to "tell their stories" (Adler 1997; Clark and Standard 1997). Cognitive-behavioral therapy (CBT) attempts to help the child alter maladaptive patterns of thinking that lead to excessive feelings of anxiety, depression, or anger; improve problem-solving and coping skills; and, in some instances, modify physiological responses to disorders such as asthma (Spirito and Kazak 2006; Szigethy et al. 2007). Using cognitive restructuring, behavioral activation, and problem-solving skills, CBT attempts to change the maladaptive cognitions that are producing exaggerated or inappropriate emotional responses.

Behavior therapy may be used to improve the child's functional ability and decrease unwanted, negative behaviors (Spirito and Kazak 2006). Behavioral programs with appropriate incentives and an effective system of monitoring and rewards can be used to reinforce desired behaviors such as medication adherence. Biofeedback, relaxation training, and hypnosis may play a role in reducing emotional distress and autonomic arousal and, in some instances, improving the child's physical condition (e.g., asthma, diabetes mellitus, headache, hypertension) (McQuaid and Nassau 1999).

Individual therapy with medically ill children and adolescents frequently incorporates aspects of several therapeutic modalities. An adolescent with spina bifida, for example, may enter into therapy because of a sense of dependency and hopelessness for the future that leads to recurrent bouts of anxiety and depression. Therapy encourages the patient to recount the challenges of his or her disability while providing support, perspective, and practical solutions. Behavioral interventions are structured for the patient and family as a means of encouraging progress and clarifying the goals of treatment.

Family Therapy

Clearly, a child's illness is a total family experience. While the physically ill child who develops behavioral or emotional problems may enter treatment as the identified patient, providing all family members the opportunity to tell their stories about their experience with the illness can be important. Parents' emotional health and functioning play a major role in helping the child maintain his or her emotional well-being and can affect adherence to medical regimens. Family therapy can play a critical role in helping with the child's, parents', and siblings' adjustment to the illness (for reviews, see Eccleston et al. 2012; Shaw and DeMaso 2006; Spirito and Kazak 2006).

Group Therapy

Group therapy has been used with patients experiencing a variety of physical diagnoses (Eccleston et al. 2003; Shaw and DeMaso 2006; Stauffer 1998). Group therapy can take the form of support groups or psychoeducational groups providing information to participants about the diagnosis, treatment, and psychosocial aspects of a particular disorder, while other groups may focus on decreasing physical symptoms (Shaw and DeMaso 2006).

Adherence

As many as 33% of patients with acute conditions and 55% of those with chronic illnesses do not adhere to recommended treatment plans (Sabaté 2003; Shaw et al. 2003), making nonadherence a significant health issue (La Greca and Bearman 2003; Sabaté 2003). Children are at greater risk for noncompliance when they have a history of psychological distress, including symptoms of depression, oppositional behavior, and poor impulse control. These children tend to be patients who deny the significance of the medical illness and have a history of nonadherence. Families that have high levels of conflict and low levels of cohesion, communication, support, and parental responsibility are at higher risk of nonadherence. Low socioeconomic status further complicates the situation. Illnesses that require long periods of follow-up with little optimism are associated with lower levels of adherence. Similarly, without strong evidence of efficacy, patients are less likely to comply with treatments that are complex, invasive, and expensive. Interventions to improve adherence typically involve increasing parental participation in care and treatment, educating patient and family on the need for adequate medical supervision and follow-up, and initiating indicated behavioral, individual, and family therapies (Shaw et al. 2003). Spirito and Kazak (2006) recommend specific family therapy techniques that address nonadherence by normalizing adolescent rebellion, improving family communication, and implementing family problem-solving strategies.

Pain Management

Pain management in pediatric patients is affected by developmental as well as physiological factors. Young patients may not communicate their needs effectively and are frightened by the hospital environment and the physical intensity of their symptoms. Caregivers may either inadvertently reinforce the pain symptoms with continuous attention or become frustrated and angry over the child's complaints and physical limitations (Shaw and DeMaso 2006; Spirito and Kazak 2006). Clinicians should avoid decisions based on a need to better "manage" the patient without properly assessing the presence, extent, and degree of pain. In these instances, children may be considered anxious or manipulative, prompting either inadequate pain treatment or oversedation. Pain should be treated aggressively and early in the patient's treatment course with family, behavioral, and pharmacological interventions (Shaw and DeMaso 2006). Clinicians should assess the child's level of pain, address the reasons for his or her requests or objections, and prescribe symptomatic treatment appropriately. Pain management is typically handled through a multidisciplinary team of medical and mental health professionals.

Procedural Preparation and Play Strategies

Children with chronic illnesses or disabilities may experience many invasive medical procedures. Prevention strategies have focused either on identifying risk factors for emotional distress (DeMaso et al. 1995) or on preparing patients for procedures or hospitalizations (Kain et al. 1996). Procedures designed to reduce the anxiety or pain associated with an invasive medical procedure (e.g., preadmission programs, bibliotherapy, support groups) tend to provide information relevant to the illnesses or treatment that might reduce unfamiliarity with the child's situation in the hospital and provide coping models to express anticipatory anxiety and then master it (Fielding and Duff 1999; Kain et al. 1996). During a painful procedure, a distraction involving video games can be useful. Their use requires minimal staff participation and costs are low (Vasterling et al. 1993). Various resources are available to help parents and professionals in the use of such procedures (DeMaso 2007; Stuber et al. 2006).

Coping strategies such as breathing, deep muscle relaxation, distraction, behavioral rehearsal, positive reinforcement, modeling, visual imagery, and hypnosis can be used during procedures (Blount et al. 2003; Spirito and Kazak 2006) and have been shown to reduce procedural distress. Local anesthetics (e.g., lidocaine-prilocaine cream) can play a useful role in needle-related procedures.

Psychosocial Interventions With Specific Disorders: Empirical Support

There are too many chronic physical disorders to review the psychological treatment literature for all of them. Instead, we have chosen to examine the treatment of six conditions: asthma, diabetes, cancer, juvenile rheumatoid arthritis, delirium, and HIV and AIDS. Asthma was chosen because of its prevalence and status as a chronic condition that has attracted research designed to alter symptoms of the disease as well as overall psychological adjustment. Diabetes is a chronic disorder with a wide range of psychological issues involved in its treatment. Cancer represents disorders that, despite improvements in life expectancy, nonetheless remain life-threatening. Delirium is an example of the neurological sequelae that may be associated with a variety of chronic physical disorders.

Asthma

Studies of psychological intervention with asthma have attempted to reduce the symptoms of the disease, reduce the impact of disease (e.g., "morbidity," such as school absences), improve adherence to the medication regimen, improve psychological adjustment of asthma patients, or some combination. Drotar (2006) found that there are some indications that psychological interventions can have an impact in each of these areas for asthma.

A review by McQuaid and Nassau (1999) concluded that frontalis electromyographic biofeedback was probably efficacious for reducing asthma symptoms, relaxation training was probably efficacious, and family therapy was a promising treatment. Lemanek et al. (2001) concluded that interventions emphasizing behavioral and educational strategies improved both adherence and health outcome, such as peak flow rate and asthma symptoms. Perrin et al. (1992) demonstrated that a multicomponent intervention using education, stress management, and coping interventions improved the adjustment of children with asthma compared with controls, reflected in fewer behavior problems and fewer internalizing symptoms. A large multisite study compared a group of inner-city children with asthma with nontreated control subjects, in which the treated-group participants were assigned a case manager who provided education and intervention for behavior management, training in ways to reduce allergen exposure, and help getting access to health care. Over a 2-year period, the treated group showed fewer days with symptoms and fewer hospitalizations (Evans et al. 1999). While these results are promising, overall, studies of psychological treatment for asthma have been judged to be of relatively poor quality, and conclusions about their efficacy are likely to be premature (Yorke et al. 2005).

Diabetes

Numerous studies of psychological interventions for insulin-dependent diabetes mellitus have been conducted. While studies vary in quality, systematic reviews suggest that these interventions have an impact in several areas. Hampson et al. (2000, 2001) reviewed behavioral interventions with adolescents with type 1 diabetes. Larger effect sizes (around 0.39) were noted for studies designed to reduce psychological adjustment problems and somewhat lower effect sizes (around 0.33) for improving blood glucose control, while effect sizes were lowest (0.15) for improving diabetic self-management. Delamater et al. (2001) found that psychoeducational intervention improved glycemic control. Wysocki et al. (2008) reported that behavioral family systems therapy improved mother-adolescent, but not father-adolescent, communication. Multicomponent interventions emphasizing self-management skills have been described as probably efficacious (Lemanek et al. 2001).

Cancer

The research literature on psychological treatments of pediatric cancer has most commonly addressed ways to reduce procedural pain and distress. Kuppenheimer and Brown (2002) found that CBT had some success in the treatment of procedure pain, although a variety of methodological problems limit the generalization of results. In other areas, psychological interventions with pediatric cancer patients showed effects in improving social skills of children with brain tumors (Barakat et al. 2003) and improving school adjustment on reentry to school (Katz et al. 1988).

Juvenile Rheumatoid Arthritis

Compared with the literature on diabetes, asthma, and cancer, there have been relatively few studies of psychological interventions for juvenile rheumatoid arthritis. Small-scale studies show promising results for reducing pain associated with juvenile rheumatoid arthritis (Lavigne et al. 1992; Walco and Ilowite 1992; Walco et al. 1992). Single-subject designs show that behavioral interventions (e.g., behavioral monitoring, verbal feedback reinforcement) can improve adherence.

Delirium

Delirium is characterized by impairments in attention and orientation, deficits in language and visuospatial skills, and deterioration in cognition not explained by an underlying dementia (Murphy 2000). Symptoms tend to fluctuate throughout the day, and the onset appears as a consequence of an illness or its treatment. Before making a diagnosis, clinicians should evaluate patients several times over an extended period. Pediatric patients seem to be especially vulnerable to delirium following toxic, metabolic, or traumatic CNS insults and fever regardless of the etiology. The most common causes of delirium are CNS infections (e.g., meningitis) or medication toxicity. The evaluation of young patients for the presence of delirium is affected by the developmental limitations of the child, particularly in the areas of communication and cognition. Only the most severe cases are identified; the remainder are either ignored or mismanaged under incorrect diagnoses. In one such case, a 14-year-old girl had a 4-week history of irritability, aggression, disorganization, and paranoia in a presentation consistent with bipolar disorder. The pediatrician immediately referred the case to a psychiatrist and informed the family that she would require long-term therapy and possibly medications. The child and adolescent psychiatrist elicited a history of a viral illness immediately preceding the mental status change. There was no family history of mood disorder, and the patient's symptoms were exacerbated when she was given diphenhydramine for sleeplessness. The psychiatrist suspected delirium secondary to viral encephalitis, treated the patient symptomatically, and told the family that she would gradually improve without symptom recurrence.

The adult literature cites increasing complication rates and longer hospital stays in patients with delirium, but few studies examine delirium in pediatric patients. The effect of the diagnosis on pediatric care is poorly understood; thus, clinicians are less motivated to assess or treat the disorder. Hypoactive delirium is often misdiagnosed as depression when children appear distant, unresponsive, and isolative. Psychiatric consultations are more frequently recommended for patients with paranoia, hallucinations, and aggression. Unfortunately, these patients are often considered oppositional and defiant and are labeled as having behavior problems. Cases can also be very complicated, with multifactorial causes of delirium that include aspects of treatment as well as illness (Lawlor and Bruera 2002). The most effective treatment for delirium is the identification and management of the cause. When this is not immediately possible, care involves environmental changes that orient and calm the patient, with the addition of pharmacotherapy (antipsychotic medications) when necessary (Breitbart et al. 1996; Martini 2005).

HIV and AIDS

More than 190,000 children died of AIDS in 2013 (Avert 2014). Approximately 40% of all new HIV cases occur among people ages 15–24. Consistent with the reports for many other chronic disorders in children and adolescents, the rate of psychological problems is elevated for children and adolescents with HIV (Betancourt et al. 2013). Among children and adolescents with HIV, passive coping was most strongly associated with depression and was more common among adolescents experiencing medication-related stressors. Higher levels of parental monitoring and better quality parent-child relationship were associated with greater resilience among African American adolescents with HIV (Dutra et al. 2000).

Obesity

Definition, Epidemiology, and Comorbidity

Assessment of obesity in most settings is done via calculation of body mass index (BMI). In youth, BMI percentiles for age and gender are based on Centers for Disease Control and Prevention growth charts. A child with a BMI within the 85th to 95th percentiles is considered overweight, a child with a BMI at or above the 95th percentile is considered obese, and a child with a BMI at or above the 99th percentile is considered to have severe childhood obesity (Barlow and Expert Committee 2007).

In 1963–1970, approximately 17.1% of children and adolescents in the United States were *at risk for overweight* or *overweight* (terms that have now been replaced with *overweight* and *obese,* respectively). By 2011–2012, approximately 31.8% of children and adolescents were overweight or obese (Ogden et al. 2014). Children and adolescents who are overweight or obese are at risk for many common psychological comorbidities, including depression, eating-disordered behaviors, diminished self-esteem, body dissatisfaction, peer victimization, decreased quality of life, and higher experiences of stigma (Lowry 2010).

Psychotropic Medications as a Contributing Factor

The use of certain psychotropic medications is a strong risk factor for the development of obesity. Medications commonly associated with this effect include antipsychotics, mood stabilizers, and antidepressants (Martínez-Ortega et al. 2013). Patients and their parents should be informed prior to medication initiation of the potential risk for weight gain. Careful baseline evaluation and monitoring for weight gain and metabolic changes are required. (Please refer to Table 19–1 for specific assessment considerations.) A preventive weight maintenance or management program may be suggested at the onset of the medication trial. If problematic weight gain occurs, alternative medications may be considered, and the prescribing physician should consider the benefits of psychotropic medication carefully along with the possible medical and psychological consequences of excessive weight gain (Zametkin et al. 2004). Other treatment options may be available, such as dose adjustment or switching to an alternative medication in the same class that is less associated with weight gain (Martínez-Ortega et al. 2013).

Preliminary research has been conducted on the use of metformin to prevent excessive weight gain and/or metabolic changes associated with psychotropic medications (Jarskogt et al. 2013). More research on the safety and effectiveness of metformin in treating medication-induced obesity in youth is needed.

Psychiatric Evaluation

Mental health professionals may work with obese youth for whom weight may or may not be the primary presenting problem or even a concern of the parent or youth. It is important for the mental health professional to inquire if the child has recently completed a medical evaluation to screen for medical comorbidities and to refer if necessary, particularly if there are metabolic, sleep-disordered, or cardiovascular symptoms (e.g., acanthosis, nocturia, elevated blood pressure). Please refer to Barlow and Expert Committee (2007) for full Expert Committee recommendations regarding medical assessment.

The psychiatric evaluation of an obese youth should screen for symptoms of depression, anxiety, and eating-disordered behaviors, including "loss of control" when eating. If these symptoms are clinically significant, it is recommended that the youth undergo psychiatric treatment first or concurrently with participation in a weight management program, as untreated mental illness could adversely affect the youth's ability to effectively participate in a weight management program (Zametkin et al. 2004). In addition to a brief overview of child or adolescent functioning, overweight and obese children and teens should be screened for psychological comorbidities, including poor self-esteem and body dissatisfaction, experiences of peer victimization and stigma, and decreased quality of life. When clinically indicated, assessment of the presence of substance use is also recommended (Zametkin et al. 2004). A final area of assessment is that of parent and youth readiness to change. Many parents misperceive their child's weight status and risk and thus may fail to recognize their child as being overweight or obese (Eckstein et al. 2006). Parents and families who do not perceive risk or report concerns may not be ready to participate in interventions to change family dietary and physical activity habits. Instead, education regarding risk and motivational counseling (see Chapter 45, "Motivational Interviewing") may be a

TABLE 19–1. Obesity-related assessment considerations when prescribing psychotropic medication to youth

Baseline assessment	Ongoing assessment
Height and weight (to calculate BMI)	Height and weight (to calculate BMI)
Blood pressure	Blood pressure
Resting heart rate	Resting heart rate
Family history of weight concerns and/or medical comorbidities	Inquire for changes such as the following:
Refer for baseline lab values if clinically indicated	• More frequent urination • Unintended weight loss • Acanthosis

Note. BMI=body mass index.

more appropriate intervention until the parent and/or youth is ready to commit to more rigorous treatment (Schwartz et al. 2007; Zametkin et al. 2004).

Treatment

Treatment options for overweight or obese youth include psychotherapeutic, pharmacological, and surgical options. Most psychotherapeutic interventions include a combination of dietary changes, physical activity changes, and behavioral techniques. Evidence exists for the short- and long-term efficacy of multicomponent behavioral treatment (Janicke et al. 2014). Successful interventions often include behavior modification strategies such as self-monitoring, stimulus control, contingency management goal setting, reinforcement, problem solving, and promotion of non-food-based interests. The inclusion of parents in treatment is also encouraged.

As is the case with most pharmacological development, weight loss medications have been much more extensively studied in adults than in youth. At the time of this publication, only orlistat is approved by the FDA for use in patients ages 12 years and older.

Bariatric surgery represents a new area of research and treatment for obese youth. Mental health professionals may be involved in the medical teams as part of the presurgical evaluation process. Evaluation should include discussion of perioperative risks, postprocedural nutritional risks, and a lifelong commitment to altered dietary practices. Attendance at support group meetings prior to and following surgery has been recommended, and surgical candidates should be provided with nutritional and psychological support after surgery (Barlow and Expert Committee 2007; Inge et al. 2004).

Summary Points

- Children and adolescents with chronic illness are at increased risk for emotional adjustment problems, particularly from internalizing syndromes, including depressive and anxiety disorders that appear early and persist over time.
- The young patient's ability to cope with physical illness is affected by the interplay of personal, psychosocial, and biological factors, as well as exposure to negative life events.

- Adaptation to illness is also determined by the patient's developmental level, history of medical illness, and temperament, in addition to parental and family factors.
- Psychiatric disorders in physically ill children can affect compliance, lifestyle, and adjustment to illness and can have a direct impact on physiology and the disease process.
- Family members may be affected individually with higher rates of irritability, anxiety, depression, and somatic complaints than the general population and may become overinvolved in aspects of medical care at the expense of family needs. The demands of caring for an ill child can change relationships between parents and among parents, patient, and siblings.
- Psychopharmacological interventions are instituted when the medical team believes that the psychiatric symptoms in the child are affecting the patient's care. The physician should be aware of possible interactions between the illness and the treatment.
- Psychosocial interventions, including individual, group, and family therapies, provide an opportunity for the patient and family to express their concerns and feelings about the illness or disability.
- When treating a child with chronic physical illness, the mental health clinician should routinely address adherence, pain management, and procedural preparation.
- Pediatric obesity is associated with significant medical and psychological comorbidities, including depression, eating-disordered behaviors, poor self-esteem, peer victimization, poorer quality of life, and stigma.
- Many psychotropic medications have significant weight-gain side effects. Pediatric patients taking such medications should be carefully monitored for weight gain and obesity-related comorbidities.

References

Adler HM: The history of the present illness as treatment: who's listening, and why does it matter? J Am Board Fam Pract 10(1):28–35, 1997 9018660

American Academy of Pediatrics Committee on Children With Disabilities and Committee on Psychosocial Aspects of Child and Family Health: Psychosocial risks of chronic health conditions in childhood and adolescence. Pediatrics 92(6):876–878, 1993 8233757

Avert: Children, HIV, and AIDS, 2014. Available at www.avert.org/children-and-hiv-aids.htm. Accessed March 29, 2015.

Band EB, Weisz JR: How to feel better when it feels bad: children's perspectives on coping with everyday stress. Dev Psychol 24(2):247–253, 1988

Barakat LP, Hetzke JD, Foley B, et al: Evaluation of a social-skills training group intervention with children treated for brain tumors: a pilot study. J Pediatr Psychol 28(5):299–307, 2003 12808006

Barlow SE, Expert Committee: Expert committee recommendations regarding the prevention, assessment, and treatment of child and adolescent overweight and obesity: summary report. Pediatrics 120(suppl 4):S164–S192, 2007 18055651

Beliles KE: Psychopharmacokinetics in the medically ill, in Psychiatric Care of the Medical Patient, 2nd Edition. Edited by Stoudemire A, Fogel BS, Greenberg DB. Oxford, UK, Oxford University Press, 2000, pp 272–394

Betancourt TS, Meyers-Ohki SE, Charrow A, et al: Research review: mental health and resilience in HIV/AIDS-affected children: a review of the literature and recommendations for future research. J Child Psychol Psychiatry 54(4):423–444, 2013 22943414

Blount RL, Piira T, Cohen LL: Management of pediatric pain and distress due to medical procedures, in Handbook of Pediatric Psychology, 3rd Edition. Edited by Roberts MC. New York, Guilford, 2003, pp 216–233

Breitbart W, Marotta R, Platt MM, et al: A double-blind trial of haloperidol, chlorpromazine, and lorazepam in the treatment of delirium in hospitalized AIDS patients. Am J Psychiatry 153(2):231–237, 1996 8561204

Campis LB, DeMaso DR, Twente AW: The role of maternal factors in the adaptation of children with craniofacial disfigurement. Cleft Palate Craniofac J 32(1):55–61, 1995 7727488

Campo JV, Bridge J, Ehmann M, et al: Recurrent abdominal pain, anxiety, and depression in primary care. Pediatrics 113(4):817–824, 2004 15060233

Chow V, Feijo I, Trieu J, et al: Successful rechallenge of clozapine therapy following previous clozapine-induced myocarditis confirmed on cardiac MRI. J Child Adolesc Psychopharmacol 24(2):99–101, 2014 24521168

Clark MC, Standard PL: The caregiving story: how the narrative approach informs caregiving burden. Issues Ment Health Nurs 18(2):87–97, 1997 9256689

Dahlquist LM, Gil KM, Armstrong FD, et al: Preparing children for medical examinations: the importance of previous medical experience. Health Psychol 5(3):249–259, 1986 3527692

Delamater AM, Jacobson AM, Anderson B, et al: Psychosocial therapies in diabetes: report of the Psychosocial Therapies Working Group. Diabetes Care 24(7):1286–1292, 2001 11423517

DeMaso DR (ed): The Experience Journals. Boston, MA, Children's Hospital Boston, 2007. Available at: http://www.experiencejournal.com. Accessed May 4, 2009.

DeMaso DR, Beardslee WR, Silbert AR, et al: Psychological functioning in children with cyanotic heart defects. J Dev Behav Pediatr 11(6):289–294, 1990 2289960

DeMaso DR, Campis LK, Wypij D, et al: The impact of maternal perceptions and medical severity on the adjustment of children with congenital heart disease. J Pediatr Psychol 16(2):137–149, 1991 2061786

DeMaso DR, Twente AW, Spratt EG, et al: Impact of psychologic functioning, medical severity, and family functioning in pediatric heart transplantation. J Heart Lung Transplant 14(6 Pt 1):1102–1108, 1995 8719457

DeMaso DR, Douglas Kelley S, Bastardi H, et al: The longitudinal impact of psychological functioning, medical severity, and family functioning in pediatric heart transplantation. J Heart Lung Transplant 23(4):473–480, 2004 15063408

Drotar D: Psychological Interventions in Childhood Chronic Illness. Washington, DC, American Psychological Association, 2006

Dutra R, Forehand R, Armistead L, et al: Child resiliency in inner-city families affected by HIV: the role of family variables. Behav Res Ther 38(5):471–486, 2000 10816906

Eccleston C, Malleson PN, Clinch J, et al: Chronic pain in adolescents: evaluation of a programme of interdisciplinary cognitive behaviour therapy. Arch Dis Child 88(10):881–885, 2003 14500306

Eccleston C, Palermo TM, Fisher E, et al: Psychological interventions for parents of children and adolescents with chronic illness. Cochrane Database Syst Rev 8(8):CD009660, 2012 22895990

Eckstein KC, Mikhail LM, Ariza AJ, et al: Parents' perceptions of their child's weight and health. Pediatrics 117(3):681–690, 2006 16510647

Evans R 3rd, Gergen PJ, Mitchell H, et al: A randomized clinical trial to reduce asthma morbidity among inner-city children: results of the National Cooperative Inner-City Asthma Study. J Pediatr 135(3):332–338, 1999 10484799

Fielding D, Duff A: Compliance with treatment protocols: interventions for children with chronic illness. Arch Dis Child 80(2):196–200, 1999 10325743

Fisher L, Weihs KL: Can addressing family relationships improve outcomes in chronic disease? Report of the National

Working Group on Family Based Interventions in Chronic Disease. J Fam Pract 49(6):561–566, 2000 10923558

Folkman S, Lazarus RS: The relationship between coping and emotion: implications for theory and research. Soc Sci Med 26(3):309–317, 1988 3279520

Frank NC, Blount RL, Smith AJ, et al: Parent and staff behavior, previous child medical experience, and maternal anxiety as they relate to child procedural distress and coping. J Pediatr Psychol 20(3):277–289, 1995 7595816

Freeman MP, Freeman SA: Clinical considerations in internal medicine. Am J Med 119(6):478–481, 2006 16750958

Garrison MM, Katon WJ, Richardson LP: The impact of psychiatric comorbidities on readmissions for diabetes in youth. Diabetes Care 28(9):2150–2154, 2005 16123482

Green SA: Principles of medical psychotherapy, in Psychiatry Care of the Medical Patient. Edited by Stoudemire A, Fogel BS, Greenberg DB. Oxford, UK, Oxford University Press, 2000, pp 3–15

Gucuyener K, Erdemoglu AK, Senol S, et al: Use of methylphenidate for attention-deficit hyperactivity disorder in patients with epilepsy or electroencephalographic abnormalities. J Child Neurol 18(2):109–112, 2003 12693777

Haddad PM, Dursun SM: Neurological complications of psychiatric drugs: clinical features and management. Hum Psychopharmacol 34 (suppl 1):15–26, 2008 18098217

Hampson SE, Skinner TC, Hart J, et al: Behavioral interventions for adolescents with type 1 diabetes: how effective are they? Diabetes Care 23(9):1416–1422, 2000 10977043

Hampson SE, Skinner TC, Hart J, et al: Effects of educational and psychosocial interventions for adolescents with diabetes mellitus: a systematic review. Health Technol Assess 5(10):1–79, 2001 11319990

Hemmer SA, Pasternak JF, Zecker SG, et al: Stimulant therapy and seizure risk in children with ADHD. Pediatr Neurol 24(2):99–102, 2001 11275457

Hocking MC, Lochman JE: Applying the transactional stress and coping model to sickle cell disorder and insulin-dependent diabetes mellitus: identifying psychosocial variables related to adjustment and intervention. Clin Child Fam Psychol Rev 8(3):221–246, 2005 16151619

Holmbeck GN, Westhoven VC, Phillips WS, et al: A multimethod, multi-informant, and multidimensional perspective on psychosocial adjustment in preadolescents with spina bifida. J Consult Clin Psychol 71(4):782–796, 2003 12924683

Hubert NC, Jay SM, Saltoun M, et al: Approach-avoidance and distress in children undergoing preparation for painful medical procedures. J Clin Child Adolesc Psychol 17(3):194–202, 1988

Inge TH, Krebs NF, Garcia VF, et al: Bariatric surgery for severely overweight adolescents: concerns and recommendations. Pediatrics 114(1):217–223, 2004 15231931

Jacobs J: Family therapy in chronic medical illness, in Psychiatric Care of the Medical Patient, 2nd Edition. Edited by Stoudemire A, Fogel BS, Greenberg DB. Oxford, UK, Oxford University Press, 2000, pp 31–39

Janicke DM, Steele RG, Gayes LA, et al: Systematic review and meta-analysis of comprehensive behavioral family lifestyle interventions addressing pediatric obesity. J Pediatr Psychol 2014 Epub ahead of print

Jarskog LF, Hamer RM, Stewart DD, et al: Metformin for weight loss and metabolic control in overweight outpatients with schizophrenia and schizoaffective disorder. Am J Psychiatry 170(9):1032–1040, 2013 23846733

Kain ZN, Mayes LC, Caramico LA: Preoperative preparation in children: a cross-sectional study. J Clin Anesth 8(6):508–514, 1996 8872693

Katz ER, Rubenstein CL, Hubert NC, et al: School and social reintegration of children with cancer. J Psychosoc Oncol 6(3–4):123–140, 1988

Kazak AE, Rourke MT, Crump TA: Families and other systems in pediatric psychology, in Handbook of Pediatric Psychology, 3rd Edition. Edited by Roberts MC. New York, Guilford, 2003, pp 159–175

Knapp PK, Harris ES: Consultation-liaison in child psychiatry: a review of the past 10 years. Part I: clinical findings. J Am Acad Child Adolesc Psychiatry 37(1):17–25, 1998 9444895

Kovacs M, Mukerji P, Drash A, et al: Biomedical and psychiatric risk factors for retinopathy among children with IDDM. Diabetes Care 18(12):1592–1599, 1995 8722057

Kovacs M, Obrosky DS, Goldston D, et al: Major depressive disorder in youths with IDDM. A controlled prospective study of course and outcome. Diabetes Care 20(1):45–51, 1997 9028692

Kuppenheimer WG, Brown RT: Painful procedures in pediatric cancer. A comparison of interventions. Clin Psychol Rev 22(5):753–786, 2002 12113204

La Greca A, Bearman KJ: Adherence to pediatric treatment regimens, in Handbook of Pediatric Psychology, 3rd Edition. Edited by Roberts MC. New York, Guilford, 2003, pp 119–140

Lavigne JV, Faier-Routman J: Psychological adjustment to pediatric physical disorders: a meta-analytic review. J Pediatr Psychol 17(2):133–157, 1992 1534367

Lavigne JV, Faier-Routman J: Correlates of psychological adjustment to pediatric physical disorders: a meta-analytic review and comparison with existing models. J Dev Behav Pediatr 14(2):117–123, 1993 8473527

Lavigne JV, Ross CK, Berry SL, et al: Evaluation of a psychological treatment package for treating pain in juvenile rheumatoid arthritis. Arthritis Care Res 5(2):101–110, 1992 1390962

Lawlor PG, Bruera ED: Delirium in patients with advanced cancer. Hematol Oncol Clin North Am 16(3):701–714, 2002 12170576

Lemanek KL, Kamps J, Chung NB: Empirically supported treatments in pediatric psychology: regimen adherence. J Pediatr Psychol 26(5):253–275, 2001 11390568

Lewis M, Vitulano LA: Biopsychosocial issues and risk factors in the family when the child has a chronic illness. Child Adolesc Psychiatr Clin N Am 12(3):389–399, v, 2003 12910814

Logan DE, Scharff L: Relationships between family and parent characteristics and functional abilities in children with recurrent pain syndromes: an investigation of moderating effects on the pathway from pain to disability. J Pediatr Psychol 30(8):698–707, 2005 16093517

Lowry KW: Obesity, in Dulcan's Textbook of Child and Adolescent Psychiatry. Edited by Dulcan MK. Washington, DC, American Psychiatric Publishing, 2010, pp 383–396

Mackin P: Cardiac effects of psychiatric drugs. Hum Psychopharmacol 23 (suppl 1):3–14, 2008 18098218

Martínez-Ortega JM, Funes-Godoy S, Díaz-Atienza F, et al: Weight gain and increase of body mass index among children and adolescents treated with antipsychotics: a critical review. Eur Child Adolesc Psychiatry 22(8):457–479, 2013 23503976

Martini DR: Commentary: the diagnosis of delirium in pediatric patients. J Am Acad Child Adolesc Psychiatry 44(4):395–398, 2005 15782088

McQuaid EL, Nassau JH: Empirically supported treatments of disease-related symptoms in pediatric psychology: asthma, diabetes, and cancer. J Pediatr Psychol 24(4):305–328, 1999 10431495

Mehndiratta P, Sajatovic M: Treatments for patients with comorbid epilepsy and depression. Epilepsy Behav 28(1):36–40, 2013 23651914

Melamed BG: Putting the family back in the child. Behav Res Ther 31(3):239–247, 1993 8476398

Melamed BG, Robbins RL, Fernandez J: Factors to be considered in psychological preparation for surgery, in Advances in Developmental and Behavioral Pediatrics. Edited by Routh D, Wolraich M. New York, JAI, 1982, pp 51–72

Murphy BA: Delirium. Emerg Med Clin North Am 18(2):243–252, 2000 10767881

Newacheck PW, McManus MA, Fox HB: Prevalence and impact of chronic illness among adolescents. Am J Dis Child 145(12):1367–1373, 1991 1669662

Noeker M, Haverkamp-Krois A, Haverkamp F: Development of mental health dysfunction in childhood epilepsy. Brain Dev 27(1):5–16, 2005 15626535

Ogden CL, Carroll MD, Kit BK, et al: Prevalence of childhood and adult obesity in the United States, 2011–2012. JAMA 311(8):806–814, 2014 24570244

Pederson C, Harbaugh BL: Children's and adolescents' experiences while undergoing cardiac catheterization. Matern Child Nurs J 23(1):15–25, 1995 7791378

Perrin JM, MacLean WE Jr, Gortmaker SL, et al: Improving the psychological status of children with asthma: a randomized controlled trial. J Dev Behav Pediatr 13(4):241–247, 1992 1506461

Pinquart M, Shen Y: Behavior problems in children and adolescents with chronic physical illness: a meta-analysis. J Pediatr Psychol 36(9):1003–1016, 2011 21810623

Pless IB, Pinkerton P: Chronic Childhood Disorder: Promoting Patterns of Adjustment. Chicago, IL, Henry Kimpton, 1975

Pliszka S, American Academy of Child and Adolescent Psychiatry Work Group on Quality Issues: Practice parameter for the assessment and treatment of children and adolescents with attention-deficit/hyperactivity disorder. J Am Acad Child Adolesc Psychiatry 46(7):894–921, 2007 17581453

Robinson MD, Owen JA: Psychopharmacology, in The American Psychiatric Publishing Textbook of Psychosomatic Medicine. Edited by Levenson JL. Washington, DC, American Psychiatric Publishing, 2005, pp 871–922

Rolland JS, Walsh F: Facilitating family resilience with childhood illness and disability. Curr Opin Pediatr 18(5):527–538, 2006 16969168

Rudolph KD, Dennig MD, Weisz JR: Determinants and consequences of children's coping in the medical setting: conceptualization, review, and critique. Psychol Bull 118(3):328–357, 1995 7501740

Sabaté E (ed): Adherence to Long-Term Therapies: Evidence for Action. Geneva, Switzerland, World Health Organization, 2003

Schwartz RP, Hamre R, Dietz WH, et al: Office-based motivational interviewing to prevent childhood obesity: a feasibility study. Arch Pediatr Adolesc Med 161(5):495–501, 2007 17485627

Shaw RJ, DeMaso DR: Clinical Manual of Pediatric Psychosomatic Medicine: Mental Health Consultation With Physically Ill Children and Adolescents. Washington, DC, American Psychiatric Publishing, 2006

Shaw RJ, Palmer L, Blasey C, et al: A typology of non-adherence in pediatric renal transplant recipients. Pediatr Transplant 7(6):489–493, 2003 14870900

Siemon M: Siblings of the chronically ill or disabled child. Meeting their needs. Nurs Clin North Am 19(2):295–307, 1984 6233538

Simeonsson RJ, Buckley L, Munson L: Conceptions of illness causality in hospitalized children. J Pediatr Psychol 4:77–84, 1979

Spirito A, Kazak AE: Effective and Emerging Treatments in Pediatric Psychology. Oxford, UK, Oxford University Press, 2006

Stauffer MH: A long-term psychotherapy group for children with chronic medical illness. Bull Menninger Clin 62(1):15–32, 1998 9524378

Stuber ML, Shemesh E: Post-traumatic stress response to life-threatening illnesses in children and their parents. Child Adolesc Psychiatr Clin N Am 15(3):597–609, 2006 16797441

Stuber ML, Schneider S, Kassam-Adams N, et al: The medical traumatic stress toolkit. CNS Spectr 11(2):137–142, 2006 16520691

Szigethy E, Kenney E, Carpenter J, et al: Cognitive-behavioral therapy for adolescents with inflammatory bowel disease and subsyndromal depression. J Am Acad Child Adolesc Psychiatry 46(10):1290–1298, 2007 17885570

Thompson RJ: Coping with the stress of chronic childhood illness, in Management of Chronic Disorders of Childhood. Edited by O'Quinn AN. Boston, MA, GK Hall, 1985, pp 11–41

Thompson RJ, Gustafson KE: Adaptation to Chronic Childhood Illness. Washington, DC, American Psychological Association, 1996

Vasterling J, Jenkins RA, Tope DM, et al: Cognitive distraction and relaxation training for the control of side effects due to cancer chemotherapy. J Behav Med 16(1):65–80, 1993 8433358

Vitulano LA: Psychosocial issues for children and adolescents with chronic illness: self-esteem, school functioning and sports participation. Child Adolesc Psychiatr Clin N Am 12(3):585–592, 2003 12910824

Voican C, Naveau S, Corruble E, et al: Antidepressant-induced liver injury: A review for clinicians. Am J Psychiatry 171(4):404–415, 2014 24362450

Walco GA, Ilowite NT: Cognitive-behavioral intervention for juvenile primary fibromyalgia syndrome. J Rheumatol 19(10):1617–1619, 1992 1464878

Walco GA, Varni JW, Ilowite NT: Cognitive-behavioral pain management in children with juvenile rheumatoid arthritis. Pediatrics 89(6 Pt 1):1075–1079, 1992 1594351

Wallander JL, Varni JW: Adjustment in children with chronic physical disorders: programmatic research on a disability-stress-coping model, in Stress and Coping in Child Health. Edited by La Greca AM, Siegel LJL, Wallander JL, et al. New York, Guilford, 1992, pp 279–299

Wallander JL, Thompson RJ, Alriksson-Schmidt A: Psychosocial adjustment of children with chronic physical conditions, in Handbook of Pediatric Psychology, 3rd Edition. Edited by Roberts MC. New York, Guilford, 2003, pp 141–158

Wamboldt MZ, Fritz G, Mansell A, et al: Relationship of asthma severity and psychological problems in children. J Am Acad Child Adolesc Psychiatry 37(9):943–950, 1998 9735613

Waxmonsky J, Wood BL, Stern T, et al: Association of depressive symptoms and disease activity in children with asthma: methodological and clinical implications. J Am Acad Child Adolesc Psychiatry 45(8):945–954, 2006 16865037

Wood BL, Miller BD, Lim J, et al: Family relational factors in pediatric depression and asthma: pathways of effect. J Am Acad Child Adolesc Psychiatry 45(12):1494–1502, 2006 17135995

Wright B: Physical Disability: A Psychosocial Approach. New York, Harper and Row, 1960

Wysocki T, Harris MA, Buckloh LM, et al: Randomized, controlled trial of behavioral family systems therapy for diabetes: maintenance and generalization of effects on parent-adolescent communication. Behav Ther 39(1):33–46, 2008 18328868

Yorke J, Fleming S, Shuldham C: Psychological interventions for children with asthma. Cochrane Database Syst Rev (4):CD003272, 2005 16235317

Zametkin AJ, Zoon CK, Klein HW, et al: Psychiatric aspects of child and adolescent obesity: a review of the past 10 years. J Am Acad Child Adolesc Psychiatry 43(2):134–150, 2004 14726719

CHAPTER 20

Eating and Feeding Disorders

Kamryn T. Eddy, Ph.D.
Helen B. Murray, B.A.
Daniel Le Grange, Ph.D.

Eating and feeding disorders are characterized by aberrations in eating or feeding behaviors and occur across the age spectrum. Eating disorders are most often observed in late adolescent and young adult females, with typical onset during adolescence (ages 12–18 years). Eating disorders may be chronic and relapsing conditions and are often associated with significant medical morbidity and psychiatric comorbidity. Feeding disorders can be diagnosed across the lifespan, with childhood onset being particularly common. The etiology, maintaining factors, and treatment of eating and feeding disorders have been understudied. In DSM-5 (American Psychiatric Association 2013), eating and feeding disorders are classified together and include 1) anorexia nervosa (AN), 2) bulimia nervosa (BN), 3) binge-eating disorder (BED), 4) avoidant/restrictive food intake disorder (ARFID), 5) pica, 6) rumination disorder, 7) other specified feeding or eating disorder (OSFED), and 8) unspecified feeding or eating disorder (UFED). OSFED is a heterogeneous diagnosis replacing DSM-IV (American Psychiatric Association 1994) eating disorder not otherwise specified and capturing other specific clinically significant eating disorder presentations. UFED is a residual diagnosis capturing clinically significant feeding or eating disorder presentations for which not enough information is available to classify elsewhere.

In this chapter, we describe the diagnostic criteria for the eating and feeding disorders and consider their application to children and adolescents. We describe the epidemiology, comorbidity, and etiology of these disorders; methods of prevention; developmental course and outcome; and assessment and treatment. While we include other eating and feeding disorders where data are available, we focus on AN, BN, and BED because the most research has been conducted with these eating disorders.

Diagnosis

Anorexia Nervosa

In DSM-5, AN is described as a restriction of food intake leading to a weight that is less than minimally expected or normal. This occurs in the context of an overriding fear of weight gain or engagement in behaviors that impede weight gain as well as a lack of recognition of the physical changes that result from malnutrition (body image distortion or denial of the seriousness of the consequences of malnutrition) (Box 20–1).

Box 20–1. DSM-5 Diagnostic Criteria for Anorexia Nervosa

A. Restriction of energy intake relative to requirements, leading to a significantly low body weight in the context of age, sex, developmental trajectory, and physical health. *Significantly low weight* is defined as a weight that is less than minimally normal or, for children and adolescents, less than that minimally expected.

B. Intense fear of gaining weight or of becoming fat, or persistent behavior that interferes with weight gain, even though at a significantly low weight.

C. Disturbance in the way in which one's body weight or shape is experienced, undue influence of body weight or shape on self-evaluation, or persistent lack of recognition of the seriousness of the current low body weight.

Coding note: The ICD-9-CM code for anorexia nervosa is **307.1,** which is assigned regardless of the subtype. The ICD-10-CM code depends on the subtype (see below).

Specify whether:

(F50.01) Restricting type: During the last 3 months, the individual has not engaged in recurrent episodes of binge eating or purging behavior (i.e., self-induced vomiting or the misuse of laxatives, diuretics, or enemas). This subtype describes presentations in which weight loss is accomplished primarily through dieting, fasting, and/or excessive exercise.

(F50.02) Binge-eating/purging type: During the last 3 months, the individual has engaged in recurrent episodes of binge eating or purging behavior (i.e., self-induced vomiting or the misuse of laxatives, diuretics, or enemas).

Specify if:

In partial remission: After full criteria for anorexia nervosa were previously met, Criterion A (low body weight) has not been met for a sustained period, but either Criterion B (intense fear of gaining weight or becoming fat or behavior that interferes with weight gain) or Criterion C (disturbances in self-perception of weight and shape) is still met.

In full remission: After full criteria for anorexia nervosa were previously met, none of the criteria have been met for a sustained period of time.

Specify current severity:

The minimum level of severity is based, for adults, on current body mass index (BMI) (see below) or, for children and adolescents, on BMI percentile. The ranges below are derived from World Health Organization categories for thinness in adults; for children and adolescents, corresponding BMI percentiles should be used. The level of severity may be increased to reflect clinical symptoms, the degree of functional disability, and the need for supervision.

Mild: BMI $\geq$ 17 kg/m^2

Moderate: BMI 16–16.99 kg/m^2

Severe: BMI 15–15.99 kg/m^2

Extreme: BMI < 15 kg/m^2

Source. Reprinted from the *Diagnostic and Statistical Manual of Mental Disorders,* 5th Edition. Arlington, VA, American Psychiatric Association, 2013. Used with permission.

Bulimia Nervosa

In DSM-5, BN is characterized by recurrent episodes of binge eating and inappropriate compensatory behaviors (e.g., self-induced vomiting; misuse of laxatives, diuretics, enemas; excessive exercising; strict dieting or fasting). In addition to the behavioral component, individuals with BN are marked by beliefs and attitudes that overemphasize shape and weight as the sole or major way self-worth and self-esteem are maintained (Box 20–2).

Box 20–2. DSM-5 Diagnostic Criteria for Bulimia Nervosa

307.51 (F50.2)

A. Recurrent episodes of binge eating. An episode of binge eating is characterized by both of the following:
   1. Eating, in a discrete period of time (e.g., within any 2-hour period), an amount of food that is definitely larger than what most individuals would eat in a similar period of time under similar circumstances.
   2. A sense of lack of control over eating during the episode (e.g., a feeling that one cannot stop eating or control what or how much one is eating).

B. Recurrent inappropriate compensatory behaviors in order to prevent weight gain, such as self-induced vomiting; misuse of laxatives, diuretics, or other medications; fasting; or excessive exercise.

C. The binge eating and inappropriate compensatory behaviors both occur, on average, at least once a week for 3 months.

D. Self-evaluation is unduly influenced by body shape and weight.

E. The disturbance does not occur exclusively during episodes of anorexia nervosa.

Specify if:

In partial remission: After full criteria for bulimia nervosa were previously met, some, but not all, of the criteria have been met for a sustained period of time.

In full remission: After full criteria for bulimia nervosa were previously met, none of the criteria have been met for a sustained period of time.

Specify current severity:

The minimum level of severity is based on the frequency of inappropriate compensatory behaviors (see below). The level of severity may be increased to reflect other symptoms and the degree of functional disability.

Mild: An average of 1–3 episodes of inappropriate compensatory behaviors per week.

Moderate: An average of 4–7 episodes of inappropriate compensatory behaviors per week.

Severe: An average of 8–13 episodes of inappropriate compensatory behaviors per week.

Extreme: An average of 14 or more episodes of inappropriate compensatory behaviors per week.

Source. Reprinted from the *Diagnostic and Statistical Manual of Mental Disorders*, 5th Edition. Arlington, VA, American Psychiatric Association, 2013. Used with permission.

Binge-Eating Disorder

Formerly a research diagnosis in DSM-IV-TR (American Psychiatric Association 2000a), in DSM-5 BED is a full-threshold eating disorder characterized by recurrent episodes of binge eating that are associated with distress and impairment and occur in the absence of inappropriate compensatory behavior (Box 20–3).

Box 20–3. DSM-5 Diagnostic Criteria for Binge-Eating Disorder

307.51 (F50.8)

A. Recurrent episodes of binge eating. An episode of binge eating is characterized by both of the following:
   1. Eating, in a discrete period of time (e.g., within any 2-hour period), an amount of food that is definitely larger than what most people would eat in a similar period of time under similar circumstances.
   2. A sense of lack of control over eating during the episode (e.g., a feeling that one cannot stop eating or control what or how much one is eating).

B. The binge-eating episodes are associated with three (or more) of the following:
   1. Eating much more rapidly than normal.
   2. Eating until feeling uncomfortably full.
   3. Eating large amounts of food when not feeling physically hungry.
   4. Eating alone because of feeling embarrassed by how much one is eating.
   5. Feeling disgusted with oneself, depressed, or very guilty afterward.

C. Marked distress regarding binge eating is present.

D. The binge eating occurs, on average, at least once a week for 3 months.

E. The binge eating is not associated with the recurrent use of inappropriate compensatory behavior as in bulimia nervosa and does not occur exclusively during the course of bulimia nervosa or anorexia nervosa.

Specify if:

In partial remission: After full criteria for binge-eating disorder were previously met, binge eating occurs at an average frequency of less than one episode per week for a sustained period of time.

In full remission: After full criteria for binge-eating disorder were previously met, none of the criteria have been met for a sustained period of time.

Specify current severity:

The minimum level of severity is based on the frequency of episodes of binge eating (see below). The level of severity may be increased to reflect other symptoms and the degree of functional disability.

Mild: 1–3 binge-eating episodes per week.

Moderate: 4–7 binge-eating episodes per week.

Severe: 8–13 binge-eating episodes per week.

Extreme: 14 or more binge-eating episodes per week.

Source. Reprinted from the *Diagnostic and Statistical Manual of Mental Disorders*, 5th Edition. Arlington VA, American Psychiatric Association, 2013. Used with permission.

Avoidant/Restrictive Food Intake Disorder

DSM-5 ARFID is a reformulation of DSM-IV *feeding disorder of infancy or early childhood*. In DSM-5, ARFID is characterized by a failure to meet energy or nutritional requirements through restriction or food avoidance in the absence of body image disturbance or fat phobia. Avoidant/restrictive eating behavior in ARFID may be motivated by lack of interest in eating or foods, sensitivity (e.g., to tastes, textures, smells), or traumatic experience (e.g., choking).

Pica

In DSM-5, pica is described as the persistent consumption of "nonnutritive, nonfood" substances, such as chalk or paper, that is not developmentally appropriate and is not culturally or socially normative. Although a diagnosis of pica can be made in conjunction with another feeding or eating disorder, to warrant independent diagnosis the ingestion of nonfood items must not primarily be for appetite reduction or weight control purposes.

Rumination Disorder

Rumination disorder is the recurrent regurgitation of food that frequently is described as involuntary or habitual. Weight loss, lack of expected weight gain, or malnutrition may occur, particularly in infants. The diagnosis should be differentiated from other gastrointestinal conditions that may present similarly and cannot be made in conjunction with AN, BN, BED, or ARFID.

Other Specified Feeding or Eating Disorder and Unspecified Feeding or Eating Disorder

OSFED is a diagnostic category comprising individuals with a range of clinically significant eating disorder symptom presentations. DSM-5 names five example presentations: atypical anorexia nervosa, bulimia nervosa (of low frequency and/or limited duration) (hereinafter referred to as subthreshold BN), binge-eating disorder (of low frequency and/or limited duration) (hereinafter referred to as subthreshold BED), purging disorder, and night eating syndrome. Individuals with OSFED other have a specific feeding or eating presentation that does not fall into one of the five example types. For cases in which there is not enough information to confer a diagnosis, such as in an emergency department setting, a diagnosis of UFED can be used.

Application of DSM-5 Criteria to Younger Populations

Children and adolescents can have a wide range of symptom presentations that may differ from those observed in adults (Eddy et al. 2008a). In DSM-5 there are specific provisions for the diagnosis of eating and feeding disorders in children and adolescents.

Eating Disorders

Within the diagnosis of AN, DSM-5 language regarding definition of low weight and operationalization of fat phobia and body image disturbance is sensitive to developmental variations. While the DSM-5 text description provides an example of low weight in children and adolescents as a BMI-for-age that is below the 5th percentile, AN criterion A is designed to allow for clinical judgment without specifying a firm cutoff for operationalizing low weight. This provision allows for the recognition of low weight in an individual who has fallen off of his or her growth curve, even if he or she has not reached the 5th percentile. Further, report of fat phobia (criterion B) no longer needs to be explicit; instead, DSM-5 allows for clinical judgment and inference of cognitive symptoms. For example, unlike older adolescent or adult patients who may explicitly endorse drive for thinness, younger patients may have limited insight into the motives for their behavior or report wishes to be healthy rather than to be thin. A clinician may infer presence of eating disorder cognitions if the individual is engaging in behaviors that interfere with weight gain. In addition, while youth often do not report body image distortion or fat phobia, they more clearly deny—through their actions and/or words—the seriousness of their current low weight, which is captured in criterion C. However, although DSM-5 broadened the criteria for AN to allow for clinical judgment regarding fat phobia and body image disturbance, BN criteria require explicit endorsement of body image disturbance. Interestingly, BED has no criteria regarding body image concerns.

Across the eating disorders, the definition of and frequency criteria for binge eating in children and adolescents can be complicated (Kelly et al. 2014), and there are no specific provisions for ascertaining whether an overeating episode constitutes a binge in youth. For example, it can be difficult to assess whether the quantity of food is objectively large for a growing child or adolescent, and the importance of size of episode (amount of food eaten) might not be as good of an indicator as the presence of loss of control (Shomaker et al. 2010). Further, binge episodes may occur less frequently in children and adolescents than in adults. These challenges in applying BN or BED criteria to youth are important and suggest that overeating-type disturbances may be significant even if threshold criteria are not met.

Feeding Disorders

DSM-IV captured feeding disorders within the section "Disorders Usually First Diagnosed in Infancy, Childhood, or Adolescence," implying that feeding disorders must have onset in youth. The DSM-5 reorganization unifies feeding and eating disorders into a single category, allowing for the recognition that the feeding disorders can have onset at any age. DSM-5 includes descriptions of a few diagnostic considerations specific to children and adolescents: 1) "picky" eating in young children can be normative and should be differentiated carefully from ARFID; 2) a minimum age of 2 years is suggested for diagnosis of pica; and 3) rumination in infants is typically described as the head arched back with tongue sucking movements and associated irritability between episodes. Additionally, an important distinction between ARFID and AN is that ARFID presents with neither endorsement of fat phobia/body image disturbance nor engagement in weight-driven behaviors.

Epidemiology

Epidemiological research in child and adolescent eating and feeding disorders is limited, and existing data are based on DSM-IV-TR diagnostic categories. Research describing the DSM-5 prevalence, demographic characteristics, and clinical characteristics—particularly in the case of OSFED, ARFID, pica, and rumination disorder—is needed.

Eating Disorders

The National Comorbidity Survey Replication (NCS-R), which included a representative sample of males and females ages 15–18 years, reported the lifetime prevalence of DSM-IV AN, BN, and BED to be 0.3%, 0.9%, and 1.6%, respectively. Although subthreshold AN and subthreshold BED were categorized by DSM-IV as *eating disorder not otherwise specified*, the study reported lifetime prevalence rates of 0.8% and 2.5%, respectively (Swanson et al. 2011). While AN typically has onset during mid to late adolescence, the age of onset of BN tends to be in later adolescence (Fairburn et al. 2000; Le Grange et al. 2004). The age of onset in BED is not as well studied, but development of some features of BED, such as loss of control over eating in youth, might be prodromal to development of full-threshold BED. Note that for all eating disorders, onset can occur at any age. Interestingly, there is some suggestion that BN has decreased in prevalence within the last decade for females (Keel et al. 2006).

Feeding Disorders

Prevalence data on feeding disorders are currently limited to clinical samples. In adolescent medicine clinics, 14% of individuals seeking initial eating disorder evaluations received a diagnosis of ARFID (Fisher et al. 2014; Ornstein et al. 2013), and in a sample of pediatric gastroenterology patients, 1.5% of consecutive referrals were identified as ARFID cases (Eddy et al. 2014). The prevalence of DSM-5 pica and rumination is even less studied in both adults and youth. A recent study of 149 adolescent females in a residential treatment center for patients with eating disorders found low rates of DSM-5 pica and no cases of DSM-5 rumination disorder, but the frequency of "pica eating" (i.e., eating ice, uncooked pasta) and rumination behavior each was 7.4% (Delaney et al. 2014).

Comorbidity

Eating Disorders

Several studies of adults suggest that comorbid psychiatric illness is common in patients with eating disorders. Estimates of the lifetime prevalence of mood disorders range from 50% to 80%, and comorbid anxiety disorders are seen in 30%–65% of individuals with AN and BN (Herzog et al. 1996; Johnson et al. 2002). While less is known about comorbidity among adolescents with eating disorders, preliminary research suggests that similar patterns apply. Data from the NCS-R reported a pervasive lifetime psychiatric comorbidity for adolescents with eating disorders, particularly associated with diagnoses of BN and BED. In clinical samples, common comorbidities include anxiety and depression. Substance use or abuse may also occur (Fischer and le Grange 2007; Lock et al. 2006). Of note, one study reported higher rates of substance abuse and posttraumatic stress disorder in women who developed binge-eating behavior in youth (Brewerton et al. 2014). More longitudinal research is needed to assess the relationship between onset of child and adolescent eating disorder and psychiatric comorbidity.

Further, some researchers have described three personality subtypes among individuals with eating disorders (regardless of diagnosis): 1) a group of high-functioning and perfectionistic individuals, 2) a group of individuals who tend to be more constricted and overcontrolled, and 3) a group that tends to be more emotionally dysregulated and undercontrolled (Westen and Harnden-Fischer 2001). Inquiry into personality differences has suggested that different personality subtypes exist among adolescents with eating disorders (e.g., Thompson-Brenner et al. 2008). Adolescents with AN tend to be more avoidant, inhibited, and constricted with regard to personality style, while those with bulimic symptoms tend to be more affectively labile and undercontrolled (Thompson-Brenner et al. 2008).

Feeding Disorders

Limited research exists on comorbidity in feeding disorders. ARFID is often comorbid with anxiety disorders, neurodevelopmental disorders including autism spectrum disorders, and gastrointestinal complaints (American Psychiatric Association 2013; Fisher et al. 2014). Individuals diagnosed with pica may also present with a co-occurring intellectual disability or autism spectrum disorder and might exhibit symptoms of ARFID. Rumination disorder, on the other hand, might present concurrently with a medical condition or symptoms of an anxiety disorder or other mental disorder. Pica often co-occurs with intellectual disability or autism spectrum disorder and to a lesser degree with schizophrenia or obsessive-compulsive disorder. Rumination disorder similarly often co-occurs with intellectual disability. Across the feeding disorders coexisting medical problems may precede or be coincident with the feeding or eating difficulty.

Etiology and Risks for Adolescent Eating Disorders

While the pathogenesis of eating and feeding disorders remains unknown, it is likely multidimensional and influenced by biological, psychological, and sociocultural factors. A developmental psychopathological perspective on eating disorders postulates that certain biological vulnerabilities interact with the individual's exposure to a range of experiences (e.g., parenting that overemphasizes physical appearance, abuse, popular or social media) that then influence beliefs and behaviors that support the development of eating disorders (Lock et al. 2001; Steiner et al. 2003). A convergence of these biological, familial, and sociocultural influences reaches a critical threshold for those adolescents who develop an eating disorder. Importantly, less is known about the etiology of feeding disorders; therefore, in this section we focus on etiological models of eating disorders.

Vulnerability to the development of an eating disorder may be due to underlying biological factors. Heritable causation is suggested by familial clustering of eating disorders and eating attitudes (Kendler et al. 1995). There are no adequate longitudinal studies that control for shared and nonshared environments. Even so, a recent review suggests that heritability estimates range from 22% to 76% for AN and subthreshold AN, from 52% to 62% for BN and subthreshold BN, and 57% in the single study of BED (Mitchison and Hay 2014). Investigation of specific genes requires large samples and has focused to date on genes involved in reward function, mood, and appetite. Neurobiological research has also demonstrated hormonal and neurohormonal systems differences in adult and late adolescent individuals with eating disorders (Kaye et al. 2013). The degree to which these differences represent premorbid risk factors as opposed to secondary effects of disordered eating and starvation remains unclear, particularly as some of these differences normalize after refeeding. Further, there is less research in adolescents. Neuroimaging studies suggest that there may be differences in serotonergic activity between individuals with AN and those with BN, although these findings are not definitive. For example, low levels of the neurotransmitter 5-hydroxytryptamine (serotonin) appear to be associated with binge-eating behaviors (Steiger et al. 2001). Dysregulated serotonin levels persist after recovery in individuals with AN (Frank et al. 2004) and BN (Kaye et al. 1998). Further, the monoamine deficiencies in BN also persist following recovery. These persistent neurobiological findings suggest that neurochemical alterations may contribute to the development of eating disorders.

Early experiences in one's family have been postulated to increase the developmental risk for eating disorders. Some research suggests that families of patients with AN are more controlling and organized compared with the families of patients with BN, which by comparison appear to be more chaotic, conflicted, and critical (Hoste and le Grange 2008). However, comparisons with families with other psychopathology or nonclinical families have shown that these features are not uniquely associated with eating disorders (Casper and Troiani 2001). Further, high levels of emotionality may also be a natural response in the context of the family of an individual with an eating disorder; thus, it can be difficult to make inferences about cause and effect. Any potential role played by the family process in the etiology of eating disorders remains undetermined.

Interestingly, there appears to be no clear continuity between eating problems in early childhood, such as failure to thrive or picky eating, or frank feeding disorders, and the development of eating disorders during adolescence. Epidemiological research suggests that a significant minority of children express the desire to be thinner and try to lose weight. However, less than 10% of these children score in the pathological range on a standard questionnaire of eating disorder pathology (Schur et al. 2000). Generally, girls endorse a desire to be thinner, while boys' weight/shape concerns are more focused on wishes to be bigger or more muscular (Field et al. 2014). These observations are consistent with gender-specific weight and shape concerns among adolescents, suggesting continuity between school-age children and adolescents in this respect.

A somewhat exaggerated focus on weight, shape, and dieting may be normative for many adolescents and could give rise to experimentation with various weight loss strategies, which may then increase risk for the development of eating disorders (Steiner et al. 2003). This increased focus on bodily appearance comes at a time when sexual attractiveness, social acceptance, and the ability to undertake actions related to these issues, independently of parents, are taking center stage and probably increase the likelihood of adolescents developing eating disorders. As adolescent girls grow older, they appear to be less satisfied with their weight. This dissatisfaction is compounded by perceived media preference for lower weight (McCabe et al. 2002). It is therefore not surprising that dieting behaviors increase from middle school years (11–13 years of age) through adolescence, and it is estimated that dieting behavior may be as high as 60%–70% among high school girls. In a test of the hypothesis that the development of eating problems is related to the onset of puberty, Attie and Brooks-Gunn (1989) prospectively followed 193 girls (seventh to tenth grade) for 2 years. They found that eating problems emerged in response to pubertal change, in particular the associated adipose accumulation, and that girls who were most dissatisfied with their bodies at puberty were at the highest risk for the development of eating difficulties. Other challenges typical of adolescence may also contribute to the development of an eating disorder (e.g., teasing by peers, discomfort in discussing problems with parents, maternal preoccupation with dietary restriction).

Sociocultural risk factors such as the influence of the media, especially the thin ideal of the fashion industry, may be relevant to the development of eating disorders (McCabe et al. 2002). Exposure to these thin ideals may give rise to body dissatisfaction and disordered eating behaviors among young females (Ohring et al. 2002), while an increased emphasis on muscularity and lower body fat leads to increased shape and weight concerns and eating disorders in males (Leit et al. 2001). Migrating to a Western culture and the associated acculturation stress also pose some risk (Gunewardene et al. 2001; Le Grange et al. 2006). Eating-disordered behaviors serve to increase social acceptance and provide comfort in this new environment.

Prevention

Ciao et al. (2014) provide a concise summary of the published controlled studies that have evaluated the mostly school-based eating disorder prevention programs. Several research-based interventions have been able to bring about improved knowledge about eating disorders and positive changes in eating attitudes. Programs that focus on addressing changes in specific risk factors (i.e., thin-ideal internalization, body dissatisfaction, negative affect) have shown improvement in or prevention of eating disorder behaviors. One project reviewed is the Body Project, which has shown reliable long-term reductions in thin-ideal internalization, body dissatisfaction, and risk for future eating disorder onset (Stice et al. 2008). The Body Project is a manualized dissonance-based prevention program that has been implemented in high school and college settings, but preliminary findings also show promise for implementation both in the middle school setting (Rohde et al. 2014) and via the Internet (Stice et al. 2012).

Prevention of feeding disorders is less studied. As neglect may increase risk for pica and rumination disorder, parental supervision and guidance around parenting and feeding practices may be useful.

Developmental Course and Outcomes

The longitudinal course of the eating and feeding disorders in children and adolescents suggests that the prognosis is generally favorable. While course of illness can be protracted or relapsing, particularly in adults, in children and adolescents improvement and recovery are expected, especially with early intervention. The literature on adults demonstrates diagnostic crossover among the eating disorders (Eddy et al. 2008b). Fewer data on the natural course of the feeding disorders are available.

Eating Disorders

By definition, AN is associated with low weight and, in turn, significant medical sequelae. Malnutrition is accompanied by evidence of physiological compromise (e.g., lowered body temperature, amenorrhea, hypotension, changes in skin and hair texture and growth), along with changes in growth hormone, hypothalamic hypogonadism, bone marrow hypoplasia, structural brain abnormalities, cardiac dysfunction, and gastrointestinal difficulties. For children and adolescents, these changes are more pronounced because of their occurrence during significant stages of physical (and psychological) development. For adolescents with AN, the potential for significant growth retardation, pubertal delay or interruption, and peak bone mass reduction is significant. Osteopenia and osteoporosis are common—secondary to low weight in AN—and although bone mineral density improves somewhat with weight gain, osteopenia often persists (Misra and Klibanski 2006). Acutely, bradycardia (very slow heart rate), hypothermia (very low body temperature), and dehydration may become life threatening (Fisher et al. 1995). Along with the physical effects of the illness come a range of psychological and social impairments, even if academic and vocational functioning are good.

Longitudinal research in adults with AN demonstrates mixed findings. Meta-analytic review of 119 studies including nearly 6,000 patients with AN indicated that over long-term follow-up, less than half of surviving patients achieve full recovery, one-third improve but continue to experience eating disorder symptoms, and one-fifth remain chronically ill (Steinhausen 2002). For adolescents, however, the course and outcome seem to be more favorable. In one longitudinal study of adolescents receiving inpatient treatment for AN, the vast majority (approximately 75%) achieved full recovery, with a median time to recovery of 5 years following participation in an intensive 6-month inpatient treatment (Strober et al. 1997). Further, follow-up studies of children and adolescents participating in family-based therapy for AN indicate substantial improvement and recovery with treatment (Le Grange and Lock 2005).

In adults with AN, premature mortality risk is increased. Meta-analyses indicate that they are approximately 5 times more likely to die prematurely and 18 times more likely to die by suicide. (Franko et al. 2013; Keshaviah et al. 2014).

BN is similarly associated with significant medical morbidity and may in addition lead to social impairment secondary to shame and the secrecy of the bulimic behaviors. While weight in patients with BN may fluctuate, it generally remains in the healthy range. Instead, complications are secondary to binge/purge behaviors and include hypokalemia, esophageal tears, gastric disturbances, dehydration, and severe changes in blood pressure or heart rate when standing or sitting (orthostasis), which may require intermittent hospitalization (Fisher et al. 2001). Reported mortality rates are not increased in BN, although death may occur as a result of any of the above factors. In terms of the social impairment, with increased entrenchment of the disorder, a significant portion of the adolescent's day-to-day life is organized around the management of binge eating and the compensatory activities related to it. The adolescent may become more irritable, exhibit social withdrawal, demonstrate a decline in school performance, and report an increase in depressed mood. Further adding to the burden of BN is the frequently reported occurrence of other impulsive behaviors, such as alcohol use and shoplifting.

Longitudinal research indicates that the course of BN is unstable, with the vast majority of individuals with BN achieving some symptom relief over time and approximately 50% reaching full recovery (for a review, see Keel and Mitchell 1997). Currently, long-term outcome studies are not available for adolescents with BN. Treatment studies show that with cognitive-behavioral guided self-care, fewer than 20% of patients are binge and purge abstinent at the end of treatment (Schmidt et al. 2007), compared with an abstinence rate of 39% for participants in family-based treatment (FBT; Le Grange et al. 2007). Diagnostic crossover from BN to AN is less common, occurring in up to one-quarter of patients (Eddy et al. 2002, 2008b).

Feeding Disorders

Less is known about the course and prognosis of the feeding disorders. ARFID often has onset in early childhood and can persist into adulthood. By definition it is associated with nutritional or psychosocial consequences, which substantiate the need for treatment. Pica can be associated with significant medical complications, including obstructions or poisoning depending on the substances ingested. The course of rumination disorder can be episodic or protracted, and the malnutrition associated with regurgitation or restriction can be severe.

Evaluation of Patients With Eating and Feeding Disorders

Children and adolescents with eating and feeding disorders are often referred by a concerned pediatrician, although both parents and pediatricians may be reluctant to make a referral to psychiatric services. This reluctance may be due to a resistance to ascribe the eating behaviors to psychological factors that may incite feelings of shame or guilt in parents or due to a difficulty finding adequate or affordable mental health services. Youth with eating disorders often deny or minimize symptoms—either unconsciously, because of a distorted perception of their behavior and attitudes, or consciously, in an effort to keep clinicians and parents from recognizing the severity of their symptoms. Similarly, youth with feeding disorders may have limited insight into the problematic nature of their behaviors or be resistant to endorsing them as such. Consequently, it is always necessary for the clinician to meet with the child or adolescent as well as his or her parents in order to obtain a more complete perspective on the referral.

Interview With the Child or Adolescent

The assessment should start with a meeting with the child or adolescent. This meeting provides a developmentally appropriate "entry" into the family and demonstrates respect for the adolescent's developing identity. While many patients with an eating disorder might present a hostile, defensive, or challenging stance, the assessor should communicate support and warmth and ask open-ended questions to facilitate a better understanding of the individual patient and his or her family. The aims of this evaluation should include obtaining an understanding of some of the potential triggers that gave rise to eating or feeding disorder behavior—for example, exposure to weight-related comments (e.g., teasing), onset of menses, experience with dating, family environment (e.g., quarrels or conflicts), experience with transitions (e.g., academic milestones, friendship or romantic relationship breakups, losses, traumas), exposure to dieting (e.g., in social circle, in family), or an aversive experience with food. For patients with eating disorders, a comprehensive assessment should include information about history of weight loss efforts, including calorie counting, restricting fat intake, restricting protein or meats, fasting or skipping meals, limiting fluid consumption, increased physical activity, avoidance of eating with others, eating in secret, hoarding food, binge eating, secretive eating, purging, and use of stimulants or diet pills. Additionally, intake evaluation should include inquiry about cognitions related to eating, weight, and shape (e.g., degree of body dissatisfaction).

Determining pretreatment levels of restriction, binge eating, compensatory behaviors, severity of weight and shape concerns, and preoccupation with eating is important, as these become targets of intervention. AN is characterized by a cascade of restricting activities that typically starts with the exclusion of fats and sugars from the diet. Restricting proteins and meats follows and, finally, restricting amounts. Although BN is also characterized by periods of dietary restriction, among individuals with BN these periods are less prolonged and are interrupted by lapses into binge eating and subsequently compensatory behaviors. For individuals with BN, patterns of failed dietary restriction, binge eating, and compensatory behaviors become cyclic. A binge may be *objective* (eating an amount in a finite period that is significantly more than for the average person) or *subjective* (eating a normal amount of food but feeling out of control at the time of eating) (American Psychiatric Association 2013). While patients can present with both types of binge eating, AN patients are more likely than the typical BN patient to report exclusively subjective binge eating.

Interview With Parents

Once the meeting with the child or adolescent has concluded, the parents should be interviewed with and without the patient. In two-parent families, it is preferable for both to be present. The parents are able to provide more general information about the patient's development, such as complications during pregnancy, early feeding patterns, timing of developmental milestones, attachment style, transitions to preschool and elementary school, early temperament and personality, and family and peer relationships. The clinician should use the information obtained during the interview with the child or adolescent, compare it with the parents' version of events, and explore commonalties as well as differences. Together, both perspectives generate a comprehensive narrative of the events leading up to and sustaining the current clinical presentation.

Medical Examination

Because eating and feeding disorders can have profound medical complications, both medical and nutritional assessments are imperative. Clinicians conducting these assessments should be well versed in the medical aspects of malnutrition and binge-eating and purging behaviors to assess any medical problems that may be present. Patients with eating disorders often complain of dizziness, headaches, fainting spells, weakness, poor concentration, stomach and abdominal pain, and amenorrhea. Individuals who engage in binge eating and purging commonly report throat pain or blood in emesis and are observed to have small dotlike lesions in the sclera of the eyes and swollen neck glands.

Standard medical assessment of an adolescent with an eating disorder would include 1) a complete physical to screen for signs of malnutrition or purging (e.g., dehydration, tooth erosion, lanugo) and 2) laboratory tests to identify any abnormalities in blood, liver, and thyroid functioning. For individuals with feeding disorders a gastrointestinal investigation may also be useful. Medical assessment is helpful in determining the severity and chronicity of illness, and it is also needed to determine a differential diagnosis. Physical disorders such as diabetes mellitus, colitis, thyroid disease, Addison disease, and brain tumors, among others, all may display clinical symptoms similar to those of AN. Similarly, neurological disorders that affect appetite regulation and eating patterns, gastrointestinal conditions, and hormonal disorders affecting metabolism may manifest symptoms similar to those of BN. When conducting a physical assessment of individuals with eating disorders, these medical conditions should be evaluated and ruled out before proceeding with treatment targeting AN or BN.

A consultation between parents and a dietitian with expertise in working with children and adolescents with eating and feeding disorders can be helpful in providing educational advice (to the parents) about the requirements of proper nutrition for restoring optimal health.

Psychometric Assessment

Specific structured interviews to evaluate eating disorder symptoms and confirm diagnosis are available. The most common screening instrument, the Eating Disorder Examination (EDE), is available for adults and older adolescents (Cooper and Fairburn 1987), as well as a version designed for use with children and young adolescents (Bryant-Waugh et al. 1996). Several self-report and parent report measures of eating and feeding disorder psychopathology are available. Such standardized interview and questionnaire assessments are clinically useful, as they allow for the monitoring of progress over time, particularly with regard to specific symptoms.

Treatment for Children and Adolescents With Eating and Feeding Disorders

Children and adolescents with eating and feeding disorders require comprehensive psychiatric and medical care (Commission on Adolescent Eating Disorders 2005). Generally, a team approach is recommended to provide mental health care, medical treatment, and nutritional guidance. Level and intensity of treatment vary from outpatient treatment to partial hospitalization to inpatient treatment. While decisions about level of care should be made on the basis of clinical severity, they may also be driven by availability of resources and third-party coverage.

Currently, there are relatively few clinical treatment guidelines for eating disorders. Methods of effective intervention differ somewhat according to the eating disorder diagnosis, and there are no clinical treatment guidelines for feeding disorders. For AN, inpatient treatment as well as one of two established outpatient approaches (FBT and adolescent-focused therapy) are generally implemented. In contrast, for adolescent BN, cognitive-behavioral therapy (CBT) and FBT are the only therapy approaches that have been investigated. Overall, pharmacotherapy for adolescent eating and feeding disorders has received little, if any, attention. Investigation into the effective treatment of eating disorders has accumulated substantial evidence for the efficacy of CBT and interpersonal therapy (IPT) for adult BN and BED but has lagged behind in the study of treatments for adult AN. No randomized controlled trials (RCTs) have been conducted in the treatment of the feeding disorders, and, consequently, less is known about best treatments for these problems. CBT, behavioral modification approaches, and family-based or parent guidance approaches are most often implemented.

Eating Disorders

Inpatient Treatment

A subset of patients will require inpatient treatment on the basis of physical or psychological health. The American Psychiatric Association (2000b) and the Society for Adolescent Medicine (Golden et al. 2003) have articulated the criteria for admission to an inpatient setting. Admission to a pediatric ward is warranted in the presence of severe and persistent medical complications that include, but are not limited to, weight 75% or less of ideal body weight, hypoglycemic syncope, fluid and electrolyte imbalance, cardiac arrhythmia, and severe dehydration. Medium-term (a few weeks) and longer-term (a month or more) admissions to a psychiatric facility that specializes in the treatment of eating disorders should be considered for severely underweight patients, particularly those who have been unresponsive to outpatient efforts at weight restoration, as well as those patients who present with serious comorbid psychiatric conditions that warrant more intensive supervision and treatment. For a more detailed description of inpatient treatment for eating disorders, see Golden et al. (2003), and for a more detailed description of appropriate refeeding regimens for medically unstable adolescents with AN, see Garber et al. (2013).

Three randomized clinical trials have been conducted to evaluate the efficacy of inpatient treatment relative to outpatient psychotherapy (Gowers et al. 2007), day-patient treatment (Herpertz-Dahlmann et al. 2014), and duration of inpatient treatment (to medical stability vs. 90% of expected body weight [EBW]) (Madden et al. 2014). Each of these studies underscores the limited efficacy of inpatient treatment and emphasizes the need to examine and use outpatient care more vigorously.

Psychotherapy

Family-Based Treatment

FBT, a short-term outpatient therapy approach first developed at the Maudsley Hospital in London, has received the most empirical study and strongest support for the treatment of adolescent eating disorders. Philosophically, FBT is pragmatic and present-oriented and involves parents in taking an active approach to targeting symptoms through parent-guided behavioral change in the child or adolescent. FBT targets restrictive eating and low weight in AN and focuses on interrupting the restricting and binge/purge cycles in BN.

In adolescent AN, different forms of FBT and individual therapy have been compared in a number of studies across several academic centers internationally (Eisler et al. 2000; Le Grange et al. 1992; Lock et al. 2005, 2010; Robin et al. 1999). In the first of these studies, the Maudsley group (Eisler et al. 2000; Le Grange et al. 1992) compared conjoint FBT and separated FBT. While the treatments were similar, in the separated form the adolescent was seen independently from the parents, albeit by the same therapist. The investigators found that regardless of the type of family treatment, approximately 70% of patients had no further eating disorder symptoms at the end of treatment. Similar to the long-term outcome of the original Maudsley study (Eisler et al. 1997), patients continued to improve in Eisler's study after treatment ended (Eisler et al. 2000). Results from a 5-year follow-up show that regardless of the type of family treatment, 75% of patients had no further eating disorder symptoms, no deaths occurred in this cohort of 40 patients, and only 8% of those who achieved a healthy weight at the end of treatment reported any kind of relapse at follow-up (Eisler et al. 2007).

Following the Maudsley work, the first study of family therapy for AN in the United States (Robin et al. 1999) compared two outpatient interventions in a controlled trial in a design that resembled the Maudsley investigations. The researchers compared behavioral systems family therapy (BSFT) with an ego-oriented individual therapy (EOIT) and reported significant improvement in AN symptoms at the end of treatment, regardless of treatment. More than two-thirds (67%) of patients reached target weight, and 80% regained menstruation. Patients continued to improve, and at 1-year follow-up, approximately 75% had reached their target weight and 85% had started or resumed menses. Meaningful differences were found between the two treatments. Patients in BSFT achieved significantly greater weight gain than those in EOIT, both at the end of treatment and at follow-up. Similarly, patients who received BSFT were significantly more likely to have returned to normal menstrual functioning at the end of treatment compared with those in EOIT. Both treatments were similar in terms of improvements in eating attitudes, depression, and self-reported eating-related family conflict. Neither group reported much family-related conflict regarding eating, either before or after treatment. Robin and colleagues concluded that BSFT produced greater weight gain and higher rates of resumption of menstruation compared with EOIT. While both treatments produced comparable improvements in eating attitudes and depression, BSFT produced a more rapid treatment response.

The fourth controlled study following the original work of the Maudsley group was conducted by Lock et al. (2005). In this randomized dose study, participants were allocated to either 10 sessions of manualized family-based treatment for AN (FBT-AN) delivered over 6 months or 20 sessions of FBT-AN over 12 months. For both treatment groups, these authors found significant weight gain and improvements in psychological symptoms of AN, as measured by the EDE. A 4-year follow-up confirmed that these initial weight gains and improvements in psychological symptoms were maintained, again showing no differences between the short- and long-term treatments (Lock et al. 2006).

The fifth controlled trial to be published was conducted in a two-site collaborative study at Stanford University and the University of Chicago (Lock et al. 2010). In this study, 121 medically stable adolescents with AN were randomly assigned to FBT-AN or individual adolescent-focused therapy (AFT). (AFT is an adaptation of EOIT that was developed for the Robin et al. [1999] study.) Participants received outpatient treatment for 12 months and were followed up at 6 and 12 months. Remission was defined as at or above 95% EBW *plus* within 1 standard deviation of the community norm on the EDE global score (Cooper and Fairburn 1987). FBT-AN was superior to AFT at both 6- and 12-month follow-up. An examination of moderators of treatment outcome in this study demonstrated that participants

TABLE 20–1. Three phases of family-based treatment of anorexia nervosa

Phase 1: Restoring the adolescent's weight Treatment is focused on the eating disorder symptoms and includes a family meal. Families are encouraged, with guidance from the therapist, to work out for themselves how best to restore weight for their anorexic child.

Phase 2: Handing control over eating back to the adolescent The start of the second phase of treatment is usually signaled by the adolescent's acquiescence to the demands of the parents to increase his or her food intake and a positive change in the mood of the family. Symptoms remain central in the discussions, while weight gain with minimum tension is encouraged. All other issues that the family has had to postpone throughout the first phase of treatment can now be brought forward for review.

Phase 3: Discussion of adolescent development The third phase is usually initiated when the adolescent has achieved and maintained a healthy weight and self-starvation has abated. Central to the discussion for this part of treatment is the establishment of a healthy relationship between the adolescent or young adult and his or her parents. That is, this relationship is no longer characterized by the illness constituting the basis of interaction. Adolescent developmental issues are also now brought to the fore.

with very high scores on the EDE global score and very high scores on the Yale-Brown-Cornell Eating Disorders Scale (YBC-ED; Mazure et al. 1994) fared better at end of treatment and follow-up if they received FBT-AN as opposed to AFT. No moderators for AFT could be identified (Le Grange et al. 2012).

An important advance that evolved in tandem with the Lock et al. (2005) study was the manualization of the family therapy model that has been implemented in almost all of the Maudsley studies (Lock and Le Grange 2013) as well as a parent handbook to assist and guide parents through treatment (Lock and Le Grange 2005). This manual allows for FBT-AN to be tested more broadly in controlled *and* uncontrolled settings, and therapists now have a tool to add to their clinical armamentarium to address AN in their young patients. An outline of FBT-AN as it proceeds through three clearly defined phases is presented in Table 20–1.

Since Minuchin et al.'s (1978) seminal work, and in addition to the controlled trials, several case series of varying sample sizes have been published. These studies involved adolescents treated with family therapy, but they also included individual and inpatient treatments, albeit to a lesser extent. Most notable are three larger uncontrolled studies that have been published recently (Le Grange et al. 2005; Lock et al. 2006; Loeb et al. 2007), all of which used manualized FBT-AN. These studies add to the body of literature that supports the notion that parents are a resource and that it is feasible and useful to incorporate them into the treatment of their adolescent. Taken together, results are supportive of FBT-AN, although only provisional conclusions can be drawn from uncontrolled studies that describe a relatively small combined series of cases. However, in conjunction with Minuchin's work and the controlled studies, these preliminary investigations put forward a substantial literature in support of family-based treatment.

In contrast to AN, the NICE guidelines (National Collaborating Centre for Mental Health 2004) made no specific recommendation for the treatment of adolescents with BN, which reflects the fact that to date, systematic research in the treatment of BN has focused almost exclusively on adults. This is true

TABLE 20–2. Three phases of family-based treatment of bulimia nervosa

Phase 1: Reestablishing healthy eating Treatment aims at empowering parents to disrupt binge eating, purging, restrictive dieting, and any other pathological weight-control behaviors. It also aims to externalize and separate the disordered behaviors from the affected adolescent to promote parental action and decrease adolescent resistance to parental assistance.

Phase 2: Helping the adolescent eat independently Once abstinence from disordered eating and related behaviors has been achieved, the second stage of treatment begins when parents transition control over eating and weight-related issues back to the adolescent under their supervision.

Phase 3: Adolescent developmental issues The focus here is on ways the family can help address the effects of bulimia nervosa on adolescent developmental processes, both on the adolescent and the family as a whole.

despite the relatively common occurrence of binge-eating and purging behaviors during adolescence and the fact that many cases of BN have onset in adolescence (Stice and Agras 1998; Swanson et al. 2011). Significant progress has been made in understanding a range of efficacious treatments for adults with BN, such as CBT, IPT, and antidepressant medications. In these studies, the mean age of participants was 28.4 years, with a duration of illness of approximately 10 years, and usually a cutoff age for entry at 18 years (Agras et al. 2000). In contrast, case series data on CBT and two RCTs (Le Grange et al. 2007; Schmidt et al. 2007) are the only treatment studies with an adolescent population that have been published.

Dodge et al. (1995) first reported on the use of family therapy for BN in a small case series, demonstrating that family psychoeducation and parental coaching in disrupting binge/purge behaviors led to significant reductions in bulimic symptoms for adolescents. More recently, Le Grange and Lock (2007) described and manualized a family-based treatment for adolescents with BN (FBT-BN), derived from the approach that has demonstrated efficacy for adolescents with AN. Similar to FBT-AN, FBT-BN is agnostic about the causes of the disorder and assumes that adolescent development is negatively affected by characteristics of the eating disorder. These characteristics include secrecy, shame, and dysfunctional eating patterns, and in addition to impeding adolescent development, they are thought to have confused and disempowered parents and other family members. FBT-BN works in three stages (Table 20–2). There are several important differences between FBT-BN and FBT-AN. Notably, in FBT-BN, treatment is focused not on weight restoration but rather on the regulation of eating patterns and the elimination of purging. An additional difference is that in BN, the treatment approach is more collaborative between parents and the affected adolescent. For adolescents with BN, the secretive nature of the disorder, along with the shame and guilt associated with these symptoms, may lead to it being more easily overlooked by parents. Finally, adolescents with BN may be more likely to have psychiatric comorbidity than those with AN, which needs to be addressed in treatment.

To date, two RCTs for adolescents with BN and subthreshold BN have been published (Le Grange et al. 2007; Schmidt et al. 2007). Le Grange and colleagues compared manualized FBT-BN with individual supportive psychotherapy for adolescents (ages 12–19 years).

Both directly following treatment and at 6-month follow-up, adolescents who had received FBT-BN were more likely to be binge/purge abstinent compared with those who had received supportive psychotherapy (39% vs. 18% following treatment and 29% vs. 10% at follow-up). Schmidt et al. (2007) compared CBT guided self-care with family therapy in adolescent and young adult patients (ages 12–20 years). At 6-month follow-up, both treatments yielded significant improvements (patients receiving family therapy were 41% abstinent), without between-group differences. Notably, while the family treatments in both studies resembled each other, Schmidt et al. defined family as any close other rather than just parents. This broader definition may have been used in part because of the slightly older age of adolescents in this UK sample (17.6±0.3 years vs. 16.1±1.6 years), who may not have wanted their parents involved. Indeed, 25% of those eligible for the UK study declined participation because they did not want their parents involved in treatment (Perkins et al. 2004). While modifying "family" treatment to include other significant individuals in the patient's life may be sensible, this may not be the most effective way to approach FBT with younger adolescents, for whom parental authority is key to the success of the treatment. These preliminary studies suggest that family-based therapy may be effective for the treatment of younger patients with BN.

Cognitive-Behavioral Therapy

The cognitive-behavioral model of eating disorders assumes that an overvaluation of weight and shape is at the core of eating disorder and is a key maintaining mechanism across the eating disorders (Fairburn 2008). Overvaluation of body weight and shape may be expressed by attempts to control shape and weight by excessive dieting. Dieting can cause a sense of both psychological and physiological deprivation, leading to depressed mood. In addition, because of dietary restriction, hunger is increased, and this, in turn, increases vulnerability toward binge eating. Because of fears of weight gain associated with eating a large amount of usually calorie-dense food, inappropriate compensatory behaviors such as purging are seen as an attempt to allay these anxieties. The clinical application of CBT has been tested in numerous controlled studies and has been found to be the most effective psychotherapeutic approach to the treatment of BN in adults. CBT is more effective than any other condition, including no treatment, nondirective therapy, pill placebo, manualized psychodynamic therapy (supportive-expressive), stress management, and antidepressant treatment (Agras et al. 2000). CBT has been enhanced in order to be applied transdiagnostically by Fairburn and colleagues (e.g., Fairburn et al. 2009, 2013), and available data demonstrate its efficacy in adults with a range of eating disorders, including BN, BED, AN (albeit with a modified extended version of CBT), and the subthreshold eating disorder variants. Table 20–3 describes the four core elements of CBT for eating disorders.

There have been two published case series of adolescents with BN using CBT adapted for adolescents (Lock 2005; Schapman-Williams et al. 2006). The adolescent version of the treatment involves modifications to allow for increased parental involvement in treatment, use of concrete examples tailored for adolescents to illustrate points, and exploration of adolescent issues in the context of BN (e.g., separation/individuation). In addition to CBT for adolescents,

TABLE 20–3. Four core elements of enhanced cognitive-behavioral therapy

Stage 1: Engagement, self-monitoring, and formulation Through psychoeducation about eating disorder symptoms and self-monitoring of eating and behavior patterns and discussion thereof, this phase involves jointly creating a formulation of the eating disorder. Patients begin practice of weekly weighing and regular eating. Family members may be involved to facilitate treatment.

Stage 2: Addressing barriers to change Once regular eating is established, this phase involves the formulation to identify and target obstacles to making changes, if necessary.

Stage 3: Addressing key maintaining mechanisms The focus here is on targeting overvaluation of weight and shape; teaching problem-solving and affect regulation strategies to reduce vulnerability to engagement in eating disorder behaviors; and addressing other maintaining mechanisms when relevant, including perfectionism, low self-esteem, mood intolerance, and interpersonal difficulties.

Stage 4: Relapse prevention The focus here is on consolidation of treatment gains, establishment of realistic posttreatment expectations, and both short- and long-term plans for minimizing relapse risk.

CBT-guided self-care has been compared with family therapy in one of the two RCTs for this population (Schmidt et al. 2007). Results from this RCT suggest that CBT-guided self-care is both an acceptable and a feasible treatment for adolescents with BN and related eating disorders, with a treatment dropout rate of 29% and an abstinence rate of 36% (from both binge eating and purging) at the end of 12 months of treatment. These abstinence rates were similar to those found in more recent adult studies of CBT (Mitchell et al. 2007). Further, one recent study of enhanced CBT suggests that it is promising in the treatment of adolescent AN (Dalle Grave et al. 2013).

Pharmacotherapy

Psychopharmacological interventions for eating disorders are limited; medications may be useful in targeting comorbidities. While the efficacy of some medications has been examined in adult AN samples, the role of these agents in adolescents remains relatively unexplored. While the use of psychopharmacological agents is limited during times of acute medical compromise, low-dose atypical antipsychotics are sometimes used to address severe obsessional thinking, anxiety, and psychotic-like thinking. Several small RCTs and case reports have examined newer antipsychotic agents (e.g., olanzapine) in the treatment of adolescents and young adults with AN (Boachie et al. 2003; Dennis et al. 2006; Kishi et al. 2012). Olanzapine may be helpful in addition to psychotherapy for adolescents with AN, helping to decrease anxiety around eating and body image concerns.

Randomized controlled pharmacological clinical trials in adults with BN have largely indicated that antidepressants are superior to placebo in reduction of binge frequency (Walsh et al. 1997). Further, weight and shape concerns and mood disturbance also seem to demonstrate greater improvement with medication compared with placebo (Mitchell et al. 1993). However, controlled studies in adults directly evaluating the relative and combined effectiveness of CBT and antidepressant medication (Walsh et al. 1997) have suggested that when added to psychological treatments (e.g., CBT, IPT), medications did not generally improve treatment outcomes. Taken together, these data suggest that the use of antidepressants in adults with BN offers only a marginal advantage over CBT alone.

To date, only one open-label medication trial including adolescents (ages 12–18) with BN has been published (Kotler et al. 2003). The findings from this study suggested that 8 weeks of fluoxetine (60 mg/day) was well tolerated in conjunction with supportive psychotherapy and yielded impressive improvement rates of approximately 70%. Controlled research with adolescents is needed, however, to determine the effectiveness of this medication in younger populations, who may have different clinical profiles compared with adults with BN (Le Grange and Schmidt 2005).

Feeding Disorders

While there are no randomized clinical trials investigating efficacious treatments for the feeding disorders, the recognition that these problems can occur across the lifespan has meant that clinics are experiencing an increase in requests for services for ARFID and other feeding disorders. Clinical wisdom and case reports suggest the utility of different approaches for feeding disorders. Depending on the specific presentation of a patient with ARFID, family-based treatment strategies (Norris et al. 2014) and cognitive-behavioral approaches (Bryant-Waugh 2013) may be beneficial. In combination with aspects of these approaches, a hierarchical food exposure strategy (e.g., Fraker et al. 2007) is valuable. Habit reversal or anxiety management tools (e.g., diaphragmatic breathing) may be useful for rumination disorder (Chitkara et al. 2006; Dalton and Czyzewski 2009). However, to our knowledge, no research exists on the treatment of pica. As with all feeding and eating disorders, support from parents and family can be instrumental in treatment adherence.

Summary Points

- Eating and feeding disorders have onset in the context of social, psychological, and physical development, making a developmental perspective on diagnosis and treatment essential.
- Inpatient treatment for adolescent eating disorders is useful for acute weight restoration but is of limited use in reducing recidivism rates.
- The small number of outpatient treatment studies suggests that involving parents in treatment (i.e., family-based treatment) may be helpful.
- There are no medications that appear to be routinely helpful with AN or BN, and pharmacological therapies remain largely unexplored.
- Less research attention has been paid to the diagnosis and treatment of the feeding disorders, but with the reorganization of eating and feeding disorders in DSM-5 this work will be forthcoming.
- Taken together, the literature supports the importance of early identification of and intervention for eating and feeding disorders in order to improve outcomes.

References

Agras WS, Walsh T, Fairburn CG, et al: A multicenter comparison of cognitive-behavioral therapy and interpersonal psychotherapy for bulimia nervosa. Arch Gen Psychiatry 57(5):459–466, 2000 10807486

American Psychiatric Association: Diagnostic and Statistical Manual of Mental Disorders, 4th Edition. Washington, DC, American Psychiatric Association, 1994

American Psychiatric Association: Diagnostic and Statistical Manual of Mental Disorders, 4th Edition, Text Revision. Washington, DC, American Psychiatric Association, 2000a

American Psychiatric Association: Practice guidelines for the treatment of patients with eating disorders (revision). Am J Psychiatry 157(suppl):1–39, 2000b

American Psychiatric Association: Diagnostic and Statistical Manual of Mental Disorders, 5th Edition. Arlington, VA, American Psychiatric Association, 2013

Attie I, Brooks-Gunn J: Development of eating problems in adolescent girls: a longitudinal study. Dev Psychol 25(1):70–79, 1989

Boachie A, Goldfield GS, Spettigue W: Olanzapine use as an adjunctive treatment for hospitalized children with anorexia nervosa: case reports. Int J Eat Disord 33(1):98–103, 2003 12474205

Brewerton TD, Rance SJ, Dansky BS, et al: A comparison of women with child-adolescent versus adult onset binge eating: Results from the National Women's Study Int J Eat Disord 2014 24904009 Epub ahead of print

Bryant-Waugh R: Avoidant restrictive food intake disorder: an illustrative case example. Int J Eat Disord 46(5):420–423, 2013 23658083

Bryant-Waugh RJ, Cooper PJ, Taylor CL, et al: The use of the eating disorder examination with children: a pilot study. Int J Eat Disord 19(4):391–397, 1996 8859397

Casper RC, Troiani M: Family functioning in anorexia nervosa differs by subtype. Int J Eat Disord 30(3):338–342, 2001 11767716

Chitkara DK, Van Tilburg M, Whitehead WE, et al: Teaching diaphragmatic breathing for rumination syndrome. Am J Gastroenterol 101(11):2449–2452, 2006 17090274

Ciao AC, Loth K, Neumark-Sztainer D: Preventing eating disorder pathology: common and unique features of successful eating disorders prevention programs. Curr Psychiatry Rep 16(7):453, 2014 24821099

Commission on Adolescent Eating Disorders: Treatment of eating disorders, in Treating and Preventing Adolescent Mental Health Disorders: What We Know and What We Don't Know. A Research Agenda for Improving the Mental Health of Our Youth. Edited by Evans DL, Foa EB, Gur RE, et al. Oxford, UK, Oxford University Press, 2005, pp 283–302

Cooper Z, Fairburn CG: The Eating Disorder Examination: a semistructured interview for the assessment of the specific psychopathology of eating disorders. Int J Eat Disord 6(1):1–8, 1987

Dalle Grave R, Calugi S, Doll HA, et al: Enhanced cognitive behaviour therapy for adolescents with anorexia nervosa: an alternative to family therapy? Behav Res Ther 51(1):R9–R12, 2013 23123081

Dalton WT 3rd, Czyzewski DI: Behavioral treatment of habitual rumination: case reports. Dig Dis Sci 54(8):1804–1807, 2009 19052867

Delaney CB, Eddy KT, Hartmann AS, et al: Pica and rumination behavior among individuals seeking treatment for eating disorders or obesity. Int J Eat Disord 48(2):238–248, 2014 24729045

Dennis K, Le Grange D, Bremer J: Olanzapine use in adolescent anorexia nervosa. Eat Weight Disord 11(2):e53–e56, 2006 16809970

Dodge E, Hodes M, Eisler I, et al: Family therapy for bulimia nervosa in adolescents: an exploratory study. J Fam Ther 17(1):59–77, 1995

Eddy KT, Keel PK, Dorer DJ, et al: Longitudinal comparison of anorexia nervosa subtypes. Int J Eat Disord 31(2):191–201, 2002 11920980

Eddy K, Celio Doyle A, Hoste R, et al: Eating disorder not otherwise specified in adolescents. J Am Acad Child Adolesc Psychiatry 47:156–164, 2008a 18176335

Eddy KT, Dorer DJ, Franko DL, et al: Diagnostic crossover in anorexia nervosa and bulimia nervosa: implications for DSM-

V. Am J Psychiatry 165:(2):245–250, 2008b 18198267

Eddy KT, Thomas JJ, Hastings E, et al: Prevalence of DSM-5 avoidant/restrictive food intake disorder in a pediatric gastroenterology healthcare network. Int J Eat Disord, 2014 25142784 Epub ahead of print

Eisler I, Dare C, Russell GFM, et al: Family and individual therapy in anorexia nervosa. A 5-year follow-up. Arch Gen Psychiatry 54(11):1025–1030, 1997 9366659

Eisler I, Dare C, Hodes M, et al: Family therapy for adolescent anorexia nervosa: the results of a controlled comparison of two family interventions. J Child Psychol Psychiatry 41(6):727–736, 2000 11039685

Eisler I, Simic M, Russell GFM, et al: A randomised controlled treatment trial of two forms of family therapy in adolescent anorexia nervosa: a five-year follow-up. J Child Psychol Psychiatry 48(6):552–560, 2007 17537071

Fairburn CG: Cognitive Behavior Therapy and Eating Disorders. New York, Guilford, 2008

Fairburn CG, Cooper Z, Doll HA, et al: The natural course of bulimia nervosa and binge eating disorder in young women. Arch Gen Psychiatry 57(7):659–665, 2000 10891036

Fairburn CG, Cooper Z, Doll HA, et al: Transdiagnostic cognitive-behavioral therapy for patients with eating disorders: a two-site trial with 60-week follow-up. Am J Psychiatry 166(3):311–319, 2009 19074978

Fairburn CG, Cooper Z, Doll HA, et al: Enhanced cognitive behaviour therapy for adults with anorexia nervosa: a UK-Italy study. Behav Res Ther 51(1):R2–R8, 2013 23084515

Field AE, Sonneville KR, Crosby RD, et al: Prospective associations of concerns about physique and the development of obesity, binge drinking, and drug use among adolescent boys and young adult men. JAMA Pediatr 168(1):34–39, 2014 24190655

Fischer S, le Grange D: Comorbidity and high-risk behaviors in treatment-seeking adolescents with bulimia nervosa. Int J Eat Disord 40(8):751–753, 2007 17683094

Fisher M, Golden NH, Katzman DK, et al: Eating disorders in adolescents: a background paper. J Adolesc Health 16(6):420–437, 1995 7669792

Fisher M, Schneider M, Burns J, et al: Differences between adolescents and young adults at presentation to an eating disorders program. J Adolesc Health 28(3):222–227, 2001 11226845

Fisher M, Rosen DS, Ornstein RM, et al: Characteristics of avoidant/restrictive food intake disorder in children and adolescents: a "new disorder" in DSM-5. J Adolesc Health 55(1):49–52, 2014 24506978

Fraker C, Fishbein M, Cox S: Food Chaining: The Proven 6-Step Plan to Stop Picky Eating, Solve Feeding Problems, and Expand Your Child's Diet. Cambridge, MA, Da Capo Press, 2007

Frank GK, Bailer UF, Henry S, et al: Neuroimaging studies in eating disorders. CNS Spectr 9(7):539–548, 2004 15208513

Franko DL, Keel PK, Dorer DJ, et al: What predicts suicide attempts in women with eating disorders? Psychol Med 34(5):843–853, 2004 15500305

Garber AK, Mauldin K, Michihata N, et al: Higher calorie diets increase rate of weight gain and shorten hospital stay in hospitalized adolescents with anorexia nervosa. J Adolesc Health 53(5):579–584, 2013 24054812

Golden NH, Katzman DK, Kreipe RE, et al: Eating disorders in adolescents: position paper of the Society for Adolescent Medicine. J Adolesc Health 33(6):496–503, 2003 14642712

Gowers SG, Clark A, Roberts C, et al: Clinical effectiveness of treatments for anorexia nervosa in adolescents: randomised controlled trial. Br J Psychiatry 191:427–435, 2007 17978323

Gunewardene A, Huon GF, Zheng R: Exposure to westernization and dieting: a cross-cultural study. Int J Eat Disord 29(3):289–293, 2001 11262507

Herpertz-Dahlmann B, Schwarte R, Krei M, et al: Day-patient treatment after short inpatient care versus continued inpatient treatment in adolescents with anorexia nervosa (ANDI): a multicentre, randomised, open-label, non-inferiority trial. Lancet 383(9924):1222–1229, 2014 24439238

Herzog DB, Nussbaum KM, Marmor AK: Comorbidity and outcome in eating disorders. Psychiatr Clin North Am 19(4):843–859, 1996 9045226

Hoste RR, le Grange D: Expressed emotion among white and ethnic minority families of adolescents with bulimia nervosa. Eur Eat Disord Rev 16(5):395–400, 2008 18240126

Johnson JG, Cohen P, Kotler L, et al: Psychiatric disorders associated with risk for the development of eating disorders during adolescence and early adulthood. J Consult Clin Psychol 70(5):1119–1128, 2002 12362962

Kaye W, Gendall K, Strober M: Serotonin neuronal function and selective serotonin reuptake inhibitor treatment in anorexia and bulimia nervosa. Biol Psychiatry 44(9):825–838, 1998 9807638

Kaye WH, Wierenga CE, Bailer UF, et al: Nothing tastes as good as skinny feels: the neurobiology of anorexia nervosa. Trends Neurosci 36(2):110–120, 2013 23333342

Keel PK, Mitchell JE: Outcome in bulimia nervosa. Am J Psychiatry 154(3):313–321, 1997 9054777

Keel PK, Heatherton TF, Dorer DJ, et al: Point prevalence of bulimia nervosa in 1982, 1992, and 2002. Psychol Med 36(1):119–127, 2006 16202192

Kelly NR, Shank LM, Bakalar JL, et al: Pediatric feeding and eating disorders: current state of diagnosis and treatment. Curr Psychiatry Rep 16(5):446, 2014 24643374

Kendler KS, Walters EE, Neale MC, et al: The structure of the genetic and environmental risk factors for six major psychiatric disorders in women. Phobia, generalized anxiety disorder, panic disorder, bulimia, major depression, and alcoholism. Arch Gen Psychiatry 52(5):374–383, 1995 7726718

Keshaviah A, Edkins K, Fairburn CG, et al: Re-examining premature mortality in anorexia nervosa: A meta-analysis redux. Compr Psychiatry 55(8):1773–1784, 2014 25214371

Kishi T, Kafantaris V, Sunday S, et al: Are antipsychotics effective for the treatment of anorexia nervosa? Results from a systematic review and meta-analysis. J Clin Psychiatry 73(6):e757–e766, 2012 22795216

Kotler LA, Devlin MJ, Davies M, et al: An open trial of fluoxetine for adolescents with bulimia nervosa. J Child Adolesc Psychopharmacol 13(3):329–335, 2003 14642021

Le Grange D, Lock J: The dearth of psychological treatment studies for anorexia nervosa. Int J Eat Disord 37(2):79–91, 2005 15732072

Le Grange D, Lock J: Treating Bulimia in Adolescents: A Family Based Approach. New York, Guilford, 2007

Le Grange D, Schmidt U: The treatment of adolescents with bulimia nervosa. J Ment Health 14:587–597, 2005

Le Grange D, Eisler I, Dare C, et al: Evaluation of family treatments in adolescent anorexia nervosa: a pilot study. Int J Eat Disord 12(4):347–357, 1992

Le Grange D, Loeb KL, Van Orman S, et al: Bulimia nervosa in adolescents: a disorder in evolution? Arch Pediatr Adolesc Med 158(5):478–482, 2004 15123482

Le Grange D, Binford R, Loeb KL: Manualized family based treatment for anorexia nervosa: a case series. J Am Acad Child Adolesc Psychiatry 44(1):41–46, 2005 15608542

Le Grange D, Binford RB, Peterson CB, et al: DSM-IV threshold versus subthreshold bulimia nervosa. Int J Eat Disord 39(6):462–467, 2006 16715488

Le Grange D, Crosby RD, Rathouz PJ, et al: A randomized controlled comparison of family based treatment and supportive psychotherapy for adolescent bulimia nervosa. Arch Gen Psychiatry 64(9):1049–1056, 2007 17768270

Le Grange D, Lock J, Agras WS, et al: Moderators and mediators of remission in family based treatment and adolescent focused therapy for anorexia nervosa. Behav Res Ther 50(2):85–92, 2012 22172564

Leit RA, Pope HG Jr, Gray JJ: Cultural expectations of muscularity in men: the evolution of playgirl centerfolds. Int J Eat Disord 29(1):90–93, 2001 11135340

Lock J: Adjusting cognitive behavior therapy for adolescents with bulimia nervosa: results of case series. Am J Psychother 59(3):267–281, 2005 16370133

Lock J, Le Grange D: Help Your Teenager Beat an Eating Disorder. New York, Guilford, 2005

Lock J, Le Grange D: Treatment Manual for Anorexia Nervosa: A Family Based Approach, Second Edition. New York, Guilford, 2013

Lock J, Reisel B, Steiner H: Associated health risks of adolescents with disordered eating: how different are they from their peers? Results from a high school survey. Child Psychiatry Hum Dev 31(3):249–265, 2001 11196014

Lock J, Agras WS, Bryson S, et al: A comparison of short- and long-term family therapy for adolescent anorexia nervosa. J Am Acad Child Adolesc Psychiatry 44(7):632–639, 2005 15968231

Lock J, Couturier J, Agras WS: Comparison of long-term outcomes in adolescents with anorexia nervosa treated with family therapy. J Am Acad Child Adolesc Psychiatry 45(6):666–672, 2006 16721316

Lock J, Le Grange D, Agras WS, et al: Randomized clinical trial comparing family based treatment with adolescent-focused individual therapy for adolescents with anorexia nervosa. Arch Gen Psychiatry 67(10):1025–1032, 2010 20921118

Loeb KL, Walsh BT, Lock J, et al: Open trial of family-based treatment for full and partial anorexia nervosa in adolescence: evidence of successful dissemination. J Am Acad Child Adolesc Psychiatry 46(7):792–800, 2007 17581443

Madden S, Miskovic-Wheatley J, Wallis A, et al: A randomized controlled trial of inpatient treatment for anorexia nervosa in medically unstable adolescents Psychol Med 14:1–13, 2014 25017941 Epub ahead of print

Mazure CM, Halmi KA, Sunday SR, et al: The Yale-Brown-Cornell Eating Disorder Scale: development, use, reliability and validity. J Psychiatr Res 28(5):425–445, 1994 7897615

McCabe MP, Ricciardelli LA, Finemore J: The role of puberty, media and popularity with peers on strategies to increase weight, decrease weight and increase muscle tone among adolescent boys and girls. J Psychosom Res 52(3):145–153, 2002 11897233

Minuchin S, Rosman B, Baker I: Psychosomatic Families: Anorexia Nervosa in Context. Cambridge, MA, Harvard University Press, 1978

Misra M, Klibanski A: Anorexia nervosa and osteoporosis. Rev Endocr Metab Disord 7(1–2):91–99, 2006 16972186

Mitchell JE, Raymond N, Specker S: A review of the controlled trials of pharmacotherapy and psychotherapy in the treatment of bulimia nervosa. Int J Eat Disord 14(3):229–247, 1993 8275060

Mitchell JE, Agras S, Wonderlich S: Treatment of bulimia nervosa: where are we and where are we going? Int J Eat Disord 40(2):95–101, 2007 17080448

Mitchison D, Hay PJ: The epidemiology of eating disorders: genetic, environmental, and societal factors. Clin Epidemiol 6:89–97, 2014 24728136

National Collaborating Centre for Mental Health: Eating Disorders: Core Interventions in the Treatment and Management of Anorexia Nervosa, Bulimia Nervosa and Related Eating Disorders. London, British Psychological Society and Gaskell, 2004

Norris ML, Robinson A, Obeid N, et al: Exploring avoidant/restrictive food intake disorder in eating disordered patients: a descriptive study. Int J Eat Disord 47(5):495–499, 2014 24343807

Ohring R, Graber JA, Brooks-Gunn J: Girls' recurrent and concurrent body dissatisfaction: correlates and consequences over 8 years. Int J Eat Disord 31(4):404–415, 2002 11948645

Ornstein RM, Rosen DS, Mammel KA, et al: Distribution of eating disorders in children and adolescents using the proposed DSM-5 criteria for feeding and eating disorders. J Adolesc Healh 53(2):303–305, 2013 23684215

Perkins S, Winn S, Murray J, et al: A qualitative study of the experience of caring for a person with bulimia nervosa. Part 1: The emotional impact of caring. Int J Eat Disord 36(3):256–268, 2004 15478131

Robin AL, Siegel PT, Moye AW, et al: A controlled comparison of family versus individual therapy for adolescents with anorexia nervosa. J Am Acad Child Adolesc Psychiatry 38(12):1482–1489, 1999 10596247

Rohde P, Auslander BA, Shaw H, et al: Dissonance-based prevention of eating disorder risk factors in middle school girls: results from two pilot trials. Int J Eat Disord 47(5):483–494, 2014 24590419

Schapman-Williams AM, Lock J, Couturier J: Cognitive-behavioral therapy for adolescents with binge eating syndromes: a case series. Int J Eat Disord 39(3):252–255, 2006 16511836

Schmidt U, Lee S, Beecham J, et al: A randomized controlled trial of family therapy and cognitive behavior therapy guided self-care for adolescents with bulimia nervosa and related disorders. Am J Psychiatry 164(4):591–598, 2007 17403972

Schur EA, Sanders M, Steiner H: Body dissatisfaction and dieting in young children. Int J Eat Disord 27(1):74–82, 2000 10590451

Shomaker LB, Tanofsky-Kraff M, Elliott C, et al: Salience of loss of control for pediatric binge episodes: does size really matter? Int J Eat Disord 43(8):707–716, 2010 19827022

Steiger H, Gauvin L, Israël M, et al: Association of serotonin and cortisol indices with childhood abuse in bulimia nervosa. Arch Gen Psychiatry 58(9):837–843, 2001 11545666

Steiner H, Kwan W, Shaffer TG, et al: Risk and protective factors for juvenile eating disorders. Eur Child Adolesc Psychiatry 12(suppl 1):I38–6, 2003 12567214

Steinhausen HC: The outcome of anorexia nervosa in the 20th century. Am J Psychiatry 159(8):1284–1293, 2002 12153817

Stice E, Agras WS: Predicting onset and cessation of bulimic behaviors during adolescence. Behav Ther 29(2):257–276, 1998

Stice E, Marti CN, Spoor S, et al: Dissonance and healthy weight eating disorder prevention programs: long-term effects from a randomized efficacy trial. J Consult Clin Psychol 76(2):329–340, 2008 18377128

Stice E, Rohde P, Durant S, et al: A preliminary trial of a prototype Internet dissonance-based eating disorder prevention program for young women with body image concerns. J Consult Clin Psychol 80(5):907–916, 2012 22506791

Strober M, Freeman R, Morrell W: The long-term course of severe anorexia nervosa in adolescents: survival analysis of recovery, relapse, and outcome predictors over 10–15 years in a prospective study. Int J Eat Disord 22(4):339–360, 1997 9356884

Swanson SA, Crow SJ, Le Grange D, et al: Prevalence and correlates of eating disorders in adolescents. Results from the national comorbidity survey replication adolescent supplement. Arch Gen Psychiatry 68(7):714–723, 2011 21383252

Thompson-Brenner H, Eddy KT, Satir DA, et al: Personality subtypes in adolescents with eating disorders: validation of a classification approach. J Child Psychol Psychiatry 49(2):170–180, 2008 18093115

Walsh BT, Wilson GT, Loeb KL, et al: Medication and psychotherapy in the treatment of bulimia nervosa. Am J Psychiatry 154(4):523–531, 1997 9090340

Westen D, Harnden-Fischer J: Personality profiles in eating disorders: rethinking the distinction between Axis I and Axis II. Am J Psychiatry 158(4):547–562, 2001 11282688

CHAPTER 21

Tic Disorders

Kenneth E. Towbin, M.D.

Tics are sudden, quick, repetitive, stereotypic, relatively involuntary muscle contractions that can occur in any part of the body. Tic disorders are highly prevalent in children and adolescents but cause severe impairment in only a small minority. However, tic disorders also are model neuropsychiatric conditions that provide a unique window into the interplay of genetic risk, psychology, experience, and environment. Exploring tic disorders has led to a deeper understanding of neural pathways and circuits in the brain that subserve sensory and motor function, linking the frontal lobes, striatum, and thalamus. The study of tic disorders has increased our knowledge of the relationship between cognition and motor activity and illuminated the role of the striatum in motor planning and execution. Treatments now include interventions that draw directly on this preclinical and clinical work.

The term *tic disorders* comprises four diagnostic entities in DSM-5 (American Psychiatric Association 2013): provisional (previously called *transient*) tics, persistent (or chronic) motor or vocal tics, and Tourette's disorder. Tourette's disorder (also called Tourette syndrome, hereinafter called *Tourette's*) takes its name from Georges Gilles de la Tourette (1982), who, while a student under Jean-Martin Charcot, first described the condition.

Symptoms and Comorbidity

Tics are repetitive, brief, sudden, stereotypic movements that can occur in any voluntary muscle. Tics affect the same muscles over days and hours but also migrate to different parts of the body and may spread to include more regions over months and years. Specific tics appear and disappear or reappear after a long hiatus. Generally, tics appear in the face first (e.g., eye blinks, grimaces) and then progress to more caudal muscles in

This work was funded by the NIMH Intramural Research Program.

the neck, shoulders, arms, trunk, back, and legs.

Tics are best understood as "relatively involuntary." They may be suppressed successfully for minutes to hours, but they cannot be constrained indefinitely. The capacity to postpone tics varies throughout the day and across situations. One measure of tic severity is how much effort a person must exert in order to suppress a tic and how successfully he can inhibit tics. Tics may be unwittingly influenced by suggestion. It is common for someone with tics to experience more symptoms while describing them. Tics also can mimic others' movements (echopraxia) or words (echolalia) or sounds in the environment. It is common for a new tic to begin with a stimulus, such as a temporary physical irritation or a forceful emotional experience, and to continue long after that stimulus has ended.

Tics characteristically show variable frequency and intensity throughout the day, across months, and through years. This waxing and waning is not random. Tics occur in clusters and bundles of clusters that have been described as *bouts* and *bouts of bouts* (Peterson and Leckman 1998). Tics may also occur during sleep, unlike other movement disorders (Kostanecka-Endress et al. 2003).

Tics often increase in association with emotionally stimulating events, whether exciting and pleasing or stressful or distressing events. Some individuals find that their symptoms cease during effortful acts such as public performances, executing skilled procedures, or athletic competition but are worse just before or afterward.

Tics are often categorized as either simple or complex. *Simple tics* are those confined exclusively to one or a few muscle groups and are very brief, such as a grimace, shoulder shrug, a cough, or a sniffing sound. *Complex tics* involve multiple muscle groups and integrated actions, such as thrusting one arm forward while slapping the contralateral thigh with the corresponding hand or repeatedly uttering the first line of a jingle. Complex tics may entail many serial movements and/or sounds, such as stopping midstride and in succession touching a hand to the floor, hopping once, barking, and completing a pirouette. These distinctions do not carry diagnostic or prognostic implications, although a display of complex repetitive behavior without simple tics should lead one to question the presence of a tic disorder.

Individuals with tics commonly report two types of mental events: *premonitory urges* (Leckman et al. 1993) and *obsessions and/or compulsions* (OCs; see Chapter 17, "Obsessive-Compulsive Disorder"). OCs are reported in 50%–90% of persons with Tourette's (Gaze et al. 2006). OCs involving obsessions with symmetry and compulsions of counting, arranging, ordering, and repeating until "just right" appear to be more prevalent in persons with tic disorders plus obsessive-compulsive disorder (OCD) than those with only OCD (Leckman et al. 2001; Nestadt et al. 2003). In comparison to people with only OCD, persons with OCD plus Tourette's more commonly may have aggressive, sexual, and religious obsessions (Leckman et al. 2001; Zohar et al. 1997) and less commonly have obsessions about contamination, germs, neatness, and cleanliness and compulsions of hoarding, cleaning, and washing.

Premonitory urges, reported by 75%–80% of persons with chronic tic disorders (CTDs) and Tourette's (Leckman et al. 1993; Reese et al. 2014), precede tics and may have a physical quality, such as localized tingling, itch-like sensations, or tensions in muscles, or an ideational feature such as thoughts or urges related to making sounds, movements, or gestures. Acknowledging these mental events has resulted in a blurring of the distinction between compulsions and complex tics. It is now recognized that many people with complex tics report thoughts, mental events, or unpleasant sensations prior to tics, and these thoughts, urges, or tensions are analogous to the thoughts and urges experienced by people with compulsions (Reese et al. 2014).

Comorbid diagnoses are common with Tourette's. Among children and adults with Tourette's disorder, attention-deficit/hyperactivity disorder (ADHD) is seen in 21%–90%. Among those who are school age with Tourette's the rate is roughly 25% (Robertson 2006). In non-clinic populations with Tourette's, ADHD has been observed in 40%–60% (Kadesjö and Gillberg 2000; Kurlan et al. 2002; Robertson et al. 2006), and 10%–80% have OCD (McNaught and Mink 2011; Kurlan et al. 2002). Among those with Tourette's seeking clinical care, 30% have comorbid anxiety disorders (Coffey et al. 2000) and 10%–75% have major depression (Robertson et al. 2006).

Other impairments common in clinically referred children with Tourette's and CTD are aggressive behaviors and temper outbursts, oppositional behavior, behavioral inflexibility, and problems with social understanding and reciprocity. Despite their common association, these are not considered "core" features of Tourette's. Interestingly, Tourette's and tics are more common among individuals with autism spectrum disorders (Simonoff et al. 2008), and, conversely, autism spectrum disorders may be more common among those with Tourette's. Reports of elevated rates of behavioral problems are more likely a result of ascertainment bias than Tourette's itself and are more closely related to comorbid ADHD symptoms (Budman et al. 2000).

The typical onset of tic disorders is during childhood and early adolescence. The peak incidence is during ages 4–7 years, and symptoms often are at their worst during late childhood and early adolescence (Knight et al. 2012). For 85% of individuals, late adolescence and early adulthood bring relief as tics become quieter (Bloch et al. 2006a). Most adults who continue to have tics have no more than mild symptoms, although there are exceptions in individuals who continue to have severe tics.

Differential Diagnosis

The DSM-5 criteria for Tourette's disorder, persistent (chronic) motor or vocal tic disorder, and provisional tic disorder are shown in Box 21–1. If tics are present for a year, then the diagnosis is persistent tic disorder (PTD) (motor or phonic) or Tourette's disorder. Differentiating Tourette's disorder from PTD is straightforward. If during the course of the disorder there have been both phonic and motor tics, even if they are not present at the same time, the diagnosis is Tourette's disorder. If during the individual's lifetime tics are exclusively motor or exclusively phonic, the diagnosis is a persistent tic disorder, specified as motor or phonic, respectively. Tics occurring for less than a year are provisional tic disorder. In DSM-5 an individual is not required to have impairment or distress from tics in order to receive a tic disorder diagnosis.

Box 21–1. DSM-5 Diagnostic Criteria for Tic Disorders

Note: A tic is a sudden, rapid, recurrent, nonrhythmic motor movement or vocalization.

Tourette's Disorder 307.23 (F95.2)

A. Both multiple motor and one or more vocal tics have been present at some time during the illness, although not necessarily concurrently.
B. The tics may wax and wane in frequency but have persisted for more than 1 year since first tic onset.
C. Onset is before age 18 years.
D. The disturbance is not attributable to the physiological effects of a substance (e.g., cocaine) or another medical condition (e.g., Huntington's disease, postviral encephalitis).

Persistent (Chronic) Motor or Vocal Tic Disorder 307.22 (F95.1)

A. Single or multiple motor or vocal tics have been present during the illness, but not both motor and vocal.
B. The tics may wax and wane in frequency but have persisted for more than 1 year since first tic onset.
C. Onset is before age 18 years.
D. The disturbance is not attributable to the physiological effects of a substance (e.g., cocaine) or another medical condition (e.g., Huntington's disease, postviral encephalitis).
E. Criteria have never been met for Tourette's disorder.

Specify if:

With motor tics only
With vocal tics only

Provisional Tic Disorder 307.21 (F95.0)

A. Single or multiple motor and/or vocal tics.
B. The tics have been present for less than 1 year since first tic onset.
C. Onset is before age 18 years.
D. The disturbance is not attributable to the physiological effects of a substance (e.g., cocaine) or another medical condition (e.g., Huntington's disease, postviral encephalitis).
E. Criteria have never been met for Tourette's disorder or persistent (chronic) motor or vocal tic disorder.

Source. Reprinted from the *Diagnostic and Statistical Manual of Mental Disorders*, 5th Edition. Arlington, VA, American Psychiatric Association, 2013. Used with permission.

The differential diagnosis of tic disorders is summarized in Table 21–1.

In clinical settings some patients report experiencing sudden onset or exacerbation of symptoms in association with streptococcal or other infections. The preponderance of evidence leaves doubt about whether a separate entity called PANDAS (pediatric autoimmune neurological disorders associated with streptococcal infection) is a valid one (Martino et al. 2014), and controlled longitudinal studies offer strong evidence against poststreptococcal infection being an etiology for tic disorders (Leckman et al. 2011). The evidence is so strong that recent proposals removed tics as a symptom of this postinfectious syndrome and renamed it PANS (pediatric acute-onset neuropsychiatric syndrome) (Swedo et al. 2012). Nevertheless, a diverse array of immune and inflammatory mechanisms could play a role in the etiology or exacerbation of tic disorders (Martino et al. 2014).

TABLE 21–1. Differential diagnosis of Tourette's and tics

Disorder	Movement type	Migration?	Suppressible?	Wax and wane?	Stimulus response?	Comment
Tics	Sudden simple or complex clonic	Yes	Yes	Yes	Yes/No	Increase with attention
Dystonias	Sudden, simple clonic	No	No	No	No	Increase with effort
Myoclonus	Simple clonic					Increase with effort
Dyskinesia	Complex slow choreiform	Yes	No	No	No	Increase with distraction
Restless legs	Complex slow	No	No	No	No	Movement relieves tension
Chorea	Slow, continuous	No	No	Yes/No	No	Increase with effort
Akathisia	Complex	No	Briefly	Yes	No	Relieved by movement
Stereotypy	Slow complex	Yes	Yes	Yes	Yes/No	Often pleasurable
Hyperekplexia	Sudden complex	No	No	No	Yes	Excessive reaction to startle
Parkinson's disease	Tremor					Gait disturbance, hyperreflexia, family history
Huntington disease	Chorea					Prominent behavioral and mental changes acquired

Epidemiology

Meta-analysis of 35 epidemiological studies of Tourette's disorder gives a lifetime prevalence rate of 0.77% (Knight et al. 2012). Early studies were flawed by failures to ascertain representative community populations, and more recent ones are difficult to compare because they apply different definitions and methods to arrive at the diagnosis. These analyses yielded a 1.61% rate for lifetime chronic tics (motor or phonic) and 2.99% for transient tics (Knight et al. 2012).

The prevalence of Tourette's in boys is four times that of girls (1.06% vs. 0.25%) (Knight et al. 2012), but for chronic motor tics and transient tics meta-analysis yields equal prevalence rates for boys and girls (Knight et al. 2012). Tourette's has been observed in all races, but rates and symptoms may differ among ethnic groups (Freeman et al. 2000; Jin et al. 2005; Mathews et al. 2007).

Genetics

Twin and family studies provide sturdy evidence that Tourette's and CTD are fundamentally genetic conditions. The twin concordance rates for Tourette's are 53%–56% for monozygotic pairs and 8% in dizygotic siblings (State 2011). When criteria are broadened to allow for a co-twin having either Tourette's or CTD, the concordance rates climb to 77%–94% for monozygotic and 23% for dizygotic pairs, strongly pointing to a genetic etiology. However, one cannot presume that genetic factors are the exclusive cause when the concordance rate for monozygotic twins is less than 100%.

Further support from many family studies (State 2011) in different sites, countries, and ethnic groups confirms high prevalence rates among family members. In families of European origin ascertained by the presence of a Tourette's proband, the prevalence of Tourette's or CTD in first-degree relatives ranges from 15% to 53%. Studies find rates of OCD and OC symptoms among relatives of Tourette's probands that are 10–20 times the general population prevalence (Bloch et al. 2006a).

Despite strenuous efforts, no reproducible findings have identified any single gene or specific multiple genes acting together to produce Tourette's disorder (Deng et al. 2012; State 2011). As a result, genetic research has shifted to the study of noncoding chromosomal regions, copy number variations, parametric linkage studies, gene-by-environment interactions, and epigenetic contributions (Deng and Jankovic 2012; State 2011). Great hope remains for exome and whole genome sequencing using genome-wide association studies (GWAS).

Neuroanatomy and Neurophysiology

Tics are associated with abnormal functioning in cortico-striatal-thalamo-cortical (CSTC) loop circuits (Parent and Hazrati 1995). Cortical fibers end in somatotopically arranged segments of the striatum (caudate nucleus and putamen) and subthalamic nucleus. The striatum and subthalamic nucleus send efferents to the globus pallidus (interna and externa), which in turn sends fibers to the globus pallidus interna (GPi). From the GPi, the pathway courses to the thalamus, which completes the loop with separate, parallel efferents to the cortex. Circuits originating in the motor and dorsolateral cortex are considered to be the most important for tic disorders.

At the cellular level in the striatum, medium-size spiny neurons and dopamine play a key role in producing tics. Medium-size spiny neurons (MSPNs) receive afferents using glutamate (excitatory), γ-aminobutyric acid (GABA; inhibitory), dopamine (D_1 excitatory, D_2 inhibitory), and serotonin (Leckman et al. 2010) and send inhibitory GABA efferents to the GPi. Interneurons acting on these MSPNs, in particular fast-spiking GABAergic interneurons, and cholinergic tonically active neurons may play a pivotal role in tic generation (Leckman et al. 2010). There are data suggesting that impaired embryonic neuronal migration of these interneurons leads to an imbalance in their density and number (Leckman et al. 2010). Decreased density of these interneurons in critical regions of the basal ganglia neurotransmitter systems would affect MSPN function. This could lead to an imbalance in the relationship between sensorimotor regions and the basal ganglia, producing movements (Leckman et al. 2010). It also would explain the influence of dopamine and serotonin synapses on tic expression and findings of hypoactivation of the basal ganglia and excessive activation of sensorimotor regions in those with Tourette's (McNaught and Mink 2011).

The association of tics and dysregulation of CSTC circuits is supported by data from magnetic resonance imaging (Rothenberger and Roessner 2013; Wang et al. 2011), positron emission tomography (Albin et al. 2003; Jeffries et al. 2002), and deep brain stimulation (Visser-Vandewalle et al. 2003). Although the ventral striatum appears to be a critical region in the neuropathology of Tourette's, CSTC dysregulation also could arise from, or be a partial compensation for, flawed signaling in the other regions such as the cerebellum, operculum, insula, or thalamus (Butler et al. 2006; Lerner et al. 2007). Current theory (Leckman et al. 2006) suggests that the normal relationship between striatum and thalamus is disrupted by malfunctioning "pacemaker" firings of interneurons in the striatum. Disorganizing thalamic discharges (Leckman et al. 2006) subsequently lead to excessive activation in the frontal cortex (Leckman et al. 2006) or excessive disorganized intercommunication between motor and orbitofrontal CSTC loops (Jeffries et al. 2002), leading to motor, premonitory, and emotional symptoms (Leckman et al. 2006).

Assessment

Since tic symptoms wax and wane, assessment and reevaluation are a routine part of treatment. The initial evaluation requires time to understand the patient in order to learn what he knows about his symptoms, his impairment, and his adaptation. Tics may influence physical, mental, familial, cultural, academic/occupational, and community realms. Focusing on each of these domains is crucial in thinking about the severity of symptoms and the kinds of interventions that are likely to be helpful. People with tic disorders often find conversations about their symptoms to be uncomfortable and may attempt to camouflage, minimize, and suppress tics. For some, focusing on tics may immediately increase symptoms, while others may be only vaguely aware of them.

Severity is deduced from the frequency and intensity of and impairment resulting from each type of tic. This requires clinical judgment, however, because there is an imperfect correlation of impairment with frequency or intensity. For example, a frequent tic, such as eye blinking, may be hardly noticeable and cause no interference, while audible coprolalia, even if very rare, may be quite impairing. A patient may have pain from repeated movements that are hardly visible to anyone else. A complex movement that demands removing both hands from the steering wheel during highway driving, even if infrequent, can be life-threatening. Thus, cataloging the entire array of tics—motor and phonic—is vital. Valid and reliable rating scales, such as the Yale Global Tourette Severity Scale (Leckman et al. 1989), Hopkins Motor and Vocal Tic Scale (Walkup et al. 1992), or the combined Tic Rating Scale (Goetz and Kompoliti 2001) may be helpful. These scales include a global measure that allows a clinician to summarize the observations into a single rating.

A comprehensive assessment should include asking about inner phenomena such as premonitory urges and obsessive-compulsive symptoms, which can be distracting and intrusive (Reese et al. 2014). The details of obsessions and the recognized senselessness of their elaborate, rule-governed behaviors often are embarrassing and a burden for the patient to discuss. Patients often regard their sexual, aggressive, or religious (often contrareligious) thoughts to be disgraceful. Checklists and standard self-report measures such as the Children's Yale-Brown Obsessive Compulsive Scale (Storch et al. 2004), the Leyton Obsessional Inventory (Berg et al. 1986; Cooper 1970), and a modified form of the Child Behavior Checklist (Hudziak et al. 2006) can promote gathering this information, but questionnaires should facilitate, not supplant, conversation. It may take multiple meetings before children or adolescents will feel enough trust and reassurance to fully reveal their symptoms.

It is important to assess for concurrent problems that are common in those with tics such as learning, mood, and anxiety disorders. Patients with Tourette's often have executive function problems that interfere with learning and work. Impairment from symptoms can lead to depression and secondary anxiety, including profound fears about competence (generalized anxiety) and social acceptance/embarrassment (social anxiety).

A patient's symptoms may cause as much stress for the family as for the individual. Tic disorders are familial in three ways: they are biologically genetic, they can affect the relationships among immediate family members, and they can influence how the family relates to the community and extended family members. A child with Tourette's is highly likely to have a parent who is wrestling with the same or a similar disorder; 15%–60% of first-degree family members of children with Tourette's have tic disorders or OCD (Robertson and Cavanna 2007; State 2011). The family may be directly affected by the child's symptoms. Frequent, loud vocalizations or noisy, forceful motor tics such as stomping or banging can disturb everyone at home and interfere with family activities. Siblings may become angry and distance themselves from the patient. The demands on parents to give time and energy to assure optimal academic and therapeutic care for one child can mean less attention and patience for others at home. Parents can develop anxiety disorders or depression as they encounter barriers to care or support. With increasing stress there may be more friction between spouses, between parents and children, and between siblings. There may be effects on the family's relationship with the wider community and extended family members who do not understand the symptoms of Tourette's and wrongly view the child with Tourette's as rude or unruly. The parents may be criticized for their responses, resulting in increasing isolation and loss of social and emotional support.

For children with the triad of tics, learning problems, and ADHD symptoms, neuropsychological assessment can focus recommendations for school accommodations. Obstacles to assistance for youth with Tourette's can force parents and school staff into adversarial exchanges and mar the child's relationships with classmates and teachers. When symptoms are covert, it may be difficult for teachers and peers to understand why the patient needs accommodations or does not act like other students. Teachers (and some parents) may find it difficult to believe that disruptive symptoms are biological, brain-based, and difficult to control and create a burden for the patient. It is pivotal to explain to parents and teachers that disruptive behaviors arise for many reasons that can be biological and/or psychological. A "team approach" that includes the child to sort out what could be driving these behaviors is a necessary part of the assessment. Simply cataloging surface manifestations is insufficient. Choosing the best intervention depends on understanding the behavior. As examples, attempts to avoid embarrassment or ridicule, concerns about inadequacy, irritable outbursts accompanied by major depression, loud disruptive vocal tics accompanied by premonitory urges, and efforts to thwart authority will each call for different interventions.

Treatment

General Comments

The cornerstone of treatment is observation. Clinicians, patients, parents, and teachers benefit from knowing what symptoms are present and how they change over time and with different circumstances (Himle et al. 2006), how much a child struggles with his or her symptoms, and what strategies he or she uses to reduce them. Observing can be as simple as a log or diary of the most prominent tics, when they change, and what efforts the child has made to contain them. Targeted behavioral approaches rely on self-monitoring, with detailed observations at specific periods (Piacentini et al. 2010). Observation alone can have a potent effect on reducing symptoms by raising awareness and increasing helpful coping responses. However, in unusual circumstances, observation can "backfire"—i.e., increase tics—by reminding the patient about symptoms or by expanding parental anxiety, increasing scrutiny, and leading the patient to feel greater pressure to contain and monitor his symptoms.

The initial focus should be on providing accurate information to patients and parents and assuring that they comprehend the problem. This includes hearing the patient's and family's conceptions about the etiology and nature of symptoms, revising them as necessary, and teaching about the course and outcome of tic disorders. Education aims to reduce fears about the future, decrease blame, and promote cohesion in the family's efforts to resolve problems that arise from the patient's symptoms.

Specific Interventions

Behavioral Interventions

There is growing evidence that behavioral interventions can reduce the severity and frequency of tics. In addition, it is recognized that medication may not be effective for everyone, and for some patients undesirable side effects can offset an otherwise good result.

In adults, randomized controlled studies suggest that habit reversal training can be more successful than wait list conditions (McGuire et al. 2014) or active treatment, such as supportive therapy (Piacentini et al. 2010). Habit reversal relies on a *competing response procedure*—an action that when carried out makes it impossible to produce the tic, can be sustained for several minutes, and would not be readily visible to someone who is casually observing the patient. A premier example would be isometric tensing of muscles in opposition to a tic or rhythmic breathing to subvert a vocal tic (Piacentini et al. 2010). Tics with premonitory urges are perfect candidates for this kind of behavioral maneuver, although the number of children treated with these methods remains small.

Behavioral treatments require time, practice, determination, and dedication. A course of treatment typically takes several months or 8–10 sessions (Piacentini et al. 2010). Behavioral treatments generally work best for motivated patients who can form a strong relationship with the behavioral therapist.

Pharmacological Treatment

The approach to treating tic disorders with medication requires the clinician to think about more than whether tics are present and what medication should be used to reduce them. First, tic severity should be considered broadly. The burden of tics is not exclusively related to frequency or severity. The impact tics are having on the individual, the family, and the patient's social environment all must be weighed. Two patients with the same level of tic severity can have radically different treatment plans. The foremost objective is to maintain a strong working relationship with each patient, because treatment of tics is usually a long-term endeavor. Reducing tics at the expense of a patient's sense of control over her treatment, her comfort, and self-image is too costly. A child who feels "worked on" rather than working in collaboration with her doctor will not continue the relationship or the medication.

The objective of treatment is to reduce, not eliminate, tics. Determining when a sufficient reduction of tics has been reached is a subjective judgment that balances the patient's needs and quality of life against side effects and the risks of each medication. Weighing the risk-to-benefit ratio should always include the patient. For example, a lean patient may prefer the least sedating medication possible even if it might cause slight weight gain. The opposite may be true for a patient who is watching in horror as his weight rises. Waxing and waning of tics creates uncertainty about whether changes in symptoms are results of medication or natural variation. When patients have mild tics, the decision is among drug treatment with α-adrenergic agonists, no medication, and perhaps behavioral treatments. Starting with symptom monitoring is the best first intervention. Decisions about medication can then be tailored to the patient's pattern of symptoms. When tics are moderate to severe, a patient might prefer and do better with low doses of risperidone or pimozide than a higher dose of an α-adrenergic agonist. Clearly, no one drug or dose fits everyone. When titrating doses, the clinician must proceed gradually and use small increments.

The side effect profile and the timing of starting or increasing medication are critically important. An art of caring for patients with tics is to learn the triggers and pattern of tic severity and work prospectively, when possible, to manage medication doses. For example, if the patient starts medication during final exams or at the start of summer camp, the passing of the initial stress may lead to a natural reduction in symptoms that could be falsely attributed to the drug. Moreover, increased sedation during exams may be costly for the patient. When patients are uncomfortable, clinicians may be pressed to quickly increase the dose, but doing so can produce side effects that neutralize whatever relief was sought by reducing tics.

Another principle of treatment is constant reevaluation. If symptoms are well controlled for a sufficient period, perhaps 6–9 months, it is important to consider reducing medication. This is particularly helpful starting in mid to late adolescence, since tics may naturally wane during this time. It is also important when there are medication side effects that are difficult to tolerate. As with dose increases, decrements should be taken in small steps and with an eye toward timing and consequences. Since the majority of patients with tics will have only minor residual symptoms by late adolescence or early adulthood, it is incumbent on clinicians to attempt reducing medications in patients of this age who are doing well. Rebound symptoms may be observed when doses are reduced, so educating patients and families about this and allowing sufficient time to elapse to reestablish equilibrium before the next decrement are important.

Dopamine Antagonists

Medications that block dopamine are the mainstay of treatment for moderate to severe tics. These medications are the most studied for tic disorders and provide the most consistent, robust, and positive results. Chapter 38, "Antipsychotic Medications," has a detailed discussion of the use and side effects of these drugs. Pimozide is a dopamine-blocking agent used frequently in Tourette's that carries the risks and side effects of other agents in this class. Pimozide, like ziprasidone, can produce changes in cardiac conduction leading to QTc prolongation. In clinical trials using dopamine-blocking agents for tic disorders, intolerance of side effects led to discontinuation in 10%–40% of participants.

α_2-Adrenergic Agonists

These agents are discussed in Chapter 35, "Medications used for Attention-Deficit/Hyperactivity Disorder." The more benign side effect profile of clonidine (compared with antipsychotic agents) has led many authorities to consider it the first-line pharmacological agent for treatment of mild to moderate tics (Kurlan 2014; McNaught and Mink 2011). However, many prescribers and patients are dissuaded by problems of sedation, cognitive dulling, more modest reductions in symptoms, decreased blood pressure (and the risk of rebound hypertension), and risk of depression Nevertheless, clonidine does not produce extrapyramidal side effects, weight gain, or tardive dyskinesia.

The other major α_2-adrenergic agonist, guanfacine, has some, though limited, evidence to support its use for tics (Kurlan 2014; McNaught and Mink 2011).

Table 21–2 summarizes the randomized controlled clinical drug trials in Tourette's (see recent review papers by Kurlan 2014; McNaught and Mink 2011). All these agents possess risks and side effects that require close monitoring and include cardiac and neurological assessments. Dopamine antagonists also require attention to metabolic disorders.

Surgical Intervention

Surgically implanting electrodes into the globus pallidus, internal capsule, nucleus accumbens, or thalamus for control of intractable tics (Piedad et al.

TABLE 21–2. Pharmacological treatment of tic disorders: agents that have randomized placebo-controlled trials

Drug	Relevant studies	Typical dosage range, mg/day	Significant side effects	Efficacy	Comments
Dopamine antagonists			All in this group carry risks of sedation, cognitive dulling, elevation in serum prolactin, extrapyramidal side effects, and TD.		
Haloperidol	Ross and Moldofsky 1978; Sallee et al. 1997	0.25–8		25%–30% reduction in symptoms	
Metoclopramide	Nicolson et al. 2005	20–40	Sedation; may have lower risk for adverse cognitive effects	39% reduction in symptoms	Exceedingly small study
Pimozide	Bruggeman et al. 2001; Gilbert et al. 2004	0.5–8	Higher risk of QTc prolongation; less severe sedation and extrapyramidal effects compared with haloperidol; less weight gain than with risperidone (Gilbert et al. 2004)	22%–53% reduction in symptoms	
Risperidone	Gaffney et al. 2002; Gilbert et al. 2004; Scahill et al. 2003	0.25–4	Risk of weight gain, 0.75–1 lb/week; prolactin elevation; possibly lower risk of TD compared with pimozide, haloperidol	26%–56% reduction in symptoms	
Ziprasidone	Sallee et al. 2000	10–100	Particularly increased risk of QTc prolongation.	40% reduction in tics compared with 16% on placebo	
Aripiprazole	Yoo et al. 2013	2-20	Decreased prolactin; weight gain	53% reduction in tics compared with 32% on placebo; 65.6% response rate on drug compared with 45% on placebo	

TABLE 21–2. Pharmacological treatment of tic disorders: agents that have randomized placebo-controlled trials *(continued)*

Drug	Relevant studies	Typical dosage range, mg/day	Significant side effects	Efficacy	Comments
α_2-Adrenergic agonists			All display sedation and risk of hypotension. Effect is greater on ADHD symptoms than on tics.		
Clonidine	Bloch et al. 2009; Gaffney et al. 2002; Leckman et al. 1991	0.15–0.25		Mixed: 20%–30% reduction in tics reported; Gaffney et al. 2002 compared with risperidone and found no difference in efficacy; Goetz et al. 1987 found no difference from placebo	Requires 0.05–0.1 mg doses given 3–5 times/day
Guanfacine	Bloch et al. 2009; Scahill et al. 2001	0.5–4		Contradictory studies: Scahill et al. 2001 reported 31% reduction	Twice a day divided dosing needed

Note. ADHD=attention-deficit/hyperactivity disorder; TD=tardive dyskensia.

2012) has been done. Which sites are optimal for relief are not yet clear (Cannon et al. 2012; Piedad et al. 2012). The role for deep brain stimulation in the care of severe Tourette's and tic disorders has yet to be discerned, and utility of this invasive treatment for children and youth remains questionable.

Treatment of Associated Symptoms

The treatment of ADHD symptoms and OCD is discussed in Chapter 10, "Attention-Deficit/Hyperactivity Disorder," and Chapter 17, "Obsessive-Compulsive Disorder," respectively. In OCD, there is good evidence that obsessions and compulsions in persons with a personal or family history of tic disorders may not respond as well to behavioral or pharmacological treatment as those in persons without such a history. First-line intervention using cognitive-behavioral therapy (CBT) or a combination of serotonin reuptake inhibitors (SRIs) with CBT is recommended. There is evidence that those who do not respond to SRIs may benefit from augmentation with low doses of dopamine antagonists (e.g., risperidone, haloperidol, pimozide) (Bloch et al. 2006b; Goodman et al. 2006; Skapinakis et al. 2007).

The treatment of ADHD symptoms in the context of Tourette's or chronic tics has been revised in the last decade. Tics may be observed in patients receiving standard stimulant medications such as methylphenidate (MPH) or dextroamphetamine (d-AMP), and they may increase in patients with preexisting tics. Initially, case reports led some experts to recommend against using stimulants in patients with ADHD and Tourette's, and the U.S. Food and Drug Administration asserted that stimulants are contraindicated in children with tics and Tourette's. Experts have recommended α-adrenergic agonists such as clonidine or guanfacine as the first-line agents for ADHD symptoms in patients with Tourette's (Bloch et al. 2009; McNaught and Mink 2011; Roessner et al. 2011). However, longitudinal studies found that tics did not increase with MPH or d-AMP treatment, that any increases are clinically trivial (Roessner et al. 2011; Tourette's Syndrome Study Group 2002), and that tics may even decrease with stimulant treatment (Tourette's Syndrome Study Group 2002). Thus, current guidelines now indicate that stimulants are the first-line agents for ADHD comorbid with Tourette's (Bloch et al. 2009; Gilbert 2006; Kurlan 2014). α-Adrenergic agonists may be effective but carry greater risk of sedation. MPH and d-AMP appear to be more effective than clonidine or guanfacine for ADHD symptoms (Scahill et al. 2001; Tourette's Syndrome Study Group 2002). Worsening of tics is seen in about 25% of Tourette's patients whether they are given stimulants, clonidine, a combination, or placebo (Tourette's Syndrome Study Group 2002). Tics that arise after starting stimulants may decline over 3 months (Castellanos et al. 1997). Data also support the use of atomoxetine for patients with tic disorders (Bloch et al. 2009; Pringsheim and Steeves 2011).

Advocacy

The Tourette Syndrome Association (TSA) has been providing solid information, legislative advocacy, family support, research, and education on behalf of patients and families since 1972. It can be useful for families to learn about the TSA by visiting its Web site (www.tsa-usa.org) and for health care providers and teachers to be aware of TSA-sponsored professional programs.

Summary Points

- Tics are repetitive, brief, sudden, stereotyped movements that can occur in any voluntary muscle. Tics characteristically wax and wane, often migrate through the body, and can range in severity from very mild to quite severe.
- Tics can be transient or chronic. Chronic tics that include both phonic and motor elements, even if they occur at different times, are called Tourette's disorder.
- Tic disorders often co-occur with ADHD and with OCD. Impairment caused by these disorders can be greater than that from the tics.
- Tics often are preceded by mental or sensory events called premonitory urges.
- Tics are associated with abnormal functioning in CSTC loop circuits.
- Tics and Tourette's disorder are genetic disorders and probably result from multiple genes acting together.
- Tics affect physical, mental, familial, and academic/occupational domains.
- There is evidence that cognitive behavioral therapies, such as habit reversal training, can be effective in the treatment of tic disorders and that the most effective drug treatment is dopamine-blocking agents, although these have serious side effects.

References

Albin RL, Koeppe RA, Bohnen NI, et al: Increased ventral striatal monoaminergic innervation in Tourette syndrome. Neurology 61(3):310–315, 2003 12913189

American Psychiatric Association: Diagnostic and Statistical Manual of Mental Disorders, 5th Edition. Arlington, VA, American Psychiatric Association, 2013

Berg CJ, Rapoport JL, Flament M: The Leyton Obsessional Inventory-Child Version. J Am Acad Child Psychiatry 25(1):84–91, 1986 3950272

Bloch MH, Peterson BS, Scahill L, et al: Adulthood outcome of tic and obsessive-compulsive symptom severity in children with Tourette syndrome. Arch Pediatr Adolesc Med 160(1):65–69, 2006a 16389213

Bloch MH, Landeros-Weisenberger A, Kelmendi B, et al: A systematic review: antipsychotic augmentation with treatment refractory obsessive-compulsive disorder. Mol Psychiatry 11(7):622–632, 2006b 16585942

Bloch MH, Panza KE, Landeros-Weisenberger A, et al: Meta-analysis: treatment of attention-deficit/hyperactivity disorder in children with comorbid tic disorders. J Am Acad Child Adolesc Psychiatry 48(9):884–893, 2009 19625978

Bruggeman R, van der Linden C, Buitelaar JK, et al: Risperidone versus pimozide in Tourette's disorder: a comparative double-blind parallel-group study. J Clin Psychiatry 62(1):50–56, 2001 11235929

Budman CL, Bruun RD, Park KS, et al: Explosive outbursts in children with Tourette's disorder. J Am Acad Child Adolesc Psychiatry 39(10):1270–1276, 2000 11026181

Butler T, Stern E, Silbersweig D: Functional neuroimaging of Tourette syndrome: advances and future directions. Adv Neurol 99:115–129, 2006 16536357

Cannon E, Silburn P, Coyne T, et al: Deep brain stimulation of anteromedial globus pallidus interna for severe Tourette's syndrome. Am J Psychiatry 169(8):860–866, 2012 22772329

Castellanos FX, Giedd JN, Elia J, et al: Controlled stimulant treatment of ADHD and comorbid Tourette's syndrome: effects of stimulant and dose. J Am Acad Child Adolesc Psychiatry 36(5):589–596, 1997 9136492

Coffey BJ, Biederman J, Smoller JW, et al: Anxiety disorders and tic severity in juveniles with Tourette's disorder. J Am Acad Child Adolesc Psychiatry 39(5):562–568, 2000 10802973

Cooper J: The Leyton obsessional inventory. Psychol Med 1(1):48–64, 1970 5526113

Deng H, Gao K, Jankovic J: The genetics of Tourette syndrome. Nat Rev Neurol 8(4):203–213, 2012 22410579

Freeman RD, Fast DK, Burd L, et al: An international perspective on Tourette syndrome: selected findings from 3,500 individuals in 22 countries. Dev Med Child Neurol 42(7):436–447, 2000 10972415

Gaffney GR, Perry PJ, Lund BC, et al: Risperidone versus clonidine in the treatment of children and adolescents with Tourette's syndrome. J Am Acad Child Adolesc Psychiatry 41(3):330–336, 2002 11886028

Gaze C, Kepley HO, Walkup JT: Co-occurring psychiatric disorders in children and adolescents with Tourette syndrome. J Child Neurol 21(8):657–664, 2006 16970866

Gilbert D: Treatment of children and adolescents with tics and Tourette syndrome. J Child Neurol 21(8):690–700, 2006 16970870

Gilbert DL, Batterson JR, Sethuraman G, et al: Tic reduction with risperidone versus pimozide in a randomized, double-blind, crossover trial. J Am Acad Child Adolesc Psychiatry 43(2):206–214, 2004 14726728

Gilles de la Tourette G: Étude sur une affection nerveuse caractérisée par l'incoordination motrice, accompagnée d'écholalie et de coprolalia, in Gilles de la Tourette Syndrome. Edited by Friedhoff AJ, Chase TN. New York, Raven, 1982, pp 1–16

Goetz CG, Kompoliti K: Rating scales and quantitative assessment of tics. Adv Neurol 85:31–42, 2001 11530438

Goetz CG, Tanner CM, Wilson RS, et al: Clonidine and Gilles de la Tourette's syndrome: double-blind study using objective rating methods. Ann Neurol 21(3):307–310, 1987 3300518

Goodman WK, Storch EA, Geffken GR, et al: Obsessive-compulsive disorder in Tourette syndrome. J Child Neurol 21(8):704–714, 2006 16970872

Himle MB, Chang S, Woods DW, et al: Establishing the feasibility of direct observation in the assessment of tics in children with chronic tic disorders. J Appl Behav Anal 39(4):429–440, 2006 17236340

Hudziak JJ, Althoff RR, Stanger C, et al: The Obsessive Compulsive Scale of the Child Behavior Checklist predicts obsessive-compulsive disorder: a receiver operating characteristic curve analysis. J Child Psychol Psychiatry 47(2):160–166, 2006 16423147

Jeffries KJ, Schooler C, Schoenbach C, et al: The functional neuroanatomy of Tourette's syndrome: an FDG PET study III: functional coupling of regional cerebral metabolic rates. Neuropsychopharmacology 27(1):92–104, 2002 12062910

Jin R, Zheng RY, Huang WW, et al: Epidemiological survey of Tourette syndrome in children and adolescents in Wenzhou of P.R. China. Eur J Epidemiol 20(11):925–927, 2005 16284870

Kadesjö B, Gillberg C: Tourette's disorder: epidemiology and comorbidity in primary school children. J Am Acad Child Adolesc Psychiatry 39(5):548–555, 2000 10802971

Knight T, Steeves T, Day L, et al: Prevalence of tic disorders: a systematic review and meta-analysis. Pediatr Neurol 47(2):77–90, 2012 22759682

Kostanecka-Endress T, Banaschewski T, Kinkelbur J, et al: Disturbed sleep in children with Tourette syndrome: a polysomnographic study. J Psychosom Res 55(1):23–29, 2003 12842228

Kurlan RM: Treatment of Tourette syndrome. Neurotherapeutics 11(1):161–165, 2014 24043501

Kurlan R, Como PG, Miller B, et al: The behavioral spectrum of tic disorders: a community-based study. Neurology 59(3):414–420, 2002 12177376

Leckman JF, Riddle MA, Hardin MT, et al: The Yale Global Tic Severity Scale: initial testing of a clinician-rated scale of tic severity. J Am Acad Child Adolesc Psychiatry 28(4):566–573, 1989 2768151

Leckman JF, Hardin MT, Riddle MA, et al: Clonidine treatment of Gilles de la Tourette's syndrome. Arch Gen Psychiatry 48(4):324–328, 1991 2009034

Leckman JF, Walker DE, Cohen DJ: Premonitory urges in Tourette's syndrome. Am J Psychiatry 150(1):98–102, 1993 8417589

Leckman JF, Zhang H, Alsobrook JP, et al: Symptom dimensions in obsessive-compulsive disorder: toward quantitative phenotypes. Am J Med Genet 105(1):28–30, 2001 11424988

Leckman JF, Vaccarino FM, Kalanithi PS, et al: Annotation: Tourette syndrome: a relentless drumbeat—driven by misguided brain oscillations. J Child Psychol Psychiatry 47(6):537–550, 2006 16712630

Leckman JF, Bloch MH, Smith ME, et al: Neurobiological substrates of Tourette's disorder. J Child Adolesc Psychopharmacol 20(4):237–247, 2010 20807062

Leckman JF, King RA, Gilbert DL, et al: Streptococcal upper respiratory tract infections and exacerbations of tic and obsessive-compulsive symptoms: a prospective longitudinal study. J Am Acad Child Adolesc Psychiatry 50(2):108–118, e3, 2011 21241948

Lerner A, Bagic A, Boudreau EA, et al: Neuroimaging of neuronal circuits involved in tic generation in patients with Tourette syndrome. Neurology 68(23):1979–1987, 2007 17548547

Martino D, Zis P, Buttiglione M: The role of immune mechanisms in Tourette syndrome. Brain Res 2014 24845720 Epub ahead of print

Mathews CA, Jang KL, Herrera LD, et al: Tic symptom profiles in subjects with Tourette syndrome from two genetically isolated populations. Biol Psychiatry 61(3):292–300, 2007 16581034

McGuire JF, Piacentini J, Brennan EA, et al: A meta-analysis of behavior therapy for Tourette syndrome. J Psychiatr Res 50:106–112, 2014 24398255

McNaught KS, Mink JW: Advances in understanding and treatment of Tourette syndrome. Nat Rev Neurol 7(12):667–676, 2011 22064610

Nestadt G, Addington A, Samuels J, et al: The identification of OCD-related subgroups based on comorbidity. Biol Psychiatry 53(10):914–920, 2003 12742679

Nicolson R, Craven-Thuss B, Smith J, et al: A randomized, double-blind, placebo-controlled trial of metoclopramide for the treatment of Tourette's disorder. J Am Acad Child Adolesc Psychiatry 44(7):640–646, 2005 15968232

Parent A, Hazrati LN: Functional anatomy of the basal ganglia. I. The cortico-basal ganglia-thalamo-cortical loop. Brain Res Brain Res Rev 20(1):91–127, 1995 7711769

Peterson BS, Leckman JF: The temporal dynamics of tics in Gilles de la Tourette syndrome. Biol Psychiatry 44(12):1337–1348, 1998 9861477

Piacentini J, Woods DW, Scahill L, et al: Behavior therapy for children with Tourette disorder: a randomized controlled trial. JAMA 303(19):1929–1937, 2010 20483969

Piedad JC, Rickards HE, Cavanna AE: What patients with Gilles de la Tourette syndrome should be treated with deep brain stimulation and what is the best target? Neurosurgery 71(1):173–192, 2012 22407075

Pringsheim T, Steeves T: Pharmacological treatment for Attention Deficit Hyperactivity Disorder (ADHD) in children with comorbid tic disorders. Cochrane Database Syst Rev 4:CD007990, 2011 DOI: 10.1002/14651858.CD007990.pub2

Reese HE, Scahill L, Peterson AL, et al: The premonitory urge to tic: measurement, characteristics, and correlates in older adolescents and adults. Behav Ther 45(2):177–186, 2014 24491193

Robertson MM: Attention deficit hyperactivity disorder, tics and Tourette's syndrome: the relationship and treatment implications. A commentary. Eur Child Adolesc Psychiatry 15(1):1–11, 2006 16514504

Robertson MM, Cavanna AE: The Gilles de la Tourette syndrome: a principal component factor analytic study of a large pedigree. Psychiatr Genet 17(3):143–152, 2007 17417057

Robertson MM, Williamson F, Eapen V: Depressive symptomatology in young people with Gilles de la Tourette Syndrome: a comparison of self-report scales. J Affect Disord 91(2–3):265–268, 2006 16464507

Roessner V, Plessen KJ, Rothenberger A, et al: European clinical guidelines for Tourette syndrome and other tic disorders. Part II: pharmacological treatment. Eur Child Adolesc Psychiatry 20(4):173–196, 2011 21445724

Ross MS, Moldofsky H: A comparison of pimozide and haloperidol in the treatment of Gilles de la Tourette's syndrome. Am J Psychiatry 135:585–587, 1978 347954

Rothenberger A, Roessner V: Functional neuroimaging investigations of motor networks in Tourette syndrome. Behav Neurol 27(1):47–55, 2013 23187141

Sallee FR, Nesbitt L, Jackson C, et al: Relative efficacy of haloperidol and pimozide in children and adolescents with Tourette's disorder. Am J Psychiatry 154(8):1057–1062, 1997 9247389

Sallee FR, Kurlan R, Goetz CG, et al: Ziprasidone treatment of children and adolescents with Tourette's syndrome: a pilot study. J Am Acad Child Adolesc Psychiatry 39(3):292–299, 2000 10714048

Scahill L, Chappell PB, Kim YS, et al: A placebo-controlled study of guanfacine in the treatment of children with tic disorders and attention deficit hyperactivity disorder. Am J Psychiatry 158(7):1067–1074, 2001 11431228

Scahill L, Leckman JF, Schultz RT, et al: A placebo-controlled trial of risperidone in Tourette syndrome. Neurology 60(7):1130–1135, 2003 12682319

Simonoff E, Pickles A, Charman T, et al: Psychiatric disorders in children with autism spectrum disorders: prevalence, comorbidity, and associated factors in a population-derived sample. J Am Acad Child Adolesc Psychiatry 47(8):921–929, 2008 18645422

Skapinakis P, Papatheodorou T, Mavreas V: Antipsychotic augmentation of serotonergic antidepressants in treatment-resistant obsessive-compulsive disorder: a meta-analysis of the randomized controlled trials. Eur Neuropsychopharmacol 17(2):79–93, 2007 16904298

State MW: The genetics of Tourette disorder. Curr Opin Genet Dev 21(3):302–309, 2011 21277193

Storch EA, Murphy TK, Geffken GR, et al: Psychometric evaluation of the Children's Yale-Brown Obsessive-Compulsive Scale. Psychiatry Res 129(1):91–98, 2004 15572188

Swedo SE, Leckman JF, Rose NR: From research subgroup to clinical syndrome: modifying the PANDAS criteria to describe PANS (pediatric acute-onset neuropsychiatric syndrome). Pediatrics & Therapeutics 2:113, 2012

Tourette's Syndrome Study Group: Treatment of ADHD in children with tics: a randomized controlled trial. Neurology 58(4):527–536, 2002 11865128

Visser-Vandewalle V, Temel Y, Boon P, et al: Chronic bilateral thalamic stimulation: a new therapeutic approach in intractable Tourette syndrome. Report of three cases. J Neurosurg 99(6):1094–1100, 2003 14705742

Walkup JT, Rosenberg LA, Brown J, et al: The validity of instruments measuring tic severity in Tourette's syndrome. J Am Acad Child Adolesc Psychiatry 31(3):472–477, 1992 1592779

Wang Z, Maia TV, Marsh R, et al: The neural circuits that generate tics in Tourette's syndrome. Am J Psychiatry 168(12):1326–1337, 2011 21955933

Yoo HK, Joung YS, Lee JS, et al: A multicenter, randomized, double-blind, placebo-controlled study of aripiprazole in children and adolescents with Tourette's disorder. J Clin Psychiatry 74(8):e772–e780, 2013 24021518

Zohar AH, Pauls DL, Ratzoni G, et al: Obsessive-compulsive disorder with and without tics in an epidemiological sample of adolescents. Am J Psychiatry 154(2):274–276, 1997 9016283

CHAPTER 22

Elimination Disorders

Edwin J. Mikkelsen, M.D.

Enuresis

Enuresis has been described throughout recorded history. A comprehensive summary by Glicklich (1951) found descriptions going back to the Papyrus Ebers of 1550 B.C.E. The history of enuresis is also rich with regard to the various treatment modalities that have been used over the years. Unfortunately, many of these would now appear to be sadistic in nature, given our current base of knowledge.

Definition and Clinical Description

The word *enuresis* is derived from the Greek word *enourein,* meaning "to void urine." A pathological connection is not inherent in the derivation but has been acquired over time. The word has come to denote nocturnal events, but that also is not inherent in the original derivation.

The phenomenology of enuresis is simply the voiding of urine, which usually occurs during sleep. However, it can also occur during the day while the individual is awake. The word *diurnal* is used to describe events that occur during the day. Individuals who have episodes during both the day and the night are referred to as having diurnal and nocturnal enuresis. The volume of urine that is voided is not specified and technically could vary considerably while still being considered an *enuretic event.* The concrete nature of the enuretic event makes data collection relatively simple. It also makes it possible to quantify the magnitude of treatment effects by comparing the pre- and post-treatment weekly averages.

Diagnosis

The DSM-5 (American Psychiatric Association 2013) criteria for enuresis are reproduced in Box 22–1. There are two subtypes of enuresis, based on the natural history of the disorder. The term *primary enuresis* is used to describe those individuals who have never achieved continence,

The author wishes to thank Ms. Patsy Kuropatkin for her invaluable assistance with preparation of this manuscript.

whereas *secondary enuresis* refers to those who were able to achieve continence but then subsequently resumed wetting. A time period of 6 months to 1 year is usually accepted as the length of time continence must have been maintained, although the DSM-5 criteria do not specify the required duration of continence. The vast majority of children with enuresis wet involuntarily. The DSM-5 notation that the wetting may be "involuntary or intentional" is unfortunate, as those whose events are intentional clearly differ in many ways.

Box 22–1. DSM-5 Diagnostic Criteria for Enuresis

307.6 (F98.0)

A. Repeated voiding of urine into bed or clothes, whether involuntary or intentional.
B. The behavior is clinically significant as manifested by either a frequency of at least twice a week for at least 3 consecutive months or the presence of clinically significant distress or impairment in social, academic (occupational), or other important areas of functioning.
C. Chronological age is at least 5 years (or equivalent developmental level).
D. The behavior is not attributable to the physiological effects of a substance (e.g., a diuretic, an antipsychotic medication) or another medical condition (e.g., diabetes, spina bifida, a seizure disorder).

Specify whether:

Nocturnal only: Passage of urine only during nighttime sleep.
Diurnal only: Passage of urine during waking hours.
Nocturnal and diurnal: A combination of the two subtypes above.

Source. Reprinted from the *Diagnostic and Statistical Manual of Mental Disorders,* 5th Edition. Arlington VA, American Psychiatric Association, 2013. Used with permission.

Epidemiology

The epidemiology of enuresis has proven to be relatively consistent in large, cross-sectional national studies. Although these studies vary with regard to the frequency of the enuretic events and the ages of the cross-sectional samples, they are similar enough to be compared. The first comprehensive epidemiological investigation was in Rutter's Isle of Wight Study (Rutter 1989), which found that the prevalence of enuresis diminished with advancing age, as only 1.1% of 14-year-old males were wetting once a week. The corresponding frequency for 14-year-old females was 0.5%. Subsequent large epidemiological studies have been generally consistent with these initial findings (Söderstrom et al. 2004). In general, the prevalence for 5-year-olds is in the 5%–10% range and drops to 3%–5% by age 10. All of the studies document the disproportionate occurrence in males.

Medical Comorbidity

The primary concern with regard to medical comorbidity is the presence of a urinary tract infection. This is most relevant in females. The possible presence of structural urinary tract abnormalities has been extensively investigated. Although some studies report a small percentage of children for whom this may be a factor, the consensus is that there is not enough evidence to warrant routinely subjecting children to these invasive studies. Enuresis has also been reported as a side effect of treatment with selective serotonin reuptake inhibitors (Hergüner et al. 2007). The potential medical causes of enuresis are outlined in Table 22–1.

TABLE 22–1. Medical causes of enuresis

Urinary tract infection
Diabetes insipidus
Diabetes mellitus
Urethritis
Seizure disorder
Sickle cell trait
Sleep apnea
Neurogenic bladder
Sleep disorders
Genitourinary malformation or obstruction
Side effect of or idiosyncratic reaction to a medication[a]

Note. [a]Per case reports regarding selective serotonin reuptake inhibitors, be vigilant for chronological correlations.

Source. Adapted from Dulcan MK, Martini DR, Lake MB: *Concise Guide to Child and Adolescent Psychiatry,* 3rd Edition. Washington, DC, American Psychiatric Publishing, 2003.

Psychological Comorbidity

Children with secondary enuresis are more apt to present with comorbid psychiatric disorders than children with primary enuresis (Mikkelsen 2001). The other major area of investigation has been with comorbid attention-deficit/hyperactivity disorder (ADHD; Baeyens et al. 2004). These studies support the hypothesis that the enuresis is comorbid with the ADHD and is not secondarily related to the ADHD. Other than the association of enuresis with ADHD, the primary finding has been that behavioral disorders in children with enuresis are nonspecific (Mikkelsen et al. 1980). This finding is consistent with a number of studies that link enuresis with a generalized developmental delay in maturation (Touchette et al. 2005).

Etiology, Mechanism, and Risk Factors

There have been discrete historical periods of research concerning the etiology and pathophysiology of enuresis. Early psychodynamic theories, which conceived of enuresis as an unconscious expression of anger or resentment, have been largely abandoned. The development of all-night polysomnographic studies led to research that focused on enuresis as a sleep disorder that was characterized as a "disorder of arousal," with the enuretic events occurring in "deep sleep." However, subsequent studies with larger sample sizes indicated that enuretic events occurred during phases of the sleep cycle in direct proportion to the amount of time spent in that phase (Mikkelsen 2001).

The success of various pharmacological treatments (which will be discussed in more detail in the subsection "Pharmacological Treatments") has also led to speculation regarding etiology. The first widely demonstrated effective pharmacological treatment was imipramine. Initially, it was thought that the efficacy of imipramine could be related to its anticholinergic effects on the urinary sphincter, as urinary retention can be a side effect of tricyclic agents. However, a large double-blind study that compared imipramine with methscopolamine (an anticholinergic agent that does not cross the blood-brain barrier) found imipramine to be significantly more effective, suggesting a central effect, although a precise mechanism could not be elucidated (Mikkelsen et al. 1980). In a more recent study, Hunsballe et al. (1997) suggested that imipramine produced a decrease in osmolar clearance and urinary output, which might contribute to its well-documented efficacy in enuresis.

The most recent era in pharmacological treatment with desmopressin acetate (DDAVP) has generated a number of hypotheses concerning the child's levels of plasma atrial natriuretic peptide (ANP) and the ability to concentrate urine during the night. Rittig et al. (1991) compared 15 children with nocturnal enuresis and 11 matched control subjects with regard to the circadian variation of ANP, creatinine clearance, and the excretion of sodium and potassium. Although the two groups did not differ in ANP levels, the children with enuresis demonstrated increased natriuresis, kalioresis, and polyuria during the initial hours of sleep. As the abnormalities did not correlate with differing levels of ANP, the authors speculated that the difference might be related to an abnormal tubular factor. Subsequent research has supported this hypothesis (Natochin and Kuznetsova 1999).

Another line of investigation has focused on the circadian production of plasma arginine vasopressin (AVP), as abnormalities with the production of this peptide could explain both the response to DDAVP and the pathophysiology of enuresis. A study by Medel et al. (1998) investigated morning levels of AVP in control subjects and in children with enuresis and found significant differences. Also of interest was the observation that these levels correlated with response or lack of response to DDAVP. However, the recognition that AVP is secreted in a pulsatile manner suggested that frequent sampling of plasma levels would be needed to draw any firm conclusions regarding the significance of AVP levels. Subsequent studies, which have used more frequent sampling of AVP, have not produced consistent results (Läckgren et al. 1997). The most detailed series of investigations with regard to AVP secretion used hourly measurements for 24 hours (Aikawa et al. 1999). The first group of studies found that children with enuresis had significantly lower AVP levels than control subjects in the 11:00 P.M. to 4:00 A.M. time period. The authors then identified two subgroups of children with enuresis on the basis of urinary osmotic pressure and volume of nocturnal urine production. One subgroup of children had low urinary osmotic pressure coupled with large nocturnal urine production, while the other had normal osmotic pressure and relatively small nocturnal urine production. The authors report that the first group had significantly lower mean nocturnal AVP levels. The AVP levels were also measured after treatment with DDAVP, and a significant increase in AVP levels was found. However, this was a group effect and was not found in every child. A recent study with a somewhat different design also implicated lower nocturnal AVP as a significant factor in a subset of individuals (Rittig et al. 2008).

The child's inherent bladder capacity is an obvious potential contributor to enuresis. In an early study, Shaffer et al. (1984) investigated the relationship between bladder capacity and behavioral disturbance as they related to the development of enuresis. The results were suggestive of a general underlying developmental delay, in that the children who were identified as having a behavioral disturbance also had more developmental delays and smaller functional bladder capacity.

Studies involving ultrasound to determine both the bladder capacity and the thickness of the bladder wall did suggest that these factors were significantly related to response to DDAVP (Sreedhar et al. 2008). However, a study that investigated a number of factors that might be predictive of response, including functional bladder capacity, indicated that functional bladder capacity is correlated with daytime fluid intake, suggesting no simple explanation for DDAVP responders and nonresponders (Dehoorne et al. 2007).

It has long been known that enuresis tends to run in families. The advent of the modern era of genetic linkage studies has led to several large pedigree studies. All of the linkage studies involve families with a history of multiple affected generations with high rates of enuresis. Loeys et al. (2002) reported heterogeneous results in a genetic linkage study of 32 families with pedigrees that were positive for multiple individuals with primary nocturnal enuresis. The results indicated linkage to chromosome 12q (four families), 13q 13–14 (six families), and 22q 11 (nine families). Other studies have also implicated multiple chromosomes. Thus, although this line of research is promising, it appears that there will not be a simple parsimonious genetic explanation for the well-documented, multigenerational transmission of enuresis.

A family history of enuresis continues to be the most significant risk factor for primary enuresis. A Scandinavian epidemiological study found that the risk of enuresis for a child was 7.1 times greater if the father had enuretic events beyond age 4 (Järvelin et al. 1988).

Course and Prognosis

Typically, there is a relatively high rate of spontaneous remission between ages 5–7 years and after age 12 years. Yearly remission rates as high as 14%–16% have been reported (Fritz et al. 2004). Thus, enuresis is usually a self-limited disorder, and the vast majority of children who are affected will eventually experience a spontaneous remission. The persistence of enuresis into late adolescence is rare.

Evaluation

The evaluation of the child with enuresis should include a thorough history obtained from both the parents and the child. This will include historical data with regard to the major developmental milestones, as well as prior attempts at toilet training. The toilet training history should include a description of the techniques used, the duration of the trials, and the results. This interview will also provide an opportunity to explore for possible environmental and emotional contributions to the enuresis. For example, is the child afraid of the dark, and does he or she wet the bed because of fear of getting up to go to the bathroom? Another example would be the child with attentional problems and daytime wetting because he or she puts off going to the bathroom until it is too late.

The objective nature of the enuretic event simplifies the evaluation process. It is useful to approach the problem in a nonjudgmental manner that emphasizes that the enuretic events are not voluntary. A simple calendar-tracking method can be used to record the frequency of enuretic events. This will both establish the diagnosis and provide a baseline for measuring treatment effects. Both the parents and the child should be instructed to collect frequency data. It will also be useful to note the time of day in addition to the date for children with daytime wetting. A urinalysis should be obtained to rule out a urinary tract infection. Invasive diagnostic studies are usually not warranted unless there is some reason to suspect an anatomical abnormality.

Behavioral disturbances that accompany enuresis may represent either an emotional reaction to having enuresis or a comorbid psychiatric disorder. The primary psychological effect related to enuresis is a decrease in self-esteem, which will often improve with effective treatment.

Treatment

The primary consideration with regard to treatment is that enuresis is a self-limited disorder with a substantial rate of spontaneous remission with each successive year. The frequency of the enuretic events should also be a consideration. A child who experiences enuretic episodes virtually every night is in a different category than the child who barely meets the threshold for diagnosis.

Pharmacological Treatments

The first era of pharmacological treatment followed MacLean's (1960) observation that imipramine was an effective treatment, which was subsequently supported by multiple double-blind studies. The treatment was generally found to be safe, although there were some tragic reports of fatal overdoses in children who thought that if taking a few pills would make the enuresis go away for a night, then taking the whole bottle would completely cure them. Treatment guidelines for imipramine suggest cardiac monitoring and periodic blood levels to guard against toxicity at higher doses. The usual protocol for imipramine treatment is to obtain a baseline electrocardiogram and to begin at 25 mg at bedtime with a slow titration of 25 mg increments at weekly intervals until continence is achieved. If doses in the 75–125 mg range have not produced a positive response, it becomes less likely that the child will respond to imipramine. A dosage of 5 mg/kg/day is considered to be the upper limit. As the rate of spontaneous remission is significant, it makes sense to withdraw (tapering from doses larger than 25 mg) the medication every 3 months to determine if the enuresis has remitted. Multiple large studies have reported that the efficacy of imipramine correlated with the steady-state concentration of imipramine combined with its active metabolite, desipramine (Rapoport et al. 1980). The variation in serum levels of children receiving the same dose of imipramine has been reported to be as great as sevenfold (Mikkelsen 2001). Imipramine is still used for children who are refractory to other methods of treatment, either as an adjunctive or a stand-alone treatment.

The advent of treatment with DDAVP largely supplanted the use of imipramine. Initially, DDAVP was administered by nasal inhalation, although an oral formulation was later developed. Moffatt et al. (1993) published a review article that identified 18 randomized controlled studies including 689 subjects. Many of these subjects had not responded to prior treatment. The range of efficacy, as measured by the decrease in frequency of enuretic events, was 10%–91%. In most subjects, wetting resumed after DDAVP was discontinued; only 5.7% were reported to maintain continence after discontinuation of DDAVP.

The most common side effects of the nasal spray formulation were abdominal pain, headaches, epistaxis, and nasal stuffiness. In general, children whose enuretic events were less frequent and those who were older than age 9 years had better outcomes.

The most significant side effect that has been identified with intranasal use of DDAVP is hyponatremia and related seizures. Excess fluid intake has been identified as a contributing factor, leading to a recommendation that children not ingest more than 8 ounces of fluid on nights when DDAVP is used (Robson et al. 1996). The risk appears to be greater during the initial stage of treatment, and younger children appear to be at a greater risk. It is thought that greater bioavailability related to prolonged half-life may contribute to the development of side effects (Dehoorne et al. 2006b). It also appears that the oral preparation may present less risk of hyponatremia. Robson et al. (2007) reported that post-marketing data revealed 151 cases of DDAVP-related hyponatremia; 145 of these were related to the nasal preparation, as compared with 6 cases of children who were receiving the oral form. In recognition of the risk of hyponatremic seizures, some of which were fatal, the U.S. Food and Drug Administration (FDA) has issued a warning that the intranasal preparation of DDAVP should no longer be used for the treatment of primary nocturnal enuresis. The alert also indicated that treatment with the oral formulation should be interrupted during acute illness that could produce a fluid or electrolyte imbalance.

The observation that wetting will usually resume after DDAVP is discontinued has led to long-term follow-up studies of chronic use. A large, multicenter Swedish study involving 399 children ages 6–12 with primary nocturnal enuresis used a 4-week baseline observational period, followed by a 6-week dose titration period, and then 1 year of long-term treatment that included a week without treatment every 3 months to identify children who had a spontaneous remission. Daily doses ranged from 20 μg to 40 μg. The average weekly frequency of wet nights during the last 3-month treatment period was 0.8, as compared with 5.3 nights during the baseline phase of the study. As in other studies, older age correlated significantly with positive response (Hjälmås et al. 1998).

The introduction of the oral form of DDAVP has made it much easier to administer. Also, as noted earlier, the FDA no longer approves of the use of the nasal formulation for enuresis because of an increased risk of hyponatremia and seizures. A large multicenter study that compared 20 μg of the nasal spray with 200 μg and 400 μg doses of oral DDAVP found no significant differences in treatment response, although the 400 μg oral preparation appeared to be superior to the 200 μg dose (Janknegt et al. 1997).

A randomized placebo-controlled study using 200 μg, 400 μg, and 600 μg doses of oral DDAVP suggested a linear dose response with increasing dose correlated with the decrease in frequency of enuretic events (Skoog et al. 1997). The long-term use of oral DDAVP was found to be safe in a large Canadian study (Wolfish et al. 2003).

A recent innovation in treatment with DDAVP has been the development of a sublingual oral lyophilisate formulation referred to as MELT, which is well tolerated and preferred by many children (Juul et al. 2013).

A number of studies have attempted to determine the pretreatment factors that are associated with a positive response to DDAVP. Those that have been repeatedly identified include lower frequency of baseline enuretic events, older age, and greater bladder capacity (Kruse et al. 2001). An extensive investigation by Dehoorne et al. (2006a) involving children who were nonresponsive to DDAVP suggested that this was due to increased urinary osmolality and nocturnal polyuria, which could be related to their dietary habits and fluid intake.

Psychotherapeutic Treatment

There is no evidence that a traditional psychotherapeutic approach will produce any benefit for primary enuresis, although it may be helpful in ameliorating the child's embarrassment and diminished self-esteem. A therapeutic-educational approach is useful in helping the family to initiate treatment in a nonjudgmental, supportive manner.

Children who have secondary enuresis are more apt to have psychological stressors contributing to the loss of continence and may be more likely to benefit from psychotherapy (Fritz et al. 2004). A psychotherapeutic approach may also be useful for comorbid psychiatric disorders.

Other Treatment Modalities

Behavioral treatment with the bell and pad method of conditioning was first described in 1904 and has been an accepted treatment strategy for several decades. In this method of treatment, the child sleeps on a pad that has wires attached to an alarm. When an enuretic event occurs, the urine completes the electrical circuit and the alarm sounds. A comprehensive review of the literature (Glazener et al. 2003) found an initial response rate of approximately two-thirds, with the rate of sustained remission close to 50%. It has long been known that there are two distinct subgroups of children who experience remission with the bell and pad: those who learn to wake up to urinate and those who sleep through the night without wetting. Butler et al. (2007) undertook a pre- and post-alarm treatment study to investigate possible physiological explanations for success. Seventy-five percent of their subjects met success criteria, and of these, 89% predominantly slept through the night on dry nights. Those who experienced success manifested an increase in posttreatment ability to concentrate urine. In approximately half of these subjects, this appeared to be due to an increase in vasopressin. The most recent innovation in this behavioral methodology uses an externally attached ultrasonic monitor that sounds an alarm at a specific threshold of bladder capacity (Pretlow 1999).

A number of other behavioral strategies have been reported, including retention-control training, evening fluid restriction, reward systems, and nighttime awakening to urinate. A thorough review of the published literature regarding these interventions (Glazener and Evans 2004) indicated that the methodology and small sample size of these reports precluded a rigorous meta-analysis.

Combined Treatment Methods

The concomitant use of the bell and pad method of treatment with DDAVP has produced variable results. A study by Leebeek-Groenewegen et al. (2001) indicated that the combination produced a more rapid response but did not improve the overall success rate. However, a study that paired imipramine with the alarm or DDAVP with the alarm found that neither was superior to the alarm alone (Naitoh et al. 2005). Another approach has been to add DDAVP after 6 weeks of bell and pad treatment that was not completely effective or after 2 weeks for children with no response at that point and multiple nocturnal events (Kamperis et al. 2008). The authors note that those children who required the addition of DDAVP had greater nocturnal urine production.

Comparison of Treatments

In a large, longitudinal study, Monda and Husmann (1995) compared the results of observation only with treatment with imipramine, DDAVP, or the bell and pad method. The length of follow-up was 12 months. However, treatment was weaned after 6 months so that the response at 6 months represents the effects of active treatment and the 12-month data represent the frequency with which continence was maintained after cessation of active treatment. These results clearly indicate the superiority of the bell and pad method of treatment with regard to the degree of relapse after the cessation of active treatment. A subsequent systematic review of the literature involving the alarm, imipramine, and DDAVP confirmed this finding (Glazener and Evans 2002).

Encopresis

The history of encopresis is less well documented than that of enuresis. There are also far fewer research studies investigating the cause of encopresis, as compared with the interest in enuresis.

Definition and Clinical Description

Encopresis is defined as the passage of feces into inappropriate places by a child who has reached a chronological age or developmental level at which he or she could be reasonably expected to be able to control the expulsion of feces. A distinction is made between retentive encopresis, which usually involves constipation with overflow incontinence, and nonretentive encopresis. An important distinction can also be made between involuntary and voluntary encopresis.

Diagnosis

DSM-5 criteria for encopresis are reproduced in Box 22–2. A distinction is not made in DSM-5 whether the encopresis is involuntary or voluntary. As with enuresis, a distinction is made between *primary* and *secondary encopresis,* with the latter term referring to those who have developed fecal continence and then relapse. The categorization of encopresis into two subtypes is clinically quite significant. The category *with constipation and overflow incontinence* represents *retentive encopresis,* whereas the category *without constipation and overflow incontinence* corresponds to *nonretentive encopresis.* The frequency required to establish the diagnosis is at least one event per month, for 3 months. The age required is a chronological age of 4 years, or equivalent developmental level.

Box 22–2. DSM-5 Diagnostic Criteria for Encopresis

307.7 (F98.1)

A. Repeated passage of feces into inappropriate places (e.g., clothing, floor), whether involuntary or intentional.
B. At least one such event occurs each month for at least 3 months.
C. Chronological age is at least 4 years (or equivalent developmental level).
D. The behavior is not attributable to the physiological effects of a substance (e.g., laxatives) or another medical condition except through a mechanism involving constipation.

Specify whether:

With constipation and overflow incontinence: There is evidence of constipation on physical examination or by history.

Without constipation and overflow incontinence: There is no evidence of constipation on physical examination or by history.

Source. Reprinted from the *Diagnostic and Statistical Manual of Mental Disorders,* 5th Edition. Arlington, VA, American Psychiatric Association, 2013. Used with permission.

Epidemiology

Encopresis is less prevalent than enuresis. Unfortunately, the sampling strategy and frequency of encopretic episodes vary considerably in large cross-sectional studies. However, there is enough consistency to warrant comparison. The first large study (Bellman 1966) found a prevalence of 1.5% among a cohort of 8,863 children ages 7–8 years. The male-to-female ratio was 3:1. Subsequent epidemiological studies have been generally consistent with these initial findings (Heron et al. 2008). As with enuresis, the prevalence of encopresis decreases as the child ages.

Medical and Psychological Comorbidity

There are occasionally children who present with both enuresis and encopresis (Rutter et al. 1981). Chronic constipation is usually present in those who have retentive encopresis, as this is part of the underlying pathophysiology of this disorder. Children with encopresis have more behavioral difficulties than control subjects, although there is no specific pattern. Obviously, children who voluntarily defecate in inappropriate places will likely have a comorbid psychiatric disorder. Voluntary encopresis and hoarding of feces may be seen as a sequel of sexual abuse, but this symptom is not diagnostic of sexual abuse (Mellon et al. 2006). Potential medical causes of encopresis appear in Table 22–2.

TABLE 22–2. Medical causes of encopresis

Constipation
Hirschsprung disease
Medical conditions producing diarrhea
Side effect or idiosyncratic reaction to a medication (maintain vigilance for chronological correlation)
Painful lesion
Hemorrhoids (contributing to constipation)
Thyroid disease
Hypercalcemia
Lactase deficiency
Pseudo-obstruction
Spina bifida
Cerebral palsy with hypotonia
Rectal stenosis
Anal fissure
Anorectal trauma, including sexual abuse

Source. Adapted from Dulcan MK, Martini DR, Lake MB: *Concise Guide to Child and Adolescent Psychiatry,* 3rd Edition. Washington, DC, American Psychiatric Publishing, 2003.

Etiology, Mechanism, and Risk Factors

Retentive Encopresis

Chronic constipation is, by definition, the major factor in the evolution of retentive encopresis. The fecal incontinence that is observed is overflow incontinence from the retained fecal mass. Loening-Baucke (2004) has extensively investigated the physiological correlates of retentive encopresis with regard to the child's ability to defecate a rectal balloon. In general, these studies support the hypothesis that children with this type of encopresis may have an inherent physiological predisposition to develop constipation. For example, in one of these studies, 56% of the subjects were unable to defecate the rectal balloon (Loening-Baucke 2004). The follow-up component of this study indicated that 64% of those who could defecate the rectal balloon were improved at 1 year of follow-up, as opposed to only 14% of those who could not defecate the balloon. Related studies by the same research group have also revealed abnormalities with regard to the functioning of the anal sphincter. However, it is also possible that the physiological difficulties with expulsion are the result of chronic constipation.

Nonretentive Encopresis

The pathophysiology of nonretentive encopresis is less clear and has not received the research attention that has been devoted to retentive encopresis. Presumably, the mechanism would be related to the child not sensing the need to defecate until it is too late and/or abnormalities of anal sphincter physiological function.

Course and Prognosis

The natural history of encopresis indicates that for the majority of individuals the disorder will eventually resolve, and reports of encopresis continuing into adolescence are rare. However, the rate of spontaneous remission is not well documented.

The concrete nature of the encopretic event makes the diagnosis relatively straightforward. The major distinction will be between retentive and nonretentive encopresis. This can usually be determined by clinical history, including a description of the encopretic events. A simple X-ray flat plate of the abdomen will reveal the presence of extensive constipation. The physiological studies discussed earlier in the chapter, which investigated the bowel and anal sphincter physiology, were research studies and are not used on a routine clinical basis. Etiologies such as Hirschsprung disease are rare but should be considered. In those situations where the defecation appears to be voluntary, more extensive psychological investigation is required. Even though the encopretic event is usually clearly defined, a thorough history is required to discern if a more benign explanation (such as poor cleaning after defecation) accounts for the apparent soiling. Other emotional environmental factors could include the child's reluctance to use the toilets at school or attentional problems that may predispose him or her to wait until it is too late to get to the bathroom. As with enuresis, a calendar that tracks the frequency and time of day and date will be useful.

Treatment

Pharmacological Treatment

Case reports anecdotally describe the efficacy of tricyclic antidepressants, such as imipramine and amitriptyline, for nonretentive encopresis (Mikkelsen 2001). Presumably, this is due to anticholinergic effects on the anal sphincter, as the therapeutic effect is usually described as occurring before the antidepressant effect would be expected to occur.

Psychotherapeutic Treatments

Psychotherapy may be indicated for those children who voluntarily defecate feces in inappropriate places and/or hoard the feces, depending on the dynamics and psychiatric comorbidity.

Behaviorally Based Treatment

Levine and Bakow (1976) described a treatment approach that involves educational, psychological, behavioral, and physiological components. The educational and psychological components are designed to inform the family about the functioning of the bowel and to address any interpersonal issues related to the encopresis. The physiological component involves bowel catharsis, accomplished with stool softeners, enemas, and laxatives, followed by daily administration of laxatives. Daily timed intervals on the toilet, coupled with rewards for success, represent the behavioral aspects of the treatment plan. The success rate for this overall treatment strategy was reported to be 78%. A comparison study that investigated variations of this approach found little additional benefit from augmenting the basic strategy with biofeedback or enhanced toilet training (Borowitz et al. 2002). This approach continues to be a primary treatment modality.

Loening-Baucke (1995) developed a treatment approach using biofeedback that was derived from his physiological studies discussed earlier (see subsection "Retentive Encopresis"). The purpose of the biofeedback was to improve defecation dynamics, and the results indicated that the biofeedback was superior to traditional approaches. A subsequent long-term follow-up study involved 129 children with constipation, encopresis, and abnormal defecation dynamics who were treated with conventional treatment and 63 children who received conventional treatment plus biofeedback training. The length of follow-up was 4.1±1.5 years. The success rates were remarkably similar for both groups, with 86% of the conventionally treated children showing improvement, as compared with 87% of those who also received biofeedback. The most significant finding of the follow-up phase of the study was that complete remission was significantly correlated with length of time at follow-up for both treatment groups. These findings led the author to conclude that biofeedback treatment was not significantly more effective than conventional treatment and that the natural course of the disorder was to resolve over time (Loening-Baucke 1995). Subsequent reviews of biofeedback treatment have reached similar conclusions (Brazzelli and Griffiths 2001).

Summary Points

Enuresis

- Enuresis is ultimately a self-limited disorder with relatively high rates of spontaneous remission of 12%–14%.
- Pharmacological treatment with imipramine or DDAVP is equally effective, although DDAVP has fewer side effects and a wider margin of safety and is the most widely used intervention.
- An FDA alert drew attention to the risk of hyponatremia, seizures, and, in some cases, death related to DDAVP. The notification stated that the nasal preparation should no longer be used for enuresis and that the use of the oral preparation should be interrupted during illnesses that would disrupt fluid balance.
- Behavioral treatment with the bell and pad method of conditioning is as effective as pharmacological treatment, and relapse is significantly less apt to occur after the cessation of active behavioral treatment compared with drug treatment.
- Children with secondary enuresis are more apt to have a psychological or stressful underlying condition than those with primary enuresis.

- Treatment decisions for primary nocturnal enuresis should be predicated on the severity of the enuresis, the response of the child and family to the enuretic events, the possibility of spontaneous remission, the reported efficacy of the intervention, the rate of relapse after active treatment is stopped, and the side effect risk related to the intervention. This equation will usually indicate that the bell and pad method of treatment is the most appropriate first choice for treatment.

Encopresis

- There are two primary subtypes of encopresis: retentive, which involves constipation and related overflow incontinence, and nonretentive encopresis. A third category would be youth who voluntarily defecate in inappropriate places, although this group is not formally recognized in DSM-5.
- A distinction is made between primary and secondary encopresis, with the latter term referring to youth who achieve continence and then relapse.
- Retentive encopresis has been more extensively studied with regard to physiology and treatment. The most accepted form of treatment is a protocol that contains educational, psychological, behavioral, and physiological components.
- Those children whose encopresis is of a voluntary nature clearly require full psychological evaluation and may respond to psychotherapeutic interventions or treatment of the underlying and/or comorbid psychopathology.
- The natural history of encopresis is to move toward continence. However, the natural history and rate of spontaneous remission are not as well understood as those of enuresis.

References

Aikawa T, Kasahara T, Uchiyama M: Circadian variation of plasma arginine vasopressin concentration, or arginine vasopressin in enuresis. Scand J Urol Nephrol Suppl 202:47–49, 1999 10573793

American Psychiatric Association: Diagnostic and Statistical Manual of Mental Disorders, 5th Edition. Arlington, VA, American Psychiatric Association, 2013

Baeyens D, Roeyers H, Hoebeke P, et al: Attention deficit/hyperactivity disorder in children with nocturnal enuresis. J Urol 171(6 Pt 2):2576–2579, 2004 15118422

Bellman M: Studies on encopresis. Acta Paediatr Scand 56(suppl 170):S1–S151, 1966 5958527

Borowitz SM, Cox DJ, Sutphen JL, et al: Treatment of childhood encopresis: a randomized trial comparing three treatment protocols. J Pediatr Gastroenterol Nutr 34(4):378–384, 2002 11930093

Brazzelli M, Griffiths P: Behavioural and cognitive interventions with or without other treatments for defaecation disorders in children. Cochrane Database Syst Rev 4(4):CD002240, 2001 11687154

Butler RJ, Holland P, Gasson S, et al: Exploring potential mechanisms in alarm treatment for primary nocturnal enuresis. Scand J Urol Nephrol 41(5):407–413, 2007 17957577

Dehoorne JL, Raes AM, van Laecke E, et al: Desmopressin resistant nocturnal polyuria secondary to increased nocturnal osmotic excretion. J Urol 176(2):749–753, 2006a 16813935

Dehoorne JL, Raes AM, van Laecke E, et al: Desmopressin toxicity due to prolonged half-life in 18 patients with nocturnal enuresis. J Urol 176(2):754–757, discussion 757–758, 2006b 16813936

Dehoorne JL, Walle CV, Vansintjan P, et al: Characteristics of a tertiary center enuresis population, with special emphasis on the relation among nocturnal diuresis, functional bladder capacity and desmopressin response. J Urol 177(3):1130–1137, 2007 17296432

Fritz G, Rockney R, Bernet W, et al: Practice parameter for the assessment and treatment of children and adolescents with enuresis. J Am Acad Child Adolesc Psychiatry 43(12):1540–1550, 2004 15564822

Glazener CM, Evans JH: Desmopressin for nocturnal enuresis in children. Cochrane Database Syst Rev 3(3):CD002112, 2002 12137645

Glazener CM, Evans JH: Simple behavioural and physical interventions for nocturnal enuresis in children. Cochrane Database Syst Rev 2(2):CD003637, 2004 15106210

Glazener CM, Evans JH, Peto RE: Alarm interventions for nocturnal enuresis in children. Cochrane Database Syst Rev 2:CD002911, 2003

Glicklich LB: An historical account of enuresis. Pediatrics 8(6):859–876, 1951 14911258

Hergüner S, Kilinçaslan A, Görker I, et al: Serotonin-selective reuptake inhibitor-induced enuresis in three pediatric cases. J Child Adolesc Psychopharmacol 17(3):367–369, 2007 17630870

Heron J, Joinson C, Croudace T, et al: Trajectories of daytime wetting and soiling in a United Kingdom 4 to 9-year-old population birth cohort study. J Urol 179(5):1970–1975, 2008 18355863

Hjälmås K, Hanson E, Hellström AL, et al: Long-term treatment with desmopressin in children with primary monosymptomatic nocturnal enuresis: an open multicentre study. Br J Urol 82(5):704–709, 1998 9839587

Hunsballe JM, Rittig S, Pedersen EB, et al: Single dose imipramine reduces nocturnal urine output in patients with nocturnal enuresis and nocturnal polyuria. J Urol 158(3 Pt 1):830–836, 1997 9258093

Janknegt RA, Zweers HM, Delaere KP, et al: Oral desmopressin as a new treatment modality for primary nocturnal enuresis in adolescents and adults: a double-blind, randomized, multicenter study. J Urol 157(2):513–517, 1997 8996345

Järvelin MR, Vikeväinen-Tervonen L, Moilanen I, et al: Enuresis in seven-year-old children. Acta Paediatr Scand 77(1):148–153, 1988 3369293

Juul KV, Van Herzeele C, De Bruyne P, et al: Desmopressin melt improves response and compliance compared with tablet in treatment of primary monosymptomatic nocturnal enuresis. Eur J Pediatr 172(9):1235–1242, 2013 23677249

Kamperis K, Hagstroem S, Rittig S, et al: Combination of the enuresis alarm and desmopressin: second line treatment for nocturnal enuresis. J Urol 179(3):1128–1131, 2008 18206924

Kruse S, Hellström AL, Hanson E, et al: Treatment of primary monosymptomatic nocturnal enuresis with desmopressin: predictive factors. BJU Int 88(6):572–576, 2001 11678753

Läckgren G, Nevéus T, Stenberg A: Diurnal plasma vasopressin and urinary output in adolescents with monosymptomatic nocturnal enuresis. Acta Paediatr 86(4):385–390, 1997 9174225

Leebeek-Groenewegen A, Blom J, Sukhai R, et al: Efficacy of desmopressin combined with alarm therapy for monosymptomatic nocturnal enuresis. J Urol 166(6):2456–2458, 2001 11696811

Levine MD, Bakow H: Children with encopresis: a study of treatment outcome. Pediatrics 58(6):845–852, 1976 995511

Loening-Baucke V: Biofeedback treatment for chronic constipation and encopresis in childhood: long-term outcome. Pediatrics 96(1 Pt 1):105–110, 1995 7596696

Loening-Baucke V: Functional fecal retention with encopresis in childhood. J Pediatr Gastroenterol Nutr 38(1):79–84, 2004 14676600

Loeys B, Hoebeke P, Raes A, et al: Does monosymptomatic enuresis exist? A molecular genetic exploration of 32 families with enuresis/incontinence. BJU Int 90(1):76–83, 2002 12081775

MacLean RE: Imipramine hydrochloride (Tofranil) and enuresis. Am J Psychiatry 117:551, 1960 13764959

Medel R, Dieguez S, Brindo M, et al: Monosymptomatic primary enuresis: differences between patients responding or not responding to oral desmopressin. Br J Urol 81(suppl 3):46–49, 1998 9634019

Mikkelsen EJ: Enuresis and encopresis: ten years of progress. J Am Acad Child Adolesc Psychiatry 40(10):1146–1158, 2001 11589527

Mikkelsen EJ, Rapoport JL, Nee L, et al: Childhood enuresis. I. Sleep patterns and psychopathology. Arch Gen Psychiatry 37(10):1139–1144, 1980 7425798

Moffatt ME, Harlos S, Kirshen AJ, et al: Desmopressin acetate and nocturnal enuresis: how much do we know? Pediatrics 92(3):420–425, 1993 8361796

Monda JM, Husmann DA: Primary nocturnal enuresis: a comparison among observation, imipramine, desmopressin acetate and bed-wetting alarm systems. J Urol 154(2 Pt 2):745–748, 1995 7609169

Naitoh Y, Kawauchi A, Yamao Y, et al: Combination therapy with alarm and drugs for monosymptomatic nocturnal enuresis not superior to alarm monotherapy. Urology 66(3):632–635, 2005 16140092

Natochin YV, Kuznetsova AA: Defect of osmoregulatory renal function in nocturnal enuresis. Scand J Urol Nephrol Suppl 202:40–43, discussion 43–44, 1999 10573791

Pretlow RA: Treatment of nocturnal enuresis with an ultrasound bladder volume controlled alarm device. J Urol 162(3 Pt 2):1224–1228, 1999 10458472

Rapoport JL, Mikkelsen EJ, Zavadil A, et al: Childhood enuresis. II. Psychopathology, tricyclic concentration in plasma, and antienuretic effect. Arch Gen Psychiatry 37(10):1146–1152, 1980 7000030

Rittig S, Knudsen UB, Nørgaard JP, et al: Diurnal variation of plasma atrial natriuretic peptide in normals and patients with enuresis nocturna. Scand J Clin Lab Invest 51(2):209–217, 1991 1828306

Rittig S, Schaumburg HL, Siggaard C, et al: The circadian defect in plasma vasopressin and urine output is related to desmopressin response and enuresis status in children with nocturnal enuresis. J Urol 179(6):2389–2395, 2008 18433780

Robson WL, Nørgaard JP, Leung AK: Hyponatremia in patients with nocturnal enuresis treated with DDAVP. Eur J Pediatr 155(11):959–962, 1996 8911897

Robson WL, Leung AK, Norgaard JP: The comparative safety of oral versus intranasal desmopressin for the treatment of children with nocturnal enuresis. J Urol 178(1):24–30, 2007 17574054

Rutter M: Isle of Wight revisited: twenty-five years of child psychiatric epidemiology. J Am Acad Child Adolesc Psychiatry 28(5):633–653, 1989 2676960

Rutter M, Tizard J, Whitmore K (eds): Education, Health and Behavior. New York, Krieger, Huntington, 1981

Shaffer D, Gardner A, Hedge B: Behavior and bladder disturbance of enuretic children: a rational classification of a common disorder. Dev Med Child Neurol 26(6):781–792, 1984 6083889

Skoog SJ, Stokes A, Turner KL: Oral desmopressin: a randomized double-blind placebo controlled study of effectiveness in children with primary nocturnal enuresis. J Urol 158(3 Pt 2):1035–1040, 1997 9258137

Söderstrom U, Hoelcke M, Alenius L, et al: Urinary and faecal incontinence: a population-based study. Acta Paediatr 93(3):386–389, 2004 15124844

Sreedhar B, Yeung CK, Leung VY, et al: Ultrasound bladder measurements in children with severe primary nocturnal enuresis: pretreatment and posttreatment evaluation and its correlation with treatment outcome. J Urol 179(4):1568–1572, discussion 1572, 2008 18295261

Touchette E, Petit D, Paquet J, et al: Bed-wetting and its association with developmental milestones in early childhood. Arch Pediatr Adolesc Med 159(12):1129–1134, 2005 16330736

Wolfish NM, Barkin J, Gorodzinsky F, et al: The Canadian Enuresis Study and Evaluation—short- and long-term safety and efficacy of an oral desmopressin preparation. Scand J Urol Nephrol 37(1):22–27, 2003 12745738

CHAPTER 23

Sleep Disorders

Anna Ivanenko, M.D., Ph.D.
Kyle P. Johnson, M.D.

Child and adolescent mental health clinicians are on the front line of recognizing sleep disorders in children and adolescents since so many children assessed by clinicians have sleep complaints. These sleep problems may represent either 1) primary sleep disorders, such as obstructive sleep apnea (OSA), restless legs syndrome (RLS), or narcolepsy, or 2) insomnia comorbid with psychiatric conditions, such as depression or anxiety. Mental health professionals must keep sleep disorders in mind when assessing children with neurocognitive, emotional, behavioral, and motivational problems because chronic sleep disruption can cause these difficulties.

Epidemiology

Sleep disorders are highly prevalent across the life span. Numerous epidemiological studies have been conducted using parental and self reports. Fewer studies have used objective sleep measurements such as actigraphy or polysomnography. Most of the surveys refer to symptoms of disrupted sleep, such as problems initiating and maintaining sleep, frequent nocturnal awakenings, delayed sleep onset, and restless sleep; behaviors associated with sleep, such as sleepwalking, sleeptalking, snoring, and witnessed apneas with gasping for air; and excessive daytime sleepiness.

Approximately 25% of children will experience sleep-related problems at some point of their development. A number of surveys completed by the parents of a community sample of children found sleep problems in 20% of 5-year-old children and 6% of 11-year-olds (Rona et al. 1998) and a 37%–50% prevalence of sleep problems in school-age children (Blader et al. 1997; Owens et al. 2000b). A high rate of problems in sleep initiation, sleep maintenance, and excessive daytime sleepiness due to chronic sleep loss has been reported by adolescents. A survey of 1,014 adolescents revealed a 10.7% lifetime prevalence of insomnia with a median age at onset of 11 years (Johnson et al. 2006). Of interest,

52.8% of the adolescents with insomnia had a comorbid psychiatric disorder.

Children with chronic medical, neurodevelopmental, and psychiatric disorders present with a much higher rate of sleep disorders. Between 30% and 80% of children with intellectual disability and from 50% to 70% of children with autism spectrum disorders have been reported to have sleep problems (Cortesi et al. 2010; Johnson 1996; Stores and Wiggs 1998).

Classification of Sleep Disorders

There are two major classification systems for sleep disorders: *International Classification of Sleep Disorders,* Third Edition (ICSD-3; American Academy of Sleep Medicine 2014), and DSM-5 (American Psychiatric Association 2013). Sleep behavior disorder and regulatory disorder with sleep problem are also included in the *Diagnostic Classification, Zero to Three* (DC: 0–3R; Zero to Three 2005).

According to DSM-5, sleep-wake disorders are divided into several categories:

- Insomnia disorder
- Hypersomnolence disorder
- Narcolepsy
- Breathing-related sleep disorders
- Circadian rhythm sleep-wake disorders
- Rapid eye movement sleep behavior disorder
- Restless legs syndrome
- Parasomnias
- Substance/medication-induced sleep disorder
- Other specified insomnia disorder
- Unspecified insomnia disorder
- Other specified hypersomnolence disorder
- Unspecified hypersomnolence disorder
- Other specified sleep-wake disorder
- Unspecified sleep-wake disorder

ICSD-3 is a more comprehensive classification of sleep disorders that includes a wide variety of sleep-related conditions, including a revised definition of primary insomnia that includes behavioral insomnia of childhood subdivided into sleep-onset association type and limit-setting type.

Evaluation

Sleep History

Taking a sleep history is the first and most important step in assessing children and adolescents for sleep disorders. Because of a high rate of sleep comorbidities with other psychiatric disorders, it is essential to obtain a sleep history in pediatric patients as they present to the clinician's office with behavioral and emotional problems.

BEARS is an easy-to-remember mnemonic introduced to help clinicians inquire about sleep symptoms. It stands for Bedtime, Excessive daytime sleepiness, Awakenings, Regularity, and Snoring (Mindell and Owens 2003). It is important to understand a child's customary sleep habits and patterns, during both weekdays and weekends; night-to-night variability in sleep duration; number of nocturnal awakenings; and sleep-related behaviors.

Medical history, physical examination, and neurodevelopmental and psychiatric history are required parts of a comprehensive sleep evaluation.

Questionnaires

Several questionnaires have been developed and validated to assess for the most common sleep problems in children and adolescents. The Pediatric Sleep Questionnaire has been validated for the assessment of sleep-disordered breathing, daytime sleepiness, snoring, and behavioral problems such as hyperactivity, impulsivity, and inattention in children ages 2–18 years (Chervin et al. 2000). The Children's Sleep Habits Questionnaire yields eight subscales that reflect the major domains of behavioral and medical sleep disorders and a total score indicating the extent and severity of sleep-related problems (Owens et al. 2000a). The Sleep Disorders Inventory for Students (SDIS) is a validated parent- and self-report questionnaire for children ages 2–10 years (SDIS-C) and adolescents ages 11–18 years (SDIS-A) that can be used for screening of sleep disorders in a variety of clinical and school settings (available at Child Uplift, Inc., P.O. Box 146, Fairview, WY 83119; www.sleepdisorderhelp.com).

The Epworth Sleepiness Scale is a clinical tool recently modified for use in children and adolescents (Drake et al. 2003) that is very helpful for screening the subjective propensity to fall asleep in certain situations and for measuring treatment outcome.

A sleep log/sleep diary (Figure 23–1) is a valuable tool that provides nightly information on the child's bedtime, sleep-onset time, rise time, and number of nocturnal awakenings. It is usually recommended to be completed for a period of 2 weeks. Sleep logs are usually filled out by parents or caregivers of younger children and by the adolescents themselves. However, sleep logs are based on observations and/or self-perception and lack objective assessment of sleep.

Actigraphy uses a small, portable motion sensor that counts and stores movements per minute using a specially designed algorithm. The device is typically worn on the nondominant wrist and collects continuous objective sleep-wake data, including total amount of sleep, sleep efficiency, and number and duration of awakenings. It is a very valuable tool to assess night-to-night variability of sleep and can detect subtle circadian sleep disturbances.

Nocturnal polysomnography (PSG) is currently the gold standard procedure for studying sleep-disordered breathing and other types of intrinsic sleep disorders in children. It includes recordings of electroencephalogram, electro-oculogram, electromyogram, airflow, respiratory and abdominal efforts, oxygen saturation, end-tidal carbon dioxide, and limb muscle activity and requires the child and one of the parents or caregivers to spend a night in a sleep laboratory. PSG is indicated for the diagnosis of OSA, central apnea, alveolar hypoventilation, snoring, and upper airway resistance syndrome in children. PSG is also used to establish the diagnosis of periodic limb movement disorder (PLMD) and to evaluate for nocturnal seizures and parasomnias, such as rapid eye movement (REM) behavior sleep disorder.

The Multiple Sleep Latency Test (MSLT) is used to assess daytime sleepiness and includes a series of four to five naps conducted at 2-hour intervals, with the first nap beginning 2 hours after the final morning awakening. The MSLT is routinely preceded the night before by a PSG. The MSLT is a routine part of the sleep laboratory assessment of narcolepsy and idiopathic hypersomnia and helps to measure objectively the degree of somnolence due to sleep apnea or resulting from chronic sleep loss.

The Maintenance of Wakefulness Test is similar to the MSLT procedure, but the patient is asked to remain awake while sleep latency is measured. The test is used in adolescents with disorders of

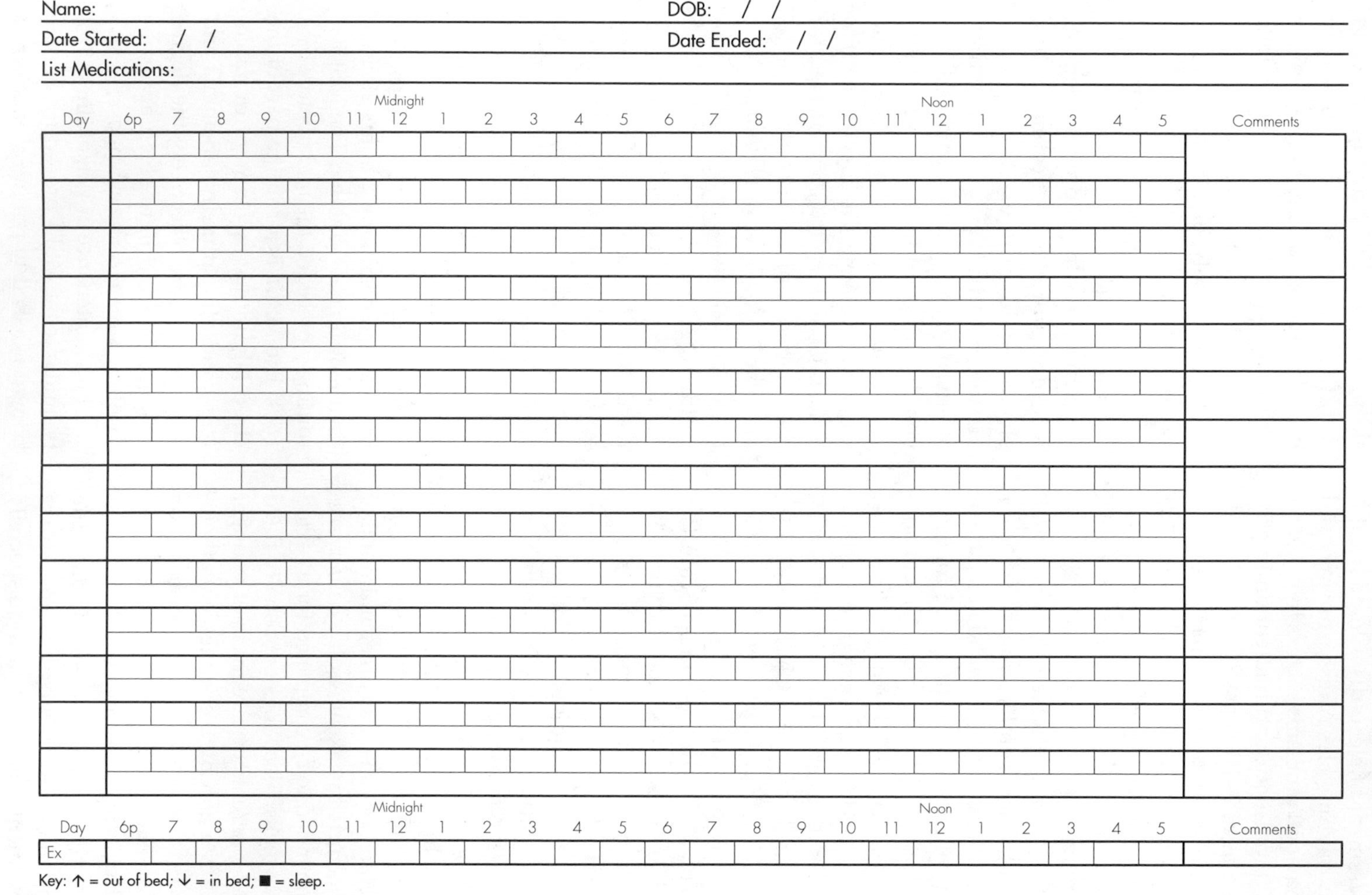

Name: DOB: / /

Date Started: / / Date Ended: / /

List Medications:

Day	6p	7	8	9	10	11	Midnight 12	1	2	3	4	5	6	7	8	9	10	11	Noon 12	1	2	3	4	5	Comments

Day	6p	7	8	9	10	11	Midnight 12	1	2	3	4	5	6	7	8	9	10	11	Noon 12	1	2	3	4	5	Comments
Ex																									

Key: ↑ = out of bed; ↓ = in bed; ■ = sleep.

FIGURE 23–1. Sleep log/sleep diary.

excessive daytime sleepiness to assess their ability to maintain adequate levels of alertness, especially when they are beginning to drive.

Insomnia Disorder

The DSM-5 criteria for primary insomnia are presented in Box 23–1.

Box 23–1. DSM-5 Diagnostic Criteria for Insomnia Disorder

780.52 (G47.00)

A. A predominant complaint of dissatisfaction with sleep quantity or quality, associated with one (or more) of the following symptoms:
   1. Difficulty initiating sleep. (In children, this may manifest as difficulty initiating sleep without caregiver intervention.)
   2. Difficulty maintaining sleep, characterized by frequent awakenings or problems returning to sleep after awakenings. (In children, this may manifest as difficulty returning to sleep without caregiver intervention.)
   3. Early-morning awakening with inability to return to sleep.

B. The sleep disturbance causes clinically significant distress or impairment in social, occupational, educational, academic, behavioral, or other important areas of functioning.

C. The sleep difficulty occurs at least 3 nights per week.

D. The sleep difficulty is present for at least 3 months.

E. The sleep difficulty occurs despite adequate opportunity for sleep.

F. The insomnia is not better explained by and does not occur exclusively during the course of another sleep-wake disorder (e.g., narcolepsy, a breathing-related sleep disorder, a circadian rhythm sleep-wake disorder, a parasomnia).

G. The insomnia is not attributable to the physiological effects of a substance (e.g., a drug of abuse, a medication).

H. Coexisting mental disorders and medical conditions do not adequately explain the predominant complaint of insomnia.

Specify if:

With non–sleep disorder mental comorbidity, including substance use disorders
With other medical comorbidity
With other sleep disorder

Coding note: The code 307.42 (F51.01) applies to all three specifiers. Code also the relevant associated mental disorder, medical condition, or other sleep disorder immediately after the code for insomnia disorder in order to indicate the association.

Specify if:

Episodic: Symptoms last at least 1 month but less than 3 months.
Persistent: Symptoms last 3 months or longer.
Recurrent: Two (or more) episodes within the space of 1 year.

Note: Acute and short-term insomnia (i.e., symptoms lasting less than 3 months but otherwise meeting all criteria with regard to frequency, intensity, distress, and/or impairment) should be coded as an other specified insomnia disorder.

Source. Reprinted from the *Diagnostic and Statistical Manual of Mental Disorders,* 5th Edition. Arlington, VA, American Psychiatric Association, 2013. Used with permission.

Prevalence

Sleep initiation and maintenance insomnia—including bedtime resistance, disruptive nocturnal awakenings, and other behavioral sleep problems—are most commonly observed in young children, with a prevalence of 25%–50% in preschool-age children.

Clinical Characteristics

The revised edition of ICSD-3 introduced two diagnostic entities of behavioral insomnia of childhood: limit-setting type and sleep-onset association type. Limit-setting type refers to parental difficulties establishing behavioral limits and enforcing bedtimes and is commonly associated with the child's stalling and refusing to go to bed. Sleep-onset association type is characterized by maladaptive sleep-onset associations such as rocking, feeding, watching TV, or parental presence. Behavioral sleep problems result in delayed sleep onset, fragmented nocturnal sleep, insufficient sleep time, and daytime sleepiness. They also contribute to nighttime awakenings because once the child wakes up at night, he or she is unable to reinitiate sleep without re-creating the same sleep association.

Treatment

Nonpharmacological interventions are the first choice of treatment. Behavioral interventions include parental education, sleep hygiene, extinction, graduated extinction, scheduled awakenings, and positive bedtime routines and cognitive-behavioral therapy (Kuhn and Elliott 2003; Kuhn and Roane 2011; Mindell 1999). Intervention for insomnia in children should start with establishing appropriate and realistic parent and child expectations and treatment goals. Age-appropriate sleep duration and bedtime should be discussed with the parents.

For example, preschool children may require 11–12 hours of total sleep time and a daytime nap, school-age children sleep on average 10 hours per night, and adolescents need 8.5–9 hours of sleep according to their physiological requirements. School schedule and extracurricular activities should be taken into consideration when establishing the treatment protocol. It is very important to set and reinforce regular bedtime and rise time. Introducing a positive relaxing bedtime routine is an important step in preparing a child to fall asleep. Morning rise time is especially important as a powerful environmental cue for entrainment of the sleep-wake cycle. The sleeping environment should be controlled to exclude television, video games, computers, and cell phones. Children should be encouraged to sleep in their own bed on a consistent basis. In younger children, establishment of appropriate nap time is very important since it will affect nocturnal sleep onset and sleep duration time. The majority of children no longer have a daytime nap after 5 years of age. Numerous behavioral techniques have been described for childhood sleep disorders and are summarized in Table 23–1. A large 5-year follow-up study demonstrated that behavioral sleep interventions can reduce the short- to medium-term burden of infant sleep problems and maternal depression without causing long-term harm (Price et al. 2012). Cognitive therapy has been successfully implemented to treat insomnia in older children and adolescents. Cognitive strategies include restructuring of thoughts and attitudes, systemic desensitization, positive reinforcement, and relaxation techniques (Kuhn and Roane 2011).

There are no well-designed controlled studies of sedative-hypnotics in children, and there are no pharmacological agents approved by the U.S. Food

TABLE 23–1. Behavioral interventions for pediatric insomnia

Intervention	Method
Sleep education	Provide information on purpose of sleep, organization of sleep states, and sleep norms for different age groups
Positive bedtime routine	Establish relaxing, low-stress interactions between a parent and a child before lights out; introduce a transitional object
Sleep hygiene	Educate the child and parent about engaging in sleep-conducive behaviors prior to bedtime; eliminate environmental stimulation
Appropriate sleep scheduling	Select age-appropriate sleep schedule for the child and teach parents how to implement it; keep bedtimes and rise times constant
Unmodified extinction	Instruct parents to consistently ignore a child's disruptive behavior at bedtime
Graduated extinction	Gradually reduce parental presence in the bedroom or parental attention to inappropriate bedtime behaviors; can be combined with periodic "check-ins"
Extinction with parental presence	The parent remains in the child's bedroom while ignoring disruptive behavior at bedtime
Scheduled awakenings (for parasomnias)	Establish a pretreatment pattern of nocturnal awakenings, then instruct parents to awaken the child 15–30 minutes prior to the anticipated spontaneous awakenings
Relaxation training	Identify symptoms associated with increased somatic and cognitive tension; teach progressive muscle relaxation and deep and diaphragmatic breathing

and Drug Administration (FDA) for use in pediatric insomnia. For the current status of knowledge on pharmacological treatment of pediatric insomnia, see the Consensus Statement by Mindell et al. (2006) as well as a recent review article by Pelayo and Yuen (2012).

Insomnia can be primary or can be a symptom of a number of medical and psychiatric conditions as well as other sleep disorders (secondary or comorbid insomnia). It is important to use sedating pharmacological agents only when behavioral interventions have been tried and found to be ineffective. The underlying diagnosis causing insomnia should influence the choice of medication. In many cases, treating the underlying condition will lead to improvement and resolution of insomnia. For example, use of a serotonin reuptake inhibitor in a child with major depressive disorder may be all that is necessary to treat the child's insomnia. However, the insomnia associated with a medical or psychiatric condition may be severe enough to warrant its own pharmacological treatment, at least in the short term. Patients and their parents must understand that there are no FDA-approved drugs for pediatric insomnia; therefore, medicines prescribed for this purpose are being used off-label. A careful discussion of the risks, benefits, and alternatives is in order. The drugs are summarized in Table 23–2.

Narcolepsy and Hypersomnolence Disorder

The DSM-5 criteria for narcolepsy are presented in Box 23–2.

TABLE 23–2. Pharmacological agents for pediatric insomnia

Drug	Dose range	Mechanism of action	Side effects	Effects on sleep	Uses in children[a]
Clonazepam	0.25–2.0 mg	GABA-agonist	Strong abuse potential	Suppresses SWS; reduces frequency of arousals	Parasomnias (sleepwalking, night terrors, confusional arousals, REM sleep behavior disorder)
Clonidine	0.025–0.3 mg	α_2-agonist	Narrow therapeutic index; dry mouth, bradycardia, hypotension; hypertension following abrupt discontinuation	Decreases SOL	Sleep onset and maintenance insomnia; ADHD
Guanfacine	0.5–2 mg	α_2-agonist	Same as clonidine but less sedating	Decreases SOL	Sleep onset and maintenance insomnia; ADHD
Diphenhydramine	12.5–50 mg	H1 agonist; crosses blood-brain barrier	In overdose may cause hallucinations, seizures, agitation	Reduces SOL; reduces frequency of arousals in children	Mild sedative effect
Trazodone	25–100 mg	5-HT serotonin agonist and reuptake inhibitor; blocks histamine receptors	Priapism, orthostatic hypotension, dizziness	Increases SWS, reduces SOL	Insomnia associated with comorbid depression and anxiety disorders
Mirtazapine	7.5–15 mg	5-HT_2, 5-HT_3 antagonist, muscarinic antagonist, H_1 receptor antagonist	Weight gain, appetite increase, dry mouth	Reduces SOL, increases sleep duration	Insomnia associated with comorbid depression and anxiety disorders

TABLE 23–2. Pharmacological agents for pediatric insomnia *(continued)*

Drug	Dose range	Mechanism of action	Side effects	Effects on sleep	Uses in children[a]
Melatonin	0.3–6 mg (up to 10 mg in adolescents)	Melatonin receptor agonist (MT-1, MT-2)	Generally well tolerated	Decreases SOL	Insomnia with comorbid autism spectrum disorder, developmental disabilities, ADHD, blindness, neurological impairments
Zolpidem	5–10 mg	BZRA	Abuse potential; sleep-related behaviors, retrograde amnesia, headaches, dizziness,	Decreases SOL	At a dosage of 0.25 mg/kg (max 10 mg) failed to reduce latency to persistent sleep in children and adolescents with insomnia associated with ADHD (Blumer et al. 2009)
Eszopiclone	1–3 mg	BZRA	Same as above	Decreases SOL and WASO	At a doses up to 3 mg was generally well tolerated by pediatric patients but failed to reduce latency to persistent sleep in children ages 6–17 years with ADHD-associated insomnia (Zammit et al. 2012)
Ramelteon	8 mg	Melatonin receptor agonist	Well tolerated; very limited data in children	Decreases SOL	

Note. [a]Not approved for these uses by the U.S. Food and Drug Administration.
ADHD=attention-deficit/hyperactivity disorder; BZRA=benzodiazepine receptor agonist; REM=rapid eye movement; SWS=slow wave sleep; SOL=sleep onset latency; WASO=wake after sleep onset.

Box 23–2. DSM-5 Diagnostic Criteria for Narcolepsy

A. Recurrent periods of an irrepressible need to sleep, lapsing into sleep, or napping occurring within the same day. These must have been occurring at least three times per week over the past 3 months.

B. The presence of at least one of the following:

   1. Episodes of cataplexy, defined as either (a) or (b), occurring at least a few times per month:

      a. In individuals with long-standing disease, brief (seconds to minutes) episodes of sudden bilateral loss of muscle tone with maintained consciousness that are precipitated by laughter or joking.

      b. In children or in individuals within 6 months of onset, spontaneous grimaces or jaw-opening episodes with tongue thrusting or a global hypotonia, without any obvious emotional triggers.

   2. Hypocretin deficiency, as measured using cerebrospinal fluid (CSF) hypocretin-1 immunoreactivity values (less than or equal to one-third of values obtained in healthy subjects tested using the same assay, or less than or equal to 110 pg/mL). Low CSF levels of hypocretin-1 must not be observed in the context of acute brain injury, inflammation, or infection.

   3. Nocturnal sleep polysomnography showing rapid eye movement (REM) sleep latency less than or equal to 15 minutes, or a multiple sleep latency test showing a mean sleep latency less than or equal to 8 minutes and two or more sleep-onset REM periods.

Specify whether:

347.00 (G47.419) Narcolepsy without cataplexy but with hypocretin deficiency: Criterion B requirements of low CSF hypocretin-1 levels and positive polysomnography/multiple sleep latency test are met, but no cataplexy is present (Criterion B1 not met).

347.01 (G47.411) Narcolepsy with cataplexy but without hypocretin deficiency: In this rare subtype (less than 5% of narcolepsy cases), Criterion B requirements of cataplexy and positive polysomnography/multiple sleep latency test are met, but CSF hypocretin-1 levels are normal (Criterion B2 not met).

347.00 (G47.419) Autosomal dominant cerebellar ataxia, deafness, and narcolepsy: This subtype is caused by exon 21 DNA (cytosine-5)-methyltransferase-1 mutations and is characterized by late-onset (age 30–40 years) narcolepsy (with low or intermediate CSF hypocretin-1 levels), deafness, cerebellar ataxia, and eventually dementia.

347.00 (G47.419) Autosomal dominant narcolepsy, obesity, and type 2 diabetes: Narcolepsy, obesity, and type 2 diabetes and low CSF hypocretin-1 levels have been described in rare cases and are associated with a mutation in the myelin oligodendrocyte glycoprotein gene.

347.10 (G47.429) Narcolepsy secondary to another medical condition: This subtype is for narcolepsy that develops secondary to medical conditions that cause infectious (e.g., Whipple's disease, sarcoidosis), traumatic, or tumoral destruction of hypocretin neurons.

Coding note (for ICD-9-CM code 347.10 only): Code first the underlying medical condition (e.g., 040.2 Whipple's disease; 347.10 narcolepsy secondary to Whipple's disease).

Specify current severity:

Mild: Infrequent cataplexy (less than once per week), need for naps only once or twice per day, and less disturbed nocturnal sleep.

Moderate: Cataplexy once daily or every few days, disturbed nocturnal sleep, and need for multiple naps daily.

Severe: Drug-resistant cataplexy with multiple attacks daily, nearly constant sleepiness, and disturbed nocturnal sleep (i.e., movements, insomnia, and vivid dreaming).

Source. Reprinted from the *Diagnostic and Statistical Manual of Mental Disorders*, 5th Edition. Arlington, VA, American Psychiatric Association, 2013. Used with permission.

Prevalence

The prevalence of narcolepsy in the adult population is approximately 2–5 per 10,000. The exact prevalence of narcolepsy in childhood is unknown. One study found that 34% of all subjects with narcolepsy had onset of symptoms prior to age 15 years (Challamel et al. 1994).

Clinical Characteristics

Narcolepsy is a rare neurological disorder characterized by daytime sleepiness, cataplexy (sudden loss of muscle tone triggered by emotional arousal such as laughter), hypnagogic hallucinations, and sleep paralysis. The classic tetrad of narcolepsy that includes all of these symptoms is rare in children. Most pediatric patients present with excessive daytime sleepiness and sleep attacks, often masked by behavioral and emotional symptoms such as irritability, hyperactivity, inattention, and increased sleep needs at younger age. A newly discovered neuropeptide, hypocretin (also known as orexin), has been linked to the pathophysiology of narcolepsy that is currently explained by a two-threshold hypothesis including both genetic and environmental factors. The diagnosis of narcolepsy requires sleep laboratory evaluation to include PSG and MSLT with evidence of pathological sleepiness and at least two sleep-onset REM periods.

Idiopathic hypersomnia is a diagnosis of exclusion and is characterized by sleepiness with long-lasting, nonrefreshing sleep that is not associated with frequent periods of sleep onset with REM.

Treatment

Treatment options for narcolepsy and idiopathic hypersomnia are similar and include pharmacotherapy and behavioral intervention. Good sleep habits with a regular sleep-wake schedule and adequate amount of nocturnal sleep are essential parts of management of excessive daytime sleepiness. Scheduled daytime naps of 25–30 minutes each are beneficial in increasing daytime alertness. Patients should avoid alcohol and recreational substances, and adolescents need to be cautioned about the risks of driving or operating machinery when sleepy. Education and support for these conditions are available through the Narcolepsy Network (www.narcolepsynetwork.org), a nonprofit organization for patients, families, and professionals.

Long-term administration of pharmacological agents is often required to reduce sleepiness and improve daytime alertness. Modafinil, a long-acting alerting medication, can provide all-day benefits following morning administration. Psychostimulants such as methylphenidate or dextroamphetamine have been used alone or in combination with modafinil or armodafinil in treating excessive sleepiness in children and are generally well tolerated. In a small sample of children with narcolepsy and idiopathic hypersomnia, modafinil at dosages of 200–600 mg/day was shown to reduce daytime sleepiness without significant side effects (Ivanenko et al. 2003). Recent studies indicated that sodium oxybate (Xyrem) was effective for the treatment of excessive daytime sleepiness associated with narcolepsy in children and adolescents (Aran et al. 2010; Murali and Kotagal 2006) and was not associated with significant side effects. Tricyclic antidepressants (clomipramine, imipramine, protriptyline), mixed action antidepressants (e.g., venlafaxine), and serotonin reuptake inhibitors may be used to treat cataplexy and other symptoms of narcolepsy, such as sleep paralysis and hypnagogic hallucinations.

Restless Legs Syndrome and Periodic Limb Movement Disorder

The DSM-5 criteria for restless legs syndrome are presented in Box 23–3.

Box 23–3. DSM-5 Diagnostic Criteria for Restless Legs Syndrome

333.94 (G25.81)

A. An urge to move the legs, usually accompanied by or in response to uncomfortable and unpleasant sensations in the legs, characterized by all of the following:
   1. The urge to move the legs begins or worsens during periods of rest or inactivity.
   2. The urge to move the legs is partially or totally relieved by movement.
   3. The urge to move the legs is worse in the evening or at night than during the day, or occurs only in the evening or at night.

B. The symptoms in Criterion A occur at least three times per week and have persisted for at least 3 months.

C. The symptoms in Criterion A are accompanied by significant distress or impairment in social, occupational, educational, academic, behavioral, or other important areas of functioning.

D. The symptoms in Criterion A are not attributable to another mental disorder or medical condition (e.g., arthritis, leg edema, peripheral ischemia, leg cramps) and are not better explained by a behavioral condition (e.g., positional discomfort, habitual foot tapping).

E. The symptoms are not attributable to the physiological effects of a drug of abuse or medication (e.g., akathisia).

Source. Reprinted from the *Diagnostic and Statistical Manual of Mental Disorders,* 5th Edition. Arlington, VA, American Psychiatric Association, 2013. Used with permission.

Prevalence

RLS is a common sensorimotor disorder with an estimated prevalence in the pediatric population of 2% (Picchietti et al. 2007).

Clinical Characteristics

RLS is defined as an urge to move the legs, usually accompanied by uncomfortable and unpleasant sensations in the legs. Periodic limb movements of sleep are characterized by episodes of repetitive stereotypic limb movements. The presence of insomnia or excessive daytime sleepiness is required to establish the diagnosis of PLMD. Children frequently report symptoms of RLS differently from adults, which makes the diagnosis of RLS in children more challenging. New diagnostic criteria have been established for children and adolescents (Picchietti et al. 2013). As RLS and PLMD have been more extensively studied, the association between these disorders and attention-deficit/hyperactivity disorder (ADHD) in children has become evident (Cortese et al. 2005). Many children with ADHD have been found to have RLS or PLMD and vice versa (Picchietti et al. 2007; Silvestri et al. 2009).

Treatment

Behavioral interventions for RLS and PLMD are mainly focused on preserving a stable sleep-wake schedule, avoiding sleep deprivation, reducing caffeine intake, eliminating tobacco and alcohol, and avoiding stimulating activities close to bedtime. Pharmacological interventions include iron supplementation (1.6–7.8 mg/kg/day), which is usually recommended if the child's serum ferritin level is below 50 ng/mL. Serum ferritin level should be monitored every 3–4 months. The goal of therapy is to achieve ferritin serum level of 80–100 ng/mL (Durmer 2011).

A controlled study of carbidopa/L-dopa 25/100 CR was shown to be safe and effective in children (England et al. 2011). Clinical evidence suggests that other dopaminergic medications such as pramipexole and ropinirole are effective in pediatric cases of RLS (Konofal et al. 2005; Walters et al. 2000). Ropinirole and pramipexole are FDA approved for RLS treatment in adults but not in children. Gabapentin is another medication known to reduce symptoms of RLS in children (Frenette 2011). Other classes of medication, such as benzodiazepines (clonazepam), α-agonists (clonidine), and carbamazepine have also been successfully used to relieve RLS symptoms in children.

Breathing-Related Sleep Disorders

The DSM-5 criteria for obstructive sleep apnea are presented in Box 23–4.

Box 23–4. DSM-5 Diagnostic Criteria for Obstructive Sleep Apnea Hypopnea

327.23 (G47.33)

A. Either (1) or (2):

1. Evidence by polysomnography of at least five obstructive apneas or hypopneas per hour of sleep and either of the following sleep symptoms:
   a. Nocturnal breathing disturbances: snoring, snorting/gasping, or breathing pauses during sleep.
   b. Daytime sleepiness, fatigue, or unrefreshing sleep despite sufficient opportunities to sleep that is not better explained by another mental disorder (including a sleep disorder) and is not attributable to another medical condition.
2. Evidence by polysomnography of 15 or more obstructive apneas and/or hypopneas per hour of sleep regardless of accompanying symptoms.

Specify current severity:

Mild: Apnea hypopnea index is less than 15.

Moderate: Apnea hypopnea index is 15–30.

Severe: Apnea hypopnea index is greater than 30.

Obstructive Sleep Apnea

Prevalence

Although habitual snoring has been reported in as many as 12% of children, the general prevalence of pediatric OSA is approximately 1%–4% (Brockmann et al. 2012; Marcus 2001). The prevalence rates are much higher among children with neuromuscular and craniofacial abnormalities. Rates approach 85% in children with some genetic syndromes (Brooks 2002).

Clinical Characteristics

Symptoms of OSA include persistent snoring, witnessed apneas with gasping for air, restless sleep, and nocturnal diaphoresis. OSA is often the result of adenotonsillar hypertrophy, obesity, sinus problems, or craniofacial abnormalities (Redline et al. 1999). Sleep-disordered breathing has been associated with subjectively reported daytime somnolence and even more commonly with neurocognitive symptoms, including inattention and hyperactivity in children (O'Brien 2014; O'Brien and Gozal 2004). OSA in children is defined as episodes of complete or partial cessation of airflow for the duration of two respiratory cycles, associated with oxygen desaturations or arousals. Polysomnography is recommended to establish a diagnosis of OSA, to assess the severity and nature of the sleep-disordered breathing, and (performed before and after treatment) to assess treatment efficacy (Section on Pediatric Pulmonology, Subcommittee on Obstructive Sleep Apnea Syndrome, American Academy of Pediatrics 2002). Because of serious neurocognitive and physical developmental consequences of OSA, it is very important to recognize and treat it early in life.

Treatment

The treatment of choice for pediatric OSA is surgery, typically adenotonsillectomy (Marcus et al. 2012; Section on Pediatric Pulmonology, Subcommittee on Obstructive Sleep Apnea Syndrome, American Academy of Pediatrics 2002). Polysomnography done after surgery demonstrates that this procedure is curative in approximately 80% of cases (Lipton and Gozal 2003). Children with allergic rhinitis and/or sinusitis may benefit from inhaled nasal steroids (Brouillette et al. 2001), antihistamines, and decongestants.

Continuous positive airway pressure (CPAP) is recommended for children who have either failed surgical intervention or are not surgical candidates (Marcus et al. 1995, 2012; Section on Pediatric Pulmonology, Subcommittee on Obstructive Sleep Apnea Syndrome, American Academy of Pediatrics 2002). The use of CPAP has been approved by the FDA for children who are 7 years and older and weigh more than 40 pounds. An attended laboratory titration of CPAP should be performed to determine the effective pressure setting. Supplemental oxygen is not recommended for routine use in children with OSA because of the risks of developing hypoventilation.

Parasomnias

Prevalence

Parasomnias are much more frequently seen in children than adults and usually represent the normal neurophysiology of sleep development. They usually appear at around the second year of life and continue into the preschool or school-age years. The prevalence of quiet sleepwalking in children ranges from 14% to 40% depending on the sample (Klackenberg 1982; Laberge et al. 2000; Petit et al. 2007). Parasomnias are much more prevalent in children with psychiatric and neurological disorders and can be also exacerbated or induced by psychopharmacological agents. Most parasomnias resolve by adolescence.

Clinical Characteristics

Parasomnias represent partial central nervous system arousals characterized by autonomic and motor activity. Parasomnias such as sleepwalking, sleeptalking, night terrors, confusional arousals, and nocturnal enuresis occur during slow-wave sleep (Table 23–3). Children usually have no recollection the next day of the nocturnal events. Nightmares and REM behavior sleep disorder occur in REM sleep and are usually associated with vivid dream recall. Sleepwalking and especially REM behavior sleep disorder are potentially dangerous conditions that are occasionally associated with injuries to self or others. Parasomnias are highly heritable and usually present in many family members. Although they usually represent a benign developmental condition, parasomnias can be associated with severe sleep disruption and may cause significant family distress and daytime sleepiness.

Treatment

The behavioral abnormalities in all of these disorders can be triggered by factors that disrupt sleep. Therefore, strict adherence to sleep hygiene principles is necessary. Children should avoid sleep deprivation, stressful situations, and caffeine close to bedtime. Treatment of other sleep, emotional, and behavioral disorders is known to reduce the frequency and intensity of parasomnias. Scheduled awakening is a behavioral treatment for confusional arousals, night terrors, and sleepwalking that has been used with some success.

In cases of likely self-injury and high parental distress, parental education and reassurance should be provided with the emphasis on preventing injury and helping the child to return to bed. In all cases, removing potentially dangerous objects close to the bedside, such as bedside tables and sharp objects; keeping knives and firearms out of the reach of a child; locking house entrance doors and windows; and installing bedroom alarm devices are examples of safety precautions.

There are no medications approved by the FDA for the treatment of disorders of arousal. In severe cases of parasomnias, medications such as clonazepam (0.01 mg/kg, usual starting dose 0.125 mg at bedtime), diazepam (0.04–0.25 mg/kg), or lorazepam (0.05 mg/kg) can be considered (Kotagal 2011; Sheldon 2004).

Circadian Rhythm Sleep-Wake Disorders

The DSM-5 criteria for circadian rhythm sleep-wake disorders are presented in Box 23–5.

TABLE 23–3. Clinical characteristics and treatment interventions for parasomnias

Clinical presentation	Parasomnia			
	Sleepwalking	**Confusional arousals**	**Sleep terrors**	**Nightmare disorder**
Peak age	4–12 years	2–10 years	1.5–10 years	3–6 years; less frequent among school-age children
Prevalence	15% of children have occasional episodes; 1%–6% have frequent ones	17% of children ages 3–13 years	3%–6% in children; less frequent in adolescents or adults	10%–50% among children ages 3–6 years
Time of the night	First third	First third	First third	Second half
Sleep state	NREM	NREM	NREM	REM
Clinical characteristics	Sits up, walks with glazed eyes, can become agitated; lasts 5 seconds to 30 minutes; amnesia the next day	Starts moving; moaning in sleep; gets agitated, confused; may become violent, combative; lasts 5–30 minutes; amnesia the next day	Sudden scream, glassy eyes wide open, tachycardia, sweating, rapid respiration; lasts 30 seconds to 3 minutes; partial or full amnesia the next day	Sudden arousal from sleep due to disturbing frightening dreams; usually fully awake; has recollection the next day
Treatment	Take safety precautions; avoid sleep deprivation; schedule awakenings prior to usual time of sleepwalking episode occurrence; take medication: benzodiazepines (clonazepam 0.25–1 mg at bedtime)	Same as sleepwalking; do not attempt to awaken the person, as he may become more agitated; gently redirect back to bed	Same as sleepwaking	Sleep hygiene; stress reduction; CBT and systemic desensitization with relaxation and imagery rehearsal; in severe cases medication may be warranted

Note. CBT=cognitive-behavioral therapy; NREM=non–rapid eye movement; REM=rapid eye movement.

Box 23–5. DSM-5 Diagnostic Criteria for Circadian Rhythm Sleep-Wake Disorders

A. A persistent or recurrent pattern of sleep disruption that is primarily due to an alteration of the circadian system or to a misalignment between the endogenous circadian rhythm and the sleep–wake schedule required by an individual's physical environment or social or professional schedule.
B. The sleep disruption leads to excessive sleepiness or insomnia, or both.
C. The sleep disturbance causes clinically significant distress or impairment in social, occupational, and other important areas of functioning.

Coding note: For ICD-9-CM, code **307.45** for all subtypes. For ICD-10-CM, code is based on subtype.

Specify whether:

307.45 (G47.21) Delayed sleep phase type: A pattern of delayed sleep onset and awakening times, with an inability to fall asleep and awaken at a desired or conventionally acceptable earlier time.

Specify if:

Familial: A family history of delayed sleep phase is present.

Specify if:

Overlapping with non-24-hour sleep-wake type: Delayed sleep phase type may overlap with another circadian rhythm sleep-wake disorder, non-24-hour sleep-wake type.

307.45 (G47.22) Advanced sleep phase type: A pattern of advanced sleep onset and awakening times, with an inability to remain awake or asleep until the desired or conventionally acceptable later sleep or wake times.

Specify if:

Familial: A family history of advanced sleep phase is present.

307.45 (G47.23) Irregular sleep-wake type: A temporally disorganized sleep-wake pattern, such that the timing of sleep and wake periods is variable throughout the 24-hour period.

307.45 (G47.24) Non-24-hour sleep-wake type: A pattern of sleep-wake cycles that is not synchronized to the 24-hour environment, with a consistent daily drift (usually to later and later times) of sleep onset and wake times.

307.45 (G47.26) Shift work type: Insomnia during the major sleep period and/or excessive sleepiness (including inadvertent sleep) during the major awake period associated with a shift work schedule (i.e., requiring unconventional work hours).

307.45 (G47.20) Unspecified type

Specify if:

Episodic: Symptoms last at least 1 month but less than 3 months.

Persistent: Symptoms last 3 months or longer.

Recurrent: Two or more episodes occur within the space of 1 year.

Source. Reprinted from the *Diagnostic and Statistical Manual of Mental Disorders*, 5th Edition. Arlington, VA, American Psychiatric Association, 2013. Used with permission.

Prevalence

It is estimated that circadian rhythm sleep disorders affect more than 10% of children. Delayed sleep phase syndrome (DSPS) occurs in 5%–10% of adolescents but may begin at a much younger age. Advanced sleep phase syndrome is more common in preschoolers.

Clinical Characteristics

Circadian rhythm sleep disorders are the disruption of the internal body rhythms that regulate sleep-wakefulness and are characterized by normal sleep that occurs at the "wrong" time relative to social demands.

DSPS is normally associated with changes seen during puberty in the regulation of sleep homeostasis and the circadian clock. These changes result in the delay of sleep phase in relation to the dark and light cycle. Early rise times on school days create significant sleep deficiency. Adolescents with DSPS present with excessive daytime sleepiness, especially in the morning hours, that results in academic impairment, mood problems, attentional deficits, and family conflict. A national survey of sleep patterns and habits among adolescents revealed chronic insufficient sleep during the school week, with a high correlation between sleep loss and depressive symptoms (National Sleep Foundation 2006).

Treatment

Sleep hygiene, family and child education, and the gradual advancement of sleep phase are essential parts of treatment for DSPS. Bright light therapy (5,000–10,000 lux) with morning exposure usually produces phase advancement in several days. Blue light therapy has demonstrated efficacy in several studies with 20 minutes to an hour exposure shortly after wake-up time (Revell et al. 2012). Melatonin administered approximately an hour before bedtime helps to facilitate sleep phase advancement. Gradual advancement of bedtime can be used to reset the biological clock in patients with DSPS. Chronotherapy, another behavioral technique that may be applied to adolescents with severe DSPS, is a gradual delay in bedtime by 3-hour increments until the desired bedtime is reached. Patients are usually instructed to maintain daily sleep logs as they delay their bedtime. Parents may need to be involved to help adolescents with the unusual sleep and wake times. The American Academy of Pediatrics has recently published a policy statement recognizing insufficient sleep in adolescents as an important public health issue (American Academy of Pediatrics 2014). It encourages school districts to improve sleep in students by delaying school start times to allow optimal levels of sleep (8.5–9 hours).

Sleep Problems in Children With Psychiatric Disorders

Attention-Deficit/Hyperactivity Disorder

Children with ADHD have a high prevalence of sleep disorders, based on subjective parental reports and self-reports and objective instrumental assessments of sleep (Cortese et al. 2009). Difficulty settling down to sleep, delayed sleep onset with frequent nocturnal awakenings, restless sleep, and reduced total amount of sleep have been reported in children with ADHD. Both behavioral and intrinsic sleep disorders have been associated with symptoms of ADHD.

Snoring and OSA have been implicated in the possible pathophysiology of ADHD symptoms in some children, an association supported by evidence that adenotonsillectomy for sleep-disordered breathing can improve inattention and hyperactivity (Chervin et al. 2006; Dillon et al. 2007; Wei et al. 2009). A strong association among RLS, PLMD, and ADHD was found in a number of studies, with 26%–64% of children with ADHD meeting criteria for PLMD on polysomnography (Picchietti et al. 1998, 1999) and more than 44% of children with PLMD having a clinical diagnosis of ADHD (Crabtree et al. 2003).

Administration of melatonin in the evening has demonstrated improvement in sleep-onset delay among children with ADHD, although the exact dose range has not been established (Cortese et al. 2013).

Sleep assessment is an important part of evaluation and treatment of ADHD. Most importantly, the clinician should screen for sleep-disordered breathing symptoms such as habitual snoring and witnessed apneas and inquire about restless legs symptoms and family history of RLS.

Mood Disorders

Problems with sleep initiation, sleep maintenance, and hypersomnia are some of the most prevalent symptoms among children and adolescents with depressive disorders. Early studies of children with major depression indicated that up to two-thirds of depressed youth reported sleep-onset and sleep-maintenance insomnia, with more than half of these children having early morning awakenings with inability to return to sleep (Ivanenko et al. 2005). A longitudinal study of 1,710 adolescents showed that 88% of those with major depressive disorder reported sleep disturbances (Roberts et al. 1995). A study of 553 depressed children assessed with the Interview Schedule for Children and Adolescents—Diagnostic Version revealed that 72.7% had sleep disturbance, 53.5% had insomnia alone, 9% had hypersomnia, and 10.1% had both insomnia and hypersomnia. The degree of sleep dysfunction correlated with the severity of depression, with more sleep-disturbed children having more depressive symptoms and anxiety disorders (Liu et al. 2007). Several recent surveys conducted among adolescents demonstrated association between sleep problems and suicidality (Fitzgerald et al. 2011; Messias and Buysse 2011; Wong et al. 2011). This emphasizes the importance of sleep screening as part of the suicide assessment.

Sleep laboratory studies examining polysomnographic characteristics in children and adolescents with major depressive disorder have found more sleep abnormalities such as longer sleep latency and shorter REM latency in adolescents than in prepubertal children, indicating that maturational factors play a significant role in the pathophysiology of sleep dysfunction associated with major depression.

Sleep complaints are frequent among youth with early onset bipolar disorders, including insomnia, excessive daytime sleepiness, night wakings, parasomnias, bedtime resistance, and nocturnal anxiety. Almost all children with bipolar disorder are reported to require pharmacological and/or nonpharmacological interventions for sleep disorder symptoms because of negative impact on their emotional and behavioral functioning (Lofthouse et al. 2008, 2010).

Autism Spectrum Disorders

Sleep difficulties are estimated to occur in 44%–86% of children with autism spectrum disorder (ASD; Richdale 1999; Stores and Wiggs 1998). The most frequently reported sleep problems in ASD are difficulty falling asleep; frequent nocturnal and early morning awakenings; irregular sleep-wake cycle; restless sleep; and parasomnias such as sleepwalking, night terrors, confusional arousals, and REM behavior sleep disorder. Sleep problems in children with ASD have been associated with disrupted daytime behavior (Goldman et al. 2011; Sikora et al. 2012). Several hypotheses have been proposed to explain these sleep difficulties, including disrupted and poorly entrained circadian rhythms due to failure to recognize social and environmental cues, neurostructural and neurochemical abnormalities involving systems regulating sleep, and altered melatonin production (Cortesi et al. 2010). Recent research suggests that bedroom access to a television or computer is more strongly associated with reduced sleep among boys with ASD compared with boys with ADHD or typically developing boys (Engelhardt et al. 2013).

Effective behavioral treatments of sleep disorders in children with ASD include sleep hygiene, stimulus control, scheduled nocturnal awakenings, positive bedtime routine, daytime nap restriction, and graduated extinction. Several studies have demonstrated the effectiveness of melatonin in improving sleep continuity and reducing sleep-onset latency (Garstang and Wallis 2006; Malow et al. 2012a; Wasdell et al. 2008; Wright et al. 2011). A recent study demonstrated a benefit to adding cognitive-behavioral treatment to melatonin when treating children with ASD and persistent insomnia (Cortesi et al. 2012). The Sleep Committee of the Autism Treatment Network has developed a practice pathway for insomnia based on expert consensus (Malow et al. 2012b).

Substance Abuse

Sleep complaints are highly prevalent among adolescents using illicit drugs, alcohol, and cigarettes. The most common sleep-related symptoms in adolescents abusing substances are excessive daytime sleepiness, insomnia, and DSPS. Johnson and Breslau (2001) surveyed 13,831 adolescents ages 12–17 years. Almost 6% of study participants reported sleep problems, with a dose-dependent relationship between alcohol and illicit drug use and severity and frequency of sleep disturbances. Other psychiatric disorders are frequently comorbid with sleep disorders and substance abuse, making this relationship even more complicated, especially when it comes to treatment options. However, the same study indicated that adolescents with illicit drug abuse history experienced more persistent sleep problems, regardless of other psychiatric comorbidities. A six-session group therapy for adolescents with substance use disorders and sleep problems included stimulus control instructions, bright light exposure, sleep hygiene, cognitive therapy, and mindfulness-based stress reduction (Bootzin and Stevens 2005). The results of this study suggested effectiveness of this complex approach.

Anxiety Disorders

Anxiety and sleep problems are closely tied together, especially during childhood. A longitudinal study of sleep and behavioral and emotional problems revealed that the presence of sleep problems at age 4 is significantly correlated with the development of depression and anxiety by age 15 (Gregory and O'Connor 2002). Children with secure affective attachments to their primary caregivers are significantly less likely to develop sleep problems and will have fewer nighttime awakenings, fewer problems at bedtime, and less excessive daytime sleepiness. It has been shown that higher-functioning families with fewer psychiatric difficulties tend to have children who are more cooperative at bedtime and show longer sleep throughout the night (Seifer et al. 1996).

Children with generalized anxiety disorder and obsessive-compulsive disorder demonstrated longer sleep onset latency and less total sleep with reduced sleep efficiency (Alfano and Kim 2011; Alfano et al. 2013). While many children experience some fears at bedtime, children with anxiety disorders experience far more fear and anxiety at bedtime. Nightmares occur in 75% of 4- to 12-year-old children. However, children who have been exposed to major stressors, including trauma and abuse, have more persistent nightmares, frequently representing flashbacks of their traumatic experiences, with increased levels of autonomic arousal causing awakenings. In addition, children who were abused have significantly poorer sleep efficiency, less quiet sleep, and more nocturnal activity on sleep studies than nonabused children, even when controlling for psychiatric disorders. Presence of sleep problems 2 years after trauma predicted the maintenance of existing PTSD symptoms in children exposed to hurricane Katrina and the emergence of new symptoms 6 months later (Brown et al. 2011).

Systemic desensitization to fears, imagery rehearsal therapy with positive bedtime routines, and cognitive-behavioral therapy have demonstrated efficacy in the treatment of sleep symptoms associated with anxiety disorders.

Summary Points

- Sleep disorders are highly prevalent in children of all ages.
- Children and adolescents with psychiatric conditions have a higher prevalence of sleep disorders.
- Primary sleep disorders may manifest with symptoms of inattention, academic difficulties, poor impulse control, mood changes, excessive daytime sleepiness, and fatigue—resembling symptoms of ADHD, depressive disorders, and learning disabilities.
- Early identification and treatment of sleep disorders are important in improving negative developmental outcomes.
- Referral to the sleep laboratory is indicated for children with suspected sleep-disordered breathing, excessive daytime sleepiness, and parasomnias.
- The first-choice treatment for children with nocturnal anxiety, behavioral insomnia of childhood, and nightmares includes behavioral interventions.
- Pharmacological interventions for children with sleep disturbances should be considered only in the context of behavioral interventions and should preferably be short term.

References

Alfano CA, Kim KL: Objective sleep patterns and severity of symptoms in pediatric obsessive compulsive disorder: a pilot investigation. J Anxiety Disord 25(6):835–839, 2011 21570250

Alfano CA, Reynolds K, Scott N, et al: Polysomnographic sleep patterns of non-depressed, non-medicated children with generalized anxiety disorder. J Affect Disord 147(1–3):379–384, 2013 23026127

American Academy of Pediatrics: School start times for adolescents: policy statement. Pediatrics 134(3):642–649, 2014

American Academy of Sleep Medicine: International Classification of Sleep Disorders, 3rd Edition. Westchester, IL, American Academy of Sleep Medicine, 2014

American Psychiatric Association: Diagnostic and Statistical Manual of Mental Disorders, 4th Edition, Text Revision. Washington, DC, American Psychiatric Association, 2013

Aran A, Einen M, Lin L, et al: Clinical and therapeutic aspects of childhood narcolepsy-cataplexy: a retrospective study of 51 children. Sleep 33(11):1457–1464, 2010 21102987

Blader JC, Koplewicz HS, Abikoff H, et al: Sleep problems of elementary school children. A community survey. Arch Pediatr Adolesc Med 151(5):473–480, 1997 9158439

Blumer JL, Findling RL, Shih WJ, et al: Controlled clinical trial of zolpidem for the treatment of insomnia associated with attention-deficit/hyperactivity disorder in children 6 to 17 years of age. Pediatrics 123(5):e770–e776, 2009 19403468

Bootzin RR, Stevens SJ: Adolescents, substance abuse, and the treatment of insomnia and daytime sleepiness. Clin Psychol Rev 25(5):629–644, 2005 15953666

Brockmann PE, Urschitz MS, Schlaud M, et al: Primary snoring in school children: prevalence and neurocognitive impairments. Sleep Breath 16(1):23–29, 2012 21240656

Brooks LJ: Genetic syndromes affecting breathing during sleep in children, in Sleep Medicine. Edited by Lee-Chiong TL, Sateia MJ, Carskadon MA. Philadelphia, PA, Hanley and Belfus, 2002, pp 305–314

Brouillette RT, Manoukian JJ, Ducharme FM, et al: Efficacy of fluticasone nasal spray for pediatric obstructive sleep apnea. J Pediatr 138(6):838–844, 2001 11391326

Brown TH, Mellman TA, Alfano CA, et al: Sleep fears, sleep disturbance, and PTSD symptoms in minority youth exposed to Hurricane Katrina. J Trauma Stress 24(5):575–580, 2011 21898601

Challamel MJ, Mazzola ME, Nevsimalova S, et al: Narcolepsy in children. Sleep 17(8 suppl):S17–S20, 1994 7701194

Chervin RD, Hedger K, Dillon JE, et al: Pediatric Sleep Questionnaire (PSQ): validity and reliability of scales for sleep-disordered breathing, snoring, sleepiness, and behavioral problems. Sleep Med 1(1):21–32, 2000 10733617

Chervin RD, Ruzicka DL, Giordani BJ, et al: Sleep-disordered breathing, behavior, and cognition in children before and after adenotonsillectomy. Pediatrics 117(4):e769–e778, 2006 16585288

Cortese S, Konofal E, Lecendreux M, et al: Restless legs syndrome and attention-deficit/hyperactivity disorder: a review of the literature. Sleep 28(8):1007–1013, 2005 16218085

Cortese S, Faraone SV, Konofal E, et al: Sleep in children with attention-deficit/hyperactivity disorder: meta-analysis of subjective and objective studies. J Am Acad Child Adolesc Psychiatry 48(9):894–908, 2009 19625983

Cortese S, Brown TE, Corkum P, et al: Assessment and management of sleep problems in youths with attention-deficit/hyperactivity disorder. J Am Acad Child Adolesc Psychiatry 52(8):784–796, 2013 23880489

Cortesi F, Giannotti F, Ivanenko A, et al: Sleep in children with autistic spectrum disorder. Sleep Med 11(7):659–664, 2010 20605110

Cortesi F, Giannotti F, Sebastiani T, et al: Controlled-release melatonin, singly and combined with cognitive behavioural therapy, for persistent insomnia in children with autism spectrum disorders: a randomized placebo-controlled trial. J Sleep Res 21(6):700–709, 2012 22616853

Crabtree VM, Ivanenko A, O'Brien LM, et al: Periodic limb movement disorder of sleep in children. J Sleep Res 12(1):73–81, 2003 12603789

Dillon JE, Blunden S, Ruzicka DL, et al: DSM-IV diagnoses and obstructive sleep apnea in children before and 1 year after adenotonsillectomy. J Am Acad Child Adolesc Psychiatry 46(11):1425–1436, 2007 18049292

Drake C, Nickel C, Burduvali E, et al: The pediatric daytime sleepiness scale (PDSS): sleep habits and school outcomes in middle-school children. Sleep 26(4):455–458, 2003 12841372

Durmer J: Restless legs syndrome, periodic limb movements and periodic limb movement disorder, in Therapy in Sleep Medicine. Edited by Barkoukis TJ, Matheson J, Ferber R, et al. Philadelphia, PA, Elsevier, 2011, pp 337–350

Engelhardt CR, Mazurek MO, Sohl K: Media use and sleep among boys with autism spectrum disorder, ADHD, or typical development. Pediatrics 132(6):1081–1089, 2013 24249825

England SJ, Picchietti DL, Couvadelli BV, et al: L-Dopa improves restless legs syndrome and periodic limb movements in sleep but not attention-deficit-hyperactivity disorder in a double-blind trial in children. Sleep Med 12(5):471–477, 2011 21463967

Fitzgerald CT, Messias E, Buysse DJ: Teen sleep and suicidality: results from the youth risk behavior surveys of 2007 and 2009. J Clin Sleep Med 7(4):351–356, 2011 21897771

Frenette E: Restless legs syndrome in children: a review and update on pharmacological options. Curr Pharm Des 17(15):1436–1442, 2011 21476956

Garstang J, Wallis M: Randomized controlled trial of melatonin for children with autistic spectrum disorders and sleep problems. Child Care Health Dev 32(5):585–589, 2006 16919138

Goldman SE, McGrew S, Johnson KP, et al: Sleep is associated with problem behaviors in children and adolescents with autism spectrum disorders. Res Autism Spectr Disord 5(3):1223–1229, 2011

Gregory AM, O'Connor TG: Sleep problems in childhood: a longitudinal study of developmental change and association with behavioral problems. J Am Acad Child Adolesc Psychiatry 41(8):964–971, 2002 12162632

Ivanenko A, Tauman R, Gozal D: Modafinil in the treatment of excessive daytime sleepiness in children. Sleep Med 4(6):579–582, 2003 14607353

Ivanenko A, Crabtree VM, Gozal D: Sleep and depression in children and adolescents. Sleep Med Rev 9(2):115–129, 2005 15737790

Johnson CR: Sleep problems in children with mental retardation and autism. Child Adolesc Psychiatr Clin N Am 5(3):673–681, 1996

Johnson EO, Breslau N: Sleep problems and substance use in adolescence. Drug Alcohol Depend 64(1):1–7, 2001 11470335

Johnson EO, Roth T, Schultz L, et al: Epidemiology of DSM-IV insomnia in adolescents: lifetime prevalence, chronicity, and an emergent gender difference. Pediatrics 117:e247–e256, 2006 16452333

Klackenberg G: Somnambulism in childhood—prevalence, course and behavioral correlations. A prospective longitudinal study (6–16 years). Acta Paediatr Scand 71(3):495–499, 1982 7136663

Konofal E, Arnulf I, Lecendreux M, et al: Ropinirole in a child with attention-deficit hyperactivity disorder and restless legs syndrome. Pediatr Neurol 32(5):350–351, 2005 15866437

Kotagal S: Parasomnias, periodic limb movements, and restless legs in children. In Therapy in Sleep Medicine. Edited by Barkoukis T, Matheson J, Ferber R, et al. Philadelphia, PA, Elsevier, 2011, pp 475–484

Kuhn BR, Elliott AJ: Treatment efficacy in behavioral pediatric sleep medicine. J Psychosom Res 54(6):587–597, 2003 12781314

Kuhn BR, Roane BM: Pediatric Insomnia and Behavioral Interventions, in Therapy in Sleep Medicine. Edited by Barkoukis T, Matheson J, Ferber R, et al. Philadelphia, PA, Elsevier, 2011, pp 448–456

Laberge L, Tremblay RE, Vitaro F, et al: Development of parasomnias from childhood to early adolescence. Pediatrics 106(1 Pt 1):67–74, 2000 10878151

Lipton AJ, Gozal D: Treatment of obstructive sleep apnea in children: do we really know how? Sleep Med Rev 7(1):61–80, 2003 12586531

Liu X, Buysse DJ, Gentzler AL, et al: Insomnia and hypersomnia associated with depressive phenomenology and comorbidity in childhood depression. Sleep 30(1):83–90, 2007 17310868

Lofthouse N, Fristad M, Splaingard M, et al: Web survey of sleep problems associated with early onset bipolar spectrum disorders. J Pediatr Psychol 33(4):349–357, 2008 18192301

Lofthouse N, Fristad MA, Splaingard M, et al: Web-survey of pharmacological and non-pharmacological sleep interventions for children with early onset bipolar spectrum disorders. J Affect Disord 120(1–3):267–271, 2010 19740548

Malow B, Adkins KW, McGrew SG, et al: Melatonin for sleep in children with autism: a controlled trial examining dose, tolerability, and outcomes. J Autism Dev Disord 42(8):1729–1737, author reply 1738, 2012a 22160300

Malow BA, Byars K, Johnson K, et al: A practice pathway for the identification, evaluation, and management of insomnia in children and adolescents with autism spectrum disorders. Pediatrics 130(suppl 2):S106–S124, 2012b 23118242

Marcus CL: Sleep-disordered breathing in children. Am J Respir Crit Care Med 164(1):16–30, 2001 11435234

Marcus CL, Ward SL, Mallory GB, et al: Use of nasal continuous positive airway pressure as treatment of childhood obstructive sleep apnea. J Pediatr 127(1):88–94, 1995 7608817

Marcus CL, Brooks LJ, Draper KA, et al: Diagnosis and management of childhood obstructive sleep apnea syndrome. Pediatrics 130(3):e714–e755, 2012 22926176

Messias E, Buysse DJ: Teen sleep and suicidality: results from the youth risk behavior surveys of 2007 and 2009. J Clin Sleep Med 7(4):351–356, 2011 21897771

Mindell JA: Empirically supported treatments in pediatric psychology: bedtime refusal and night wakings in young children. J Pediatr Psychol 24(6):465–481, 1999 10608096

Mindell JA, Owens JA: Sleep problems in pediatric practice: clinical issues for the pediatric nurse practitioner. J Pediatr Health Care 17(6):324–331, 2003 14610449

Mindell JA, Emslie G, Blumer J, et al: Pharmacologic management of insomnia in children and adolescents: consensus statement. Pediatrics 117(6):e1223–e1232, 2006 16740821

Murali H, Kotagal S: Off-label treatment of severe childhood narcolepsy-cataplexy with sodium oxybate. Sleep 29(8):1025–1029, 2006 16944670

National Sleep Foundation: Sleep in America poll, 2006. Washington, DC, National Sleep Foundation, 2006. Available at: http://sleepfoundation.org/sleep-polls-data/sleep-in-america-poll/2006-teens-and-sleep. Accessed March 24, 2015.

O'Brien LM: Cognitive and behavioral consequences of obstructive sleep apnea, in Principles and Practice of Pediatric Sleep Medicine, 2nd Edition. Edited by Sheldon S, Ferber R, Kryger M, et al. Philadelphia, PA, Elsevier, 2014, pp 231–238

O'Brien LM, Gozal D: Neurocognitive dysfunction and sleep in children: from human to rodent. Pediatr Clin North Am 51(1):187–202, 2004 15008589

Owens JA, Spirito A, McGuinn M: The Children's Sleep Habits Questionnaire (CSHQ): psychometric properties of a survey instrument for school-aged children. Sleep 23(8):1043–1051, 2000a 11145319

Owens JA, Spirito A, McGuinn M, et al: Sleep habits and sleep disturbance in elementary school-aged children. J Dev Behav Pediatr 21(1):27–36, 2000b 10706346

Pelayo R, Yuen K: Pediatric sleep pharmacology. Child Adolesc Psychiatr Clin N Am 21(4):861–883, 2012 23040905

Petit D, Touchette E, Tremblay RE, et al: Dyssomnias and parasomnias in early childhood. Pediatrics 119(5):e1016–e1025, 2007 17438080

Picchietti DL, England SJ, Walters AS, et al: Periodic limb movement disorder and restless legs syndrome in children with attention-deficit hyperactivity disorder. J Child Neurol 13(12):588–594, 1998 9881529

Picchietti DL, Underwood DJ, Farris WA, et al: Further studies on periodic limb movement disorder and restless legs syndrome in children with attention-deficit hyperactivity disorder. Mov Disord 14(6):1000–1007, 1999 10584676

Picchietti D, Allen RP, Walters AS, et al: Restless legs syndrome: prevalence and impact in children and adolescents—the

Peds REST study. Pediatrics 120(2):253–266, 2007 17671050

Picchietti DL, Bruni O, de Weerd A, et al: Pediatric restless legs syndrome diagnostic criteria: an update by the International Restless Legs Syndrome Study Group. Sleep Med 14(12):1253–1259, 2013 24184054

Price AM, Wake M, Ukoumunne OC, et al: Five-year follow-up of harms and benefits of behavioral infant sleep intervention: randomized trial. Pediatrics 130(4):643–651, 2012 22966034

Redline S, Tishler PV, Schluchter M, et al: Risk factors for sleep-disordered breathing in children. Associations with obesity, race, and respiratory problems. Am J Respir Crit Care Med 159(5 Pt 1):1527–1532, 1999 10228121

Revell VL, Molina TA, Eastman CI: Human phase response curve to intermittent blue light using a commercially available device. J Physiol 590(Pt 19):4859–4868, 2012 22753544

Richdale AL: Sleep problems in autism: prevalence, cause, and intervention. Dev Med Child Neurol 41(1):60–66, 1999 10068053

Roberts RE, Lewinsohn PM, Seeley JR: Symptoms of DSM-III-R major depression in adolescence: evidence from an epidemiological survey. J Am Acad Child Adolesc Psychiatry 34(12):1608–1617, 1995 8543532

Rona RJ, Li L, Gulliford MC, et al: Disturbed sleep: effects of sociocultural factors and illness. Arch Dis Child 78(1):20–25, 1998 9534671

Section on Pediatric Pulmonology, Subcommittee on Obstructive Sleep Apnea Syndrome, American Academy of Pediatrics: Clinical practice guideline: diagnosis and management of childhood obstructive sleep apnea syndrome. Pediatrics 109(4):704–712, 2002 11927718

Seifer R, Sameroff AJ, Dickstein S, et al: Parental psychopathology and sleep variation in children. Child Adolesc Psychiatr Clin N Am 5(3):715–727, 1996

Sheldon SH: Parasomnias in childhood. Pediatr Clin North Am 51(1):69–88, vi, 2004 15008583

Sikora DM, Johnson K, Clemons T, et al: The relationship between sleep problems and daytime behavior in children of different ages with autism spectrum disorders. Pediatrics 130(suppl 2):S83–S90, 2012 23118258

Silvestri R, Gagliano A, Arico I, et al: Sleep disorders in children with attention-deficit/hyperactivity disorder (ADHD) recorded overnight by video-polysomnography. Sleep Med 10(10):1132–1138, 2009 19527942

Stores G, Wiggs L: Abnormal sleep patterns associated with autism. Autism 2(2):157–169, 1998

Walters AS, Mandelbaum DE, Lewin DS, et al: Dopaminergic therapy in children with restless legs/periodic limb movements in sleep and ADHD. Pediatr Neurol 22(3):182–186, 2000 10734247

Wasdell MB, Jan JE, Bomben MM, et al: A randomized, placebo-controlled trial of controlled release melatonin treatment of delayed sleep phase syndrome and impaired sleep maintenance in children with neurodevelopmental disabilities. J Pineal Res 44(1):57–64, 2008 18078449

Wei JL, Bond J, Mayo MS, et al: Improved behavior and sleep after adenotonsillectomy in children with sleep-disordered breathing: long-term follow-up. Arch Otolaryngol Head Neck Surg 135(7):642–646, 2009 19620583

Wong MM, Brower KJ, Zucker RA: Sleep problems, suicidal ideation, and self-harm behaviors in adolescence. J Psychiatr Res 45(4):505–511, 2011 20889165

Wright B, Sims D, Smart S, et al: Melatonin versus placebo in children with autism spectrum conditions and severe sleep problems not amenable to behaviour management strategies: a randomised controlled crossover trial. J Autism Dev Disord 41(2):175–184, 2011 20535539

Zammit G, Huang H, Sangal RB, et al. A randomized, placebo-controlled double-blind, fixed-dose study of the efficacy and safety of eszopicline in children (6 to 11 years) and adolescents (12 to 17 years) with attention deficit/hyperactivity disorder (ADHD)-associated insomnia. Sleep, 35 Abstract Suppl, A354. 2012

Zero to Three: Diagnostic Classification, 0–3R: Diagnostic Classification of Mental Health and Developmental Disorders of Infancy and Early Childhood, Revised Edition. Arlington, VA, Zero To Three, 2005

PART IV

Special Topics

CHAPTER 24

Evidence-Based Practice

John Hamilton, M.D.
Eric Daleiden, Ph.D.
Eric Youngstrom, Ph.D.

Defining Evidence-Based Practice(s)

In the last quarter of the twentieth century, evidence-based medicine (EBM), as originally conceived by David Sackett and others at McMaster University in Canada and Archie Cochrane and the virtual library named after him in the United Kingdom, grew into a widespread movement that influenced the practice of medicine worldwide, including child and adolescent psychiatry. The first electronic presentation of systematic reviews of interventions in medicine was *The Oxford Database of Perinatal Trials* (Starr et al. 2009, p. 182). Indeed, the United Kingdom and other countries based their national health services on the principles of evidence-based medicine. During this same time period, the American Psychological Association developed clear guidelines for what interventions could be called evidence-based, as did professional groups in dentistry, social work, and physical therapy. The American Psychiatric Association and the American Academy of Child and Adolescent Psychiatry (AACAP) have developed many practice parameters for disorders and clinical techniques. When multiple professional groups came together to work as teams, the term *evidence-based practice* became useful. It is in the spirit of multiprofessionalism that we use the term evidence-based practice in this chapter.

Evidence-based practice is a process in which "decisions about health care are based on the best available, current, valid and relevant evidence. These decisions should be made by those receiving care, informed by the tacit and explicit knowledge of those providing care, within the context of available resources" (Dawes et al. 2005, p. 4). The plural term EBPs refers to those processes that woven together create EBP. The singular term EBP is an umbrella term referring to a way of practice based on those processes.

EBPs in child mental health can be defined as *those processes that reduce uncertainty in clinical practice by aligning with the most valid, relevant, and bias-free empirical results from studies of outcome in similar youth, as applied to the goals of improved symptomatic and/or functional outcomes achieved by a higher proportion of youth more quickly for longer durations with fewer adverse events at less cost using methods acceptable to (or ideally sought after by) the youth and his/her parent or guardian, with outcome tracking to assess the results.* This sprawling and ambitious definition emphasizes the desired goals while recognizing that what is "best" is often open to debate on the basis of values. The construct used to define outcome, the size of the effect, its duration, adverse effects, the speed of response, cost, availability, convenience, patient and parent preferences, and a provider's capabilities may all enter a debate on the value of a study or choice of a treatment. EBP can also be defined by what it is *not:* loyalty to the status quo that lacks assessment of whether routine practices align with the current best evidence and also lacks empirical outcome measurement.

Evidence-Based Practice and the Movement to Reduce Errors in Medical Practice

During the rapid growth of EBP in the last decades of the twentieth century, another movement—the movement to reduce errors in medical practice—also grew rapidly, although much more slowly in child mental health. Searching PubMed using the medical subject headings (MeSH) term "medical errors" retrieves a torrent of studies from internal medicine and surgery, for example, yet almost none using both MeSH terms "child psychiatry" and "medical errors." In this movement an *error* is defined as "a mistake in performance or thought which caused an adverse event," that is, "an unintended injury that was caused by medical management and that resulted in measurable disability" (Leape et al. 1991, p. 377). In child mental health, *functional impairment* refers to interference with normative activities or failure to keep pace with peers developmentally and is a useful synonym for the term *disability* as used by the error reduction movement.

At first glance, *error* seems to imply gross mistakes, but the authors' classification of errors is revealing: they clearly mean much more. Leape and colleagues (1991) classify errors into errors of performance, prevention, diagnosis, drug treatment, or systemic functioning. It is not difficult for clinicians to imagine their own errors in each category. Under *performance,* using solely supportive treatment for an abuse victim would be an error ("use of inappropriate or outmoded form of therapy"), as would maintaining a wait list ("avoidable delay in treatment") in a system with underutilized capacity. Under *diagnosis,* use of an instrument with unknown or inadequate reliability or validity if a better one is available could be considered "use of inappropriate or outmoded diagnostic tests." Examples in the category of *drug treatment* would include any errors in drug choice, dose, or recognizing drug interactions or inadequate monitoring for side effects (Leape et al. 1991). All these errors would be likely to result in measurable functional impairment (e.g., in the first example, the gap between outcome for proven trauma-specific interventions and that of supportive treatment). *Using an outmoded practice or outmoded diagnostic approach is scored as an error if it results in a measurable functional impairment that likely could have been avoided with feasible EBPs.*

Such errors can have serious consequences and are undoubtedly common in child mental health. Errors are extremely common in the practice of medicine, but currently there are few methods for identifying or preventing them (Gawande 2014). Errors of omission easily imagined in clinical practices include failure to use indicated diagnostic tests, use of inappropriate or outmoded diagnostic tests, an avoidable delay in diagnosis, use of inappropriate or outmoded therapy, and practicing outside one's area of expertise (Leape et al. 1991). With this broad definition, clinician errors are an everyday experience but often "invisible" to the parent, the clinical system (e.g., hospital, agency), and even the clinician. For example, if an anxious child does not receive exposure as a key proven treatment element and fails to improve, most clinical organizations do not identify this as an error. Similarly, an adolescent receiving only supportive treatment rather than cognitive-behavioral therapy (CBT) or interpersonal psychotherapy for a serious depression and achieving a poor functional outcome may not be identified as an error. Quality-monitoring organizations like the National Committee for Quality Assurance would also fail to note either of these failures as errors because they do not track meaningful outcome measures in child psychiatry (Hamilton et al. 2011). However, recent examples of system-wide practice monitoring and feedback efforts are emerging (e.g., Higa-McMillan et al. 2011).

EBP is even more valuable when considered in the context of the error reduction movement. EBP detects a poor functional outcome because it monitors outcome. Furthermore, EBP has the potential to reduce errors by focusing on those domains (e.g., diagnosis, treatment, system) outlined as crucial in error reduction. EBP has the benefit of being positively focused, avoiding at least some of the inevitable backlash resulting from a focus only on errors. In a sense, EBP incorporates and anticipates many of the issues in the error reduction movement by "doing it right" the first time: using reliable diagnostic instruments, avoiding outmoded therapies, and tracking outcomes.

We now turn to implementation of EBPs in multidisciplinary organizations to make effective treatments available. *Implementation* refers to a purposeful set of specific activities for putting defined programs or professional behaviors into practice such that "independent observers can detect its presence and strength" (Fixsen et al. 2005). Although effective implementation of effective treatments is complex, it can lead to substantial improvements in youth outcomes (Daleiden et al. 2006).

Conceptualizing Evidence-Based Practice: A Guiding Framework

Modern health systems provide a context in which service delivery typically occurs as a set of care processes involving interactions between a developing patient (and family) and a developing provider (or team of providers). The EBP movement calls attention to the notion that a developing body of empirical knowledge is a key piece of the context of care and that each individual and care process offers a potential point of contact where facts from the body of knowledge may influence the nature and outcomes of health care. Metaphorically, how do we evolve care so that science becomes an integral part of the collaboration between patients and providers?

Stated another way, what mechanisms are effective at communicating (e.g., sending messages) from the body of scientific knowledge to the actors in the therapeutic change process? To date, the field of child and adolescent psychiatry has offered two dominant approaches to answering this question. The *evidence-based treatment model* has emphasized the packaging of scientific knowledge into specific protocols that are tested in the laboratory and disseminated to the field (Rounsaville et al. 2001); *the individualized care model* has emphasized the establishment of social processes (e.g., family treatment teams) to use the expertise of knowledgeable individuals in plans of care that may be implemented and monitored (Burchard et al. 2002).

These approaches emphasize integration of knowledge and procedural control at different points in the treatment development and delivery process (see Chorpita and Daleiden 2014). The development and dissemination of specific protocols emphasize integration of evidence at the time of protocol design and deliver that knowledge to the process of care through the nature and order of the procedures in the protocol, with controls emphasizing integrity to the treatment model. The development of individualized treatment plans emphasizes integration of evidence via expert knowledge and delivers that knowledge to the process of care through individual recall and social communication with controls that emphasize accountability to attain patient goals. Each approach has strengths and highlights opportunities for integrating knowledge and empirically guiding care.

Implementation Within a Specific Context

Just as Donald Winnicott noted that there is no baby without a mother, there is no clinician without a system. The *context* of a clinician's system is central to implementing EBP. Aspects of context include the regulatory, funding, and working environments where the patient and provider meet. Just as the clinician may strive to change a patient's behavior, forces within systems (e.g., culture, regulations, financial goals, resources) influence how clinicians conduct treatment. For example, a large health maintenance organization may find "report card" ratings from quality assurance groups important in retaining market share and pass on to the clinician the values of those quality assurance groups via behavioral rewards. Or a clinician operating within an outpatient system whose culture emphasizes long-term treatment may routinely create patient expectations of long-term treatment. Even within a system, however, it is almost always feasible for a clinician to introduce in her own work core EBP practices such as assessment instruments with known validity and outcome tracking. This by itself can lead to significant improvements in care or even lead to an invitation from the system to inject EBPs into a much larger context that includes multiple clinicians.

Funding mechanisms and access pressures differ markedly across contexts and need to be considered in planning system-wide implementation of EBPs. Similarly, what is considered "quality care" may differ across contexts, with one system rewarding rapid access and another rewarding low hospitalization readmissions or high customer satisfaction or client retention. Such differences in how an organization defines the construct "quality" will affect efforts to implement EBPs. The central point is that each clinician operates within a complex system that tends to push and pull clinical decision making and choices, just as the clinician actively tries to shape the behavior of his or her patients.

Because forces within systems (e.g., insistence on group treatment, preference for or avoidance of psychopharmacological intervention) are powerful and because systems vary enormously, attention to these systemic forces (*context*) is pivotal in bringing EBPs into a practice. For example, will a specific assessment instrument be well accepted at a specific day treatment program? Will a particular outcome measure make sense to clinicians with a special interest in autism spectrum disorder? Attention to such issues is critical to bringing EBPs to life in a sustainable fashion.

Studies of implementation suggest that several factors are critical for success: strong leadership with a clear strategy, visionary staff in key positions, openness to experimentation and risk taking, available "extra" resources, accessible staff training and coaching, a culture that includes knowledge sharing, and effective monitoring and feedback systems (Fixsen et al. 2005; Greenhalgh et al. 2004). Building these features into the context of care may help support effective transfer of knowledge into clinical operations of health systems.

Encouraging Patients to Support Evidence-Based Practices at the Initial Orientation

Integrating evidence-based content into frontline presentations where potential patients and care systems initially make contact can create demand for EBPs and promote a match between patient characteristics and effective treatments. For example, some clinics offer an orientation session for parents before their child sees a clinician. The orientation explains eligibility rules and educates and motivates parents and adolescents, shapes expectations, and explains treatment modalities available for common disorders. Youth and families may then help maintain EBPs by asking for and expecting services supported by evidence when they arrive at clinicians' offices. Such an orientation can also emphasize the value of patients bringing their own experiences and knowledge base to the evaluation process and respects patients as the experts on their own experiences, values, preferences, and history.

Provider Development and Preparation

Patient-clinician interactions remain at the heart of behavioral health care practices. Supportive contexts, program policies, and integrated information delivery are organizational tools for increasing the use of evidence. These tools capitalize on the unique expertise that both patients (experts in their goals and histories) and clinicians (experts in assessment, psychopathology, and treatment) bring to this interaction. Continuing education and active communication with networks of professional peers help clinicians maintain their expertise and bring it to patient encounters (Davis 1998; Rogers and Rogers 2003).

Clinicians create their own context by giving meanings to what they perceive within their work setting and by choosing what to initiate and how to respond to expectations within their organizational culture (Dopson and Fitzgerald 2005). The meanings that clinicians assign to events (in this case, efforts to implement EBPs) are crucial. However, even if well-defined evidence-based programs do not exist within a clinician's organization or practice, individual professionals can nevertheless strive to align their knowledge, skills, and behaviors with state-of-the-art practices as well to place their work in better alignment with the evidence.

Assessment

Assessment instruments are readily available to improve the assessment of general functioning and psychopathology and to reduce the likelihood of errors of omission (e.g., failing to recognize a comorbid anxiety disorder or substance use disorder) (Jensen-Doss et al. 2014). Thus, one obvious application of the evidence base to the assessment process is the selection of well-validated instruments, since assessment is essential for developing a patient-specific evidence base and evaluating care (Straus et al. 2011; Youngstrom 2013). The assessment process itself is an opportunity to introduce EBP recommendations into the care process and to define intervention targets for monitoring.

Adopting an evidence-based approach to assessment offers opportunities to organize practice to work more efficiently. Clinicians can start by evaluating the clinical context where they work: What are the most common presenting problems? What are the common diagnoses? The prevalence of mood disorder or the likely sources of stress and anxiety are likely to vary depending on whether the clinician is working in the community, a forensic setting, or an inpatient unit (Youngstrom et al. 2014). Knowing the "base rates" of common disorders—the proportion of all youth presenting in that setting who have a specific disorder—will help clinicians calibrate diagnoses and case formulations (Meehl 1954).

These benchmarks can also guide assessment practices. Does the standard intake procedure provide enough information to detect the most common problems? Does the clinician have the tools and methods in place to distinguish between major differential diagnoses? The clinician can configure the assessment tool kit to contain the best tools for working with common scenarios. Clinicians too often rely on informal, unstructured interviews and typically agree on formulations at levels only slightly better than chance. Contrary to clinicians' beliefs, patients actually tend to prefer structured approaches to interviewing and diagnoses, perceiving these as more comprehensive and building rapport rather than damaging it (Bruchmüller et al. 2011; Suppiger et al. 2009).

Evidence-based assessment often starts with broad measures of major problem dimensions. If an early adolescent presents with some conduct symptoms and some depressive symptoms, for example, the resulting data can be combined with base rates (i.e., the proportion of youth presenting to an outpatient clinic who meet Schedule for Affective Disorders and Schizophrenia for School-Age Children [K-SADS] criteria for major depressive disorder [MDD]) to get a sense of which of the presenting problems may need further assessment and which are unlikely to meet diagnostic criteria for a categorical diagnosis (Youngstrom 2013). More specialized rating scales and supplemental testing then focus on the hypotheses that are in the *assessment zone*—the region where the probability of a disorder does not definitively either rule in or rule out a specific diagnosis, suggesting the need for more testing. The next assessment findings raise or lower the probability until it is either functionally ruled out or clearly established as a treatment target. The most formal way of combining the information is via Bayes' theorem, using tools such as a probability nomogram (Figure 24–1) or online calculators (e.g., http://araw.mede.uic.edu/cgi-bin/testcalc.pl) to integrate base rates and clinical impressions with the diagnostic likelihood ratios attached to the assessment results or clinical findings (Straus et al. 2011). These methods are straightforward to learn, and they can produce large improvements in consistency and accuracy of clinical decisions (Jenkins et al. 2011) that generalize across clinical settings (Jenkins et al. 2012). Online calculators facilitate using likelihood ratios and eliminate the need for a paper nomogram.

A well-designed approach to assessment avoids the pitfalls of too much testing as well as too little. Too much assessment adds time and expense without improving clarity about treatment; it actually can lead to worse decisions and outcomes (Kraemer 1992). There are costs to the patient when mistakes are made. Errors of commission assign invalid diagnoses and lead to treatment choices with less chance of benefit while still carrying the full risk of harm. Errors of omission lead to failure to intervene early and effectively, as well as increasing the chances of misattributing the sources of the problem to some other diagnosis or mechanism.

The diagnosis and case formulation processes guide decisions about what and how to treat. The wide-scale adoption of structured diagnostic systems has promoted a literature with meta-analyses and systematic reviews and funding structures often organized around diagnostic categories (e.g., Cohen et al. 2010; Rettew et al. 2009). Although diagnosis is often a good place to start in matching treatments to a particular patient's circumstances, careful consideration of the match between what patients say is important to them and outcomes documented in studies is essential to serve patients' interests. In choosing an appropriate treatment, it is important to know what the youth and family want to achieve (e.g., better grades, fewer tantrums) and choose treatments likely to achieve that outcome. Noting both the target population (e.g., adolescents with MDD) and the chosen outcome domain (e.g., improved school functioning) facilitates finding and applying the intervention literature. In addition to specifying treatment targets, case formulation should specify the working etiological model of the patient's symptoms. Fortunately, well-supported EBPs are often associated with specific causal models of change.

Treatment Planning and Selection

Pharmacological Treatment

Good medication treatment adheres to several principles, including a comprehensive evaluation of both psychosocial factors and the symptoms to be addressed pharmacologically, a medical history, a clear plan for psychosocial and medication treatment based on the best evidence, and a plan for how to monitor outcomes, including *specifically targeted symptoms and deficits in functioning* as well as adherence and side effects and how to educate parents and youth regarding the disorders (Walkup and

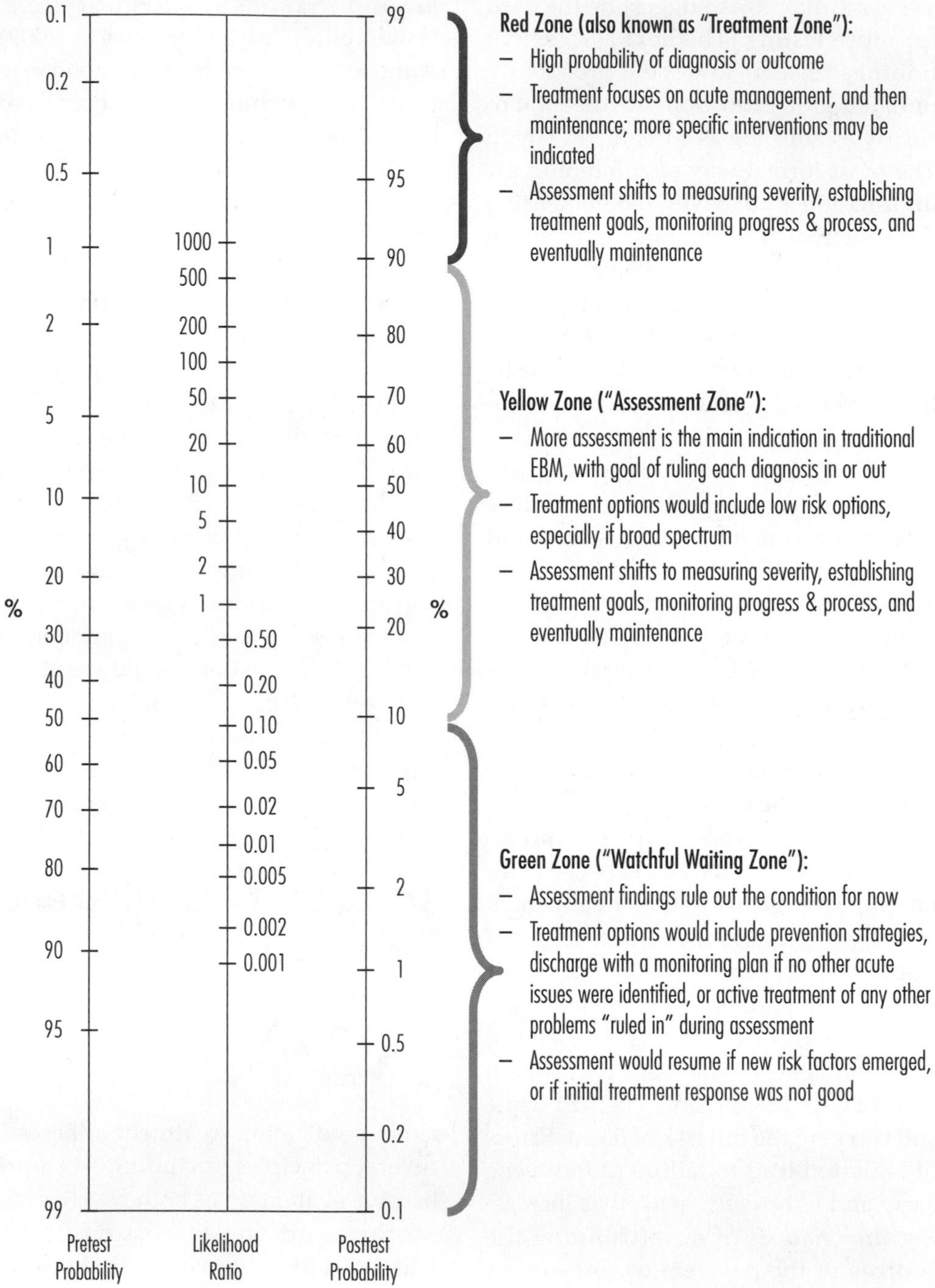

0.1
0.2
0.5
1
2
5
10
20
30
40
50
60
70
80
90
95
99
%
1000
500
200
100
50
20
10
5
2
1
0.50
0.20
0.10
0.05
0.02
0.01
0.005
0.002
0.001
99
95
90
80
70
60
50
40
30
20
10
5
2
1
0.5
0.2
0.1
%
Pretest Probability
Likelihood Ratio
Posttest Probability
Red Zone (also known as "Treatment Zone"):
– High probability of diagnosis or outcome
– Treatment focuses on acute management, and then maintenance; more specific interventions may be indicated
– Assessment shifts to measuring severity, establishing treatment goals, monitoring progress & process, and eventually maintenance
Yellow Zone ("Assessment Zone"):
– More assessment is the main indication in traditional EBM, with goal of ruling each diagnosis in or out
– Treatment options would include low risk options, especially if broad spectrum
– Assessment shifts to measuring severity, establishing treatment goals, monitoring progress & process, and eventually maintenance
Green Zone ("Watchful Waiting Zone"):
– Assessment findings rule out the condition for now
– Treatment options would include prevention strategies, discharge with a monitoring plan if no other acute issues were identified, or active treatment of any other problems "ruled in" during assessment
– Assessment would resume if new risk factors emerged, or if initial treatment response was not good

FIGURE 24–1. Probability nomogram for combining assessment findings with risk factors and patient probability of diagnosis, mapping onto zones of next clinical action (including treat, assess more, or watchful waiting).

Jenkins et al. (2011) and Youngstrom et al. (2014) illustrate using the nomogram to integrate risk factors and assessment findings in making decisions about a patient. EBM=evidence-based medicine.
Source. Adapted from Straus et al. 2011 and Youngstrom 2013.

American Academy of Child and Adolescent Psychiatry 2009).

Common errors of omission occur in the evaluation process, in treatment planning (insufficient use of existing evidence), and when outcome tracking is absent. Evaluating clinicians commonly omit comorbid disorders and are reluctant to assign "no disorder." Agreement between diagnoses made by clinicians and structured interviews is poor (Jensen and Weisz 2002; Rettew et al. 2009). As in other specialties, clinicians often do not search existing evidence or dismiss it as irrelevant or infeasible (Hamilton et al. 2011). Finally, many youth are treated without ongoing tracking of a targeted domain using a validated instrument.

Psychotropic medications have the capacity to do significant harm. The most feasible solutions to common errors in using psychotropics are the routine use of validated low-burden online resources (many in the public domain) *to improve diagnostic processes* (e.g., modules of the K-SADS [Kaufman et al. 1997], available at http://www.psychiatry.pitt.edu/node/8233, or Achenbach System of Empirically Based Assessment [ASEBA] instruments [Achenbach and Rescorla 2001], available at www.aseba.org), *to find evidence* (e.g., PubMed at http://www.ncbi.nlm.nih.gov/pubmed/ and PsycINFO abstracts at http://www.apa.org/pubs/databases/psycinfo/index.aspx), and *to track outcome* (e.g., NIH's PROMIS instruments at www.nihpromis.org/).

Combining Pharmacological and Psychosocial Treatments

Evidence supports the combining of pharmacological and psychosocial treatments for many of the most common disorders, including anxiety disorders and major depression (March et al. 2004; Pediatric OCD Treatment Study Team 2004; Swanson et al. 2001). However, the reality of clinical practice is that individual youth are not assigned a treatment on the basis of randomization, as in a research study, but rather arrive with their own ideas about treatment, while clinicians arrive with their own prejudices, loyalties, professional identities, and defined skill sets. Organizations have their own limitations of what fits within their boundaries. The result is that treatment proceeds via a negotiation between clinician and patient, a negotiation that is partially rational and evidence based but also contains the prejudices and loyalties of each party as well as issues of feasibility, workload, availability, and organizational culture.

Evidence can create common ground for reaching consensus in negotiations about treatment. Reviewing evidence together can build collaboration and reduce conflict. For example, a psychotherapist, after learning about the large effect size in youth with obsessive-compulsive disorder treated with exposure and response prevention (Pediatric OCD Treatment Study Team 2004), successfully resumed CBT treatment and stopped pressuring the physician to change medications during a treatment stalled by the child's refusal to be exposed to school attendance. In another situation, a clinician decided not to recommend a trial of stimulants, partly because of parent preference and partly on the basis of a search discovering a behavioral, skills-based approach for a child with attention-deficit/hyperactivity disorder (ADHD) whose academic failures involved problems in organization and planning (Abikoff et al. 2013).

Psychosocial Treatments

As with pharmacological and combined treatments, many factors are relevant to selecting psychosocial treatments. One dimension meriting careful consideration is the level of analysis at which psychosocial treatments are defined (Chorpita et al. 2005). Common examples include defining practice as *clusters of similar treatments* (e.g., all treatments for children that teach parents behavioral management skills or all treatments using a CBT or psychodynamic psychotherapy), as a *treatment program* (e.g., a Maudsley eating disorder clinic, therapeutic foster care, or assertive community treatment), as a *protocol or manual* (e.g., coping with depression, parent-child interaction therapy, or dry bed training), or as a *common element or core component present in multiple protocols* (e.g., behavioral contracting, exposure, support networking). Different levels of analysis have different strengths and limitations that make them appropriate for different patient and context configurations. For example, in a triage and referral context, selecting a clinic with an established service array may be efficient. Within the context of such a clinic, selecting a specific protocol may fruitfully guide delivery and quality assurance. In the context of failure to make progress with a selected protocol, recommending or selecting common elements may help enhance treatment while remaining grounded in evidence.

Treatment Implementation

Selecting a good treatment is not the same as doing a treatment well. The litmus test for treatment implementation is whether an independent observer reviewing a session can detect the occurrence of the evidence-based activities (Fixsen et al. 2005). Thus, a treatment protocol or practice needs to translate into specific clinician behaviors. Clinicians must have the capacity to perform the behaviors (e.g., knowledge, materials, tools) and the discipline to execute the behaviors in each session. How does a single person or group of individuals motivated to use EBPs move toward that goal?

Establishing a readily accessible library of relevant treatment materials is a cornerstone of EBP infrastructure. In addition to material access, clinicians must become knowledgeable about the content of treatment protocols and implement that knowledge during the treatment session. Knowledge may be developed by reading materials and searching the Internet as well as attending training and role-playing treatment practices. For example, a Web site applicable to youth exposed to trauma (http://tfcbt.musc.edu/) includes specific, step-by-step instructions for each component of therapy, printable sample scripts for introducing concepts and techniques to patients, streaming video demonstrations of the therapy procedures, and continuing education credits (MUSC 2007). Finally, recalling knowledge and applying skills within treatment sessions may be facilitated through the use of prepared materials, memory tickler systems (e.g., checklists), and on-the-job coaching.

Treatment developers have also worked to redesign treatment protocols to increase their accessibility and adaptability within treatment sessions. For example, a well-studied manualized treatment for depression, the Adolescent Coping With Depression course, provides a curriculum and detailed specification for each treatment session and is available in the public domain (Lewinsohn et al. 1990). Another approach, core components, was developed to increase clinician knowledge about the content of treatment protocols and to support EBP implementation by promoting learning of reusable practices (Chorpita and Daleiden 2009). Using modular design techniques, a modern manual for treatment of multiple common problems (anxiety, depression, trauma, conduct) using a single system brings the core components of empirically supported treatments into busy clinics in a feasible way, including reproducible handouts, records, and worksheets as well as online learning (Chorpita and Weisz 2009). These new resources make many more EBPs feasible in most settings. These include Internet-based continuing education with streaming videos (the Medical University of South Carolina, or the MUSC Web site cited in the previous paragraph), Internet-based sophisticated workbooks for depressed adolescents available at no cost (http://www.kpchr.org/research/public/acwd/acwd.html), and a focus on core components rather than lengthy full-scale manuals (Chorpita and Weisz 2009).

Patients' gains reinforce initial efforts to learn EBPs. In one example, acceptance of trauma-focused CBT increased over time as clinicians and supervisors both gained experience and saw patients improve (Hoagwood et al. 2007). Parent management training (PMT) trainers report similar results: once clinicians try showing parents of youth with oppositional defiant disorder how to praise their children effectively for the "positive opposite" (i.e., desired behavior) and children begin to change, therapists become enthusiastic about PMT.

Monitoring and Supervision

Routine use of low-burden tracking of relevant symptoms and functioning is essential. Monitoring refers to the measurement and review of not only patient progress but also treatment practices, including fidelity to empirically supported practices. The resulting data can be directly used by clinicians to facilitate successful implementation. Preliminary evidence suggests that large-scale implementation of EBPs within a system of care, including monitoring of individual cases, may significantly improve youth and family outcomes (Daleiden et al. 2006). Monitoring can be done by self-report, chart review, observation, or recording of sessions to assess the type and quality of the practices implemented and adherence of actual care practices to the planned treatment.

Many research studies but few clinical systems are designed with ongoing patient monitoring and supervision of clinicians. Fixsen et al. (2005) review striking evidence that on-the-job coaching is a vital component in generalizing behavior from training and role-play sessions to actual intervention sessions. For example, direct supervision by an expert in the specific treatments being administered is ideal, but peer consultation, periodic self-review of session audiotapes or videotapes, targeted searching and reading in the context of specific clinical decisions, targeted input from lecturers at regional and national meetings, training videos, and instructional Web sites are also useful and are likely more feasible in clinical settings.

Progress monitoring is also helpful for the patient. Tracking events, cognitions, and emotions on three- or five-column charts in CBT, using sticker charts in behavioral therapy, or logging mood and energy on paper life charts or on smartphone apps all play a role analogous to the scale when dieting: they help quantify progress. Not only do these tools offer guidance about whether treatment is working, they also indirectly inform about the quality of treatment implementation. A treatment that never checks mood logs or behavior charts is no more likely to be helpful than a diet without a scale. With a little thought, many of the homework assignments and exercises in treatment can be turned into progress measures, or patient checklists can be designed to track key indicators (Weisz et al. 2011). Ideally, tools used to track progress are brief and convenient enough to be used regularly and are clearly tied to the causal model underpinning the intervention. Many rating scales and checklists also are sensitive to treatment effects and can be used intermittently as "midterm" or "final exam" outcome evaluations. There are several models for looking at clinically significant change at the individual patient level that consider both the precision of the tool (e.g., is there *reliable change* on the scale) along with normative benchmarks (Jacobson and Truax 1991). Public domain rating scales often are as sensitive to treatment effects as are much longer and expensive interviews (Youngstrom et al. 2013), making it feasible to do more outcome assessment in a range of clinical settings. Tracking methods can also help in monitoring relapse, identifying when the patient might benefit from booster sessions or early intervention to maintain gains.

Conclusion

An array of instruments, both for initial assessment and outcome tracking, as well as relevant databases in the public domain make EBP increasingly feasible for both individual clinicians and entire systems. Databases such as PubMed and PsycINFO offer abstracts, and many clinicians enjoy access to full text for at least some databases (e.g., membership in AACAP offers full text access to the *Journal of the American Academy of Child and Adolescent Psychiatry* Web site). The electronic medical record can assist in low-burden tracking of ADHD symptoms, depressive symptoms, or a simple measure of functioning, and systems can aggregate data more easily than in the past using readily available software such as Excel.

Child and adolescent psychiatry may benefit from embracing these ideas within the umbrella of error reduction, a concept widely validated in medicine and surgery and a good fit for understanding our common errors and especially errors of omission. Injecting these processes into systems is increasingly feasible but requires an understanding of the forces within the organization affecting clinician behaviors. Studies of systems reducing diagnostic errors and improving the alignment of clinicians' behavior with the best evidence and patients' values and preferences document significantly improved outcomes for youth, the ultimate goal of clinicians' work. The "loop" of valid assessment, evidence-based interventions, and monitoring outcomes creates a system of one or more clinicians capable of steadily refining their efforts, reducing their errors, and improving their results, as is becoming more common in other specialties of medicine.

Summary Points

- Evidence-based practice (EBP) is not an end in itself but rather a tool to achieve better outcomes more often and more quickly.
- Start somewhere—anywhere—but consider starting by refining assessment.
- Errors of omission are as common in psychiatry as in medicine or surgery; they are an everyday occurrence.
- Reduce errors of omission using feasible standardized instruments during the assessment process.
- Effective implementation understands organizational context, aligns the implementation with the values of high-level authority, and includes practice-based coaching and access to a relevant knowledge base: it is a social process.
- Track relevant outcomes using low-burden instruments in the public domain such as the revised Swanson, Nolan, and Pelham (SNAP-IV) questionnaire for ADHD symptoms (http://www.adhd.net/snap-iv-form.pdf), the Columbia Impairment Scale for functioning, or one of the Patient Reported Outcomes Measurement Information System (PROMIS) measures (www.nihpromis.org/patients/measures).
- Treatment integrity—delivering the treatment recommended and planned—is enhanced via treatment monitoring using observation, tapes, self-monitoring, and chart review.
- Anticipate disputes about what is evidence.
- Overly rigid and perfectionistic definitions of EBP alienate clinicians and generate a reputation for infeasibility.
- A guide to searching for evidence and essential EBP statistics is available at http://iacapap.org/wp-content/uploads/A.6-EVIDENCE-BASED-PRACTICE-072012.pdf.

References

Abikoff H, Gallagher R, Wells KC, et al: Remediating organizational functioning in children with ADHD: immediate and long-term effects from a randomized controlled trial. J Consult Clin Psychol 81(1):113–128, 2013 22889336

Achenbach TM, Rescorla LA: Manual for the ASEBA School-Age Forms and Profiles. Burlington, University of Vermont, 2001

Bruchmüller K, Margraf J, Suppiger A, et al: Popular or unpopular? Therapists' use of structured interviews and their estimation of patient acceptance. Behav Ther 42(4):634–643, 2011 22035992

Burchard JD, Bruns EJ, Burchard SN: The wraparound approach, in Community Treatment for Youth: Evidence-based Interventions for Severe Emotional and Behavioral Disorders. Edited by Burns BJ, Hoagwood K. New York, Oxford University Press, 2002, pp 69–90

Chorpita BF, Daleiden EL: Mapping evidence-based treatments for children and adolescents: application of the distillation and matching model to 615 treatments from 322 randomized trials. J Consult Clin Psychol 77(3):566–579, 2009 19485596

Chorpita BF, Daleiden EL: Structuring the collaboration of science and service in pursuit of a shared vision. J Clin Child Adolesc Psychol 43(2):323–338, 2014 23981145

Chorpita BF, Weisz JR: MATCH ADTC: Modular Approach to Therapy for Children With Anxiety, Depression, Trauma, or Conduct Problems. Satellite Beach, FL, PracticeWise, 2009

Chorpita BF, Daleiden EL, Weisz JR: Identifying and selecting the common elements of evidence based interventions: a distillation and matching model. Ment Health Serv Res 7(1):5–20, 2005 15832690

Cohen JA, Bukstein O, Walter H, et al: Practice parameter for the assessment and treatment of children and adolescents with posttraumatic stress disorder. J Am Acad Child Adolesc Psychiatry 49(4):414–430, 2010 20410735

Daleiden EL, Chorpita BF, Donkervoet C, et al: Getting better at getting them better: health outcomes and evidence-based practice within a system of care. J Am Acad Child Adolesc Psychiatry 45(6):749–756, 2006 16721326

Davis D: Does CME work? An analysis of the effect of educational activities on physician performance or health care outcomes. Int J Psychiatry Med 28(1):21–39, 1998 9617647

Dawes M, Summerskill W, Glasziou P, et al: Sicily statement on evidence-based practice. BMC Med Educ 5(1):1, 2005 15634359

Dopson S, Fitzgerald L: The active role of context, in Knowledge to Action? Evidence-Based Health Care in Context. Edited by Dopson S, Fitzgerald L. Oxford, UK, Oxford University Press, 2005, pp 79–103

Fixsen D, Naoom S, Blase K, et al: Implementation Research: A Synthesis of the Literature. Tampa, University of South Florida, 2005. Available at: http://nirn.fpg.unc.edu/sites/nirn.fpg.unc.edu/files/resources/NIRN-MonographFull-01-2005.pdf. Accessed January 2, 2006.

Gawande A: When Doctors Make Mistakes (video), 2014. Available at: http://prezi.com/ghqkhkmpmwec/when-doctors-make-mistakes-by-atul-gawande/. Accessed June 10, 2014.

Greenhalgh T, Robert G, Bate P, et al: How to Spread Good Ideas. Southampton, UK, National Co-ordinating Centre for NHS Service Delivery and Organisation R & D, 2004. Available at: http://www.cs.kent.ac.uk/people/staff/saf/share/great-missenden/reference-papers/Overviews/NHS-lit-review.pdf. Accessed March 30, 2015.

Hamilton J, Daleiden E, Dopson S: Implementing evidence-based practices for youth in an HMO: the roles of external ratings and market share. Adm Policy Ment Health 38(3):203–210, 2011 21461777

Higa-McMillan CK, Kimhan Powell CK, Daleiden E, et al: Pursuing an evidence-based culture through contextualized feedback: Aligning youth outcomes and practices. Prof Psychol Res Pr 42(2):137–144, 2011

Hoagwood KE, Vogel JM, Levitt JM, et al: Implementing an evidence-based trauma treatment in a state system after September 11: the CATS project. J Am Acad Child Adolesc Psychiatry 46(6):773–779, 2007 17513990

Jacobson NS, Truax P: Clinical significance: a statistical approach to defining meaningful change in psychotherapy research. J Consult Clin Psychol 59(1):12–19, 1991 2002127

Jenkins MM, Youngstrom EA, Washburn JJ, et al: Evidence-based strategies improve assessment of pediatric bipolar disorder by community practitioners. Prof Psychol Res Pr 42(2):121–129, 2011 21625392

Jenkins MM, Youngstrom EA, Youngstrom JK, et al: Generalizability of evidence-based assessment recommendations for pediatric bipolar disorder. Psychol Assess 24(2):269–281, 2012 22004538

Jensen AL, Weisz JR: Assessing match and mismatch between practitioner-generated and standardized interview-generated diagnoses for clinic-referred children and adolescents. J Consult Clin Psychol 70(1):158–168, 2002 11860042

Jensen-Doss A, Youngstrom EA, Youngstrom JK, et al: Predictors and moderators of agreement between clinical and research diagnoses for children and adolescents. J Consult Clin Psychol 82(6):1151–1162, 2014 24773574

Kaufman J, Birmaher B, Brent D, et al: Schedule for Affective Disorders and Schizophrenia for School-Age Children-Present and Lifetime Version (K-SADS-PL): initial reliability and validity data. J Am Acad Child Adolesc Psychiatry 36(7):980–988, 1997 9204677

Kraemer HC: Evaluating Medical Tests: Objective and Quantitative Guidelines. Newbury Park, CA, Sage, 1992

Leape LL, Brennan TA, Laird N, et al: The nature of adverse events in hospitalized patients. Results of the Harvard Medical Practice Study II. N Engl J Med 324(6):377–384, 1991 1824793

Lewinsohn P, Clarke G, Hops H, et al: Cognitive-behavioral group treatment of depression in adolescents. Behav Ther 21(4):385–401, 1990

March J, Silva S, Petrycki S, et al: Fluoxetine, cognitive-behavioral therapy, and their combination for adolescents with depression: Treatment for Adolescents With Depression Study (TADS) randomized controlled trial. JAMA 292(7):807–820, 2004 15315995

Meehl PE: Clinical Versus Statistical Prediction: A Theoretical Analysis and a Review of the Evidence. Minneapolis, University of Minnesota Press, 1954

MUSC: TF-CBT Web: A Web-Based Learning Course for Trauma-Focused Cognitive-Behavioral Therapy, 2007. Available at: http://tfcbt.musc.edu. Accessed August 9, 2007.

Pediatric OCD Treatment Study Team: Cognitive-behavior therapy, sertraline, and their combination for children and adolescents with obsessive-compulsive disorder: the Pediatric OCD Treatment Study (POTS) randomized controlled trial. JAMA 292(16):1969–1976, 2004 15507582

Rettew DC, Lynch AD, Achenbach TM, et al: Meta-analyses of agreement between diagnoses made from clinical evaluations and standardized diagnostic interviews. Int J Methods Psychiatr Res 18(3):169–184, 2009 19701924

Rogers EM, Rogers E: Diffusion of Innovations. New York, Free Press, 2003

Rounsaville BJ, Carroll KM, Onken LS: A stage model of behavioral therapies research: getting started and moving on from stage 1. Clin Psychol Sci Pract 8(2):133–142, 2001

Starr M, Chalmers I, Clarke M, et al: The origins, evolution, and future of The Cochrane Database of Systematic Reviews. Int J Technol Assess Health Care 25 (suppl 1):182–195, 2009 19534840

Straus SE, Glasziou P, Richardson WS, et al: Evidence-Based Medicine: How to Practice and Teach EBM. New York, Churchill Livingstone, 2011

Suppiger A, In-Albon T, Hendriksen S, et al: Acceptance of structured diagnostic interviews for mental disorders in clinical practice and research settings. Behav Ther 40(3):272–279, 2009 19647528

Swanson JM, Kraemer HC, Hinshaw SP, et al: Clinical relevance of the primary findings of the MTA: success rates based on severity of ADHD and ODD symptoms at the end of treatment. J Am Acad Child Adolesc Psychiatry 40(2):168–179, 2001 11211365

Walkup J, American Academy of Child and Adolescent Psychiatry: Practice parameter on the use of psychotropic medication in children and adolescents. J Am Acad Child Adolesc Psychiatry 48(9):961–973, 2009 19692857

Weisz JR, Chorpita BF, Frye A, et al: Youth Top Problems: using idiographic, consumer-guided assessment to identify treatment needs and to track change during psychotherapy. J Consult Clin Psychol 79(3):369–380, 2011 21500888

Youngstrom EA: Future directions in psychological assessment: combining evidence-based medicine innovations with psychology's historical strengths to enhance utility. J Clin Child Adolesc Psychol 42(1):139–159, 2013 23153181

Youngstrom E, Zhao J, Mankoski R, et al: Clinical significance of treatment effects with aripiprazole versus placebo in a study of manic or mixed episodes associated with pediatric bipolar I disorder. J Child Adolesc Psychopharmacol 23(2):72–79, 2013 23480324

Youngstrom EA, Choukas-Bradley S, Calhoun CD, et al: Clinical guide to the evidence-based assessment approach to diagnosis and treatment. Cogn Behav Pract 2014 Epub ahead of print

CHAPTER 25

Child Abuse and Neglect

Paramjit T. Joshi, M.D.
Lisa M. Cullins, M.D.
Cathy A. Southammakosane, M.D.

Child abuse continues to be a serious pediatric and social problem worldwide. Although earlier studies attempted to separate the impact of physical abuse from the impact of sexual abuse, contemporary research is focusing on the impact of polyvictimization, as it is the rare child who experiences only one type of abuse. It has become clear that the worst outcomes, including poor mental and physical health, are seen in children who experience a multitude of adversities. Prevention efforts, timely intervention, and fostering resiliency of abused children can help mitigate some of the long-term effects of abuse.

Definitions

In the Child Abuse Prevention, Adoption, and Family Services Act of 1988, *physical abuse* was defined as "the physical injury of a child under 18 years of age by a person who is responsible for the child's welfare, under circumstances which indicate that the child's health or welfare is harmed or threatened" (Kaplan et al. 1998). For the National Incidence Study, physical abuse was defined as a child younger than age 18 years experiencing nonaccidental injury (harm standard) or risk of injury (endangerment standard) as a result of having been hit with a hand or other object or having been kicked, shaken, thrown, burned, stabbed, or choked by a parent or parent substitute (Sedlak and Broadhurst 1996). *Child neglect* is differentiated from child abuse and refers to the failure of the responsible caretaking adults to provide adequate physical care and supervision.

Sexual abuse most commonly refers to activity on a spectrum ranging from inappropriate physical touching to sexual intercourse or rape. For decades, child sexual abuse has eluded specific definition, despite the efforts of researchers, therapists, and child advocates (Haugaard 2000). Important considerations in assessment include the wide range of normal sexual behavior and development among children and adolescents (Ryan 2000). Children may exhibit a wide range of sexual behaviors, even in circumstances where abuse may not be present (Friedrich et al. 1998). Eroticized behavior, increased sexual interest, and sexual play may result from numerous influences beyond potential abuse, including inadvertent observation of adults engaged in sexual activity, oedipal fantasies, manic or hypomanic states, or exposure to pornographic materials and television (Yates 1997). *Sexual play* generally involves mutually interested children at similar ages and developmental stages and does not involve coercion (American Academy of Pediatrics Committee on Child Abuse and Neglect 1999). *Incest* refers to the sexual abuse of children within the context of the nuclear family, generally involving sexual activity between a parent and child or among siblings.

Legal definitions of sexual abuse generally involve sexual contact between an adult and a minor child (Green 1997). If both the perpetrator and the victim are minors, abuse can be understood to have occurred if there is a significant discrepancy in age or there is coercion. Some have defined age discrepancies of 4–5 years as being more definitive for an abuse scenario, but there is not a commonly accepted age difference defining abuse of a minor by another minor.

Epidemiology

The work of Kempe et al. (1962), who first described the battered child syndrome, led to the recognition of child abuse as a major pediatric, psychiatric, and social problem. By 1965, child protective services were established throughout the United States, and laws were passed that required medical reporting and legal investigation of child abuse and neglect. However, maltreatment still appears to be significantly underreported. Parents continue to be the main perpetrators. In 2010, the Centers for Disease Control and Prevention found 4% of children suffering from neglect, 1% from sexual assault, 9% from physical abuse, and 12% from emotional abuse. The U.S. Department of Health and Human Services National Child Abuse and Neglect Data System confirmed that one in eight children suffered from some form of maltreatment (Wildeman et al. 2014). The lifetime costs of this victimization of children approximated $124 billion, attributable to lost productivity over the lifetime, health care, special education, and child welfare and criminal justice costs (Fang et al. 2012).

The number of child fatalities caused by maltreatment remains unchanged, with younger children at greatest risk, especially those under age 3 years and boys (Kaplan et al. 1999). Other risk factors include having been born to a mother under 21 years of age, having non–European American ethnicity, or being the product of multiple births. Homicides occurring during the first week of life are almost exclusively perpetrated by mothers. Mothers and fathers were equally likely to fatally injure their children ages 1 week to 13 years. However, fathers committed 63% of parent-perpetrated homicides among 13- to 15-year-olds and were responsible for 80% of those occurring in 16- to 19-year-olds (Kunz and Bahr 1996).

Some studies report that 10%–25% of girls are sexually victimized in some manner before age 18 (Fergusson et al. 1996). The most common age of initial sexual abuse is 8–11 years. Male parents or male parent figures continue to be the most common perpetrators of sexual abuse. Women are reported as abusers in a distinct minority of cases, and adolescents are reported to be the perpetrators in 20% of cases (American Academy of Pediatrics Committee on Child Abuse and Neglect 1999).

Sexual abuse of boys has been less well studied and may be even more significantly underreported and untreated. Boys seem less likely to disclose sexual abuse, generally for fear of disbelief, retribution, or social stigma and reluctance to admit vulnerability (Holmes and Slap 1998). Perpetrators of sexual abuse against boys are most likely to be male and unrelated to the victim.

Risk Factors

Most experts believe that physical and sexual abuse results from a combination of factors within both parents and children, in multiproblem families with significant instability. Significant family risk factors include parental mental illness or substance abuse, lack of social support, poverty, minority ethnicity, presence of four or more children in a family, young parental age, parental history of abuse, stressful events, and exposure to family violence (Chemtob et al. 2013). While sexual abuse is prevalent in all socioeconomic classes, physical abuse and neglect may be more common in lower socioeconomic classes. However, abusers have racial, religious, and ethnic distributions similar to those of the general population (Fergusson et al. 1996; Ryan 2000). Risk factors in the child include prematurity, intellectual disabilities, and physical handicaps (Cicchetti and Toth 1995). Children with cognitive deficits may have impaired judgment and decreased ability to verbally communicate feelings.

Perpetrators have a wide variety of character and personality pathology. Abusers have been described as passive and inadequate in most aspects of their lives; contact with children gives them feelings of power and control. Abusers may seek to "groom" victims, offering them gifts or money in order to gain their trust prior to engaging in any abusive behavior. Victimization by known perpetrators is generally more common than sexual abuse from an unknown or extrafamilial source.

Polyvictimization is more the rule than the exception; in addition to sexual and physical abuse, it includes bullying, property damage, witnessing peer or sibling victimization, and witnessing others (such as parents) being victimized. The Adverse Childhood Experiences (ACE) and National Comorbidity Replication Studies, among others, demonstrated that cumulative adversities correlate with greater risk of mental illness and suicide, substance abuse, unintended pregnancies and fetal death, risky health behaviors, medical injury and illness, and premature death (Hodges et al. 2013). Whether a child has been sexually abused versus physically abused, for example, matters less in the long term compared with the overall level of adversity and the number of victimizations experienced by the child (Leventhal 2007). Poor outcomes are more likely in individuals who have experienced greater adversity. It is not adequate to simply ask about physical or sexual abuse. Instead, the clinician needs to explore the depth of adversity that a child has experienced in order to gauge the risk of subsequent psychopathology and to identify and guide needed treatment interventions. Remarkably, many of these maltreated children grow up to be competent, nonabusive parents if they have the emo-

TABLE 25–1. Behavioral observations

The clinician needs to be sensitive to and aware of certain frequently observed behaviors that have been associated with abuse in children:

- Unusually fearful and docile, distrustful, and/or guarded
- Wary of physical contact
- On the alert for danger
- Attempts to meet parents' needs by role reversal
- Afraid to go home
- Angry reactions and delinquent behaviors
- Hypersexual behavior, self-exposing
- Artwork or play with themes of sexual activity or aggression
- Substance abuse
- Suicidality
- Fire-setting behavior
- Sleep difficulties, nightmares

tional support of a safe, nurturing adult in their lives.

Clinical Presentation

Clinicians must consider the possibility of physical abuse in every child who presents with an injury. Photographic documentation of all injuries is crucial. The clinician should obtain a careful and thorough history and complete a comprehensive physical examination, including radiological and laboratory studies, in every injured child. Indicators suggesting possible abuse include lack of a reasonable explanation for the injury; contradictory, changing, or vague history of the injury; observation of an inappropriate history for the injury; excessive or inadequate level of concern; and delay in seeking medical attention (Cheung 1999). In addition, a parent blaming an injury on a sibling, claiming that a child's injury was self-inflicted, or having unrealistic and premature expectations of the child could also be suggestive of abuse. The behavioral observations and findings on clinical examination are described in Tables 25–1, 25–2, and 25–3.

Special attention needs to be paid when examining an infant or toddler for physical abuse. In 1972, pediatric radiologist John Caffey coined the term *whiplash shaken baby syndrome* to describe a constellation of clinical findings in infants and toddlers, including retinal hemorrhages, subdural or subarachnoid hemorrhages, and little or no evidence of external cranial trauma. It was postulated that whiplash forces caused subdural hematomas by tearing cortical bridging veins. Serious injuries in infants are rarely accidental unless there is a clear explanation. Head injuries are the leading cause of traumatic childhood death and of child abuse fatalities.

Radiological documentation of skeletal injuries may be the best early evidence of alleged abuse. A skeletal survey to identify recent and old fractures is indicated in a child less than age 2 years with suspicious bruising or fractures. Such surveys are not as helpful in children older than age 5 years (American Academy of Pediatrics Committee on Child Abuse and Neglect 2001). Bone scans should be

TABLE 25–2. Medical findings after physical abuse

The physician should closely examine an injured child for suspicious physical findings suggesting abuse (Cheung 1999):

Cutaneous injuries, such as bruises or lacerations in the shape of an object or multiple bruises in areas that are difficult to injure in play (e.g., upper arms, medial thighs)

Stocking-glove distribution burns, suggesting immersion, burns on the perineum, burns in recognizable shapes (e.g., an iron), cigarette burns, and especially multiple burns in various stages of healing

Head injuries, including complex skull fractures with intracranial hemorrhage, retinal hemorrhage, bilateral ocular injury, dental injury, or traumatic hair loss with scalp hematomas

Ear injuries, including twisting injuries of the lobe and ruptured tympanic membranes

Skeletal injuries, including posterior rib fractures (especially when there are multiple fractures), multiple fractures in different stages of healing, metaphyseal fractures in long bones of infants, spiral fractures, and femur fractures in a nonambulatory child; also, radiological signs of subperiosteal hemorrhage, epiphyseal separation, periosteal shearing, and periosteal calcification

Abdominal injuries, including hepatic hematoma, laceration, or hemorrhage and duodenal hematoma or perforation

Chest injuries, such as pulmonary contusion, pneumothorax, and pleural effusion

TABLE 25–3. Medical findings of sexual abuse

Vague somatic complaints such as abdominal pain and headaches

Secondary enuresis and/or encopresis

Redness or irritation of the vulva; anogenital injuries such as lacerations, scarring, or bruising of genitalia; anal dilatation or scarring

Repeated urinary tract infections and/or hematuria

Anal fissures or blood in the stool

performed to identify subtle fractures in children younger than age 5 years. A magnetic resonance imaging (MRI) study can better identify epiphyseal separations if they are suspected from the plain films. Ultrasound may also be indicated to identify epiphyseal injury. However, thoracoabdominal trauma is best initially evaluated by computed tomographic (CT) scanning. Both MRI and CT scans can assist in determining when the injuries occurred and can also substantiate repeated injuries by documenting changes in the chemical states of hemoglobin in affected areas. In the event of suspected brain or head injury, a CT scan is the first-line imaging investigation, with its sensitivity to intraparenchymal, subarachnoid, subdural, and epidural hemorrhage and also to mass effect. Because of its relative insensitivity to subarachnoid blood and fractures, an MRI study is considered complementary to a CT scan and should ideally be obtained 2–3 days later if possible. Because MRI may fail to detect acute bleeding, its use should be delayed for 5–7 days in acutely ill children (American Academy of Pediatrics Section on Radiology 2000; Cheung 1999).

Specific findings such as a dilated, bruised, or scarred hymen or anus or perianal tearing are important findings to discern and to document appropriately (Shaw and American Academy of Child and Adolescent Psychiatry Working Group on Quality Issues 1999). The presence of sexually transmitted diseases may or may not confirm the occurrence of sexual activity or abuse. Generally, gonorrhea, genital herpes, or syphilis definitively diagnosed in a child outside of the perinatal period usually confirms the occurrence of sexual activity and possible sexual abuse. The presence of HIV, chlamydia, or anogenital condylomata acuminata should raise suspicion for sexual abuse but does not confirm the diagnosis. Pregnancy or the presence of semen confirms sexual activity. Pregnancy in an adolescent should always lead to an inquiry as to the possibility of sexual abuse.

Emergency department physicians are commonly called on to perform acute evaluations that include a physical examination, evidence collection, and crisis management. However, if the abuse has occurred in the previous 72 hours, physical examinations should be performed immediately with the goal of obtaining reliable physical evidence. It is recommended that a physician trained in conducting sexual abuse evaluations perform the examination. The examination should be done a minimum number of times by the smallest possible number of clinicians. The assessment should be done as part of a comprehensive physical examination to avoid emphasizing to the child the genital exam. Sexually abused children frequently do not have corroborating physical findings. Obtaining evidence from a physical examination is exquisitely important; if physical evidence is present, perpetrators are 2.5 times more likely to receive legal consequences (American Academy of Child and Adolescent Psychiatry 1997).

The American Academy of Pediatrics Committee on Child Abuse and Neglect (1999) has outlined comprehensive guidelines for the necessary physical examination after sexual abuse; among them are the following:

- The examination should not cause additional emotional trauma. Appropriate time must be allowed to account for the child's anxiety.
- Careful explanation of every step should precede the examination.
- Particular attention needs to be given to examination of the mouth, genitals, perineal region, anus, buttocks, and thighs.
- A supportive adult known to the child as well as a nursing chaperone should be present.
- The examination should be thorough, including developmental, growth, mental, and emotional factors as well as physical findings.
- History taking should be thorough and ideally should be obtained before the physical examination. Care should be taken not to suggest answers to questions.
- If collection of forensic samples is imperative and the child is unable to cooperate, use of sedation should be considered.
- Appropriate agency reporting and thorough documentation of findings, including the child's statements and behavior, are essential.
- The physician should offer reassurance about healing and recovery.

Diagnostic Considerations and Comorbidity

Children who are victims of abuse exhibit a variety of emotional and behavioral symptoms. Increasing evidence suggests that children who are victims of abuse have varying symptoms and sequelae, stemming from the variability in timing, duration, frequency, and specific characteristics of the abuse as well as an individual child's resilience and vulnerability to mental illness. In reviewing the psychological effects of abuse, Cicchetti and Toth (1995) noted a wide range of effects, including affective dysregulation, disruptive and aggressive behaviors, insecure and atypical attachment patterns, impaired peer relationships with either increased aggression or social withdrawal, and academic underachievement. High rates of other comorbid psychiatric disorders have been reported and include major depression, conduct disorder, oppositional defiant disorder (ODD), agoraphobia, overanxious disorder, attention-deficit/hyperactivity disorder (ADHD), and substance abuse (Kaplan et al. 1998).

McCrae et al. (2006) evaluated data on children investigated for sexual abuse from the National Survey of Child and Adolescent Well-Being, looking at not only abuse rates but also characteristics of abuse (such as penetration) and co-occurring family problems. They found that among 3- to 7-year-olds, behavioral symptoms were associated with caregiver domestic violence and mental illness. Among 8- to 11-year-olds, depressive symptoms were associated with severe abuse and multiple family problems, and posttraumatic stress was associated with chronic unresolved abuse. Characteristics of sexual abuse related to poor outcomes include longer duration, use of force, penetration, and a perpetrator who is close to or related to the child. The highest rates of symptoms other than depression were observed in children with severe sexual abuse, such as intercourse or oral sex. More girls than boys suffered from depression. African American children ages 8–11 years showed elevated behavioral symptoms regardless of socioeconomic class. This suggests that cultural views of sexual abuse may heighten shame in victims and that lower health care utilization and disparities or help-seeking differences may lead to greater psychological problems.

Impact of Abuse

Traumatic events are overwhelming and lead to disrupted brain homeostasis and a maladaptive compensatory response (Perry and Pollard 1998). Sustained stress leads to overstimulation of the hypothalamic-pituitary-adrenal (HPA) axis and subsequently to elevated cortisol levels (Bremner et al. 2003). Theoretically, all parts of the brain—cortex, limbic system, midbrain, and brainstem—may be affected, and powerful traumatic memories may be created. Altered cortical homeostasis impacts cognitive or narrative memory, altered limbic homeostasis impacts emotional memory, altered midbrain homeostasis impacts motor memory, and altered brainstem homeostasis may impact physiological-state memories (Perry and Pollard 1998).

Altered brain homeostasis overall impacts natural stress responses of hyperarousal and dissociation. Hyperarousal, or a fight-or-flight state, naturally involves activation of the sympathetic nervous system via norepinephrine-specific neurons stemming from the locus coeruleus of the midbrain. Interaction between the locus coeruleus and the HPA axis results in increased release of adrenocorticotropin and cortisol to prepare the body for defense (Perry and Pollard 1998). Arousal, startle responses, vigilance, irritability, and sleep are all affected by this activation. Abused youth exhibit impaired sleep efficiency and prolonged sleep latency. Chronic activation of the HPA axis and resulting cortisol system alteration may damage the hippocampus. Adults with posttraumatic stress disorder (PTSD) due to severe sexual or physical abuse have decreased hippocampal size, detected with MRI and positron emission tomographic scans (Bremner et al. 2003). Such findings may explain the memory impairment often present in victims of abuse. Studies of abused children have revealed hippocampal and limbic abnormalities, which may predispose these children to memory deficits and emotional dysregulation. Following the acute fear response, the brain may create a set of memories that can be rapidly triggered by reminders of the trauma. Affected children thus remain in a persistent state of fear, with hypersensitivity and emotional overreactivity. In many cases, the most adaptive response to the pain of the abuse may be to activate dissociative mechanisms involving disengagement from the external world by using primitive psychological defenses such as depersonalization, derealization, numbing, and—in extreme cases—catatonia. Dissociation may then be protective, allowing the child to psychologically survive the abuse. Over time, the defense often becomes maladaptive, emerging at inappropriate times (Perry and Pollard 1998).

Cognitive, academic, and language delays have been consistently documented in maltreated youth. Studies of preschool children report significantly lower intelligence compared with control subjects (Vondra et al. 1990). Wodarski et al. (1990) studied a group of physically abused youth and found that 60% of the neglected youth and 55% of the abused youth had repeated at least one grade, compared with 24% of the comparison group. A 3-year follow-up study of this population found that language and mathematics scores dropped in the abused group. In severely abused children, frontotemporal and anterior brain electroencephalographic abnormalities have been noted as well.

Attachment Dysregulation

A child's internal representation of his or her attachment figure(s) depends on the availability and responsiveness of the caregiver. Research has shown that the way a child thinks about his or her relationship with primary caregivers is related to the child's self-esteem, social competence, peer relationships, arousal, distress, and psychopathology. Over time, the infant develops a set of expectations about future interactions based on previous experiences and interactions with the primary caregiver (Bowlby 1982). An infant securely attaches to a mother who is sensitive to the infant's needs. Insensitive or unresponsive parenting leads to insecure attachments that have been subcategorized as anxious/avoidant, anxious/ambivalent, and disorganized attachment. Abusive parenting is associated with insecure attachments, often of the disorganized type, which in turn often lead to later psychopathology in the infant. In a review of the impact of child maltreatment on subsequent attachment patterns (Morton and Browne 1998), 11 of 13 controlled studies found that significantly more maltreated infants displayed insecure attachments. Children exposed to abusive parenting are excessively sensitized in their arousal level, emotional regulation, and behavioral reactivity and are at risk for later developing neuropsychiatric problems (Perry and Pollard 1998). Conversely, Gunnar (1998) suggests that the security of attachment between an infant and the caregiver buffers stress by downregulating the HPA axis. Compared with insecurely attached infants, 18-month-old children with secure attachments to their mothers were found to have lower cortisol levels when frightened by a clown (Nachmias et al. 1996). The work of Lyons-Ruth et al. (1990) and Beardslee et al. (1997) has shown that healthy infant-parent attachment promotes optimal development and protects against adverse outcomes.

Aggression

The most frequent outcome of abuse is aggression. At all developmental stages abused children are more likely to be aggressive (Herrenkohl et al. 1997). Pathological defense mechanisms may also play a role, including identification with the aggressor. Lewis (1996) writes that abusive experiences provide a model for violence, teach aggression through reinforcement, inflict pain, and cause central nervous system injuries associated with impulsivity, emotional lability, and impaired judgment. Furthermore, this experience creates a sense of being endangered and thus increases distrustful feelings and diminishes the child's capacity to recognize feelings and put them into words, not actions.

Substance Abuse and Self-Injurious Behavior

Children may resort to behaviors that facilitate opioid-mediated dissociation, such as rocking, head banging, and self-mutilation, with these painful stimuli activating the brain's endogenous opiates. Abused children are also more likely to develop substance abuse, likely in a self-medicating fashion. Alcohol serves to reduce anxiety, opiates trigger soothing dissociation, and stimulants activate mesolimbic dopaminergic reward areas in children deprived of true rewards in their lives (Perry and Pollard 1998).

Glassman et al. (2007) noted that emotional and sexual abuse had the strongest link to nonsuicidal self-injury (NSSI). In exploring the etiology, the authors suggest that emotional abuse may lead to a self-critical cognitive style, which in turn leads to NSSI as a form of self-punishment. Underlying depression may intensify NSSI behaviors.

Attention-Deficit/ Hyperactivity Disorder

Several studies have documented a higher prevalence of ADHD in abused children and adolescents. It is possible that children who have ADHD are more likely to provoke abusive behaviors in adults. Impulsive parents could directly transmit ADHD genetically to their children. However, it is also proposed that the trauma of abuse itself plays a causal role in the development of ADHD symptoms (Weinstein et al. 2000).

Depression and Suicide

Abused infants are prone to affective withdrawal and diminished capacity for pleasure and have a tendency to exhibit negative affect such as sadness and distress (Green 1997). Major depression or dysthymia was reported in 27% of children of latency age who had been abused (Green 1997). One study reports that approximately 8% of children and adolescents with documented abuse have a current diagnosis of major depressive disorder (MDD), 40% have lifetime MDD diagnoses, and at least 30% have lifetime disruptive disorder diagnoses (ODD or conduct disorder). These prevalence rates are several times higher than those found in community samples of children and adolescents (Kaplan et al.

1999). Depression may be a consequence of abuse or may result in a child being more vulnerable to abuse. Studies also report an association between abuse in childhood and subsequent suicidal behavior and risk taking (Kaplan et al. 1999). Furthermore, Green (1997) reported increased self-mutilation and suicidal ideation or attempts in children subjected to parental beatings or threatened by abandonment by their adult caretakers. Depression and suicidal behavior are overrepresented among adolescent inpatients with a history of sexual abuse. Further, sexually abused girls may be particularly at risk for suicide attempts, independent of other psychopathology (Bergen et al. 2003).

Danielson et al. (2005) studied differences in adolescent depression severity and symptoms on the basis of the type of abuse (e.g., sexual abuse, physical abuse, both combined) and gender. Results showed differences in depression severity and symptoms based on the type of abuse and gender. Adolescents who experienced both sexual and physical abuse were more likely to be depressed, have suicidal ideation, or have PTSD than those who experienced physical abuse only or those who did not experience any abuse at all. Longer duration of abuse was related to greater depression severity, sleep disturbances, and greater anxiety. Consistent with prior research, greater guilt was experienced by those who were abused by a relative. Such youth also endorsed more problems with appetite and thoughts of death, which may be related to underlying hopelessness and anger in children abused by a relative. Finally, female adolescents were more depressed than males. A prospective study of depression in abused and neglected children grown up found that abuse and neglect were associated with increased risk for MDD in adulthood (Widom et al. 2007). Children who were physically abused or experienced multiple types of abuse were at increased risk of lifetime major depression, whereas neglect increased risk for current major depression. Surprisingly, childhood sexual abuse was not associated with increased risk of major depression. Significantly more of the abused and neglected children who met criteria for major depression in adulthood also met the criteria for at least one other lifetime diagnosis, including PTSD, substance use disorder, antisocial personality disorder, and dysthymia.

The authors urge clinicians to explore for underlying abuse histories in patients with mood disorders, given the clear link between trauma and the later development of depression and that any form of child maltreatment correlates with higher rates of suicidal ideation and attempts (Miller et al. 2013). Such an assessment is imperative, as it may lead to the identification of a child currently in an abusive environment and/or a child who is at high risk for self-harm and suicidality.

Dissociative and Psychotic Disorders

Dissociative disorders may result from abuse. Children who dissociate may experience brief psychotic symptoms such as hearing command auditory hallucinations. Severely abused children commonly hear voices commanding them to harm themselves or others. As a result, they may be misdiagnosed with a psychotic disorder such as schizophrenia. A dissociating child may also be misdiagnosed with an externalizing disorder—ADHD, ODD, or impulse control disorder. A study of a group of severely abused youngsters in residential treatment facilities found that 23% of the boys met criteria for dissociative identity disorder (Yeager and Lewis 2000). Dissociative disorders are difficult to discern in younger children, especially prior to age 7 when faculties of concrete reasoning are less well developed. Dissociation may be present in victims of sexual abuse more often than in victims of physical abuse. Some children may have dissociative experiences as defense mechanisms or as a manner of reexperiencing or gaining understanding and mastery over the abusive experience.

Literature and clinical experience support an association between child maltreatment and psychosis (Dvir et al. 2013). One study involving young people who were deemed clinically high risk for psychosis found greater trauma history in these subjects relative to controls. These individuals also endorsed greater levels of depression and anxiety (Addington et al. 2013). It remains to be elucidated exactly how maltreatment and psychosis are related; however, it is feasible that bidirectional influence and epigenetics may underlie this association.

Anxiety Disorders and Posttraumatic Stress Disorder

Anxiety disorders may take many forms, including phobias, social anxiety, generalized anxiety disorder, and PTSD. Symptoms of PTSD include fear reactions, reexperiencing phenomena, flashbacks, sleep disruption, exaggerated startle response, and hyperacuity, as well as general anxiety and deterioration of functioning. The chronicity and severity of abuse increase the likelihood of a PTSD diagnosis. Children often display disorganized or agitated behavior rather than the fear, helplessness, and horror described in adults. Repetitive play involving themes of the trauma is common rather than the classic flashbacks or recurrent and intrusive recollections of the trauma.

In her review of trauma leading to PTSD, Terr (1996) wrote that traumatic events, including physical abuse, cause psychic trauma when the child understands that something terrible is happening and that he or she is in danger, senses his or her own helplessness, and registers and stores an implicit or explicit traumatic memory. Soon after a traumatic event, play can be "grim, monotonous, and at times, dangerous." The child often does not make a connection between the play and the trauma. Terr cites protective factors, including intelligence, humor, and relatedness. Only later does the clinician see more clearly intrusive thoughts, fears, and repeated dreams. A foreshortened sense of the future is common in abused children and can lead to reckless risk taking. Unconscious reenactment of the trauma can lead to retraumatization of the child. In some cases, this reenactment can be dangerous to the child or to others. Pelcovitz et al. (1994) studied the prevalence of PTSD in physically abused adolescents and found that these youth may be more at risk for behavioral, emotional, and social difficulties than for clear PTSD. This is in contrast to the previous work of Green (1997), who found that physically abused adolescents were at risk for developing PTSD. Pelcovitz et al. (1994) suggested that physically abused adolescents may "enact" their victimization rather than express their reactions to the abuse via symptoms of PTSD. The authors point out the differences between physical and sexual assaults, with sexual abuse often accompanied by a higher level of secrecy and shame, which may reinforce emergent PTSD symptoms. External signs of physical abuse, such as bruises and fractures, may lead to more support, facilitating integration of the trauma. Pelcovitz et al. add that an alternative possibility is that the physically abused youth in their study did not manifest PTSD symptoms because they remained in an abusive environment. There may be a delay in the onset of PTSD symptoms until after the trauma has ended.

Multiple Somatic Health Problems

An association has been found between childhood abuse and adult health problems, including poor self-rated health, pain, physical disabilities, and frequent emergency department and health professional visits (Springer et al. 2007). Sexual risk taking leads to increased teenage pregnancy and exposure to HIV and other sexually transmitted diseases (Kaplan et al. 1999).

Prevention

The Centers for Disease Control and Prevention developed important summary recommendations to raise awareness and improve efforts for primary prevention (McMahon and Puett 1999). Primary prevention includes educating children about "bad touch" and empowering them to resist abusers. School-based primary prevention programs have been shown to be effective in raising awareness, particularly when used over the long term and with older as well as younger children (Hébert et al. 2001). Efforts have also included providing outreach to adults who are abusers or victims themselves.

The cornerstone of treatment of children who are victims of abuse is first to make certain that the child is protected and safe from further injury and abuse. Making a report to child protective services needs to occur as soon as possible, preferably in the context of the initial evaluation or first disclosure. Kaplan et al. (1998) review three types of child abuse primary prevention strategies: 1) competency enhancement with parent education programs; 2) media campaigns, hotlines, and parent socialization programs; and 3) targeting of high-risk groups, such as single parents and teenage parents, parents of low socioeconomic status, and parents with neurocognitively compromised children. Research has shown that maltreated children with healthier ego resiliency, ego overcontrol, and higher self-esteem fared better in their overall adjustment (Glaser 2000). A focus of treatment should therefore be helping abused youth gain better control over their urges and actions and better self-awareness, ultimately creating a coherent narrative of their life story. This is a complex undertaking, due in part to the likelihood that ego control and ego resilience are in part temperamentally determined and that self-esteem is influenced by nurturance (Glaser 2000). Because brain development is related to environmental forces, intense and early intervention offers the greatest hope for healthier outcomes.

Leventhal (2001) described two home-based models for preventing child abuse and neglect. Both models focus on high-risk families. The Healthy Families model uses the Kempe Family Stress Inventory to identify high-risk families, covering areas such as parental history of abuse, violence, substance abuse, mental illness, or criminal acts. In the Olds model, first-time mothers are eligible if they have two of the following characteristics: 1) they have fewer than 12 years of education, 2) they are unmarried, or 3) they are of low socioeconomic status. Research on the effectiveness of these two models has shown that there is a resulting stronger alliance with the parents and that the effects are sustained over many years. However, when high levels of domestic violence are present, it is difficult for parents to improve their parenting by the use of home visits.

Lyons-Ruth et al. (1990) examined attachment patterns among infants at social risk, measuring development, mother-infant interaction, and maternal depression and social contacts while also evaluating the efficacy of home visits in improving the security of a child's attachment to the caregiver. The home-visiting service had four goals:

1. Provide an accepting relationship
2. Increase the family's competence in accessing resources
3. Model and reinforce more interactive, positive, and developmentally appropriate exchanges between mother and infant, emphasizing the mother's dual role as teacher and source of emotional security for her infant
4. Decrease social isolation with a weekly parenting group or a monthly social hour using psychodynamic and behavioral interventions

At age 18 months, infants of depressed mothers who received home-visiting services scored a mean of 10 points higher on the Bayley Mental Development Index than unserved infants of depressed mothers. They were also twice as likely to be classified as securely attached in their relationships with their mothers. Because a secure attachment has been associated with lower risk of abuse, this could be a powerful intervention to decrease the risk of physical maltreatment.

Triple P (Positive Parenting Program) is an evidence-based system with multiple layers of intervention focusing on parent management skills; interventions range from a broad public health, media communication aspect to group parenting didactic sessions to individualized support by a trained professional. Triple P demonstrated decreased rates of child maltreatment (Prinz et al. 2009).

McCrae et al. (2006) suggest that rather than a one-size-fits-all intervention, treatment should be tailored according to the overall level of adversity experienced by the child, avoiding assumptions that all children with a certain type of abuse need a certain type of treatment. Services need to be anchored in a comprehensive understanding of the individual child's life experience, his or her current needs, and an understanding of the impact of the trauma on the child.

Child and Parent Treatment

The major goals of treatment are first to protect the child and strengthen the family and then to address the impact of past abuse in treatment of the child and the family. The ecological model calls for a focus on the multidimensional aspects of child abuse rather than just on the abusive parent. Attachment theory has emphasized the interactive aspects of maltreatment and the importance of intervening in changing the parent-child relationship, with the hope of facilitating a more secure attachment between child and parent. Therapeutic techniques vary depending on the developmental level of the child. Treatment of ensuing psychiatric disorders such as major depression and PTSD should be done promptly and should involve consultation with a child and adolescent psychiatrist. In any abuse-specific therapy, it is important to consider the notion of retraumatization. Therapists must be exceedingly sensitive to issues of resistance and the pace necessary for successful treatment. Many victims may not directly confront the realities of their abuse but instead may benefit sufficiently from a problem-oriented or supportive approach. Despite this fact, it is prudent for the therapist early on to make clear the reason for the initiation of the therapy and to point out behavior patterns that may be maladaptive as a result.

Family-based therapy needs to improve the parent's devalued self-image, reverse distortions of his or her child that can lead to scapegoating, interpret any links between the current abuse and the parent's own abuse history, and provide the parent with a positive model of raising children. Green (1997) suggests using therapeutic nurseries to treat infants and pathological parent-child interactions, with dyadic parent-child therapy serving as the foundation of treatment. Psychotherapy of the child should include creating a therapeutic environment, in either individual or group settings, that allows the child to master the trauma, in part through controlled repetitions of the event using symbolic reenactments with dolls, puppets, drawings, or other expressive media.

The child must be told that the abuse is not his or her fault and that he or she is not to blame. Terr (1996) reminds clinicians of the need to explore issues of betrayal, overexcitement, and personal responsibility, especially in children who have been abused within their own families. Play therapy may be useful in the treatment of a traumatized young child (Terr 1996). Play and drawing allow for safe displacement of the complex thoughts and feelings stemming from the abuse and help the child to use nonverbal and symbolic expressions of events that are too painful to be expressed in words. A goal of therapy should be helping the child use healthier coping responses. (See also Chapter 16, "Posttraumatic Stress Disorder and Persistent Complex Bereavement Disorder.")

Clinicians should be sensitive to the consequences that may ensue following the results of abuse disclosure and should not make impossible promises regarding reporting events to the appropriate authorities. Adolescent girls may be more resistant to discussing certain topics of abuse with a male counselor. Individual cases merit specific consideration in terms of the mode, duration, and frequency of therapy; flexibility on the part of the therapist is essential. The overall goals of treatment have to be clearly focused on behavioral and functional issues that need improvement.

Group therapy may benefit older adolescents who have relatively positive self-esteem. It is crucial that a safe space is created before group or individual therapy begins. This population can be easily retraumatized by overzealous therapists who neglect first building a trusting and safe alliance with the patient. Ideal candidates for group therapy have emotional and cognitive capacities to benefit from the experience and not to impair the treatment of others. Specific activities, including role-playing and games to improve communication skills, can be effective in group settings (Celano et al. 1996). Before recommending group treatment, the clinician should consider any pending legal proceedings involving the patient. It may be inadvisable to involve a victim in group treatment before the individual is to give legal testimony because the information may be rejected or perceived as having been contaminated by suggestion from others.

Family therapy or individual therapy for parents is often necessary to assist caregivers in coming to terms with their own responses to the child's victimization. Nonoffending parents often have issues of guilt or depression regarding the fact that they were unable to prevent the child's victimization. Treatment that includes individual therapy for nonoffending parents can improve the psychosocial functioning of the abused child (Celano et al. 1996). Furthermore, a parent's own issues of childhood sexual abuse may emerge and may ultimately be disclosed coincidentally with the child's treatment. Family therapy can help to establish appropriate boundaries and roles for family members and can help avoid scapegoating the victim (Hilton and Mezey 1996).

Cognitive-behavioral therapy has been shown to be superior to supportive counseling in a 12-month follow-up study (Cohen et al. 2004). Randomized controlled trials show that trauma-focused cognitive-behavioral therapy (TF-CBT) improves not only PTSD symptoms but also the attributions of abuse, shame, depression, and other behavior problems. TF-CBT has also been found to be superior to comparison and control conditions in improving comorbid depression, anxiety, and externalizing symptoms (Cohen et al. 2004).

Medications may improve the outcome of abused children, especially if they are manifesting symptoms of PTSD (see Chapter 16). However, in childhood PTSD adding sertraline to TF-CBT did not yield additional benefit (Cohen et al. 2007). For most children with PTSD, including those with major depressive disorder, a trial of initial TF-CBT or other trauma-focused psychotherapy alone is warranted before adding medication. According to anecdotal reports (Kaplan et al. 1999; Terr 1991), propranolol decreased hyperarousal and hypervigilance in abused children. Clonidine has also helped to reduce symptoms of hyperarousal, aggression, and insomnia in abused preschool children with PTSD (Harmon and Riggs 1996). Guanfacine was found to help alleviate sleep disturbances in patients with PTSD (Leonard 1999).

Positive outcomes can be enhanced with rapid, early, and effective psychotherapeutic interventions, and positive outcomes are possible despite egregious abuse scenarios. Prognosis after abuse depends on many factors, including familial, demographic, and treatment characteristics. A degree of stability within the family plays an important role. In general, parent support and involvement in treatment with the affected child yield a significantly better outcome.

Resilience

Heller et al. (1999) reviewed the literature on resilience to the effects of child maltreatment. Dispositional or temperamental attributes of the child include above-average intelligence, high self-esteem, internal locus of control, external attribution of blame, presence of spirituality, ego resilience, and high ego control. Familial cohesion, including competent foster care, has been related to developing resilience in children. Extrafamilial support such as a positive school experience promotes resilience, which in turn likely increases individual self-worth and a sense of control over one's destiny. Rutter (1990) has argued that the field must move beyond focusing on single resilience factors to considering the developmental processes that promote adaptive functioning. Rutter has also suggested that resilience is probably not a fixed state but is rather a malleable and organic trait that can be enhanced with a nurturing environment; resilience may buffer the impact of abuse and promote a positive sense of one's worth.

The ecological model of recovery involves integrating affects and cognitions related to the trauma within a coherent and continuous sense of self, a particularly key task for adolescent identity formation. After a sense of safety and security is established, the next crucial step is to develop improved self-esteem and a safe attachment with an adult. It is postulated that this promotes the integration of trauma-related memories, affects, and cognitions within a coherent sense of self and then leads to the active establishment of healthy interpersonal relationships where abusive experiences can be renegotiated. Daigneault et al. (2007) suggest that this path likely leads to resilience in certain adolescents.

Furthermore, Daigneault et al. (2007) studied four factors that could predict resilience: interpersonal trust, maternal conflicts, family violence, and out-of-home placements. Interpersonal trust emerged as the most predictive of resilience. Similarly, Masten (2011) proposed a framework fostering resilience: using a strengths-based approach, promoting competence, establishing positive goals, reducing conditions that threaten function and development and enhancing factors that foster adaptations, tailoring interventions to developmental level, and collaborating in a multidisciplinary fashion. Clinicians treating such youth need to develop a trusting relationship and promote a sense of empowerment and self-efficacy. Traumatized individuals often reexperience feelings of powerlessness within their psychotherapy, and on the basis of this research, providing a degree of control and power over treatment is important, after a safe space has been created in the therapy, in order to promote underlying resilience.

Legal Considerations

Legal considerations are important in the initial stages of evaluation. Physicians and mental health clinicians are mandated by all 50 states to report suspected cases of child physical and sexual abuse. The specific requirements in terms of timing, level of suspicion, and other details vary according to state guidelines. Most important is prompt referral to a child protective services organization to ensure appropriate collection and validation of forensic information.

The forensic evaluation should be performed by a clinician who is trained in forensic assessment; this individual should not be the physician or therapist who is involved in ongoing treatment (Yuille et al. 1993). Confidentiality issues must be clarified before a forensic evaluation. The fact that an evaluation is being done for purposes of court proceedings needs to be made clear to the parents and child from the outset. Treating clinicians should document direct statements of disclosure in the medical record, preferably as quotations. Depending on specific legal circumstances, such information may obviate the need for direct testimony from the child victim. Guidelines for forensic evaluation of children have been published by the American Academy of Child and Adolescent Psychiatry (Kraus et al. 2011) and by the American Professional Society on the Abuse of Children (1990).

Summary Points

- Child abuse and neglect continue to be serious problems worldwide, with estimates of prevalence up to 20% or higher.
- Family structure, child mental or physical illness, caregiver psychopathology, and disadvantaged environments are key risk factors for abuse.
- Multiple instances of abuse or polyvictimization are more common than previously thought and may be more associated with subsequent impaired function.
- Evaluation of abused children must include thorough physical examination, appropriate documentation, and exclusion of other potential causes of injury.
- Child sexual abuse is linked to future high-risk sexual behaviors.
- The most frequent behavioral outcome of child abuse is dysregulated aggression.
- Childhood abuse is linked to adult health problems, including frequent emergency department and health professional visits.
- Treatment focus should include protecting the child, strengthening the family, and understanding the impact of the trauma on the child.
- Treatment approaches that capitalize on individual strengths and improve interpersonal trust are the most predictive of resilience and improved outcome following abuse.

References

Addington J, Stowkowy J, Cadenhead KS, et al: Early traumatic experiences in those at clinical high risk for psychosis. Early Interv Psychiatry 7(3):300–305, 2013 23343384

American Academy of Child and Adolescent Psychiatry: Practice parameters for the forensic evaluation of children and adolescents who may have been physically or sexually abused. J Am Acad Child Psychiatry 36(3):423–442, 1997 9055524

American Academy of Pediatrics Committee on Child Abuse and Neglect: Guidelines for the evaluation of sexual abuse of children: subject review. Pediatrics 103(1):186–191, 1999 9917463

American Academy of Pediatrics Committee on Child Abuse and Neglect: Shaken baby syndrome: rotational cranial injuries-technical report. Pediatrics 108(1):206–210, 2001 11433079

American Academy of Pediatrics Section on Radiology: Diagnostic imaging of child abuse. Pediatrics 105(6):1345–1348, 2000 10835079

American Professional Society on the Abuse of Children: Guidelines for Psychosocial Evaluation of Suspected Sexual Abuse in Young Children. Chicago, IL, American Professional Society on the Abuse of Children, 1990

Beardslee WR, Salt P, Versage EM, et al: Sustained change in parents receiving preventive interventions for families with depression. Am J Psychiatry 154(4):510–515, 1997 9090338

Bergen HA, Martin G, Richardson AS, et al: Sexual abuse and suicidal behavior: a model constructed from a large community sample of adolescents. J Am Acad Child Adolesc Psychiatry 42(11):1301–1309, 2003 14566167

Bowlby J: Attachment and Loss, Vol I: Attachment, 2nd Edition. London, Hogarth, 1982

Bremner JD, Vythilingam M, Vermetten E, et al: MRI and PET study of deficits in hippocampal structure and function in women with childhood sexual abuse and posttraumatic stress disorder. Am J Psychiatry 160(5):924–932, 2003 12727697

Celano M, Hazzard A, Webb C, et al: Treatment of traumagenic beliefs among sexually abused girls and their mothers: an evaluation study. J Abnorm Child Psychol 24(1):1–17, 1996 8833025

Chemtob CM, Gudiño OG, Laraque D: Maternal posttraumatic stress disorder and depression in pediatric primary care: association with child maltreatment and frequency of child exposure to traumatic events. JAMA Pediatr 167(11):1011–1018, 2013 23999612

Cheung KK: Identifying and documenting findings of physical child abuse and neglect. J Pediatr Health Care 13(3 Pt 1):142–143, 1999 10531908

Cicchetti D, Toth SL: A developmental psychopathology perspective on child abuse and neglect. J Am Acad Child Adolesc Psychiatry 34(5):541–565, 1995 7775351

Cohen JA, Deblinger E, Mannarino AP, et al: A multisite, randomized controlled trial for children with sexual abuse-related PTSD symptoms. J Am Acad Child Adolesc Psychiatry 43(4):393–402, 2004 15187799

Cohen JA, Mannarino AP, Perel JM, et al: A pilot randomized controlled trial of combined trauma-focused CBT and sertraline for childhood PTSD symptoms. J Am Acad Child Adolesc Psychiatry 46(7):811–819, 2007 17581445

Daigneault I, Hébert M, Tourigny M: Personal and interpersonal characteristics related to resilient developmental pathways of sexually abused adolescents. Child Adolesc Psychiatr Clin N Am 16(2):415–434, x, 2007 17349516

Danielson CK, de Arellano MA, Kilpatrick DG, et al: Child maltreatment in depressed adolescents: differences in symptomatology based on history of abuse. Child Maltreat 10(1):37–48, 2005 15611325

Dvir Y, Denietolis B, Frazier JA: Childhood trauma and psychosis. Child Adolesc Psychiatr Clin N Am 22(4):629–641, 2013 24012077

Fang X, Brown DS, Florence CS, et al: The economic burden of child maltreatment in the United States and implications for prevention. Child Abuse Negl 36(2):156–165, 2012 22300910

Fergusson DM, Horwood LJ, Lynskey MT: Childhood sexual abuse and psychiatric disorder in young adulthood: II. Psychiatric outcomes of childhood sexual abuse. J Am Acad Child Adolesc Psychiatry 35(10):1365–1374, 1996 8885591

Friedrich WN, Fisher J, Broughton D, et al: Normative sexual behavior in children: a contemporary sample. Pediatrics 101(4):E9, 1998 9521975

Glaser D: Child abuse and neglect and the brain—a review. J Child Psychol Psychiatry 41(1):97–116, 2000 10763678

Glassman LH, Weierich MR, Hooley JM, et al: Child maltreatment, non-suicidal self-injury, and the mediating role of self-criticism. Behav Res Ther 45(10):2483–2490, 2007 17531192

Green AH: Physical abuse of children, in Textbook of Child and Adolescent Psychiatry, 2nd Edition. Edited by Weiner JM. Washington, DC, American Psychiatric Press, 1997, pp 687–697

Gunnar MR: Quality of early care and buffering of neuroendocrine stress reactions: potential effects on the developing human brain. Prev Med 27(2):208–211, 1998 9578997

Harmon RJ, Riggs PD: Clonidine for posttraumatic stress disorder in preschool children. J Am Acad Child Adolesc Psychiatry 35(9):1247–1249, 1996 8824068

Haugaard JJ: The challenge of defining child sexual abuse. Am Psychol 55(9):1036–1039, 2000 11036706

Hébert M, Lavoie F, Piché C, et al: Proximate effects of a child sexual abuse prevention program in elementary school children. Child Abuse Negl 25(4):505–522, 2001 11370723

Heller SS, Larrieu JA, D'Imperio R, et al: Research on resilience to child maltreatment: empirical considerations. Child Abuse Negl 23(4):321–338, 1999 10321770

Herrenkohl RC, Egolf BP, Herrenkohl EC: Preschool antecedents of adolescent assaultive behavior: a longitudinal study. Am J Orthopsychiatry 67(3):422–432, 1997 9250343

Hilton MR, Mezey GC: Victims and perpetrators of child sexual abuse. Br J Psychiatry 169(4):408–415, 1996 8894189

Hodges M, Godbout N, Briere J, et al: Cumulative trauma and symptom complexity in children: a path analysis. Child Abuse Negl 37(11):891–898, 2013 23643387

Holmes WC, Slap GB: Sexual abuse of boys: definition, prevalence, correlates, sequelae, and management. JAMA 280(21):1855–1862, 1998 9846781

Kaplan SJ, Pelcovitz D, Salzinger S, et al: Adolescent physical abuse: risk for adolescent psychiatric disorders. Am J Psychiatry 155(7):954–959, 1998 9659863

Kaplan SJ, Pelcovitz D, Labruna V: Child and adolescent abuse and neglect research: a review of the past 10 years. Part I: Physical and emotional abuse and neglect. J Am Acad Child Adolesc Psychiatry 38(10):1214–1222, 1999 10517053

Kempe CH, Silverman FN, Steele BF, et al: The battered-child syndrome. JAMA 181:17–24, 1962 14455086

Kraus LJ, Thomas CR, Bukstein OG, et al: Practice parameters for the forensic evaluation of children and adolescents who may have been physically or sexually abused. J Am Acad Child Adolesc Psychiatry 50:1299–1312, 2011 22115153

Kunz J, Bahr SJ: A profile of parental homicide against children. J Fam Violence 11(4):347–362, 1996

Leonard H: Guanfacine alleviates sleep disorders in boys with PTSD. Brown Univ Child Adolesc Psychopharmacol Update (October):1, 1999

Leventhal JM: The prevention of child abuse and neglect: successfully out of the blocks. Child Abuse Negl 25(4):431–439, 2001 11370718

Leventhal JM: Children's experiences of violence: some have much more than others. Child Abuse Negl 31(1):3–6, 2007 17212970

Lewis DO: Development of the symptom of violence, in Child and Adolescent Psychiatry: A Comprehensive Textbook, 2nd Edition. Edited by Lewis M. Baltimore, MD, Williams and Wilkins, 1996, pp 334–344

Lyons-Ruth K, Connell DB, Grunebaum HU, et al: Infants at social risk: maternal depression and family support services as mediators of infant development and security of attachment. Child Dev 61(1):85–98, 1990 2307048

Masten AS: Resilience in children threatened by extreme adversity: frameworks for research, practice, and translational synergy. Dev Psychopathol 23(2):493–506, 2011 23786691

McCrae JS, Chapman MV, Christ SL: Profile of children investigated for sexual abuse: association with psychopathology symptoms and services. Am J Orthopsychiatry 76(4):468–481, 2006 17209715

McMahon PM, Puett RC: Child sexual abuse as a public health issue: recommendations of an expert panel. Sex Abuse 11(4):257–266, 1999 10597642

Miller AB, Esposito-Smythers C, Weismoore JT, et al: The relation between child maltreatment and adolescent suicidal behavior: a systematic review and critical examination of the literature. Clin Child Fam Psychol Rev 16(2):146–172, 2013 23568617

Morton N, Browne KD: Theory and observation of attachment and its relation to child maltreatment: a review. Child Abuse Negl 22(11):1093–1104, 1998 9827314

Nachmias M, Gunnar M, Mangelsdorf S, et al: Behavioral inhibition and stress reactivity: the moderating role of attachment security. Child Dev 67(2):508–522, 1996 8625725

Pelcovitz D, Kaplan S, Goldenberg B, et al: Post-traumatic stress disorder in physically abused adolescents. J Am Acad Child Adolesc Psychiatry 33(3):305–312, 1994 8169174

Perry BD, Pollard R: Homeostasis, stress, trauma, and adaptation. A neurodevelopmental view of childhood trauma. Child Adolesc Psychiatr Clin N Am 7(1):33–51, viii, 1998 9894078

Prinz RJ, Sanders MR, Shapiro CJ, et al: Population-based prevention of child maltreatment: the U.S. Triple p system population trial. Prev Sci 10(1):1–12, 2009 19160053

Rutter M: Psychosocial resilience and protective mechanisms, in Risk and Protective Factors in the Development of Psychopathology. Edited by Rolf J, Masten AS, Cicchetti K, et al. New York, Cambridge University Press, 1990, pp 181–214

Ryan G: Childhood sexuality: a decade of study. Part I—research and curriculum development. Child Abuse Negl 24(1):33–48, 2000 10660008

Sedlak AJ, Broadhurst DD: The Third National Incidence Study of Child Abuse and Neglect. Washington, DC, U.S. Department of Health and Human Services, 1996

Shaw JA, American Academy of Child and Adolescent Psychiatry Working Group on Quality Issues: Practice parameters for the assessment and treatment of children and adolescents who are sexually abusive of others. J Am Acad Child Adolesc Psychiatry 38(12 suppl):55S–76S, 1999 10624085

Springer KW, Sheridan J, Kuo D, et al: Long-term physical and mental health consequences of childhood physical abuse: results from a large population-based sample of men and women. Child Abuse Negl 31(5):517–530, 2007 17532465

Terr LC: Childhood traumas: an outline and overview. Am J Psychiatry 148(1):10–20, 1991 1824611

Terr LC: Acute responses to external events and posttraumatic stress disorder, in Child and Adolescent Psychiatry: A Comprehensive Textbook, 2nd Edition. Edited by Lewis M. Baltimore, MD, Williams and Wilkins, 1996

Vondra JI, Barnett D, Cicchetti D: Self-concept, motivation, and competence among preschoolers from maltreating and comparison families. Child Abuse Negl 14(4):525–540, 1990 2289183

Weinstein D, Staffelbach D, Biaggio M: Attention-deficit hyperactivity disorder and posttraumatic stress disorder: differential diagnosis in childhood sexual abuse. Clin Psychol Rev 20(3):359–378, 2000 10779899

Widom CS, DuMont K, Czaja SJ: A prospective investigation of major depressive disorder and comorbidity in abused and neglected children grown up. Arch Gen Psychiatry 64(1):49–56, 2007 17199054

Wildeman C, Emanuel N, Leventhal JM, et al: The prevalence of confirmed maltreatment among US children, 2004–2011. JAMA Pediatr 168(8):706–713, 2014

Wodarski JS, Kurtz PD, Gaudin JM Jr, et al: Maltreatment and the school-age child: major academic, socioemotional, and adaptive outcomes. Soc Work 35(6):506–513, 1990 2284600

Yates A: Sexual abuse of children, in Textbook of Child and Adolescent Psychiatry, 2nd Edition. Edited by Wiener JM. Washington, DC, American Psychiatric Press, 1997, pp 699–709

Yeager CA, Lewis DO: Mental illness, neuropsychologic deficits, child abuse, and violence. Child Adolesc Psychiatr Clin N Am 9(4):793–813, 2000 11005007

Yuille JC, Hunter R, Joffe R, et al: Interviewing children in sexual abuse cases, in Child Witnesses: Understanding and Improving Testimony. Edited by Goodman GS, Bottoms BL. New York, Guilford, 1993, pp 95–115

CHAPTER 26

Cultural and Religious Issues

Mary Lynn Dell, M.D., D.Min.

North America is experiencing unparalleled changes in the ethnicities and backgrounds that residents claim as their primary identities. Racial groups officially recognized by the 2010 U.S. Census included white, black or African American, American Indian or Alaska Native, Asian, Native Hawaiian or other Pacific Islander, and other. Of 308,745,538 individuals counted in 2010, 72% (223.6 million) declared themselves to be white, 13% (38.9 million) black, 5% (14.7 million) Asian, 0.9% (2.9 million) American Indian or Alaska Native, and 0.2% (0.5 million) Native Hawaiian or other Pacific Islander. The U.S. population grew by 9.7% (29.3 million) between 2000 and 2010, with the percentage of the majority white population declining relative to increasing percentages of minority groups. After 2025, international migration, not the number of births and deaths, is anticipated to be the most significant factor in U.S. population growth, yielding a more diverse and younger population. Especially relevant to child and adolescent mental health is the fact that by 2020 the majority of the population under age 18 is projected to be from nonwhite, minority racial groups (U.S. Census Bureau 2011, 2013, 2014). A substantial and growing percentage of children and families, whether permanent residents or transients, live in a home with a family of origin culture surrounded by a variety of other U.S. cultural influences. This array of cultural, ethnic, and religious diversity and its implications for patient care require special attention and cultural competence from child and adolescent mental health care providers.

History of Cultural Psychiatry and Key Definitions

The roots of cultural psychiatry are in eighteenth-century observations that immigrant groups from Europe presented different types of emotional problems than those born and living in the continental United States. By the late nineteenth and early twentieth centuries, clinical case reports detailed unusual symptom patterns in numerous minority, indigenous, and tribal groups from around the world. Emil Kraepelin, father of comparative psychiatry, described differences he observed in non-Western societies in the late 1800s. Beginning with Sigmund Freud and continuing with Jung, Adler, and Horney, psychoanalysts highlighted the importance of cultural factors in neuroses and psychotherapy. By the mid-twentieth century, anthropologists, social workers, psychologists, and even theologians shared an overlapping interest in culture and mental health. Academic psychiatry departments on both U.S. coasts and in Hawaii led the way in research, writing, and training. The American Psychiatric Association established the Transcultural Psychiatry Committee, which has authored statements since the 1960s. The inclusion of sections on "Cultural Formulation" and "Glossary of Cultural Concepts of Distress" in DSM-5 (American Psychiatric Association 2013) attests to the relevance of this discipline to psychiatric practice (Ton and Lim 2015; Tseng 2001).

Several terms are used interchangeably, although with somewhat different meanings, in this multidisciplinary mental health specialty and thus require definition. The Committee on Cultural Psychiatry of the Group for the Advancement of Psychiatry (2002) defines *culture* as

> a set of meaning, behavioral norms, and values used by members of a particular society as they construct their unique view of the world. These…include social relationships, language, nonverbal expression of thoughts and emotions, religious beliefs, moral thought, technology, and financial philosophy. (pp. 6–7)

Culture is dynamic, and it shapes and is shaped by individuals and evolves over time as it is passed on to succeeding generations. It shapes meanings and expressions of disease, illness, pain, and suffering, which in turn influence a people's receptivity to medical and psychiatric care. *Ethnicity* encompasses one's identity with a group of people sharing common origins, history, customs, and beliefs. Ethnicity may include geographical, national, and religious identities, such as Irish Catholic, Vietnamese American, or Greek Orthodox. *Race* refers to physical, biological, and genetic qualities of humans, particularly as these features lead to categorization of visible similarities or differences. Race as a concept is not scientifically valid and does not lend itself well to objective, reliable description, yet it is a powerful factor not only in human politics but also in psychiatric diagnosis, access to care, and therapeutic relationships. *Cultural psychiatry,* then, is the discipline concerned with matters of culture, ethnicity, and race as they affect description, assessment, diagnosis, biopsychosocial formulation, treatment planning, and training in all aspects of psychiatric practice (Group for the Advancement of Psychiatry 2002; Ton and Lim 2015).

Cultural Aspects of Typical Child Development and Family Life

In virtually all cultures, marriage and family are the foundational units in which children are conceived, grow, and develop. Marriage is the socially sanctioned unit, usually intended to be long lasting, if not permanent, from which a family is created and nurtured. Families, in turn, function as groups through which individuals grow physically, emotionally, and socially; learn to relate to the outside world; and transmit cultural beliefs, histories, and behaviors to the next generation.

Family life cycles emerge from biology and childbearing yet are influenced significantly by cultural patterns and religious beliefs and rituals. Many cultures worldwide now follow the stages of a Western family life cycle, including marriage, childbearing, childrearing, empty nest, and widowhood. However, the time spent in each stage is affected by gender roles, education, acceptable ages for marriage and parenthood, number and autonomy of offspring, remarriage, and occupational and work lives. In addition, particular cultures and religious traditions celebrate and react to family and individual life cycle events differently. For instance, Judaism's emphasis on a child's transition into adulthood at age 13 is shared by many cultures. American funerals can be either very solemn or celebratory occasions depending on the history and ethnicity of the family and cultural group (Kaslow et al. 1995; Tseng 2001).

Theory and practical study of individual child and adolescent development have been dominated by Western schemas, especially Freud's psychosexual, Piaget's cognitive, and Erikson's psychosocial frameworks. Methodologically sound studies of development outside of Western Europe and North America are few, although scholarship on cross-cultural child development generally spans a continuum. On one end is the position that because children are biologically humans and thus very similar, cultural influences are minimal, if any. The other extreme is that culture is such a huge factor in the family, social, and psychological makeup of children that few, if any, generalizations can be made across cultures (Koss-Chioino and Vargas 1992; Tseng 2001). Cross-cultural studies have consistently documented that certain qualities of temperament and mother-child interactions are found more often in certain cultures than in others. Later in development, different cultures mark adulthood at varying times, some with unique rites or rituals of passage often tied temporally to puberty. Young people tend to take on adult roles and responsibilities after such a public acknowledgment of their maturation, especially in non-Western cultures (Tseng 2001).

Culture Competence and DSM-5

Exact psychiatric diagnosis in culturally diverse children living in the United States is difficult, primarily because of factors beyond the simple counting of symptoms on a checklist. Poverty, suboptimal living conditions, language and communication issues with children and their caregivers, value differences across generational lines, poor health care, and excessive stresses of daily living blur lines between usual and understandable emotional reactions, adjustment problems, coping mechanisms, expectable cultural variation, and genuine psychiatric illness. Physicians must remember to consider medical problems with neuropsychiatric manifestations as they work with culturally diverse children. Children born in other countries and adopted by families in the United States may have been exposed to infectious agents or toxins, in utero or early infancy, with central nervous system sequelae.

The poverty and trying living conditions of some cultural minorities increase the possibility of limited or no prenatal and subsequent pediatric care. Many cultural minorities are suspicious of majority health care providers, and even when desirous of evaluation and treatment, they may face considerable challenges with transportation, child care, missed work for appointments, language, and navigation of the American health care system. The effects of violence on culturally diverse youth cannot be underestimated. Many children immigrating from other countries have witnessed and suffered through war, persecution, refugee camps, natural disasters, and grave illnesses. Frequently, children have more than one DSM diagnosis. At other times, they may not meet strict criteria for any DSM diagnosis, but symptoms and the overall clinical picture beg nonetheless for therapeutic intervention.

DSM-5 was updated with significant attention to cultural elements of case formulation, mentioning these explicitly in the manual's introductory chapter (American Psychiatric Association 2013, pp. 14–15). The term *culture-bound syndrome* has been retired in favor of three more clinically useful constructs. *Cultural syndromes* are consistent and specific symptoms occurring in cultural groups or contexts. *Cultural idiom of distress* refers to a way of conceptualizing and communicating about suffering experienced by individuals within a cultural group. *Cultural explanation or perceived cause* provides a reason or reasons for symptoms or distress. These are helpful in devising a *cultural formulation.* DSM-5 offers an updated formulation outline, requiring consideration of 1) cultural identity of the individual, 2) cultural conceptualizations of distress, 3) psychosocial stressors and cultural features of vulnerability and resilience, 4) cultural features of the relationship between the individual and the clinician, and 5) overall cultural assessment (pp. 749–750). New to DSM-5 is the Cultural Formulation Interview (pp. 750–759). Child and adolescent mental health clinicians will find these resources very helpful in understanding patients, their families, and cultural aspects of their care (American Psychiatric Association 2013).

The Culture and Diversity Committee of the American Academy of Child and Adolescent Psychiatry (AACAP) has been an effective leader and advocate for culturally competent assessment and care of multicultural youth across life domains. Leaders of this group have partnered with the AACAP Committee on Quality Issues to develop a Practice Parameter for Cultural Competence in Child and Adolescent Psychiatric Practice (Pumariega et al. 2013). Key points of this important document are summarized in Table 26–1.

Religion, Spirituality, and Culture

Basic Definitions and Relevance to Care

In a sense, religion and spirituality can be considered as a subset or category of culture. Unlike other cultural elements, this topic transcends diverse societies and deals with individual and collective values, norms, core beliefs, and relationships with the divine—matters of ultimate importance to members of a culture. This unique role of religion and spirituality in virtually all cultures and their pervasive influences on mental health and illness merit special consideration.

Religion is an organized system of beliefs, principles, rituals, practices, and related symbols that brings individuals

TABLE 26–1. Culturally competent child and adolescent mental health clinicians

Recognize and address obstacles to mental health services for culturally diverse populations
Provide care in patients' preferred language when possible
Appreciate the implications of dual or multiple languages for a child's acculturation and development
Are insightful regarding the cultural biases they bring to their work
Appreciate cultural influences on development, distress, and symptom expression
Ask about individual and group trauma associated with immigration
Address different degrees of acculturation and associated stress in multigenerational families
Include extended family members and important others in assessment and treatment
Include cultural strengths in assessment and treatment
Work with culturally diverse families in familiar community settings when possible
Use evidence-based practices in ethnic/cultural psychopharmacology, behavioral management, and psychosocial treatments

Source. Adapted from Pumariega et al. 2013.

and groups to sacred or ultimate reality and truth. It includes relationships with others, whether inside a community of individuals with shared beliefs or external to a like-minded community. *Spirituality* includes religion and faith communities but is not restricted to organized religion and group membership. It may encompass an individual's understandings of and quest for ultimate meaning in life's deepest, most perplexing questions and mysteries (Koenig et al. 2001). One can be religious only, spiritual only, both religious and spiritual, or neither and can pass between these descriptions on multiple occasions in a lifetime.

Two terms important to understanding religion and spirituality in North America, especially regarding Protestantism, are *evangelicalism* and *fundamentalism.* Evangelicals are Protestants with a conservative approach to the Bible, believing that one must have a close, personal relationship with Jesus Christ in order to be a Christian. Typically, although not always, evangelical Christians believe that all aspects of life should be guided by biblical teachings, including family life, major life decisions, politics, and entertainment, to name but a few. Fundamentalists are a subset of evangelicals, noted for literal interpretation of scripture or a belief in the absolute authority of the Bible. Modernism, especially science, may be suspect unless it is compatible with strict biblical precepts. Fundamentalists, compared with more liberal evangelicals, are less likely to participate in secular society without wanting, or even insisting, that society change to conform to their values. In the United States, the term fundamentalism primarily is applied to very conservative Protestantism. However, the concept of *fundamentalism,* including strict interpretation of sacred writings, traditional lifestyle practices guided by religious teachings, and suspicion of or resistance to modernity, may be found worldwide in Judaism, Islam, Hinduism, and other major world faith traditions (Ammerman 1991; Hood et al. 2005; Wentz 2003).

Ironically, Sigmund Freud, often caricatured as unfriendly to religion and spirituality, coined a term that is helpful in understanding this potentially sensitive subject matter and its importance in psychiatry and culture. *Weltanschauung,* or *worldview,* refers to a philosophy of life or belief system that addresses life's most common, basic questions. These include the meaning and purpose of life, life direction and goals, what is good and desirable in life, happiness, relationships with others, suffering, and death. A worldview may or may not include or share aspects with an organized religious tradition (Freud 1933/1962).

Many, if not most, practical elements in the lives of children and families are influenced to varying degrees by religious convictions, practices, or values stemming from spiritual beliefs. Examples include childrearing practices and attitudes toward medical and psychiatric care, substance use, sexuality, dating, and money. Seemingly mundane matters, such as choice of which clothing is appropriate for school and what children are permitted to view on television and the Internet, are rooted in core values formed by religious beliefs or lack thereof. Even children, adolescents, and families who claim no religious or spiritual belief are immersed in a secular culture that reflects majority values shaped or influenced by religious principles. As these issues are often identified as concerns by children and families presenting to child and adolescent psychiatrists and influence diagnosis and treatment planning, clinicians are well advised to attune themselves to both the overt and the subtle religious and spiritual themes in the lives of their patient populations (Josephson and Dell 2004).

Religious and Spiritual Diversity in North American Culture

Psychiatrists are treating increasingly diverse patients from many cultural and religious backgrounds. While mental health clinicians do not need to be experts in comparative religion, more psychiatrists are seeking familiarity with basic beliefs and daily rituals of faith traditions found in geographical areas where they practice. Table 26–2 summarizes basic facts regarding seven major traditions commonly encountered today.

Beliefs and practices are diverse both within major world faith traditions and between them. The concept of *continuum of belief and practice* is helpful clinically and refers to the following observations:

1. Most major world faith traditions have subgroups, branches, or denominations that identify themselves as a distinct subgroup of the larger tradition. These subgroups may be distinguished by the nature and extent of their religious practices and observances. For example, the three largest groups within Judaism—Orthodox, Conservative, and Reform—generally fall on a continuum from orthodox belief and strict observance of religious law and custom to less defined and ritualized belief and practice.
2. Most major faith traditions consist of followers or members who, as both individuals and local faith communities, fall on a continuum from observant to nonobservant, politically conservative to liberal, and rigid and excluding of others to open and welcoming of those who have differing viewpoints. For example, in any single Protestant denomination are members who believe that homosexuality is sinful and others who believe that sexual orientation is biologically determined and same-sex relationships are acceptable—with both groups self-identifying as faithful members of the same denomination.

As already noted, the relationships among religion, spirituality, and culture are complex, always influencing and shaping each other. For instance, what does it mean when a patient claims a

TABLE 26–2. Major faith traditions: important facts

Christianity

Three major groups: Catholic (Roman, others), Orthodox (Greek, Russian, others), Protestant

80% of U.S. adults (51% Protestant, 24% Catholic, 0.6% Orthodox, ~3% other)

Abrahamic, monotheistic, early members from Jewish and non-Jewish backgrounds

Based on life and teachings of Jesus, son of God

Sacred text is the Bible, including Old (Hebrew Scriptures) and New Testaments

Judaism

12 million worldwide

6 million in the United States, 1.7% of U.S. adults

Originated in ancient Mesopotamia; traces heritage to patriarch Abraham

Can refer to both a religion and an ethnicity

Defined primarily by practices and ethics found in sacred texts instead of doctrines

Three major groups in the United States: Orthodox (10%), Conservative (35%), Reform (40%)

Islam (Muslim)

Second-largest world religion, 20% of world's population (Indonesia, Middle East, Bangladesh, Pakistan, Nigeria)

0.6% of U.S. adults, >6 million people, and third-largest religion in the United States

Abrahamic—shares historical and theological elements with Judaism and Christianity

Muhammad viewed as last messenger of God (Allah)

Sacred text is the Qur'an

Important practices (five pillars): profession of belief, prayer, fasting, charity, pilgrimage to Mecca

Three major branches: Sunni, Shi'a, Sufi

Buddhism

Fourth-largest religious tradition in the world (Tibet, Sri Lanka, Thailand, China, Korea, Japan)

0.7% of U.S. adults

Originated in 5th century B.C.E. India with teachings of Siddhartha Gautama, the Buddha

Three branches: East Asian, Tibetan, Theravada

Elements include nonextremism (Middle Way), teachings of Buddha (dharma), view of suffering (Four Noble Truths), and state of complete selflessness and dissolution of self's boundaries (nirvana)

Emphasizes right living, compassion, morality, self-discipline

Hinduism

83% of population in India; not widespread in rest of world

0.4% of U.S. adults, primarily of Asian Indian lineage

No clear historical beginning, but roots identifiable as early as 3000 B.C.E.

Complex system of beliefs, ideals, practices; God and Truth are one; many gods and goddesses represent truth and divinity

Key concepts: cycle of birth, death, rebirth in another body (reincarnation); current experiences are fruits of past actions (karma); ethical teachings (dharma); social class system (castes)

Important duties: personal cleanliness, food preparation and eating habits, marriage and family relationships, quiet meditation

TABLE 26–2. Major faith traditions: important facts *(continued)*

African American religious traditions
More African Americans claim formal religious affiliation than all other ethnic groups
Predominantly Christian, with both predominantly black denominations and black churches in predominantly white denominations
Two-thirds of historically black Protestant churches in the United States are Baptist
Centers of community life: education, social justice, social work, culture
Churches and clergy were leaders in civil rights movement
Nation of Islam: organized African American Muslim group founded in 1930
Native American religion and spirituality
<0.3% U.S. adults
Nearly as many forms as nations, tribes, cultures
Spirituality is a personal relationship connecting individual's spirit to creation, present world, sense of place, other people, and animals
Many rituals involving nature, human development, and rites of passage
Modern expressions may be admixed with traditional aspects of Christianity
Opposition to majority consumerism, materialism, politics, economics, and environmental abuse and neglect is also attractive to many non–Native Americans

Source. Cutting 2006; Eckel 2003; Esposito 2003; Gill 2003; Johnson 2006; Larson 2003; Neusner 2003; Pew Research Center 2008; Raman 2006; Scarlett 2006.

Baptist religious preference on her clinic registration form? The twelfth edition of the authoritative *Handbook of Denominations in the United States* (Mead et al. 2005) lists 31 distinct Baptist denominations, 11 more than recognized 4 years previously in the eleventh edition (Mead et al. 2001). Is her family Southern Baptist, upper middle class, Euro-American, and suburban with conservative political leanings? Or is the patient African American and active in a smaller, historically black, poorer denomination whose theology and beliefs are rooted in the Deep South long before the Civil War? The geographical area of the country, the characters of the civil communities in which we live, and extended-family histories, myths, and legends can tell practitioners as much or more about priorities, values, and clinically relevant lifestyle issues as one's religious affiliation. In the context of the increasing multiculturalism and ethnic diversity of the early twenty-first century, the intertwining of religion, ethnicity, and immigration/acculturation must be appreciated. For instance, three different families may identify themselves as Catholic on hospital registration forms: a family from the Bronx whose two sets of grandparents moved from Puerto Rico as teenagers but whose present-day grandchildren know little to no Spanish; a second-generation Italian Catholic family from south Philadelphia whose children attend parochial schools and whose non-English-speaking grandmother attends daily morning Mass and provides most of the after-school child care; and a bilingual Mexican American family in El Paso, Texas, whose adult members go back and forth to Mexico on the basis of visa or work status and affordability of necessary medical care. Catholicism may be important to all but is lived out differently in their radically different life circumstances.

In 2007, the Pew Research Center interviewed 35,000 Americans ages 18 years and older in an effort to explore the contemporary U.S. religious landscape (Pew Research Center 2008). Their findings support the importance of religion and spirituality in the United States. Approximately 84% of the sample claimed a religious affiliation, with an additional 6% stating they were religious but not affiliated. While the study documented increasing religious diversity both in major traditions claimed (i.e., Buddhism, Hinduism, Islam) and in denominational or subgroup differences within the larger religions, Protestantism just barely remained the majority tradition at 51.3%. Of importance for medical and psychiatric history taking are the findings that 1) 28% of Americans have left the tradition in which they were raised for a different religion or none at all, 2) 25% of Americans younger than the age of 30 claim no religious affiliation at all, and 3) more than half of adults who were unaffiliated as a child have chosen a faith tradition to claim as an adult. In addition, ongoing Latino immigration is increasing the absolute number of Catholics in the United States (Pew Research Center 2008).

Religion, Spirituality, and Culture in Assessment and Treatment Planning

Obviously, if time permits, a wealth of helpful clinical information can be obtained in individual work with the child and in family sessions regarding religion and spirituality and their roles in pathology and treatment (Moncher and Josephson 2004; Sexson 2004). Several tools have been developed (primarily for adults) to inquire about religion and spirituality in clinical settings (Fitchett 1993; Puchalski and Romer 2000). While some measures have been used in particular pediatric settings (Barnes et al. 2000; McEvoy 2003), no single instrument has been developed for children that can be used across inpatient, outpatient, emergency, medical, and long-term treatment and other settings. However, the following are questions that may be used across the age spectrum that may be helpful for beginning discussions in clinical encounters.

Questions for young children:

1. Do you go to church/synagogue/mosque? What is it like? What do you learn there?
2. What is God like?
3. What do you pray for?
4. If you could ask God to change just one thing, what would it be?
5. What is your favorite Bible (sacred text) story? Why do you like it?
6. What happens when a person (you) dies?

Questions for older youth and parents or adult caregivers:

1. Is religion or personal faith an important part of your life? Would you describe yourself as religious or spiritual?
2. What is your value system? How do you live out your faith or beliefs in daily life?
3. What kinds of things do you pray about?
4. Are you a part of a faith community, such as a church, synagogue, or mosque?
5. With what beliefs and practices of your faith community do you agree or disagree? Why?
6. Who or what do you turn to when in trouble, scared, sick, or alone?
7. What has your religious education been?
8. What does your faith community teach and what do you believe about health, illness, pain, and suffering?

9. What religious practices, rituals, and holidays are important to you and why?
10. What do you believe happens after death?

Inadvertently, clinicians and the families they treat often overlook treatment resources available through local religious institutions and faith-based organizations. These resources include food pantries, clothes closets, emergency cash assistance, shelters, health clinics, transportation to medical appointments, English as a second language classes, day care for children and elders, recreational activities, and practical training in areas such as job interviewing and computer skills. These services are becoming increasingly valuable as government and health care funds diminish in amount and availability (Dell 2004).

Summary Points

- The population of North America is increasing in diversity at an astounding rate. By 2020, the majority of the population under age 18 is projected to comprise individuals from nonwhite, minority racial groups.
- Child, adolescent, and family development are influenced by both genetics and the psychological and experiential aspects of culture.
- DSM-5 is attentive to cultural elements of psychiatric diagnosis. It contains an updated Outline for Cultural Formulation, a 16-question Cultural Formulation Interview, and a Glossary of Cultural Concepts of Distress.
- Religion and spirituality form a subset of culture that affects and is affected by all other elements of culture. These relationships are becoming increasingly complex and important as the United States increases in ethnic and religious pluralism.
- Familiarity with general facts about major world faith traditions is helpful in clinical practice. However, there is considerable variation in individual belief and practice, so clinicians are well advised to inquire about the belief systems and customs of specific patients and families.
- Religion, spirituality, and religious/spiritual professionals and institutions can provide resources for coping with illness and stresses, as well as assistance with practical needs associated with health and wellness.

References

American Psychiatric Association: Diagnostic and Statistical Manual of Mental Disorders, 5th Edition. Arlington, VA, American Psychiatric Association, 2013

Ammerman NT: North American Protestant fundamentalism, in Fundamentalisms Observed. Edited by Marty ME, Appleby RS. Chicago, IL, University of Chicago Press, 1991, pp 1–65

Barnes LL, Plotnikoff GA, Fox K, et al: Spirituality, religion, and pediatrics: intersecting worlds of healing. Pediatrics 106(4 suppl):899–908, 2000 11044142

Cutting C: Islam, in Encyclopedia of Religious and Spiritual Development. Edited by Dowling EM, Scarlett WG. Thousand Oaks, CA, Sage, 2006, pp 212–217

Dell ML: Religious professionals and institutions: untapped resources for clinical care. Child Adolesc Psychiatr Clin N Am 13(1):85–110, 2004 14723302

Eckel MD: Buddhism in the world and in America, in World Religions in America, 3rd Edition. Edited by Neusner J. Louisville, KY, Westminster John Knox, 2003, pp 142–153

Esposito JL: Islam in the world and in America, in World Religions in America, 3rd Edition. Edited by Neusner J. Louisville, KY, Westminster John Knox, 2003, pp 172–185

Fitchett G: Assessing Spiritual Needs: A Guide for Caregivers. Minneapolis, MN, Augsburg Fortress, 1993

Freud S: The question of a weltanschauung (1933), in The Standard Edition of the Complete Psychological Works of Sigmund Freud, Vol 22. Translated and edited by Strachey J. London, Hogarth, 1962, pp 158–167

Gill S: Native Americans and their religions, in World Religions in America, 3rd Edition. Edited by Neusner J. Louisville, KY, Westminster John Knox, 2003, pp 9–23

Group for the Advancement of Psychiatry: Committee on Cultural Psychiatry: Cultural Assessment in Clinical Psychiatry. Washington, DC, American Psychiatric Publishing, 2002

Hood RW Jr, Hill PC, Williamson WP: The Psychology of Religious Fundamentalism. New York, Guilford, 2005

Johnson T: Native American Indian spirituality, in Encyclopedia of Religious and Spiritual Development. Edited by Dowling EM, Scarlett WG. Thousand Oaks, CA, Sage, 2006, pp 313–315

Josephson AM, Dell ML: Religion and spirituality in child and adolescent psychiatry: a new frontier. Child Adolesc Psychiatr Clin N Am 13(1):1–15, v, 2004 14723297

Kaslow NJ, Celano M, Dreelin ED: A cultural perspective on family theory and therapy. Psychiatr Clin North Am 18(3):621–633, 1995 8545271

Koenig HG, McCullough ME, Larson DB: Handbook of Religion and Health. New York, Oxford University Press, 2001

Koss-Chioino JD, Vargas LA: Through the cultural looking glass: a model for understanding culturally responsive psychotherapies, in Working With Culture. Edited by Vargas LA, Koss-Chioino JD. San Francisco, CA, Jossey-Bass, 1992, pp 1–22

Larson GJ: Hinduism in India and in America, in World Religions in America, 3rd Edition. Edited by Neusner J. Louisville, KY, Westminster John Knox, 2003, pp 124–141

McEvoy M: Culture and spirituality as an integrated concept in pediatric care. MCN Am J Matern Child Nurs 28(1):39–43, quiz 44, 2003 12514355

Mead FS, Hill SS, Atwood CD: Handbook of Denominations in the United States, 11th Edition. Nashville, TN, Abingdon Press, 2001

Mead FS, Hill SS, Atwood CD: Handbook of Denominations in the United States, 12th Edition. Nashville, TN, Abingdon Press, 2005

Moncher FJ, Josephson AM: Religious and spiritual aspects of family assessment. Child Adolesc Psychiatr Clin N Am 13(1):49–70, vi, 2004 14723300

Neusner J: Judaism in the world and in America, in World Religions in America, 3rd Edition. Edited by Neusner J. Louisville, KY, Westminster John Knox, 2003, pp 106–123

Pew Research Center: The U.S. religious landscape survey reveals a fluid and diverse pattern of faith, in Pew Forum on Religion and Public Life. Washington, DC, Pew Research Center, 2008. Available at: http://pewresearch.org/pubs/743/united-states-religion. Accessed March 8, 2008.

Puchalski C, Romer AL: Taking a spiritual history allows clinicians to understand patients more fully. J Palliat Med 3(1):129–137, 2000 15859737

Pumariega AJ, Rothe E, Mian A, et al: Practice parameter for cultural competence in child and adolescent psychiatric practice. J Am Acad Child Adolesc Psychiatry 52(10):1101–1115, 2013 24074479

Raman VV: Hinduism, in Encyclopedia of Religious and Spiritual Development. Edited by Dowling EM, Scarlett WG. Thousand Oaks, CA, Sage, 2006, pp 199–203

Scarlett WG: Buddhism, in Encyclopedia of Religious and Spiritual Development. Edited by Dowling EM, Scarlett WG. Thousand Oaks, CA, Sage, 2006, pp 59–60

Sexson SB: Religious and spiritual assessment of the child and adolescent. Child Adolesc Psychiatr Clin N Am 13(1):35–47, vi, 2004 14723299

Ton H, Lim RF: Assessment of culturally diverse individuals, in Clinical Manual of Cultural Psychiatry, 2nd Edition. Edited by Lim RF. Arlington, VA, American Psychiatric Publishing, 2015, pp 1–41

Tseng W-S: Handbook of Cultural Psychiatry. San Diego, CA, Academic Press, 2001

U.S. Census Bureau: 2010 Census Shows America's Diversity. March 14, 2011. Available at: http://www.census.gov/2010census/news/releases/operations/cb11-cn125.html. Accessed August 3, 2014.

U.S. Census Bureau: International Migration is Projected to Become Primary Driver of U.S. Population Growth for First Time in Nearly Two Centuries. May 15, 2013. Available at: http://www.census.gov/newsroom/releases/archives/population/cb13-89.html. Accessed August 3, 2014.

U.S. Census Bureau: USA Quick Facts from the US Census Bureau. July 8, 2014. Available at: http://quickfacts.census.gov/qfd/states/00000.html. Accessed August 3, 2014.

Wentz RE: American Religious Traditions: The Shaping of Religion in the United States. Minneapolis, MN, Fortress Press, 2003

CHAPTER 27

Youth Suicide

Tina R. Goldstein, Ph.D.
David A. Brent, M.D.

Definitions

The most currently accepted definitions of different types of suicide-related behaviors are the Columbia Classification Algorithm for Suicide Assessment (C-CASA, Posner et al. 2007; see Table 27–1).

Epidemiology

In the United States in 2010, suicide was the third leading cause of death among youth and young adults and accounted for 11% of the mortality in this age group (Centers for Disease Control and Prevention 2010). Results from a recent survey of adolescents in the United States indicate the lifetime prevalence of suicide attempts is 4.1%, suicidal ideation with plan is 4%, and any suicidal ideation is 12.1% (Nock et al. 2013). Yet the Youth Risk Behavior Surveillance Study of high school students in the United States recently reported substantially higher incidences: 7.8% of youth reported attempting suicide within the prior year, 2.4% of whose attempts were medically serious; 12.8% of youth reported suicidal ideation with plan over the prior year; and 15.8% endorsed suicidal ideation (Eaton et al. 2012).

Characteristics

Age

The rates of attempted and completed suicide increase dramatically with age throughout childhood into adolescence. Various explanations may account for this relationship, including elevated risk for psychopathology during adolescence, increased cognitive capacity to prepare and execute a suicide plan, and decreased supervision with age. Although prepubertal children do endorse suicidal ideation, their cognitive immaturity appears to limit their ability to plan and execute lethal suicide attempts. Recent data suggest suicidal ideation is rare before age 10 years (less than 1%), increases slowly through age 12 years, and then increases more rapidly through age 17, whereas plans and attempts increase linearly from age 12 to

TABLE 27–1. Suicide terminology

Term	Definition
Completed suicide	Suicide attempt that results in death
Suicide attempt	A potentially self-injurious behavior with some evident intent to die (may be inferred from the behavior)
Suicidal ideation	Thoughts of death without actually engaging in the behavior; can range from "passive," in which the person thinks about wanting to be dead, to active thoughts about killing oneself
Aborted attempt	The person begins to make a suicide attempt but stops himself or herself prior to experiencing injury
Interrupted attempt	The person begins to make a suicide attempt but is interrupted by another person or circumstance prior to experiencing injury
Nonsuicidal self-injurious behavior	A self-injurious behavior performed without intent to die (other intent may be, for example, to relieve distress, effect change in others or the environment)

age 15 years and then more slowly through age 17 (Nock et al. 2013).

Gender and Sexual Orientation

The rate of completed suicide among youth is significantly higher for males than females, with a ratio of nearly 5 to 1 in 2010 (Centers for Disease Control and Prevention 2010). However, females endorse higher rates of suicidal ideation (19.3% vs. 12.5%) and have higher suicide attempt rates than males (9.8% vs. 5.8%; Eaton et al. 2012). The higher rate of completed suicide among male youth may be attributable to higher rates of associated risk factors, including substance use and antisocial behaviors and the tendency for males to employ more violent and lethal means of attempting suicide. As compared with heterosexual youth, sexual minority youth are at greater risk of attempted suicide and suicidal ideation. This disparity may be explained in part by higher rates of previous abuse, peer victimization, and parental rejection (Marshal et al. 2011).

Race and Socioeconomic Status

In general, the suicide rate in the United States is higher among white than nonwhite youth. However, American Indians/Alaska Natives exhibit the highest suicide rate of all ethnic groups in the United States (Centers for Disease Control and Prevention 2010). With regard to suicide attempt, 1-year incidence rates are greater among black (8.3%) and Hispanic (10.2%) youth than among white youth (6.2%), whereas white (15.5%) and Hispanic (16.7%) youth endorse greater rates of suicidal ideation as compared with black youth (13.2%; Eaton et al. 2012).

With regard to socioeconomic status, in the United States increased suicide risk is associated with lower socioeconomic status. Suicide attempts are more common among youth with a parent who only graduated from high school and among youth with a parent who completed some college as compared with youth with a parent with either more or less education (Nock et al. 2013).

Risk Factors

Suicidal Ideation

Approximately 33% of youth with suicidal ideation go on to make a suicide plan; of these, the majority of youth (63.1%) experience progression of ideation within 1 year of ideation onset. Similarly, of the 33% of youth whose suicidal ideation progresses to attempt, 86.1% will make the attempt within 1 year of ideation onset (Nock et al. 2013).

Previous Suicidal Behavior

The strongest predictor of future suicidal behavior is a history of suicidal behavior (Brent et al. 1999). Follow-up studies of adolescent suicide attempters report a reattempt rate within 1 year of 6.8% in first-time attempters and 24.6% in those with a history of attempts (Hultén et al. 2001), with the greatest risk period for reattempt occurring within 3 months of the initial attempt (Goldston et al. 1999). The period immediately following discharge from an inpatient psychiatric unit appears to be associated with particularly high risk (Kjelsberg et al. 1994). Youth with a history of attempting suicide using methods high in medical lethality, such as hanging, shooting, or jumping, are at especially high risk for eventual completed suicide (Beautrais 2004). However, it is not necessarily the case that an attempt of low lethality reflects low suicidal intent, particularly among younger children who may overestimate the lethality of means.

Availability of Lethal Means

In 2010, nearly 45% of young people who completed suicide in the United States died by firearm (Centers for Disease Control and Prevention 2010). Indeed, evidence from case control studies indicates that firearms are much more common in the homes of suicide completers than in those of attempters and control subjects. If a loaded gun is in the home, it is highly likely to be selected as a means of suicide. In one study, a loaded gun in the home was associated with a thirtyfold increased risk for completed suicide, even among youth with no apparent psychopathology (Brent and Bridge 2003). Thus, assessment of both presence and storage/accessibility of firearms and ammunition in the homes of young people is recommended.

Psychiatric Disorders

The overwhelming majority—nearly 90%—of youth who die by suicide have evidence of serious psychopathology (Brent et al. 1988).Youth who attempt suicide also demonstrate high rates of psychopathology, with recent estimates as high as 96% (Nock et al. 2013). Mood disorders convey the most potent risk, with more than 80% of attempters and 60% of completers meeting criteria for at least one major mood disorder (Brent 1993). Depressed youth with a chronic course of illness lasting 2 years or more are at particularly elevated risk for both attempted and completed suicide.

Other psychiatric conditions frequently associated with youth suicide and suicide attempt include disruptive, anxiety, and substance use disorders. Comorbidity is the rule rather than the exception among youth who attempt and complete suicide, with comorbid mood, disruptive, and substance use disorders associated with substantially elevated risk (Cash and Bridge 2009).

Psychological Factors

Psychological factors linked to suicide risk include impulsive aggression in response to frustration or provocation (McGirr et al. 2008). Hopelessness also correlates strongly with suicidal intent and predicts risk for reattempt and completed suicide beyond its association with depression (Goldston et al. 2001).

In terms of personality traits, *neuroticism*—the tendency to experience prolonged and severe negative affect in response to stress—has repeatedly been associated with suicide attempts in youth, above and beyond its association with other risk factors (Roy 2002). Although perfectionism is another personality trait associated with suicide attempts in youth, studies have failed to find a link between perfectionism and completed suicide (Shaffer et al. 1996).

Medical Disorders

Chronic medical conditions affecting the central nervous system (e.g., epilepsy, migraine) and those involving inflammation (e.g., asthma, inflammatory bowel disease) are associated with increased risk for suicidal ideation and behavior in pediatric populations (Scott et al. 2010).

Family Factors

Research suggests both environmental and genetic mechanisms for the familial transmission of suicidal behavior, and evidence suggests that suicidal behavior is transmitted in families distinct from its association with familial psychiatric illness. The first-degree relatives of adolescent suicide attempters and completers exhibit a suicide attempt rate two to six times higher than that found in the general population, even after controlling for higher rates of psychopathology (Brent and Melhem 2008). Likewise, the offspring of mood-disordered adults with a history of suicide attempt are at four to six times greater risk for suicide attempt as compared with offspring of mood disordered adults with no history of suicide attempt (Melhem et al. 2007). Greater familial loading has been found to be specifically associated with earlier age at onset of suicidal behavior in offspring, suggesting that early onset suicidality may be a particularly familial form that is mediated by impulsive aggression (McGirr et al. 2008; Brent and Melhem 2008).

The family environments of suicide attempters are characterized by high levels of discord and violence and are perceived as less supportive and more conflictual than those of nonattempters (Wagner et al. 2003); conversely, a supportive and warm parent-child relationship can buffer against suicidal behavior in otherwise high-risk adolescents (Borowsky et al. 2001). Both physical and sexual abuse also have a potent association with attempted and completed suicide in youth, as does parental loss or absence (King and Merchant 2008).

Assessment

Suicidal ideation should be assessed according to both severity (intent) and pervasiveness (frequency and intensity). Suicidal ideation characterized by a high degree of severity and pervasiveness is associated with greater likelihood of suicide attempt in adolescents (Lewinsohn et al. 1996). In addition, prior suicidal behavior should be carefully reviewed. At present, the Columbia Suicide Severity Rating Scale (C-SSRS; Posner et al. 2011) is a widely used and accepted tool for suicide assessment (www.cssrs.columbia.edu).

Suicidal Intent

Suicidal intent is the extent to which the individual wishes to die. Given findings that adolescents may disclose suicidal ideation on self-report ratings but deny this information during interviews, assessment of suicidal risk should incorporate both means of assessment. The individual's behavior should also be carefully assessed.

With regard to suicidal intent, four components should be explored (Kingsbury 1993): 1) belief about intent (i.e., the extent to which the individual is wishing to die); 2) preparatory behavior (e.g., giving away prized possessions, writing a suicide note); 3) prevention of discovery (i.e., planning the attempt so that rescue is unlikely); and 4) communication of suicidal intent. High intent—as evidenced by expressing a wish to die, planning the attempt ahead of time, timing the attempt to avoid detection, and confiding suicide plans prior to the attempt—is associated with recurrent suicide attempts and with suicide completion.

Suicide Plan and Access to Means

Assessment should include inquiry regarding specific plans for inflicting self-harm, as well as access to means considered (see the subsection "Means Restriction" in the "Treatment" section later in this chapter).

Medical Lethality

Suicide attempts of high medical lethality (e.g., hanging, shooting) are frequently characterized by high suicidal intent, and individuals who use more medically lethal means are at higher risk to complete suicide. However, evidence also indicates that an impulsive attempter with relatively low intent but ready access to lethal means may also engage in a medically serious and even fatal attempt (Brent et al. 1999).

It is important to differentiate nonsuicidal self-injurious behavior from suicide attempt (see terminology in Table 27–1) by expressly inquiring about intent. Given that the risk factors for nonsuicidal self-harm and suicidal behavior overlap, many youth engage in both behaviors, and therefore the presence of one should alert the clinician to inquire about the other.

Precipitants

The most common precipitant for adolescent suicidal behavior is interpersonal conflict or loss, most often involving a parent or a romantic relationship. Legal and disciplinary problems also frequently precipitate suicidal behavior, particularly among youth with conduct disorder and substance abuse. Precipitants that are chronic and ongoing, especially recurrent physical or sexual abuse, are associated with poorer outcomes, including recurrence of suicidal behavior and even subsequent completion (Brent et al. 1999).

Motivation

Motivation is the reason the individual cites for his or her suicidality. Individuals with high suicidal intent indicate that their primary motivation is either to die or to permanently escape an emotionally painful situation, and these youth are at elevated risk for reattempt (Boergers et al. 1998). Many youth who attempt suicide report they are motivated by the desire to influence others or to communicate a feeling. Understanding the motivation for the suicide attempt has important implications for treatment, as intervention may focus on helping youth explicitly identify their needs and find less dangerous ways to get their needs met.

Consequences

The consequences of suicidality refer to any environmental contingencies that occur in response to suicidality. Particularly salient is whether there are naturally occurring contingencies in the environment that reinforce suicidal communications and behaviors (e.g., increased attention and support, decreased demands and responsibilities). However, positive reinforcement from the environment does not necessarily indicate that the individual acted purposefully to gain the reinforcement.

Treatment

Few clinical trials have examined the treatment of adolescent suicidal behavior. In fact, most treatment studies of depressed adolescents exclude suicidal youth and do not report outcomes related to suicidality. Data from psychosocial and pharmacological studies suggest that the treatment of depression may not be sufficient to reduce suicidal risk; rather, specific treatments targeting suicidality may be required (Emslie et al. 2006).

Approaches to the treatment of youth suicidality that show promise include clinical interventions such as safety planning and hospitalization, as well as psychosocial treatment packages that involve cognitive, emotion regulation, family, and interpersonal approaches. Although no pharmacological treatment has demonstrated efficacy in treating suicidality per se in youth, medications that target aggression and emotional dysregulation such as lithium and atypical (second-generation) antipsychotics may hold promise.

Clinical Management

Safety Plans

Safety planning is considered best practice for suicide prevention with at-risk individuals (Suicide Prevention Resource Center 2012). The creation of a safety plan involves working with the patient and family to collaboratively create a list of strategies that the patient agrees to use when a suicidal crisis occurs (Brent et al. 2011; Stanley et al. 2009). The first step in safety planning is elimination of the availability of lethal means. Next, an agreement with the adolescent is negotiated whereby he or she agrees to some action in the event of suicidal thoughts and/or urges. Such actions may include implementing coping skills and contacting a responsible adult and/or a professional or crisis line. Next, triggers and warning signs (including cognitive, emotional, and behavioral) of a pending suicidal crisis are identified such that the adolescent can identify when it would be necessary to implement the plan. Specific steps in the plan, arranged hierarchically, are then collaboratively identified. Steps in the plan begin with strategies the adolescent can employ without the assistance of others (e.g., listening to music, watching a movie); if ideation/urges persist, external strategies should then be identified that include responsible adults (along with their contact information) the adolescent can turn to for help. Family members are invited to provide input during development of the plan. Few studies have examined the effectiveness of safety plans. One quasi-experimental study showed a reduction in suicide attempts among youth at high risk for suicide in a runaway shelter after implementing a one-session intervention that included a written safety plan with a no-harm contract (Rotheram-Borus and Bradley 1991). A recent review found that no-harm contracts alone are not a sufficient method for suicide prevention (Lewis 2007).

Means Restriction

Few studies have evaluated the effectiveness of restriction of access to lethal means. However, removal of guns from the homes of at-risk youth is strongly recommended. Studies in psychiatric and pediatric outpatient settings have not found a significant effect of parental psychoeducation on minimizing youth access to lethal means (Brent et al. 2000). Specific elements of psychoeducation regarding access to lethal means—insisting on removal of the gun (rather than merely minimizing access such as by locking it up), speaking directly to the gun owner, and ascertaining the perceived risks of removing the gun—may be critical in decreasing risk. Some parents are unwilling to remove guns but are willing to store them securely. Therefore, risk reduction may be achieved by exploring alternatives to removal, including storing guns locked, unloaded, and/or disassembled.

Inpatient Hospitalization

Although psychiatric hospital admission is believed to provide a safe environment for suicidal patients to resolve acute suicidal crises, there is no research to support the efficacy of inpatient hospitalization in reducing suicidality. Among individuals hospitalized for a suicide attempt, the highest-risk period for suicide and reattempt occurs after discharge from the hospital (Kjelsberg et al. 1994), making the transition particularly important.

Several studies have attempted to target this risk period. Carter et al.'s (2005) "Postcards From the Edge" study demonstrated that adolescents and adults who were randomly assigned to receive written contact via postcard during the year following self-poisoning exhibited fewer suicide reattempts and fewer days hospitalized as compared with those who did not receive written contact. For adolescent suicide attempters, adherence with treatment following hospitalization may be maximized by having hospital staff schedule the initial outpatient appointment.

Psychotherapy Approaches

Cognitive-Behavioral Therapy

Brent et al.'s (1997) study of depressed adolescents included suicidal teens; findings indicated that cognitive-behavioral therapy (CBT) was superior to both family and supportive therapies in the treatment of depressive symptoms, but all three treatments were associated with similar reductions in suicidality. In the multisite Treatment for Adolescents With Depression Study (TADS) in which fluoxetine, CBT, and the combination were compared with each other and with placebo, both fluoxetine and the combination produced substantial improvements in depression relative to placebo and CBT alone, but only the combination was associated with decreased suicidal ideation compared with placebo (March et al. 2004).

Rotheram-Borus et al. (2000) compared brief family CBT alone to an "enhanced" CBT condition in which an additional family psychoeducation session was delivered in the emergency room for female adolescent suicide attempters. The enhanced CBT group showed increased adherence to CBT treatment and lower suicidal ideation at posttreatment. At 18-month follow-up, the rates of attempts and suicidal ideation were not different between the two groups.

Esposito-Smythers et al. (2011) examined an integrated model combining CBT with motivational interviewing and family therapy for suicidal substance-abusing adolescents. In a randomized trial, they found fewer suicide attempts and hospitalizations, as well as fewer arrests and episodes of heavy drinking and marijuana use at 18-month follow-up among adolescents receiving the CBT intervention as compared with treatment as usual.

Dialectical Behavior Therapy

Dialectical behavior therapy (DBT)—a treatment that focuses on enhancing mindfulness, emotional regulation, distress tolerance, and interpersonal skills—has been shown to reduce recurrent suicidal and self-harm behavior in personality disordered adults. To date, multiple open and quasi-experimental trials with suicidal adolescents indicate significant reductions in suicidal ideation and behavior among adolescents receiving DBT (for a review, see MacPherson et al. 2013).

Family Interventions

Pineda and Dadds (2013) recently adapted the Resourceful Adolescent Parent Program (RAP-P)—an intervention that aims to target parents' and families' strengths by focusing on managing parental stress, understanding adolescence, and promoting communication—for the parents of suicidal adolescent outpatients. In the randomized study, the addition of RAP-P to usual care was associated with greater reductions in adolescent suicidal behavior than usual care alone, and these decreases were mediated by changes in family functioning.

Diamond et al. (2010) compared attachment-based family therapy (ABFT) with clinical management for suicidal adolescents and found that AFBT resulted in more rapid and complete resolution of suicidal ideation as well as depression.

Harrington et al. (1998) compared a five-session home-based family therapy plus routine care with routine care alone for adolescent suicide attempters. Overall, the home-based family therapy intervention was no better than routine care for reducing ideation or reattempt. However, among the subgroup of suicide attempters in the sample who were not depressed, the home-based treatment reduced suicidal ideation more than did routine care.

Multisystemic Therapy

Huey et al. (2004) compared multisystemic therapy (MST)—an intensive family-based treatment delivered in the patient's natural environment that involves case management and both individual and family treatment—with psychiatric hospitalization and usual care for youth presenting to the emergency room with suicidal ideation, suicide attempt, homicidal ideation, or psychosis. Rates of reattempt were significantly lower in the MST group than in the usual-care group at 1-year follow-up. However, high rates of hospitalization in the MST group render these findings difficult to interpret. Additionally, there were no group differences for suicidal ideation, depression, or hopelessness.

Mentalization-Based Treatment

Rossouw and Fonagy (2012) examined mentalization-based treatment for adolescents (MBT-A), a year-long psychodynamic psychotherapy, versus routine community-based mental health care (treatment as usual [TAU]) for adolescents with self-harm behavior (including both suicidal and nonsuicidal self-injury) and depression. While both groups showed a decline in self-harm behavior with treatment, this effect was greater in the MBT-A group; 43% of the MBT-A group and 68% of the TAU group endorsed self-harm behavior at posttreatment (12 months). MBT-A was also associated with greater reductions in depressive symptoms, with most prominent between-group differences at 9 months.

Youth-Nominated Support Teams

Youth-Nominated Support Team for Suicidal Adolescents (Version 1; YST-1) intervention aims to augment the connection between suicidal adolescents and individuals in their social network by providing psychoeducation to those individuals nominated by suicidal adolescents as supportive (most commonly parents, nonparental relatives, nonadult relatives, peers, teachers) and facilitating weekly contact between the nominated individuals and the suicidal adolescents (King et al. 2006). A randomized study comparing YST-1 plus usual care to usual care alone for adolescents hospitalized for suicidal ideation or attempt found no between-group differences in the rate of suicide attempt. Suicidal ideation declined in both groups, but among girls, the YST-1 group showed a greater decline in suicidal ideation. However, the low (35%) acceptance rate into randomization, as well as the high attrition rate in the experimental condition because of adolescents' unwillingness or inability to involve at least two supportive individuals, may limit the utility of this approach.

Developmental Group Therapy

Wood et al. (2001) compared a six-session skills-based group therapy plus usual care to usual care alone for adolescents who had engaged in at least two episodes of self-harm within the past year. The developmental group therapy approach focused on family conflict, problem solving, interpersonal relationships, anger management, school problems, depression, and hopelessness. As compared with usual care, the experimental treatment group showed an overall reduction in conduct and school problems as well as repeated self-harm episodes.

Skills-Based Therapy

Donaldson et al. (2005) conducted a randomized trial comparing a brief skills-based therapy (SBT), including problem-solving and emotion regulation skills, with supportive relationship therapy (SRT) for adolescent suicide attempters. Both groups showed similar improvements in depression and suicidal ideation. A trend emerged for subjects receiving SBT to have a higher rate of reattempts than those in SRT at 3 and 6 months and a higher dropout rate. This study suggests SRT might be at least as efficacious as the experimental treatment.

School-Based Prevention

Eggert et al. (1995) developed a semester-long personal growth class focused on enhancing protective factors against suicide (e.g., school attendance, self-esteem, personal control, prosocial peer group). They compared the class plus screening for suicidality with a more intensive version of the class (two semesters) and suicidality screening alone. All three groups received school-based case management. Surprisingly, the brief screening intervention was as efficacious as both class interventions in reduction of suicidal ideation and associated risk factors, with one exception: the personal growth class resulted in greater improvements in self-rated personal control. Brief screening and contact with a case manager may be an effective and sufficient intervention to reduce suicidal risk, although this approach awaits replication. One school-based educational intervention, Signs of

Suicide (SOS), was found to reduce the incidence of suicide attempts in high school students by around half (Aseltine et al. 2007). SOS teaches students to recognize signs of suicidal risk, especially depression and alcohol abuse, in themselves and peers, and to seek help or encourage others to do so.

Pharmacological Approaches

No studies have expressly examined the effect of fluoxetine or any other selective serotonin reuptake inhibitors (SSRIs) on impulsive aggression in youth. Findings from the TADS indicate that fluoxetine is superior to placebo for the treatment of depression in youth but is not associated with greater decreases in suicidal ideation. It is important to note, however, that all groups exhibited a significant decrease in suicidal ideation (March et al. 2004). Findings from the Treatment of Resistant Depression in Adolescents (TORDIA) study of teens who did not respond to an adequate initial SSRI trial indicate that switching to a different SSRI was just as efficacious as switching to venlafaxine; there were no differences in rates of suicidality between groups (Brent et al. 2008).

There is concern regarding a possible association between SSRI treatment and emergent suicidality in children and adolescents. Indeed, TADS documented a twofold increase in suicide-related adverse events among youth receiving active medication as compared with those taking placebo. Similarly, the U.S. Food and Drug Administration's meta-analysis of short-term placebo-controlled trials of SSRIs and other antidepressants in youth also indicated an increased risk of suicidal ideation or attempt in patients taking antidepressants. Most commonly, suicidality occurred early in treatment and consisted of increased or new-onset suicidal ideation, with very few suicide attempts and no suicide completions. The mechanism by which SSRIs might increase risk for suicidal behavior is not known; possible explanations include increased irritability and agitation, disinhibition, and potentiation of a mixed state in those with a preexisting bipolar diathesis.

It is imperative to consider the public health implications of these data from a broader perspective. Although causation has not been demonstrated, there is a significant correlation in time between an increase in SSRI prescriptions and sales and a decline in both the overall suicide rate and the suicide rate among adolescents (Ludwig and Marcotte 2005). Additionally, the decrease in SSRI prescriptions following the public health warning of a possible association between SSRIs and suicide in youth was associated with a marked increase in youth suicide in the United States (Gibbons et al. 2007). Furthermore, one meta-analysis supports the assertion that 11 times more depressed youth will show a good clinical response to SSRIs than will become suicidal (Bridge et al. 2007).

Conclusion

The public health implications of youth suicide in this country are serious. Although progress has been made in improving our understanding of risk and protective factors for suicidality in youth, a great deal remains to be known about the effective prevention and treatment of suicidality in this population.

Summary Points

- The strongest predictor of future suicide is a history of suicide attempts.
- The majority of youth who die by suicide have evidence of serious psychopathology, with mood disorders conveying the most potent risk for attempt and completion.
- Psychological factors associated with suicidality include hopelessness and a tendency toward impulsive aggression.
- Assessment of suicidal ideation should include attention to both severity (intent) and pervasiveness (frequency and intensity).
- Assessment with suicidal individuals should include explicit questions regarding plans for self-harm, as well as determination of access to lethal means.
- Clinical management of suicidal youth includes safety planning with the adolescent and family members, means restriction, and inpatient hospitalization when warranted.
- Despite recent concerns regarding increased suicide risk among children and adolescents taking SSRIs, research indicates that more youth will show a good clinical response to SSRIs than will become suicidal.
- Data from psychosocial and pharmacological studies suggest that treatment of depression may not be sufficient to reduce suicidal risk in youth; rather, specific treatments targeting suicidality may be required and may include pharmacological and psychosocial interventions.

References

Aseltine RH Jr, James A, Schilling EA, et al: Evaluating the SOS suicide prevention program: a replication and extension. BMC Public Health 7:161, 2007 17640366

Beautrais AL: Further suicidal behavior among medically serious suicide attempters. Suicide Life Threat Behav 34(1):1–11, 2004 15106883

Boergers J, Spirito A, Donaldson D: Reasons for adolescent suicide attempts: associations with psychological functioning. J Am Acad Child Adolesc Psychiatry 37(12):1287–1293, 1998 9847501

Borowsky IW, Ireland M, Resnick MD: Adolescent suicide attempts: risks and protectors. Pediatrics 107(3):485–493, 2001 11230587

Brent DA: Depression and suicide in children and adolescents. Pediatr Rev 14(10):380–388, 1993 8255818

Brent DA, Bridge J: Firearms availability and suicide: evidence, interventions, and future directions. Am Behav Sci 46(9):1192–1210, 2003

Brent DA, Melhem N: Familial transmission of suicidal behavior. Psychiatr Clin North Am 31(2):157–177, 2008 18439442

Brent DA, Perper JA, Goldstein CE, et al: Risk factors for adolescent suicide. A comparison of adolescent suicide victims with suicidal inpatients. Arch Gen Psychiatry 45(6):581–588, 1988 3377645

Brent DA, Holder D, Kolko D, et al: A clinical psychotherapy trial for adolescent depression comparing cognitive, family, and supportive therapy. Arch Gen Psychiatry 54(9):877–885, 1997 9294380

Brent DA, Baugher M, Bridge J, et al: Age- and sex-related risk factors for adolescent suicide. J Am Acad Child Adolesc Psychiatry 38(12):1497–1505, 1999 10596249

Brent DA, Baugher M, Birmaher B, et al: Compliance with recommendations to remove firearms in families participating in a clinical trial for adolescent depression. J Am Acad Child Adolesc Psychiatry 39(10):1220–1226, 2000 11026174

Brent DA, Emslie GJ, Clarke GN, et al: Switching to another SSRI or to venlafaxine with or without cognitive behavioral therapy for adolescents with SSRI-resistant depression: the TORDIA randomized controlled trial. JAMA 299(8):901–913, 2008 18314433

Brent DA, Poling KD, Goldstein TR: Treating Depressed and Suicidal Adolescents. New York, Guilford, 2011

Bridge JA, Iyengar S, Salary CB, et al: Clinical response and risk for reported suicidal ideation and suicide attempts in pediatric antidepressant treatment: a meta-analysis of randomized controlled trials. JAMA 297(15):1683–1696, 2007 17440145

Carter GL, Clover K, Whyte IM, et al: Postcards from the EDge project: randomised controlled trial of an intervention using postcards to reduce repetition of hospital treated deliberate self-poisoning. BMJ 331(7520):805, 2005 16183654 Epub

Cash SJ, Bridge JA: Epidemiology of youth suicide and suicidal behavior. Curr Opin Pediatr 21(5):613–619, 2009 19644372

Centers for Disease Control and Prevention: Web-based Injury Statistics Query and Reporting System (WISQARS). Atlanta, GA, Centers for Disease Control and Prevention, 2010. Available at: http://www.cdc.gov/ncipc/wisqars. Accessed May 29, 2014.

Diamond GS, Wintersteen MB, Brown GK, et al: Attachment-based family therapy for adolescents with suicidal ideation: a randomized controlled trial. J Am Acad Child Adolesc Psychiatry 49(2):122–131, 2010 20215934

Donaldson D, Spirito A, Esposito-Smythers C: Treatment for adolescents following a suicide attempt: results of a pilot trial. J Am Acad Child Adolesc Psychiatry 44(2):113–120, 2005 15689724

Eaton DK, Kann L, Kinchen S, et al: Youth risk behavior surveillance—United States, 2011. MMWR Surveill Summ 61(4):1–162, 2012 22673000

Eggert LL, Thompson EA, Herting JR, et al: Reducing suicide potential among high-risk youth: tests of a school-based prevention program. Suicide Life Threat Behav 25(2):276–296, 1995 7570788

Emslie G, Kratochvil C, Vitiello B, et al: Treatment for Adolescents with Depression Study (TADS): safety results. J Am Acad Child Adolesc Psychiatry 45(12):1440–1455, 2006 17135989

Esposito-Smythers C, Spirito A, Kahler CW, et al: Treatment of co-occurring substance abuse and suicidality among adolescents: a randomized trial. J Consult Clin Psychol 79(6):728–739, 2011 22004303

Gibbons RD, Brown CH, Hur K, et al: Early evidence on the effects of regulators' suicidality warnings on SSRI prescriptions and suicide in children and adolescents. Am J Psychiatry 164(9):1356–1363, 2007 17728420

Goldston DB, Daniel SS, Reboussin DM, et al: Suicide attempts among formerly hospitalized adolescents: a prospective naturalistic study of risk during the first 5 years after discharge. J Am Acad Child Adolesc Psychiatry 38(6):660–671, 1999 10361783

Goldston DB, Daniel SS, Reboussin BA, et al: Cognitive risk factors and suicide attempts among formerly hospitalized adolescents: a prospective naturalistic study. J Am Acad Child Adolesc Psychiatry 40(1):91–99, 2001 11195570

Harrington R, Kerfoot M, Dyer E, et al: Randomized trial of a home-based family intervention for children who have deliberately poisoned themselves. J Am Acad Child Adolesc Psychiatry 37(5):512–518, 1998 9585653

Huey SJ Jr, Henggeler SW, Rowland MD, et al: Multisystemic therapy effects on attempted suicide by youths presenting psychiatric emergencies. J Am Acad Child Adolesc Psychiatry 43(2):183–190, 2004 14726725

Hultén A, Jiang GX, Wasserman D, et al: Repetition of attempted suicide among teenagers in Europe: frequency, timing and risk factors. Eur Child Adolesc Psychiatry 10(3):161–169, 2001 11596816

King CA, Merchant CR: Social and interpersonal factors relating to adolescent suicidality: a review of the literature. Arch Suicide Res 12(3):181–196, 2008 18576200

King CA, Kramer A, Preuss L, et al: Youth-Nominated Support Team for Suicidal Adolescents (Version 1): a randomized controlled trial. J Consult Clin Psychol 74(1):199–206, 2006 16551158

Kingsbury SJ: Clinical components of suicidal intent in adolescent overdose. J Am Acad Child Adolesc Psychiatry 32(3):518–520, 1993 8496114

Kjelsberg E, Neegaard E, Dahl AA: Suicide in adolescent psychiatric inpatients: incidence and predictive factors. Acta Psychiatr Scand 89(4):235–241, 1994 8023689

Lewinsohn PM, Rohde P, Seeley JR: Adolescent suicidal ideation and attempts: prevalence, risk factors, and clinical implications. Clin Psychol Sci Pract 3(1):25–46, 1996

Lewis LM: No-harm contracts: a review of what we know. Suicide Life Threat Behav 37(1):50–57, 2007 17397279

Ludwig J, Marcotte DE: Anti-depressants, suicide, and drug regulation. J Policy Anal Manage 24(2):249–272, 2005 15776534

MacPherson HA, Cheavens JS, Fristad MA: Dialectical behavior therapy for adolescents: theory, treatment adaptations, and empirical outcomes. Clin Child Fam Psychol Rev 16(1):59–80, 2013 23224757

March J, Silva S, Petrycki S, et al: Fluoxetine, cognitive-behavioral therapy, and their combination for adolescents with depression: Treatment for Adolescents With Depression Study (TADS) randomized controlled trial. JAMA 292(7):807–820, 2004 15315995

Marshal MP, Dietz LJ, Friedman MS, et al: Suicidality and depression disparities between sexual minority and heterosexual youth: a meta-analytic review. J Adolesc Health 49(2):115–123, 2011 21783042

McGirr A, Renaud J, Bureau A, et al: Impulsive-aggressive behaviours and completed suicide across the life cycle: a predisposition for younger age of suicide. Psychol Med 38(3):407–417, 2008 17803833

Melhem NM, Brent DA, Ziegler M, et al: Familial pathways to early onset suicidal behavior: familial and individual antecedents of suicidal behavior. Am J Psychiatry 164(9):1364–1370, 2007 17728421

Nock MK, Green JG, Hwang I, et al: Prevalence, correlates, and treatment of lifetime suicidal behavior among adolescents: results from the National Comorbidity Survey Replication Adolescent Supplement. JAMA Psychiatry 70(3):300–310, 2013 23303463

Pineda J, Dadds MR: Family intervention for adolescents with suicidal behavior: a randomized controlled trial and mediation analysis. J Am Acad Child Adolesc Psychiatry 52(8):851–862, 2013 23880495

Posner K, Oquendo MA, Gould M, et al: Columbia Classification Algorithm of Suicide Assessment (C-CASA): classification of suicidal events in the FDA's pediatric suicidal risk analysis of antidepressants. Am J Psychiatry 164(7):1035–1043, 2007 17606655

Posner K, Brown GK, Stanley B, et al: The Columbia-Suicide Severity Rating Scale: initial validity and internal consistency findings from three multisite studies with adolescents and adults. Am J Psychiatry 168(12):1266–1277, 2011 22193671

Rossouw TI, Fonagy P: Mentalization-based treatment for self-harm in adolescents: a randomized controlled trial. J Am Acad Child Adolesc Psychiatry 51(12):1304–1313, e3, 2012 23200287

Rotheram-Borus MJ, Bradley J: Triage model for suicidal runaways. Am J Orthopsychiatry 61(1):122–127, 1991 2006668

Rotheram-Borus MJ, Piacentini J, Cantwell C, et al: The 18-month impact of an emergency room intervention for adolescent female suicide attempters. J Consult Clin Psychol 68(6):1081–1093, 2000 11142542

Roy A: Family history of suicide and neuroticism: a preliminary study. Psychiatry Res 110(1):87–90, 2002 12007597

Scott KM, Hwang I, Chiu WT, et al: Chronic physical conditions and their association with first onset of suicidal behavior in the world mental health surveys. Psychosom Med 72(7):712–719, 2010 20498290

Shaffer D, Gould MS, Fisher P, et al: Psychiatric diagnosis in child and adolescent suicide. Arch Gen Psychiatry 53(4):339–348, 1996 8634012

Stanley B, Brown G, Brent DA, et al: Cognitive-behavioral therapy for suicide prevention (CBT-SP): treatment model, feasibility, and acceptability. J Am Acad Child Adolesc Psychiatry 48(10):1005–1013, 2009 19730273

Suicide Prevention Resource Center: Best practices registry, 2012. Available at: http://www.sprc.org. Accessed May 29, 2014.

Wagner BM, Silverman MA, Martin CE: Family factors in youth suicidal behaviors. Am Behav Sci 46(9):1171–1191, 2003

Wood A, Trainor G, Rothwell J, et al: Randomized trial of group therapy for repeated deliberate self-harm in adolescents. J Am Acad Child Adolesc Psychiatry 40(11):1246–1253, 2001 11699797

CHAPTER 28

Gender Dysphoria and Nonconformity

Scott Leibowitz, M.D.
Diane Chen, Ph.D.
Marco A. Hidalgo, Ph.D.

Key Concepts and Terminology

This chapter begins with a brief review of key concepts and terminology related to sex, gender, and sexuality. Terminology described and used here mostly reflects that which is defined within the American Academy of Child and Adolescent Psychiatry's Practice Parameter on lesbian, gay, bisexual, transgender, and gender-nonconforming youth (Adelson and American Academy of Child and Adolescent Psychiatry Committee on Quality Issues 2012) unless noted otherwise. It is important to first distinguish sex from gender. An individual's *sex* refers to anatomical aspects associated with reproduction, including reproductive tracts (e.g., vas deferens, fallopian tubes, uterus), gonads (e.g., testes, ovaries), and observed genitalia (e.g., penis, vaginal labia). In most cases, infants are assigned at birth a *natal sex* of male or female on the basis of a physician's visual assessment of their genitalia. The presence of a penis indicates male natal sex, whereas the presence of a vagina indicates female natal sex.

In contrast to sex, *gender identity* refers to an individual's personal sense of self as male or female, which is not assigned but is psychologically rooted. According to cognitive theories of gender development, the majority of children have a sense of gender identity by age 3 years, with most establishing a lifelong male or female gender identity consistent with their natal sex by age 5 or 6 years (Martin et al. 2002). An important aspect of gender is *gender expression,* which refers to the way in which individuals communicate their gender identity within a given culture (American Psychological Association 2009). In North America (and worldwide) social norms dictate that males and females conform to *gender role behavior* defined as personal and social attributes that are recognized as masculine (in males) or feminine (in females). It is important to note that expectations associated with gender expression vary across cultures (e.g., in some cultures men wear kilts, skirts, or waist-wraps) and over time (e.g., women in the United States were once strongly discouraged from wearing trousers).

Gender nonconformity (sometimes used synonymously with *gender variance*) refers to gender role behavior that does not conform to culturally defined norms. Although some individuals communicate their internal sense of gender identity via gender expression, this is not always the case. Others may express gender nonconformity without exhibiting *gender discordance,* which is incongruence between anatomical sex and gender identity. The term *gender dysphoria* refers to the affective disturbance or distress that individuals with gender discordance may experience (Coleman et al. 2011). Gender dysphoria (GD) is also now included in DSM-5[1] (American Psychiatric Association 2013) as a psychiatric disorder. It should be noted that not all individuals with gender discordance experience the affective distress that defines gender dysphoria.

The term *transsexual* describes individuals with gender discordance and gender dysphoria who identify as the "opposite" gender and who may pursue some form of social, medical, and/or surgical gender reassignment to decrease their gender discordance and dysphoria. Because not all gender-variant individuals identify as either male or female, express their gender as exclusively masculine or feminine, or experience gender discordance or dysphoria, transgender has become an intentionally all-inclusive term for individuals who exhibit any combination of gender nonconformity, gender discordance, and/or gender dysphoria, including those formerly described as transsexual (American Psychological Association 2009). *Sexual orientation* refers to the sex of a person "to whom an individual is erotically attracted and comprises several components including sexual fantasy, patterns of physiological arousal, sexual behavior, sexual identity, and social role" (Adelson and American Academy of Child and Adolescent Psychiatry Committee on Quality Issues 2012, p. 6). *Heterosexual* (opposite-gender sexual orientation), *lesbian* (same-gender sexual orientation in females), gay (same-gender sexual orientation in males), and *bisexual* (same- and opposite-gender sexual orientation) are all examples of sexual orientation identities. The acronym *LGBT* (lesbian, gay, bisexual, and transgender) has been used to broadly describe all individuals who fit within these categories of sexual orientation (i.e., LGB) and gender identity/expression (i.e., T). A list of additional relevant terms can be found in Table 28–1.

Clinical Presentations and Diagnostic Classification of Gender

The diagnosis of GD, which is new in DSM-5, comprises separate criteria for children and adolescents/adults (American Psychiatric Association 2013). The criteria for these diagnoses are listed in Box 28–1. Gender identity variants per se are no longer conceptualized as psychiatric pathology. The nomenclature has

[1] Henceforth in this chapter, the abbreviation GD will be used to distinguish the DSM-5 diagnosis of gender dysphoria from the phenomenon of gender dysphoria.

Table 28–1. Terminology related to sex and gender

Disorder/difference of sex development (DSD) Congenital medical conditions in which there is lack of agreement between a person's genetic sex and the appearance of the external or internal reproductive structures. DSDs may include conditions such as congenital adrenal hyperplasia, 46 XY DSD, or hypospadias.

Cisgender Refers to individuals whose affirmed gender matches their natal sex

Genderqueer Refers to individuals who defy all categories of culturally defined gender and prefer to self-identify as gender-free, gender neutral, or completely outside gender; more common in adolescents. The term transcends the male-female gender binary and/or sexual orientation identity labels (Ehrensaft 2012).

Pansexual A colloquial term used by youth who are attracted to individuals along all lines of the gender spectrum, not necessarily within the male-female gender binary

shifted from DSM-IV-TR's classification of gender-specific phenomena as identity *disorders* (American Psychiatric Association 2000) to a state of affective distress for some individuals whose gender identity is incongruent with anatomical aspects of their natal sex. More details of the evolution of these diagnoses since the removal of homosexuality from DSM in 1973 are described by Drescher (2010).

Box 28–1. DSM-5 Diagnostic Criteria for Gender Dysphoria

Gender Dysphoria in Children 302.6 (F64.2)

A. A marked incongruence between one's experienced/expressed gender and assigned gender, of at least 6 months' duration, as manifested by at least six of the following (one of which must be Criterion A1):

1. A strong desire to be of the other gender or an insistence that one is the other gender (or some alternative gender different from one's assigned gender).
2. In boys (assigned gender), a strong preference for cross-dressing or simulating female attire; or in girls (assigned gender), a strong preference for wearing only typical masculine clothing and a strong resistance to the wearing of typical feminine clothing.
3. A strong preference for cross-gender roles in make-believe play or fantasy play.
4. A strong preference for the toys, games, or activities stereotypically used or engaged in by the other gender.
5. A strong preference for playmates of the other gender.
6. In boys (assigned gender), a strong rejection of typically masculine toys, games, and activities and a strong avoidance of rough-and-tumble play; or in girls (assigned gender), a strong rejection of typically feminine toys, games, and activities.
7. A strong dislike of one's sexual anatomy.
8. A strong desire for the primary and/or secondary sex characteristics that match one's experienced gender.

B. The condition is associated with clinically significant distress or impairment in social, school, or other important areas of functioning.

Specify if:

With a disorder of sex development (e.g., a congenital adrenogenital disorder such as 255.2 [E25.0] congenital adrenal hyperplasia or 259.50 [E34.50] androgen insensitivity syndrome).

Coding note: Code the disorder of sex development as well as gender dysphoria.

Gender Dysphoria in Adolescents and Adults **302.85 (F64.1)**

A. A marked incongruence between one's experienced/expressed gender and assigned gender, of at least 6 months' duration, as manifested by at least two of the following:
   1. A marked incongruence between one's experienced/expressed gender and primary and/or secondary sex characteristics (or in young adolescents, the anticipated secondary sex characteristics).
   2. A strong desire to be rid of one's primary and/or secondary sex characteristics because of a marked incongruence with one's experienced/expressed gender (or in young adolescents, a desire to prevent the development of the anticipated secondary sex characteristics).
   3. A strong desire for the primary and/or secondary sex characteristics of the other gender.
   4. A strong desire to be of the other gender (or some alternative gender different from one's assigned gender).
   5. A strong desire to be treated as the other gender (or some alternative gender different from one's assigned gender).
   6. A strong conviction that one has the typical feelings and reactions of the other gender (or some alternative gender different from one's assigned gender).

B. The condition is associated with clinically significant distress or impairment in social, occupational, or other important areas of functioning.

Specify if:

With a disorder of sex development (e.g., a congenital adrenogenital disorder such as 255.2 [E25.0] congenital adrenal hyperplasia or 259.50 [E34.50] androgen insensitivity syndrome).

Coding note: Code the disorder of sex development as well as gender dysphoria.

Specify if:

Posttransition: The individual has transitioned to full-time living in the desired gender (with or without legalization of gender change) and has undergone (or is preparing to have) at least one cross-sex medical procedure or treatment regimen—namely, regular cross-sex hormone treatment or gender reassignment surgery confirming the desired gender (e.g., penectomy, vaginoplasty in a natal male; mastectomy or phalloplasty in a natal female).

Source. Reprinted from the *Diagnostic and Statistical Manual of Mental Disorders,* 5th Edition. Arlington, VA, American Psychiatric Association, 2013. Used with permission. Copyright © American Psychiatric Association.

Gender Variance in Children

Gender-variant children are those who have an affinity for toys, dress, and/or activities that are stereotypically associated with the opposite gender. For natal girls this might include an aversion to wearing dresses or having a feminine hairstyle, a desire to play exclusively with boys, and/or a preference for rough-and-tumble play. For natal boys, this might include an aversion to rough-and-tumble play, a desire to wear stereotypically feminine clothing (e.g., dresses) or simulate a feminine hairstyle, and/or an exclusive preference for female playmates. Some children insistently express a transgender identity, display a preoccupation with anatomical features associated with the opposite gender, and/or experience gender dysphoria. The parents of these children may seek social gender transition (e.g., living fully or partially as the other gender through adoption of a different name and use of different pronouns), although parents vary widely in their degree of acceptance of gender nonconformity. Other gender-variant children may express gender-nonconforming behaviors along with acceptance of their natal sex. While not empirically studied, some children do not fit within the strict male-female gender binary roles that society often reinforces (Ehrensaft 2012). These children may periodically express a desire to be a gender different from that assigned at birth and may lack the persistent insistence that they are, in fact, another gender.

Gender Variance in Adolescents

Gender-variant adolescents may exhibit only gender nonconformity; however, they may also express gender dysphoria that can be precipitated by the phenotypic changes of puberty. For natal males, distress related to gender dysphoria may increase as they grow taller; their shoulders broaden; and they experience growth of body and facial hair, deepening voice, and/or physiological genital changes (e.g., erections). Natal females with gender dysphoria may experience distress due to breast development, onset of menstruation, lack of significantly advancing height, and/or absent facial and body hair. Adolescents with gender dysphoria may exhibit a strong desire to develop physical characteristics associated with the other gender and often seek some form of gender reassignment, which may involve social gender transition, a desire to suppress the further development of secondary sexual characteristics associated with their natal sex (i.e., pubertal suppression), a desire to phenotypically appear and be perceived as their affirmed gender (e.g., by initiating cross-sex hormones such as testosterone or estrogen), and/or desire for future surgical procedures. Other adolescents may wish to be affirmed outside a male-female gender binary model and adopt the use of gender-neutral words when referring to themselves (e.g., their affirmed first name, a plural pronoun set "they/them/their," or the use of other colloquial pronouns such as "ze") (Ehrensaft 2012).

Epidemiology

Epidemiological studies examining sexual orientation estimate that the prevalence of homosexuality (including bisexuality) emerging during adolescence does not exceed 10% across cultures (Hill et al. 2013). Gender identity variants are relatively less understood. Within the United States, no population-based studies have examined the prevalence of gender-variant identity or behavior phenomena in children, adolescents, or adults. Prevalence estimates of adult transsexualism in Asia, Western Europe, and the United States differ among countries and by natal gender, suggesting a range between 1 in 2,900–30,400 natal males and 1 in 8,300–100,000 natal females (American Psychiatric Association 2000; Bakker et al. 1993; Tsoi 1988). These estimates are based on samples comprising only adult transsexuals pursuing hormonal treatment and/or sex reassignment surgery and therefore significantly underestimate the prevalence of the broader phenomenon of gender variance in children and adolescents.

As noted by Zucker and Lawrence (2009), in the absence of epidemiological studies examining childhood gender variance, parent report studies of non-clinic-referred Canadian and Dutch children ages 4–11 years find that natal girls are more often rated as having any behavior "like [the] opposite sex" than are natal boys (8.3% vs. 3.8%) (van Beijsterveldt et al. 2006; Zucker et al. 1997). However, relatively fewer parents report that their children have a strong desire to be of the opposite gender. Rates are similar between natal girls and boys (around 1.0%). In treatment referral rates in children, natal gender differences are found. Natal boys are more often referred for treatment in the context of gender variance than natal girls (ratio of 5.78–2.9:1) (Cohen-Kettenis et al. 2003). Adolescent rates of referral are lower and nearly equal (1.75:1 natal boys to natal girls) (Cohen-Kettenis and Pfäfflin 2003 as cited by Zucker and Lawrence 2009).

Mental Health Vulnerabilities for LGBT Youth and Comorbidity with Gender Dysphoria

LGBT individuals are exposed to bias and discrimination within society in general and in health care settings at much higher rates than the general population (Graham et al. 2011). For youth, this is particularly challenging given that LGBT adolescents face psychosocial challenges associated with identity exploration and physical maturation. A report by the Institute of Medicine (Graham et al. 2011) summarized the poor health outcomes observed among LGBT youth, including higher rates of suicidal ideation, nonsuicidal self-injury, suicide attempts, mental health disorders (e.g., anxiety and depression), and health risk behaviors (e.g., substance abuse, high-risk sexual behaviors that could lead to sexually transmitted disease). Within the last decade, there has been a conceptual shift to attribute these associations to the result of psychosocial challenges, including rejection, discrimination, victimization, and bias.

Youth who are, or are perceived to be, LGBT, including those who are gender-nonconforming, are at increased risk for bullying, peer nonacceptance, and family rejection (Ryan et al. 2009; Toomey et al. 2010). Among LGB youth, those who come from "rejecting families" are at an eight to nine times greater risk for suicidal behavior and have significantly increased risk for illegal drug use, unprotected sex, and depression when compared with LGB youth whose families are not rejecting (Ryan et al. 2009).

Given the adversity they may experience because of their gender expression, gender-nonconforming children are susceptible to the development of psychological symptoms, regardless of the presence or absence of gender dysphoria. For example, studies have found that gender-nonconforming youth who are subject to psychological abuse in childhood are at increased risk for depression (Roberts et al. 2013) and have increased rates of major depression and suicidality in adolescence (Nuttbrock et al. 2010) and that when victimized in school, these youth have lower rates of life satisfaction in young adulthood (Toomey et al. 2010). About 50% of children (Wallien et al. 2007) and adolescents (Spack et al. 2012) with gender dysphoria who presented for care at specialized gender identity clinics who met diagnostic criteria for DSM-IV-TR gender identity disorder (GID) also met diagnostic criteria for at least one comorbid psychiatric illness. Across childhood and adolescence, internalizing disorders such as anxiety disorders predominate (Cohen-Kettenis et al. 2003; de Vries et al. 2011; Spack et al. 2012; Zucker and Bradley 1995). When externalizing disorders were present, children were at higher risk of social ostracism (Wallien et al. 2007). Among adolescents with GID, increased risk of suicidality (Grossman and D'Augelli 2007) and self-mutilation (Spack et al. 2012) have been observed. Interestingly, recent research has found a higher than expected rate of gender variance among children presenting to a neurodevelopmental clinic for treatment related to autism spectrum disorder (ASD) and attention-deficit/hyperactivity disorder (Strang et al. 2014) as well as approximately eight times greater prevalence of ASD in gender-variant children presenting to a specialized gender clinic than in the general population (de Vries et al. 2010). The coexistence of ASD and gender dysphoria introduces additional clinical complexity in decision making, particularly when these adolescents seek irreversible medical interventions such as cross-sex hormone therapy.

Overview of Gender and Sexuality Development

According to prospective research on trajectories of childhood gender variance, gender dysphoria "desists" during early adolescence in the majority of youth. These youth as adults are more likely to express a gender identity consistent with their natal sex and more often identify as gay, lesbian, or bisexual than as heterosexual (Steensma et al. 2013; van Beijsterveldt et al. 2006; Wallien and Cohen-Kettenis 2008; Zucker and Bradley 1995; Zucker and Lawrence 2009). Adolescents for whom gender dysphoria does not desist around puberty are more likely to experience persistent gender dysphoria into adulthood (de Vries and Cohen-Kettenis 2012). While additional research is needed to more fully understand gender development in gender-variant youth, recent findings from a clinic-referred sample of youth in the Netherlands highlight possible childhood markers of subsequent young adulthood transgender identity. Transgenderism in early adulthood may be predicted by a high degree of childhood gender dysphoria that persists into adolescence, as well as a child's cognitive ("I am a [girl/boy]") versus affective ("I feel like or wish I was a [girl/boy]") statements regarding gender (Steensma et al. 2011, 2013).

Research examining the etiology of gender-variant phenomena in adults, including gender dysphoria, has explored both psychological and biological underpinnings. Psychological research examining factors such as parental involvement and coping with extreme childhood trauma has been inconclusive. While studies examining in utero exposure to sex hormones have also been inconclusive, preliminary magnetic resonance imaging research shows similarities in the brains of adult male-to-female transsexual individuals with cisgender natal females (Luders et al. 2009). This research is more thoroughly reviewed by Sánchez and Vilain (2013).

Assessment

Comprehensive assessment of gender-variant children and adolescents should be multimethod and multi-informant in nature. A clinical interview should include the child or adolescent and parents, both together and separately, focused on obtaining the necessary information to ascertain if GD is present, to consider differential diagnosis and comorbidity, and to observe the parent-child relationship. Table 28–2 highlights the key assessment aims across developmental periods. In addition to assessing gender development and the diagnostic

TABLE 28–2. Assessment aims for gender-variant youth

Patient population	Assessment aims
All gender-variant youth	Criteria for DSM-5 diagnosis of gender dysphoria (GD)
	General psychiatric and psychological functioning
	Degree of family support and/or rejection
	Presence of positive peer relationships and/or bullying
	School environment
	Positive and negative coping strategies
	Pronoun and name preference across various situations
Gender-variant children and their families	Degree of social gender transition (pronoun, name, clothing) across different settings
	How the child understands the meaning of gender (consistent with developmental stage)
	Degree of parent/guardian ability to affirm child's gender identity while allowing for open-ended exploration of future identity trajectories
Gender-variant adolescents and their families	Degree of distress (or lack thereof) resulting from maturing anatomical features that denote gender (secondary sexual characteristics)
	Sexual identity and behavior history and how this intertwines with gender
	Early gender development history
	Desire (or lack thereof) for medical gender transition interventions
	Pubertal stage (by pediatrician) to determine if medical interventions are indicated to alleviate dysphoria
	Ability to assent to medical gender transition interventions if they are indicated to alleviate dysphoria

criteria for GD, a general evaluation of emotional, behavioral, social, and cognitive functioning to determine whether comorbid psychopathology is present is recommended (Coleman et al. 2011). Ideally, questions are worded in a way that is both affirming (i.e., conveys implied empathic acceptance of all variants of gender expression and identity) and lacking assumptions of a monolithic gender identity end goal (i.e., conveys open-ended possibilities for current and future identifications). Table 28–3 includes examples of questions that could be asked in both the presence and absence of the parents or guardians.

Among those children who meet diagnostic criteria for GD, particular care should be given to assessing how long the child has asserted a cross-gender identity (persistence), degree of cross-gender identification across contexts and situations (consistency), degree of emphatic assertion of a cross-gender identity (insistence), and the perspective of cross-gender assertions (cognitive vs. affective), as these factors have been implicated in differentiating between gender dysphoric children and children who are gender nonconforming in behavior and preferences but accepting of their assigned natal gender (Ehrensaft 2012; Steensma et al. 2011).

When a gender-variant adolescent presents in clinical practice, assessing for the presence of gender dysphoria (or diagnostic criteria of GD) is important in the development of an appropriate treatment plan. If an adolescent meets criteria for GD, particular importance should be paid to detecting comorbid psychiatric diagnoses that 1) may affect the adolescent's ability to accurately describe the presence of gender dysphoria (e.g., comorbid ASD, active psychosis), 2) are not well controlled (e.g., active suicidality or mania) and might impair the ability to provide informed consent for appropriate medical interventions, and 3) may be secondary to GD and thus might be improved by social gender transition and/or hormonal interventions.

There are no specific laboratory tests or imaging procedures that can detect the presence or absence of gender dysphoria. However, should a diagnosis of GD be made, a careful physical examination by a pediatrician to evaluate the stage of phenotypic pubertal advancement would be helpful in determining the appropriateness of various hormonal interventions.

Psychometric Measures Across Development

Standardized measures have been developed to systematically assess the diagnostic criteria for GD/GID for both prepubertal children and adolescents (for a comprehensive review, see Zucker 2005). For prepubertal children, these measures include interviews (e.g., Gender Identity Interview for Children [Zucker et al. 1993]) and projective tests (e.g., Draw-A-Person [Zucker et al. 1983]) administered to the child, parent-report questionnaires assessing gender expression (e.g., Gender Identity Questionnaire for Children [Johnson et al. 2004]), and free play observation that facilitates the use of toys and clothing. These measures provide a more dimensional picture of a child's clinical presentation (i.e., degree and intensity of gender nonconformity and/or gender dysphoria) and can be used to complement the standard clinical interview, which focuses on assessing the presence or absence of symptom criteria from a categorical perspective.

Dimensional assessments are particularly relevant given research findings suggesting that severity or intensity of

TABLE 28–3. Common scenarios and suggested questions when assessing gender-variant adolescents

Scenario	Initial questions or statements for parents and adolescents presenting with gender issues
Parent(s) in either the presence or absence of the adolescent	"What would be the most appropriate name to refer to your child/adolescent?"
	"What gender does [patient name] most identify as?"
	"What gender pronoun do you feel most comfortable with me using to refer to your child/adolescent?"
	"Has [patient name] expressed any verbal desire to live life as an alternative gender? If so, please describe the statements/desires."
	"Has [name of patient] expressed any dissatisfaction with aspects of his/her [use pronoun that parent feels most comfortable with] anatomy/body? If so, what are they?"
Adolescent in the presence of the parent(s)	"I will have a chance to also ask you these questions without your parent(s), if you feel that would be helpful."
	"What name for yourself do you feel most comfortable being used in front of your parents?"
	"What pronoun do you feel most comfortable with me using in front of your parents?"
Adolescent without the parent(s) present	Name and pronoun questions:
	"What name for yourself do you feel most comfortable with?"
	What name should I use when we're meeting with your parents?"
	"How else might this change depending on who you are with?"
	"Which gender pronouns do you feel most comfortable being used to refer to you?"
	"What gender pronouns should I use when we're meeting with your parents?"
	"How else might this change depending on who is referring to you or whom you are with?"
	Gender questions:
	"What gender do you feel most comfortable identifying as?"
	"Are there aspects of the gender you were assigned since birth that you are comfortable with?"
	"Are there aspects of the gender you were assigned since birth that you are not comfortable with?"
	"Have you thought about living life as a different gender?"
	Body image questions:
	"Are there aspects of your body that you are not comfortable with or wish you could change?"
	"Are there physical aspects of another gender that you wish you could have?"

childhood gender dysphoria is predictive of persistence of these feelings into adolescence (Steensma et al. 2013; Wallien and Cohen-Kettenis 2008). Recent research has supported the predictive validity of the Gender Identity Interview for Children (GIIC; Steensma et al. 2013). The GIIC is a 12-item child informant instrument that measures two factors: cognitive gender confusion and affective gender confusion (Zucker et al. 1993). *Cognitive gender confusion* is assessed by four questions asking whether the child identifies as a boy or a girl (e.g., "When you grow up, will you be a mommy or a daddy?"). *Affective gender confusion* is assessed by eight questions such as "Are there things that you don't like about being a boy?" Higher levels of both cognitive gender confusion and affective gender confusion predicted persistence of gender dysphoria into adolescence (i.e., continuing to meet diagnostic criteria for GID) (N=127, n=47 persisters, n=80 desisters) with cognitive responses to the GIIC identified as the strongest predictor, accounting for 11% of the unique variability in persistence of gender dysphoria. This finding is consistent with published clinical case studies differentiating between gender variant children who most often declare they *are* an alternative gender from those who *wish to be* or *feel like* an alternative gender (Ehrensaft 2012).

Therapeutic Intervention and Treatment Planning

Gender-variant youth presenting for clinical care have treatment needs that vary according to their developmental stage. Generally accepted approaches are summarized in the Standards of Care of the World Professional Association for Transgender Health (Coleman et al. 2011). Four overarching points are relevant to the clinical approach toward gender-variant youth. First, there has been an ideological and clinical shift in the treatment of transgender adults from that of the *gatekeeper model* (i.e., all patients must see a mental health clinician to obtain clearance for the initiation of medical interventions) to an *informed consent model* (i.e., mental health evaluation is not necessary for patients with the cognitive capacity to provide informed consent for hormonal interventions) (Ehrbar and Gorton 2010). Second, interventions that are sometimes viewed as controversial (e.g., prepubertal social gender transition, pubertal suppression in younger adolescents) have increased in acceptance by some clinicians over the past decade (Radix and Silva 2014). Third, for children and adolescents there is increased reliance on approaches that facilitate emotional adjustment by supporting the child's affirmed gender identity (Hidalgo et al. 2013). With these *affirming approaches* increasing in use, there is sometimes debate as to how to strike the optimal balance between taking the (limited) scientific evidence base into account in clinical decision making while concurrently providing care that is affirming and supportive. Fourth, it is important to create a welcoming clinical experience for the treatment of gender-variant youth. Table 28–4 provides suggestions for clinicians.

Clinical Approaches to Gender Variance in Childhood

Evidence-based treatments for prepubertal children with GD have not been established. The literature has focused on three alternative theoretical

TABLE 28–4. Creating a welcoming office for gender dysphoric and/or nonconforming youth

Establish a system in which all staff are able to know and use the correct name and pronoun when interacting with patients (when different from the legal name and natal sex listed in the medical record).
Add a narrative "Name and Pronoun Use" section in the beginning of a note when documenting in the medical record if the name and pronoun differ from the legal name listed in the medical record.
Use the appropriate name and pronoun in documentation when referring to an individual.
Use the appropriate name in all supporting clinic materials, such as appointment cards.
Work with the pharmacist to determine the possibility of including a patient's preferred name on the medication bottle (when it differs from the legal name).
Provide a dedicated bathroom that can be used for individuals of any gender. If this is not possible, provide clear signage indicating that patients are welcome to use the bathroom assigned to their affirmed gender identity.

approaches. The first is to consider reducing gender dysphoria (and improving social acceptance) by actively using behavioral techniques (e.g., setting limits on cross-gender behaviors, encouraging gender-normative play and preferences, promoting same-sex peer relationships) to align gender expression with the child's natal sex (Zucker et al. 2012). Inherent in this approach are the beliefs that preventing adult transgenderism reduces subsequent psychosocial adversity and the need for hormonal/surgical interventions and that gender identity in childhood is malleable.

The second theoretical approach is to focus treatment on targeting concomitant emotional, behavioral, and family problems that may or may not be related to a child's gender dysphoria and "wait and see" how gender identity unfolds after the onset of puberty, neither encouraging nor discouraging cross-gender expression (de Vries and Cohen-Kettenis 2012; Menvielle 2012). Central to this approach is the belief that although gender variance is not "disordered," gender identity cannot be reliably determined among prepubertal children.

The third described approach is to assist children with GD who have been insistent, persistent, and consistent in asserting a cross-gender identity and their families in engaging in developmentally appropriate gender transition interventions, including prepubertal social gender transition (Ehrensaft 2012; Hidalgo et al. 2013). Prepubertal social gender transition refers to adoption of the affirmed cross-gender role, which may include the use of a preferred name and gender pronoun in some or all contexts. Major premises informing this third approach include the belief that gender variations are not disorders, that gender may be fluid and nonbinary, and that it is possible to differentiate children who will persist in asserting a transgender identity from children who are exploring gender nonconforming expressions but accept their assigned gender. It is important to note that prepubertal social gender transition is controversial, even among specialists treating these children (Leibowitz and Telingator 2012). Some clinicians believe that children who are perceived by their peers in the gender role that they affirm will experience less stigma and discrimination, which may have a positive impact on a child's self-esteem and minimize developing comorbid psychopathology. Alternatively, other clinicians believe that assisting children in developing coping strategies to manage varying degrees of stigma, bullying, and victimization would be less harmful than risking the possibility of a second social transition in adolescence back to the natal sex, given the high rate of desistance of childhood gender dysphoria. Additionally, the degree to which a socially transitioned child feels shame as a result of suppressing or hiding his or her natal sex has not been studied. Research evidence is lacking to support any one approach to prepubertal social gender transition, despite the increasing prevalence of children with gender dysphoria initially presenting for clinical care who have already socially transitioned and initial evidence that prepubertal social gender transition predicts persisting gender dysphoria among natal males (Steensma et al. 2013).

The lack of evidence-based treatment options for prepubertal gender-variant children highlights the need for nuanced decision making by the clinician. Regardless of the theoretical approach, Leibowitz and Telingator (2012) recommend that treatment be individualized for each child and family, recognizing the developmental capacity of the child and determining the child's understanding of the meaning of gender before making absolute intervention decisions. Treatment of prepubertal gender-variant children should aim to increase flexibility and coping strategies among children who are contending with invalidating relationships and environments by helping the child understand how others may be responding to his or her perceived gender. Facilitating parents' acceptance of gender nonconformity and tolerance of the ambiguity of their child's gender identity trajectory is key. Additionally, helping the child and parents negotiate the social complexities that result from an alternative gender identification and advocating for youth legally and in schools is often required (Adelson and American Academy of Child and Adolescent Psychiatry Committee on Quality Issues 2012).

Clinical Approaches to Gender Variance in Adolescence

Promoting positive health outcomes for gender-variant adolescents should focus on improving self-esteem and coping strategies, open-ended identity exploration, and consideration of external factors that include working with schools and family members (Adelson and American Academy of Child and Adolescent Psychiatry Committee on Quality Issues 2012). There is no evidence to suggest that encouraging an adolescent to suppress or change internal aspects of self, such as sexual orientation or gender identity, through "corrective" approaches rooted in behavioral modification is effective, and in fact this type of treatment intervention has been deemed harmful (Adelson and American Academy of Child and Adolescent Psychiatry Committee on Quality Issues 2012). Family members who may be struggling to accept their gender-nonconforming adolescent may benefit from a referral for that individual to work with his or her own therapist. Combining supportive individual, family, and parent guidance techniques may be useful in the approach to youth with gender nonconformity (Malpas 2011). Connecting adolescents to groups of other gender-nonconforming youth can also be helpful (Menvielle 2012). Clinical guidelines recommend that the clinician be familiar with community resources for LGBT youth (Adelson and American

Academy of Child and Adolescent Psychiatry Committee on Quality Issues 2012). For adolescents who meet the DSM-5 criteria for GD, additional treatment goals should be considered, in addition to those aims described for the broader population of gender-nonconforming adolescents. Many of these adolescents seek gender reassignment, requiring the clinician to be familiar with the various therapeutic options used to treat GD.

Social Gender Transition

Initiating social gender transition, including using the name and pronouns of the adolescent's affirmed gender, can help the adolescent feel supported and correctly perceived by others. This can be particularly helpful for exploring and/or ambivalent adolescents who might be seeking cues from their environment to help them recognize the degree to which living in their affirmed gender makes sense. When framed as supportive measures, these completely reversible interventions may also help ambivalent parents feel they are participating in their adolescent's gender identity exploration prior to using any form of irreversible hormonal intervention. Further ways to explore social gender transition include simulating the physical appearance of the affirmed gender through use of breast binders (for natal females) or breast pads (for natal males) and/or wearing the clothing of the affirmed gender. Sometimes, initial exploration may take place within the confines of the office to minimize fear, shame, and/or any unsafe outcomes.

Pubertal Suppression Therapy

Pubertal suppression, a medical intervention first implemented and studied in the Netherlands, relies on gonadotropin-releasing hormone agonists to suppress the development of distressing secondary sexual characteristics of the youth's natal sex. This intervention allows transgender adolescents who have matured to at least Tanner stage 2 to "buy time" to explore their gender identity before the initiation of partially or fully irreversible medical interventions (e.g., cross-sex hormones and/or surgical procedures) (Delemarre-van de Waal and Cohen-Kettenis 2006). Largely not covered by insurance in the United States, pubertal suppression can be quite costly; however, it is associated with positive psychiatric outcomes and ultimately may prevent the need for more invasive procedures (e.g., mastectomy) while promoting a more natural phenotypic appearance in the affirmed gender later on. A recent study demonstrated that when provided with ongoing psychological support during the transition, life satisfaction among a sample of young adults previously treated with pubertal suppression who are now post–gender confirmation surgery was equal to that of the general population (de Vries et al. 2014). The ability to appear as one's affirmed gender is associated with better psychiatric outcomes for transgender adults (Lawrence 2003). Careful consideration of the risks and benefits of pubertal suppression are important for the mental health clinician and multidisciplinary collaborators (endocrine, primary care, surgical).

Cross-Sex Hormone Therapy

Cross-sex hormones (i.e., estrogen for natal males and testosterone for natal females) are partially irreversible interventions that promote the development of secondary sex characteristics of the desired gender, historically used for adolescents age 16 years or older after they have explored the issues in depth within a behavioral health setting. The World Professional Association of Transgender Health Standards of Care, seventh edition (WPATH SOC7; Coleman et al. 2011) specifies the indications, risks, and benefits of cross-sex hormone therapy. Some clinics are recommending the intervention at younger ages, especially since the use of pubertal suppression in younger adolescents has increased in recent years (Olson et al. 2011; Steever 2014). Waiting until late adolescence to initiate cross-sex hormone therapy among those receiving pubertal suppression delays the important effects of sex hormones (e.g., bone development, potential effects on brain development) and ignores the potential importance of going through puberty concurrently with peers. Optimally, an adolescent would be referred for cross-sex hormone therapy only after comprehensive psychiatric assessment to ensure that the adolescent meets criteria for GD, has proper psychosocial supports in place, has any psychiatric comorbid conditions reasonably well controlled, and can understand the irreversible aspects of treatment (including possible infertility) and risks associated with treatment. When the clinical presentation lacks clarity, an important question to consider would be whether or not implementing cross-sex hormones might perpetuate or exacerbate any comorbid psychiatric conditions. Per WPATH SOC7, it is reasonable to attempt to achieve relative psychiatric stability prior to referring for cross-sex hormone treatment.

Surgical Interventions

Irreversible surgical procedures (such as metoidoplasty, phalloplasty, and vaginoplasty) are sometimes beneficial for transgender adults when transitioning to the sex that is consistent with their gender identity (Coleman et al. 2011). While potentially beneficial, some of the procedures are not ideal, and most of them have limitations and associated risks. In natal females, mastectomy (also referred to as "top surgery") has been performed for adolescents younger than age 18, particularly when this aspect of body dysphoria causes significant distress. Clinicians should not assume that all adolescents with gender dysphoria desire to pursue such interventions.

Summary Points

- Phenomenology, outcome, and approaches to assessment and treatment of gender-variant youth differ between children and adolescents. Assessing for the presence of gender dysphoria in a gender-nonconforming child or adolescent is essential for treatment planning.
- Social gender transition for prepubertal children is a controversial intervention, and a nuanced and individualized approach is required when guiding families who are considering this option.

- Medical interventions for adolescents with gender dysphoria include pubertal suppression for younger adolescents and cross-sex hormones for older adolescents. The most common surgical intervention in this age group is a mastectomy in natal females with gender dysphoria.
- Supportive and affirming approaches include minimizing shame, supporting a child or adolescent to openly explore the affirmed gender, and promoting family support.
- LGBT youth require advocacy efforts on many levels that include connection to community LGBT youth resources and coordination with schools to promote safe learning environments.

References

Adelson SL, American Academy of Child and Adolescent Psychiatry Committee on Quality Issues: Practice parameter on gay, lesbian, or bisexual sexual orientation, gender nonconformity, and gender discordance in children and adolescents. J Am Acad Child Adolesc Psychiatry 51(9):957–974, 2012 22917211

American Psychiatric Association: Diagnostic and Statistical Manual of Mental Disorders, 4th Edition, Text Revision. Washington, DC, American Psychiatric Association, 2000

American Psychiatric Association: Diagnostic and Statistical Manual of Mental Disorders, 5th Edition. Arlington, VA, American Psychiatric Association, 2013

American Psychological Association: Report of the American Psychological Association Task Force on Gender Identity and Gender Variance. Washington, DC, American Psychological Association, 2009

Bakker A, van Kesteren PJM, Gooren LJG, et al: The prevalence of transsexualism in The Netherlands. Acta Psychiatr Scand 87(4):237–238, 1993 8488743

Cohen-Kettenis PT, Pfäfflin F: Transgenderism and Intersexuality in Childhood and Adolescence: Making Choices. Thousand Oaks, CA, Sage, 2003

Cohen-Kettenis PT, Owen A, Kaijser VG, et al: Demographic characteristics, social competence, and behavior problems in children with gender identity disorder: a cross-national, cross-clinic comparative analysis. J Abnorm Child Psychol 31(1):41–53, 2003 12597698

Coleman E, Bockting W, Botzer M, et al: Standards of care for the health of a transsexual, transgender and gender non-conforming people, version 7. International Journal of Transgenderism 13:165–232, 2011, www.wpath.org

Delemarre-van de Waal HA, Cohen-Kettenis PT: Clinical management of gender identity disorder in adolescents: a protocol on psychological and paediatric endocrinology aspects. Eur J Endocrinol 155(suppl 1):S131–S137, 2006

de Vries ALC, Cohen-Kettenis PT: Clinical management of gender dysphoria in children and adolescents: the Dutch approach. J Homosex 59(3):301–320, 2012 22455322

de Vries ALC, Noens ILJ, Cohen-Kettenis PT, et al: Autism spectrum disorders in gender dysphoric children and adolescents. J Autism Dev Disord 40(8):930–936, 2010 20094764

de Vries ALC, Doreleijers TAH, Steensma TD, et al: Psychiatric comorbidity in gender dysphoric adolescents. J Child Psychol Psychiatry 52(11):1195–1202, 2011 21671938

de Vries ALC, McGuire J, Steensma T, et al: Young adult psychological outcome after puberty suppression and gender reassignment. Pediatrics 134(4):696–704, 2014

Drescher J: Queer diagnoses: parallels and contrasts in the history of homosexuality, gender variance, and the diagnostic and statistical manual. Arch Sex Behav 39(2):427–460, 2010 19838785

Ehrbar RD, Gorton RN: Exploring provider treatment models in interpreting the standards of care. International Journal of Transgenderism 12:198–201, 2010

Ehrensaft D: From gender identity disorder to gender identity creativity: true gender self child therapy. J Homosex 59(3):337–356, 2012 22455324

Graham R, Berkowitz B, Blum R, et al: The Health of Lesbian, Gay, Bisexual, and Transgender People: Building a Foundation for Better Understanding. Washington, DC, Institute of Medicine of the National Academies, 2011

Grossman AH, D'Augelli AR: Transgender youth and life-threatening behaviors. Suicide Life Threat Behav 37(5):527–537, 2007 17967119

Hidalgo MA, Ehrensaft D, Tishelman AC, et al: The gender affirmative model: what we know and what we aim to learn. Hum Dev 56(5):285–290, 2013

Hill AK, Dawood K, Puts DA: Biological foundations of sexual orientation, in The Handbook of Psychology and Sexual Orientation. Edited by Patterson CJ, D'Augelli AR. New York, Oxford University Press, 2013, pp 55–68

Johnson LL, Bradley SJ, Birkenfeld-Adams AS, et al: A parent-report gender identity questionnaire for children. Arch Sex Behav 33(2):105–116, 2004 15146143

Lawrence AA: Factors associated with satisfaction or regret following male-to-female sex reassignment surgery. Arch Sex Behav 32(4):299–315, 2003 12856892

Leibowitz SF, Telingator C: Assessing gender identity concerns in children and adolescents: evaluation, treatments, and outcomes. Curr Psychiatry Rep 14(2):111–120, 2012 22367419

Luders E, Sánchez FJ, Gaser C, et al: Regional gray matter variation in male-to-female transsexualism. Neuroimage 46(4):904–907, 2009 19341803

Malpas J: Between pink and blue: a multidimensional family approach to gender nonconforming children and their families. Fam Process 50(4):453–470, 2011 22145719

Martin CL, Ruble DN, Szkrybalo J: Cognitive theories of early gender development. Psychol Bull 128(6):903–933, 2002 12405137

Menvielle E: A comprehensive program for children with gender variant behaviors and gender identity disorders. J Homosex 59(3):357–368, 2012 22455325

Nuttbrock L, Hwahng S, Bockting W, et al: Psychiatric impact of gender-related abuse across the life course of male-to-female transgender persons. J Sex Res 47(1):12–23, 2010 19568976

Olson J, Forbes C, Belzer M: Management of the transgender adolescent. Arch Pediatr Adolesc Med 165(2):171–176, 2011 21300658

Radix A, Silva M: Beyond the guidelines: challenges, controversies, and unanswered questions. Pediatr Ann 43(6):e145–e150, 2014 24972423

Roberts AL, Rosario M, Slopen N, et al: Childhood gender nonconformity, bullying victimization, and depressive symptoms across adolescence and early adulthood: an 11-year longitudinal study. J Am Acad Child Adolesc Psychiatry 52(2):143–152, 2013 23357441

Ryan C, Huebner D, Diaz RM, et al: Family rejection as a predictor of negative health outcomes in white and Latino lesbian, gay, and bisexual young adults. Pediatrics 123(1):346–352, 2009 19117902

Sánchez FJ, Vilain E: Transgender identities: research and controversies, in The Handbook of Psychology and Sexual Orientation. Edited by Patterson CJ, D'Augelli AR. New York, Oxford University Press, 2013, pp 42–54

Spack NP, Edwards-Leeper L, Feldman HA, et al: Children and adolescents with gender identity disorder referred to a pediatric medical center. Pediatrics 129(3):418–425, 2012 22351896

Steensma TD, Biemond R, de Boer F, et al: Desisting and persisting gender dysphoria after childhood: a qualitative follow-up study. Clin Child Psychol Psychiatry 16(4):499–516, 2011 21216800

Steensma TD, McGuire JK, Kreukels BPC, et al: Factors associated with desistence and persistence of childhood gender dysphoria: a quantitative follow-up study. J Am Acad Child Adolesc Psychiatry 52(6):582–590, 2013 23702447

Steever J: Cross-gender hormone therapy in adolescents. Pediatr Ann 43(6):e138–e144, 2014 24972422

Strang JF, Kenworthy L, Dominska A, et al: Increased gender variance in autism spectrum disorders and attention deficit hyperactivity disorder. Arch Sex Behav 43(8):1525–1533, 2014 24619651

Toomey RB, Ryan C, Diaz RM, et al: Gender-nonconforming lesbian, gay, bisexual, and transgender youth: school victimization and young adult psychosocial adjustment. Dev Psychol 46(6):1580–1589, 2010 20822214

Tsoi WF: The prevalence of transsexualism in Singapore. Acta Psychiatr Scand 78(4):501–504, 1988 3265846

van Beijsterveldt CEM, Hudziak JJ, Boomsma DI: Genetic and environmental influences on cross-gender behavior and relation to behavior problems: a study of Dutch twins at ages 7 and 10 years. Arch Sex Behav 35(6):647–658, 2006 17109235

Wallien MS, Swaab H, Cohen-Kettenis PT: Psychiatric comorbidity among children with gender identity disorder. J Am Acad Child Adolesc Psychiatry 46(10):1307–1314, 2007 17885572

Wallien MSC, Cohen-Kettenis PT: Psychosexual outcome of gender-dysphoric children. J Am Acad Child Adolesc Psychiatry 47(12):1413–1423, 2008 18981931

Zucker KJ: Measurement of psychosexual differentiation. Arch Sex Behav 34(4):375–388, 2005 16010461

Zucker KJ, Bradley SJ: Gender Identity Disorder and Psychosexual Problems in Children and Adolescents. New York, Guilford, 1995

Zucker KJ, Lawrence AA: Epidemiology of Gender Identity Disorder: recommendations for the Standards of Care of the World Professional Association for Transgender Health. Int J Transgenderism 11:8–18, 2009

Zucker KJ, Finegan JA, Doering RW, et al: Human figure drawings of gender-problem children: a comparison to sibling, psychiatric, and normal controls. J Abnorm Child Psychol 11(2):287–298, 1983 6352776

Zucker KJ, Bradley SJ, Sullivan CB, et al: A gender identity interview for children. J Pers Assess 61(3):443–456, 1993 8295110

Zucker KJ, Bradley SJ, Sanikhani M: Sex differences in referral rates of children with gender identity disorder: some hypotheses. J Abnorm Child Psychol 25(3):217–227, 1997 9212374

Zucker KJ, Wood H, Singh D, et al: A developmental, biopsychosocial model for the treatment of children with gender identity disorder. J Homosex 59(3):369–397, 2012 22455326

CHAPTER 29

Aggression and Violence

Jeffrey H. Newcorn, M.D.
Iliyan Ivanov, M.D.
Anil Chacko, Ph.D.
Shabnam Javdani, Ph.D.

Aggression is one of the most frequent indications for child and adolescent psychiatric referral, often in association with severe and urgent symptoms—yet aggression is a normal behavior, present in all people to some extent. The nature, meaning, and prevalence of aggression in children differ as a function of developmental level and context, and it is important to distinguish *pathological, maladaptive,* or *antisocial* manifestations of aggression from *prosocial* or adaptive behaviors (e.g., self-defense). Aggression is generally considered to be a highly stable behavioral trait. Nevertheless, only half of school-age children who are aggressive continue to manifest this behavior in adolescence. When aggression persists, it is highly impairing and often carries severe consequences for academic achievement and occupational attainment, family and peer relationships, and psychological development, as well as risk for dire outcomes—including antisocial personality disorder, substance abuse, and criminality.

Definition and Clinical Description

Pathological or maladaptive aggression occurs outside an expectable social context and occurs in the absence of antecedent social cues and/or with an intensity, frequency, duration, and/or severity that is disproportionate to its causes. It generally does not terminate in an appropriate time frame and/or in response to feedback. Pathological aggression can occur in the context of specific psychiatric disorders, or it can be a nonspecific manifestation of anger or frustration. Numerous subtypes of aggression have been described, but most classification schemes dichotomize aggression with respect to the ability to modulate and control the behavior and/

or the intended goal. Examples of subtypes include the following:

- *Proactive* (i.e., goal-directed, usually associated with leadership skills and positive peer perceptions) versus *reactive* (i.e., responding to a threat, retaliating)
- *Predatory* (i.e., deliberate, controlled) versus *affective* (i.e., impetuous, poorly controlled)
- *Instrumental* (implies goal-directed behavior that offers some benefit to the aggressor) versus *hostile* (attempting to cause pain to the victim with no independent gain)

However, in actuality, most children exhibit a combination of these behaviors.

Epidemiology

Aggression and violence among youth represent a major public health concern. A 1997 U.S. Office of Juvenile Justice and Delinquency Prevention survey found that 9% of high school students carried a weapon to school within the past 30 days; 44% of guns used in crimes were owned by persons younger than age 25, with 11% belonging to juveniles younger than 17; and an estimated 1,400 homicides involved a juvenile offender (Center for Disease Control and Prevention, National Center for Chronic Disease Prevention and Health Promotion 2000). Moreover, there has been an explosion in school-based violence; in the decade following the 1999 Columbine shooting, at least 40 similar events were documented internationally. These events have raised questions regarding the availability and use of mental health services for early identification and treatment of individuals at risk for conducting such heinous aggressive acts.

Most research on youth violence has focused on boys, since males commit violent acts more frequently than females. This robust gender bias is seen worldwide, as documented by a recent survey in 20 countries showing that boys are more likely to report frequent fighting than girls, with the highest prevalence rates in the Eastern Mediterranean (Swahn et al. 2013). The underidentification of aggression in girls may be related to its later age at onset (Monuteaux et al. 2007) and its "relational" nature—perhaps reflecting the vulnerability of girls to family dysfunction and/or traumatic experiences. However, aggression in girls is more prominent than previously believed, with prevalence estimates ranging from 4% to 9%. An Office of Juvenile Justice and Delinquency Prevention survey found that in the 1990s there was a 23% increase in the number of violent crime arrests in adolescent females (vs. 11% increase in males) and an increase in the severity of adolescent female crime (Center for Disease Control and Prevention, National Center for Chronic Disease Prevention and Health Promotion 2000). Aggressive girls exhibit more covert aggression and less intense behavioral disturbance than boys—yet despite these apparently less intense characteristics, aggression in girls predicts substantial subsequent impairment. One important difference between aggression in girls and in boys is the relatively higher rate of posttraumatic stress disorder (PTSD) symptoms in females. Of interest are new findings that gender differences in violent behavior are less pronounced in gender-equalitarian neighborhoods compared with those characterized by gender inequality (Lei et al. 2014). The narrowing of the gender gap in those neighborhoods appears related to decreased rates of violence in boys, while girls' rates remain relatively low.

Aggression frequently occurs in the context of specific psychiatric diagnoses. Although it is a defining characteristic for only one disorder (i.e., conduct disorder [CD]), aggression may be an associated feature in youth with attention-deficit/hyperactivity disorder (ADHD), oppositional defiant disorder (ODD), substance use disorders, depression, bipolar disorders, anxiety disorders, PTSD, psychotic disorders (including but not limited to schizophrenia), autism spectrum disorder, Tourette's disorder, and organic mental disorders (see chapters on these disorders in this book). Further, a large subgroup of aggressive youth does not meet criteria for any specific psychiatric diagnosis.

Etiology, Mechanisms, and Risk Factors

The different types of aggression appear to be associated with distinct neurobiological mechanisms. Prosocial aggression (e.g., male dominance) appears to be heavily influenced by testosterone, while impulsive aggression is more consistently related to serotonin (5-HT). Findings from neuroimaging studies implicate the orbital prefrontal cortex (which inhibits limbic and other subcortical regions), anterior cingulate cortex (which manages incoming affective stimuli), and ventromedial prefrontal cortex (which regulates emotion processing). Studies in youth with CD have shown deactivation of the anterior cingulate cortex and reduced activation in the left amygdala in response to negative stimuli, as well as reduced right temporal lobe volume, reflecting possible impairments in the recognition and cognitive control of emotional stimuli (Cappadocia et al. 2009).

Neurochemistry

Convergent data from studies in animals and human adults have linked aggressive behaviors to abnormalities in neurotransmission mediated by serotonin and the catecholamines (i.e., dopamine and norepinephrine). Inhibition of 5-HT synthesis, depletion of 5-HT stores, or destruction of 5-HT neurons can produce aggressive behavior. Cerebrospinal fluid levels of the 5-HT metabolite 5-hydroxyindoleacetic acid (5-HIAA) have been inversely correlated with measures of aggressive behavior in both male and female primates. In addition, low 5-HT function early in life predicts excessive aggression, risk taking, and premature death in nonhuman male primates. However, less convincing evidence exists with regard to childhood aggression. One study reported elevated prolactin response to fenfluramine challenge (indicative of elevated 5-HT activity) in association with aggression in younger brothers of convicted delinquents (Pine et al. 1997) and a positive association of 5-HT responsivity and adverse rearing circumstances. Nevertheless, other investigators found that blunted prolactin response to fenfluramine at ages 7–11 was associated with increased aggression in adolescence and increased risk for antisocial personality disorder (ASPD) and borderline personality disorder in adulthood (Flory et al. 2007). The role of catecholamines in pathological aggression is likely attributable to norepinephrine receptors in both the central nervous system and the autonomic nervous system, with characteristic findings in relation to physiological measures of arousal. Low heart rate, an indicator of low autonomic activity, has been shown to predict aggressive and delinquent behavior in adults, adolescents, and school-age children. Similarly, low skin conductance, another measure of reduced autonomic reactivity, has also been associated with aggressive behaviors in childhood.

Hormones

Aggression is also associated with hormonal changes that occur in response to stress. Aggression has been linked with both elevated peripheral cortisol, which is characteristic of acute stress or anxiety states, and reduced cortisol, which may accompany chronic or posttraumatic stress. Reduced cortisol has been specifically related to the early onset and persistence of aggression (Murakami et al. 2006). It is likely that the observed associations reflect a combination of direct and indirect effects and that aggression and cortisol levels may well be related through association with one or more other factors.

Prominent gender differences in the nature and level of aggression (i.e., greater in males than females) have stimulated research examining the potential role of male sex steroids. In animals, testosterone levels generally reflect prosocial dominance behavior, not antisocial or pathological aggression. Testosterone concentration and aggressive behavior are correlated in boys only after puberty—suggesting the importance of developmental mechanisms. Moreover, testosterone is primarily associated with aggression following provocation—very likely through interactions with a variety of neurotransmitters.

Genetic Factors

Familiality/Heritability

Considerable data indicate that aggression runs in families. Twin studies consistently report higher concordance rates for aggression among monozygotic compared with dizygotic twins (Button et al. 2004), with heritability estimates ranging from 0.28 to 0.72. However, the variability in heritability across studies indicates that genes account for only a portion of the variance. A host of adverse environmental factors, including poverty, low socioeconomic status, marital discord, harsh parenting, poor supervision, parental psychopathology, and crowded living conditions, have been linked to aggressive behavior in youth. It is hypothesized that families with limited resources (e.g., psychological, cognitive, educational, social, financial) are likely to have less structured households, resulting in less parental supervision and heightened risk for aggression. However, this seemingly face valid explanation offers little insight into the interplay of biological and environmental risk factors. Both adoption and molecular genetic studies indicate that there is greater susceptibility to adverse environmental factors in genetically vulnerable individuals. For instance, among adopted-away children whose biological parents were diagnosed with ASPD, children who had both biological vulnerability (i.e., family history of ASPD) and environmental risk (i.e., adverse adoptive environment) were found to have higher levels of aggression than either children with biological vulnerability who were raised in more stable environments or those with environmental but not biological risk.

Candidate Genes

The candidate genes most consistently linked to aggression are the 5-HT transporter (*5-HTT*) gene and the genes for three enzymes that have an important role in the homeostasis, inactivation, and clearance of dopamine and norepinephrine: monoamine oxidase (MAO), catechol *O*-methyltransferase, and dopamine β-hydroxylase (Pedraza et al. 2012). Human studies have demonstrated that a rare mutation in the MAO-A gene is associated with impulsively violent behavior over multiple generations and that risk for physical aggression during adulthood may be increased by the interaction of low *MAOA* activity and exposure to early trauma. Similarly, youth homozygous for the long variant of *5-HTT* and parental antisocial behavior were shown to have high levels of antisocial behavior. The oxytocin-vasopressin neurohumoral system has also been implicated in social behavior, and genetic variants regulating its activity have been associated with childhood-onset aggression (Malik et al. 2014).

Social-Environmental Factors

Psychosocial Stress and Trauma

Research has clearly demonstrated that childhood trauma is a predictor of subsequent violent behavior. Studies have shown that childhood physical and emotional abuse and neglect are associated with aggression, with repeated and prolonged exposure related to increased risk of aggression and violence. Further, corporal punishment, compared with no punishment, is related to increased levels of antisocial behavior in adolescence as well as externalizing problems in general. Recently, Harford et al. (2014), using the National Epidemiological Survey on Alcohol and Related Condition ($n=34{,}000+$), found that childhood physical, emotional, and sexual abuse is directly related to risk for violent behavior to self and others in adulthood. The bases for this association have been elucidated using animal models (Liu et al. 1997). Rodents exposed to early environmental stress (e.g., decreased frequency of maternal licking, grooming, and arched back nursing) have altered neurophysiological and neuroendocrine parameters mediated by neural circuits linking the amygdala, hippocampus, and prefrontal cortex, affecting domains such as processing of emotional information and stress responsivity. These findings are consistent with data indicating that victims of childhood abuse and neglect often have difficulty processing and modulating emotional reactions to life events and that the inability to properly regulate physiological arousal in the context of affect-laden experiences can easily escalate to aggressive behavior (Maneta et al. 2012). Social information processing models also suggest that individuals with histories of child abuse likely misattribute ambiguous stimuli in social contexts as potentially threatening and then engage in more aggressive behavior in response to these stimuli.

Family Structure and Function

A variety of family-based risk factors contribute to the etiology or maintenance of aggression in youth, including large sibships, parental separation, single-parent households, child neglect, parental conflict, poverty, harsh discipline practices, poor supervision, and parental criminality (see Chapter 11, "Oppositional Defiant Disorder and Conduct Disorder"). Much of the research on aggression has focused on the risk conveyed by authoritarian (high hostility and low warmth) parenting style, corporal punishment (particularly in boys), low monitoring, low attachment to parents, and coercive climate theory, which posits that chronic aggression is promoted by a replacement (in part) of healthy family management practices during childhood with coercive and punishment-centered strategies that are linked with aggression during adolescence.

Peer Interactions

Delinquent peer membership and residence in a neighborhood with high rates of crime, poverty, poor language skills, and/or unemployment all increase risk for youth violence. Moreover, both bullying and being a victim of bullying set the stage for a host of negative outcomes for youth over time, including increased aggression and violence, even after taking into account other risk factors. Peer contagion theory suggests that children's peer interactions are amplified when they interact with a higher number of more deviant peers, underscoring the importance of examining children's social networks in understanding the development of aggression. While delinquent peer membership is associated with aggression for both boys and girls, several studies suggest that association with deviant opposite-sex peers is particularly risky for girls' aggression, whereas it is protective for that of boys (Javdani et al. 2011). Early peer rejection is also an important (and often underappreciated) predictor of aggression. Several studies have found that peer rejection is associated with impulsive and emotionally reactive behaviors. Essentially, the effect is that of a social stressor, which augments problem behavior in predisposed youth (who also are at increased risk for peer rejection). The impact of peer rejection is particularly evident when it occurs early in childhood—with significant effects found even after controlling for ADHD and aggression. However, interactions among multiple risk factors are the rule, and moderating variables such as hostility appear to play a predictive role (Reijntjes et al. 2011). Moreover, the direction of the effects is uncertain. For example, is peer rejection associated with increased risk for aggression, or is peer acceptance protective, perhaps by minimizing the impact of other risk factors? Emerging evidence suggests that peer victimization predicts subsequent changes in externalizing problems, and vice versa, suggesting that aggression functions as both an antecedent and consequence of peer rejection (Reijntjes et al. 2011).

Community and Social Factors

The occurrence of high-visibility incidents of youth violence in schools (e.g., Columbine High School and Heritage High School shootings) highlights the link between community factors and aggression. Studies have differentiated among multiple types of community violence exposure, including direct violence, witnessing, and hearing reports of aggression against familiars and/or strangers. Findings suggest that direct violence exposure is the most robust predictor of externalizing problems, although witnessing violence against familiars is also a robust predictor, particularly for girls (Javdani et al. 2014). Aggressive, antisocial acts occur more frequently in crowded, high-poverty, high-crime areas, and a variety of community-based factors influence their development and maintenance. Intergenerational transmission of aggression is associated with consequences of urban poverty, including the robust link between parental incarceration and children's later antisocial behavior. An important component of peer-related transmission of risk is the reciprocal, positive reinforcement of antisocial acts that occurs between deviant group members (i.e., deviancy training). The grouping of aggressive, antisocial youth in residential treatment or special education settings has therefore been questioned, with some programs found to promote increased aggression. Although deviancy training appears to be less significant in treatment settings (Weiss et al. 2005), it is clearly operative in adolescent gangs and, possibly, classroom placements in schools with high numbers of aggressive youth. However, family- and parent-related factors mediate these relationships, suggesting that intervention at multiple levels is possible. Interestingly, intervention programs that create what has been termed a positive "gang" environment can have the opposite effect, promoting loyalty and proactive goal-oriented behaviors, reducing risk for aggression.

Neurocognitive and Academic Factors

Neurocognitive deficits have been found in children at high risk for chronic aggression and violence (Eme 2009). Seminal work conducted by Moffitt (1990) suggests that neurocognitive deficits, particularly verbal deficits, appear early in development. These early neurocognitive delays set the stage for early disruptive behavior and poor academic readiness in early childhood, which become more pronounced with increased expectations for behavioral regulation and academic demands (particularly reading) over time. In early adolescence, active rejection by typically achieving peers and/or self-selection with other lower-achieving peers may occur, placing these youth at higher risk for delinquency. Others have found that over time youth with early problems go on to develop anxiety and depression through their experiences of failure with peers and academics, which further complicates longer-term functioning (Burke et al. 2005).

Environmental Toxins

Prenatal or postnatal exposure to a variety of toxins, substances of abuse, or infectious agents is associated with increased risk for aggression. Maternal use of alcohol, nicotine, and/or other drugs during pregnancy substantially increases risk for both ADHD and conduct problems in offspring because of toxic effects on neurodevelopment of catecholamine systems and/or alterations in gene expression. However, interpretation is complicated by the elevated rates of ADHD, substance abuse, and conduct and antisocial disorders in mothers who use alcohol, nicotine, or other drugs during pregnancy, suggesting that gene-environment interactions are likely involved.

Prevention

Early Intervention

A number of programs have been developed to aid in the prevention of aggression and conduct problems in children and families who are at risk given their residence in low-resource communities (e.g., Chicago Child Parent Center, Head Start, HighScope Perry Preschool Study, Houston Parent-Child Developmental Center, Early Head Start, Syracuse University Family Development Project, Yale Child Welfare Research Program). Typically, these early prevention/intervention programs are implemented during preschool, continuously over several years, with the goal of increasing social competence, social problem solving, resilience, and academic readiness. Results point to long-term benefits of many programs in reducing antisocial behavior and aggression. Characteristics of successful programs include 1) multimodal intervention for children and parents, parent support, teacher involvement, and early childhood education; 2) delivery of interventions consistently on a daily to weekly basis; 3) duration of 2 years or longer; 4) specific interventions to remediate coercive family processes and harsh and inconsistent parenting techniques through skill building and development of problem-solving and coping skills; 5) application of individual classroom management techniques; and 6) collaboration among community, school, family, and mental health professionals.

School-Based Violence Prevention Programs

School-based violence prevention programs for elementary, middle, and high school youth have been developed and disseminated (see Chapter 48, "School-Based Interventions"), particularly following highly visible violent events in schools, such as the shootings at Sandy Hook Elementary School and Columbine High School. A meta-analysis of 44 school-based violence prevention programs found at least moderate success, with effect sizes ranging from 0.36 to 0.59 (Mytton et al. 2002). Data suggest that the greatest reductions in aggression are found for higher-risk children (Multisite Violence Prevention Project 2009). School-based interventions that have shown particular promise appear to target mediating variables, such as positive school climate, which in turn reduces bullying and peer rejection (Hong and Espelage 2012). School anti-bullying programs have also received notable attention over the past few years and share many features with other school-based violence prevention programs (e.g., focusing on knowledge, attitude change, monitoring of behavior in school, discipline methods). Overall, the data suggest that anti-bullying programs can decrease bullying at school by 23% and victimization by 20%. More intensive anti-bullying programs that include key features (e.g., parent meetings, firm disciplinary methods, improved playground supervision) result in better outcomes (Ttofi and Farington 2011).

Preventive Parent Training

Several preventive parent training programs emphasize the development of social skills, problem-solving techniques, and anger management strategies in children, while also promoting parents' responsiveness, proactive discipline strategies, and ability to provide cognitive stimulation in reducing child aggression and conduct problems (e.g., Incredible Years parenting program, Playing and Learning Strategies). A meta-analysis of parent training programs suggests that the common core features of these effective programs include a focus on increasing positive parent-child interactions, emotional communication skills, parenting consistency, and the use of effective behavioral rewards systems (Kaminski et al. 2008). In addition, other more targeted parenting interventions have demonstrated promise for improving factors related to the development of aggression and conduct problems (e.g., development of empathy) through instructing parents on how to reinforce these skills in their children (Waller et al. 2013).

Course and Prognosis

Aggression is considered to be a relatively stable trait, and aggression in childhood often predicts continuation or even escalation of behavior problems over time, leading to ASPD, domestic abuse, and/or incarceration. Nevertheless, many aggressive children do not become aggressive adults. Antecedent problems present during the preschool years, including poor peer relationships and inadequate problem-solving patterns, predict the development of impulsive aggression; 20%–25% of these youth have also been physically abused. Planned aggression starts later in development and is fueled by aggressive role models and a positive valence of aggression.

Several models have attempted to describe the escalation from childhood ADHD to aggression and criminal behavior and the predictors of escalation and/or persistence. While no single theory can predict an individual course, several points are generally accepted.

1. Antisocial behavior emerges in an orderly fashion that begins with oppositionality and seemingly trivial nondelinquent antisocial acts (e.g., aggressiveness, arguing, fighting with siblings, talking back to adults, yelling, lying, noncompliance, temper tantrums) that presage more serious delinquent acts (e.g., physical fighting, stealing, fire setting).
2. Predictors of continuity include early onset, increased variety, and high frequency of problem behaviors; increases in one area (frequency) are often associated with increases in other areas (variety).
3. Children who practice both overt and covert antisocial acts (i.e., versatile offenders) differ from those who partake in only covert antisocial activities (e.g., theft only or substance abuse only). Versatile child offending is associated with increased family adversity and greater police contact.
4. Physical aggression in childhood is one of the most important predictors of later diversified offending, although family history of aggression and/or affective lability in childhood also increase the risk for persistence and escalation.

Evaluation: Clinical Assessment

Treatment planning with aggressive youth is based on a comprehensive understanding of psychological, behavioral, cognitive, and differential diagnostic considerations related to the nature, context, and severity of aggression and to the risk and protective factors that characterize the individual patient and family. There are several important components of this examination.

1. Interview the patient and relevant others to understand how and why the aggressive behavior developed, whether it is situation specific, what the consequences have been, and whether there is any current ideation or plan. Imminent risk to any individual carries a legal obligation to warn the potential target (i.e., *Tarasoff* decision), although state laws vary and advice should be sought.
2. Determine whether there are specific stresses and/or contextual factors related to the aggressive behavior, as these may be amenable to change either directly or indirectly (e.g., via psychosocial intervention).
3. Determine whether there is substance abuse and, if so, the nature

and extent of the abuse (because substances of abuse may be disinhibiting or lead to instrumental aggression).

4. Obtain information regarding individual, family, and peer risk factors—including family history of aggression, criminality, substance abuse, and personality disorders; family relationships (including parenting styles, disciplinary practices, and family violence); academic function (including ADHD, learning disabilities, and academic achievement); and current and past peer interactions—noting changes in affectively charged relationships, such as a breakup with a close friend or a romantic partner.
5. Obtain detailed information regarding ADHD and disruptive and aggressive behavior to aid in understanding the developmental trajectory of the aggressive behavior.

Mental Status Examination

The primary focus of the mental status examination should be differential diagnosis because aggression often accompanies other psychiatric diagnoses. It is also important to assess cognitive capacity, specifically verbal skills (which relate to the capacity for insight, judgment, and problem-solving skills), as well as personality characteristics such as adaptability, affect regulation, and cognitive flexibility (which are necessary for shifting focus away from affectively charged topics or events before they escalate to aggressive behavior). It is important to evaluate the capacity for empathy, the degree of connection to others, and the extent to which there is hostile attribution bias (i.e., ascribing hostile intent even when there is none) or more frank distortions of factual content, the most severe example being paranoid thinking. These factors inform not only the assessment of risk but also the patient's capacity to engage in treatment.

Psychometric Instruments

A variety of psychometric instruments can be used for assessing youth and monitoring treatment. Aggression rating scales and structured interviews can augment the unstructured clinical assessment. Broadband rating scales (e.g., Achenbach and Conners scales) can be used to get an overview of the child's or adolescent's mental health functioning and screen for aggressive behavior. However, the behavior disorder and aggression items on broad-based scales often evaluate oppositional behavior and covert aggressive behaviors rather than overt physical aggression. The latter is more easily evaluated using one of many narrowband rating scales. Table 29–1 describes frequently used aggression rating scales.

Psychological Testing

Neuropsychological testing may aid in the assessment of cognitive functions that may confer relative or specific risk for aggression—such as intellectual capacity, learning disorders, language skills, verbal reasoning, attention, vigilance, inhibitory control, and academic achievement. Projective tests may provide information relative to how the patient is likely to think in unstructured or stressful situations. Tests evaluating social information processing and measures of emotional functioning (e.g., emotional dysregulation versus callousness/unemotionality) may be particularly valuable in assessing the mechanism by which aggression occurs for a particular youth and guiding subsequent treatment planning.

TABLE 29–1. Frequently used rating scales for aggression in children and adolescents

Scale	Description/features/comments	References
Buss-Perry Hostility Inventory	Originally developed for college students; a modified version for youth with updated items, eliminated items not relevant to youth, and improved readability for youth with lower vocabulary skills	Buss and Perry 1992
Children's Aggression Scale (parent and teacher versions)	Contains five factors: verbal aggression, aggression against objects and animals, provoked physical aggression, unprovoked physical aggression, and use of weapons; distinguishes aggression 1) inside versus outside the home and 2) against children versus adults	Halperin et al. 2002, 2003
New York Teacher Rating Scale	Teacher report that includes DSM items for both oppositional defiant disorder and conduct disorder, as well as a number of other items of disruptive and/or aggressive behavior	Miller et al. 1995
Overt Aggression Scale (OAS)—Modified	Self/other modification of OAS suitable for outpatient settings; rates behavior over a 1-week interval; the same four domains of aggression are included, but a 5-point response format allows assessment of both severity and frequency	Sorgi et al. 1991

Differential Diagnosis

Aggressive behavior can be either a specific core symptom or an associated feature of a psychiatric disorder. Conditions to carefully consider include ADHD, ODD, and CD; mood disorders (including depressive and bipolar disorders); disruptive mood dysregulation disorder; anxiety disorders, obsessive-compulsive disorder, and PTSD; substance use disorders; tic disorders (including Tourette's disorder); specific learning disorder; autism spectrum disorder; psychotic disorders; somatization disorder; and a variety of medical conditions, including seizure disorders (ictal or interictal) and acute metabolic syndromes producing delirium and/or confusional states. The rationale for careful differential diagnosis is that treatment of underlying or associated conditions may lead to improvement or resolution of the aggressive behavior. This is most often seen when the underlying medical or psychiatric condition is acute, although it is less likely to occur when there is chronic physical or psychiatric illness.

Pediatric Evaluation and Laboratory Tests

Medical and neurological evaluations are required to rule out conditions (e.g., exposure to toxins, seizures, infections, head trauma, substance use) associated with reversible changes of mental state. See Chapter 6, "Neurological Examination, Electroencephalography, Neuroimaging, and Neuropsychological Testing," for further discussion.

Treatment

The treatment of aggression in children and adolescents is often challenging, as the syndrome rarely responds to a single treatment modality. Several psychosocial and pharmacological interventions have demonstrated efficacy and feasibility. Psychosocial intervention can be used for either impulsive or planned aggression; medication is generally effective only in the treatment of impulsive aggression. Improvement is often relative, and multimodal intervention is optimal.

Recently, the Center for Education and Research on Mental Health Therapeutics developed guidelines for the comprehensive treatment of maladaptive aggression in youth by primary care clinicians and mental health providers (Scotto-Rosato et al. 2012). This multistep (i.e., systematic reviews of published literature, an expert survey of recommended practices, a consensus conference of experts and family advocates) review process resulted in 11 recommendations. Key recommendations include evidence-based parent and child skills training as the first line of treatment; treatment of the underlying disorder in accordance with evidence-based guidelines; careful consideration of potential risks of and contraindications for the initiation of medications; avoiding the simultaneous use of multiple psychotropic medications; careful monitoring of treatment response with structured rating scales; and close medical monitoring for side effects, including metabolic changes.

Psychotherapeutic Treatments

Empirically supported psychosocial interventions target one or more of the behaviors that characterize (e.g., verbal aggression, property destruction, physical aggression) or serve to maintain (e.g., affect regulation, social information processing deficits, coercive parenting behaviors) aggressive behavior. Behavioral parent training (BPT; see Chapter 41, "Behavioral Parent Training") is the best-studied and best-validated treatment for youth aggression. BPT attempts to break the coercive reinforcement cycle between parents and their children that contributes to the development and proximal maintenance of aggressive behaviors. Broadly, BPT focuses on applying social learning and operational conditioning theories to support parents in modifying their own parenting behavior in order to increase children's use of prosocial, nonaggressive behavior and minimize the use of coercive, aggressive behaviors. Parents are instructed on how to manipulate antecedents (e.g., rules, commands) and consequences (e.g., rewards, time out) related to the aggressive behavior. The anticipated results are a shift away from an aversive parent-child relationship to one that is mutually reinforcing and the acquisition of prosocial nonaggressive skills by the child. Components of BPT include didactic instruction, videotaped vignettes to elicit discussion, and modeling/role-playing of specific strategies. Treatment may be conducted in either individual or group formats and may include the child (most often in families of young children). Numerous commercially available BPT programs exist for use in clinical practice (see Chapter 41).

Cognitive-behavioral therapy (CBT) has also been used successfully. Aggressive youth often have hostile attribution biases, make errors in interpreting social cues, and have positive expectations related to their aggressive behavior. CBT primarily targets these social-cognitive deficits by teaching youth to effectively recognize and interpret social cues; generate multiple interpretations for others' behavior; and implement nonaggressive, prosocial problem-solving strategies. CBT is typically conducted in groups, often using discussion, modeling, and role-playing (with feedback and reinforcement from the leader) to aid in skill development. While several studies have documented the positive effects of CBT in treating aggressive youth, the combination of CBT and BPT is often more effective than either intervention alone.

Considerable research has examined both the limitations of BPT and CBT and moderating factors. Youth with greater severity of problems, higher levels of parental psychopathology, greater family dysfunction, and/or more difficult life circumstances often do poorly with either BPT or CBT, although this is not always seen, at least in regard to BPT (Shelleby and Shaw 2014). BPT appears to be most effective for younger youth, while CBT is more effective for older youth. Motivation and other attitudinal factors likely affect treatment attendance, the ability to learn new skills, and the willingness to use skills learned in treatment. Adherence to treatment is particularly salient for BPT, as up to 40%–60% of parents drop out, and even among those who continue treatment, use of BPT skills is often not consistent. Unfortunately, the families that are most likely to discontinue BPT and have the most difficulties implementing BPT skills are the ones at highest risk for persistence of aggressive/antisocial behavior.

More recently, treatment approaches have focused on ways to allow the clinician to more flexibly address the needs of youth with comorbid psychiatric disorders or problem areas—a particularly relevant issue for youth with aggression. This is accomplished by incorporating elements of evidence-based treatments for common psychiatric disorders (e.g., anxiety, trauma, depression, conduct problems) as modular, free-standing components. These modular components are used flexibly to address specific problem areas on the basis of ongoing assessment of treatment response. A recent randomized controlled trial demonstrated enhanced benefits of this modular approach compared with single evidence-based treatments (Weisz et al. 2012).

Given the limitations of single interventions for youth with the greatest severity of aggression risk, multimodal approaches are often necessary. Substantial evidence supports the efficacy of multisystemic treatment (MST) and Multidimensional Treatment Foster Care (MTFC) for high-risk youth with aggressive, antisocial behavior—many of whom are also at risk of out-of-home placement and involvement with the juvenile justice system. MST and MTFC use well-established, developmentally appropriate strategies to target risk and support youth competence in a manner that is highly intensive and tailored to the needs of the individual child and family. Both treatments reduce rates of recidivism, arrest, criminal offenses, substance-related offenses, and out-of-home placement—even in the highest-risk youth. Importantly, despite offering intensive, multimodal interventions, both MST and MTFC have been shown to be cost-effective compared with alternative methods (e.g., psychiatric hospitalization).

Pharmacological Treatments

Although the evidence from controlled clinical trials for the pharmacological treatment of aggression remains limited, the preponderance of hospitalized children and adolescents receive pharmacotherapy to address aggression—with 40% receiving two or more medications, most commonly including second-generation antipsychotics (SGAs; see also Chapter 38, "Antipsychotic Medications"). One recent review of the overall use of SGAs reported beneficial effects of risperidone in reducing aggression in the short term in children ages 5–18 with disruptive behavior disorders (Loy et al. 2012). These positive effects of risperidone can be maintained for up to 6 months; however, the authors expressed caution regarding their recommendations because of the low number of high-quality studies. This report found no evidence supporting the use of quetiapine for disruptive behavior disorders in children and adolescents. Another recent review reported that four placebo-controlled studies support the short-term efficacy of low-dose risperidone in youth with a subaverage IQ (Pringsheim and Gorman 2012). In contrast, placebo-controlled evidence did not show efficacy of other SGAs in either youth with intellectual disabilities or those of normal IQ. The apparent disconnect between this limited evidence base and the frequent use of SGAs for aggression in clinical practice is noteworthy. Possible contributing factors include extrapolation from positive studies in youth with autism spectrum disorder or low IQ to typically developing youth, unavailability of or lack of familiarity with available psychosocial treatments, and limited familiarity with alternative pharmacological options, as well as advertisements from the pharmaceutical industry.

Aggression often develops in youth diagnosed with ADHD and/or CD. Stimulants are effective for both overt and covert aggression. For children with ADHD, treating the underlying ADHD is an important, although sometimes overlooked, approach. Nevertheless, severely aggressive youth often require additional interventions. For instance, combining a stimulant and an antipsychotic has been found to be useful in controlling physical aggression in children with ADHD (Aman et al. 2014); however, this is considered a third-line treatment, following stimulant monotherapy and combination of stimulant with behavioral interventions. There is no agreement regarding this pharmacological combination approach. One recent review (Linton et al. 2013) concluded that the existing data do not clearly demonstrate superiority of combination treatment versus monotherapy with either antipsychotic or stimulant medication. Another limitation is that there are no data that compare medication with behavioral interventions. Despite these reservations, data do not suggest significantly worse adverse effects for combination treatment compared with monotherapy. Contrary to speculation, use of stimulant medication together with an antipsychotic had no significant effect on reducing metabolic effects of the antipsychotic, although studies using the oral hypoglycemic agent metformin report benefit (Penzner et al. 2009; Shin et al. 2009). In an open-label, uncontrolled pilot study, combining the nonstimulant atomoxetine and the antipsychotic olanzapine appeared promising for treating aggression in ADHD and comorbid disruptive behavior disorder (Holzer et al. 2013), pointing to the possible value of considering nonstimulant interventions for ADHD. Initial studies using lithium carbonate in hospitalized aggressive children with CD also yielded positive results (Malone et al. 2000); however, other studies found the benefits of lithium to be less substantial than originally suggested (Pringsheim et al. 2015).

The anticonvulsant divalproex has been shown to be effective in treating impulsive aggression. Divalproex reduces the explosive aggression associated with bipolar disorder and CD and has fewer side effects and drug interactions than many other agents used for these conditions. Like the atypical antipsychotics, divalproex and other anticonvulsant mood stabilizers (see Chapter 37, "Mood Stabilizers") potentially have a dual role in the treatment of aggression—as interventions for a primary underlying disorder (e.g., bipolar and psychotic disorders) and as symptom-based treatments for aggression. Recent findings from Blader et al. (2013) indicate the beneficial effect of combined treatment with divalproex and a stimulant in youth with ADHD and aggression who are not adequately controlled with optimized stimulant monotherapy. There is also interest in the possible beneficial effects of the α_2-adrenergic agonists, clonidine and guanfacine. Published data point to ameliorative effects in youth with ADHD plus oppositional behavior (see Chapter 35, "Medications Used for Attention-Deficit/Hyperactivity Disorder"), but there are few published controlled trials in aggressive youth. Finally, beta-blockers such as propranolol (often at higher doses) have been used to treat aggression in patients with organic brain dysfunction and disruptive behavior disorders (often in combination with stimulants), but data are limited, and use of these drugs is infrequent.

Conclusion

Although we know a great deal about the psychological, interpersonal, and biological bases of aggression—and have several evidence-based psychosocial and pharmacological interventions for this condition—few of these "successes" have translated into meaningful changes in prevalence and treatment. There is an urgent need to identify effective, broadly accessible interventions that engage and retain youth and families in treatment in order to maximize outcomes. An important corollary is to study these interventions in relevant demographic and clinical groups, with a focus on community-based settings. Unfortunately, the most difficult patients to engage and treat are precisely the ones who need treatment the most. Even more important would be to improve primary and secondary prevention efforts. However, substantively changing risk for aggression will require major changes in social policy and allocation of resources, in addition to new developments in clinical science, as it is impossible to overstate the contribution of poverty and its consequences to the development and maintenance of aggression. Finally, while it is likely that psychopharmacological interventions will remain second-line interventions for aggression, research that more accurately elucidates the neurobiological bases and mechanisms of aggression holds promise for the development of safer, more effective, and more specific treatments.

Summary Points

- Aggression has origins in early childhood. Identification of young children exhibiting early aggression and/or exposed to trauma for appropriate treatment is essential to altering poor longer-term trajectories for these children.
- Minimizing a child's exposure to violence in various settings (e.g., school) is necessary. Thoughtful consideration of grouping and management of children in school settings (classrooms, lunchrooms, playgrounds, and so forth) can be helpful.

- Aggression is not a psychiatric diagnosis itself, but it can accompany many psychiatric diagnoses. With the exception of conduct disorder, aggression is not part of the defining criteria for the frequently co-occurring conditions.
- A variety of structured and semistructured assessment measures are available. Obtaining information from multiple informants is essential.
- Early intervention must target a variety of issues at multiple levels (e.g., early language abilities in children, parenting behaviors, access to high-quality preschool)
- To maximize the benefits, families who reside in socioeconomically disadvantaged communities will require support to consistently engage in and maintain intervention efforts.
- For school-age youth, behavioral parent training is the most effective psychosocial intervention to address aggression.
- For late school-age youth and adolescents, a focus on improving cognitive and information processing deficits related to aggression, peer group norms and behaviors related to aggression and violence (at school and in the community), and parental/school monitoring and consequences for aggressive behavior are essential.
- Various medications are potentially useful, although supporting evidence is limited. Differential diagnosis is key, as identifying treatable conditions accompanying the presentation of aggression can aid in directing intervention.

References

Aman MG, Bukstein OG, Gadow KD, et al: What does risperidone add to parent training and stimulant for severe aggression in child attention-deficit/hyperactivity disorder? J Am Acad Child Adolesc Psychiatry 53(1):47–60, e1, 2014 24342385

Blader JC, Pliszka SR, Kafantaris V, et al: Callous-unemotional traits, proactive aggression, and treatment outcomes of aggressive children with attention-deficit/hyperactivity disorder. J Am Acad Child Adolesc Psychiatry 52(12):1281–1293, 2013 24290461

Burke JD, Loeber R, Lahey BB, et al: Developmental transitions among affective and behavioral disorders in adolescent boys. J Child Psychol Psychiatry 46(11):1200–1210, 2005 16238667

Buss AH, Perry M: The aggression questionnaire. J Pers Soc Psychol 63(3):452–459, 1992 1403624

Button TM, Scourfield J, Martin N, et al: Do aggressive and non-aggressive antisocial behaviors in adolescents result from the same genetic and environmental effects? Am J Med Genet B Neuropsychiatr Genet 129B(1):59–63, 2004 15274042

Cappadocia MC, Desrocher M, Pepler D, et al: Contextualizing the neurobiology of conduct disorder in an emotion dysregulation framework. Clin Psychol Rev 29(6):506–518, 2009 19573964

Center for Disease Control and Prevention, National Center for Chronic Disease Prevention and Health Promotion: Assessing Health Risk Behaviors Among Young People: Youth Risk Behavior Surveillance System, At-a-Glance. Atlanta, GA, Centers for Disease Control and Prevention, 2000

Eme R: Male life-course persistent antisocial behavior: a review of neurodevelopmental factors. Aggress Violent Behav 14(5):348–358, 2009

Flory JD, Newcorn JH, Miller C, et al: Serotonergic function in children with attention-deficit hyperactivity disorder: relationship to later antisocial personality disorder. Br J Psychiatry 190:410–414, 2007 17470955

Halperin JM, McKay KE, Newcorn JH: Development, reliability, and validity of the children's aggression scale-parent version. J Am Acad Child Adolesc Psychiatry 41(3):245–252, 2002 11886018

Halperin JM, McKay KE, Grayson RH, et al: Reliability, validity, and preliminary normative data for the Children's Aggression Scale-Teacher Version. J Am Acad Child Adolesc Psychiatry 42(8):965–971, 2003 12874499

Harford TC, Yi HY, Grant BF: Associations between childhood abuse and interpersonal aggression and suicide attempt among U.S. adults in a national study. Child Abuse Negl 38(8):1389–1398, 2014 24656711

Holzer B, Lopes V, Lehman R: Combination use of atomoxetine hydrochloride and olanzapine in the treatment of attention-deficit/hyperactivity disorder with comorbid disruptive behavior disorder in children and adolescents 10–18 years of age. J Child Adolesc Psychopharmacol 23(6):415–418, 2013 23952189

Hong JS, Espelage DI: A review of research on bullying and peer victimization in school: An ecological system analysis. Aggress Violent Behav 17(4):311–322, 2012

Javdani S, Sadeh N, Verona E: Expanding our lens: female pathways to antisocial behavior in adolescence and adulthood. Clin Psychol Rev 31(8):1324–1348, 2011 22001339

Javdani S, Abdul-Adil J, Suarez L, et al: Gender differences in the effects of community violence on mental health outcomes in a sample of low-income youth receiving psychiatric care. Am J Community Psychol 53(3–4):235–248, 2014 24496719

Kaminski JW, Valle LA, Filene JH, et al: A meta-analytic review of components associated with parent training program effectiveness. J Abnorm Child Psychol 36(4):567–589, 2008 18205039

Lei MK, Simons RL, Simons LG, et al: Gender equality and violent behavior: how neighborhood gender equality influences the gender gap in violence. Violence Vict 29(1):89–108, 2014 24672996

Linton D, Barr AM, Honer WG, et al: Antipsychotic and psychostimulant drug combination therapy in attention deficit/hyperactivity and disruptive behavior disorders: a systematic review of efficacy and tolerability. Curr Psychiatry Rep 15(5):355, 2013 23539465

Liu D, Diorio J, Tannenbaum B, et al: Maternal care, hippocampal glucocorticoid receptors, and hypothalamic-pituitary-adrenal responses to stress. Science 277(5332):1659–1662, 1997 1219287218

Loy JH, Merry SN, Hetrick SE, et al: Atypical antipsychotics for disruptive behaviour disorders in children and youths. Cochrane Database Syst Rev 9:CD008559, 2012 22972123

Malik AI, Zai CC, Berall L, et al: The role of genetic variants in genes regulating the oxytocin-vasopressin neurohumoral system in childhood-onset aggression (Epub ahead of print). Psychiatr Genet 24(5):201–210, 2014 24871896

Malone RP, Delaney MA, Luebbert JF, et al: A double-blind placebo-controlled study of lithium in hospitalized aggressive children and adolescents with conduct disorder. Arch Gen Psychiatry 57(7):649–654, 2000 10891035

Maneta E, Cohen S, Schulz M, et al: Links between childhood physical abuse and intimate partner aggression: the mediating role of anger expression. Violence Vict 27(3):315–328, 2012 22852434

Miller LS, Klein RG, Piacentini J, et al: The New York Teacher Rating Scale for disruptive and antisocial behavior. J Am Acad Child Adolesc Psychiatry 34(3):359–370, 1995 7896678

Moffitt TE: The neuropsychology of juvenile delinquency: A critical review, in Crime and Justice: A Review of Research, Vol 12. Edited by Tonry M, Morris N. Chicago, University of Chicago Press, 1990, pp 99–169

Monuteaux MC, Faraone SV, Michelle Gross L, et al: Predictors, clinical characteristics, and outcome of conduct disorder in girls with attention-deficit/hyperactivity disorder: a longitudinal study. Psychol Med 37(12):1731–1741, 2007 17451627

Multisite Violence Prevention Project: The ecological effects of universal and selective violence prevention programs for middle school students: a randomized trial. J Consult Clin Psychol 77(3):526–542, 2009 19485593

Murakami S, Rappaport N, Penn JV: An overview of juveniles and school violence. Psychiatr Clin North Am 29(3):725–741, 2006 16904508

Mytton JA, DiGuiseppi C, Gough DA, et al: School-based violence prevention programs: systematic review of secondary prevention trials. Arch Pediatr Adolesc Med 156(8):752–762, 2002 12144364

Pedraza J, Ivanov I, Otoy O, et al: Functional genetic variations and their role in aggressive behavior in the context of disruptive behavior disorders, in Advances in Psychology Research, Vol 95. Edited by Columnus AM. New York, NOVA Publishing, 2012, pp 118–138

Penzer JB, Dudas M, Saito E, et al: Lack of effect of stimulant combination with second-generation antipsychotics on weight gain, metabolic changes, prolactin levels, and sedation in youth with clinically relevant aggression or oppositionality. J Child Adolesc Psychopharmacol 19(5):563–573, 2009 19877981

Pine DS, Coplan JD, Wasserman GA, et al: Neuroendocrine response to fenfluramine challenge in boys. Associations with aggressive behavior and adverse rearing. Arch Gen Psychiatry 54(9):839–846, 1997 9294375

Pringsheim T, Gorman D: Second-generation antipsychotics for the treatment of disruptive behaviour disorders in children: a systematic review. Can J Psychiatry 57(12):722–727, 2012 23228230

Pringsheim T, Hirsch L, Gardner D, et al: The pharmacological management of oppositional behaviour, conduct problems, and aggression in children and adolescents with attention-deficit hyperactivity disorder, oppositional defiant disorder, and conduct disorder: a systematic review and meta-analysis. Part 2: antipsychotics and traditional mood stabilizers. Can J Psychiatry 60(2):52–61, 2015 25886656

Reijntjes A, Thomaes S, Kamphuis JH, et al: Explaining the paradoxical rejection-aggression link: the mediating effects of hostile intent attributions, anger, and decreases in state self-esteem on peer rejection-induced aggression in youth. Pers Soc Psychol Bull 37(7):955–963, 2011 21632967

Scotto-Rosato N, Correll CU, Pappadopulos E, et al: Treatment of maladaptive aggression in youth: CERT guidelines II. Treatments and ongoing management. Pediatrics 129(6):e1577–e1586, 2012

Shelleby EC, Shaw DS: Outcomes of parenting interventions for child conduct problems: a review of differential effectiveness. Child Psychiatry Hum Dev 45(5):628–645, 2014 24390592

Shin L, Bregman H, Breeze JL, et al: Metformin for weight control in pediatric patients on atypical antipsychotic medication. J Child Adolesc Psychopharmacol 19(3):275–279, 2009 19519262

Sorgi P, Ratey J, Knoedler DW, et al: Rating aggression in the clinical setting. A retrospective adaptation of the Overt Aggression Scale: preliminary results. J Neuropsychiatry Clin Neurosci 3(2):S52–S56, 1991 1687961

Swahn MH, Gressard L, Palmier JB, et al: The prevalence of very frequent physical fighting among boys and girls in 27 countries and cities: regional and gender differences. J Environ Public Health 2013:215126, 2013 23935643

Ttofi MM, Farington DP: Effectiveness of school-based programs to reduce bullying: a systematic and meta-analytic review. Journal of Experimental Criminology 7(1):27–56, 2011

Waller R, Gardner F, Hyde LW: What are the associations between parenting, callous-unemotional traits, and antisocial behavior in youth? A systematic review of evidence. Clin Psychol Rev 33(4):593–608, 2013 23583974

Weiss B, Caron A, Ball S, et al: Iatrogenic effects of group treatment for antisocial youths. J Consult Clin Psychol 73(6):1036–1044, 2005 16392977

Weisz JR, Chorpita BF, Palinkas LA, et al: Testing standard and modular designs for psychotherapy treating depression, anxiety, and conduct problems in youth: a randomized effectiveness trial. Arch Gen Psychiatry 69(3):274–282, 2012 22065252

CHAPTER 30

Psychiatric Emergencies

Lisa L. Giles, M.D.
D. Richard Martini, M.D.

Children and adolescents with psychiatric disorders are presenting in the emergency department (ED) at ever-increasing rates. This situation is complicated by a shortage of inpatient and outpatient mental health services for pediatric patients. The ED is often the initial contact with the mental health system and is increasingly used as a safety net for diagnosing and managing psychiatric illness in children. Children and adolescents present to the ED with a wide range of mental health issues, including suicidal attempt or ideation; worsening or emerging psychiatric illness, including eating disorders; substance abuse; acute change in mental status; aggression; or other behavioral difficulties (Bridge et al. 2012; Grupp-Phelan et al. 2009). Young patients needing psychiatric services stress the system by placing unique demands on both pediatric and mental health clinicians. Psychiatric patients in the emergency room often require an inordinate amount of time and resources and have high rates of recidivism (Grupp-Phelan et al. 2009; Santiago et al. 2006). These children may be aggressive and dangerous and may need intense psychiatric services that are not immediately available. Additionally, patients may present with adults who are not the child's primary caregivers and who are unfamiliar with their history. The ED, where there may be no private or quiet area, is not the optimal setting for assessing and managing patients and families in distress. However, despite the challenges, identification and treatment of psychiatric emergencies in children and adolescents are essential parts of the "safety net" that must be available for children in crisis and for those who have not been able to appropriately access mental health services.

Common Clinical Presentations

Suicidal Behavior

The assessment of pediatric patients with self-injurious behavior is based on the review of three basic questions:

- Is the patient likely to commit suicide in the future?
- Is the patient likely to make a suicide attempt in the future?
- Will the patient follow through on a psychiatric referral on the basis of this evaluation?

Presentations to the ED for suicide-related behaviors have increased significantly over the past two decades (Dolan et al. 2011; Newton et al. 2010). Children and adolescents present with a wide range of suicidal behaviors and ideation, with varying levels of risk and severity, making appropriate care and disposition decisions essential. There is limited, but emerging, research to direct the management of pediatric suicide-related ED presentations. Details on the characteristics and epidemiology of suicidal adolescents are provided in Chapter 27, "Youth Suicide."

Assessment

The psychiatric assessment includes a careful physical examination, including mental status. Evidence of an organic illness that may cause delirium, signs of previous suicide attempts (e.g., scars from cutting, bruises on the neck from attempted asphyxiation), indicators of physical or sexual abuse, and evidence of possible substance use are included. Patients who are delirious typically present with dramatic changes in behavior and mental status that are related to the appearance or treatment of a physical illness. Dangerousness is related to the presence of mood lability as well as cognitive and perceptual distortions. A urine toxicology screen and a pregnancy test for adolescent girls are often indicated. Whether to order additional tests, including liver enzyme tests and drug and alcohol screens, depends on the method of suicide attempt and resulting physical complications. Medical illnesses can cause a variety of psychiatric symptoms, and the evaluation should screen for neurological, endocrine, gastrointestinal, autoimmune, and infectious diseases when indicated.

The assessment of the suicidal patient includes risk factors for future suicidal actions (see Table 30–1). Research consistently finds that suicidal ideation and a history of suicide attempts are among the most salient risk factors for future suicide attempts. The assessment of the suicidal patient should thus focus on the severity of ideation and the lethality and intent of the action. Recent studies suggest that using a structured assessment tool, such as the Columbia Suicide Severity Rating Scale, as an adjunct to a routine clinical interview improves the identification of high-risk patients (Horwitz et al. 2014; Newton et al. 2010; Posner et al. 2011). In pediatrics, medical lethality is not necessarily related to severity of the attempt. Patients may accidentally ingest lethal amounts of a substance or overestimate the toxicity of a small amount while making an attempt with serious intent. The latter is often followed by a trend toward more lethal means. Young patients typically have limited access to methods with a high mortality rate. They do, however, have access to drugs, both prescription and over the counter, and choose overdose as the preferred approach. Clinicians should be aware of local preferences among children and adolescents and inquire about the patient's familiarity and previous experiences with these methods during both psychiatric and pediatric assessments. The assessment of intent tends to focus on several important questions. Why was this method chosen? What were the expectations from the attempt (did the patient think that the attempt was going to kill him or her)? How potentially reversible was the

TABLE 30–1. Risk factors for a suicide attempt

Patient history
Verbalization or threats regarding suicide
Substance abuse
Poor impulse control
Recent loss or other severe stressor
Previous suicide attempt(s)
Friend or family member who has committed suicide
Exposure to recent news stories or movies about suicide
Poor social supports
Victim of physical or sexual abuse
Nature of the attempt
Accidental discovery (vs. attempt in view of others or telling others immediately)
Careful plans to avoid discovery
Hanging or gunshot
Family
Wishes to be rid of child or adolescent
Does not take child's problems seriously
Is overly angry and punitive
Depression or suicidality is present in a family member
Is unwilling or unable to provide support and supervision
Mental status examination
Depression
Hopelessness
Regret at being rescued
Belief that things would be better for self or others if dead
Wish to rejoin a dead loved one
Belief that death is temporary and pleasant
Unwillingness to promise to call before attempting suicide
Psychosis
Intoxication

attempt? Could the patient change his or her mind and quickly recover from the attempt? Does the patient demonstrate any ambivalence about living? How strong was the patient's intent to die? Was there evidence of premeditation, including preparations and precautions against discovery (Spirito et al. 1994)? The answers to these questions are found not only in the interview but also in the details of the patient's behavior. Incidents that immediately precede the attempt may provide clues about motivation and intent. In an ingestion, for example, did the patient take a large number of pills or perhaps all of the pills that were available? Did the patient tell anyone about the ingestion, particularly responsible caregivers? What did the patient do immediately after taking the pills? Did she seek help or did she simply disregard the danger of the ingestion and go to bed? When the patient experienced the physical consequences of an overdose (i.e., nausea, vomiting, abdominal pain) and was discovered, did he or she acknowledge the suicidal behavior or continue to hide the reasons for his or her discomfort?

The clinician should realize that a primary purpose of the assessment is to uncover and address the precipitants to the suicide attempt as well as other predisposing factors. Adolescents experience relationship problems with friends, family, and boyfriends or girlfriends—or school failures in academics, sports, or the arts—that produce high levels of frustration and occasionally narcissistic injury leading to suicidal behavior. Children and adolescents, regardless of age, may express a real desire to die as a means of obtaining relief or of escaping from a difficult situation. These patients are more likely to suffer from symptoms of depression and have strong perfectionistic tendencies.

Treatment

Traditionally, management of the suicidal adolescent in the ED setting usually involves the decision to psychiatrically hospitalize or to refer for outpatient care. A recommendation for psychiatric hospitalization is made when the severity of the suicidal ideation or behavior is felt to be severe, for example, if the patient actively voices suicidal ideation with intent, has frequent thoughts about suicide that occur over long periods of time, and/or describes specific plans that are not only well conceived and potentially lethal but also feasible in his or her home environment. Clinicians should be particularly concerned if during the interview the idea of suicide seems perfectly acceptable to the patient. In addition, suicidal patients who present with a history of psychiatric diagnoses unsuccessfully treated in an outpatient or day hospital setting should be considered for the inpatient unit. Youth who are intoxicated at the time of assessment or who have an active history of substance abuse are strongly considered for admission. Lack of available social support may indicate a need for inpatient psychiatric admission in order to guarantee appropriate psychiatric follow-up and a reduction in the patient's level of dangerousness. This is a much stronger indicator for admission in children than in adults.

Outpatient treatment is appropriate for patients who exhibit low levels of suicidal behavior and who are prepared to participate in outpatient sessions with the support of their caregivers. The clinician should recommend that firearms be removed from the home and that access to medications and sharp objects be prevented to decrease risk. Studies do not support the use of "no-suicide contracts" in reducing dangerousness. However, safety planning, which is focused on problem solving a plan that the patient can use during times of crisis, seems to be a helpful strategy, although research on outcomes is limited. Physicians should not prescribe for suicidal adolescents medications with overdose potential until the patient is considered stable and cooperative with treatment. Unfortunately, studies that examine the likelihood of successful follow-up after ED visits do not paint an optimistic picture (Spirito et al. 1992, 2002). A recent study examining Medicaid claims databases of all 50 states found that only 40% of youth seen in the ED after deliberate self-injury had outpatient mental health care visits within 30 days (Bridge et al. 2012). A history of previous hospitalization, higher socioeconomic status, and increased severity of suicidal behavior improve the likelihood of outpatient follow-through (Bridge et al. 2012; Spirito et al. 2002).

In addition to disposition triage and planning, emerging literature suggests that interventions in the emergency room can in and of themselves have an impact on reducing suicide-related outcomes. When families have positive experiences in the ED, they are more likely to follow up with mental health aftercare. Efforts should be made by ED staff to increase the number and frequency of positive interactions with family members, even while orienting them to the surroundings, procedures, and hectic pace that is typical in a medical setting. Treatment adherence is increased by addressing treatment barriers, discussing treatment expectations, and negotiating session attendance. The clinician should educate both the patient and the caregiver about the nature of suicidal behavior and the importance of treatment. As appropriate, comorbid psychiatric disorders and the role that substance use plays in escalating the lethality of self-destructive behavior should be reviewed. Families should understand the nature and importance of the therapeutic process in both treating the underlying psychiatric disorder and preventing a recurrence of suicidal behavior. Additionally, families can benefit when assisted in basic problem-solving strategies. A handful of studies suggest that when care initiated in the ED can be extended post-ED, such as with a rapid response team, suicidal outcomes are greatly improved (Newton et al. 2010).

Eating Disorders

Less than 30% of children and adolescents who have behavior that may be classified as an eating disorder tell their physicians (Kaye et al. 2000). The problem is frequently uncovered when the medical consequences of the behavior prompt an ED visit. Patients may present with profound weight loss, dehydration, palpitations, evidence of starvation and fatigue, and a general malaise that suggests both illness and depression. Parents and family members are typically baffled and may not realize that the patient is dieting when not at home; exercising excessively; or repeating restricting, bingeing, and purging cycles that hinder the maintenance of a healthy weight.

Patients with eating disorders experience low rates of metabolism, with evidence of lanugo, hypothermia, and cyanotic extremities, a clinical picture consistent with symptoms of hypothyroidism. Abnormalities in glucose metabolism lead to episodes of hypoglycemia and ketoacidosis, although patients who binge and purge may experience elevated glucose levels. Adolescents with diabetes may lose weight by avoiding insulin, controlling intake, and burning fat rather than carbohydrates while ignoring the dangerous consequences of ketoacidosis. Electrolyte changes that are a consequence of fluid restriction, sudden water intoxication, and restricted food intake can cause bradycardia, hypotension, and cardiac arrhythmias. Malnutrition leads to decreased muscle mass throughout the body, including the heart, with resulting decrease in contractility and cardiac output (Romano et al. 2003). Patients who weigh less than 70% of ideal body weight are at risk for life-threatening dysrhythmias, and 30%–50% of these patients experience chest pain secondary to mitral valve prolapse (de Simone et al. 1994; Mascolo et al. 2012). Gastrointestinal disturbances include constipation, obstipation, and severe abdominal pain secondary to superior mesenteric artery syndrome. Dental caries and parotitis are telltale signs of bulimia along with calluses on fingers (Russell's sign) secondary to repetitive gagging. Vomiting and diuretic abuse can lead to hypokalemia and metabolic alkalosis, otherwise referred to as pseudo-Bartter syndrome (Mitchell et al. 1988). Patients with eating disorders may present in the ED with fractures secondary to osteoporosis and osteopenia due to poor nutrition. For general discussion of eating disorders, see Chapter 20, "Eating and Feeding Disorders."

Substance Abuse

Clinicians do not recognize alcohol use in as many as 50% of the patients who eventually test positive in the ED. The inability to identify these patients is due not only to a reluctance to pursue the issue aggressively but also because ED staff do not routinely use quick and effective means of case identification. Concise screening instruments such as the Drug Abuse Screening Test (DAST) or the CRAFFT screening test must accompany the interview and any indicated laboratory studies in the ED (Burke et al. 2005; Yudko et al. 2007). Substance use should be suspected when there is a sudden change in behavior, including a decline in academic or social functioning and multiple contacts with the police. Patients may use substances in physically dangerous situations and present to the ED as trauma victims. In studies of adults, nearly 50% of all trauma victims are alcohol positive at the time of ED admission, with a nearly 50% reduction in recurrent injury and readmission rate following a brief intervention (Kelleher et al. 2013). Caregivers may report unsuccessful attempts to control access and intake along with evidence in the patient of dependence, including tolerance, withdrawal, and physical or psychological consequences of substance use. If the goal is a treatment partnership with the adolescent, the ED assessment of substance abuse requires support rather than recrimination. An appearance in the ED frequently indicates a medical complication that alerts the patient and caregivers about the need for treatment. This is a critical period for insight and change both individually for the patient and within the family system (Meyers et al. 1999). Comorbid psychiatric disorders, particularly depression, may be the presenting complaint, and in these cases the relationship between substance abuse and suicidal behavior should be assessed along with risk factors that include dysphoric mood, disinhibition, impaired judgment, and an increased level of impulsivity. Parental involvement is an essential part of any successful treatment plan. Parental supervision motivates adolescents to change their behavior and improves assessment and treatment adherence. In addition, the relationship between substance abuse and the need for subsequent medical and mental health treatment encourages caregiver participation (Barnett et al. 2002; Spirito et al. 2001). ED staff members should be aware of community resources for young patients with substance abuse problems and begin the referral process before discharge. Substance abuse is covered in Chapter 12, "Substance Use Disorders and Addictions."

Autism Spectrum Disorder

Children with autism spectrum disorder typically present with delays in language and communication; restricted, repetitive, and stereotypic patterns of behaviors, interests, and activities; deficits in socialization; and in severe cases a presentation that is characteristic of patients with severe or profound intellectual disability. Their inability to communicate effectively means that a thorough physical examination is essential when evaluating a history of aggression, agitation, or self-abuse. In addition, the exacerbation of emotional or behavioral symptoms may be the result of pain or discomfort from simple problems such as otitis media or dental caries or more complicated and serious physical disorders. The ED is an anxiety-provoking environment for any child but particularly for these patients and their parents. The sights and sounds are frequently unsettling, and there is a steady stream of medical personnel either caring for the child or monitoring his or her behavior. ED staff should provide a safe and quiet environment away from traffic where the door can close and the family can have privacy. The parent or primary caregiver understands how best to communicate with the child and establish a level of cooperation that allows for assessment and treatment. Print and electronic versions of visual communication systems can be customized to the ED environment with photographs that are specific to the site (Gordon et al. 2011). The caregiver can be a source of information on the patient's needs during the ED admission; define the parameters of calm and safe surroundings for the child; and assist in the medical management of these patients, particularly the urgent administration of medications. In the ED, clinical staff routinely check on patients while they wait for an examination as a method of ensuring quality care. For autistic patients, these interruptions can be unsettling. Instead, a small and consistent group of clinicians can develop simple yet familiar routines for the patient during even brief stays in the ED.

Because children and adolescents with autism spectrum disorder may have idiosyncratic responses to medications, drug regimens should not be started without a specific plan for follow-up. For example, benzodiazepines (e.g., 0.5–1.0 mg of lorazepam) may produce paradoxical reactions that further complicate care, and high-potency antipsychotics (e.g., 0.5–2 mg of haloperidol) may induce extrapyramidal side effects leading to a clinical preference for atypical antipsychotics to urgently manage behavior.

Delirium

Delirium is characterized by a serious decline in functioning that develops over a short period of time and is typically the consequence of a medical condition, substance use or withdrawal, or toxin exposure. The most common symptoms in pediatric patients include disorientation, irritability, inattention, memory loss, diffuse cognitive deficits, and "clouded consciousness" (Turkel and Tavaré 2003). Children and adolescents less frequently present with disorganized thinking, language abnormalities, and disturbances in sleep-wake cycle. When young patients are admitted to the ED with the sudden appearance of delusions, visual or auditory hallucinations, illusions, and affective lability, delirium is a likely diagnosis. Critically ill patients in the ED, including victims of trauma, are vulnerable to delirium secondary to the direct neurophysiological effects of the disorder, including central nervous system (CNS) injury, metabolic abnormalities, changes in oxygen saturation, and volume depletion. The relative risk of delirium is related to the severity of the insult.

Physicians do not typically screen for acute mental status changes in young patients, and when they do so, symptoms are described in ambiguous diagnostic terminology. Delirium may prolong hospitalization and increase complication rates because patients are unable to actively participate in treatment. Clinicians more easily identify the "hyperactive" form of delirium that presents with irritability, agitation, disorientation, and abnormalities of thought and perception. Although these patients may be considered oppositional early in the course of their treatment, the impact of the symptoms on their care eventually leads to a psychiatric consultation. The "hypoactive" presentation is less well recognized and understood. These patients are quietly confused and anxious and are often misdiagnosed as depressed. Delirium typically presents with fluctuating levels of severity, with lucid intervals alternating with periods of confusion and agitation, making serial assessments necessary for adequate diagnosis.

Illnesses presenting in the ED may indirectly affect the CNS through a variety of mechanisms. *Hepatic encephalopathy,* for example, causes a decrease in acetylcholine synthesis, increased levels of serotonin and dopamine, and an increase in γ-aminobutyric acid activity leading to a hypoactive-hypoalert presentation. *Burn injury* creates a hypermetabolic state with an increased turnover of glucose and inconsistent insulin secretion. The result can be either hypo- or hyperglycemia. Several case studies document acute changes in mental status in pediatric patients with *seizure disorders* (Benson and Klein 2001; Zorc and Ludwig 2004). Children may experience confusion, lethargy, emotional lability, and disorientation before losing consciousness. Among the more common etiologies for acute mental status change following the sudden onset of a seizure disorder are viral infections and cerebral vasculitis. Delirium may be an early indication of *systemic lupus erythematosus,* with changes in behavior, mood, and personality as well as evidence of social withdrawal, confusion, noncompliance, bizarre and disorganized behavior, abnormalities of thought and perception, and sleep continuity disorders. Delirium following *steroid administration* was initially described in the 1950s. There is no dose-response relationship, but symptoms in adults appear in a bimodal distribution after either 4 days or 15–25 days of treatment (Sirois 2003).

Physicians often misinterpret symptoms of delirium as indicators of inadequate pain management and aggressively treat patients with narcotic medications that may cause further deterioration in mental status. In a retrospective chart review, nondelirious adult patients received most of their pain medications during the day, while delirious patients received their medications for "breakthrough pain" at night, when mental status changes that are labeled as *sundowning* are more likely to occur (Gagnon et al. 2001).

The most effective treatment for delirium is the correction of the underlying medical cause of the disorder, although patients often present with multiple causes that are not easily identified or controlled. When resolution of the primary cause is not possible, the clinician treats the symptoms in order to ease distress in the patient and family and improve the medical outcome (American Psychiatric Association 1999). The patient is both oriented and calmed by consistent caregivers in the family or on the clinical staff. The environment in the examination room should neither overstimulate nor understimulate the patient. Antipsychotic medications are recommended when the symptoms are persistent and severe and affect the child's medical outcome. High-potency first-generation antipsychotics are known to be effective on the basis of controlled trials in adults using standardized assessments. Haloperidol is administered at a low dose of 1 mg and titrated up by 0.25–0.5 mg increments (Tabet and Howard

2001). Atypical antipsychotics are now more often recommended, primarily because of their lower risk of extrapyramidal side effects. Risperidone is the most commonly used (Preval et al. 2005; Sipahimalani and Masand 1998). Benzodiazepines alone are rarely effective in children and may complicate or exacerbate symptoms of delirium.

Management of the Aggressive Pediatric Patient

Violent behavior increases the likelihood that a patient will present in the ED. Since payment for psychiatric hospitalization by both private and public organizations is based on the level of dangerousness rather than on the need for treatment, the system supports the referral of aggressive patients to the ED for admission. The ED has become the primary treatment site for many patients with chronic and severe mental illness that is associated with aggression and agitation. In addition, agitation may be the result of an underlying medical illness or exacerbated by the ED environment. Table 30–2 lists many of the reasons pediatric patients may be agitated or aggressive in the ED. Predictors of violent behavior seem to include male sex, history of prior violence, arrival in the ED in police custody, being a victim of violence, having a history of drug or alcohol use, and a history of psychiatric illness (Marzullo 2014). Screening tools are being developed to help ED staff assess level of aggressive risk (Barzman et al. 2012). A timely assessment with targeted testing should be completed to determine the underlying cause of agitation, specifically looking for causes of delirium.

Unfortunately, the circumstances in the ED often dictate the course of treatment and the techniques used to manage the patient (Masters et al. 2002). Agitated patients require more time and attention from the ED staff in order to identify the behaviors that trigger the patient's loss of control. When evaluating children and adolescents, ED clinicians may not be aware of premorbid psychiatric histories and therefore may make decisions that affect the safety of the patient and staff solely on the basis of the urgency of the situation. Behavior that is considered dangerous to the patient and others in the ED or that interferes with the ability to complete a medical evaluation may require acute interventions. Although there are no evidence-based guidelines on how to best manage aggressive pediatric patients in the ED, management typically includes some behavioral measures, seclusion, mechanical restraints, and/or pharmacological interventions.

Behavioral Measures

Most experts agree that behavioral approaches to aggression should be used first. Ideally, all ED staff and consultants should be skilled at recognizing the early signs of agitation and be able to intervene early, before symptoms escalate. During the assessment and approach to irritable children and adolescents, it is helpful to stay calm and use simplified language, a soft voice, and slow movements. Patients should be informed of the impact of their behavior on others and the fear they are eliciting among staff members, including the interviewer. Denying the impact of the patient's behavior on others may be perceived as a provocative challenge and result in an escalation of the aggressive symptoms. Environmental stimulation

TABLE 30–2. Causes of aggression and agitation in the emergency department

Behavior disorders
Attention-deficit/hyperactivity disorder
Oppositional defiant disorder
Conduct disorder
Intellectual disability
Anxiety-provoked aggression
Separation anxiety disorder
Panic disorder
Obsessive-compulsive disorder
Acute phobic hallucinations (especially in children ages 2–6 years)
Organic delirium
Medical illness
Infection such as meningitis or encephalitis
Electrolyte imbalance
Central nervous system tumor, trauma, or vascular accident
Seizures/postictal state
Endocrine or autoimmune disorder
Hypoxia
Metabolic disorder
Adverse reaction to prescribed or over-the-counter medication
Toxic ingestion
Reaction to illicit substance
Acute intoxication or toxic reaction
Withdrawal syndromes
Psychotic reaction to chronic drug use
Psychosis
Mania
Abuse or neglect

should be reduced when possible, and the child or adolescent should remain in the company of a family member or caregiver unless this adult is provoking more agitation in the patient. When alone, the aggressive patient may ruminate about incidents that led to the admission and become increasingly anxious about the assessment and disposition from the ED. The clinician should explain what will happen in the ED and negotiate with the patient in an attempt to meet his or her immediate needs—finding something that the child can control. Since perceived ignoring may encourage escalation, clinicians should remain engaged and empathetic with young patients. At times, if the child or adolescent does not respond to a verbal reassurance, it may be necessary to provide a "show of force." This conveys a message to the patient that some external control will be placed on his or her behavior. Hospital security staff can effectively deter acting-out behaviors simply by being visible in sufficient numbers. Emerging data from pediatric psychiatric units suggest that the formal adoption of behavioral interventions across an institution can greatly reduce the need for seclusions, restraints, and medications for agitation (De Hert et al. 2011).

Seclusion and Restraint

The use of seclusion and restraints is a frequent intervention with aggressive and potentially dangerous patients; however, their effectiveness in the pediatric population is largely unknown and remains controversial (De Hert et al. 2011). Seclusion is generally defined as the placement of a patient alone in a specifically designed room in order to deescalate behaviors, assure physical safety, and achieve behavioral control. Restraint use refers to a physical intervention, either through the use of physical force by one or more staff members or using mechanical restraints to restrict the movement of the patient. Opponents of the use of seclusion and restraint question their therapeutic value and effectiveness, citing concerns about coercion, reactivating prior trauma experience, and physical side effects. However, proponents of seclusion and restraint use report that when used with proper monitoring and oversight when less restrictive interventions have failed, they are an important tool in providing safety and stabilization.

Because of concerns about the use of seclusion and restraint, the Centers for Medicare and Medicaid Services and the Joint Commission on Accreditation of Healthcare Organizations, now known as The Joint Commission, have created specific guidelines for the initiation, use, and monitoring of seclusion and restraint (Joint Commission on Accreditation of Healthcare Organizations 2006). Restraint devices should be only those that are designed specifically for this purpose. This includes limb holders, abdominal belts, and vests. Makeshift restraints are always contraindicated because the devices are typically difficult to apply, frequently are tied too tightly and ineffectively, and often are uncomfortable and even dangerous for the patient. All restraint policies recommend seclusion and restraint only after less restrictive measures have failed. Seclusion and restraint are not to be used as punishment for the patient or as a convenience for the staff. The emergency team should anticipate the need for seclusion and restraint and identify roles for clinical personnel. This avoids confusion and encourages more efficient decision making in times of crisis. For example, the clinical program identifies who makes the decision to initiate the restraint, who physically puts the patient in restraints, and who performs the required face-to-face assessments to evaluate the need for continued intervention. No clinical trials demonstrate the most effective way to release a patient from restraints. The process is best approached as an ongoing negotiation, with the clinician constantly communicating with and reassuring the patient. Restraints are gradually released one step at a time, but the patient should never be left with one limb tied down. It provides too much mobility, and should the patient suddenly become combative, the situation may rapidly escalate into a dangerous incident. When staff are trained on the management of circumstances that both precede and accompany seclusion and restraint, these interventions are used less frequently, and there are fewer incidents of patient and staff injury (Bower et al. 2003; Busch and Shore 2000).

Pharmacological Interventions

Pharmacological interventions aimed at reducing aggression in the pediatric emergency setting are quite common, although there are limited data on their use. Pharmacological management of aggression, with medication prescribed on an as needed basis, seems preferable to the use of restraints, particularly when considering potential complications. There are no evidence-based guidelines for the acute management of children or adolescents with aggression or agitation.

Historically, benzodiazepines, haloperidol, and antihistamines have been used most commonly to treat agitation in both adult and pediatric settings (Baeza et al. 2013; Dorfman and Kastner 2004; Marzullo 2014). However, in the pediatric population, there are concerns about benzodiazepines and antihistamines causing paradoxical and disinhibiting reactions. There is also a trend toward choosing second-generation atypical antipsychotics over first-generation agents because of the lower risk of extrapyramidal side effects. Atypical antipsychotics have demonstrated efficacy in the treatment of aggression and self-injurious behavior in intellectually and developmentally delayed patients as well as the treatment of adolescent aggression across psychiatric diagnoses, with number needed to treat of 2–5 (Baeza et al. 2013). Newer oral preparations that quickly dissolve in the mouth and are swallowed have become an appealing option for agitated and uncooperative patients. Risperidone and olanzapine are cited frequently in the literature as preferred oral agents to treat agitation because of their rapid onset of action and likelihood of sedation (Hilt and Woodward 2008; Marzullo 2014). Other oral atypical antipsychotics (including quetiapine, ziprasidone, and aripiprazole) are felt to be less effective for acute agitation.

Because studies suggest that oral risperidone is just as effective as intramuscular haloperidol with similar onset of action, there seems to be little reason to use intramuscular medications for agitation unless an uncooperative patient refuses to take oral medication (Yildiz et al. 2003). Intramuscular ziprasidone with or without lorazepam seems to be the intramuscular treatment of choice in the adult literature followed by haloperidol plus lorazepam (Currier and Medori 2006; Lukens et al. 2006). Although in adults the combination of benzodiazepines with either a typical or an atypical antipsychotic may produce greater efficacy for symptoms of arousal as well as faster onset of action (Yildiz et al. 2003), there are very limited studies of using combination therapy in children.

Although there is no consensus on the most appropriate medication strategy for the pediatric emergency psychiatry patient, the following are general recommendations:

- Use medications targeting the underlying illness when possible.
- Administer repeated low doses of medication rather than a single high dose when titrating the drug.
- If the patient is already taking psychiatric medications, consider an additional dose of the same medication (unless there is suspicion of toxicity). Patients have often missed a dose before coming to the ED or during the time spent in the ED, and consideration should be given to replacing this missed dose.
- Combined treatments should be used only with great caution.
- Low-dose benzodiazepines must be used very carefully because of the possibility of paradoxical reactions.

Conclusion

Children and adolescents are presenting with psychiatric emergencies with increasing frequency in medical and mental health settings. Appropriate early services may not be accessed or may not be available. Symptoms progress, and the severity of the clinical presentation escalates until the situation demands attention. As a consequence, these patients exhibit high levels of dangerousness to themselves and others. In emergency assessments, the clinician is usually unfamiliar with the patient and must obtain details about psychiatric history and social environment from an agitated youth and an anxious parent. The formulation and treatment recommendations are typically based on the current crisis and the need to ensure a safe environment for the patient and staff. The pediatric and mental health clinician should be familiar with features that identify the most problematic cases and be able to safely and effectively triage these young patients to the most appropriate care.

Summary Points

- The demand for emergency psychiatric care of children and adolescents is increasing along with the challenges of assessing and treating dangerous and volatile populations.
- Suicidal behavior can be characterized by lethality and intent, and disposition recommendations are based on risk factors for dangerousness.
- Emergency presentation of patients with eating disorders is frequently due to the presence of concomitant medical complications along with a history of failed outpatient treatment.
- Substance abuse is underrecognized in the emergency department (ED), indicating a need for specific assessment and intervention whenever substance use is suspected.
- The ED is often a threatening and anxiety-provoking setting for a young patient with autism spectrum disorder.
- Delirium should be suspected in patients who experience a sudden change in behavior as a consequence of a medical condition, substance use or withdrawal, or toxin exposure.
- Management of the agitated and aggressive child should take into account the safety of the patient and staff and follow the guidelines outlined by The Joint Commission.

References

American Psychiatric Association: Practice guideline for the treatment of patients with delirium. Am J Psychiatry 156(5 suppl):1–20, 1999 10327941

Baeza I, Correll C, Saito E, et al: Frequency, characteristics and management of adolescent inpatient aggression. J Child Adolesc Psychopharmacol 23(4):271–281, 2013 23647136

Barnett NP, Lebeau-Craven R, O'Leary TA, et al: Predictors of motivation to change after medical treatment for drinking-related events in adolescents. Psychol Addict Behav 16(2):106–112, 2002 12079248

Barzman D, Mossman D, Sonnier L, et al: Brief rating of aggression by children and adolescents: a reliability study. J Am Acad Psychiatry Law 40(3):374–382, 2012

Benson PJ, Klein EJ: New-onset absence status epilepsy presenting as altered mental status in a pediatric patient. Ann Emerg Med 37(4):402–405, 2001 11275834

Bower FL, McCullough CS, Timmons ME: A synthesis of what we know about the use of physical restraints and seclusion with patients in psychiatric and acute care settings: 2003 update. Online J Knowl Synth Nurs 10:1, 2003 12800050

Bridge JA, Marcus SC, Olfson M: Outpatient care of young people after emergency treatment of deliberate self-harm. J Am Acad Child Adolesc Psychiatry 51(2):213–222, e1, 2012 22265367

Burke PJ, O'Sullivan J, Vaughan BL: Adolescent substance use: brief interventions by emergency care providers. Pediatr Emerg Care 21(11):770–776, 2005 16280955

Busch AB, Shore MF: Seclusion and restraint: a review of recent literature. Harv Rev Psychiatry 8(5):261–270, 2000 11118235

Currier GW, Medori R: Orally versus intramuscularly administered antipsychotic drugs in psychiatric emergencies. J Psychiatr Pract 12(1):30–40, 2006 16432443

De Hert M, Dirix N, Demunter H, et al: Prevalence and correlates of seclusion and restraint use in children and adolescents: a systematic review. Eur Child Adolesc Psychiatry 20(5):221–230, 2011 21298305

de Simone G, Scalfi L, Galderisi M, et al: Cardiac abnormalities in young women with anorexia nervosa. Br Heart J 71(3):287–292, 1994 8142200

Dolan MA, Fein JA, Committee on Pediatric Emergency Medicine: Pediatric and adolescent mental health emergencies in the emergency medical services system. Pediatrics 127(5):e1356–e1366, 2011 21518712

Dorfman DH, Kastner B: The use of restraint for pediatric psychiatric patients in emergency departments. Pediatr Emerg Care 20(3):151–156, 2004 15094571

Gagnon B, Lawlor PG, Mancini IL, et al: The impact of delirium on the circadian distribution of breakthrough analgesia in advanced cancer patients. J Pain Symptom Manage 22(4):826–833, 2001 11576799

Gordon K, Pasco G, McElduff F, et al: A communication-based intervention for nonverbal children with autism: what changes? Who benefits? J Consult Clin Psychol 79(4):447–457, 2011 21787048

Grupp-Phelan J, Mahajan P, Foltin GL, et al: Referral and resource use patterns for psychiatric-related visits to pediatric emergency departments. Pediatr Emerg Care 25(4):217–220, 2009 19382317

Hilt RJ, Woodward TA: Agitation treatment for pediatric emergency patients. J Am Acad Child Adolesc Psychiatry 47(2):132–138, 2008 18216715

Horwitz AG, Czyz EK, King CA: Predicting future suicide attempts among adolescent and emerging adult psychiatric emergency patients. J Clin Child Adolesc Psychol 28:1–11, 2014 24871489

Joint Commission on Accreditation of Healthcare Organizations: Comprehensive Accreditation Manual for Hospitals: The Official Handbook. Oakbrook Terrace, IL, Joint Commission on Accreditation of Healthcare Organizations, 2006

Kaye WH, Klump KL, Frank GK, et al: Anorexia and bulimia nervosa. Annu Rev Med 51:299–313, 2000 10774466

Kelleher DC, Renaud EJ, Ehrlich PF, et al: Guidelines for alcohol screening in adolescent trauma patients: a report from the Pediatric Trauma Society Guidelines Committee. J Trauma Acute Care Surg 74(2):671–682, 2013 23354268

Lukens TW, Wolf SJ, Edlow JA, et al: Clinical policy: critical issues in the diagnosis and management of the adult psychiatric patient in the emergency department. Ann Emerg Med 47(1):79–99, 2006 16387222

Marzullo LR: Pharmacologic management of the agitated child. Pediatr Emerg Care 30(4):269–275, quiz 276–278, 2014 24694885

Mascolo M, Trent S, Colwell C, et al: What the emergency department needs to know when caring for your patients with eating disorders. Int J Eat Disord 45(8):977–981, 2012 22707235

Masters KJ, Bellonci C, Bernet W, et al: Practice parameter for the prevention and management of aggressive behavior in child and adolescent psychiatric institutions, with special reference to seclusion and restraint. J Am Acad Child Adolesc Psychiatry 41(2 suppl):4S–25S, 2002 11833634

Meyers K, Hagan TA, Zanis D, et al: Critical issues in adolescent substance use assessment. Drug Alcohol Depend 55(3):235–246, 1999 10428364

Mitchell JE, Pomeroy C, Seppala M, et al: Pseudo-Bartter's syndrome, diuretic abuse, idiopathic edema, and eating disorders. Int J Eat Disord 7(2):225–237, 1988

Newton AS, Hamm MP, Bethell J, et al: Pediatric suicide-related presentations: a systematic review of mental health care in the emergency department. Ann Emerg Med 56(6):649–659, 2010 20381916

Posner K, Brown GK, Stanley B, et al: The Columbia-Suicide Severity Rating Scale: initial validity and internal consistency findings from three multisite studies with adolescents and adults. Am J Psychiatry 168(12):1266 1277, 2011 22193671

Preval H, Klotz SG, Southard R, et al: Rapid-acting IM ziprasidone in a psychiatric emergency service: a naturalistic study. Gen Hosp Psychiatry 27(2):140–144, 2005 15763126

Romano C, Chinali M, Pasanisi F, et al: Reduced hemodynamic load and cardiac hypotrophy in patients with anorexia nervosa. Am J Clin Nutr 77(2):308–312, 2003 12540387

Santiago LI, Tunik MG, Foltin GL, et al: Children requiring psychiatric consultation in the pediatric emergency department: epidemiology, resource utilization, and complications. Pediatr Emerg Care 22(2):85–89, 2006 16481922

Sipahimalani A, Masand PS: Olanzapine in the treatment of delirium. Psychosomatics 39(5):422–430, 1998 9775699

Sirois F: Steroid psychosis: a review. Gen Hosp Psychiatry 25(1):27–33, 2003 12583925

Spirito A, Plummer B, Gispert M, et al: Adolescent suicide attempts: outcomes at follow-up. Am J Orthopsychiatry 62(3):464–468, 1992 1497112

Spirito A, Lewander WJ, Levy S, et al: Emergency department assessment of adolescent suicide attempters: factors related to short-term follow-up outcome. Pediatr Emerg Care 10(1):6–12, 1994 8177812

Spirito A, Barnett NP, Lewander W, et al: Risks associated with alcohol-positive status among adolescents in the emergency department: a matched case-control study. J Pediatr 139(5):694–699, 2001 11713449

Spirito A, Boergers J, Donaldson D, et al: An intervention trial to improve adherence to community treatment by adolescents after a suicide attempt. J Am Acad Child Adolesc Psychiatry 41(4):435–442, 2002 11931600

Tabet N, Howard R: Optimising management of delirium. Patients with delirium should be treated with care. BMJ 322(7302):1602–1603, 2001 11458900

Turkel SB, Tavaré CJ: Delirium in children and adolescents. J Neuropsychiatry Clin Neurosci 15(4):431–435, 2003 14627769

Yildiz A, Sachs GS, Turgay A: Pharmacological management of agitation in emergency settings. Emerg Med J 20(4):339–346, 2003 12835344

Yudko E, Lozhkina O, Fouts A: A comprehensive review of the psychometric properties of the Drug Abuse Screening Test. J Subst Abuse Treat 32(2):189–198, 2007 17306727

Zorc JJ, Ludwig S: A 12-year-old girl with altered mental status and a seizure. Pediatr Emerg Care 20(9):613–616, 2004 15599266

CHAPTER 31

Family Transitions

Challenges and Resilience

Froma Walsh, Ph.D.

In this chapter, the challenges posed by major family transitions for child, adolescent, and family functioning are addressed. A brief overview places family transitional dilemmas in broad societal context. Normative and nonnormative family developmental transitions are examined, with focus on the effects of highly disruptive transitions due to death, divorce and stepfamily formation, immigration, multistress conditions, and foster care. Clinical guidelines are offered to buffer stresses and strengthen resilience in youth and their families to enhance adaptation.

Family Transformations in a Changing Society

In the midst of social, economic, and political upheavals over recent decades, families have become more diverse and complex (Walsh 2012b). It is useful to highlight the following trends: 1) varied family structures and gender roles, 2) increasing cultural diversity and economic disparity, and 3) expanded and more fluid family life course.

Changing Family Structures and Gender Roles

The 1950s model family—white, middle class, intact nuclear household, headed by a breadwinner father and a homemaker mother—is now only a narrow band on the wide spectrum of families. Family structures encompass two-earner households; divorced families, single-parent families, and stepfamilies; cohabiting unmarried parents; extended kinship care; and families headed by gay and lesbian parents.

The vast majority of two-parent families today are headed by dual-earner couples who navigate stressful demands of jobs, household maintenance, childrearing, and elder care (Repetti et al. 2009). Most couples strive for an egalitarian partnership and shared involvement in childrearing. Most men carry more household and child care responsibilities than their own fathers did, although still much less than their wives' share (Bianchi and Milkie 2010; Fraenkel and Capstick 2012).

Divorce rates, after rising in recent decades, have leveled off for first marriages (Amato 2010). Most children in divorced families undergo further transition with parental remarriage and stepfamily formation. Difficulties in combining households and forging new steprelationships contribute to the high divorce rate (near 60%) for remarriages. Nearly half of all children, and more than 60% of poor, ethnic minority children, live for some time in one-parent households (nearly 90% of them headed by divorced or unmarried mothers) (Anderson 2012). Fortunately, unwed teen parenting, with high risks for long-term poverty and for health and psychosocial problems, has been declining. Children generally fare well in financially secure and stable one-parent homes with strong parental functioning. Kinship care, particularly with grandparents, is increasingly common when parents are working or unable to provide care (Engstrom 2012).

Increasing numbers of gay, lesbian, bisexual, and transgender parents are raising children. Research clearly shows that children in gender-variant families fare as well as those with heterosexual parents, although they are challenged by social stigma (Biblarz and Savci 2010; Green 2012). Adoptive families have also been increasing for couples and single parents, both gay and straight (Rampage et al. 2012). Most adoptions are now open, on the basis of findings that children benefit developmentally if they know who their birth families are, have the option for contact, and in biracial and international adoption are encouraged to develop bicultural identities and connections.

Preconceptions of "the normal family" can compound a sense of deficiency and failure for families in transition that do not conform to the intact nuclear family model (Walsh 2012b). The term *single-parent family* can blind clinicians to the important role of a nonresidential parent or a caregiving grandparent and supportive kin network. It is inadvisable to regard a stepparent or adoptive parent as not the "real" or "natural" parent.

Cultural Diversity and Socioeconomic Disparity

In our multicultural society, growing numbers of children and families are multiethnic, biracial, and multifaith (Rosenblatt 2013; Walsh 2010). Therefore, clinicians must be attuned to the diverse beliefs and practices in families, their views of healthy development and dysfunction, and their preferred pathways in solving problems. Strong kinship bonds foster resilience, particularly for African Americans, Native Americans, and immigrants struggling to overcome conditions of poverty and discrimination (Boyd-Franklin and Karger 2012; Falicov 2012).

A widening socioeconomic gap, with gross disparities, has had a significant impact on family formation and stability. Those with limited education, job skills, and employment opportunities have been hit hardest and are least likely to marry and most likely to divorce (Cherlin 2010). Declining economic conditions and job dislocation have a devastating impact on family functioning and child well-being. Persistent unemployment or recurring job transitions can fuel substance abuse, relational conflict and violence, family breakup, loss of homes, and an increase in poor single-parent households. Conditions of discrimination, neighborhood decay, poor schools, crime, violence, and inadequate health care worsen life chances.

Varying, Extended Family Life Course

With greater life expectancy, four- and five-generation families are increasingly common (Bengston 2001), as are two or more sequential committed relationships, interspersed with periods of cohabitation and single living. Our view of the family life cycle must be expanded to the varied life course that makes each family unique. Children and their parents are increasingly likely to transition in and out of several household and kinship arrangements over the life course. Some adults become first-time parents at the age when others become grandparents. Some start second families at midlife, with children even a generation apart. For resilience, families need to buffer transitions and learn how to live successfully in complex kinship arrangements.

Given the diversity of family structures, cultural and socioeconomic influences, and the timing of nodal events, no single model or sequential life trajectory should be regarded as the standard or as essential for healthy child development (Walsh 2015). There is abundant evidence that children can be raised well in a variety of family structures (Lansford et al. 2001), yet disruptive family transitions are distressing, and highly unstable relationships increase the risk for child maladaptation (Fomby and Cherlin 2007). What matters most for healthy child development and resilience are caring committed relationships and effective family processes throughout stressful transitions.

Family Systems–Oriented Practice

Family systems practice approaches are guided by a developmental, multilevel systemic perspective on human problems and processes of change, attending to the family and social context of dysfunction and resilience (Rolland and Walsh 2008). This biopsychosocial orientation addresses the complex interplay of individual, family, and social influences, including school, workplace, court, and health care systems. It attends to cultural, spiritual, and socioeconomic influences, including the impact of racism and other forms of discrimination. Regardless of the origin of problems, families can play a key role for optimal child development (Masten 2014; Masten and Monn 2015).

The family is viewed as a transactional system evolving over the life course and across the generations (McGoldrick et al., in press). Individual and family development are intertwined, with each phase posing new challenges. Shifts in family organization, roles, and boundaries are required with relationship changes and with the addition and loss of members. Child distress often occurs around major family transitions, including both predictable, normative stresses and unexpected disruptions. Stressful transitions affect the family as a functional unit, with reverberations for all members and their relationships. In turn, family processes can heighten risk or foster positive adaptation (Walsh 2003, 2015). Thus, the family is an essential partner in assessment and treatment.

A systemic lens is required to identify key relationships in the family system, including all household members, nonresidential parents and steprelations, the extended kin network, and other significant relationships (e.g., intimate partner, informal kin, caregivers). Companion animals can also be vital resources (Walsh 2009a). The *genogram* and timeline (McGoldrick et al. 2008) are essential tools to map the family system, noting relationship information and tracking system patterns to guide intervention planning. In a resilience-oriented assessment (Walsh 2003, 2006), the clinician searches for positive influences and potential resources alongside problematic patterns (e.g., substance abuse, relational conflicts, cutoffs).

Family functioning is assessed in the context of the multigenerational system over time. A timeline is useful for noting the sequence of critical events or pileup of stressors and presenting problems. For instance, a son's drop in school grades may be precipitated by family tensions around his father's recent job loss. Because family members may not mention, or even notice, such connections, the genogram and timeline can guide inquiry and reveal patterns to explore. Clinicians need to inquire about family organizational shifts and coping strategies in response to anticipated, recent, and past stressors, particularly disruptive transitions. Family strain increases exponentially if a current crisis, such as a threatened separation, reactivates past trauma or loss (McGoldrick et al., in press). Families may conflate the situations, generating catastrophic fears. It is important to identify processes that promote resilience, such as active coping and perseverance, and to draw out stories of positive adaptation in facing other life challenges.

Childrearing Phases: Expectable Developmental Transitions

Anticipated family developmental transitions are more manageable than unexpected changes, yet they are stressful because family structures must adapt to meet emerging needs and priorities. Symptoms often coincide with family developmental transitions. Families need to counterbalance continuity and change to provide stability through disruption and to maintain ongoing connections.

Transition to Parenthood and Early Childrearing

With the birth or adoption of a child, parents must reorganize their lives. For the development of secure attachments, they must be emotionally engaged and consistently attentive to innumerable demands. Raising two or more children requires even more juggling of time and resources. With the first child, transformations take place in a couple's relationship as they expand their bond from dyad to triad (Cowan and Cowan 2012). Each partner's identity and focus shift in new parental roles and the formation of a shared parental coalition. All life patterns are altered for new parents: time and space, money, work schedules, and leisure. Couples need to negotiate workplace-family strains and relational imbalances as well as childrearing values and practices, such as discipline. In many ethnic groups, as in Latino families, parent-child bonds commonly take precedence as the dominant dyad, which can generate tensions in the couple relationship (Falicov 2012).

Single parents function best when they can draw on practical, emotional, and financial resources in kinship and social networks. When grandparents provide support, intergenerational tensions can arise over issues of authority, especially in a shared household (Engstrom 2012). Problematic triangles occur if a mother and grandmother compete for a child's loyalty, affection, or obedience. Grandparents with financial or health concerns may become overburdened. Most functional is a caring, collaborative relationship, with clear coordination and communication.

Transitions With Adolescence

Family transitions with adolescence are particularly disruptive, requiring flexible shifts in family roles, rules, and relationships to fit needs for greater autonomy, separate space, and peer involvement. Parents often confront stresses on both generational sides, with financial, practical, and emotional support of their teenage or young adult children and their own aging parents. In one case, a mother's escalating conflict with her "out of control" teenage son was fueled by her anxiety that she could not provide care for her mother, whose worsening dementia was now also "out of control." In other cases, past family-of-origin issues can be reactivated. One close father-son relationship became stormy as the launching transition approached, replicating the father's unresolved conflict with his own father around leaving home.

Highly Disruptive Family Transitions

Nonnormative—unanticipated and untimely—family transitions are highly disruptive in family life, heightening risk for child and adolescent emotional and behavioral problems. The loss of a breadwinner's job or a parent's life-threatening illness can generate anxiety and family upheaval. The impact of death and loss will be considered first, followed by transitions with divorce and stepfamily formation, migration, multistress conditions, and foster care, all of which require attention to loss for positive adaptation.

Adaptation to Death and Loss

Coming to terms with loss through death is the most painful challenge a family must confront. From a family systems perspective, the transactional process involves those who die and all who survive in a shared life cycle, recognizing both the finality of death and the continuity of life (Walsh and McGoldrick 2004, 2013). A death in the family involves multiple losses: the person, the meaning of a relationship for each member, family role functions (e.g., breadwinner, caregiving grandmother), and special position (e.g., only child). Survivors experience the loss of their intact family and the loss of hopes and dreams for the future. A traumatic loss often is accompanied by shattered assumptions in family members' worldviews regarding predictability, security, and trust (Walsh 2007).

Variables in Child and Family Risk

The *nature and circumstances of loss* can increase risk of child and family dysfunction. Such situations include the following:

1. *Sudden death* leaves the child and family without time to prepare for the loss, to say good-byes, or to deal with unfinished business.

2. *Lingering death,* such as after a long illness, depletes family resources and generates both relief and guilt that a prolonged ordeal is over.
3. *Ambiguous loss* occurs when there is lack of clarity about the fate of a loved one who is missing or when there is psychological and relational loss of a loved one who is still alive, as in dementia (Boss 1999).
4. *Disenfranchised losses,* with socially unacknowledged losses (such as miscarriage, pet loss) or stigmatized deaths (as with HIV/AIDS or suicide), can produce secrecy, guilt, and estrangement.
5. *Violent deaths,* such as a fatal accident, homicide, or suicide, generate lingering anger, guilt, remorse, and forgiveness issues.

The particular *timing of a loss* in the family life cycle may heighten risk for dysfunction; these types of risk include the following:

1. *Untimely loss,* especially early loss of a parent or death of a child
2. *Concurrence of death with other loss, stressors, or transitions,* which may overload families and pose incompatible demands (e.g., grieving and attachment)
3. *Past traumatic loss and complicated mourning,* which intensify reactions to other transitions, especially with regard to attachment and separation

Transgenerational anniversary reactions can be triggered by a current developmental transition. In each situation, the state of relationships and role functions lost will interact in effects. Unresolved conflicts and cutoffs have long-lasting reverberations for survivors. Reconnection and repair foster resilience.

Death of a Parent

Children who lose a parent or primary caretaker are at risk for long-term complications, such as difficulty in forming intimate attachments or catastrophic fears of separation and abandonment (Worden 2008). Clinicians may need to mobilize the kin network to provide support, structure, and reassurance that children will be cared for and not suffer further loss. Adolescents, with their own developmental thrust for separation, may minimize the meaning of the loss and withdraw, rebuffing family efforts at closeness and mutual support. If there has been conflict over autonomy and control issues, adolescents may develop guilt or long-term patterns of conflict with authority figures. Reactions are also influenced by peer models of acting-out behavior to escape pain, such as drinking, drug use, stealing, eating disorders, sexual activity, and pregnancy. For a surviving parent, financial and childrearing demands can interfere with mourning processes. Mourning can also be blocked if children suppress their grief to support the parent or if well-meaning relatives push for premature closure and precipitous replacement of a spouse or parent.

Death of a Child or Sibling

The death of a child is especially tragic, reversing generational life cycle expectations. Families often struggle with a sense of injustice and shattered hopes and dreams for their child. Because parents are responsible for their children's well-being, their guilt and blame can be especially strong in accidental or ambiguous deaths. Miscarriages and perinatal losses, often minimized by others, involve the loss of a desired child and fear of future pregnancy complications. Well-intentioned relatives may push couples to try to have another child before they have grieved, complicating the new attachment.

Bereaved fathers commonly minimize their grief and vulnerability; too often only mothers attend support groups. The loss of a child places the parents' relationship at risk for conflict and divorce if they withdraw, grieve separately, or blame each other. Brief couples therapy or support groups can facilitate mourning, recovery, and mutual support.

With the illness and death of a child, the needs of siblings may suffer because of parental preoccupation with caring for the ill child or their own grief. In some cases, parents withdraw to avoid further vulnerability to loss or they become anxiously overprotective of surviving children and may have difficulty with later normative transitions of separation and launching. Survivor guilt, common for both siblings and parents, can block life pursuits. A sibling may be inducted into an undifferentiated replacement role for the family, sacrificing his or her own developmental needs and unique qualities. Attempts at separation and individuation can disrupt the family equilibrium and precipitate intense delayed grief in parents. When a child is in crisis, it is particularly important to note other deaths at the same age and life cycle transition (Walsh and McGoldrick 2013).

Case Example 1

After a suicide attempt, Dan, age 13, remained silent, and his parents were unable to comprehend his actions. They made no mention of a deceased older brother. A family genogram revealed that Dan's older brother had died of leukemia at age 13. Over the years, the parents never talked about their loss, to avoid their grief. Yet Dan, aware of their loss, had tried to assuage their sadness by taking his brother's place, wearing his clothes, and combing his hair to look like photos of his brother. Now turning 14 and changing physically with adolescence, he did not know "who to be," so he decided to join his brother in heaven.

The death of an adolescent can be agonizing for family members. The most common adolescent deaths are from accidents, suicide, and homicide. In cases of impulsive, risk-taking behavior, as with substance abuse or reckless driving, family members commonly carry intense anger, frustration, and despair about the senseless loss of life and future potential. Stigma and blame can block comprehension, communication, and social support. It is crucial to explore possible connections to other traumatic losses in the family and peer network. Inner-city violence takes a tragic toll on young lives, particularly in poor, blighted neighborhoods. The frequency of early violent death, especially for young males, contributes to a foreshortened expectation of their life chances and to a present focus, high-risk sex, and self-destructive substance abuse.

Facilitating Adaptation to Loss

Family adaptation to loss involves sharing grief, gaining meaning and perspective, and moving ahead with life. Bereavement has no orderly sequence, timetable, or final resolution. Facets of the grief process can resurface at such nodal points as birthdays and anniversaries. The multiple meanings of any death are transformed over the life cycle and integrated with other life experiences, particularly losses. Work with families facing loss requires respect for diverse cultural and spiritual preferences. Families may need help in tolerating members' varied reactions, coping styles, and pace. Four core family tasks facilitate immediate and long-term adaptation for children and strengthen the family as a functional unit (Walsh and McGoldrick 2004, 2013):

1. *Share acknowledgment of the reality of death and loss* through information and communication.
2. *Share experience of loss* via memorial rituals and empathic sharing of feelings and meaning-making.
3. *Reorganize family system* through restabilization and realignment of relationships and role functions to provide continuity, cohesion, and adaptive flexibility.
4. *Reinvest in relationships and life pursuits and transform bonds with the deceased* from living presence to spiritual connections, memories, and legacies.

Divorce and Stepfamily Formation

Family transitions with divorce pose a series of challenges over time and are especially painful and disruptive through the first year. However, claims that divorce inevitably damages children have been refuted by longitudinal research on risk and resilience (Greene et al. 2012). Despite some reports of a higher rate of problems for children of divorced parents than those in intact families, fewer than one in four children from divorced families shows serious or lasting difficulties. Financial strain and unreliable contact with and support by the nonresidential parent heighten risk. However, the vast majority of children adjust reasonably well, and a third do remarkably well. In high-conflict families, children whose parents divorce tend to do better than those whose families remain intact. Although grown children may have painful memories of the divorce, most have no greater difficulty developing committed intimate relationships than those whose parents stayed unhappily married. What matters most for adaptation is the quality of relationships with parents and between the parents before and after divorce (Ahrons 2004).

Longitudinal studies have tracked family processes associated with successful adaptation versus dysfunction: from an escalation of tensions in the predivorce climate, through separation, legal divorce processes, and subsequent reorganization of households, roles, and relationships (Hetherington and Kelly 2002). Divorce mediation and collaborative divorce counseling are recommended, except in extreme cases such as abusive relationships. Joint custody works well when parents can cooperate in decision making, child contact, financial support, and shared responsibilities. With serious conflict, sole custody and a primary residence are advised, with clear guidelines for support and visitation by the nonresidential parent (Kelly 2007). Clinicians should evaluate the current status and potential involvement of a parent who was unreliable, absent, or harmful in the past. If barriers can be surmounted and a child's security is protected, these parents often can become more supportive of their child's positive development.

Divorce adaptation is complicated by ambiguous loss: the family unit is dissolved, but parents move on in separate lives, forming new attachments that may include cohabitation, marriage, and families. Continuing contact between parents around child-related issues and events can arouse painful feelings. In contrast to the idealization and sorrow common in widowhood, divorce tends to highlight hurts and injustices, with anger and resentment often stoked by lengthy litigation and custody battles. Parents may need help to not disparage the other parent or triangulate a child in disputes or competition for loyalty (Bernstein 2007).

Research on risk and resilience following divorce can inform efforts to help parents plan separation decisions and custody and residential and visitation options, as well as postdivorce transitions, such as changes in residence, repartnering or remarriage, and stepfamily formation (Pasley and Garneau 2012). Clinicians need to explore previous family units, the timing and nature of transitions, and future anticipated changes. In particular, recent or impending changes in membership or household composition may precipitate a crisis related to the presenting problems. Focusing on only the current household can restrict clinical understanding.

Case Example 2

A single-parent father with custody of his two children, Matt, age 14, and Maggie, age 12, sought help for Maggie's stormy behavior with him. The therapist initially focused on the father-daughter relationship and parenting skills, without success. A developmental, systemic inquiry revealed that the father had divorced the mother 2 years earlier after learning of her infidelity. He won a bitter custody fight and continued to demonize her to the children, severely restricting their contact. He plunged into a new relationship with a divorced woman with two children, who was now pressing him to get married. Maggie was angry at having been turned against her mother, upset by her loss of contact, and resentful of the "replacement" mom in the wings. The father, in an individual session, then expressed his own anxiety about remarriage, rooted in his unresolved emotional divorce, shattered trust, and sense of betrayal. These issues required therapeutic work before moving on to consider remarriage and the complications of new steprelations.

Migration Challenges

Migration poses multiple challenges in navigating disruptive transitions and losses and adapting to a new culture and way of life. Immigrants often experience a profound loss of kin and social networks and a sense of rootlessness: between two worlds and belonging to neither. Ongoing stresses can be overwhelming—meeting practical challenges of housing, jobs, schools, and language barriers; navigating immigration laws, cultural rules, and customs; and experiencing marginalization and loss of identity and status.

Falicov (2012) has developed a multilevel model for prevention and intervention with transnational families, integrating three contexts in risk and resilience: the relational, the community, and the cultural-sociopolitical. The relational level deals with marital and parent-child interaction patterns that are a product of the migration experience. The community level addresses the loss of social networks and the reconstitution of new and old community bonds. The sociopolitical level attends to issues of cultural diversity and to encounters with prejudice and discrimination that affect adaptation. Inquiry about migration experiences should attend to both traumas and losses family members suffered and to the sources of resilience that enabled them to survive, regenerate, and make their way in a new world. Spiritual beliefs and practices should be explored, as they are commonly wellsprings for strength and endurance. Indigenous beliefs or traditional faith healing practices may not be mentioned unless a therapist inquires respectfully about them (Walsh 2009b).

It is crucial to assess the fit of children and their families with their sociocultural contexts. Families and their children do best over time when they not only acculturate to "fit into" their new world but also preserve valued connections with their kin, community, and ethnic and spiritual roots. Resilience is fostered by weaving together a bicultural identity, sustaining cultural continuities, stories and rituals, regular contact, and affective bonds that bolster health and mental health when coping with migration stresses (Falicov 2012, 2013).

Intergenerational tensions are common between immigrant parents and adolescents born and/or raised in the United States. Frequently there is a clash of gender and cultural norms (for instance, for teenage daughters in traditional Middle Eastern families who want to date and socialize). Conflict often arises around authority and autonomy.

Case Example 3

Stavros, an Eastern European immigrant, brought his 17-year-old only son, Stavros Jr., for therapy to "straighten him out." He was furious that his son was hanging around with "no-good" friends and wanted to quit school. Steve (as the son preferred to be called) defended his friends and said he felt constantly pressured by his father to succeed academically. He looked down on his father's work as a janitor and felt badgered to make up for the father's "failure" in life.

The therapist encouraged Stavros to share his migration story with his son. He described the brutal military regime that he had fled, leaving school at age 17 to escape being drafted. In the United States he took the only work he could find, adding odd jobs to send money back to his parents. In a hushed voice, he revealed his shame at his humble position and his poor English. Like many immigrants, he struggled tenaciously to enable his children to have a better life, putting away a few dollars whenever he could for his son's college education. He was so proud to have such a smart son. How could Steve not care about his future?

Despite initial disinterest in his father's story, Steve listened intently. Coming to realize his father's hardships and courage, his view of him as a failure and a tyrant shifted to admiration and appreciation. Having felt only his father's disapproval, he became aware of his father's pride in him. The sessions also helped his father gain tolerance for Steve's friends and activities as he came to understand Steve's differences less as rejection and more about finding himself and his place in American culture. He reflected that in demanding that Steve do everything *his* way, he had become like the dictator he had fled. Therapy helped to rebalance their relationship. Steve still needed his father's support in making his own choices for a good life. Cast in a new light, the very possibility of choice meant that Stavros had truly succeeded in his dream of a better life for his son, giving him the gift of freedom.

In this resilience-oriented approach, the therapist drew out the father's life story to help the son gain compassion for his father's struggles and appreciate his loving intentions. Reaching greater mutual understanding, the father became less controlling and more accepting of his son's autonomous strivings. In turn, the son became less likely to make bad choices for himself out of angry defiance.

Refugee families face myriad additional challenges, particularly overcoming experiences of physical and psychosocial trauma and loss (Walsh

2007). Many have fled persecution, brutal atrocities, or harsh conditions and have endured multiple relocations, with uncertainty about their future. Many have suffered traumatic losses of loved ones, homes, and communities. Marital and intergenerational tensions common in migration can be intensified by posttraumatic distress. Survivor guilt and anxieties about the safety of loved ones left behind can add to suffering. Refugees commonly do not use mental health services, feeling pathologized and stigmatized by labels of symptoms as mental illness. Most immigrants respond well to family-centered, community-based approaches. Resilience-oriented multifamily groups provide a respectful, supportive context in which to share their full experience of loss and suffering, as well as positive strivings for adaptation (Walsh 2013; Weine et al. 2005).

Multistressed Families and At-Risk Youth

Family vulnerability and risks for children are heightened by a pileup of stressors and chronic disruptions. Multiple traumas, losses, and dislocations can overwhelm coping efforts. Recurrent crises and persistent demands drain resources, especially for single parents. Family organization, patterns of interaction, and relationships can become fragmented and chaotic, contributing to abuse and neglect, youth substance abuse, and conduct disorder. When leadership is erratic and boundaries are weak, a child may be drawn into a parentified role such as "man of the house" to fill the void, or a child may be sexually abused. Constant stress and frustration can spark intense conflict. With inconsistent limit setting and discipline, frustration can trigger violence or threat of abandonment.

Families in poor communities, disproportionately minorities, are most likely to be destabilized by frequent crises, traumatic losses, abrupt transitions, and chronic stresses of unemployment, housing, discrimination, and health care. With neighborhood crime, violence, and drugs, parents worry constantly for their children's safety. Bleak life prospects make it hard to break the cycle of poverty and despair, leaving parents defeated by repeated frustration and failure. High instability in their lives and relationships increases youth adjustment problems (Fomby and Cherlin 2007). Intertwined family and environmental stresses contribute to school dropout, gang activity, and teen pregnancy.

Even in brief therapy, it is crucial to understand how symptoms and catastrophic fears are fueled by overwhelming stresses, trauma, and losses. When therapy is overly problem focused, it grimly replicates the family's problem-saturated experience. A resilience-oriented perspective seeks to empower struggling families to master the challenges in their stress-laden lives (Walsh, in press). Interventions that enhance positive interactions, support coping efforts, and build resources are more effective in reducing stress and enhancing pride and more effective functioning. A compassionate understanding of internal and external stressors can engage parents in efforts to break dysfunctional cycles and raise their children well. All parents want a better life for their children, even when a myriad of difficulties block their ability to act on these intentions. They often know what they need to change in their lives and will take active steps if clinicians value their potential and support their best efforts.

By strengthening the family, the home becomes a more solid foundation for at-risk youth. If parents are unable to provide this structure, it is important to recruit caregivers and positive models and mentoring relationships in the extended kin network to nurture youth resilience (Ungar 2004; Walsh 2012a). Grandfathers are often overlooked resources, as are godparents, who each have a special bond with a child. In one family that was involved in a gang prevention/youth development program (Walsh 2013), the 11-year-old son was at high risk of gang involvement, with his older brother in a gang and his father estranged. A genogram-assisted assessment of the family system noted that an uncle (mother's brother), who was previously gang involved and incarcerated, had turned his life around and was now doing well. He was contacted and gladly stepped up to actively mentor his nephew and encourage his positive strivings. Seeing the whole family together may not be feasible in overstressed or fragmented families. Maintaining a family-centered approach involves a systemic view that addresses family members' problems in context, repairs and strengthens bonds, and supports the family's efforts to thrive. By shifting focus from problems to possibilities toward a preferred future vision, risk factors are addressed as obstacles to overcome, and family members are engaged to support their child's positive aims (Madsen 2011).

A strengths-oriented assessment lays the groundwork for therapist-family collaboration by prioritizing areas of concern and identifying potential resources in kin and community networks (see Chapter 42, "Family-Based Assessment and Treatment"). Genograms and timelines are essential to diagram and plan interventions with complex family systems, such as those with unstable households, multiple fathers, foster placements, or extended kin care. Seeing everyone on the same "family tree" can bring a sense of coherence for children in fragmented families.

With a family in perpetual crisis, therapists can get caught in a reactive mode, responding to the latest crisis. Well-structured family interviews facilitate planning and proactive interventions to anticipate, avert, and buffer problem situations before they spiral out of control. The therapeutic priorities are to strengthen the family structure, stability, and leadership to provide nurturance, guidance, and protection. It is important to build positive connections in shared mealtime and pleasurable activities. Action-oriented, concrete approaches work best, with clear objectives and small manageable steps to build on successes. Tasks are designed to reduce stress and to strengthen cohesion and functioning. Therapy is present and future focused yet draws on each family's past. A parent may have been powerless as a child in a troubled family but can learn from that experience to become a better parent. Building on their potential, families gain hope and confidence that they can rise above persistent adversity.

Families and Foster or Kinship Care

When children are removed from their home to protect them from abuse or neglect, too often this transition is abrupt and traumatic, with complete cutoff from contact with parents and extended family members. Siblings may lose a vital bond when separated. Traditional approaches to foster care—rescuing children from dysfunctional families—set up parents and foster caregivers as adversaries (i.e., the bad parents vs. the good parents).

In a collaborative resilience-oriented approach, family assessment expands beyond the risk posed by an offender to potential resources in the kin network. By involving family members in placement decisions, they are more likely to support the best arrangement for children. A family council—much like a tribal council—can be convened, rallying key members (e.g., grandparents, aunts, uncles, godparents) whose input could be valuable. Together with professionals, they consider various options, taking stock of kin and community resources. This process reduces the sense that children are being removed by outside forces beyond family control, such as arbitrary court decisions. Decisions for child placement are made without robbing parents of humanity and dignity and with hope that they can turn their lives around. Involving key family members also promotes their cooperation with a foster arrangement, ongoing contact with children, and investment in a successful placement experience.

With placement, maintaining the continuity of significant relationships for children is a priority. Planning should determine how they can be nurtured and protected from abuse *and* at the same time maintain some connections with their family network and their cultural and spiritual roots. Loss issues too often go unaddressed, particularly with multiple placements. Children are less likely to feel abandoned and unloved when ways are found to sustain vital bonds through monitored contact with parents, visits with relatives, phone calls, the Internet, cards, and letters. When direct contact is not feasible (as with a parent's incarceration), photos and keepsakes, such as a favorite scarf, can be precious during separation. On the child's return to parents, photos, scrapbooks, and occasional contact (such as birthday greetings) from a former foster family help the child integrate the experience. Children can be encouraged to make drawings and keep journals to record their experiences, memories, and future hopes and dreams.

Recidivism in child placements is high. It is critical to plan the transition back to parents carefully (Minuchin et al. 2007). Clinicians need to address the disruption and shifts in role relations.

Case Example 4

Terrell, age 8, was seen in therapy for anxiety and poor concentration in school soon after he and three siblings were returned to their mother's custody following her recovery from drug addiction. They had been living with their maternal grandmother for 2 years. In regaining their mother, the children had now lost their grandmother. The mother cut off all contact, still angry that the grandmother had initiated the court-ordered transfer of the children. Now becoming overwhelmed by job and child care demands, the mother risked losing custody again.

A systemic approach was needed to guide intervention efforts. Sessions with the mother and grandmother were held to calm the transitional upheaval, repair their strained relationship, and negotiate their changing role relations. The therapist facilitated their collaboration across households, with the mother in charge as primary parent. It was crucial to reframe the grandmother's role—not rescuing the children from a deficient mother, but supporting her daughter's best efforts to succeed with her children and her job. The children's vital bond with their grandmother was renewed in her after-school child care.

Follow-up sessions are crucial. Often, after an initial "honeymoon" period in family relationships, risk increases toward the end of the first year, with substance use relapses, return of an abusive partner, or a pileup of stresses. Periodic sustaining contacts can solidify gains and prevent recurrence of serious problems.

Clinical Approaches With Family Transitions

Brief family intervention is useful when the chief complaint is a focal problem involving a family transition. A preventive early intervention or consultation with a family can avert a major crisis or spiraling of distress. More intensive family therapy may be needed if there are multiple, chronic stressors or complications of past trauma and losses. Family members involved may include 1) those affected by a stressful transition, 2) those involved in problem maintenance, and 3) those who can contribute to positive adaptation and resilience.

Family psychoeducational models (Rolland and Walsh 2008) are finding useful application with disruptive transitions and multistress conditions. Formats may include family consultations and brief or ongoing multifamily groups, which offer practical information and social support for stress reduction, management, and problem solving through transitional crises and stressful periods. Intervention "modules" can be timed with critical transitions to provide a psychosocial road map for navigating a long-term coping process, such as the initial crisis or chronic or terminal phases of a life-threatening illness (Rolland 2012). Stressors can be approached as ongoing processes with landmarks, transitions, and changing demands. Each phase poses challenges that may require varied family strengths. A brief transitional crisis demands immediate mobilization; afterward, a family may resume accustomed patterns in living. In a transition with long-term ramifications, such as divorce, families need to grieve the loss of their precrisis identity and alter familiar patterns, as well as hopes and dreams, to accommodate a new set of circumstances. Children and families chart varied pathways in adaptation and resilience, depending on their situation, values, resources, and aims. This resilience-oriented framework can guide consultations and periodic family "psychosocial checkups" to strengthen family teamwork, communication, and resourcefulness to manage stress-related crises and meet future challenges.

Summary Points

- Major family transitions are disruptive for all members and relationships; family processes can heighten risk or promote resilience for children and adolescents.
- A systemic approach addresses symptoms in the context of family and sociocultural influences and in relation to developmental challenges.
- A genogram and timeline are useful tools for noting the influence of family transitional stresses in manifesting problems and for identifying potential resources for resilience.
- Therapists work collaboratively with key family members to repair and strengthen vital bonds and tap resources for positive adaptation and resilience.

References

Ahrons C: We're Still Family. New York, HarperCollins, 2004

Amato P: Research on divorce: continuing trends and new developments. J Marriage Fam 72(3):650–666, 2010

Anderson CM: The diversity, strengths, and challenges of single-parent households, in Normal Family Processes: Growing Diversity and Complexity, 4th Edition. Edited by Walsh F. New York, Guilford, 2012, pp 128–148

Bengston VG: Beyond the nuclear family: the increasing importance of multigenerational bonds. J Marriage Fam 63(1):1–16, 2001

Bernstein AC: Re-visioning, restructuring, and reconciliation: clinical practice with complex postdivorce families. Fam Process 46(1):67–78, 2007 17375729

Bianchi S, Milkie M: Work and family research in the first decade of the 21st century. J Marriage Fam 72(3):705–725, 2010

Biblarz T, Savci E: Lesbian, gay, bi-sexual, and transgender families. J Marriage Fam 72(3):480–497, 2010

Boss P: Ambiguous Loss. Cambridge, MA, Harvard University Press, 1999

Boyd-Franklin N, Karger M: Intersections of race, class, and poverty: Challenges and resilience in African-American families, in Normal Family Processes, 4th Edition. Edited by Walsh F. New York, Guilford, 2012, pp 273–296

Cherlin A: Demographic trends in the United States: A review of research in the 2000s. J Marriage Fam 72(3):403–419, 2010 22399825

Cowan PA, Cowan CP: Normative family transitions, couple relationship quality, and healthy child development, in Normal Family Processes, 4th Edition. Edited by Walsh F. New York, Guilford, 2012, pp 428–451

Engstrom M: Family processes in kinship care, in Normal Family Processes, 4th Edition. Edited by Walsh F. New York, Guilford, 2012, pp 196–221

Falicov CJ: Immigrant family processes: a multidimensional framework, in Normal Family Processes, 4th Edition. Edited by Walsh F. New York, Guilford, 2012, pp 297–323

Falicov CJ: Latino Families in Therapy: A Guide to Multicultural Practice, 2nd Edition. New York, Guilford, 2013

Fomby P, Cherlin AJ: Family instability and child well-being. Am Sociol Rev 72(2):181–204, 2007 21918579

Fraenkel P, Capstick C: Two-parent families: navigating work and family challenges, in Normal Family Processes: Growing Diversity and Complexity, 4th Edition. Edited by Walsh F. New York, Guilford, 2012, pp 78–101

Green R-J: Gay and lesbian couples and families, in Normal Family Processes, 4th Edition. Edited by Walsh F. New York, Guilford, 2012, pp 172–195

Greene S, Anderson E, Forgatch M, et al: Risk and resilience after divorce, in Normal Family Processes, 4th Edition. Edited by Walsh F. New York, Guilford, 2012, pp 102–127

Hetherington EM, Kelly J: For Better or For Worse: Divorce Reconsidered. New York, W.W. Norton, 2002

Kelly JB: Children's living arrangements following separation and divorce: insights from empirical and clinical research. Fam Process 46(1):35–52, 2007 17375727

Lansford JE, Ceballo R, Abby A, et al: Does family structure matter? A comparison of adoptive, two-parent biological, single-mother, stepfather, and stepmother households. J Marriage Fam 63(3):840–851, 2001

Madsen WC: Collaborative helping maps: a tool to guide thinking and action in family centered services. Fam Process 50(4):529–543, 2011 22145724

Masten A: Ordinary Magic: Resilience in Development. New York, Routledge, 2014

Masten A, Monn AR: Child and family resilience: A call for integrating science, practice, and training. Fam Relat 64(1):5–21, 2015

McGoldrick M, Garcia Preto N, Carter B (eds): The Expanded Family Life Cycle, 5th Edition. New York, Pearson, in press

McGoldrick M, Gerson R, Petry S: Genograms: Assessment and Intervention, 3rd Edition. New York, W.W. Norton, 2008

Minuchin P, Colapinto J, Minuchin S: Working With Families of the Poor, 2nd Edition. New York, Guilford, 2007

Pasley K, Garneau C: Remarriage families and stepparenting, in Normal Family Processes, 4th Edition. Edited by Walsh F. New York, Guilford, 2012, pp 149–171

Rampage C, Eovaldi M, Ma C, et al: Adoptive families, in Normal Family Processes, 4th Edition. Edited by Walsh F. New York, Guilford, 2012, pp 222–246

Repetti R, Wang S, Saxbe D: Bringing it all back home. How outside stressors shape families' everyday lives. Current Psychological Directions in Science 18(2):106–111, 2009

Rolland JS: Mastering family challenges in illness, disability, and genetic conditions, in Normal Family Processes, 4th Edition. Edited by Walsh F. New York, Guilford, 2012, pp 452–482

Rolland JS, Walsh F: Family systems theory and practice, in Textbook of Psychotherapeutic Treatments. Edited by Gabbard G. Washington, DC, American Psychiatric Publishing, 2008, pp 499–531

Rosenblatt PC: Family grief in cross-cultural perspective. Family Science 4(1):12–19, 2013

Ungar M: The importance of parents and other caregivers to the resilience of high-risk adolescents. Fam Process 43(1):23–41, 2004 15359713

Walsh F: Family resilience: a framework for clinical practice. Fam Process 42(1):1–18, 2003 12698595

Walsh F: Traumatic loss and major disasters: strengthening family and community resilience. Fam Process 46(2):207–227, 2007 17593886

Walsh F: Human-animal bonds II: the role of pets in family systems and family therapy. Fam Process 48(4):481–499, 2009a 19930434

Walsh F (ed): Spiritual Resources in Family Therapy, 2nd Edition. New York, Guilford, 2009b

Walsh F: Spiritual diversity: multifaith perspectives in family therapy. Fam Process 49(3):330–348, 2010 20831764

Walsh F: Family resilience: Strengths forged through adversity, in Normal Family Processes, 4th Edition. New York, Guilford, 2012a, pp 399–427

Walsh F (ed): Normal Family Processes: Growing Diversity and Complexity, 4th Edition. New York, Guilford, 2012b

Walsh F: Community-based practice applications of a family resilience framework, in Handbook of Family Resilience. Edited by Becvar D. New York, Springer, 2013, pp 65–82

Walsh F: A family developmental framework: challenges and resilience across the life cycle, in Handbook of Family Therapy. Edited by Sexton T, Lebow J. New York, Routledge, 2015

Walsh F: Strengthening Family Resilience, 3rd Edition. New York, Guilford, in press

Walsh F, McGoldrick M (eds): Living Beyond Loss: Death in the Family, 2nd Edition. New York, W.W. Norton, 2004

Walsh F, McGoldrick M: Bereavement: a family life cycle perspective. Special Issue, Bereavement: Family Perspectives. Family Science 4(1):20–27, 2013

Weine S, Knafi K, Feetham S, et al: A mixed methods study of refugee families engaging in multiple-family groups. Fam Relat 54(4):558–568, 2005

Worden WJ: Grief Counseling and Grief Therapy, 4th Edition. New York, Springer, 2008

CHAPTER 32

Legal and Ethical Issues

John B. Sikorski, M.D.
Anlee D. Kuo, J.D., M.D.

During the past decade, legal and ethical issues regarding the mental health, psychopathology, and risk behavior of children and youth have received increased public attention, parental concern, and professional consultation and opinion. These issues range from the impact of increased use, misuse, and abuse of the Internet and electronic communications and entertainment/media devices on children's character development to eruptions of mass violence and murder by apparently disturbed youth. Increases in substance abuse and high-risk behaviors, along with high rates of academic underachievement and school failure in vulnerable youth, are also featured in the news media.

In parallel, there is an increase in scientific information and knowledge about environmental and psychosocial effects on neural networks and development and subsequent adaptation or risk behaviors for vulnerable youth. These technological and psychosocial changes highlight the need for clinicians to have training and competence at the interface of child mental health, developmental psychopathology, and relevant social and legal issues because they are called on for assessments, treatment planning, and sometimes professional opinions arising out of their clinical work or legal mandates.

The American Academy of Child and Adolescent Psychiatry (AACAP) has developed "Practice Parameters for Child and Adolescent Forensic Evaluations" (Kraus et al. 2011) to address the key components that differentiate forensic evaluations from clinical assessments. It also highlights the ethical issues in forensic as well as clinical arenas.

Clinicians working at the interface of child and adolescent psychiatry and the law are aware of the evolving natures of science and evidence-based medicine and the complex nature of the law and related ethical considerations. This warrants proceeding with thoughtful caution, maintaining a current knowledge base in the area of clinical work, maintaining awareness of relevant legal developments in the local jurisdiction, and, when in doubt, consulting with experienced colleagues or seeking the advice of one's own legal counsel. In this regard, familiarity with the changes in DSM-5, particularly involving the expansion of diagnostic criteria in autism spectrum disorder, attention-deficit/ hyperactivity disorder, and intellectual disability; disruptive, impulse-control, and conduct disorders; and the introduction of disruptive mood dysregulation disorder, is especially pertinent to current forensic evaluations (Wills 2014).

It is the intent of this chapter to 1) provide a framework for understanding the current status of rights of children and ethical issues and behavior in clinical practice and research and 2) provide an overview of legal issues involved in the clinical practice of child and adolescent mental health, including divorce and child custody, child abuse and neglect, and civil litigation involving minors, including cyberbullying and harassment, school-related legal issues, and the growing interest in adolescent competency to stand trial in juvenile court proceedings.

Evolving Concepts of the Status of Children

Current concepts and interpretations of civil rights, privacy rights, rights of minors, and family and dependency law are based on legislative enactments and appellate court interpretations and opinions that have evolved in the context of vast technological, demographic, and sociocultural changes in American society during the twentieth century. While the civil rights movement of the 1950s and 1960s was focused primarily on adults and due process, there was growing social concern about the well-being, health, education, and age-appropriate needs and rights of minors. As noted in her landmark review "Children Under the Law," Hillary Rodham (1973) stated, "Children's rights cannot be secured until some particular institution has recognized them and assumed responsibility for enforcing them" (p. 507).

Most advances in recognizing the rights of minors have been downward extrapolations of the rights of adults. Since the 1960s, states have defined the age of majority as 18 years, providing the usual range of adult rights and responsibilities at that age except for the purchase of alcoholic beverages, which is now usually age 21. However, states vary widely in their provisions for specific rights of minors in areas such as educational services, paid employment, and contractual obligations, as well as with regard to emancipation, marriage, obtaining a driver's license, and giving consent for and having access to health care.

In the United States, contemporary society's perception and treatment of minors continues to reflect the traditional legal doctrines of *parens patriae* and the twentieth-century articulation of "the best interests of the child." *Parens patriae* traditionally has empowered state initiatives to protect persons who are unable to care for or protect themselves—and also has allowed state agencies to interfere with parental prerogatives when there is evidence of neglect, inability to perform parental responsibilities, or abuse of minors. This evolving interface is reflected in the U.S. Supreme Court decision noted in *Santosky v. Kramer* (455 U.S. 745 [1982]): "So long as the child is part of a viable family his own interests are merged with those of the other members. Only after the family fails in its functions should the child's interests become a matter for state intrusion."

Articulating and prioritizing children's needs evolved at the turn of the twentieth century and was articulated by Judge Benjamin Cardozo as specifying the court's role to serve as *parens patriae* and do "what is in the best interests of the child" (*Finlay v. Finlay* [148 N.E. 624 (N.Y. ct. app. 1925)]). As the legal standard for clinical decision making, the best interests of the child was extensively studied at the Yale Child Study Center (Goldstein et al. 1996), initially focusing on child placement conflicts requiring value preferences and clinical judgment in determining in each case what is in the child's best interest. This standard became variably codified in each state as the standard for child custody determination and family law. It has been criticized as too vague and imprecise and a rationalization for adult decision makers to project their prejudices and judgments about children's futures. It has also been advocated as providing a rational framework for judgments involving the multiple factors and issues in the tension and balance between parental values and responsibilities and children's rights and needs.

Ethical Issues in Clinical Practice and Research

Ethics can be defined as the study of moral principles and values that guide and determine the conduct of individuals in particular (usually professional) circumstances and relationships (see American Academy of Psychiatry and the Law, "Ethics Guidelines for the Practice of Forensic Psychiatry," 2005, http://aapl.org/docs/pdf/ETHICSGDLNS.pdf). The awareness of ethical values and duties in the practice of medicine dates to the time of the Hippocratic oath. Ethical guidelines are evolving to highlight several principal issues: respect for the patient's autonomy, beneficence, and justice. The concept of respect for the person's autonomy includes informed consent in treatment and research, including maintaining appropriate professional boundaries and confidences, as well as factual honesty and avoidance of misrepresentations. The concept of beneficence expands the "do no harm" concept to include acting in the patient's best interests and minimizing risks and maximizing benefits in professional judgments and relationships. The concept of justice relates to the allocation of resources and fair and equitable distribution of risks and benefits.

Since psychiatric disorders may adversely affect the individual's autonomy, decision-making ability, and ability to provide informed consent, professionals have developed guidelines for ethical considerations in decision making in the practice of psychiatry. The "Principles of Medical Ethics With Annotations Especially Applicable to Psychiatry" has been revised and published in the form of an ethics primer (American Academy of Child and Adolescent Psychiatry 1995; American Psychiatric Association 2001).

Ethical tensions in child and adolescent psychiatry derive from the evolving developmental stages of the child or adolescent, the family structure, and treatment contexts. There may also be overlapping and potentially conflicting rights and responsibilities for the child and for the child's parents or guardians. The nature of clinical work with children interfaces with agencies external to the family—such as schools; courts; and specialized treatment, educational, or recreation programs that may have responsibility or authority for the child—and may require exchange of information or consultative or collateral professional work.

The ethical duty for the clinician is to provide sufficient relevant and factual information regarding the patient's condition and prognosis, the risks and benefits of types of treatments available, and recommendations, so that the patient can provide informed consent to the diagnostic procedures and treatment process. In clinical practice with children and parents, the clinician strives to articulate the issues involved in confidentiality and informed consent with both the child and the parents or legal guardian during the beginning of the evaluation process, taking into account the child's level of understanding and ability to assent to participate in the process and the treatment planning.

The ethical principle of confidentiality is considered the cornerstone for building trust and honest communication in the physician-patient relationship. This principle obligates the clinician to hold in confidence the communications with the patient, as the patient, even if a minor, is the holder of the right to confidentiality and must give consent for the release of that information. However, as with all children under legal age of maturity, the legal consent must be made by the parents or legal guardian, except where there are specific statutory exceptions, such as the mandatory child abuse reporting laws or in situations where a child is an imminent danger to self or others.

Transference and countertransference phenomena in the professional relationship may develop to blur the appropriate role and boundary, leading to inappropriate advocacy for or exploitation of the patient. Vigilance in one's usual and customary practice and consultation with one's peers is helpful in maintaining professional roles and boundaries and minimizing conflicts of interest.

The need for research to strengthen the scientific knowledge base has generated an effort to further develop ethical principles relevant to research (Munir and Earls 1992). From this perspective, the interests of the subject have priority over the interests of science and society, and voluntary informed consent is essential. In response to federal requirements, research and educational institutions have developed local institutional review boards (IRBs) to ensure legal and ethical conduct in human subject research. IRBs are made up of researchers, clinicians, members of the public, patient advocates, and experts in relevant law and ethics. Federal regulations state in part

> The IRB shall determine that adequate provisions are made for soliciting the assent of children when in the judgment of the IRB, children are capable of providing assent. In determining whether children are capable of assenting, the IRB shall take into account the ages, maturity, and psychological state of the children involved. (U.S. Department of Health and Human Services 1991)

Legal Issues in Clinical Practice

Confidentiality, Privilege, and Duty

Confidentiality and privilege are two distinct ethical and legal duties protected by state statutes to promote communication and trust between the physician and patient. *Privilege* refers to the patient's right to prevent disclosure of information obtained during treatment in judicial or quasi-judicial proceedings. The term *confidentiality* is broader and refers to the clinician's obligation to avoid disclosure of the patient's information to any person other than the patient.

The legal and ethical rights of confidentiality and privilege belong to the patient and can be waived only by the patient except as provided for by certain statutory exceptions. For example, the right of confidentiality is automatically waived when the patient is a threat to herself or others or when a reportable condition is revealed such as sexual abuse, neglect, maltreatment, or physical abuse. Frequent exceptions to privileged communications include issues arising in commitment proceedings, probate court, child custody cases, and criminal matters (Macbeth 2002). In these types of proceedings, the court may mandate the disclosure of confidential or privileged communication, such as when a person puts his or her own mental condition at issue in a lawsuit (Bernet 1998). States are not uniform in these rules regarding confidential and privileged communication and exceptions to these communications, so clinicians should familiarize themselves with the relevant statutes in their jurisdiction.

Confidentiality becomes more complicated when it involves the legal status of minors and raises the issue as to who holds the right. In general, the parent who is legally entitled to authorize treatment for the child holds the legal right to confidentiality for the child (Macbeth 2002). Some jurisdictions allow minors to hold the right to confidentiality on the basis of their age or their ability to consent to certain treatments on their own. The law has increasingly given adolescents the right and responsibilities of adults, so clinicians should be familiar with the statutory exceptions specific to each state.

Informed Consent and Competence

Minors are generally not deemed competent to give legal consent to psychiatric evaluation, treatment, or the release of information. The consent of the parent or guardian is required unless statutory exceptions exist or the minor is emancipated. The consent must also be based on an informed choice—i.e., the patient (or parent/guardian) must have the cognitive capacity and mental competence to adequately understand the nature of the condition, the recommended treatment, and the potential risks and benefits of and alternatives to the treatment. Furthermore, the patient's choice must be voluntary and not coerced. The informed consent from the parent or legal guardian should be clearly documented in the medical record.

States provide various statutory exceptions to the general requirement of parental consent. For example, emancipated minors can consent to their own treatment. This group generally includes minors who are older than age 15, living away from parents, and economically self-sufficient; married minors; minors on active duty in the U.S. armed services; and minors who have been emancipated through a specific court order. Courts can also determine that a minor is "mature" and able to appreciate the nature, extent, and consequences of a medical treatment.

State legislatures have allowed more minors to consent to certain treatment such as care related to sexual behavior and time-limited outpatient mental health treatment. This trend raises increasing concern about the lack of sufficient maturity, understanding, and experience in minors to make an informed judgment about a procedure. Clinicians should always explain relevant information at a level that is developmentally appropriate.

Recent subregulatory guidance regarding the Health Insurance Portability and Accountability Act (HIPAA) from the U.S. Department of Health and

Human Services (www.hhs.gov/ocr/privacy/hipaa/understanding/special/mhguidance.html) indicates the rules governing disclosures to parents of minor patients, including the following:

- Unless a competent person objects, the psychiatrist and other clinicians can speak with other family members who are assisting in the patient's treatment
- When psychiatric disorders or substance abuse impair a patient's capacities, mental health professionals can share patient-related information in the patient's best interest
- Certain disclosures are permissible when patients present serious and imminent threats to themselves or others (http://www.hhs.gov/ocr/privacy/hipaa/understanding/special/mhguidance.html)

In some states, however, the laws regarding mental health confidentiality are stricter than those of HIPAA.

Civil Commitment

Parents, legal guardians, and state agencies may occasionally need to hospitalize a seriously disturbed child or adolescent, and this necessity may conflict with the child's or adolescent's desire for autonomy and self-determination. The AACAP has published guidelines regarding this issue and listed the following factors to consider: 1) a qualified psychiatrist's evaluation; 2) diagnosis by DSM criteria; 3) severity of impairment in two or more areas of daily functioning; 4) likelihood of benefit from the proposed treatment; 5) prior consideration of less restrictive treatment procedures and the judgment that they are inappropriate or inadequate to meet the patient's needs; 6) encouragement of the child to voluntarily participate in the admission, treatment planning, and discharge process; and 7) the parent's full information about and participation in the hospitalization and treatment planning decisions (American Academy of Child and Adolescent Psychiatry 1989).

In the governing U.S. Supreme Court case on this issue, *Parham v. J.R.* (422 U.S. 584, 99 S. Ct. 2493, 61 L. Ed. 2d 101 [1979]), the Supreme Court granted substantial autonomy to parents in making decisions about placing their children in mental health facilities. However, an independent medical review must confirm the nature of the illness and the likelihood of benefit from the proposed treatment, and the youth may request periodic reviews of the treatment and confinement necessity. States have addressed this situation by implementing exceptions to the general rule of parental consent (Horowitz 2002).

Professional Liability

In the past few decades, child psychiatrists have become increasingly subject to malpractice suits based on matters such as alleged abandonment of patients, battery, breach of confidentiality or duty, failure to follow standards of care, failure to report or protect against abuse or harassment of patients, negligence, improper treatment, harmful effects of medications, or other alleged violations of federal or state laws regarding professional practice.

These suits are based on principles of tort law or civil wrongful behavior, in which the practitioner may be liable for the unintended consequences of alleged harm or injury to the patient or to a third party that could have or should have been prevented by the practitioner's action. The four elements of a claim of professional negligence are as follows:

1. *Duty*—a duty of care was owed to the patient by the physician
2. *Dereliction*—the duty of care was breached
3. *Damages*—the patient experienced actual damage due to the breach of duty
4. *Direct causation*—the dereliction was the direct cause of the damages

The plaintiff must demonstrate to the court the existence of these elements according to the standard of care in the community at the time. In civil cases, the standard of proof is the preponderance of evidence (i.e., more likely than not).

One area of increasing ethical and legal vulnerability involves the conflict between independent clinical judgment of attending physicians and the cost containment purposes of managed care agencies. When a managed care company denies coverage for a service for "lack of medical necessity," the physician has four duties (*Wickline v. California,* 192 Cal. App. 3d 1630, 239 Cal Rptr 810 [1986]): 1) appeal the decision, 2) discuss the issues raised by the managed care company with the patient, 3) treat the patient in an emergency even without payment, and 4) develop alternative treatment plans.

Responding to a Subpoena

A *subpoena* is a legal order requiring appearance at a specified proceeding or the production of certain documents or both. The subpoena may be issued to a clinician if either party in a legal proceeding believes that the clinician may possess information relevant to the legal dispute. If a clinician receives a subpoena, he should immediately inform the patient of the facts of the subpoena and discuss with the patient the possible responses. If the patient provides consent for the release of information, the clinician must respond or run the risk of being held in contempt. If the patient does not provide consent for release of the information requested by the subpoena, the clinician should consult with his own attorney. In special circumstances, the clinician can request to have the records reviewed in private chambers by the judge to determine their relevance to the case at hand. However, in no circumstances should a clinician ignore a valid subpoena. In institutional practice, the clinician should always immediately contact the risk management and/or legal department.

Overview of the Legal System

Structurally, the legal system is divided into two main court systems: state courts and federal courts. State courts adjudicate both civil and criminal cases arising under state law. They consist of lower courts (i.e., trial courts), higher courts (i.e., appellate courts), and the state's supreme court. The appellate and supreme courts play a supervisory role over the trial courts. Some specialized courts exercise jurisdiction over specific types of cases. For example, juvenile courts deal with juvenile delinquency and abuse and neglect. Family courts have jurisdiction over matters involving divorce and child custody issues. Probate courts handle wills and administer decedents' estates.

The federal court system presides over civil and criminal cases arising under the U.S. Constitution and federal statutes. It can also adjudicate civil actions if the parties are residents of different states. This system consists of federal trial courts, 13 U.S. Courts of Appeal, and the U.S. Supreme Court.

The appellate courts hear appeals from the trial courts, and the U.S. Supreme Court hears appeals from the federal appellate courts and exercises discretionary jurisdiction to grant review in other cases by *writ of certiorari.*

The courts of general jurisdiction preside over two types of legal proceedings: civil and criminal cases. Civil cases include breach of contract disputes; property and financial disputes; and torts, including injury, negligence, professional liability, libel, and slander. Torts are the most common civil action where a plaintiff asserts that a defendant owed her a "duty of care" and acted in a negligent manner, causing the plaintiff a foreseeable harm, loss, or injury.

The standard of proof is the level of certainty required for a certain judicial outcome, which varies depending on the type of legal proceeding. For example, the standard of a preponderance of evidence is used in most civil proceedings. The intermediate standard of "clear and convincing evidence" is required in cases where a deprivation of fundamental rights or liberty is at stake, such as termination of parental rights. The highest standard of proof, "beyond a reasonable doubt," is used in criminal proceedings as well as juvenile court and delinquency proceedings. Physicians who testify in court typically state their opinions within a reasonable degree of medical certainty. This standard reflects the level of certainty equivalent to what a physician uses when making a diagnosis and starting treatment (Rappeport 1985).

Child Psychiatrist as Expert Witness

Child psychiatrists are increasingly being called on to testify as experts in various types of legal proceedings. In the emerging subspecialty field of forensic psychiatry, the child psychiatrist applies her clinical and scientific expertise to legal issues in legal contexts. This role is distinguished from the role of treating clinician by the absence of a doctor-patient relationship. The psychiatrist's opinion may even ultimately result in harm to the child. For example, the child may be waived to an adult court or taken away from her parents in a dependency hearing. As an expert witness, a child psychiatrist will draw on her specific body of knowledge to form an opinion about a legal issue. No treatment is rendered, and the usual medical, legal, and ethical principles regarding interactions between a physician and patient do not apply. The psychiatrist's client is the attorney or the court who is hiring her to render an expert opinion. Acting as an expert witness, the psychiatrist is typically asked to read legal documents, conduct interviews, and then write a report, provide depositions, and/or testify in court.

When an attorney or the court calls on the psychiatrist's expertise for child custody evaluations, the expert typically assists the court in determining a custody and visitation schedule in accordance with the best interests of the child (Goldstein et al. 1996). In child abuse and neglect cases, the forensic evaluator often conducts assessments of the nature and extent of harm to a child, evaluates parental fitness, and makes recommendations regarding placement, treatment, or termination of parental rights. These assessments are used in dependency and guardianship proceedings, custodial disputes, termination of parental rights, and criminal and civil litigation (Barnum 2002).

Child psychiatrists can be called on to conduct assessments on adolescents in the juvenile and adult criminal courts. In these cases, they are often called on to evaluate and provide testimony regarding the juvenile's degree of dangerousness and amenability to treatment or rehabilitation and to discuss potential disposition options. One topic of increasing concern involves the juvenile's competence to stand trial or waive Miranda rights (Grisso and Schwartz 2000). Finally, the child psychiatrist can be called to evaluate children in legal issues related to special education such as compliance with state and federal disability statutes.

Practice guidelines have been developed for assessing children and youth in many of these legal proceedings (Kraus et al. 2011).

Recent Forensic Issues in Juvenile Court

States developed their own separate juvenile court procedures around the first decade of the twentieth century. However, policies and procedures must adhere to guidelines and administrative regulations from the Department of Justice following the Juvenile Justice and Delinquency Prevention Act of 1974 (and subsequent additions) in order to qualify for supplemental federal funding for their juvenile justice programs. State laws, which vary in their provisions for transfer or waiver of adolescents to adult court for serious offenses, must follow a minimum of evaluation and transfer provisions set forth in the U.S. Supreme Court decision *Kent v. United States* (383 U.S. 541 [1966]).

Recent developments in neuroscience (Pope et al. 2012), particularly with regard to the maturation of the affective and cognitive neural networks during adolescence, are beginning to influence professional evaluations and public policy regarding adolescents, including a juvenile's competency to stand trial. While the U.S. Supreme Court's decision in *Dusky v. United States* (362 U.S. 402 [1960]) set the standard for competency as "whether a defendant has sufficient present ability to consult with his lawyer within a reasonable degree of rational understanding and whether he has a rational as well as factual understanding of the proceedings against him," recent research in this area has clarified the neurodevelopmental processes relevant for adjudicative competency and provided an evaluation format for assessing these processes (Grisso 2005). This issue of developmental immaturity is also relevant in three recent U.S. Supreme Court cases: *Roper v. Simmons* (543 U.S. 551 [2005]), *Graham v. Florida* (130 S. Ct. 2011 [2010]), and *Miller v. Alabama* (132 S. Ct. 2455 [2012]) (Pope et al. 2012).

Forensic Aspects of Child Custody and Divorce

With approximately half of marriages in the United States ending in divorce, legal and ethical considerations are frequently encountered in forensic aspects of child custody and divorce work.

One of the most important ethical concepts is role clarification by the child psychiatrist. Unlike a clinician, who acts as the child's advocate for the purpose of treatment, the forensic evaluator is a neutral expert who can draw on objective facts and data to arrive at impartial and informed opinions for the family court. The evaluator should clearly communicate her role to the parent and child prior to the assessment and avoid the mistake of "wearing two hats"—i.e., acting as both clinician and forensic expert (Schetky 2007).

Forensic evaluations in child custody and divorce cases involve nonconfidential communications between the forensic mental health clinician expert and the child and parent. The information obtained from the interview will be used in a report, deposition, or testimony that is available to the judge, attorneys, and other involved legal personnel. The person(s) being evaluated should be given a clear understanding of this lack of confidentiality in the forensic setting. The potential evaluator should also guard against the pitfalls of bias and conflict of interest. Prior involvement with either party may unduly influence the evaluator and jeopardize the objectivity of the assessment. Similarly, conducting a unilateral evaluation that includes an assessment of the child interacting with only one parent inherently leads to biased opinions.

The prevailing legal doctrine of the best interests of the child is the guiding principle in deciding child custody disputes. Although the concept remains ambiguous, some clarification has been achieved through legislation and statutes. The Uniform Marriage and Divorce Act, promulgated by the National Conference of Commissioners on Uniform State Laws and approved by the American Bar Association in 1974, established the language and definition regarding the best interests criteria and includes factors such as the wishes of the parent and child; the interactions of the child with those who may significantly affect his or her best interests; the child's adjustment to his or her home, school, and community; and the mental and physical health of all individuals involved. The majority of states have adapted their statutes from the concept and language of this act.

In a child custody dispute, the legal outcome is typically either joint or sole custody. In joint legal custody, both parents have legal decision-making power for the child. Complicated issues involving joint custody or shared parenting continue to be controversial, with some parents and professionals advocating for predetermined or categorical positions while others favor using a broader range of social science data and evidence as articulated in "Closing the Gap: Research, Policy, Practice, and Shared Parenting" (Pruett and DiFonzo 2014). In sole legal custody, only one parent has the authority. For clinicians providing treatment for a child, this concept is important because in joint custody situations, treatment and medication administration must be approved by both parents. In joint physical custody, both parents share physical custody of the child, and the child typically lives in both homes, each for a percentage of the time.

To minimize the risks of the expert providing unwarranted conclusions and to promote uniformity and maintain standards of care, guidelines have been published by organizations and experts (Stahl 1999).

Forensic Aspects of Child Abuse and Neglect

Child mental health professionals are increasingly involved in the assessment and treatment of children who have been abused. Since the passage of the Child Abuse Prevention and Treatment Act in 1974 and implementation of federal guidelines, all states have passed laws mandating designated persons, such as child mental health professionals, to report child abuse and neglect.

Failure to do so can result in civil liabilities and criminal penalties.

Forensic aspects of child abuse and neglect cases can involve a broad range of functions, such as assessment of the extent of physical and emotional harm to the child; parental fitness evaluations; and recommendations regarding placement, treatment, and/or termination of parental rights. These assessments may be used in a variety of legal proceedings, including divorce and custody disputes; civil and criminal proceedings; dependency, guardianship, and termination of parental right actions; and cases related to child endangerment, cyberbullying, and child pornography (Abrams 2013). Several guidelines are available to help assist the child mental health professional conduct an appropriate forensic assessment of a child who may have been abused (Barnum 2002; Quinn 2002).

Child as Witness

Because of a frequent lack of sufficient physical evidence in cases of sexual abuse allegations, a child's testimony is often critical in determining the likelihood of truth behind an allegation of abuse. With the increase in allegations of child sexual abuse over the past several decades and the importance of a child's testimony in these legal cases, a large body of information has developed regarding children's competency, memory, suggestibility, and credibility (Clark 2002; Kulkofsky and London 2010).

A child's competency to act as a witness essentially refers to his ability to testify in court in a reliable and meaningful manner. In general, competence is determined by four criteria: the capacity to register an event, the ability to accurately recall and recount the event, the ability to distinguish truth from falsehood, and the capacity to communicate on the basis of personal knowledge of the facts.

Research exploring the accuracy of children's memory and suggestibility has found that memory and retention abilities generally begin at about age 3 years and improve with age. The literature also shows that children are highly suggestible, with preschool children being more suggestible than older children or adults (Poole and Lindsay 1995). The credibility of a child refers to the child's truthfulness and accuracy and is ultimately determined by the judge or jury. Through expert testimony, forensic experts can assist the judge and jury in this determination. The factors relevant to determining the issue of credibility include the increased likelihood of accuracy in allegations when statements are spontaneous and consistent and use of age-appropriate vocabulary (Kulkofsky and London 2010). However, these factors are not definitive in assessing credibility, since suggestive interviewing techniques and other more complicated aspects of memory can contaminate the information.

The child's own testimony as a witness may be required in criminal proceedings as well as in civil litigation against the perpetrator. The evaluation of the child in these cases may subject her to multiple assessments in the home, school, clinical, or police settings and lead to increasing concern about the effect of the process on the child witness.

The U.S. Supreme Court has decided a number of cases that balanced the best interests and the cognitive and emotional capabilities of a child witness against the constitutional rights of defendants. These rights include protection against self-incrimination (Fifth Amendment), the right to confront and cross-examine witnesses (Sixth Amendment), and the right to due process (Fourteenth Amendment.) In *White v. Illinois* (112 S. Ct. 736 [1992]), the U.S. Supreme Court recognized what amounts to a specific hearsay exception: The testimony of a physician was admitted and did not violate the defendant's Sixth Amendment rights because the child's statement to the physician was a "spontaneous declaration" made to the physician for the purpose of medical diagnosis and treatment. This area of law continues to evolve, and clinicians should be aware of current standards of assessment and legal guidelines related to their particular case.

Civil Litigation

Civil lawsuits involving children and adolescents are frequently brought by their parents or guardians in the form of a tort, which is 1) a claim that a wrong has been done by the negligence or intention of another person or entity and 2) a demand for compensation for the damage suffered by the victim (Schetky and Guyer 2002). The majority of civil litigation involving children alleging psychic trauma is the result of accidental injury, dog bites, burns, battery and violence, negligence by caregivers or product manufacturers, and toxic exposure. Aside from assessing the physical injuries the child may have sustained, the child psychiatrist or other mental health professional is called on for clinical diagnosis and treatment or for forensic examination and testimony as an expert witness (American Academy of Child and Adolescent Psychiatry 1998).

If either the clinician or the forensic expert provides both the clinical work and the forensic expert evaluation and testimony, there is an ethical violation based on conflict of interest and dual agency. The forensic evaluation, by a court-appointed expert or forensic expert hired by a party in the lawsuit, has a different set of professional and ethical duties and responsibilities from those of the treating clinician. The forensic expert is responsible for understanding the clinician's role in the evaluation and legal proceedings, knowing the limits on confidentiality, striving for honesty and objectivity, and maintaining one's competence and qualifications (see http://aapl.org/docs/pdf/ETHICSGDLNS.pdf) in that area of expertise.

Internet-Related Legal Issues

In today's rapidly changing Internet world, teenagers and children are engaging in an increasingly online social life. This participation in a cyberspace society has led to new dangers in the lives of teenagers and children. Cyberbullying has become increasingly common among teenagers, especially after the fifth grade, with some surveys indicating prevalence of 35%–40% (Englander 2012). Adolescents who may not otherwise engage in bullying behavior may engage in cyberbullying because it can occur 24 hours a day, it can be anonymous, and the perpetrator is physically and emotionally removed from the victim. Cyberbullying has been categorized as bullying through text messaging, pictures/video clips, phone calls, e-mails, chat rooms, instant messaging, and Web sites. Among these categories, posting of personal pictures and videos has been reported to have the most negative emotional impact on the victim. Other new dangers that have evolved from increasing use of the Internet include online sexual victimization (including exposure to pornography and sexual perpetrators) and the facilitation of suicide through Web sites and chat rooms that provide information on how to commit the act (Scott and Temporini 2010).

Addressing these forensic Internet issues (i.e., cyberbullying, online sexual victimization, information on suicide on the Internet) involves informed evaluation of the involved youth as well as the environment of the family, school, and community. It is important for those involved to be current on information technology, including its uses and abuses, and to have an understanding of the ever-evolving cyberspace language (i.e., knowledge of acronyms and emoticons). In assessing either the victim or the perpetrator, the evaluator should take a thorough Internet use history. Many youth victims have not told others about the online bullying, so they should be asked specific questions about online harassment. In assessing the perpetrator, there should be an inquiry into the person's online and off-line behavior and his or her social history, in addition to the standard approaches for violence risk assessments (Scott and Temporini 2010). A response to cyberbullying requires a coordinated effort from the community, school, and family. Possible actions include having an educational discussion about cyberbullying with the individuals and parents with a school officer or police officer present, implementing immediate consequences for the bullying, ensuring that the victim has a safety plan, and informing all relevant adults of the event (Englander 2012). Parents can also implement filtering and blocking of Internet software.

School-Related Legal Issues

Until the latter half of the twentieth century, the federal government played no role in the public education of children. However, the landmark U.S. Supreme Court decision Brown v. Board of Education (347 U.S. 483 [1954]) ended segregation as a legal policy in public schools. In the Rehabilitation Act of 1973, Section 504 (29 U.S.C. Sect. 794), Congress established the cornerstone of civil rights for individuals with disabilities, stating in part, "No otherwise qualified handicapped individual in the United States…shall solely by reason of her or his handicap be excluded from participation in, be denied benefits of, or be subject to discrimination under any program or activity receiving federal financial assistance." The Americans With Disabilities Act of 1990 (P.L. 101-336, 42 U.S.C. §12101 et seq.) expanded the articulation of these rights of persons with disabilities and serves as a basis for accommodations in school curricula and procedures and school-based activities. Title IX of the Education Amendments of 1972 (20 U.S.C. Sect. 1681 et seq.) also prohibits sex discrimination in any educational institution receiving federal funding.

In the landmark Education for All Handicapped Children Act of 1975 (P.L. 94-142, sec. 611, 88 Stat. 579, et seq.), Congress stated that the purpose of the act was to ensure that "All handicapped children have available to them a free appropriate public education which emphasizes special education, and related services, designed to meet their unique needs." This law provided federal definitions of these conditions, such as learning disabilities, serious emotional disturbance, intellectual disability, and speech and language disorders. The law also defined processes and procedures to be followed in special education services, including "free and appropriate public education," "related services," "individual educational program," and "least restrictive environment," along with numerous rights and procedural safeguards.

In 1991, Congress amended and changed the name of this act to the Individuals With Disabilities Education Act (IDEA, P.L. 102-119). This act, defining processes and procedures for special education for states and school districts, is modified and reauthorized periodically, most recently in 2004 (Individuals With Disabilities Education Improvement Act, P.L. 108-446).

Clinicians working with children involved in school district special education programs should be aware that the U.S. Department of Education definitions of various mental and emotional disorders may be different from DSM-5 (American Psychiatric Association 2013) diagnoses and that school districts are required to follow Department of Education diagnostic criteria and procedures (see Chapter 9, "Developmental Disorders of Learning, Communication, and Motor Skills," and Chapter 48, "School-Based Interventions").

Each state must develop its own implementing regulations. Therefore, clinicians should familiarize themselves with the criteria for their own state as well as with the DSM-5 criteria. The AACAP "Practice Parameter for Psychiatric Consultation to Schools" (Walter and Berkovitz 2005) provides the clinician with comprehensive descriptions of and references to school mental health consultation and services.

Summary Points

- Children's rights as a legal concept developed during the twentieth century, and they are reflective of continuously changing sociocultural values.
- The best interest of the child is the legal standard for decision making regarding children's needs and placement.
- Ethical guidelines for clinical practice include respect for the patient's autonomy, beneficence, and justice balanced with traditional concepts of parents' rights and responsibilities.
- The principle of confidentiality requires the clinician to hold in confidence the patient's privileged communication.
- Psychiatric evaluation, treatment, and release of information require informed consent from the parent or legal guardian of a minor except in cases that involve emancipated or mature minors or where there are specific statutory exceptions.
- Malpractice suits against clinicians follow principles of tort law.

References

Abrams DE: A primer on criminal child abuse and neglect law. Juv Fam Court J 64(3):1–27, 2013

American Academy of Child and Adolescent Psychiatry: Policy Statement: Inpatient Hospital Treatment of Children and Adolescents. Washington, DC, American Academy of Child and Adolescent Psychiatry, 1989

American Academy of Child and Adolescent Psychiatry: Annotation to American Academy of Child and Adolescent Psychiatry Ethics Code With Special References to Evolving Healthcare Delivery and Reimbursement Systems. Washington, DC, American Academy of Child and Adolescent Psychiatry, 1995

American Academy of Child and Adolescent Psychiatry: Practice parameters for the assessment and treatment of children and adolescents with posttraumatic stress disorder. J Am Acad Child Adolesc Psychiatry 37(10 suppl):4S–26S, 1998 9785726

American Psychiatric Association: Ethics Primer of the American Psychiatric Association. Arlington, VA, American Psychiatric Association, 2001

American Psychiatric Association: Diagnostic and Statistical Manual of Mental Disorders, 5th Edition. Arlington, VA, American Psychiatric Association, 2013

Barnum R: Parenting assessment in cases of neglect and abuse, in Principles and Practice of Child and Adolescent Forensic Psychiatry. Edited by Schetky D, Benedek E. Washington, DC, American Psychiatric Publishing, 2002, pp 81–96

Bernet W: The child and adolescent psychiatrist and the law, in Handbook of Child and Adolescent Psychiatry. Edited by Adams P, Bleiberg E. New York, Wiley, 1998, pp 438–468

Clark BK: Developmental aspects of memory in children, in Principles and Practice of Child and Adolescent Forensic Psychiatry. Edited by Schetky D, Benedek E. Washington, DC, American Psychiatric Publishing, 2002, pp 129–135

Englander EK: Spinning our wheels: improving our ability to respond to bullying and cyberbullying. Child Adolesc Psychiatr Clin N Am 21(1):43–55, viii, 2012 22137810

Goldstein J, Solnut AJ, Goldstein S: In the Best Interests of the Child. New York, Free Press, 1996

Grisso T: Evaluating Juvenile Adjudicative Competence: A Guide for Clinical Practice. Professional Resources Press, Sarasota, FL, 2005

Grisso T, Schwartz RG: Youth on Trial: A Developmental Perspective on Juvenile Justice. Chicago, IL, University of Chicago Press, 2000

Horowitz R: Legal rights of children. Child Adolesc Psychiatr Clin N Am 11(4):705–717, 2002 12397894

Kraus LJ, Thomas CR, Bukstein OG, et al: Practice parameter for child and adolescent forensic evaluations. J Am Acad Child Adolesc Psychiatry 50(12):1299–1312, 2011 22115153

Kulkofsky S, London K: Reliability and suggestibility of children's statements, in Principles and Practice of Child and Adolescent Forensic Mental Health. Washington, DC, American Psychiatric Publishing, 2010, pp 217–225

Macbeth J: Legal issues in the treatment of minors, in Principles and Practice of Child and Adolescent Forensic Psychiatry. Edited by Schetky D, Benedek E. Washington, DC, American Psychiatric Publishing, 2002, pp 309–323

Munir K, Earls F: Ethical principles governing research in child and adolescent psychiatry. J Am Acad Child Adolesc Psychiatry 31(3):408–414, 1992 1592771

Poole DA, Lindsay DS: Interviewing preschoolers: effects of nonsuggestive techniques, parental coaching and leading questions on reports of nonexperienced events. J Exp Child Psychol 60(1):129–154, 1995

Pope K, Luna B, Thomas CR: Developmental neuroscience and the courts: how science is influencing the disposition of juvenile offenders. J Am Acad Child Adolesc Psychiatry 51(4):341–342, 2012 22449636

Pruett MK, DiFonzo JH: Closing the gap: research, policy, practice, and shared parenting. Fam Court Rev 52(2):152–174, 2014

Quinn KM: Interviewing children for suspected sexual abuse, in Principles and Practice of Child and Adolescent Forensic Psychiatry. Edited by Schetky D, Benedek EP. Washington, DC, American Psychiatric Publishing, 2002, pp 149–159

Rappeport JR: Reasonable medical certainty. Bull Am Acad Psychiatry Law 13(1):5–15, 1985 3995190

Rodham H: Children under the law, in The Rights of Children. Harv Educ Rev 43:487–514, 1973

Schetky DH: Ethics, in Lewis's Child and Adolescent Psychiatry: A Comprehensive Textbook, 4th Edition. Edited by Martin A, Volkmar FR. Philadelphia, PA, Lippincott Williams and Wilkins, 2007, pp 17–22

Schetky DH, Guyer MJ: Psychic trauma and civil litigation, in Principles and Practice of Child and Adolescent Forensic Psychiatry. Edited by Schetky D, Benedek E. Washington, DC, American Psychiatric Publishing, 2002, pp 355–364

Scott CL, Temporini HT: Forensic issues and the Internet, in Principles and Practice of Child and Adolescent Forensic Mental Health. Washington, DC, American Psychiatric Publishing, 2010, pp 253–263

Stahl P: Complex Issues in Child Custody Evaluations. Thousand Oaks, CA, Sage Publications, 1999

U.S. Department of Health and Human Services: Protection of Human Subjects, C.F.R. Title 45, Part 46, 1991

Walter HJ, Berkovitz IH: Practice parameter for psychiatric consultation to schools. J Am Acad Child Adolesc Psychiatry 44(10):1068–1083, 2005 16175112

Wills CD: DSM-5 and neurodevelopmental and other disorders of childhood and adolescence. J Am Acad Psychiatry Law 42(2):165–172, 2014 24986343

CHAPTER 33

Telemental Health

Sharon Cain, M.D.
Eve-Lynn Nelson, Ph.D.
Kathleen Myers, M.D., M.P.H., M.S.

Technology affects many aspects of daily life, and health care is no exception. Telecommunications systems make it possible to provide health care at a distance, virtually connecting patients and providers. This method of health care delivery, generically referred to as *telemedicine,* has been used for a wide range of medical applications. As psychiatry relies predominantly on conversation and observation, it has been one of the most widely adopted disciplines in telemedicine (Shore 2013).

The American Telemedicine Association (ATA) defines *telemedicine* as "the use of medical information exchanged from one site to another via electronic communications to improve patients' health status" (www.americantelemed.org). Telemedicine falls under the telehealth umbrella, with telehealth more broadly encompassing "a collection of means or methods for enhancing health care, public health, and health education delivery and support using telecommunications technologies" (www.telehealthresourcecenter.org). Telemedicine is closely allied with health information technology (HIT), with HIT traditionally focused on electronic health records and telemedicine associated with clinical services using technology (American Telemedicine Association 2012).

Telemental health (TMH) is defined as the application of telemedicine across the range of mental and behavioral health specialties. *Telepsychiatry* and *telepsychology* refer to telemedicine applications within specific mental and behavioral health specialties. In this chapter, we limit the term TMH to the provision of mental health services using real-time, interactive videoconferencing technology. This technology is identified in the literature by the terms videoteleconferencing (VTC), videoconferencing (VC), interactive televideo (ITV), and interactive television (IATV). In this chapter, we use the acronym VC for this technology. When referring generically to a psychiatrist, psychologist, or therapist providing TMH, we use the term *teleprovider.* Additional technology terms are defined in Table 33–1.

Technical Aspects of Telemental Health

TMH focuses on live, interactive, two-way VC. Mobile health is narrowly included, specific to mobile-based VC. Technological advances in VC systems have made secure, inexpensive, user-friendly, reliable VC more available. For VC services, the teleprovider and distant site must have access to 1) modern, well-functioning VC equipment, including camera, monitor, microphone, and speakers; 2) encrypted VC software; 3) secure clinical space for the equipment setup; and 4) high-speed connectivity with consistent quality of service. VC equipment varies in expense and should be selected to meet clinical need and space considerations. It may include large room-based systems, computer-based systems, or newer mobile devices. Across all devices, high-quality cameras and microphones are essential. Consideration should be given to initial and ongoing technical support and associated costs.

The purpose of the TMH service should drive the selection of the technology. There are a daunting number of choices across VC service needs. In addition to vendor input, broad information from telehealth resource centers (www.telehealthresources.org), organizations using the system, professional organizations, and others may help inform decision making. Teleproviders often consider whether the technology system is user-friendly and whether the system is compatible with other systems or is highly proprietary. Both initial and upgrade costs should be explored. Considerations include initial purchase, lease or license costs, installation costs, costs associated with Internet access and possible additional wiring, training, maintenance, and support. Ongoing operational cost considerations include continuation lease or licensing fees, upgrades, equipment, maintenance and support, technical assistance, and Internet access fees. If multiple sites are connected, bridging costs should be considered. TMH guidelines recommend ongoing technical training across teleprovider and service sites. Ongoing, consumer-friendly technical support is often noted as a key factor in TMH program success and sustainability. Teleproviders are encouraged to consider the availability of such support at both sites and associated costs.

The available technologies fall into two broad categories: 1) standards-based applications and 2) consumer-grade software applications (Goldstein and Myers 2014). These distinctions are blurring with newer hybrid technologies. Traditionally, *standards-based applications* refer to the secure, point-to-point transmission of high-bandwidth (>386 kbits/second) signals over satellite or fiber optics (T1 lines or integrated services digital networks) that provide high-definition video and audio interactions. These systems typically include a camera with zoom and pan/tilt features that allow the examiner to look closely at a child's facial features and to follow the child's movements around the room. Standards-based applications typically allow multipoint conferencing and interoperability. Sites "purchase" bandwidth and time from a telecommunications vendor. These sophisticated systems are typically used in major medical centers or clinics and require additional infrastructure for con-

TABLE 33–1. Technology terms

Term	Definition
Interactive videoconferencing	Live video connections that transmit information in both directions during the same time period; also called synchronous or real-time videoconferencing
Store-and-forward	A type of telehealth service that relies on transmission of recorded health information through an electronic communications system to a practitioner, usually a specialist, who uses the information to provide care or a consultative opinion at a time that is after the information was recorded and thus not interactive; also called asynchronous
Remote patient monitoring	The collection of personal health data from an individual in one location that is transmitted in real time via electronic communication technologies to a provider in a different location for use in providing medical care and related support
Mobile Health (mHealth)	Practice of medicine and public health supported by mobile communication devices, such as mobile phones, tablet computers, and PDAs for health services and information
Bandwidth	A measure of the information-carrying capacity of a communications channel; a practical limit to the size, cost, and capability of a telemedicine service
Encryption	A system of encoding electronic data in which the information can be retrieved and decoded only by the person or computer system authorized to access it; often described in kbits/second
Authentication	A method of verifying the identity of a person sending or receiving information using passwords, keys, and other automated identifiers
H.323	ITU standard for videoconferencing compression that allows different equipment to interoperate via the Internet Protocol, the protocol by which data are sent from one computer to another over the Internet
Interoperability	The ability of two or more systems (computers, communication devices, networks, software, other information technology components) to interact with one another and exchange data according to a prescribed method in order to achieve predictable results
Multipoint teleconferencing	Interactive electronic communication between multiple users at two or more sites, which facilitates voice, video, and/or data transmission systems: audio, graphics, and computer and video systems; requires an MCU or bridging device to link multiple sites into a single videoconference

TABLE 33–1. Technology terms *(continued)*

Term	Definition
Patient site	Location of the patient at the time the service being furnished via a telecommunications system occurs; also known as originating site, spoke site, remote site, or rural site
Provider site	Site at which the physician or other licensed practitioner delivering the service is located at the time the service is provided via telecommunications system; also known as distant site, hub site, specialty site, provider/physician site, or referral site
Patient presenter	A clinical staff person at the patient site who is trained to "present" the patient to the provider during a telehealth encounter; this includes the presenter's management of the telehealth equipment and his or her performance of "hands-on" activities needed to successfully complete the telehealth visit; also called site coordinator

Note. ITU=International Telecommunication Union; MCU=multipoint control unit; PDAs=personal digital assistants.
Source. Adapted from definitions found at the American Telemedicine Association Web site (American Telemedicine Association 2009, 2011, 2012, 2013b, 2014) and the Telehealth Resource Center Web site (http://www.telehealthresourcecenter.org/sites/main/files/file-attachments/telehealth_definintion_framework_for_trcs_1.pdf).

necting outside of firewalls and maintenance. Generally, more expensive, standards-based systems have been viewed as being less risky for an organization, as they provide transparent encryption, can be managed by organizational technical staff, and use established and open protocols for communication.

Consumer-grade applications are provided over the Internet using software that encrypts the transmission and can be readily loaded onto desktop computers and are, therefore, much more accessible to providers and patients. Many options exist through a range of vendors who may provide downloadable software for connectivity or may provide a "virtual meeting room" with technical support (American Telemedicine Association 2013b; National Telehealth Technology Assessment Resource Center 2014). A key advantage to consumer-grade applications is the ease of use and frequently lower cost. In the past, disadvantages have included less secure transmissions and lower-quality audio and video streams, although transparency in business affiliate agreement disclosures and advances in video compression decrease these concerns in some situations. Previously, disadvantages of consumer-grade products also included lack of interoperability with existing devices, inability to support multipoint connections, limitation in the types of devices that could be connected, and lack of teleprovider control of the distant site camera such as lack of zoom and pan/tilt features. However, a number of recent advances have addressed these challenges, including increasing adoption of standards-based approaches in order to be able to communicate across systems, newer products that allow connection of multiple device types, and more advanced cameras for desktop use. Finally, consumer-grade applications are increasingly accessible through mobile devices (e.g., smartphones, tablets). With this increased flexibility and portability, teleproviders weigh advantages and disadvantages in a specific situation, balancing increased access with privacy, security, and functionality. This information is summarized in an online toolkit (National Telehealth Technology Assessment Resource Center 2014).

Development of Child and Adolescent Telemental Health Programs

The Case for Telemental Health

Over the past two decades, technological innovations have converged with mandates for mental health care reform (Patient Protection and Affordable Care Act, P.L. 111-148, 2010; President's New Freedom Commission on Mental Health 2003) to make TMH a viable service delivery model for youth who are underserved by traditional models of care. VC services are driven by the need to address the widening gap between supply and demand for child mental and behavioral health services. According to the U.S. Bureau of Health Professions, the United States will have only two-thirds of the child and adolescent psychiatrists required to meet needs in 2020, with similar workforce challenges seen across other behavioral health disciplines (Hyde 2013). The shortage particularly affects rural communities that have experienced shrinking populations, declining economies, and increasing poverty as well as delays in treatment, less access to mental health insurance, and limited transportation options. Health care reform has spurred increased interest in addressing the maldistribution of mental health care for children. New models of health care delivery will need to be developed and implemented in order to achieve the goal of improved mental health care access for rural and underserved youth.

Telemental Health Programs

Initially, TMH programs were developed to bring specialty care to patients in rural areas, often in consultation to primary care. Various models have been used for responding to referrals from primary care providers (PCPs) such as direct assessment and treatment by the teleprovider (Myers et al. 2007, 2010), assessment followed by treatment recommendations for the PCP and local therapists to carry out (Myers et al. 2007; Yellowlees et al. 2008), and a stabilization model. In this latter model, the teleprovider treats the patient until he or she is stable, after which the patient returns to care by the PCP. In a newer model, the *consultation conference,* a telepsychiatrist provides consultation over VC to one or a group of PCPs who present their cases and ask topical questions (Dobbins et al. 2011).

While TMH services initially focused on rural settings (Duncan et al. 2014), they are increasingly offered in diverse locations, including underserved parts of urban communities (Spaulding et al. 2011). Mental health centers and other child-serving facilities may provide infrastructure that facilitates the implementation of VC services (Cain and Spaulding 2006). Many schools are seeking to understand their students' mental health needs and are willing to use their VC systems to access TMH services (Grady et al. 2011). Most behavioral health diagnoses across the developmental spectrum have been evaluated through VC consistent with patients in usual outpatient practice (Myers et al. 2004). Youth living in underserved communities often differ in their racial and ethnic heritage from their clinical providers. TMH allows these youth to be evaluated in their own communities accompanied by family or community members who may provide context and perspective that are not available if services are provided in distant health centers (Savin et al. 2011).

Evidence Base Supporting the Effectiveness of Telemental Health

Although the body of literature supporting child and adolescent TMH has grown substantially since 2000, it lags behind the adult literature. Most outcome data for mental health treatment using VC technology come from the growing evidence base in the adult TMH literature. A number of adult studies have demonstrated the equivalency of VC-delivered psychiatric and psychological interventions to the same treatments delivered in person. Hilty et al. (2013) have reviewed the effectiveness of TMH care across age groups.

Acceptability of Child and Adolescent Telemental Health

A majority of the reports of TMH with children and adolescents are descriptive and address feasibility of and/or satisfaction with TMH in increasing access to service (Hilty et al. 2013; Myers et al. 2011). Attitudes toward TMH have been shown to be positive for providers (Myers et al. 2007), referring physicians

(Myers et al. 2007), families (Elford et al. 2000; Myers et al. 2004, 2008), and youth (Boydell et al. 2010; Myers et al. 2006). Individuals living in rural areas may prefer to access care via TMH because of less concern about confidentiality and stigma if the treatment professional is from outside of their community (Nelson and Bui 2010). VC approaches have also been successful in urban areas because of many of the same access concerns, particularly for underserved populations who may not be familiar with mental health services (Spaulding et al. 2011). The author of one case series argues that telepsychiatric consultation might be more effective than face-to-face consultation (Pakyurek et al. 2010). Although feasibility and/or satisfaction do not equate to efficacy, they imply perception of improvement and inform future systematic investigation and implementation. Diamond and Bloch's (2010) review concluded that there are no data to suggest that the process of TMH leads to negative outcomes.

Outcomes of Child and Adolescent Telemental Health

Although still limited, the evidence base for TMH with youth now includes outcome studies. See Table 33–2 for a summary of selected studies. Five of these studies are randomized controlled trials (RCTs). One RCT supports the validation of diagnostic evaluation using VC (Elford et al. 2000), and the other four are intervention trials. In one treatment study, Nelson et al. (2003) demonstrated that the effectiveness of cognitive-behavioral therapy for depressed youth using VC was comparable to that of in-person therapy. In another RCT, Himle et al. (2012) found no difference in response to treatment with a "comprehensive behavioral intervention for tics" between a VC treatment group and a face-to-face group. Two controlled studies addressed treatments for children with attention-deficit/hyperactivity disorder (ADHD). One showed that group parent training using VC can be as effective as traditional face-to-face sessions (Xie et al. 2013). The remaining RCT is the only study to look at the outcome of pharmacological treatment of children and adolescents delivered by VC. Myers et al. (2015) found that participants treated through VC had significantly better ADHD symptom outcomes per caregivers' reports than the group treated in primary care after a one-time telepsychiatry consultation. This study suggests the added value of providing a short-term intervention compared with a single consultation session to PCPs, both using VC.

A reasonable conclusion from the available evidence is that TMH is a viable option for bringing best practices of in-person psychiatric and psychological care to the underserved.

Clinical Practice of Telemental Health

Developmental and Clinical Considerations

Applications of TMH have been described across development and most diagnostic categories. Children as young as ages 2 years (Boydell et al. 2007) and 3 years (Elford et al. 2000; Myers et al. 2004) and those with developmental disabilities (Reese et al. 2013) have been evaluated over VC. The modal age group comprises school-age children (Myers et al. 2004, 2007; Nelson et al. 2003), and ADHD is the most com-

TABLE 33–2. Selected reports and studies in child and adolescent telemental health

Citation	Design	Sample	Telepsychiatry Findings
Elford et al. 2000	RCT (diagnostic validation)	23 children	High concordance and satisfaction between VC and in-person evaluations
Nelson et al. 2003	RCT (intervention)	28 youth with depression	CBT provided using VC comparable to in-person evaluations
Himle et al. 2012	RCT (intervention)	20 children with TD or CTD	Treatment for tic reduction equivalent to in-person evaluations
Xie et al. 2013	RCT (intervention)	22 children with behavioral disorder	Parent training equally effective as in-person training and well accepted
Myers et al. 2015	RCT (intervention)	223 youth with ADHD	Improvement in ADHD and ODD symptoms via telepsychiatry
Marcin et al. 2005	Descriptive chart review	223 patients, including psychiatry and other specialties	VC consultation led to treatment changes and symptom improvement
Boydell et al. 2007	Descriptive chart review	100 children ages 2–17, mean 11 years	Pros and cons of adherence
Fox et al. 2008	Pre-post study	190 youth in juvenile detention	Improvement in goal attainment, family relations, and behavior with treatment via VC
Yellowlees et al. 2008	Pre-post study	41 children in an e-mental health program	Improvement in affect and oppositional domains on the CBCL
Stain et al. 2011	Diagnostic validation	11 adolescents and young adults	Strong correlation of assessments using VC versus in-person evaluations
Kopel et al. 2001	Descriptive	136 children and adolescents	High satisfaction by families and health workers.
Myers et al. 2006	Descriptive	115 incarcerated youth	Successful treatment including medication management via VC
Greenberg et al. 2006	Descriptive	35 PCPs, 12 caregivers	PCP and caregiver satisfactions and frustrations with telepsychiatry
Myers et al. 2007	Descriptive	172 patients and 387 visits	PCP satisfaction with telepsychiatry
Myers et al. 2008	Descriptive	172 patients and 387 visits	Use of telepsychiatry and high satisfaction by families
Myers et al. 2010	Descriptive	701 patients 190 PCPs	Feasibility and acceptability of telepsychiatry

Note. ADHD=attention-deficit/hyperactivity disorder; CBCL=Child Behavior Checklist; CBT=cognitive-behavioral therapy; CTD=chronic tic disorder (chronic motor or vocal tic disorder); ODD=oppositional defiant disorder; PCP=primary care physician; RCT=randomized controlled trial; TD=Tourette's disorder; VC=videoconferencing.

monly treated disorder, although most diagnostic groups have been treated (Myers et al. 2004, 2007). Children who are uncooperative pose challenges, but they can be treated if there are assisting staff at the patient site. The appropriateness of a youth for care via TMH should be individualized to developmental considerations, parents' preferences, supports at the patient site, and the telepsychiatrist's resourcefulness.

Optimizing the Virtual Clinical Encounter

The main key to successful TMH practice is effective clinical care. Multiple factors may affect the quality of the clinical encounter and are worthy of consideration. Several authors have addressed these issues (Carlisle 2013; Glueck 2013b; Goldstein and Myers 2014; Onor and Misan 2005; Savin et al. 2011), and more information is available at the Web sites www.tmhguide.org, www.telehealthresourcecenter.org, and www.americantelemed.org.

Arrangement of Clinical Space at the Patient and Provider Sites

Confidentiality is a primary concern. Both the interview room at the patient site and the clinician's room at the provider site should be maintained as confidential space. Practical steps such as placing a sign on the door that alerts others that a private telemedicine session is taking place may decrease interruptions. Support staff at the patient site may assist with the flow of traffic between the clinical room and the waiting area in order to decrease the potential for "eavesdropping."

It is also crucial for the interview room at the patient site to be a safe, quiet, patient-friendly space. Whether in a medical or a nonmedical facility, the room should be cleared of potentially dangerous objects and fragile equipment that is not necessary for the VC encounter or that may distract the child (Carlisle 2013). A clinical staff person at the patient site may attend the session or be immediately available to assist with the technology, provide immediate help to maintain safety, and ensure continuity of care.

The room at the patient site should be the right size, neither too small nor too large. An ideal room is large enough to accommodate the youth, a clinical staff person, and at least two other adults (two parents or a parent and another person whom the parent might invite, such as a teacher) but not so large that it encourages distractibility or hyperactivity. The room should be large enough to evaluate children's motor skills, play, and exploration and to note abnormal movements. A table allows the child to draw or play but should not interfere with viewing of motor skills. The space that the teleprovider is operating from during the virtual visit will likely be construed as the provider's office. Thus, it is expected that the space will appear professional, and the teleprovider should reassure the patient that the space is confidential.

Technological Factors Affecting the Clinical Encounter

A high-quality video signal is crucial to the success of the virtual encounter. One important factor in determining quality is adequate bandwidth for high-resolution video. A bandwidth of greater than 384 kbits/second is thought to help to facilitate the reading of nonverbal cues and affective states (Glueck 2013b). Good lighting is also important to the quality of video conferencing (Onor and Misan 2005). Incandescent or compact fluorescent lighting appears more natural and ideally should emanate from behind the camera to avoid shadows. It is easier to control lighting in rooms with no windows. Various colors or backgrounds have been used to enhance the video quality, but with current technology, teleproviders are finding a typical office setting to be adequate. The clothing worn by the teleprovider may also affect the visual image. It is best to avoid clothing with high contrast, such as stripes and busy patterns, because of possible visual distortion.

Camera placement is another consideration. The camera is typically mounted above the monitor, causing individuals to appear to be looking downward. Conversely, a camera placed below the monitor will make individuals appear to be looking upward. These views might falsely convey difficulties in relatedness or impede rapport. Therefore, the teleprovider should alternate his or her gaze from camera to monitor to provide sufficient eye contact to convey optimal relatedness. To address this shortcoming clinically, teleproviders should query parents about the child's relatedness. Placing the camera just above the center of the computer screen can approximate the appearance of direct eye contact.

The audio component of VC is another critical component of effective communication. A high-quality audio signal is necessary for the patient and provider to understand the nuances of each other's verbal communication. The room should ideally be away from clinic and street noise, as the microphones are very sensitive and extraneous sounds can interfere with the session. Toys, although important to have on hand for young children, can produce uncomfortable levels of noise. One author (Carlisle 2013) suggests equipping the interview room with items such as foam blocks, books, markers, and papers and recommends avoiding electronic toys except under limited circumstances (e.g., allowing the child to be distracted by playing a muted electronic game when the parent needs time to talk).

The Virtual Relationship and Videoconferencing Etiquette

The virtual relationship is affected by screen presence (Onor and Misan 2005). Interpersonal style is adjusted to overcome limitations imposed by the technology. For example, more animation is generally demonstrated with broader hand gestures; however, if these gestures occur too fast, pixilation will occur. Verbal communications are more deliberate to adjust for the slight auditory lag and to clearly indicate when the teleprovider has finished speaking in order to facilitate reciprocity in communication.

Rapport is established within a space that does not physically exist, and participants may miss each other's nonverbal clues and details that are easier to read in an in-person interaction (Glueck 2013b). A more casual style may optimize rapport, and methods such as a virtual handshake or "high five" are ways to increase friendliness (Savin et al. 2011). Rapport building can also be facilitated by showing youth their own image on the full screen or in the "picture-in-picture" box on the screen and scanning the teleprovider room. VC etiquette also includes rapport-building adaptations, such as the child showing a photo over televideo or faxing to the teleprovider a picture drawn during the session.

Another consideration relating to the virtual relationship is whether to include a clinical staff coordinator at the patient site as a "presenter" who may attend part or all of the VC session. Coordinators can provide assistance with the technology, support for the patient, and immediate help in the event of safety or other emergent concerns. Additionally, they can provide educational material to the patients' families, assist with follow-through on recommendations, and help ensure continuity of care. However, the presence of a coordinator during the session may affect the therapeutic relationship with the patient and present a privacy concern. This may especially be true in small communities, when the local staff person may be known to the patient. Thus, such arrangements should be addressed in the initial needs assessment and then individually for each family.

Training for the telepresenter is encouraged and is available on the ATA Web site (American Telemedicine Association 2011).

Clinical Care

Clinical care provided via TMH should, of course, be consistent with professional practice parameters and guidelines. The American Academy of Child and Adolescent Psychiatry (AACAP) has published practice parameters on a number of topics related to psychiatric evaluation and treatment that can be found at www.aacap.org. One AACAP practice parameter specifically addresses telepsychiatry with children and adolescents (American Academy of Child and Adolescent Psychiatry, 2008). The American Psychological Association (2014) also has guidelines for the practice of telepsychology. The ATA has developed practice guidelines for VC-based TMH (American Telemedicine Association 2009) and guidelines addressing video-based online mental health (American Telemedicine Association 2013b) that are available at www.americantelemed.org.

Assessment

The psychiatric assessment of children and adolescents includes spending some time interviewing the youth alone. Older children with good impulse control, adequate verbal skills, and the ability to separate can be interviewed alone. Younger, developmentally impaired, or impulsive youth need a modified approach. Traditional play sessions may be challenging. The child may be observed interacting with staff in a structured or free play session. Some limited play with the child may be possible over the telemonitor (e.g., drawing pictures and then discussing themes or developing a play scenario with puppets).

In assessing preschoolers, it is helpful to observe the child in developmentally appropriate interactions. This should include the child's interactions with his or her parent(s) and preferably with an unfamiliar adult, perhaps a staff member. The teleprovider should also attempt direct interaction with the child, with the parent and/or a staff member in the room. This might be done by giving the child simple tasks—e.g., to distinguish colors, to point to body parts, or to count. As it may be difficult to appreciate the young child's level of attunement, pleasure in the interaction, or spontaneity in play, it is helpful to have an adult present with the child to comment on these aspects of the mental status. Another consideration is the child's level of cognitive development and his or her ability to understand the VC process. Preschool-age children may have difficulty with the concept that the teleprovider is a "real" person existing in a different location.

Treatment

Pharmacotherapy

Pharmacotherapy is one of the most commonly requested telepsychiatry services and can be accomplished with consideration of clinical, regulatory, and logistical issues (Cain and Sharp, in press).

Approaches to medication management depend on the system in which the telepsychiatrist is working. Models of care differ by whether medication is prescribed directly by the telepsychiatrist, by a collaborating midlevel clinician, or by the referring primary care physician. Regardless of the model used, it is important to maintain communication with the PCP about the treatment.

When prescribing via telepsychiatry, a procedure needs to be in place for providing prescriptions to patients. Prescriptions for noncontrolled medications can be e-prescribed, ordered by calling the pharmacy, or written and mailed through the U.S. Postal Service directly to the patient's home or to the patient site for distribution to families. Controlled medications such as schedule II stimulants can also be written and mailed but cannot be called to the pharmacy or refilled. Additionally, they can be e-prescribed in some settings. The federal government approved e-prescribing of controlled substances (EPCS) in 2010 contingent on specific security measures and the development of collaborative prescribing systems (Department of Justice 2015). In locations where state laws permit and prescribing systems are in place, EPCS may solve logistical issues for telepsychiatrists prescribing stimulants.

Managing and monitoring psychotropic medications via telepsychiatry are feasible (Myers et al. 2007, 2015; Spaulding et al. 2011). Tracking vital signs and weight, obtaining rating scales, checking metabolic laboratory work, and monitoring for adverse effects can be accomplished with coordination from staff at the patient site. When antipsychotic medications are prescribed, screening for abnormal movements can be done locally by a nurse or PCP and/or remotely by the telepsychiatrist. The Abnormal Involuntary Movement Scale (AIMS) was found to be reliable in telepsychiatry with adults (Amarendran et al. 2011).

An important aspect of medication management is providing care between TMH sessions. Patients' families need clear direction and contact numbers for interim needs such as requesting refills, asking questions, and reporting adverse effects. Depending on the logistics of the telepsychiatry service, the family may be instructed to call the patient site, the PCP office, or the telepsychiatrist's office directly. Protocols describing this process help to ensure safe monitoring of medications and to define expectations for staff at both sites, such as identifying the staff responsible for triaging patient calls and deciding when and how to contact the telepsychiatrist.

Psychotherapy

With therapy over VC, the goal is to translate the clinical site's best practices to the TMH setting using the latest evidence-based approaches (American Psychological Association 2014). In addition to translating therapy strategies to the TMH setting, the therapist gives particular attention to developing rapport with the child and family, with attention to the unique cultural context. Many different child therapy approaches have been used over VC, including individual therapy, family therapy, group therapy, and pediatric psychology interventions (American Telemedicine Association 2009). Lessons may be drawn from the more robust adult therapy literature, with roughly equivalent clinical outcomes using evidence-based practices to treat posttraumatic stress disorder, depression and anxiety, eating disorders, and substance abuse concerns and similar process findings across therapy satisfaction, alliance, attendance, and completion (Gros et al. 2013). Individual therapy using VC has also been successfully implemented with urban and rural children in a variety of settings, with reports most often using cognitive-behavioral approaches. The majority of studies have been therapy interventions for ADHD, but there are also examples in autism spectrum disorder, behavioral concerns with juvenile offenders, depression, obsessive-compulsive disorder, and tic disorders (Nelson and Patton, in press). Pediatric psychology interventions with medically ill children include pediatric cancer, congenital heart disease, cystic fibrosis, diabetes, epilepsy, feeding disorders, inflammatory bowel disease, obesity, and sleep disorders. A number of pediatric psychology interventions have been used via VC, such as cognitive-behavioral strategies to promote child and family coping as well as interventions to enhance adherence to medical regimens. As with individual therapies, findings have been positive overall for feasibility, satisfaction, and outcome, although definitive statements are difficult in light of the limited number of studies, small samples, and limited replication.

Telemental Health in a System of Care

TMH is poised to play an increasingly important role within pediatric health care systems. Services to primary care settings are anticipated to increase with national and state initiatives around the patient-centered medical home (Keller and Sarvet 2013). The essence of this model is to increase coordination and communication between PCPs and psychiatrists. TMH is one strategy for incorporating mental health treatment into primary care settings and has the added potential for increasing the PCPs' skills in caring for mental health problems.

There is also increasing emphasis on extending the reach of evidence-based mental health treatment. TMH combined with other forms of information technology may bring evidence-based services, including pharmacotherapy or psychotherapy, to communities. A psychiatrist, psychologist, or team of specialists can be telecommuted to the patient's community, or the system of care can choose from a menu of services at the provider's site. The teleprovider can readily collaborate in the child's care by meeting virtually with local team members, such as school personnel.

With an increased role for TMH, new models of service delivery and of training teleproviders in remote areas will be needed. Innovative telementoring approaches such as Project ECHO are emerging. These educational models use the same VC technologies for case-based learning between teams of specialists and rural providers in pediatric behavioral health conditions, including ADHD (Arora et al. 2014). The inclusion of TMH experiences in graduate medical education holds the promise of increasing the numbers of clinicians who are competent in and interested in serving patients through TMH. Some child and adolescent psychiatry training programs include TMH experiences as elective or required rotations.

Establishing a Telemental Health Practice

The following is a brief overview of issues for potential teleproviders to address in determining whether TMH is relevant to their clinical practice. More information can be found at www.americantelemed.org and www.telehealthresourcecenter.org.

Feasibility and Sustainability of a Telemental Health Practice

Determination of feasibility of a TMH service is based on an accurate needs assessment that identifies the mental health needs of the patient site and determines whether the proposed service is likely to meet those needs and to complement existing services. If possible, it is helpful to visit the patient site and meet with local stakeholders, including local health care and mental health care providers, for discussions and collaborative problem solving.

Sustainability of a TMH service may best be determined within the larger context of the community's needs. For example, a local medical center may not benefit financially from using telepsychiatry to provide psychiatric evaluations and pharmacotherapy services, but there could be an institutional financial benefit if use of the emergency department decreases as a result. The community as a whole might also benefit from lower expenses related to correctional or educational services for youth with mental health challenges. With technology costs lowering and an increasing number of insurers reimbursing TMH services, sustaining such a service without outside funding may become more possible. TMH providers are encouraged to review information at the Center for Medicare and Medicaid Services Web site (http://www.cms.gov/Outreach-and-Education/Medicare-Learning-Network-MLN/MLNProducts/downloads/TelehealthSrvcsfctsht.pdf) and the ATA Web site (http://www.americantelemed.org/) prior to any billing to determine any jurisdiction-specific guidelines.

Patient Population and Model of Care

The patients to be served should be identified and may be determined by the site (e.g., mental health center, primary care practice, school). Patient inclusion and exclusion criteria should be based on needs of the referring clinicians, judgment of the teleprovider, and resources at the patient site, including the ability of staff at the site to attend to acutely suicidal or agitated patients. The teleprovider should make sure there are appropriate on-site clinical resources in order to safely conduct an evaluation. Exclusion criteria may include factors such as youth without accompanying guardians, patients without a PCP, or patients with a PCP who is uncomfortable resuming care for psychiatric patients. Several models of care have been used to provide TMH (Carlisle 2013; Goldstein and Myers 2014; Hilty et al. 2006). One distinction between models is whether the service provides consultation, ongoing direct care, or collaboration with another provider. Some programs have developed specific models for consultation to primary care (Myers et al. 2007; Yellowlees et al. 2008), including one that moves flexibly between consultation and direct care (Myers et al. 2010). When ongoing direct care is offered via TMH, a PCP should be identified to provide care when the teleprovider is unavailable and to resume care when the patient becomes stable.

Private Practice Options

TMH programs are no longer solely the purview of major medical centers. Mental health clinicians in private practice have several options for implementing TMH (Glueck 2013a). Teleproviders preferring more practice support may choose to work for a company offering a virtual group practice. Multiple private companies offer a spectrum of services ranging from models that provide a high level of structure, including management of the VC technology and patient referrals, while contracting with clinicians to provide the TMH clinical service (www.americantelemed.org). An alternative strategy for teleproviders who are confident with technology and require less support is to contract with a company to simply provide a secure Web-based connection by downloading their software (Glueck 2013a). Of course, the independent provider is responsible for performing the needs assessment to determine if the new service is needed, feasible, and sustainable. It is also necessary to determine the patient population and establish protocols between the provider and the patient site, addressing clinical, business, and regulatory issues (Glueck 2013a; American Academy of Child and Adolescent Psychiatry, 2008).

Administrative Issues

Before establishing a TMH program, there are a number of administrative issues to consider. Protocols are helpful to address administrative concerns, including a business plan with start-up and sustainability considerations, and defining how information about the TMH services will be shared with potential patients. In addition, work flow and patient flow must be considered, including needs related to patient scheduling, support staff, clinical documentation, and billing.

Another consideration when establishing a TMH service is to identify an individual at the patient site who can be the "clinical champion" of the TMH program. The clinical champion contributes to the program's success by advocating for program support and providing key functions. This may include socialization of the teleprovider to the local culture and health care systems, monitoring adherence to protocols, maintaining effective communication between sites, and coordinating the response to safety or other emergent concerns.

Evaluating a Telemental Health Service

All teleproviders are encouraged to collect process and outcome data for their practices for quality improvement, patient safety, and research purposes. The demand for TMH services has outpaced the evidence base supporting their efficacy, and more outcome data are needed. When pharmacotherapy is provided, monitoring of adherence and adverse effects via TMH could be compared with in-person treatment. Evaluation of clinical outcomes may include rating scales, interviews, and functional assessments. A "lexicon of assessment and outcome measures for telemental health" is available at the ATA Web site (American Telemedicine Association 2013a). Outcome measures may include adverse events, hospitalization, adherence to the treatment plan, and equipment failures, as well as changes in caregiver burden, clinicians' practices, school staffing, and barriers to care. Exploration of the virtual relationship between the patient and teleprovider could lead to insights for improving rapport. Kramer et al. (2012) provide a model to inform overall TMH research design, with Slone et al. (2012) providing additional guidance specific to pediatric research settings.

Regulatory and Ethical Issues

At the national level, The Joint Commission (formerly The Joint Commission for the Accreditation of Healthcare Organizations) has regulations applicable to telemedicine. Locally, laws regarding involuntary commitment and reporting child maltreatment may vary across jurisdictions. Institutional requirements concerning credentialing at the patient site should be reviewed. It is also necessary for malpractice insurance to cover the telemedicine practice.

Licensure is a complex issue. Efforts toward national telemedicine licensing have so far been unsuccessful, and requirements are determined by individual state medical boards (Center for Telehealth and e-Health Law 2014). National organizations differ somewhat in how they address licensure in policies and guidelines. The Federation of State Medical Board's "model" telemedicine policy requires physicians to be licensed in the state where the patient is located (SMART Workgroup 2014), and ATA guidelines require "health professionals" to comply with all laws and regulations related to their practice in both the patient site and provider site jurisdictions (American Telemedicine Association 2014). It is wise to review local and state-specific guidelines and check with licensure boards prior to starting a new TMH service. Individuals employed through the government (e.g., military, Veterans Affairs) should refer to federal regulations.

When a teleprovider sees a patient for an initial encounter over VC, it is necessary for the teleprovider to collect identifying information about the patient and to confirm the location of the patient (American Telemedicine Association 2013b). If the patient site is a medical office or other facility, the site may assist with this verification. If the patient is in a nonclinical setting, such as a home, the teleprovider may request documents to confirm identity. It is equally important for the teleprovider to inform the patient of the teleprovider's location (exact address is not required) and credentials. One suggestion for the teleprovider is to begin the initial clinical session by stating his or her own name and the city and state where the provider site is located.

Other important factors to consider include the patient's privacy and compliance of the VC transmission with the Health Insurance Portability and Accountability Act and state law regarding confidentiality of mental health information. Informed consent for treatment may include an additional consent to receive services through VC. A review of the potential limitations and acknowledgment of the patients' right to refuse treatment via VC is part of informed consent as well as clarification of whether the sessions will be recorded and/or stored in any way.

Just as in on-site clinical settings, the core ethical concern to protect the patient remains paramount for VC settings (Nelson et al. 2013). In addition, guidelines addressing therapy using VC are emerging to inform "reasonable steps" for TMH practice across clinical, administrative, and technical considerations. This includes guidelines from the ATA (2009. 2013b), the American Psychological Association (2014), and the AACAP (American Academy of Child and Adolescent Psychiatry, 2008).

Summary Points

- Child and adolescent telemental health has been practiced successfully in diverse settings, for most psychiatric disorders, across development, with youth of various ethnicities.
- Treatments, including pharmacotherapy and psychotherapy, have been provided successfully using interactive videoconferencing.
- While evidence is emerging concerning the efficacy of telemental health, telepsychiatric care should adhere to evidence-based guidelines and best practices as summarized in the practice parameters of the American Academy of Child and Adolescent Psychiatry.
- In general, telemental health providers adapt the same evidence-based treatment approaches for care delivery and patient safety when using videoconferencing.
- Modest modifications in usual practice space and techniques can be used to optimize telemental health care.
- Before a telemental health practice is established, a careful assessment of need, business plan and sustainability, the existing system of care, and stakeholders' interests will best ensure success.
- Technical decisions should be based on the specific clinical needs, using the highest bandwidth that is financially and technologically feasible to optimize the clinical experience.
- Telepsychiatrists should know and comply with all federal, state, and local regulations pertaining to their practice of telehealth.
- Teleproviders should obtain informed consent for care to be delivered over videoconferencing in addition to consent for treatment. They should also take steps to confirm the identity and location of the person receiving treatment.

References

Amarendran V, George A, Gersappe V, et al: The reliability of telepsychiatry for a neuropsychiatric assessment. Telemed J E Health 17(3):223–225, 2011 21443440

American Academy of Child and Adolescent Psychiatry: Practice Parameter for Telepsychiatry With Children and Adolescents. Washington, DC, American Academy of Child and Adolescent Psychiatry, 2008. Available at: http://www.aacap.org/aacap/Resources_for_Primary_Care/Practice_Parameters_and_Resource_Centers/Practice_Parameters.aspx. Accessed March 30, 2015.

American Psychological Association: Guidelines for the Practice of Telepsychology, 2013. Available at: http://www.apa.org/practice/guidelines/telepsychology.aspx. Accessed September 19, 2014.

American Telemedicine Association: Practice Guidelines for Videoconferencing-Based Telemental Health. Washington, DC, American Telemedicine Association, 2009. Available at: http://www.americantelemed.org/resources/standards/ata-standards-guidelines/videoconferencing-based-telemental-health. Accessed June 29, 2014.

American Telemedicine Association: Expert Consensus Recommendations for Videoconferencing-Based Telepresenting. Washington, DC, American Telemedicine

Association, 2011. Available at: http://www.americantelemed.org/docs/default-source/standards/expert-consensus-recommendations-for-videoconferencing-based-telepresenting.pdf?sfvrsn=4. Accessed June 29, 2014.

American Telemedicine Association: ATA telemedicine nomenclature, 2012. Available at: http://www.americantelemed.org/resources/nomenclature#.U6utCfldWSo. Accessed June 29, 2014.

American Telemedicine Association: Lexicon of Assessment and Outcome Measures for Telemental Health. Washington, DC, American Telemedicine Association, 2013a. Available at: http://www.americantelemed.org/docs/default-source/standards/a-lexicon-of-assessment-and-outcome-measurements-for-telemental-health.pdf?sfvrsn=2. Accessed September 19, 2014.

American Telemedicine Association: Practice Guidelines for Video-Based Online Mental Health Services. Washington, DC, American Telemedicine Association, 2013b. Available at: http://www.americantelemed.org/docs/default-source/standards/practice-guidelines-for-video-based-online-mental-health-services.pdf?sfvrsn=6. Accessed June 29, 2014.

American Telemedicine Association: Core operational guidelines for telehealth services involving provider-patient Interactions, 2014. Available at: http://www.americantelemed.org/resources/standards/ata-standards-guidelines. Accessed September 17, 2014.

Arora S, Thornton K, Komaromy M, et al: Demonopolizing medical knowledge. Acad Med 89(1):30–32, 2014 24280860

Boydell KM, Volpe T, Kertes A, et al: A review of the outcomes of the recommendations made during paediatric telepsychiatry consultations. J Telemed Telecare 13(6):277–281, 2007 17785023

Boydell KM, Volpe T, Pignatiello A: A qualitative study of young people's perspectives on receiving psychiatric services via televideo. J Can Acad Child Adolesc Psychiatry 19(1):5–11, 2010 20119561

Cain S, Spaulding R: Telepsychiatry: Lessons from two models of care. Presented at the 53rd Annual Meeting of the American Academy of Child and Adolescent Psychiatry, San Diego, CA, October 2006

Cain S, Sharp S: Telepharmacotherapy for children and adolescents. J Child Adolesc Psychopharmacol (in press)

Carlisle LL: Child and adolescent telemental health, in Telemental Health: Clinical, Technical and Administrative Foundations for Evidence-Based Practice. Edited by Myers K, Turvey C. London, Elsevier, 2013, pp 197–221

Center for Telehealth and e-Health Law: Breaking down telemedicine licensure process: CTeL surveys landscape. August 4, 2014. Available at: http://ctel.org/2014/08/breaking-down-telemedicine-licensure-process-ctel-surveys-landscape/. Accessed September 16, 2014.

Department of Justice: Electronic Prescriptions for Controlled Substances (EPCS). Washington, DC, Drug Enforcement Administration Office of Diversion Control, 2015. Available at: http://www.deadiversion.usdoj.gov/ecomm/e_rx. Accessed January 29, 2015.

Diamond JM, Bloch RM: Telepsychiatry assessments of child or adolescent behavior disorders: a review of evidence and issues. Telemed J E Health 16(6):712–716, 2010 20575615

Dobbins MI, Roberts N, Vicari SK, et al: The consultation conference: a new model of collaboration for child psychiatry and primary care. Acad Psychiatry 35(4):260–262, 2011 21804048

Duncan AB, Velasquez SE, Nelson EL: Using videoconferencing to provide psychological services to rural children and adolescents: a review and case example. J Clin Child Adolesc Psychol 43(1):115–127, 2014 24079653

Elford R, White H, Bowering R, et al: A randomized, controlled trial of child psychiatric assessments conducted using videoconferencing. J Telemed Telecare 6(2):73–82, 2000 10824374

Fox KC, Connor P, McCullers E, et al: Effect of a behavioural health and specialty care telemedicine programme on goal attainment for youths in juvenile detention. J Telemed Telecare 14(5):227–230, 2008 18632995

Glueck DA: Business aspects of telemental health in Private Practice, in Telemental

Health: Clinical, Technical and Administrative Foundations for Evidence-Based Practice. Edited by Myers K, Turvey C. London, Elsevier, 2013a, pp 111–133

Glueck D: Establishing therapeutic rapport in telemental health practice, in Telemental Health: Clinical, Technical and Administrative Foundations for Evidence-Based Practice. Edited by Myers K, Turvey C. London, Elsevier, 2013b, pp 29–46

Goldstein F, Myers K: Telemental health: a new collaboration for pediatricians and child psychiatrists. Pediatr Ann 43(2):79–84, 2014 24512157

Grady BJ, Lever N, Cunningham D, et al: Telepsychiatry and school mental health. Child Adolesc Psychiatr Clin N Am 20(1):81–94, 2011 21092914

Greenberg N, Boydell KM, Volpe T: Pediatric telepsychiatry in Ontario: Caregiver and service provider perspectives. J Behav Health Serv Res 33(1):105–111, 2006 16636911

Gros DF, Morland LA, Greene CJ, et al: Delivery of evidence-based psychotherapy via video telehealth. J Psychopathol Behav Assess 35(4):506–521, 2013

Hilty DM, Yellowlees PM, Cobb HC, et al: Models of telepsychiatric consultation—liaison service to rural primary care. Psychosomatics 47(2):152–157, 2006 16508028

Hilty DM, Ferrer DC, Parish MB, et al: The effectiveness of telemental health: a 2013 review. Telemed J E Health 19(6):444–454, 2013 23697504

Himle MB, Freitag M, Walther M, et al: A randomized pilot trial comparing videoconference versus face-to-face delivery of behavior therapy for childhood tic disorders. Behav Res Ther 50(9):565–570, 2012 22743661

Hyde PS: Report to Congress on the Nation's Substance Abuse and Mental Health Workforce Issues. Rockville, MD, U.S. Department of Health and Human Services, Substance Abuse and Mental Health Services Administration, 2013

Keller D, Sarvet B: Is there a psychiatrist in the house? Integrating child psychiatry into the pediatric medical home. J Am Acad Child Adolesc Psychiatry 52(1):3–5, 2013 23265627

Kopel H, Nunn K, Dossetor D: Evaluating satisfaction with a child and adolescent psychological telemedicine outreach service. J Telemed Telecare 7(suppl 2):35–40, 2001 11747654

Kramer GM, Shore JH, Mishkind MC, et al: A standard telemental health evaluation model: the time is now. Telemed J E Health 18(4):309–313, 2012 22424077

Marcin JP, Nesbitt TS, Cole SL, et al: Changes in diagnosis, treatment, and clinical improvement among patients receiving telemedicine consultations. Telemed J E Health 11(1):36–43, 2005 15785219

Myers KM, Sulzbacher S, Melzer SM: Telepsychiatry with children and adolescents: are patients comparable to those evaluated in usual outpatient care? Telemed J E Health 10(3):278–285, 2004 15650522

Myers K, Valentine J, Morganthaler R, et al: Telepsychiatry with incarcerated youth. J Adolesc Health 38(6):643–648, 2006 16730590

Myers KM, Valentine JM, Melzer SM: Feasibility, acceptability, and sustainability of telepsychiatry for children and adolescents. Psychiatr Serv 58(11):1493–1496, 2007 17978264

Myers KM, Valentine JM, Melzer SM: Child and adolescent telepsychiatry: utilization and satisfaction. Telemed J E Health 14(2):131–137, 2008 18361702

Myers KM, Vander Stoep A, McCarty CA, et al: Child and adolescent telepsychiatry: variations in utilization, referral patterns and practice trends. J Telemed Telecare 16(3):128–133, 2010 20197356

Myers KM, Palmer NB, Geyer JR: Research in child and adolescent telemental health. Child Adolesc Psychiatr Clin N Am 20(1):155–171, 2011 21092919

Myers K, Vander Stoep A, Zhou C, et al: Effectiveness of a telehealth service delivery model for treating attention-deficit/hyperactivity disorder: a community-based randomized controlled trial. J Am Acad Child Adolesc Psychiatry 54(4):263–274, 2015 25791143

National Telehealth Technology Assessment Resource Center: Desktop video applications toolkit, 2014. Available at: http://www.telehealthtechnology.org/toolkits/desktop-video-applications. Accessed June 29, 2014.

Nelson EL, Bui T: Rural telepsychology services for children and adolescents. J Clin Psychol 66(5):490–501, 2010 20306524

Nelson E, Patton S: Using videoconferencing to deliver individual therapy and pediatric psychology interventions with children. J Child Adolesc Psychopharmacol (in press)

Nelson EL, Barnard M, Cain S: Treating childhood depression over videoconferencing. Telemed J E Health 9(1):49–55, 2003 12699607

Nelson EL, Davis K, Velasquez S: Ethical considerations in providing mental health services over videoconferencing in telemental health in Clinical, Technical and Administrative Foundations for Evidence-Based Practice. Edited by Myers K, Turvey C. New York, Elsevier, 2013, pp 47–60

Onor ML, Misan S: The clinical interview and the doctor-patient relationship in telemedicine. Telemed J E Health 11(1):102–105, 2005 15785228

Pakyurek M, Yellowlees P, Hilty D: The child and adolescent telepsychiatry consultation: can it be a more effective clinical process for certain patients than conventional practice? Telemed J E Health 16(3):289–292, 2010 20406115

President's New Freedom Commission on Mental Health: Achieving the Promise: Transforming Mental Health Care in America. Rockville, MD, Substance Abuse and Mental Health Services Administration, 2003

Reese RM, Jamison R, Wendland M, et al: Evaluating interactive videoconferencing for assessing symptoms of autism. Telemed J E Health 19(9):671–677, 2013 23870046

Savin D, Glueck DA, Chardavoyne J, et al: Bridging cultures: child psychiatry via videoconferencing. Child Adolesc Psychiatr Clin N Am 20(1):125–134, 2011 21092917

Shore JH: Telepsychiatry: videoconferencing in the delivery of psychiatric care. Am J Psychiatry 170(3):256–262, 2013 23450286

Slone NC, Reese RJ, McClellan MJ: Telepsychology outcome research with children and adolescents: a review of the literature. Psychol Serv 9(3):272–292, 2012 22867120

SMART Workgroup: Model Policy for the Appropriate Use of Telemedicine Technologies in the Practice of Medicine. Washington, DC, Federation of State Medical Boards, April 2014. Available at: http://www.fsmb.org/Media/Default/PDF/FSMB/Advocacy/FSMB_Telemedicine_Policy.pdf. Accessed September 16, 2014.

Spaulding R, Cain S, Sonnenschein K: Urban telepsychiatry: uncommon service for a common need. Child Adolesc Psychiatr Clin N Am 20(1):29–39, 2011 21092910

Stain HJ, Payne K, Thienel R, et al: The feasibility of videoconferencing for neuropsychological assessments of rural youth experiencing early psychosis. J Telemed Telecare 17(6):328–331, 2011 21844174

Xie Y, Dixon JF, Yee OM, et al: A study on the effectiveness of videoconferencing on teaching parent training skills to parents and children. Telemed J E Health 19(3):192–199, 2013 23405952

Yellowlees PM, Hilty DM, Marks SL, et al: A retrospective analysis of a child and adolescent eMental Health program. J Am Acad Child Adolesc Psychiatry 47(1):103–107, 2008 18174831

PART V

Somatic Treatments

CHAPTER 34

Principles of Psychopharmacology

Esther S. Lee, M.D.
Robert L. Findling, M.D., M.B.A.

When clinicians contemplate the therapeutic options for psychiatric disorders, the use of medications is often considered. There are many factors to take into account when treating a child or adolescent with psychiatric illness, many of which differ significantly from those in a psychiatrically ill adult, or even in other children with general medical conditions. Some of these distinguishing factors include the following:

- Differences between children and adults in drug metabolism
- Differences in psychotropic drug efficacy and tolerability between young people and adults
- Limitations of current psychiatric nosology when diagnosing psychiatric disorders in younger patients
- Relative paucity of research data on pediatric psychopharmacology
- Involvement of outside parties in treatment planning (e.g., parents, relatives, teachers, counselors, therapists, pediatricians, neurologists)
- Multidisciplinary nature of child and adolescent psychiatric treatment
- Chronic nature of most childhood psychiatric illnesses

Despite the unique challenges that accompany pediatric psychopharmacology, the use of such medications is often considered in the treatment of a substantial number of children and adolescents who present with psychiatric illnesses. Untreated psychiatric illness in this population is not without its own inherent risks, and when these potential negative outcomes are balanced against both the known and potentially unknown risks of psychotropic medications, many times it is the former concern that compels clinicians into action (Vitiello 2008).

Once the decision has been made to employ treatment with medication, clinicians must continue to exercise caution and thoughtfulness in their prescribing practices in order to maximize potential benefits while minimizing the possibility of a harmful outcome. Such diligence can be achieved when treating these vulnerable youth by looking beyond the principles of pharmacokinetics and pharmacodynamics and considering additional clinically important principles such as child and adolescent development, drug efficacy and safety, regulatory issues, ethical considerations, and multimodal treatment. With all of this information in hand, clinicians can then have a thoughtful, comprehensive discussion with patients and families about whether or not psychiatric medication should be prescribed. This decision should be based on the results of a thorough assessment using current evidence-based practice guidelines (when available), as well as a biopsychosocial approach to the treatment of youth and their families. Assessment at each developmental period is covered in this book in "Part I: Assessment and Diagnosis." Please see the subsequent chapters in "Part V: Somatic Treatments" for the use of specific medications.

Brief History of Pediatric Psychopharmacology

Many consider the field of child and adolescent psychopharmacology to have begun in the late 1930s, when Charles Bradley published a landmark study on the salutary effects of racemic amphetamine (Benzedrine) in children with behavioral disturbances (Bradley 1937). Over the next 50 years, with the exception of the psychostimulants for treatment of attention-deficit/hyperactivity disorder (ADHD), there were few methodologically stringent studies pertaining to psychopharmacology in pediatric populations. Clinicians treating psychiatric disorders in the young were frequently obliged to extrapolate from adult psychopharmacology research, and, with rigorous pediatric data on dosing, safety, and efficacy seldom available, the use of psychotropics in this population was often problematic (Bourgeois et al. 2012).

By the mid-1980s, pediatric research began extending beyond ADHD to include treatment of early onset psychiatric disorders such as pervasive developmental disorders, depressive disorders, bipolar disorder, obsessive-compulsive disorder, schizophrenia, and conduct disorder. Improved experimental design and assessment methods paved the way for this increase in pediatric psychopharmacology research. In 1997, U.S. federal legislation further promoted the study of drugs in children by providing new financial incentives to pharmaceutical companies. As a result, by the end of the 1990s, pediatric psychopharmacology grew into a substantial and independent field of study (Connor and Meltzer 2006).

Although the field of child and adolescent psychiatry has experienced rapid growth since that time, there continue to be many barriers to the further advancement of knowledge in the field. The World Health Organization's 2004 Global Burden of Disease study showed that depression, schizophrenia, and bipolar disorder represent three of the top five conditions causing the highest disease burden among children in high-income countries. For children living in middle-income and lower-income countries, depression is also a serious concern, ranking immediately behind lower respiratory tract infections, diarrheal disease, malaria, and HIV/AIDS. On the basis of this information, Bourgeois et al. (2012) found that although children represent a significant proportion of the disease burden for these medical conditions, their representation among clinical drug trials worldwide is less than 15%.

General Principles of Psychopharmacological Assessment, Diagnosis, and Treatment

The clinical implementation of child and adolescent psychopharmacology differs considerably from clinical practice in adults. The initial steps that clinicians take in completing this evaluation generally include performing a complete psychiatric assessment of the patient and the family, arriving at a psychiatric diagnosis, crafting a biopsychosocial case formulation, and developing a comprehensive, evidence-based treatment plan.

Psychiatric Assessment

The completion of a thorough patient assessment is the first step in the successful psychiatric treatment of a child or adolescent. This initial evaluation has several goals, one of which is for the clinician to identify psychiatric symptoms that may indicate one or more underlying psychiatric disorders. The clinician can then decide which elements of these disorders might best be addressed by psychopharmacological treatments, which might respond to psychosocial treatments and/or environmental interventions, and which elements require a combination approach. Another goal of the psychiatric assessment is to uncover relevant patient and family historical information that may determine which modalities of psychiatric treatment or which psychotropic medications might be most suitable for that particular patient.

During the initial assessment, the clinician becomes acquainted with the patient while trying to understand the patient's concerns and level of functioning in multiple contexts, including the home/family environment, school, and peer groups. This evaluation is also an opportunity to initiate a positive relationship with the patient and family that can eventually translate into a more effective therapeutic alliance. Good rapport between the clinician, patient, and family is generally beneficial to all participants, allowing for a more honest exchange of relevant information, higher likelihood of treatment adherence, and improved clinic attendance.

Sources of Assessment Information

The primary source of information is usually the patient and his or her family, all of whom should ideally be included in a comprehensive psychiatric assessment. If the patient is younger than age 18 years, then the parents or legal guardians (hereinafter referred to as *parents*) generally need to be present and to consent to the evaluation. It is important to remain up to date on the state laws that govern individual practices regarding exceptions to this rule, as some states allow underage consent in certain situations such as substance abuse treatment, brief counseling, and emergency situations.

Additional sources of information may include other individuals who also spend significant time with the patient, such as classroom teachers, relatives, and other caretakers. It is also important to reach out to any other providers of medical or mental health care, such as pediatricians, neurologists, therapists, and counselors, in order to promote better understanding of the patient and consistency of treatment goals. These individuals may be contacted with the written permission of the patient's parents and, depending on age and state law, the patient.

To supplement the information gathered during the assessment interview, psychiatric rating scales are typically used. These questionnaires can be completed by the patient, parents, and/or teachers prior to the assessment, allowing clinicians to review the results during the interview. Some examples of commonly used rating scales that have been found to be valid and reliable are the Child Behavior Checklist (CBCL; Achenbach and Rescorla 2001; Ivanova et al. 2007) and the Conners 3rd Edition (Conners 3; Conners 2008), which screen for multiple types of psychopathology. The CBCL and the Conners 3 allow for the calculation of a standardized score, therefore allowing comparison of reported symptoms to those in age- and gender-matched counterparts who do not suffer from a psychiatric disorder. Rating scales directed toward specific areas of concern may also be used, including the Screen for Childhood Anxiety Related Emotional Disorders (SCARED) and Multidimensional Anxiety Scale for Children (MASC) addressing anxiety, the Beck Depression Inventory for Youth (BDI-Y) and Center for Epidemiological Studies Depression Scale for Children (CES-DC) addressing depression, and the Vanderbilt ADHD Diagnostic Parent/Teacher Rating Scales and the revised Swanson, Nolan, and Pelham IV (SNAP-IV-R) rating scale for ADHD. Although psychometric scales can be useful in supplementing clinical psychiatric diagnoses by providing information about symptom severity, one must remember that they cannot diagnose psychiatric disorders per se. Results may be helpful in highlighting particular areas of concern, but they do not substitute for a comprehensive clinical evaluation done by an appropriately trained professional.

Assessment Interview

During the assessment interview, a clinician asks questions and gathers information about key aspects of a patient's history and presentation (Table 34–1). As clinicians gather this clinical information, they typically concentrate on the data that will help establish the psychiatric diagnosis and determine the best options for treatment, including possible psychopharmacotherapy.

Interviewing pediatric patients can be challenging, owing to their developmental variability in psychological and cognitive characteristics. Younger children may have relatively limited verbal abilities and may be less experienced than adults at recognizing their emotions and feelings, thus leading to difficulty talking about their mood or thoughts. It is not until late childhood or early adolescence that children generally become more proficient at recognizing their emotions and feelings and verbally communicating that information to others. Younger children may also have difficulty accurately estimating time increments, and references to specific events (e.g., holidays, birthdays) and significant life experiences (e.g., the birth of a sibling, a move to a new house, a specific year in school) can be useful when asking a child about the onset and duration of symptoms.

While older children typically have better verbal skills, they may not understand psychiatric terms such as *irritability, euphoria,* or *paranoia.* Similarly, there may be difficulty differentiating the clinical meaning of certain words or phrases

TABLE 34–1. Selected areas of the psychiatric assessment that are important to pediatric psychopharmacology

Area of psychiatric assessment	Relevance to pediatric psychopharmacology
Chief complaint	The parents' principal areas of concern help define the goals for psychiatric pharmacotherapy.
History of present illness	Certain psychiatric symptoms and responses to psychosocial stressors may be amenable to psychopharmacological treatment. Target symptoms can be identified and monitored to determine drug effectiveness.
Psychiatric review of systems	Comorbid disorders may require modified psychopharmacological treatment.
Past psychiatric history	Information on past psychotropic medication trials (reason prescribed, highest dose achieved, effectiveness, side effects, duration of treatment, reason for discontinuation) can guide future medication choices and dosing. Current psychotropic medications may need to be adjusted or discontinued if new medications are initiated in order to prevent toxicity and minimize drug-drug interactions.
Suicidality and homicidality history	Past and current safety concerns may require certain precautions as pharmacotherapy is initiated (choosing drugs that are less toxic in overdose, prescribing limited amounts of medication, monitoring patient particularly closely for behavioral changes).
Substance abuse and chemical dependency history	Past or current substance use may necessitate caution when prescribing controlled substances. Current abuse of medications, illicit drugs, or alcohol can cause drug-drug interactions with psychotropic medications. Current chemical dependency may require detoxification. Comprehensive chemical dependency treatment may be necessary before psychopharmacotherapy for comorbid psychiatric disorders is initiated.
Developmental and early childhood history	A patient's slow growth may raise concern over potential negative effects on stature associated with the long-term use of certain psychotropic medications.
General medical history	Known drug allergies may limit psychopharmacotherapy options. Past and current medical conditions may also affect choice of psychotropic medications (avoiding psychostimulants in youth with cardiac problems, valproic acid in children with hepatic disease, or lithium in those with renal insufficiency).
Family history	Family history may highlight other possible diagnostic concerns, heritable conditions, and/or comorbid illnesses.
School history	Younger children or older children with low intellectual functioning may require increased monitoring of medication administration and effects. The timing of a child's ADHD symptoms throughout the school day may require adjustments in dosing the child's psychostimulant medication. Adverse medication effects such as sedation may interfere with academic performance.
Social history	Peer relationships and attitudes may affect a youth's adherence to psychotropic medication. Adverse medication effects such as sedation may interfere with leisure activities.

from the colloquial meaning, and a clinician should always seek to clarify what is being said by the patient to ensure that the child's words are being correctly understood. In order to foster better understanding and rapport, the clinician should also take into account the patient's language skills and vocabulary and adapt his or her own language to the level best understood by the patient. If there is suspicion that a patient does not fully comprehend what is being discussed, the clinician should assess the patient's understanding and present the information again using different language or examples if necessary.

Mental Status Examination

When assessing a child or adolescent patient, clinicians typically conduct a mental status examination by observing the key features of a patient's appearance, behavior, speech, language, mood, affect, thought process, thought content, cognition, and social relatedness. These observations, when added to the data from the patient interview, can help the clinician establish a diagnosis and decide on possible pharmacological treatment options. Also, certain psychiatric symptoms that are observed during the mental status examination may be used by the clinician as a baseline to subsequently assess the effectiveness of a chosen treatment option.

Variability in mental status is common in children and adolescents. An appreciation of such variability is important because different circumstances can influence a patient's mood or behavior during the initial psychiatric assessment. For example, a child with ADHD symptoms that are typically well controlled with a psychostimulant may appear to have difficulty with hyperactivity or concentration during the mental status examination if he or she did not receive medication that day. Alternatively, a child with untreated ADHD may appear to have good attention and concentration in the office during the first visit with a new clinician, owing to the unfamiliarity and novelty of the encounter. Similarly, a youth who is experiencing symptoms of an upper respiratory infection may present with low energy and irritable mood, which to a clinician may appear to be symptomatic of depression. Thus, it is advisable for clinicians to consider any suspected influences on a patient's mental status examination while the diagnosis and options for possible psychopharmacological treatment are being considered.

Physical Evaluation

A patient's physical condition is also typically assessed during a psychiatric assessment. The clinician's decision about which components to include in this focused physical evaluation depends on the patient's general physical health and the type of psychotropic medication that the clinician is considering for treatment. There are several key reasons to evaluate a young patient's physical health prior to definitively ascribing a psychiatric diagnosis or making treatment recommendations. One reason is that general medical conditions may manifest with psychiatric symptoms, such as in the case of depressive symptoms presenting in a patient with hypothyroidism. Additionally, the presence of certain general medical conditions might influence decisions about the prescription of psychotropic agents, such as when determining the role of a psychostimulant in the treatment of a patient with a structural cardiac abnormality.

Examining the physical well-being of patients and measuring selected physical parameters prior to the initiation of pharmacotherapy also provide a baseline with which subsequent evaluations can be compared, thus facilitating the assessment of possible adverse effects of treatment. It is also important for mental health clinicians to collaborate with the patient's primary medical doctor throughout the patient's psychiatric care, as the mental health clinician can thus remain informed of changes in the patient's general medical status and of nonpsychotropic medications being prescribed. Such communication also provides the general medical physician with an appraisal of changes in the child's diagnosis and psychiatric care.

Physical Examination

Ideally, a pediatric patient will have been seen by his or her primary medical doctor for a physical examination within the year prior to the psychiatric assessment. If not, it is often advisable that the patient be evaluated before psychotropic medication is administered.

Other Physical Parameters

Clinicians may check a patient's vital signs, height, and weight during the psychiatric assessment in order to screen for any immediate medical concerns, such as obesity or hypertension, prior to initiating psychotropic medication. Comparison of such baseline measurements to future physical parameters can aid clinicians in monitoring for potential adverse medication effects, including possible changes in growth trajectory. Monitoring growth is generally advisable since, with the exception of psychostimulants, there are relatively little data available on the long-term effects of psychopharmacotherapy on the growth and development of children.

Laboratory Tests

Laboratory tests can supplement the data gathered from the physical examination and other diagnostic procedures, helping to rule out certain underlying medical conditions and guiding the clinician's choice of possible psychotropic medication. Furthermore, establishing certain baseline laboratory values prior to initiating psychotropic medication can aid in monitoring for potential adverse medication effects. Common tests that a clinician may choose are included in Table 34–2 (Zametkin et al. 1998).

Electrocardiogram and Other Diagnostic Procedures

In patients with current symptoms, personal history, or family history of cardiovascular illness, clinicians may elect to obtain a baseline electrocardiogram (ECG) (preferably read by a pediatric cardiologist) to assess current cardiac status before initiating psychotropic medication. Certain medications may either prolong the QTc interval or substantively affect cardiovascular functioning at therapeutic doses. Cardiovascular implications must be considered when prescribing psychotropic medications such as the following (McNally et al. 2007):

- α_2-Adrenergic agonists such as clonidine or guanfacine
- First-generation antipsychotics (neuroleptics), especially pimozide
- Atypical (second-generation) antipsychotics such as clozapine and ziprasidone
- Tricyclic antidepressants
- Lithium
- Stimulants such as methylphenidate and amphetamine

Additional diagnostic procedures that clinicians may wish to obtain for certain pediatric patients prior to psychopharmacotherapy include an electroencephalogram (EEG) and a computed tomography (CT) or magnetic resonance imaging (MRI) scan of the brain. An EEG

TABLE 34–2. Laboratory tests to check during the psychopharmacological assessment of a pediatric patient

Laboratory test	Psychopharmacological reasons for obtaining test
Complete blood count with differential	Screening for anemia, which can cause decreased energy; baseline for drugs that may affect blood counts
Serum electrolytes	Screening for purging or restricting of food for patients in whom an underlying eating disorder is suspected
Blood urea nitrogen, creatinine	Screening for renal dysfunction, which may alter psychopharmacotherapy options; baseline for lithium treatment
Liver function tests (aspartate aminotransferase, alanine aminotransferase, alkaline phosphatase, bilirubin)	Screening for hepatic problems, which may affect psychopharmacotherapy options; baseline for subsequent monitoring
Fasting glucose level	Screening and baseline for metabolic syndrome and/or diabetes mellitus, especially if second-generation antipsychotics are being considered
Fasting lipid profile (high-density and low-density cholesterol, triglycerides)	Screening and baseline for hyperlipidemia and/or hypercholesterolemia, especially if weight gain–inducing agents are being considered
Urinalysis	Screening for renal disease and/or diabetes mellitus
Urine toxicology screen	Screening for illicit drug use
Thyroid-stimulating hormone (TSH) level	Screening for thyroid dysfunction, which can contribute to symptoms of depression, anxiety, and psychosis; baseline for lithium treatment
Urine pregnancy test	Screening for pregnancy in females of reproductive age, particularly if a teratogenic medication is being considered
Serum lead level	Screening for lead toxicity, especially in children who are younger than age 7 years or have a history of pica or recent exposure

may be considered for patients who have a history of seizure disorder and are being considered for treatment with psychotropic medications that potentially lower the seizure threshold (e.g., antipsychotics such as clozapine, tricyclic antidepressants, or lithium). Clinicians may decide to obtain a CT or MRI of the brain to either confirm or refute the presence of an anatomic abnormality that may be a potential etiology of psychiatric symptoms in certain young patients.

Diagnosis

Following the psychiatric assessment, the clinician is next faced with the task of identifying the primary psychiatric diagnosis (if one exists), as well as recognizing any comorbid disorders. An accurate psychiatric diagnosis is important because it helps to identify appropriate treatment options, often via evidence-based treatment guidelines that have been developed for many disorders.

In DSM-5 (American Psychiatric Association 2013), constellations of emotional, thought, and behavioral symptoms are recognized, and these sets of symptoms are classified into various categories of psychiatric disorders. In the recently updated DSM-5, some of the limitations in the current nosology for diagnosing psychiatric disorders in the young are addressed, which is complicated by the fact that many disorders, including ADHD and mood disorders, manifest differently in children than in adults.

It is important for clinicians to successfully identify any comorbid diagnoses since psychiatric comorbidity can influence pharmacological management. Although there are more data on the treatment of individual primary psychiatric disorders than on the treatment of comorbid psychiatric disorders, clinicians can consult empirically based treatment guidelines while adhering to the general principles of pediatric psychopharmacology.

It is also important to discuss the patient's diagnoses with the patient and parents because a well-informed family can better make educated, responsible decisions about treatment. Patients and their parents frequently have questions about the diagnoses, including possible causes of the disorders, typical symptoms associated with the disorders, treatment options for the primary disorder and its comorbidities, and expected prognosis. After answering these questions, clinicians may refer families to sources of information, such as reputable books and Web sites. A good starting point for families is the Web site for the American Academy of Child and Adolescent Psychiatry (www.aacap.org).

Biopsychosocial Formulation and Treatment Planning

In addition to a DSM-5 diagnosis, there are many other factors that can affect a youth's emotions and behaviors. These include comorbid medical conditions, level of development, psychological distress, family relationships, social relationships, environmental stressors, and educational functioning. A biopsychosocial formulation supplements the diagnosis by describing the predisposing, precipitating, perpetuating, and protective factors that have shaped the patient's clinical presentation.

Once this formulation has been constructed, the next task for the clinician, patient, and family is to develop a treatment plan. Treatment planning for young patients typically involves multiple people, including parents, relatives, teachers, and pediatricians. A multidisciplinary and multimodal treatment approach is commonly used, which may include pharmacotherapy as well as individual psychotherapy, group psychotherapy, family psychotherapy, parental counseling, and educational interventions. Psychopharmacological treatment should generally not be initiated without the consideration of accompanying psychotherapeutic interventions.

Treating Psychiatric Disorders Rather Than Target Symptoms

It is important to note that clinical guidelines do not recommend psychiatric pharmacotherapy solely to address specific target psychiatric symptoms. Rather, clinicians generally treat psychiatric syndromes and then measure treatment response by tracking specified target symptoms. This principle is also seen in general pediatric practice. For instance, fever is not necessarily treated with antibiotics. However, bacterial pneumonia is treated with antibiotics, and fever is one of several parameters that may be monitored to see if the antibiotic treatment is effective. Fever may also be treated symptomatically while the underlying cause receives specific treatment or resolves spontaneously. In the field of child and adolescent psychiatry, it is not generally recommended that a specific agent be prescribed to a child with an impairing irritable mood. This is because there are multiple potential causes of irritability in children, including major depressive disorder, disruptive mood dysregulation disorder, bipolar disorder, generalized anxiety disorder, and posttraumatic stress disorder, as well as developmental, cognitive, medical, and environmental causes. Addressing irritability depends on the accurate identification of the most likely cause. Once an accurate diagnosis has been identified by thorough assessment, the success of the selected course of treatment can be monitored by tracking the patient's level of irritability.

Therapeutic Alliance

In order to reach an agreement with the parents on a treatment plan, a clinician may use certain styles of presenting the information and answering the family's questions. This can generally be either authoritative (presenting the options and asking the family to choose one) or authoritarian (being more directive with the family regarding which option or options they should choose). In many treatment settings, it is advisable for clinicians to take an authoritative approach to the family. By being thorough and comprehensive in the assessment and diagnosis of a patient, a clinician can develop positive rapport and a strong therapeutic alliance with the patient and parents. Furthermore, by making reasonable and appropriate treatment recommendations and by taking the time to adequately answer the family's questions, a clinician can help the patient and family develop a sense of confidence in both the provider and the selected treatment option. A family may be more likely to cooperate with treatment and remain adherent to the recommendations of such a positively regarded authoritative clinician. There are some instances, however, when a more authoritarian approach is necessary, such as when families are having difficulty making treatment choices, requesting treatment approaches that are likely to be ineffective or even harmful, or resisting treatments that may be important for the safety of the patient or others.

Selecting Psychopharmacological Agents

Clinicians typically rely on several principles when selecting and dosing psychotropic medications for children and adolescents. These considerations include the differences in drug metabolism between children and adults, data on the efficacy and safety of psychotropic medications in children, regulatory issues associated with the off-label use of psychotropic medications, and ethical issues surrounding the psychopharmacological treatment of children and adolescents.

Drug Metabolism and Disposition

Children are not merely "little adults" when it comes to the metabolism of drugs. This fact is a result of physiological differences between youth and adults that affect drug dosing, therapeutic effect, and safety.

Pharmacokinetics

The primary differences in drug metabolism between children and adults are the results of two key pharmacokinetic factors:

1. When adjusted for body weight, youth have proportionally more liver tissue. As a result, this population may have more rapid hepatic drug metabolism, and thus more rapid elimination, of drugs that use hepatic pathways (Kearns et al. 2003).
2. When adjusted for body weight, children may have higher glomerular filtration rates than adults, possibly resulting in more rapid excretion of drugs that use renal pathways (Chen et al. 2006).

As a result of these pharmacokinetic differences, children may require larger weight-adjusted doses of psychiatric medications than adults in order to attain comparable serum drug levels. In addition, these patients may also benefit from more frequent drug dosing in order to compensate for shorter drug half-lives (Jatlow 1987).

Drugs are also absorbed and distributed differently in children as compared with adults, requiring further adjustments in dosing. These pharmacokinetic differences include the following (Funk et al. 2012; Kearns et al. 2003):

- Children have proportionally more extracellular and total-body water than adults, which may lead to lower plasma concentrations of hydrophilic drugs. As a result, some drugs (e.g., lithium) may require higher weight-based dosing in youth.
- Many children have proportionally less fat tissue than adults, so there has historically been concern for the possibility of higher plasma concentrations of some lipophilic drugs (e.g., paroxetine), although these agents generally do not show a lower volume of distribution in infants and young children.
- The functioning of the gastrointestinal tract does not fully mature until 10–12 years of age. This phenomenon may lead to greater variability of oral drug absorption in the young when compared with adults.

The physiological changes experienced by developing children contribute to drug disposition, and a thorough understanding of these changes can lead to more effective use of pharmacological agents in this population. These age-dependent differences in drug disposition appear to gradually diminish throughout childhood, with a clear decline typically occurring during puberty. At approximately 15 years of age, a child's pharmacokinetic characteristics begin to become more like those of an adult. Accordingly, clinicians can generally assume that adult drug doses may be employed in youth once they reach midadolescence (Jatlow 1987).

Pharmacodynamics

Some psychiatric medications do not have the same efficacy or tolerability in children and adolescents as in adults. For example, the tricyclic antidepressants, which are an effective treatment for depression in adults, have been found to be ineffective for depressed children and adolescents (Hazell et al. 2002). One factor that may play a role in the age-related differences seen for drug effect and tolerability is the stage of maturation of certain neurotransmitter systems. The serotonin and catecholamine (norepinephrine, epinephrine, dopamine) networks of the central nervous system play important roles in regulating mood, thought, and behavior. As such, these networks are also the primary targets of psychiatric medications. It has been found that these neural pathways are not fully developed in the young and do not reach full adult functionality until the third decade of life (Murrin et al. 2007).

Drug Efficacy and Safety

As outlined earlier in the section "Brief History of Pediatric Psychopharmacology," there are historical reasons for the current paucity of pediatric drug efficacy data, including limitations in experimental design and assessment methods prior to the 1980s. There are also practical limitations to conducting this research, which include the greater level of difficulty generally associated with conducting research in children compared with adults, the scarcity of funding to support psychopharmacological research in children, and the ethical issues that surround pediatric clinical research. Currently available pediatric psychopharmacology data typically address the efficacy of pharmacotherapy for the acute phases of psychiatric illnesses, with much less information on long-term efficacy. Since many psychiatric disorders first manifest during childhood and are chronic in nature, there is a great need for more information about the effectiveness and risks of long-term pharmacological management of these disorders.

The safety of medications is an important consideration. Safety is a comparative notion, as the risks of pharmacotherapy are not considered in isolation but are instead measured against the risks of untreated psychiatric illness. All medications carry some risk of adverse events. It is important for clinicians to educate young patients and their parents about not only a drug's potential side effects but also the potential benefits of effective intervention.

Most psychotropic medications have warnings, precautions, and contraindications that are included in each drug's labeling information. Some psychotropic medications have more serious warnings, commonly referred to as *black box* warnings. A black box warning that has greatly affected the practice of pediatric psychopharmacology is the "increased suicidality in children and adolescents" warning that was added to all antidepressants by the U.S. Food and Drug Administration (FDA; U.S. Food and Drug Administration 2004). A similar warning has been added to the labeling for anticonvulsants (U.S. Food and Drug Administration 2008). Clinicians must be aware of these safety warnings and discuss safety issues with patients and families. Specific medication safety issues are covered in the subsequent chapters of Part V.

Clinicians should also be aware of potentially dangerous drug-drug interactions and take a careful inventory of all prescription and over-the-counter medications, vitamins, and herbal preparations during the assessment interview. In addition, the prescribing physician should review these concerns with families prior to the addition of a new medication and throughout the course of its use.

Regulatory Considerations

Because a large percentage of psychotropic medications have not been adequately studied in youth, many of these compounds do not have FDA-approved indications for pediatric patients. Therefore, medications are frequently used "off-label" in children and adolescents. The FDA does not regulate physician prescribing practices and therefore does not prohibit the off-label use of medication. However, as FDA-approved indications are generally the result of methodologically stringent evidence, clinicians should first consider FDA-approved medication options whenever available and feasible.

One key means by which the dearth of research in pediatric drugs is being addressed is through federal legislation on drug studies in children and adolescents (www.fda.gov). The U.S. Food and Drug Administration Modernization Act of 1997 (FDAMA) gave pharmaceutical companies greater financial incentives to voluntarily conduct clinical trials of medications in children and adolescents. In 2002, the Best Pharmaceuticals for Children Act (BPCA) renewed the financial incentives previously provided by the FDAMA while authorizing the National Institutes of Health to fund pediatric studies of older, off-patent medications. One year later, the Pediatric Research Equity Act (PREA) of 2003 required pharmaceutical companies to begin conducting pediatric studies of drugs in development if those drugs had potential for use in the young. These initiatives were further strengthened in 2012 by the Food and Drug Administration Safety and Innovation Act, which, in addition to making BPCA and PREA permanent, empowered the FDA to ensure that requirements were being met by manufacturers in a timely manner (U.S. Food and Drug Administration 2012). The passage of these federal laws has driven an increase in the number of pediatric clinical studies, resulting in improved data about the efficacy of several medications in children. As a result, there is less need for off-label drug use as more medications are given FDA approval for use in pediatric patients. Data derived from these multicenter studies have also led to a better characterization of these agents' tolerability profiles and, in some instances, have led to new warnings pertaining to drug safety.

Ethical Issues

Since children and adolescents are a particularly vulnerable population, certain ethical principles guide the practice of pediatric psychopharmacotherapy. These include obtaining informed consent and assent prior to prescribing psychotropic medications and continuing discussions with the patient and family about the treatment over time.

Informed Consent and Assent

As treatment options are presented to the patient and parents, the clinician provides education to help the family understand the purpose of the therapeutic interventions and the potential risks and benefits associated with each treatment option. This initiates both an informed consent process with the parents and an assent process with the patient that generally occur before beginning psychopharmacological treatment. Informed consent to initiate or continue a psychotropic medication generally requires the patient's parents to be competent, to demonstrate adequate knowledge about the proposed medication, and to make the treatment decision freely without coercion. "Adequate knowledge" about a psychotropic medication usually includes an understanding of the nature of the patient's psychiatric disorder, the potential risks, benefits, and side effects of the proposed psychopharmacological treatment, the possible alternatives to the proposed treatment, and the patient's expected prognosis both with and without the proposed treatment. Published information on pediatric psychotropic medications can be useful when shared with parents as part of the discussion (see, e.g., Dulcan and Ballard 2015).

Children generally have a limited capacity to fully understand the issues surrounding medical treatment, which is why decisions about medical treatment are usually made by a child's parents. However, many children can still provide assent for their psychopharmacological treatment. Informed assent generally requires a child to demonstrate an age-appropriate awareness of the psychiatric diagnosis and both an understanding and acceptance of the recommended treatment (including possible diagnostic procedures). Once the general requirements for informed consent are met, the parents can then decide whether to accept or decline the proposed psychopharmacological treatment.

Explaining Psychotropic Medication to Children and Adolescents

When prescribing psychotropic medication for a pediatric patient, clinicians are encouraged not only to discuss the medication with the patient to obtain informed assent but also to help the patient feel like a participant in the treatment planning process. By helping to monitor the effects of psychotropic medication on psychiatric symptoms, providing information about internal experiences such as mood and thought content, and watching for possible adverse side effects, the patient can feel a greater sense of control over his or her own treatment. Active participation can be a positive experience for many youth, especially those at a developmental stage in which autonomy is an especially important consideration. In addition, encouraging a pediatric patient's active participation in treatment can strengthen the therapeutic alliance and possibly improve future treatment adherence.

Management of Psychopharmacotherapy

Psychopharmacotherapy generally consists of three phases: initiation of psychotropic medication, medication maintenance, and discontinuation of the medication (if there are clinical indications to do so). Each phase of treatment is accompanied by its own set of potential complications. These may be related to the medication itself, such as side effects or insufficient therapeutic effect, or may represent challenges in medication management, including the treatment of comorbid psychiatric conditions and treatment nonadherence.

Initiating and Titrating Psychotropic Medication

The first task after selecting a specific psychotropic medication is to select the starting dose. It is often recommended that treatment be started at relatively low doses and, after tolerability has been established, cautiously titrated upward to a level that is expected to be therapeutic. The choice of medication, the starting dose, the rate at which it is increased, the target dose, and the maximum total daily dose should all be based as much as possible on scientific evidence derived from patients of similar age. As both side effects and benefits are frequently increased at higher doses, patients should generally be treated with the dose that provides for them the best balance of symptom amelioration and tolerability.

Symptom Response

The effectiveness of psychopharmacological treatment is typically measured by the patient, family, clinician, and other involved observers, who all monitor for improvement in selected target symptoms. Various symptom rating scales can be used to assist in assessing psychiatric symptom improvement or worsening. Additionally, serum levels of certain psychotropic medications (such as lithium and valproic acid) can be measured to guide the clinician in choosing a therapeutic dose while avoiding drug toxicity.

Side Effects

Patients must be monitored for possible side effects throughout the course of their psychotropic treatment. Some side effects (such as sedation or appetite increase) may become apparent soon after medication initiation, while others (such as tardive dyskinesia) may occur later in the treatment course. The monitoring of certain adverse effects may require the serial measurement of various physical parameters such as vital signs, growth, laboratory tests, and ECGs. For example, a pediatric patient who is taking medication that can cause weight gain may require periodic checks of fasting glucose level and lipid profile in order to monitor for the onset of metabolic syndrome or diabetes mellitus.

When side effects do occur, several courses of action may be taken, including lowering the drug dose or changing the drug dosing schedule to minimize side effects. For example, a once-a-day medication causing sedation within the first few hours after administration might be given at bedtime in an effort to minimize the disruption to the patient's daytime routine. Other adverse effects may improve after the co-administration of an additional agent, such as the use of an anticholinergic drug to alleviate extrapyramidal muscular side effects secondary to an antipsychotic medication. Proper management of adverse effects may prevent premature discontinuation of a psychopharmacological agent that has been otherwise effective.

Medication Maintenance

If the medication has been adequately effective and well tolerated, the patient next enters the maintenance phase. The primary goal of maintenance treatment is to prevent a recurrence of symptoms. As the majority of psychiatric disorders are chronic in nature, the continued use of psychotropic medication for prolonged periods of time may be necessary in order to reduce the risk of symptom recurrence. The continuation of psychotropic medications, sometimes for years, can help optimize a patient's functioning throughout adolescence and into adulthood.

Adequacy of a Medication Trial

A common mistake made by clinicians is to discontinue a psychotropic medication for lack of effectiveness before a trial of the medication at an adequate dose for an adequate length of time has been completed. The dose and length of treatment required for an adequate trial depend on both the drug being used and the condition being treated. For example, for a disorder such as ADHD, only a few weeks of psychostimulant treatment at an appropriate dose are needed on a trial basis, while for a diagnosis such as major depressive disorder, up to 2–3 months of antidepressant treatment may be necessary before making a determination of whether the medication is effective. If the medication in question is found to be ineffective after an adequate trial, the medication may be discontinued and a new psychotropic medication and/or other treatment options considered. Adding a second agent to one with questionable effectiveness is generally not recommended.

Changing Medications

When a psychotropic medication is not effective or causes intolerable side effects, a clinician may recommend replacing the currently prescribed drug with another psychotropic agent, weighing the empirical evidence when choosing which medication to try next. Although a different drug from the same therapeutic family may be considered, a trial of a medication from a different therapeutic family may be warranted. In instances where treatment with a psychotropic medication results in a partial therapeutic response, augmentation with an additional agent may be considered. However, except for ADHD, data on combination medication treatment strategies for psychiatric disorders are generally limited, particularly in children and adolescents.

Discontinuing Psychotropic Medication

At some point, it may become clinically indicated or medically necessary to discontinue a psychotropic medication. For example, a child's ADHD symptoms may naturally improve as the child matures into an adolescent, or side effects may limit a drug's dosing to subtherapeutic levels. Prior to discontinuing a psychotropic medication, a clinician generally discusses with the patient and parents the possible risks (psychiatric symptom recurrence) and benefits (decreased risk of medication-related side effects) associated with medication discontinuation. Drugs that are more rapidly metabolized or medications that can result in drug tolerance may require a gradual tapering of the dosage in order to prevent "rebound" effects or withdrawal syndromes.

Challenges in Pediatric Psychopharmacotherapy

Treatment of Comorbid Diagnoses

The psychotropic treatment of comorbid psychiatric disorders presents challenges because of the dearth of relevant clinical research. Clinicians may choose to treat certain comorbidities (e.g., ADHD and oppositional defiant disorder) with a single psychotropic agent, while in other cases (e.g., mania and ADHD) comorbid disorders may require a stepwise approach, with the clinician first treating the primary (or more disabling) psychiatric disorder with one psychotropic medication and then addressing the remaining comorbid disorder(s) with separate agent(s).

Treatment Adherence

Nonadherence to psychopharmacological treatment is a commonly observed problem. Reasons may include a perceived lack of drug efficacy on the part of the patient or family, the patient experiencing adverse drug effects, misperceptions about the possible effects of psychotropic medications, peer pressure to avoid taking psychiatric medication, social stigma associated with mental illness, pressure from family or outside sources, or the patient's resistance to following directions from parents and other adults. A positive therapeutic alliance among the clinician, patient, and parents may reduce the likelihood of treatment nonadherence by facilitating open communication between all parties and better educating the patient and family regarding psychiatric conditions and treatment.

Summary Points

- Psychopharmacological treatment of children and adolescents begins with a meticulous diagnostic assessment.
- Differences in drug biodisposition in children and adolescents compared with adults may substantively affect drug dosing in the young.
- Psychotropic medications that are safe and effective in adults may be neither effective nor well tolerated in pediatric patients.
- Fastidious measurement of target symptoms and thoughtful monitoring of side effects can facilitate rational drug therapy.
- Clinicians should employ evidence-based treatments, as they are available, in the clinical practice of pediatric psychopharmacology.
- The risk-benefit deliberations associated with psychopharmacological treatment decisions in children should include a consideration of the risks associated with untreated psychiatric illnesses.

References

Achenbach TM, Rescorla LA: Manual for the ASEBA School-Age Forms and Profiles. Burlington, University of Vermont, Research Center for Children, Youth, and Families, 2001

American Psychiatric Association: Diagnostic and Statistical Manual of Mental Disorders, 5th Edition. Arlington, VA, American Psychiatric Association, 2013

Bourgeois FT, Murthy S, Pinto C, et al: Pediatric versus adult drug trials for conditions with high pediatric disease burden. Pediatrics 130(2):285–292, 2012 22826574

Bradley C: The behavior of children receiving Benzedrine. Am J Orthopsychiatry 94:577–585, 1937

Chen N, Aleksa K, Woodland C, et al: Ontogeny of drug elimination by the human kidney. Pediatr Nephrol 21(2):160–168, 2006 16331517

Conners CK: Conners 3rd Edition. North Tonawanda, NY, Multi-Health Systems, 2008

Connor D, Meltzer B: A brief history of the field, in Pediatric Psychopharmacology Fast Facts. New York, WW Norton, 2006, pp 4–6

Dulcan MK, Ballard R: Helping Parents and Teachers Understand Medications for Behavioral and Emotional Problems: A Resource Book of Medication Handouts, 4th Edition. Washington, DC, American Psychiatric Publishing, 2015

Funk RS, Brown JT, Abdel-Rahman SM: Pediatric pharmacokinetics: human development and drug disposition. Pediatr Clin North Am 59(5):1001–1016, 2012 23036241

Hazell P, O'Connell D, Heathcote D, et al: Tricyclic drugs for depression in children and adolescents. Cochrane Database Syst Rev (2):CD002317, 2002 12076448

Ivanova MY, Dobrean A, Dopfner M, et al: Testing the 8-syndrome structure of the child behavior checklist in 30 societies. J Clin Child Adolesc Psychol 36(3):405–417, 2007 17658984

Jatlow PI: Psychotropic drug disposition during development, in Psychiatric Pharmacosciences of Children and Adolescents. Edited by Popper C. Washington, DC, American Psychiatric Press, 1987, pp 27–44

Kearns GL, Abdel-Rahman SM, Alander SW, et al: Developmental pharmacology—drug disposition, action, and therapy in infants and children. N Engl J Med 349(12):1157–1167, 2003 13679531

McNally P, McNicholas F, Oslizlok P: The QT interval and psychotropic medications in children: recommendations for clinicians. Eur Child Adolesc Psychiatry 16(1):33–47, 2007 16944043

Murrin LC, Sanders JD, Bylund DB: Comparison of the maturation of the adrenergic and serotonergic neurotransmitter systems in the brain: implications for differential drug effects on juveniles and adults. Biochem Pharmacol 73(8):1225–1236, 2007 17316571

U.S. Food and Drug Administration: Public Health Advisory: Suicidality in Children and Adolescents Being Treated with Antidepressant Medications. Silver Spring, MD, U.S. Food and Drug Administration, October 15, 2004. Available at: http://www.fda.gov/drugs/drugsafetypostmarketdrugsafetyinformationforpatientsandproviders/ucm161679.htm. Accessed June 23, 2009.

U.S. Food and Drug Administration: Safety Alerts for Human Medical Products: Antiepileptic Drugs. Silver Spring, MD, U.S. Food and Drug Administration, January 31, 2008. Available at: http://www.fda.gov/Safety/Med Watch/SafetyInformation/SafetyAlertsforHumanMedicalProducts/ucm074939.htm. Accessed June 23, 2009.

U.S. Food and Drug Administration: Regulatory Information: Fact Sheet: Pediatric provisions in the Food and Drug Administration Safety and Innovation Act (FDASIA). Silver Spring, MD, U.S. Food and Drug Administration, July 9, 2012. Available at: http://www.fda.gov/RegulatoryInformation/Legislation/FederalFoodDrugandCosmeticActFDCAct/SignificantAmendmentstotheFDCAct/FDASIA/ucm311038.htm. Accessed on May 26, 2014.

Vitiello B: Developmental aspects of pediatric psychopharmacology, in Clinical Manual of Child and Adolescent Psychopharmacology. Edited by Findling RL. Washington, DC, American Psychiatric Publishing, 2008, pp 1–31

Zametkin AJ, Ernst M, Silver R: Laboratory and diagnostic testing in child and adolescent psychiatry: a review of the past 10 years. J Am Acad Child Adolesc Psychiatry 37(5):464–472, 1998 9585646

CHAPTER 35

Medications Used for Attention-Deficit/ Hyperactivity Disorder

Thomas J. Spencer, M.D.
Joseph Biederman, M.D.
Timothy E. Wilens, M.D.

Attention-deficit/hyperactivity disorder (ADHD) is one of the major clinical and public health problems in the United States in terms of morbidity and disability in children and adolescents. It is estimated to affect 5%–10% of school-age children. Its impact on society is enormous in terms of the financial cost, the stress to families, the impact on schools, and the damaging effects on self-esteem (see Chapter 10, "Attention-Deficit/Hyperactivity Disorder").

ADHD is a heterogeneous disorder of unknown etiology. It has been viewed as a "frontal" disorder because of associated deficits in executive function. Executive function deficits include problems with planning and organization, cognitive flexibility, working memory, and response inhibition/impulse control. Individuals with ADHD often have impaired performance on one or more tasks of vigilance, search, and attention; working memory (ability to retain information while processing new information); response inhibition (ability to juggle competing or distracting tasks); verbal learning (encoding); and delay aversion (the need to have immediate gratification).

Imaging studies have documented diffuse abnormalities in children and adults with ADHD. Sonuga-Barke (2003) articulated a dual-pathway model consisting of an executive circuit and a reward circuit. The reward circuit involves maintaining interest in a task and the ability to tolerate delayed rewards. The executive, cognitive circuit involves directed attention and the ability to keep an innate goal in mind while working on the details of a task. In concert with these tasks are different, parallel feedback control loops that regulate executive control, inhibition and emotional regulation, and motivation and reward (Cummings 1993). Additionally, medication may attenuate abnormalities in some of these functional deficits (Spencer et al. 2013).

The frontosubcortical pathways are rich in catecholamines. In addition, catecholamines are implicated in ADHD because of the mechanism of action of stimulants. Notably, in both childhood and adulthood, ADHD symptoms respond favorably to drugs that block the dopamine transporter and/or the norepinephrine transporter.

Data from family genetic, twin, and adoption studies as well as segregation analysis suggest a genetic origin for some forms of the disorder (Li et al. 2014). The majority of candidate genes are related to monoamine neurotransmission, including monoamine metabolic biosynthesis and monoamine transmission, including transporters and receptors (Li et al. 2014). Increasingly, there has been recognition that ADHD is highly heterogeneous with significant levels of psychiatric, cognitive, and social disability comorbidity.

Stimulant Treatments

Stimulant drugs are the first class of compounds reported to be effective in the treatment of children with ADHD. Stimulants are sympathomimetic drugs structurally similar to endogenous catecholamines. The most commonly used compounds in this class include methylphenidate (e.g., Ritalin, Concerta), *d*-methylphenidate (Focalin), *d*-amphetamine (Dexedrine), a mixed amphetamine salts product (Adderall), and a *d*-amphetamine prodrug (Vyvanse). These drugs have been shown to enhance dopaminergic and noradrenergic neurotransmission in the central nervous system and peripherally (Volkow et al. 2001). Since the various stimulants have somewhat different mechanisms of action, some patients may respond preferentially to one or another (Greenhill et al. 1999).

Stimulant Dosing

The usual dosage range is 0.3–2 mg/kg/day for methylphenidate and approximately half of that for dexmethylphenidate and amphetamine compounds since they are roughly twice as potent as methylphenidate (Table 35–1). Because of their short half-life, the short-acting, immediate-release stimulants (methylphenidate and dextroamphetamine) are given in divided doses throughout the day, typically 4 hours apart. The starting dosage is generally 5 mg/day, given in the morning, with the dose being increased if necessary every few days by 5 mg in a divided dose schedule. Because of the appetite-reducing effects of the stimulants, it may be beneficial to administer the medicine after meals. Dextroamphetamine and mixed amphetamine salts can last up to 6 hours; thus, for full coverage they are typically given twice daily (such as 8:00 A.M. and 2:00 P.M.) in dosages of 1–1.5 mg/kg/day. Typically, stimulants have a rapid onset of action, so clinical response will be evident when a therapeutic dose has been obtained.

Stimulant Efficacy

An extensive literature has clearly documented the short-term efficacy of methylphenidate treatment, mostly in latency-age white boys (Spencer et al. 1997). Recently, there has been a more robust literature in adults, and a growing literature exists for the use of stimu-

TABLE 35–1. Immediate-release stimulants

Medication	Daily dosage, mg/kg	Daily dose schedule
Dextroamphetamine (Dexedrine)	0.3–1.0	Two or three times
Mixed salts of levoamphetamine and dextroamphetamine (Adderall)	0.5–1.5	Once or twice
Methylphenidate (e.g., Ritalin, Methylin)	1.0–2.0	Two or three times
Dexmethylphenidate (Focalin)	0.5–1.0	Twice

Note. Doses are general guidelines. All doses must be individualized with appropriate monitoring. Weight-corrected doses are less appropriate for obese children. FDA-approved total daily doses: methylphenidate, 60 mg; dexmethylphenidate, 20 mg; mixed amphetamine salts, 30 mg.

lants at other ages, for females, and for ethnic minorities. Studies of stimulants in adolescents reported rates of response highly consistent with those seen in latency-age children. In contrast, the few studies on preschoolers appear to indicate that young children respond less well to stimulant therapy, suggesting that in preschoolers ADHD may be more treatment refractory.

A large multicenter controlled trial (the Preschool ADHD Treatment Study [PATS]) investigated the efficacy and safety of immediate-release methylphenidate (MPH-IR), given three times daily to children ages 3–5.5 years with ADHD (Greenhill et al. 2006b). The 8-phase, 70-week PATS protocol included two double-blind controlled phases and a crossover titration trial followed by a placebo-controlled parallel trial. Of 303 preschoolers enrolled, 165 were randomly assigned in the titration trial. Compared with placebo, significant decreases in ADHD symptoms were found with MPH-IR at 2.5 mg (P<0.01), 5 mg (P<0.001), and 7.5 mg (P<0.001) dosages thrice daily but not for 1.25 mg (P<0.06) dosages. The mean optimal MPH-IR total daily dose for the entire group was 14.2±8.1 mg (0.7±4 mg/kg/day). For the preschoolers later randomly assigned in the parallel phase (n=114), only 21% on best-dose MPH-IR and 13% on placebo achieved the categorical criterion for remission (as defined by the Multimodal Treatment Study of Children With ADHD [MTA]) for school-age children with ADHD. Thirty percent of parents spontaneously reported moderate to severe adverse events in all study phases after baseline (Wigal et al. 2006). These included emotional outbursts, difficulty falling asleep, repetitive behaviors/thoughts, appetite decrease, and irritability. During maintenance treatment, trouble sleeping and appetite loss persisted and other MPH-related adverse events decreased. There were transient one-time pulse and blood pressure elevations in five children. Twenty-one children (11%) discontinued treatment because of drug-attributed adverse events. Of the serious adverse events reported, only one was possibly related to MPH.

The literature clearly documents that treatment with stimulants improves not only abnormal impulsive and hyperactive behaviors of ADHD but also self-esteem and cognitive, social, and family function, thus supporting the importance of treating patients with ADHD beyond school or work hours to include evenings, weekends, and vacations. Controlled clinical trials have documented the efficacy of methylphenidate and amphetamine in adults with ADHD (Wilens et al. 2011).

Treatment with stimulants improves a wide variety of cognitive abilities (Barkley 1977; Gittelman-Klein 1987; Rapport et al. 1988), increases school-based productivity (Famularo and Fenton 1987), and improves performance in academic testing (Scheffler et al. 2009). However, despite these beneficial cognitive effects, it is important to be aware that patients with ADHD may have comorbid learning disabilities that are not responsive to pharmacotherapy (Bergman et al. 1991) but may respond to educational remediation.

The early concern that optimal clinical efficacy is attained at the cost of impaired learning ability has not been confirmed (Gittelman-Klein 1987). In fact, the majority of studies indicate that both behavior and cognitive performance improve with stimulant treatment in a dose-dependent fashion (Barr et al. 1999; Douglas et al. 1988; Gittelman-Klein 1987; Kupietz et al. 1988; Pelham et al. 1985; Rapport et al. 1987, 1989). The literature on the association between clinical benefits in ADHD and plasma levels of stimulants has been equivocal and complicated by large inter- and intraindividual variability in plasma levels at constant oral doses (Gittelman-Klein 1987).

Stimulant Side Effects and Risks

The U.S. Food and Drug Administration (FDA) reviewed the prescribing information on stimulants in an effort to clarify risks and benefits. After this careful review, the only black box warning for stimulants concerns their abuse potential. While misuse for treating fatigue can be accomplished by oral administration, abuse for euphoria typically requires snorting or injecting, and thus there is greater risk in immediate-release formulations that can be crushed. Despite the concern that ADHD may increase the risk of drug abuse in adolescents and young adults (or their associates), to date there is no clear evidence that youth with ADHD treated with stimulants abuse prescribed medication when they are appropriately diagnosed and carefully monitored. Moreover, the most commonly abused substance in adolescents and adults with ADHD is marijuana, not stimulants (Biederman et al. 1995). A recent meta-analysis of longitudinal studies reported that stimulant treatment was not associated with an increase in the risk of substance use disorders (Humphreys et al. 2013). Moreover, a large (n=25,656) Swedish registry study found that stimulant-treated subjects had significantly lower rates of criminality: 32% less for men and 41% less for women. A significant portion of the criminal incidents were drug related, suggesting that the use of medication reduces the risk of drug use in adults with ADHD (Lichtenstein et al. 2012).

The most commonly reported side effects associated with the administration of stimulant medication are appetite suppression and sleep disturbances. Delay of sleep onset is commonly reported and usually accompanies late afternoon or early evening administration of the stimulant medications. Preexisting sleep disturbance is common because of oppositional defiant disorder, separation anxiety, environmental overstimulation, and so forth. Less commonly reported are mood disturbances ranging from increased tearfulness and social withdrawal to a full-blown major depression–like syndrome (Wilens and Biederman 1992). Other fairly common side effects include headaches and abdominal discomfort and, more rarely, increased lethargy and fatigue.

Regarding adverse cardiovascular effects of stimulants, studies have consistently documented stimulant-induced mild increases in pulse and blood pressure of unclear clinical significance (Brown et al. 1984). Cardiovascular concerns have led to several large studies. The association between stimulant medication and blood pressure and heart rate over 10 years was examined in the MTA. In the MTA, 579 children were randomly assigned to 14 months of medication treatment, behavioral therapy, the combination of the two, or usual community treatment. The controlled trial was followed by naturalistic treatment with periodic assessments. Associations between cumulative stimulant exposure and blood pressure or heart rate were assessed. Stimulant treatment did not increase the risk for prehypertension or hypertension over the 10-year period of observation. Stimulants had a persistent adrenergic effect on heart rate at the end of the 14-month controlled trial but not thereafter. Stimulant medication did not increase the risk for tachycardia. However, greater cumulative stimulant exposure was associated with a higher heart rate at years 3 and 8 but not at year 10. Additionally, in a large pharmacoepidemiological study, Cooper et al. (2011) conducted a retrospective cohort study with automated data from four health plans with 1,200,438 children and young adults between the ages of 2 and 24 years with 2,579,104 person-years of follow-up, including 373,667 person-years of current use of ADHD drugs. Risk for serious cardiovascular events was not increased for stimulant users or for current users as compared with former users.

However, because it appeared that patients with underlying heart defects might be at increased risk for sudden death, the labeling for all stimulants was changed to include a warning that these patients might be at particular risk and that these patients should ordinarily not be treated with stimulants. While at this time there is little concern about the general cardiovascular safety of psychostimulants, the American Heart Association (AHA) issued guidelines stating that caution should be used in the treatment of patients presenting with a family history of early cardiac death or arrhythmias or a personal history of structural abnormalities, chest pain, palpitations, shortness of breath, or fainting episodes of unclear etiology, especially during exercise or during treatment with stimulants (Gutgesell et al. 1999). Before initiating treatment, patients should have a careful history taken to assess for the presence of preexisting cardiac disease. In such cases, consultation with a cardiologist is recommended. Stimulant cardiovascular risk guidelines were reviewed by the AHA (Vetter et al. 2008). Recommendations were unchanged from the 1999 report except for a new recommendation for routine use of electrocardiograms (ECGs) in prescreening. A subsequent clarification was issued by the AHA:

> It is reasonable for a physician to consider obtaining an ECG as part of the evaluation of children being considered for stimulant drug therapy, but this should be at the physician's judgment, and it is not mandatory to obtain one. (http://www2.aap.org/pressroom/aap-ahastatement.htm)

In addition, the American Academy of Pediatrics published a policy statement that an ECG is *not* routinely indicated prior to stimulant treatment in otherwise healthy youth (Perrin et al. 2008). Although less of an immediate clinical concern in pediatric care, blood pressure and pulse should be monitored with stimulant treatment and may be of greater clinical significance in the treatment of adults with ADHD.

Stimulant-associated toxic psychosis has been very rarely observed, usually in the context of either a rapid rise in the dose or very high doses. This reported psychosis in children resembles a toxic phenomenon (i.e., visual hallucinosis) and is dissimilar to the psychotic symptoms present in schizophrenia. The development of psychotic or manic symptoms in a child exposed to stimulants requires careful evaluation to rule out the presence of a preexisting psychotic or bipolar disorder. Aggressive behavior is often observed in children or adolescents with ADHD, and stimulants are often effective treatments for aggression in that context (Blader et al. 2013; Connor et al. 2002). However, all patients beginning treatment should be monitored for the appearance or worsening of aggressive behavior or hostility.

Early reports indicated that children with a personal or family history of tic disorders were at greater risk for developing a tic disorder when exposed to stimulants (Lowe et al. 1982). However, more recent work has increasingly challenged this view. In a controlled study of 34 children with ADHD and tics, Gadow et al. (1995) reported that methylphenidate effectively reduced ADHD symptoms with only a weak effect on the frequency of tics. In addition, in a study of 128 boys with ADHD, Spencer et al. (1999) reported no evidence of earlier onset, greater rates, or worsening of tics in the subgroup exposed to stimulants. Moreover, a multisite placebo-controlled trial of methylphenidate in children with ADHD found that the proportion of individual subjects reporting a worsening of tics as an adverse effect was no higher in those treated with MPH (20%) than those being administered placebo (22%) (Tourette's Syndrome Study Group 2002). Although this work is reassuring, clearly, more information is needed in a larger number of subjects over longer periods of time to obtain closure on this issue. Until more is known, it seems prudent to weigh risks and benefits in individual cases with appropriate discussion with the child and family about the benefits and pitfalls of the use of stimulants in children with ADHD and tics.

Persistent concerns remain about the effects of stimulants on growth in children. To address this issue, Faraone et al. (2008) published a meta-analysis of growth effects in a large number of longitudinal stimulant studies. These studies provide strong evidence that for most patients, treatment with stimulant medication into adolescence leads to, at worst, modest delays in growth. Weight deficits were greater than height deficits, and the two were only modestly associated with one another. This effect is greatest for taller and heavier children and is greater for children compared with adolescents. The studies reviewed suggest that these deficits attenuate over time, even with continued treatment, and do not differ between methylphenidate and amphetamine or between long- and short-acting formulations. Some studies suggest that ADHD itself, not its treatment, is associated with dysregulation of growth and that final adult height is not affected (Klein and Mannuzza 1988; Spencer et al. 1998b). Thus, although treatment with stimulants can lead to some reductions in expected growth velocity in height and weight, these reductions are, on average, small, attenuate with time, and do not cause a greater proportion of children to become extremely short or thin.

While growth does need to be monitored in children treated with stimulants, the data on growth would not support the routine practice of "drug holidays" in ADHD children. However, it seems prudent in children suspected of stimulant-associated growth deficits to provide them with unmedicated periods or alternative treatment. This recommendation should be carefully weighed against the risk for exacerbation of symptoms due to drug discontinuation. In some children, transient behavioral deterioration can occur on the abrupt discontinuation of stimulant medications. The prevalence of this phenomenon and the etiology are unclear. Rebound phenomena can occur in some children between doses or following the final dose of the day, creating an uneven, often disturbing clinical course. In those cases, consideration should be given to alternative or supplementary medications, including use of additional doses or long-acting formulations of stimulants. Presumed "rebound" from medications may actually represent return of ADHD symptoms or the environmental effects of late afternoon and early evening fatigue, hunger, homework, and so forth.

New-Generation Stimulants

Stimulant Stereoenantiomers

Methylphenidate has four optical isomers: *d*-threo, *l*-threo, *d*-erythro, and *l*-erythro. There is stereoselectivity in receptor site binding and its relationship to response. The standard preparation is composed of the threo, *d,l* racemate. Data suggest that the *d*-methylphenidate isomer is the active form. In a positron emission tomography study, *d*-threo-methylphenidate was found to bind specifically to the basal ganglia, which is rich in dopamine transporter receptors, whereas *l*-threo-methylphenidate was widely distributed with only nonspecific binding (Ding et al. 1995). This led to the development of a purified *d*-threo-methylphenidate compound, dexmethylphenidate (Focalin). Studies have documented similar pharmacokinetic profiles of *d*-threo-methylphenidate and *d,l*-threo-methylphenidate when given in equimolar doses. Thus, the time to maximum concentration (T_{max}), the maximum concentration (C_{max}) of *d*-threo-methylphenidate, and the half-life were the same between *d* and *d,l*-threo-methylphenidate.

The efficacy of Focalin was established in two controlled studies. In the first trial, 132 children and adolescents were randomly assigned to receive *d*-threo-methylphenidate, *d,l*-threo-methylphenidate, or placebo at 8:00 A.M. and noon for 4 weeks. At week 4, teacher ratings on the Swanson, Nolan, and Pelham (SNAP) rating scale revealed robust improvement in both active treatments. The average improvement from baseline was equivalent to one standard deviation on the SNAP, a magnitude of change that is clinically important. Parent ratings on the SNAP revealed superiority of both treatments to placebo 3 hours after dosing but superiority of only *d*-methylphenidate and not *d,l*-methylphenidate 6 hours after dosing (Wigal et al. 2004). In a second controlled study, investigators tested the specificity of response to *d*-threo-methylphenidate (Arnold et al. 2004). Patients were treated openly with *d*-threo-methylphenidate (N=116) to determine the optimal dose. At the end of 6 weeks, 75 responders were randomly assigned to blinded treatment with *d*-threo-methylphenidate or placebo over 2 weeks. Subjects randomly assigned to placebo had a high rate (62%) of relapse compared with those who continued on *d*-threo-methylphenidate (17%). In addition, the parent SNAP ratings indicated persistent effect of *d*-threo-methylphenidate 6 hours after dosing. In both studies, adverse effects of *d*-threo-methylphenidate were consistent with those of *d,l*-threo-methylphenidate. These studies have shown Focalin to be as effective as the racemate at half the dose. Focalin is available in 2.5, 5, and 10 mg to approximate 5, 10, and 20 mg of *d,l*-methylphenidate.

Long-Acting Stimulant Formulations

A generation of highly sophisticated, well-developed, safe, and effective long-acting preparations of stimulant drugs has reached the market and revolutionized the treatment of ADHD (Table 35–2). These compounds employ novel delivery systems to allow a reduced number of doses per day. In a number of these medications, an analogue classroom paradigm was used to test the fine-grained pharmacodynamic and pharmacokinetic profiles of these medications. Developed by Swanson and colleagues, these settings simulate real-life demands and distractions of a typical classroom (Swanson et al. 2000). Hour-by-hour ratings are made by trained observers recording frequency counts of behaviors as well as academic production and accuracy. Sequential serum sampling (using venous catheters) allows correlation of blood levels to behavioral activity.

The first of these medications developed was Concerta, which uses an osmotic pump mechanism to create an ascending level of methylphenidate in the blood. This provides effective extended treatment that approximates thrice daily dosing of MPH-IR. Concerta is available in 18, 27, 36, and 54 mg to approximate 5, 7.5, 10, and 15 mg tid dosing of MPH-IR. A laboratory classroom study of 68 children found that a single morning dose of Concerta was effective for 12 hours on social and on-task behaviors, as well as academic performance (Pelham et al. 2001).

A large multicenter randomized clinical trial was used to determine the safety and efficacy of Concerta in an outpatient setting (Wolraich et al. 2001). Children with ADHD (ages 6–12 years; N=282) were randomly assigned to placebo, MPH-IR three times a day, or Concerta once a day in a double-blind, 28-day trial. Children in the Concerta and MPH-IR groups showed significantly greater reductions in core ADHD symptoms than did children on placebo throughout the study. Concerta was well tolerated, with mild appetite suppression but no sleep abnormalities.

Metadate CD is a capsule with a mixture of immediate- and delayed-release beads containing methylphenidate, 30% of which are immediate release and 70% of which are delayed release. It is designed to provide effective treatment for 6–8 hours. The efficacy and safety of Metadate CD were tested in a multicenter randomized, double-blind, placebo-controlled trial conducted at 32 sites on 316 children with ADHD. There was a 1-week single-blind placebo run-in, followed by a 3-week double-blind titration and treatment period.

Improvement with treatment versus placebo was equally good morning and afternoon as rated by teachers on the Conners' Global Index. The medication was well tolerated, with relatively low rates of decreased appetite (9.7% vs. 2.5%) and insomnia (7.1% vs. 2.5%) in active treatment versus placebo. Metadate CD is available in 10, 20, 30, 40, 50, and 60 mg capsules (Greenhill et al. 2002). The bioavailability and tolerability of Metadate CD are not altered when the capsule is opened and the beads are sprinkled on food (Pentikis et al. 2002). This is useful for children who do not swallow capsules.

TABLE 35–2. Long-acting stimulants

Medication	Daily dosage, mg/kg	Daily dose schedule	Duration of behavioral effect	Comments
Methylphenidate	1.0–2.0	Once or twice		
Concerta			10–12 hours	Ascending profile, OROS technology Capsules with IR and DR beads
Ritalin LA			8–9 hours	50:50 ratio (IR:DR)
Metadate CD			6–8 hours	30:70 ratio (IR:DR)
Focalin XR			10–12 hours	50:50 ratio (IR:DR)
Daytrana			12 hours with 9-hour wear time	Patch with variable wear time
Quillivant XR			10–12 hours	Extended-release oral suspension 20:80 ratio (IR:DR)
Mixed salts of levoamphetamine and dextroamphetamine (Adderall XR)	0.5–1.5	Once or twice	10–12 hours	Capsule with IR and DR beads 50:50 ratio (IR:DR)
Lisdexamfetamine (Vyvanse)	0.5–1.5	Once	12 hours	Prodrug; continuous conversion of nonactive prodrug to active *d*-amphetamine

Note. Doses are general guidelines. All doses must be individualized with appropriate monitoring. Weight-corrected doses are less appropriate for obese children. FDA-approved total daily doses: methylphenidate, 60 mg; OROS, 72 mg; dexmethylphenidate, 20 mg; dexmethylphenidate XR, 40 mg; amphetamine mixed salts, 30 mg; amphetamine mixed XR 30 mg children, 20 mg adults; ER oral suspension MPH, 60 mg; lisdexamfetamine, 70 mg.
DR=delayed release; ER=extended release; FDA=U.S. Food and Drug Administration; IR=immediate release; MPH=methylphenidate; OROS= osmotic controlled-release oral delivery system.

Ritalin LA has been developed to provide effective methylphenidate treatment for 8–9 hours. It uses a bimodal release system that produces pharmacokinetic characteristics that in single-dose administration resemble those of two doses of Ritalin immediate-release tablets administered 4–5 hours apart. Ritalin LA consists of a mixture of immediate- and delayed-release beads in a 50:50 ratio. The delayed-release beads are coated with an absorption-delaying polymer. Ritalin LA is available in 10, 20, 30, and 40 mg capsules to approximate 10, 15, and 20 mg bid dosing of MPH-IR. Ritalin LA may be used as a sprinkle preparation for children unable to swallow pills. An analogue classroom study evaluated the pharmacodynamic (efficacy) profile, safety, and tolerability of Ritalin LA (Spencer et al. 2000). One-time administration of Ritalin LA was effective relative to placebo in improving classroom behavior and academic productivity over the subsequent 9-hour period. Ritalin LA had a rapid onset of effect, and the improvement relative to placebo was statistically significant during both the morning (0–4 hours after dosing) and the afternoon (4–9 hours after dosing).

Ritalin LA was further tested in a multicenter double-blind trial of 160 children (Biederman et al. 2003). There was an initial 2–4 week titration to optimal dose followed by a 1-week placebo washout period. Subjects with persistent ADHD symptoms during the washout (n=137) were randomly assigned to Ritalin LA or placebo. Children on Ritalin LA were rated as greatly improved over placebo by teachers and parents on the Conners' ADHD/DSM-IV Scales (CADS). Improvements were equally robust in the subscales of inattention and hyperactivity. Significant drug-specific improvement was also noted by clinicians on the Clinical Global Impressions–Improvement (CGI-I) scale. Ritalin LA was well tolerated with minimal side effects. Rates of mild appetite suppression and mild insomnia were both low (3.1%).

Adderall XR is a capsule with a 50:50 ratio of immediate- to delayed-release beads designed to release drug content in a time course similar to that of Adderall given twice a day (0 and 4 hours). Adderall XR is available in 5, 10, 15, 20, 25, and 30 mg capsules. An analogue classroom study compared various doses of Adderall XR with Adderall given twice daily and placebo (McCracken et al. 2003). Behavioral and academic improvements were documented to 12 hours postdose. The efficacy and safety of Adderall XR were further tested in a multicenter randomized, double-blind, placebo-controlled trial conducted at 47 sites (Biederman et al. 2002). Children with ADHD (N=584) were randomly assigned to receive single daily morning doses of placebo or Adderall XR 10 mg, 20 mg, or 30 mg for 3 weeks. Continuous significant improvement in morning and afternoon assessments was found by teachers and in morning, afternoon, and late afternoon assessments by parents on the Conners' Global Index Scale for Teachers and Parents. All active treatment groups showed significant dose-related improvement in behavior from baseline. The medication was well tolerated, with rates of adverse events similar for active treatments and placebo. A 1-year follow-up of 411 children on Adderall XR examined long-term safety and efficacy (McGough et al. 2005). Efficacy was maintained for 12 months as measured by the Conners' Global Index Scale. The medication was safe and well tolerated with a low frequency of mild adverse events and no evidence of untoward cardiovascular effects.

An extended-release dosage form of Focalin (Focalin XR) has been developed to provide effective methylphenidate treatment for 10–12 hours. Focalin XR uses the same bimodal release system as Ritalin LA, producing pharmacokinetic characteristics that in single-dose administration resemble those of two doses of Focalin tablets administered 4–5 hours apart. Similarly, Focalin XR consists of a mixture of immediate- and delayed-release beads in a 50:50 ratio. The delayed-release beads are coated with an absorption-delaying polymer. Focalin XR is available in 5, 10, 15, 20, 25, 30, 35, and 40 mg capsules. Focalin XR was found to be effective in children, adolescents, and adults and is FDA approved for all three age groups.

Focalin XR was tested in a multicenter randomized, double-blind study of 103 patients ages 6–17 years (Greenhill et al. 2006a). The patients were flexibly dosed to receive 5–30 mg capsules or placebo once daily for 7 weeks. Doses were titrated to optimal levels during the first 5 weeks and maintained for the final 2 weeks. Efficacy was evaluated weekly at school and at home using the CADS. Drug-specific improvement was documented on each scale. At final visit, 67.3% of patients receiving Focalin XR and 13.3% receiving placebo were "very much improved" or "much improved" on the CGI-I ($P<0.001$) scale. Focalin XR was well tolerated, with adverse event rates similar to those reported with immediate-release dexmethylphenidate.

A transdermal delivery system (methylphenidate transdermal system [MTS]) contains methylphenidate within a multipolymeric adhesive layer attached to a transparent backing. Patches are applied once daily and deliver a consistent amount of methylphenidate during the time the patch is worn. The drug does not go through first-pass metabolism in the liver; therefore, more methylphenidate is bioavailable. Transdermal delivery of methylphenidate might represent a useful treatment option for patients who have difficulty swallowing or tolerating oral formulations (e.g., nausea) or for patients who need flexible duration of medication effect. An initial randomized, double-blind study of MTS conducted in a summer treatment program (Pelham et al. 2005) demonstrated significant improvement on measures of social behavior in recreational settings, classroom functioning, and parent ratings of evening behavior. However, patch wear times of at least 12 hours resulted in insomnia for many of the participants. Ensuing trials (Pelham et al. 2005) used MTS with a wear time of 9 hours. A classroom analogue study (McGough et al. 2006) demonstrated effectiveness over 12 hours for a wear time of 9 hours.

A large 5-week randomized, double-blind multicenter study of MTS and osmotic controlled-release oral delivery system methylphenidate was conducted in children ages 6–12 years diagnosed with ADHD ($n=282$; Findling et al. 2008). Treatment with MTS was effective at reducing the symptoms of ADHD as assessed by clinicians, teachers, and parents and was generally well tolerated. Skin redness or itching at the application site is common and does not necessitate discontinuation. More severe rashes, as indicated by swelling, bumps, or blisters around the application site, may indicate a skin allergy to MTS and may require discontinuation and may signal a new allergy to all forms of MPH. Because of differences in bioavailability, a 10 mg MTS patch is approximately equivalent to 5 mg of MPH-IR tid, and 20 mg MTS is equivalent to about 10 mg MPH-IR tid. The manufacturer recommends against cutting a patch. MTS is available in dose strengths of 10, 15, 20, and 30 mg.

Lisdexamfetamine dimesylate (LDX) is a novel prodrug in which *d*-amphetamine is covalently bound to the amino acid L-lysine. This chemical bond renders the amphetamine component therapeutically inactive. Following oral administration, LDX is converted in the body to the active *d*-amphetamine after enzymatic hydrolysis in a rate-limited manner, at or following absorption. The saturable rate-limited hydrolysis releases active amphetamine slowly, creating predictable long-acting delivery of the active drug (*d*-amphetamine). Saturation of enzymatic hydrolysis at supratherapeutic doses suggests that LDX may be associated with diminished risk for abuse and toxicity. LDX dose strengths of 30 mg, 50 mg, and 70 mg were developed to provide an amphetamine base approximately equivalent to mixed amphetamine salts—10 mg, 20 mg, and 30 mg, respectively. While adequately powered comparison studies have not been done, in a classroom analogue study, these doses of LDX were at least as effective and long lasting as the comparable mixed amphetamine salts doses (Biederman et al. 2007b). In a large 4-week double-blind study of children (ages 6–12) with ADHD (N=290), single daily doses of LDX (30 mg, 50 mg, or 70 mg) were effective and well tolerated (Biederman et al. 2007a). Improvements were observed throughout the day up to 6:00 P.M. The tolerability profile was similar to the other currently marketed extended-release stimulants. LDX is available in 20, 30, 40, 50, 60, and 70 mg.

Extended-release oral suspension of methylphenidate (ER oral suspension MPH) is supplied as a powder that is reconstituted with water by the pharmacist prior to dispensing. The resulting ER MPH oral suspension has a concentration of 25 mg/5 mL (5 mg/mL) and does not require refrigeration. It is composed of cationic polymer matrix particles that bind *d,l*-threo-methylphenidate racemic mixture via an ion exchange mechanism. A proprietary coating of various thicknesses is applied to the particles to confer extended-release properties. ER oral suspension MPH is a blend of uncoated and coated particles that is composed of 20% immediate-release (IR) and 80% ER methylphenidate. A pharmacokinetic (PK) study in adults found that a single dose of 60 mg ER oral suspension MPH is equally bioavailable to two 30-mg doses of IR MPH 6 hours apart. In adults the T_{max} was 5 hours and the half-life of ER oral suspension MPH was 5.65 hours. In a further PK study in children ages 9–15 years, there were no age-related PK differences after oral administration. Over the dose range of methylphenidate used in this study (0.45–3.3 mg/kg), the pharmacokinetics of ER oral suspension MPH were linear and dose proportional.

ER oral suspension MPH was studied in an analogue laboratory school model over 12 hours in children with ADHD (Wigal et al. 2013). Efficacy measures included Swanson, Kotkin, Agler, M-Flynn and Pelham (SKAMP) Rating Scale–Combined and Permanent Product Measure of Performance (PERMP) mathematics tests measured at predose and at 0.75, 2, 4, 8, 10, and 12 hours postdose on each laboratory classroom day. Significant separation from placebo occurred at each time point tested (0.75, 2, 4, 8, 10, 12 hours), with onset of action of ER oral suspension MPH at 45 minutes postdose and duration of efficacy extending to 12 hours postdose. Adverse events and changes in vital signs following ER oral suspension MPH treatment were generally mild and consistent with the known safety profile of MPH. The authors concluded that ER oral suspension MPH treatment effectively reduced symptoms of ADHD in children beginning at 45 minutes and continuing for 12 hours postdose and that ER oral suspension MPH was well tolerated.

Nonstimulants

While there is no doubt that the stimulants are effective in the treatment of ADHD, it is estimated that at least 30% of affected individuals do not adequately respond to or cannot tolerate stimulant medication (Barkley 1977; Gittelman 1980; Spencer et al. 1996). In addition, immediate-release stimulants are short-acting drugs that require multiple administrations during the day, with their attendant impact on compliance and need to take treatment during school or work hours. Although the problem of multiple doses may be offset by the use of long-acting stimulants, this class of drugs may adversely affect sleep, making use in the evening hours difficult when symptom control is still needed. The fact that stimulants are controlled substances continues to fuel worries in children, families, and the treating community that inhibit their use. These fears are based on lingering concerns about the abuse potential of stimulant drugs by the child, family member, or associates; the possibility of diversion; and safety concerns regarding the use of a controlled substance by patients who are impulsive and may have antisocial tendencies (Goldman et al. 1998). Similarly, the controlled nature of stimulant drugs poses medicolegal concerns to the treating community that further increase the barriers to treatment. In addition, because of controlled substance restrictions, use is often inconvenient.

Specific Norepinephrine Reuptake Inhibitors

Atomoxetine (Strattera) is one of a newer class of compounds known as specific norepinephrine reuptake inhibitors (Table 35–3). Initial encouraging results in an adult trial (Spencer et al. 1998a), coupled with extensive safety data, fueled efforts in developing this compound in the treatment of pediatric ADHD. An open-label dose-ranging study of this compound in pediatric ADHD documented strong clinical benefits with excellent tolerability, including a safe cardiovascular profile, and provided dosing guidelines for further controlled studies (Spencer et al. 2001).

Atomoxetine Efficacy

Further controlled trials have led to FDA approval of atomoxetine for both children and adults with ADHD. In the first pediatric controlled studies, 291 children ages 7–13 with ADHD were randomly assigned to treatment in two trials (combined: atomoxetine, $n=129$; placebo, $n=124$; and methylphenidate, $n=38$) (Spencer et al. 2002b). The acute treatment period was 9 weeks. The stimulant-naive stratum patients were randomly assigned to double-blind treatment with atomoxetine, placebo, or methylphenidate. Patients in the stimulant prior exposure stratum (prior exposure to any stimulant) were randomly assigned to double-blind treatment with atomoxetine or placebo. Atomoxetine significantly reduced total scores on an investigator-rated DSM-IV (American Psychiatric Association 1994) ADHD rating scale. The definition of response was a ≥25% decrease in the ADHD rating scale, and the response rates were greater on atomoxetine than placebo (61.4% vs. 32.3%, respectively; $P<0.05$). In the stimulant-naive stratum subjects, 69.1% of

TABLE 35–3. Specific noradrenergic reuptake inhibitor atomoxetine

Medication	Daily dosage, mg/kg/day	Daily dose schedule	Main indications	Common adverse effects/Comments
Atomoxetine (Strattera)	0.5–1.4	Once or twice	ADHD	Mechanism of action: noradrenergic-specific reuptake inhibitor
			ADHD plus enuresis	Mild/moderate appetite decrease
			Tic disorders	Gastrointestinal symptoms
			Anxiety disorders	Mild initial weight loss
				Cardiovascular effects (mild increase in blood pressure, pulse)
				No ECG conduction or repolarization delays
				Not abusable
				Rare serious hepatotoxicity
				Uncommon increase in suicidal thoughts

Note. Doses are general guidelines. All doses must be individualized with appropriate monitoring. Weight-corrected doses are less appropriate for obese children. When high doses are used, serum levels may be obtained in order to avoid toxicity. FDA-approved total daily dose: 1.4 mg/kg (≤100 mg). ADHD=attention-deficit/hyperactivity disorder; ECG=electrocardiogram.

atomoxetine patients, 73% of methylphenidate patients, and 31.4% of placebo patients were considered responders.

In an additional controlled study, 297 children and adolescents were randomly assigned to different doses of atomoxetine or placebo for 8 weeks (Michelson et al. 2001). Atomoxetine was associated with a graded dose response. Response was best at 1.2 or 1.8 mg/kg/day and was superior to 0.5 mg/kg/day, which was superior to placebo. In close parallel was found a dose-dependent enhancement of social and family function. The Child Health Questionnaire was used to assess the well-being of the child and family. Parents of children on atomoxetine reported fewer emotional difficulties and behavioral problems as well as greater self-esteem in their children and less emotional worry and limitation in their own personal time.

Atomoxetine Side Effects and Risks

Atomoxetine was well tolerated in pediatric studies (Spencer et al. 2002b). Mild appetite suppression was reported in 22% of patients receiving atomoxetine versus 32% receiving methylphenidate and 7% receiving placebo. Compared with methylphenidate, there was less insomnia with atomoxetine (7.0% vs. 27.0%; $P<0.05$). Mild increases in diastolic blood pressure and heart rate were noted in the atomoxetine treatment group, with no significant differences between atomoxetine and placebo in laboratory parameters and ECG intervals.

A year-long open follow-up of children and adolescents treated with atomoxetine ($N=325$) found that atomoxetine treatment continued to be effective and well tolerated. The acute mild increases in diastolic blood pressure and heart rate persisted without worsening. Growth in height and weight was normal, and there were no significant differences between atomoxetine and placebo in laboratory parameters or ECG intervals (Kratochvil et al. 2001; Spencer et al. 2005).

Rare cases of severe liver injury have been reported in a denominator of greater than 3 million patients who have taken atomoxetine since approval. Several patients have recovered with normal liver function after discontinuing the medication. While cases were rare and several of the patients recovered, severe drug-related liver injury might progress to acute liver failure resulting in death or the need for a liver transplant. Eli Lilly (www.lilly.com) added a warning in bold to the product label for atomoxetine that indicates that the medication should be discontinued in patients with jaundice (yellowing of the skin or whites of the eyes) or laboratory evidence of liver injury. Patients on atomoxetine are cautioned to contact their doctor immediately if they develop pruritus, jaundice, dark urine, upper right-side abdominal tenderness, or unexplained "flu-like" symptoms. It will be important to remain current on any new information on this risk.

There is now a black box warning for the increased risk of suicidal ideation with atomoxetine use in children and adolescents. Pooled analyses of short-term (6–18 weeks) placebo-controlled trials of atomoxetine in children and adolescents (a total of 12 trials involving more than 2,200 patients, including 11 trials in ADHD and 1 trial in enuresis) revealed a greater risk of suicidal ideation early during treatment in those receiving atomoxetine compared with placebo. The average risk of suicidal ideation in patients receiving atomoxetine was 0.4% (5 of 1,357 patients), compared with none in placebo-treated patients (851 patients). No completed suicides occurred in these trials.

Atomoxetine has been shown to have low abuse potential (Heil et al. 2002).

Atomoxetine Dosing

Current dosing guidelines recommend that atomoxetine be initiated at 0.5 mg/kg/day for 2 weeks and increased to a target dosage of 1.2 mg/kg/day, with a recommended maximum dosage of 1.4 mg/kg/day or 100 mg/day. While higher doses are not FDA approved, clinicians familiar with the medication have reported further improvement at dosages up to 1.8 mg/kg/day, a dose maximum used in both the juvenile and adolescent studies. While atomoxetine is effective at once-a-day dosing, divided doses twice a day can provide a better tolerability profile and potentially a more robust effect later in the day on oppositional defiant symptoms (Waxmonsky et al. 2011). Since atomoxetine is metabolized by the hepatic 2D6 enzymatic system, care should be taken with co-administration with medications that inhibit 2D6 (e.g., fluoxetine, paroxetine). Atomoxetine is available in 10, 18, 25, 40, 60, 80, and 100 mg capsules.

Noradrenergic Modulators: Clonidine and Guanfacine

Clonidine

Clonidine is an imidazoline derivative with α-adrenergic (2a,b,c) agonist properties that has been primarily used in the treatment of hypertension. At low doses, it appears to stimulate inhibitory, presynaptic autoreceptors in the central nervous system. The most common past use of clonidine in pediatric psychiatry was for the treatment of Tourette's disorder and other tic disorders (Leckman et al. 1991), ADHD, and ADHD-associated sleep disturbances (Hunt et al. 1990; Prince et al. 1996).

Clonidine Efficacy

Immediate-release clonidine does not have an FDA-approved indication for the treatment of ADHD. However, immediate-release clonidine has been widely used in children with ADHD, despite a paucity of studies (*n*=6 studies [4 controlled], *N*=292 children) (Gunning 1992; Hunt 1987; Hunt et al. 1985; Singer et al. 1995; Steingard et al. 1993; Tourette's Syndrome Study Group 2002) supporting the safety and efficacy of clonidine for this use. An important early study that compared clonidine with methylphenidate in a sample of children with ADHD and Tourette syndrome (Tourette's Syndrome Study Group 2002) found that clonidine worked as well as methylphenidate on teacher ratings of ADHD, but clonidine was most helpful for impulsivity and hyperactivity and not as helpful for inattention. Moreover, sedation was a common side effect, occurring in 28% of subjects.

Clonidine Dosing

Immediate-release clonidine is a relatively short-acting compound despite a relatively long plasma half-life (up to 12 hours). Daily doses should be titrated and individualized. Usual daily dosage ranges from 3 to 10 mcg/kg, given generally in divided doses, typically two, three, or four times a day depending on intended duration of coverage. Clonidine is usually started at the low dose of a full or half 0.1 mg tablet, depending on the size of the child (approximately 1–2 µg/kg) and increased depending on clinical response and adverse effects. The initial dose is often given in the evening hours or before bedtime because of sedation.

Clonidine Side Effects and Risks

The most common short-term adverse effect of clonidine is sedation. It can also produce, in some cases, hypotension, dry mouth, depression, and confusion. Clonidine is not known to be associated with long-term adverse effects. In hypertensive adults, abrupt withdrawal of clonidine has been associated with rebound hypertension. Thus, it requires slow tapering when discontinued. Clonidine should not be administered concomitantly with beta-blockers since adverse interactions have been reported.

Guanfacine

Studies have shown the more selective α_2-agonist (immediate release) guanfacine to have a similar spectrum of benefits to those of clonidine with less sedation and longer duration of action (Chappell et al. 1995; Horrigan and Barnhill 1995; Hunt et al. 1995). Immediate-release guanfacine does not have an FDA indication for the treatment of ADHD. There are three open studies (*n*=36 total) and one controlled study (*n*=34) of immediate-release guanfacine in children and adolescents with ADHD (Chappell et al. 1995; Horrigan and Barnhill 1995; Hunt et al. 1995; Scahill et al. 2001). In these studies, beneficial effects on hyperactive behaviors and attentional abilities were reported. In the controlled study of children with tic disorders and ADHD, guanfacine improved attention on teacher ratings and performance on a continuous performance test (Scahill et al. 2001). The usual daily dose ranges from 42 to 86 µg/kg, typically given in divided doses, two or three times daily, depending on intended duration of coverage.

New Generation Formulations of α-Adrenergic Agents

Clonidine Extended Release

An extended-release (12-hour) formulation of clonidine hydrochloride (CLON-XR) (Kapvay) was developed for the treatment of ADHD in children and adolescents. CLON-XR has a C_{max} that is 50% lower than immediate-release clonidine and a longer T_{max} of 3–5 hours. CLON-XR is designed to be given twice daily. FDA approval was granted on the basis of an 8-week, placebo-controlled, fixed-dose trial in patients ages 6–17 years with ADHD that evaluated the efficacy and safety of CLON-XR 0.2 mg/day or CLON-XR 0.4 mg/day versus placebo in three separate treatment arms (Jain et al. 2011). Patients (n=236) were randomly assigned to receive placebo (n=78), CLON-XR 0.2 mg/day (n=78), or CLON-XR 0.4 mg/day (n=80). Improvement from baseline in ADHD Rating Scale-IV (ADHD-RS-IV) total score was significantly greater in both CLON-XR groups versus placebo at week 5. A significant improvement in ADHD-RS-IV total score occurred between groups as soon as week 2 and was maintained throughout the treatment period. The most common treatment-emergent adverse event was mild to moderate somnolence. Changes on electrocardiogram were minor and reflected the known pharmacology of clonidine. CLON-XR comes in tablets of either 0.1 or 0.2 mg. Recommended dosage is from 0.1 mg once a day up to 0.2 mg bid.

Guanfacine Extended Release

Similarly, an extended-release formulation of guanfacine hydrochloride (GXR) (Intuniv) was developed for the treatment of ADHD in children and adolescents. GXR has a lower C_{max} and a longer half-life than immediate-release guanfacine and was designed to be given once daily. There were two large (n=345; n=324) 8–9 week randomized, double-blind, multicenter studies of GXR in children ages 6–17 years diagnosed with ADHD (Biederman et al. 2008). Doses of 1 mg, 2 mg, 3 mg, and 4 mg were tested. Efficacy for ADHD was substantial and proportionate to weight-corrected dose. Adverse events were mild to moderate in severity, with most common events related to somnolence, sedation, or fatigue. Small to moderate changes in blood pressure and pulse rate were observed as expected for a medication with antihypertensive properties. The results of this study led to the FDA approval of GXR in doses of 1, 2, 3, and 4 mg.

α_2-Adrenergic Medications Combined With Stimulants

While psychostimulants are generally first-line pharmacotherapy for ADHD, symptom improvement is suboptimal in some patients. In these patients, clinicians have frequently used a combination of psychostimulants and nonscheduled medications to manage ADHD, although, until recently, published evidence supporting this practice was relatively scarce. A series of studies were conducted that examined the efficacy and safety of the combination of α-adrenergic medications and stimulants (Table 35–4).

Clonidine Extended Release Plus Stimulants

A large study assessed the efficacy and safety of CLON-XR combined with stimulants (i.e., methylphenidate or amphet-

TABLE 35–4. Noradrenergic Modulators

Drug	Daily dose	Daily dose schedule	Main indications	Common adverse effects
Immediate-acting noradrenergic modulators				
α_2-Agonists				
Clonidine (Catapres)	0.003–0.010 mg/kg	tid or qid	ADHD and/or Tourette's disorder Aggression/self-abuse Severe agitation Opioid withdrawal syndromes	Sedation (very frequent) Hypotension (rare) Dry mouth Confusion (with high dose) Depression Rebound hypertension Localized irritation with transdermal preparation
Guanfacine (Tenex)	0.015–0.05 mg/kg	bid or tid		Same as clonidine Less sedation, hypotension
Long-acting noradrenergic modulators				
α_2-Agonists				
Clonidine extended-release (Kapvay)	0.1–0.4 mg (divided doses)	bid	ADHD and/or Tourette's disorder Aggression/self-abuse Severe agitation Withdrawal syndromes	Sedation (very frequent) Hypotension (rare) Dry mouth Confusion (with high dose) Depression Rebound hypertension
Guanfacine extended-release (Intuniv)	1–4 mg	Once (morning or evening)		Same as clonidine Less sedation, hypotension

Note. Doses are general guidelines; bid= two times daily; qid=four times daily; tid=three times daily. All doses must be individualized with appropriate monitoring. Weight-corrected doses are less appropriate for obese children.

amine) for ADHD (Kollins et al. 2011). In this double-blind placebo-controlled trial, children and adolescents with hyperactive- or combined-subtype ADHD who had an inadequate response to their stable stimulant regimen were randomly assigned to receive CLON-XR or placebo in combination with their baseline stimulant medication. Of 198 patients, 102 received CLON-XR plus stimulant and 96 received placebo plus stimulant. At week 5, statistically significant greater improvement from baseline was reported in ADHD-RS-IV total score and ADHD-RS-IV hyperactivity and inattention subscale scores in the CLON-XR plus stimulant group versus the placebo plus stimulant group. Adverse events and changes in vital signs in the CLON-XR group were generally mild. The results of this study suggested that CLON-XR in combination with stimulants is useful in treating ADHD in children and adolescents with partial response to stimulants. The results of this study led to the FDA approval of combined CLON-XR plus stimulant for treatment of ADHD.

Guanfacine Extended Release Plus Stimulants

GXR, a selective α_2-adrenoceptor agonist, has been studied as an adjunctive therapy to psychostimulant medications. Drug-drug interaction studies demonstrate that the adjunctive administration of GXR with a long-acting methylphenidate preparation or LDX does not change exposure to the active components of either medication (e.g., *d*-amphetamine, *d,l*-methylphenidate, or guanfacine) in a clinically meaningful way compared with either treatment alone. Data supporting the potential efficacy of GXR adjunctive added to a psychostimulant was preliminarily observed in a 9-week, open-label, dose escalation study and subsequent extension study (24 months) in subjects ages 6–17 years with suboptimal control of ADHD symptoms on psychostimulant monotherapy (Spencer et al. 2009). The safety and efficacy of adjunctive GXR was more thoroughly evaluated in a 9-week, randomized, double-blind, placebo-controlled study. Among subjects ages 6–17 years with a suboptimal response to a long-acting, extended-release oral psychostimulant, adjunctive GXR (administered in the morning or evening) was associated with significantly greater symptom reduction than placebo plus psychostimulant (ADHD-RS-IV total score, GXR AM [P=0.002]; GXR PM [0.001]) (Wilens et al. 2012). Across multiple studies, the safety and tolerability profile of GXR administered adjunctively to a psychostimulant has been consistent with the known profiles of each medication. The results of this study led to the FDA approval of use of combined GXR plus stimulant treatment.

Antidepressants

Of nonstimulants, noradrenergic and dopaminergic compounds, including monoamine oxidase inhibitors (Zametkin et al. 1985), secondary amine tricyclic antidepressants (TCAs; Biederman et al. 1989), and bupropion (Conners et al. 1996), have been found to be superior to placebo in controlled clinical trials. However, none of them are FDA approved for treatment of ADHD. Possible advantages of these compounds over stimulants include a longer duration of action without symptom rebound or insomnia, the option of monitoring plasma drug levels, and minimal risk of abuse or dependence as well as the potential treatment of comorbid internalizing symptoms and tics.

Tricyclic Antidepressants

Historically, the first nonstimulant treatments for ADHD that were extensively evaluated were the TCAs. Out of 33 studies (21 controlled, 12 open) evaluating TCAs in children and adolescents (*N*=1,139) and adults (*N*=78), 91% reported positive effects on ADHD symptoms (Spencer et al. 1997). In a controlled study, Spencer et al. (2002a) reported that desipramine had a beneficial effect on ADHD and tic symptoms. The mechanism of action of the antidepressants appears to be due to various effects on the release and reuptake of brain neurotransmitters, including norepinephrine, serotonin, and dopamine. Common short-term adverse effects of the TCAs include anticholinergic effects, such as dry mouth, blurred vision, and constipation. Gastrointestinal symptoms and vomiting may occur when these drugs are discontinued abruptly; thus, slow tapering of these medications is recommended. Since the anticholinergic effects of TCAs limit salivary flow, they may promote tooth decay.

Several case reports in the 1980s of sudden death in children being treated with desipramine raised concern about the potential cardiotoxic risk associated with TCAs in the pediatric population (Riddle et al. 1991). Although of unclear hemodynamic significance, the development of conduction defects on ECG in children receiving TCA treatment merits closer ECG and clinical monitoring, especially when relatively high doses of these medicines are used. Therefore, treatment with a TCA should be preceded by a baseline ECG, with serial ECGs at regular intervals throughout treatment. In the context of cardiac disease, conduction defects may have potentially more serious clinical implications. When in doubt about the cardiovascular state of the patient, before starting treatment with a TCA a more comprehensive cardiac evaluation is suggested, including 24-hour ECG and cardiac consultation, to help determine the risk-benefit ratio of such an intervention. Because of the potential lethality of TCA overdose, parents should be advised to carefully store the medication in a place inaccessible to children.

Bupropion

Bupropion hydrochloride is a novel-structured antidepressant of the aminoketone class related to the phenylisopropylamines but pharmacologically distinct from other antidepressants (see also Chapter 36, "Antidepressants"). Although its specific site and mechanism of action remains unknown, bupropion seems to have an indirect mixed agonist effect on dopamine and norepinephrine neurotransmission. Bupropion has been shown to be effective for ADHD in children (Conners et al. 1996) and in adults (Wilens et al. 1999, 2005). Bupropion is rapidly absorbed, with peak plasma levels usually achieved after 2 hours. The average elimination half-life is 14 hours (8–24 hours). The usual dosage range is 4.0–6.0 mg/kg/day in divided doses. Side effects include irritability, anorexia, insomnia, and, rarely, edema, rashes, and nocturia. Exacerbation of tic disorders also has been reported with bupropion. While bupropion has been associated with a slightly increased risk (0.4%) for drug-induced seizures relative to other antidepressants, this risk has been linked to high doses and patients with a previous history of seizures or eating disorders. Bupropion has been formulated into long-acting preparations (SR, XR) that can be administered twice daily.

Selective Serotonin Reuptake Inhibitors

At present, expert opinion does not support the usefulness of selective serotonin reuptake inhibitors (SSRIs) in the treatment of core ADHD symptoms (National Institute of Mental Health 1996). Nevertheless, because of the high rates of comorbidity in ADHD, these compounds are frequently combined with effective anti-ADHD agents. Since many psychotropics are metabolized by the cytochrome P450 system (Nemeroff et al. 1996), which in turn can be inhibited by the SSRIs, caution should be exercised when combining agents such as the TCAs with SSRIs.

Other Compounds

Modafinil

Modafinil is an antinarcoleptic agent that is structurally and pharmacologically different from other agents approved to treat ADHD. While the mechanism of action is unknown, it may improve symptoms of ADHD via the same mechanism by which it improves wakefulness. Preclinically, modafinil selectively activates the cortex without causing widespread central nervous system stimulation (Engber et al. 1998). Modafinil does not appear to activate areas of the brain that mediate reward and abuse and has a low potential for abuse (Myrick et al. 2004).

While initial studies demonstrated significant improvement in ADHD symptoms, recent studies reported increased efficacy with higher dosages (340–425 mg/day) in children and adolescents (Swanson et al. 2006).

The most commonly reported adverse events of modafinil are insomnia (29%), headache (20%), and decreased appetite (16%). While there is evidence of the effectiveness of modafinil in ADHD, the drug was not FDA approved for ADHD because of concerns about a few potentially serious Stevens-Johnson–like rashes in these trials. When used off-label for ADHD in children, the risk-benefit evaluation should take into account the possibility of a rash of this type.

Typical Antipsychotics

While an old literature suggested that typical (first-generation) antipsychotics were effective in the treatment of children with ADHD, their spectrum of adverse effects, both short-term (extrapyramidal reactions) and long-term (tardive dyskinesia), greatly limits their usefulness.

Conclusion

ADHD is a heterogeneous disorder with a strong neurobiological basis that afflicts millions of individuals of all ages worldwide. Although the stimulants remain the mainstay of treatment for this disorder, a newer generation of nonstimulant drugs provides viable alternatives for patients and families.

Summary Points

- There is a substantial body of literature documenting the efficacy of multiple unrelated pharmacological agents in individuals with ADHD.
- Pharmacological treatment leads to improvement not only on core behavioral (ADHD, oppositional defiant disorder) symptoms but also on associated impairments including cognition, social skills, and family function.
- Anti-ADHD compounds include not only the stimulants but also a specific norepinephrine reuptake inhibitor (atomoxetine), α-adrenergic agents (clonidine, guanfacine), and several antidepressants (off-label).
- Effective pharmacological treatments for ADHD seem to share noradrenergic and dopaminergic mechanisms of action.
- Despite great progress, less is known about the treatment of ADHD in preschoolers, adolescents, females, and minorities.
- There are limited data on the differential response of medications in comorbid ADHD, the effects of combined pharmacotherapy, or the effects of combined pharmacotherapy and psychotherapy.
- Risks of stimulant use include their abuse potential; (rare) cardiac risk in individuals with preexisting structural cardiac abnormalities; and precipitation or exacerbation of anxiety, agitation, aggression, manic symptoms, and psychotic symptoms.
- Risks of atomoxetine use include possible suicidal ideation; (rare) risk of severe liver injury; (rare) cardiac risk in individuals with preexisting structural cardiac abnormalities; and precipitation or exacerbation of agitation, aggression, manic symptoms, and psychotic symptoms.

References

American Psychiatric Association: Diagnostic and Statistical Manual of Mental Disorders, 4th Edition. Washington, DC, American Psychiatric Association, 1994

Arnold LE, Lindsay RL, Conners CK, et al: A double-blind, placebo-controlled withdrawal trial of dexmethylphenidate hydrochloride in children with attention deficit hyperactivity disorder. J Child Adolesc Psychopharmacol 14(4):542–554, 2004 15662146

Barkley RA: A review of stimulant drug research with hyperactive children. J Child Psychol Psychiatry 18(2):137–165, 1977 326801

Barr CL, Wigg K, Malone M, et al: Linkage study of catechol-O-methyltransferase and attention-deficit hyperactivity disorder. Am J Med Genet 88(6):710–713, 1999 10581494

Bergman A, Winters L, Cornblatt B: Methylphenidate: effects on sustained attention, in Ritalin: Theory and Patient Management. Edited by Greenhill L, Osman B. New York, Mary Ann Liebert, 1991, pp 223–231

Biederman J, Baldessarini RJ, Wright V, et al: A double-blind placebo controlled study of desipramine in the treatment of ADD: I. Efficacy. J Am Acad Child Adolesc Psychiatry 28(5):777–784, 1989 2676967

Biederman J, Wilens T, Mick E, et al: Psychoactive substance use disorders in adults with attention deficit hyperactivity disorder (ADHD): effects of ADHD and psychiatric comorbidity. Am J Psychiatry 152(11):1652–1658, 1995 7485630

Biederman J, Lopez FA, Boellner SW, et al: A randomized, double-blind, placebo-controlled, parallel-group study of SLI381 (Adderall XR) in children with attention-deficit/hyperactivity disorder. Pediatrics 110(2 Pt 1):258–266, 2002 12165576

Biederman J, Quinn D, Weiss M, et al: Efficacy and safety of Ritalin LA, a new, once daily, extended-release dosage form of methylphenidate, in children with attention deficit hyperactivity disorder. Paediatr Drugs 5(12):833–841, 2003 14658924

Biederman J, Krishnan S, Zhang Y, et al: Efficacy and tolerability of lisdexamfetamine dimesylate (NRP-104) in children with attention-deficit/hyperactivity disorder: a phase III, multicenter, randomized, double-blind, forced-dose, parallel-group study. Clin Ther 29(3):450–463, 2007a 17577466

Biederman J, Boellner SW, Childress A, et al: Lisdexamfetamine dimesylate and mixed amphetamine salts extended-release in children with ADHD: a double-blind, placebo-controlled, crossover analog classroom study. Biol Psychiatry 62(9):970–976, 2007b 17631866

Biederman J, Melmed RD, Patel A, et al: A randomized, double-blind, placebo-controlled study of guanfacine extended release in children and adolescents with attention-deficit/hyperactivity disorder. Pediatrics 121(1):e73–e84, 2008 18166547

Blader JC, Pliszka SR, Kafantaris V, et al: Callous-unemotional traits, proactive aggression, and treatment outcomes of aggressive children with attention-deficit/hyperactivity disorder. J Am Acad Child Adolesc Psychiatry 52(12):1281–1293, 2013 24290461

Brown RT, Wynne ME, Slimmer LW: Attention deficit disorder and the effect of methylphenidate on attention, behavioral, and cardiovascular functioning. J Clin Psychiatry 45(11):473–476, 1984 6386794

Chappell PB, Riddle MA, Scahill L, et al: Guanfacine treatment of comorbid attention-deficit hyperactivity disorder and Tourette's syndrome: preliminary clinical experience. J Am Acad Child Adolesc Psychiatry 34(9):1140–1146, 1995 7559307

Conners CK, Casat CD, Gualtieri CT, et al: Bupropion hydrochloride in attention deficit disorder with hyperactivity. J Am Acad Child Adolesc Psychiatry 35(10):1314–1321, 1996 8885585

Connor DF, Glatt SJ, Lopez ID, et al: Psychopharmacology and aggression. I: A meta-analysis of stimulant effects on overt/covert aggression-related behaviors in ADHD. J Am Acad Child Adolesc Psychiatry 41(3):253–261, 2002 11886019

Cooper WO, Habel LA, Sox CM, et al: ADHD drugs and serious cardiovascular events in children and young adults. N Engl J Med 365(20):1896–1904, 2011 22043968

Cummings JL: Frontal-subcortical circuits and human behavior. Arch Neurol 50(8):873–880, 1993 8352676

Ding YS, Fowler JS, Volkow ND, et al: Carbon-11-d-threo-methylphenidate binding to dopamine transporter in baboon brain. J Nucl Med 36(12):2298–2305, 1995 8523123

Douglas VI, Barr RG, Amin K, et al: Dosage effects and individual responsivity to methylphenidate in attention deficit disorder. J Child Psychol Psychiatry 29(4):453–475, 1988 3063718

Engber TM, Koury EJ, Dennis SA, et al: Differential patterns of regional c-Fos induction in the rat brain by amphetamine and the novel wakefulness-promoting agent modafinil. Neurosci Lett 241(2–3):95–98, 1998 9507929

Famularo R, Fenton T: The effect of methylphenidate on school grades in children with attention deficit disorder without hyperactivity: a preliminary report. J Clin Psychiatry 48(3):112–114, 1987 3818551

Faraone SV, Biederman J, Morley CP, et al: Effect of stimulants on height and weight: a review of the literature. J Am Acad Child Adolesc Psychiatry 47(9):994–1009, 2008 18580502

Findling RL, Bukstein OG, Melmed RD, et al: A randomized, double-blind, placebo-controlled, parallel-group study of methylphenidate transdermal system in pediatric patients with attention-deficit/hyperactivity disorder. J Clin Psychiatry 69(1):149–159, 2008 18312050

Gadow K, Sverd J, Sprafkin J, et al: Efficacy of methylphenidate for attention-deficit hyperactivity disorder in children with tic disorder. Arch Gen Psychiatry 52(6):444–455, 1995 7771914

Gittelman R: Childhood disorders, in Drug Treatment of Adult and Child Psychiatric Disorders. Edited by Klein D, Quitkin F, Rifkin A, et al. Baltimore, MD, Williams and Wilkins, 1980, pp 576–756

Gittelman-Klein R: Pharmacotherapy of childhood hyperactivity: an update, in Psychopharmacology: The Third Generation of Progress. Edited by Meltzer HY. New York, Raven, 1987, pp 1215–1224

Goldman LS, Genel M, Bezman RJ, et al: Diagnosis and treatment of attention-deficit/hyperactivity disorder in children and adolescents. Council on Scientific Affairs, American Medical Association. JAMA 279(14):1100–1107, 1998 9546570

Greenhill LL, Halperin JM, Abikoff H: Stimulant medications. J Am Acad Child Adolesc Psychiatry 38(5):503–512, 1999 10230181

Greenhill LL, Findling RL, Swanson JM, et al: A double-blind, placebo-controlled study of modified-release methylphenidate in children with attention-deficit/hyperactivity disorder. Pediatrics 109(3):E39, 2002 11875167

Greenhill LL, Muniz R, Ball RR, et al: Efficacy and safety of dexmethylphenidate extended-release capsules in children with attention-deficit/hyperactivity disorder. J Am Acad Child Adolesc Psychiatry 45(7):817–823, 2006a 16832318

Greenhill L, Kollins S, Abikoff H, et al: Efficacy and safety of immediate-release methylphenidate treatment for preschoolers with ADHD. J Am Acad Child Adolesc Psychiatry 45(11):1284–1293, 2006b 17023867

Gunning B: A Controlled Trial of Clonidine in Hyperkinetic Children. Thesis, Department of Child and Adolescent Psychiatry, Academic Hospital Rotterdam–Sophia Children's Hospital. Rotterdam, The Netherlands, 1992

Gutgesell H, Atkins D, Barst R, et al: Cardiovascular monitoring of children and adolescents receiving psychotropic drugs: A statement for healthcare professionals from the Committee on Congenital Cardiac Defects, Council on Cardiovascular Disease in the Young, American Heart Association. Circulation 99(7):979–982, 1999 10027824

Heil SH, Holmes HW, Bickel WK, et al: Comparison of the subjective, physiological, and psychomotor effects of atomoxetine and methylphenidate in light drug users. Drug Alcohol Depend 67(2):149–156, 2002 12095664

Horrigan JP, Barnhill LJ: Guanfacine for treatment of attention-deficit hyperactivity disorder in boys. J Child Adolesc Psychopharmacol 5(3):215–223, 1995

Humphreys KL, Eng T, Lee SS: Stimulant medication and substance use outcomes: a meta-analysis. JAMA Psychiatry 70(7):740–749, 2013 23754458

Hunt RD: Treatment effects of oral and transdermal clonidine in relation to methylphenidate: an open pilot study in ADD-H. Psychopharmacol Bull 23(1):111–114, 1987 3602304

Hunt RD, Capper L, O'Connell P: Clonidine in child and adolescent psychiatry. J Child Adolesc Psychopharmacol 1(1):87–102, 1990 19630604

Hunt RD, Arnsten AF, Asbell MD: An open trial of guanfacine in the treatment of attention-deficit hyperactivity disorder. J Am Acad Child Adolesc Psychiatry 34(1):50–54, 1995 7860456

Hunt RD, Minderaa RB, Cohen DJ: Clonidine benefits children with attention deficit disorder and hyperactivity: report of a double-blind placebo-crossover therapeutic trial. J Am Acad Child Psychiatry 24(5):617–629, 1985 3900182

Jain R, Segal S, Kollins SH, et al: Clonidine extended-release tablets for pediatric patients with attention-deficit/hyperactivity disorder. J Am Acad Child Adolesc Psychiatry 50(2):171–179, 2011 21241954

Klein RG, Mannuzza S: Hyperactive boys almost grown up. III. Methylphenidate effects on ultimate height. Arch Gen Psychiatry 45(12):1131–1134, 1988 3058089

Kollins SH, Jain R, Brams M, et al: Clonidine extended-release tablets as add-on therapy to psychostimulants in children and adolescents with ADHD. Pediatrics 127(6):e1406–e1413, 2011 21555501

Kratochvil CJ, Bohac D, Harrington M, et al: An open-label trial of tomoxetine in pediatric attention deficit hyperactivity disorder. J Child Adolesc Psychopharmacol 11(2):167–170, 2001 11436956

Kupietz SS, Winsberg BG, Richardson E, et al: Effects of methylphenidate dosage in hyperactive reading-disabled children: I. Behavior and cognitive performance effects. J Am Acad Child Adolesc Psychiatry 27(1):70–77, 1988 3343209

Leckman JF, Hardin MT, Riddle MA, et al: Clonidine treatment of Gilles de la Tourette's syndrome. Arch Gen Psychiatry 48(4):324–328, 1991 2009034

Li Z, Chang SH, Zhang LY, et al: Molecular genetic studies of ADHD and its candidate genes: a review. Psychiatry Res 219(1):10–24, 2014 24863865

Lichtenstein P, Halldner L, Zetterqvist J, et al: Medication for attention deficit-hyperactivity disorder and criminality. N Engl J Med 367(21):2006–2014, 2012 23171097

Lowe TL, Cohen DJ, Detlor J, et al: Stimulant medications precipitate Tourette's syndrome. JAMA 247(8):1168–1169, 1982 6120250

McCracken JT, Biederman J, Greenhill LL, et al: Analog classroom assessment of a once-daily mixed amphetamine formulation, SLI381 (Adderall XR), in children with ADHD. J Am Acad Child Adolesc Psychiatry 42(6):673–683, 2003 12921475

McGough JJ, Biederman J, Wigal SB, et al: Long-term tolerability and effectiveness of once-daily mixed amphetamine salts (Adderall XR) in children with ADHD. J Am Acad Child Adolesc Psychiatry 44(6):530–538, 2005 15908835

McGough JJ, Wigal SB, Abikoff H, et al: A randomized, double-blind, placebo-controlled, laboratory classroom assessment of methylphenidate transdermal system in children with ADHD. J Atten Disord 9(3):476–485, 2006 16481664

Michelson D, Faries D, Wernicke J, et al: Atomoxetine in the treatment of children and adolescents with attention-deficit/hyperactivity disorder: a randomized, placebo-controlled, dose-response study. Pediatrics 108(5):E83, 2001 11694667

Myrick H, Malcolm R, Taylor B, et al: Modafinil: preclinical, clinical, and post-marketing surveillance—a review of abuse liability issues. Ann Clin Psychiatry 16(2):101–109, 2004 15328903

National Institute of Mental Health: Alternative Pharmacology of ADHD. Bethesda, MD, National Institute of Mental Health, 1996

Nemeroff CB, DeVane CL, Pollock BG: Newer antidepressants and the cytochrome P450 system. Am J Psychiatry 153(3):311–320, 1996 8610817

Pelham WE, Bender ME, Caddell J, et al: Methylphenidate and children with attention deficit disorder. Dose effects on classroom academic and social behavior. Arch Gen Psychiatry 42(10):948–952, 1985 3899046

Pelham WE, Gnagy EM, Burrows-Maclean L, et al: Once-a-day Concerta methylphenidate versus three-times-daily methylphenidate in laboratory and natural settings. Pediatrics 107(6):E105, 2001 11389303

Pelham WE, Burrows-Maclean L, Gnagy EM, et al: Transdermal methylphenidate, behavioral, and combined treatment for children with ADHD. Exp Clin Psychopharmacol 13(2):111–126, 2005 15943544

Pentikis HS, Simmons RD, Benedict MF, et al: Methylphenidate bioavailability in adults when an extended-release multiparticulate formulation is administered sprinkled on food or as an intact capsule. J Am Acad Child Adolesc Psychiatry 41(4):443–449, 2002 11931601

Perrin JM, Friedman RA, Knilans TK, et al: Cardiovascular monitoring and stimulant drugs for attention-deficit/hyperactivity disorder. Pediatrics 122(2):451–453, 2008 18676566

Prince JB, Wilens TE, Biederman J, et al: Clonidine for sleep disturbances associated with attention-deficit hyperactivity disorder: a systematic chart review of 62 cases. J Am Acad Child Adolesc Psychiatry 35(5):599–605, 1996 8935206

Rapport MD, Jones JT, DuPaul GJ, et al: Attention deficit disorder and methylphenidate: group and single-subject analyses of dose effects on attention in clinic and classroom settings. J Clin Child Psychol 16(4):329–338, 1987

Rapport MD, Stoner G, DuPaul GJ, et al: Attention deficit disorder and methylphenidate: a multilevel analysis of dose-response effects on children's impulsivity across settings. J Am Acad Child Adolesc Psychiatry 27(1):60–69, 1988 3343208

Rapport MD, DuPaul GJ, Kelly KL: Attention deficit hyperactivity disorder and methylphenidate: the relationship between gross body weight and drug response in children. Psychopharmacol Bull 25(2):285–290, 1989 2602521

Riddle MA, Nelson JC, Kleinman CS, et al: Sudden death in children receiving Norpramin: a review of three reported cases and commentary. J Am Acad Child Adolesc Psychiatry 30(1):104–108, 1991 2005044

Scahill L, Chappell PB, Kim YS, et al: A placebo-controlled study of guanfacine in the treatment of children with tic disorders and attention deficit hyperactivity disorder. Am J Psychiatry 158(7):1067–1074, 2001 11431228

Scheffler RM, Brown TT, Fulton BD, et al: Positive association between attention-deficit/hyperactivity disorder medication use and academic achievement during elementary school. Pediatrics 123(5):1273–1279, 2009 19403491

Singer HS, Brown J, Quaskey S, et al: The treatment of attention-deficit hyperactivity disorder in Tourette's syndrome: a double-blind placebo-controlled study with clonidine and desipramine. Pediatrics 95(1):74–81, 1995 7770313

Sonuga-Barke EJ: The dual pathway model of AD/HD: an elaboration of neurodevelopmental characteristics. Neurosci Biobehav Rev 27(7):593–604, 2003 14624804

Spencer T, Biederman J, Wilens T, et al: Pharmacotherapy of attention-deficit hyperactivity disorder across the life cycle. J Am Acad Child Adolesc Psychiatry 35(4):409–432, 1996 8919704

Spencer T, Biederman J, Wilens T: Pharmacotherapy of ADHD: a life span perspective, in American Psychiatric Press Review of Psychiatry, Vol 16. Edited by Dickstein LJ, Riba MB, Oldham JM. Washington, DC, American Psychiatric Press, 1997, pp IV87–IV127

Spencer T, Biederman J, Wilens T, et al: Effectiveness and tolerability of tomoxetine in adults with attention deficit hyperactivity disorder. Am J Psychiatry 155(5):693–695, 1998a 9585725

Spencer T, Biederman J, Wilens T: Growth deficits in children with attention deficit hyperactivity disorder. Pediatrics 102(2 Pt 3):501–506, 1998b 9685453

Spencer T, Biederman M, Coffey B, et al: The 4-year course of tic disorders in boys with attention-deficit/hyperactivity disorder. Arch Gen Psychiatry 56(9):842–847, 1999 12884890

Spencer T, Swanson J, Weidenman M, et al: Pharmacodynamic profile of Ritalin LA, a new extended-release dosage form of Ritalin, in children with ADHD. Presented at the 47th annual meeting of the American Academy of Child and Adolescent Psychiatry, New York, October 2000

Spencer T, Biederman J, Heiligenstein J, et al: An open-label, dose-ranging study of atomoxetine in children with attention deficit hyperactivity disorder. J Child Adolesc Psychopharmacol 11(3):251–265, 2001 11642475

Spencer T, Biederman J, Coffey B, et al: A double-blind comparison of desipramine and placebo in children and adolescents with chronic tic disorder and comorbid attention-deficit/hyperactivity disorder. Arch Gen Psychiatry 59(7):649–656, 2002a 12090818

Spencer T, Heiligenstein JH, Biederman J, et al: Results from 2 proof-of-concept, placebo-controlled studies of atomoxetine in children with attention-deficit/hyperactivity disorder. J Clin Psychiatry 63(12):1140–1147, 2002b 12523874

Spencer T, Newcorn J, Kratochvil CJ, et al: Effects of atomoxetine on growth after 2-year treatment among pediatric patients with attention-deficit/hyperactivity disorder. Pediatrics 116(1):e74–e80, 2005 15995021

Spencer TJ, Greenbaum M, Ginsberg LD, et al: Safety and effectiveness of coadministration of guanfacine extended release and psychostimulants in children and adolescents with attention-deficit/hyperactivity disorder. J Child Adolesc Psychopharmacol 19(5):501–510, 2009 19877974

Spencer TJ, Brown A, Seidman LJ, et al: Effect of psychostimulants on brain structure and function in ADHD: a qualitative literature review of magnetic resonance imaging-based neuroimaging studies. J Clin Psychiatry 74(9):902–917, 2013 24107764

Steingard R, Biederman J, Spencer T, et al: Comparison of clonidine response in the treatment of attention-deficit hyperactivity disorder with and without comorbid tic disorders. J Am Acad Child Adolesc Psychiatry 32(2):350–353, 1993 8444764

Swanson J, Agler D, Fineberg E, et al: University of California, Irvine, laboratory school protocol for pharmacokinetic and pharmacodynamic studies, in Ritalin: Theory and Practice, 2nd Edition. Edited by Greenhill L, Osman BB. Larchmont, NY, Mary Ann Liebert, 2000, pp 405–430

Swanson JM, Greenhill LL, Lopez FA, et al: Modafinil film-coated tablets in children and adolescents with attention-deficit/hyperactivity disorder: results of a randomized, double-blind, placebo-controlled, fixed-dose study followed by abrupt discontinuation. J Clin Psychiatry 67(1):137–147, 2006 16426100

Tourette's Syndrome Study Group: Treatment of ADHD in children with tics: a randomized controlled trial. Neurology 58(4):527–536, 2002 11865128

Vetter VL, Elia J, Erickson C, et al: Cardiovascular monitoring of children and adolescents with heart disease receiving medications for attention deficit/hyperactivity disorder [corrected]: a scientific statement from the American Heart Association Council on Cardiovascular Disease in the Young Congenital Cardiac Defects Committee and the Council on Cardiovascular Nursing. Circulation 117(18):2407–2423, 2008 18427125

Volkow ND, Wang G, Fowler JS, et al: Therapeutic doses of oral methylphenidate significantly increase extracellular dopamine in the human brain. J Neurosci 21(2):RC121(1–5), 2001 11160455

Waxmonsky JG, Waschbusch DA, Akinnusi O, et al: A comparison of atomoxetine administered as once versus twice daily dosing on the school and home functioning of children with attention-deficit/hyperactivity disorder. J Child Adolesc Psychopharmacol 21(1):21–32, 2011 21288121

Wigal S, Swanson JM, Feifel D, et al: A double-blind, placebo-controlled trial of dexmethylphenidate hydrochloride and d,l-threo-methylphenidate hydrochloride in children with attention-deficit/hyperactivity disorder. J Am Acad Child Adolesc Psychiatry 43(11):1406–1414, 2004 15502600

Wigal SB, Childress AC, Belden HW, et al: NWP06, an extended-release oral suspension of methylphenidate, improved attention-deficit/hyperactivity disorder symptoms compared with placebo in a laboratory classroom study. J Child Adolesc Psychopharmacol 23(1):3–10, 2013 23289899

Wigal T, Greenhill L, Chuang S, et al: Safety and tolerability of methylphenidate in preschool children with ADHD. J Am Acad Child Adolesc Psychiatry 45(11):1294–1303, 2006 17028508

Wilens TE, Biederman J: The stimulants. Psychiatr Clin North Am 15(1):191–222, 1992 1347939

Wilens T, Spencer T, Biederman J, et al: A Controlled Trial of Bupropion SR for Attention Deficit Hyperactivity Disorder in Adults. Boca Raton, FL, New Clinical Drug Evaluation Unit Program, 1999

Wilens T, Haight BR, Horrigan JP, et al: Bupropion XL in adults with attention-deficit/hyperactivity disorder: a randomized, placebo-controlled study. Biol Psychiatry 57(7):793–801, 2005 15820237

Wilens TE, Morrison NR, Prince J: An update on the pharmacotherapy of attention-deficit/hyperactivity disorder in adults. Expert Rev Neurother 11(10):1443–1465, 2011 21955201

Wilens TE, Bukstein O, Brams M, et al: A controlled trial of extended-release guanfacine and psychostimulants for attention-deficit/hyperactivity disorder. J Am Acad Child Adolesc Psychiatry 51(1):74–85, 2012 22176941

Wolraich ML, Greenhill LL, Pelham W, et al: Randomized, controlled trial of OROS methylphenidate once a day in children with attention-deficit/hyperactivity disorder. Pediatrics 108(4):883–892, 2001 11581440

Zametkin A, Rapoport JL, Murphy DL, et al: Treatment of hyperactive children with monoamine oxidase inhibitors. I. Clinical efficacy. Arch Gen Psychiatry 42(10):962–966, 1985 3899047

CHAPTER 36

Antidepressants

Graham J. Emslie, M.D.
Paul Croarkin, D.O.
Meredith R. Chapman, M.D.
Taryn L. Mayes, M.S.

Antidepressants are widely used in children and adolescents for a variety of disorders, with significant increases over the past 20 years. Primarily, antidepressants have been used for the same disorders as in adults (depression, anxiety), with additional potential use for attention-deficit/hyperactivity disorder (ADHD), repetitive behaviors (e.g., autism spectrum disorders), and reactive aggression. Newer antidepressants, particularly selective serotonin reuptake inhibitors (SSRIs), have demonstrated efficacy and safety in children and adolescents, with the greatest effect seen in obsessive-compulsive disorder (OCD) and anxiety disorders, followed by major depressive disorder (MDD). Yet limited data are available on pharmacokinetics and dosing in this age group. For example, it is not known whether lower doses may be sufficient in children or whether this age group does, in fact, require adult dosing. Theoretically, children may metabolize medications more quickly because of their proportionally larger liver mass.

Prior to 1995, fewer than 250 children and adolescents with depression had been studied in randomized controlled trials (RCTs). Clearly, widespread use of antidepressants despite lack of evidence of efficacy or safety was a major concern. To address the issue, the U.S. Food and Drug Administration (FDA), through the U.S. Food and Drug Administration Modernization Act of 1997 (U.S. Food and Drug Administration 1997), began requiring additional pediatric data for new compounds that were likely to be used in the pediatric population and encouraging pediatric research on medications with FDA indications for adults that were commonly used for youth. This process substantially increased the amount of research in pediatric pharmacology in general, and with antidepressants in particular. However, problems with the new data included limited research infrastructure (trials included sites with limited pediatric psychiatry experience) and lack of clarity on optimal study design. Furthermore, many of these earlier studies were conducted with short timelines because of limited remaining medication patent time; thus, the incentive was simply to complete the trials, with less emphasis on proving efficacy. Regardless of these limitations, there is now substantial information on use of antidepressants in the pediatric age group, with more than 5,500 children and adolescents participating in antidepressant RCTs by 2009.

Evaluating Antidepressant Studies

It has become increasingly clear that it is not possible to extrapolate from adult data to determine effectiveness and safety of antidepressants in the pediatric population. In evaluating efficacy in the pediatric age group, there appears to be continuity between the child and adult versions of the same disorder in, for example, OCD. This has allowed effectiveness of antidepressants to be proven on the basis of extrapolating from adults and conducting only one bridging study in children (although issues still remain about dosing). Similarly, the effect size in treatment of pediatric anxiety disorders with antidepressants generally has been large (Bridge et al. 2007). However, the lack of efficacy of tricyclic antidepressants (TCAs; the previous gold standard in adults) raised questions about extrapolating from adult efficacy data for MDD in spite of continuity across the life span on the basis of phenomenology and pathophysiology (Birmaher et al. 2007). Thus, in MDD, two positive trials are required in the pediatric population for the medication to receive an FDA pediatric indication.

Pharmacodynamics

Pediatric drug development needs to move beyond the concept of children being "little adults," particularly regarding dosing. The majority of pediatric antidepressant trials were conducted with limited preliminary data on dosing for children. Doses for trials were often determined by adjusting from adult doses on the basis of weight. It is possible that some differences seen in children between antidepressants reflect wrong choice of doses for the trial rather than different levels of effectiveness. Because antidepressants are metabolized primarily in the liver and children have a proportionately large liver mass, half-lives of antidepressants are generally shorter in children. In addition, clinical trials frequently use forced titration of medication, so it remains unclear whether equal effectiveness can be achieved at a lower dose.

Outcome Assessments

Use of outcome assessments as part of routine clinical care is increasingly recommended in adults (Trivedi et al. 2007). However, adult rating scales are not appropriate for children. Thus, child- and adolescent-specific outcome measures have been developed to assess efficacy. For clinicians to interpret clinical trial data, it is necessary to have some familiarity with what is being measured and whether the criterion (e.g., 25% decrease in the Children's Yale-Brown Obsessive Compulsive Scale [CY-BOCS]) is a clinically meaningful change.

Safety

RCTs are the gold standard for assessing not only efficacy but also safety. Without a placebo control, it is very difficult to identify whether adverse events are related to the medication, especially if they occur relatively frequently (e.g., headaches). In large clinical trials of newer antidepressants (both SSRIs and atypical antidepressants) in children and adolescents, rates of discontinuation due to adverse events have generally been low, especially compared with older antidepressants. For example, in the paroxetine adolescent trial, discontinuation from the study was equivalent in the paroxetine and placebo groups (9.7% and 6.9%, respectively) but was substantially higher in the imipramine group (31.5%; Keller et al. 2001).

Antidepressant adverse events in children and adolescents are not the same as in adults. It appears, for example, that increased rates of suicidality reported in children and adolescents treated with antidepressants relative to placebo (Hammad et al. 2006) extend only to age 24 (Friedman and Leon 2007).

The controversy around increases in suicidality in children and adolescents treated with antidepressants also highlighted problems in assessing adverse effects in clinical trials. When the initial reports suggesting increased activation, agitation, and suicidal behavior became available, it became evident that the process of eliciting these events (spontaneous report) and definition of the events (what constitutes a suicide attempt or increased suicidal ideation) were inconsistent across trials and across sites. This resulted in the FDA requesting an independent reanalysis of the adverse event data. Even with the reanalysis and the findings that suicidality (not suicide) occurred in 4% of children on antidepressants compared with 2% on placebo on the basis of spontaneous report, the prospectively collected rating scales from those studies did not demonstrate any difference in suicidality between active treatment and placebo (Bridge et al. 2007; Hammad et al. 2006). These findings highlight the need to assess possible antidepressant-specific adverse events both before and during treatment.

Selective Serotonin Reuptake Inhibitors

The primary mode of action for SSRIs as a class is thought to be presynaptic inhibition of serotonin reuptake. Chronic treatment also down-regulates serotonin receptors in most cases and modulates serotonergic transmission. However, mechanisms extend further than this and vary among SSRIs. For example, some SSRIs inhibit dopamine and norepinephrine transporters as well. They also have differences in antagonism at a variety of receptor sites. SSRIs display a lower side effect profile than TCAs and monoamine oxidase inhibitors (MAOIs), are relatively safe in overdose, and are easily absorbed from the gastrointestinal tract. Table 36–1 provides the formulations and dosing of SSRIs.

General Side Effects

Most side effects manifest within the first few weeks of treatment with an SSRI, but many of these adverse effects will resolve with time. Known side effects of SSRIs include nausea, vomiting, diarrhea, headaches, dizziness, bruxism, somnolence, vivid or strange dreams, changes in appetite, weight loss, weight gain, tremors, akathisia, skin rashes, increased sweating, and mania; how-

TABLE 36–1. Formulations and dosing for selective serotonin reuptake inhibitors

			Target dose, mg		
Medication	**Formulations**	**Initial dose, mg**	**Children**	**Adolescents**	**Maximum dose**
Citalopram	Tablet: 10 mg, 20 mg, 40 mg Solution: 10 mg/5 mL	10	20–40	20–40	40
Escitalopram	Tablet: 5 mg, 10 mg, 20 mg Solution: 5 mg/5 mL	5–10	10–20	10–20	20
Fluoxetine	Capsule: 10 mg, 20 mg, 40 mg Tablet: 10 mg Solution: 20 mg/5 mL	10	20	20–40	60
Fluvoxamine	Tablet: 25 mg, 50 mg, 100 mg	25	50–200	50–200	200 300
Paroxetine	Tablet: 10 mg, 20 mg, 30 mg, 40 mg Tablet CR: 12.5 mg, 25 mg, 37.5 mg Suspension: 10 mg/5 mL	10	10–30	20–40	50
Sertraline	Tablet: 25 mg, 50 mg, 100 mg Solution: 20 mg/mL	12.5–25	50–200	50–200	200

Note. CR=controlled release.

ever, there is a great deal of individual variation among patients. SSRIs may increase the risk of bleeding, especially in patients taking aspirin or nonsteroidal anti-inflammatory medications. Sexual side effects are also common, including decreased libido, anorgasmia, and erectile dysfunction. As noted, SSRIs, along with all antidepressants, carry a risk of increased suicidal thinking and behaviors. Therefore, careful monitoring of suicidality, especially during initial stages of treatment and following dose adjustments, is necessary.

Flu-like discontinuation symptoms (e.g., headache, diarrhea, nausea, vomiting, chills, dizziness, fatigue) may occur when suddenly stopping SSRI medications. This is more common in agents with short half-lives. Fortunately, SSRIs also have a higher margin of safety in overdose compared with TCAs and MAOIs. However, deaths have been reported with large ingestions of SSRIs (either alone or in combination with other medications).

Contraindications

SSRIs should not be taken with any of the MAOIs, as this combination may lead to confusion, high blood pressure, tremor, and hyperactivity. In addition, tryptophan can cause headaches, nausea, sweating, and dizziness when taken with an SSRI. Patients taking pimozide also should not take SSRIs. Although rare, co-administration with tramadol hydrochloride (a centrally acting analgesic sometimes used for chronic pain) can cause seizures.

Efficacy

SSRIs are the first-line medication treatment for youth with MDD, OCD, and other anxiety disorders (Birmaher et al. 2007; Cheung et al. 2007; Connolly et al. 2007; Hughes et al. 2007). In a meta-analysis of all newer antidepressants, Bridge and colleagues found that pooled benefit-risk difference favored SSRIs for MDD (11%; 95% confidence interval [CI], 6%–15%), OCD (19.8%; 95% CI, 13%–26.6%), and other anxiety disorders (40%; 95% CI, 31%–48%) (Bridge et al. 2007). Table 36–2 lists the approved indications for SSRIs. SSRIs also have potential utility in several other areas, including OCD spectrum disorders, autism spectrum disorders, aggression, eating disorders, ADHD, and psychiatric symptoms related to medical conditions. However, few controlled trials have been conducted in these areas. Information on specific SSRI antidepressants is detailed in the following sections.

Citalopram

Chemical Structure and Pharmacology

Citalopram is a racemic bicyclic phthalane derivative. Its structure is chemically unrelated to other antidepressants. It is the most selective of all SSRIs. It has a greater than 3,000-fold potency for inhibiting serotonin reuptake as compared with norepinephrine and a greater than 20,000-fold potency compared with dopamine reuptake (Hyttel et al. 1995). Citalopram's S-(+) enantiomer inhibits serotonin reuptake. Its R-(-) enantiomer is inactive. In animal studies, there is an increase in extracellular serotonin following administration. This, in turn, activates serotonin type 1A (5-HT_{1A}) autoreceptors. It is thought that this leads to a feedback inhibition of the raphe nuclei and downregulation of autoreceptors, with an increase in serotonergic activity.

Pharmacokinetics

Citalopram is easily absorbed after oral intake, with a bioavailability of 80%. Food does not affect its absorption. Peak

TABLE 36–2. U.S. Food and Drug Administration (FDA) indications for selective serotonin reuptake inhibitors

Medication	FDA-approved indication	Indication age range
Citalopram (Celexa)	Depression	Adults
Escitalopram (Lexapro)	Depression	12 years to adult
	GAD	Adults
Fluoxetine (Prozac)	Bulimia	Adults
	Depression	8 years to adult
	OCD	7 years to adult
	PD	Adults
	Depressive episodes (bipolar disorder)	Adults
Fluvoxamine (Luvox)	OCD	8 years to adult
Paroxetine (Paxil)	Depression	Adults
	GAD	Adults
	OCD	Adults
	PD	Adults
	PMDD	Adults
	PTSD	Adults
	SOC	Adults
Sertraline (Zoloft)	Depression	Adults
	OCD	6 years to adult
	PD	Adults
	PMDD	Adults
	PTSD	Adults
	SOC	Adults

Note. GAD=generalized anxiety disorder; OCD=obsessive-compulsive disorder; PD=panic disorder; PMDD=premenstrual dysphoric disorder; PTSD=posttraumatic stress disorder; SOC=social anxiety disorder.

plasma levels are achieved after 2–4 hours with single or multiple doses (Bezchlibnyk-Butler et al. 2000). The mean peak plasma concentration (C_{max}) with a dose of 40 mg daily at steady state is 311 nmo/L. Its volume of distribution (V_d) is 12–16 L/kg. Citalopram is estimated to be 80% protein bound, which is less than other SSRIs. Citalopram is thought to have a low liability for drug interactions via protein-binding interactions, P-glycoprotein, or renal clearance. It is also believed to have a wide margin of safety if plasma levels rise. It is affected little by first-pass metabolism and drug-drug interactions involving protein binding (Baumann and Larsen 1995). Table 36–3 provides the pharmacodynamic and pharmacokinetic data for citalopram and other SSRIs.

There are two pharmacokinetic studies of citalopram in children and adolescents, with varying results. The first study, which compared the pharmacokinetic data of adolescents and adults, found that citalopram's half-life was 38.4 hours in adolescents and 44 hours in adults. A second study, which included children and adolescents (ages 9–17 years), displayed a half-life of 16.9 hours after a 20 mg dose and 19.2 hours after multiple doses, which was substantially shorter than in

TABLE 36–3. Pharmacodynamics and pharmacokinetics of selective serotonin reuptake inhibitors

Medication	Half-life	Time to steady state	CYP enzyme inhibited	Kinetics
Citalopram	20 hours	6–10 days	2D6 (weak)	Linear
Escitalopram	27–32 hours	7 days	2D6 (weak)	Linear
Fluoxetine	4–6 days	>4 weeks	1A2 (weak) 2B6 (moderate) 2C9 (moderate) 3A4 (moderate) 2C19 (potent) 2D6 (potent)	Nonlinear
Fluvoxamine	15 hours	10 days	2D6 (weak) 3A4 (moderate) 2C9 (moderate) 2B6 (moderate) 2C19 (moderate) 1A2 (potent)	Nonlinear
Paroxetine	21 hours	7–14 days	1A2 (weak) 2C9 (weak) 2C19 (weak) 3A4 (moderate) 2B6 (potent) 2D6 (potent)	Nonlinear
Sertraline	26 hours	5–7 days	1A2 (weak) 3A4 (moderate) 2B6 (moderate) 2D6 (moderate at low doses, potent at high doses)	Linear

Note. CYP=cytochrome P450.

previous studies of drug half-life in adults. Investigators have questioned whether twice daily dosing for youth may improve efficacy, although this has not yet been studied (Findling et al. 2006a).

Adverse Effects Profile

Citalopram is generally safe and well tolerated at dosages of 20–40 mg/day. Because of its low liability for drug interactions, it is an ideal choice for patients requiring multiple medications. However, use with any other serotonergic agent should be undertaken only with caution given the potential for serotonin syndrome. Citalopram is relatively safe with large ingestions, although fatal ingestions of 840–4,000 mg have been reported in adults (Luchini et al. 2005). Convulsions can develop with doses exceeding 600 mg, and ventricular fibrillation occurred in a 2 g ingestion (Personne et al. 1997).

The FDA has recommended that citalopram should no longer be used at doses greater than 40 mg because of potential electrical activity abnormalities in the heart. Furthermore, because of potential QT prolongation, citalopram is not recommended for individuals with certain heart conditions that could lead to torsade de pointes, a potentially fatal abnormal heart rhythm (U.S. Food and Drug Administration 2012).

Efficacy

The only two RCTs conducted in pediatric patients with MDD had inconsistent findings. Wagner et al. (2004b) reported greater improvement of depressive symptoms with citalopram compared with placebo as early as week 1, which persisted throughout the study. A second study, however, showed no difference between citalopram and placebo on any outcome measures. In this study, which was conducted internationally, both inpatients and outpatients were enrolled in the study, suggesting a potentially more severe population. In addition, approximately two-thirds of subjects were receiving psychotherapy during the study. Although not powered to detect a significant difference in the subgroup of subjects who did not receive psychotherapy, citalopram treatment showed greater response rate than placebo (41% vs. 25%). On the other hand, in subjects receiving psychotherapy, there was no significant difference between active medication and placebo (44% vs. 53%). The results are difficult to interpret because of the limited available data, the fact that both inpatients and outpatients were used, and the inclusion of psychotherapy for most patients (von Knorring et al. 2006).

Escitalopram

Chemical Structure and Pharmacology

Escitalopram is the active (S)-enantiomer of citalopram, which has been shown to be twice as potent as citalopram with respect to serotonin inhibition (Aronson and Delgado 2004). With oral administration of 10 mg, it is rapidly and almost entirely absorbed and achieves peak plasma concentrations of 10–30 ng/mL in approximately 2–6 hours (Table 36–3) (Rao 2007). Its affinity for dopamine and norepinephrine receptors is negligible. Like citalopram, escitalopram inhibits serotonin reuptake. Radioligand single-photon emission computed tomography studies of patients receiving escitalopram or citalopram indicated that serotonin transporter occupancy in the midbrain was higher with escitalopram (Klein et al. 2007).

Pharmacokinetics

The pharmacokinetics of escitalopram are very similar to those of citalopram. Pharmacokinetic studies in pediatrics are limited. One study with a single dose of 10 mg given to 11 teenagers and 12 adults found that the half-life of escitalopram was 19 hours in adolescents and 28.9 hours in adults. Total blood levels were 15% greater in adults than adolescents (Findling et al. 2006a).

Adverse Effects Profile

Escitalopram's adverse event profile is similar to that of other SSRIs. It is relatively safe with large ingestions, and there have been no deaths or adverse events in published reports of overdoses up to 300 mg (LoVecchio et al. 2006).

Efficacy

Two RCTs have been conducted with escitalopram in youth with MDD. Although the first study, which included both children and adolescents, was negative, there was some evidence of efficacy for the adolescent subgroup on several secondary outcomes (Wagner et al. 2006). As a result of the potential utility in adolescents, a trial of adolescents only (*N*=312) was completed. Results demonstrated positive efficacy on several outcomes (Emslie et al. 2009). A recent study of continuation treatment in adolescents with depression (ages 12–17 years) also showed greater improvement with escitalopram over placebo during 24 weeks of continuation treatment (Findling et al. 2013). In 2009 escitalopram received an FDA-approved indication for treatment of depression in adolescents. No placebo-controlled RCTs of escitalopram have been conducted in any other pediatric psychiatric disorders.

Fluoxetine

Chemical Structure and Pharmacology

Fluoxetine's chemistry is similar to that of diphenhydramine, but its pharmacological activity is very different. Its structure is unique among antidepressants. However, like other SSRIs, fluoxetine appears to target the serotonin transporter, thereby inhibiting serotonin reuptake. Fluoxetine's inhibition decreases further release of serotonin, inhibits firing in the dorsal raphe nuclei, down-regulates serotonin autoreceptors, and increases serotonergic transmission in the hippocampus. Fluoxetine does not have clinically significant noradrenergic or dopaminergic activity. Its binding at muscarinic, histaminergic, and α_1-adrenergic receptors is minimal and much less than that of TCAs (DeVane 1998).

Pharmacokinetics

Fluoxetine is almost totally absorbed with oral administration. Food can decrease the rate but not the degree of absorption. Its bioavailability is less than 90% because of first-pass effect. It is lipophilic and has a volume of distribution of 14–100 L/kg. This surpasses all other SSRIs. Fluoxetine's long half-life (Table 36–4) makes withdrawal or discontinuation effects unlikely, but it requires an extensive washout period before starting medications with drug-drug interactions. Patients with renal failure have little difficulty metabolizing this drug; however, liver damage reduces plasma clearance of fluoxetine (Hiemke and Härtter 2000).

One pharmacokinetic study of 10 children (ages 6–12) and 11 adolescents (ages 13–18) with OCD or MDD demonstrated higher concentrations of fluoxetine and norfluoxetine in children than adolescents. After correcting for weight, this difference was not significant. Population analysis also indicated that oral clearance, absorption rate constant, and volume of distribution were not significantly different from those of adults (Findling et al. 2006a). No relationship

TABLE 36–4. U.S. Food and Drug Administration (FDA) indications for atypical antidepressants

Medication	Drug class	FDA-approved indication (adults only)
Bupropion (Wellbutrin)	NDRI	Depression
Desvenlafaxine (Pristiq)	SNRI	Depression, vasomotor symptoms associated with menopause
Duloxetine (Cymbalta)	SSNRI	Depression, GAD, diabetic peripheral neuropathic pain, fibromyalgia, chronic musculoskeletal pain
Levomilnacipran (Fetzima)	SSNRI	Depression
Mirtazapine (Remeron)	NaSSA	Depression
Trazodone (Desyrel)	SARI	Depression
Venlafaxine (Effexor)	SSNRI	Depression, GAD
Vilazodone (Viibryd)	SSRI and partial 5-HT_{1A} agonist	Depression
Vortioxetine (Brintellix)	SMS	Depression

Note. GAD=generalized anxiety disorder; NaSSA=noradrenergic and specific serotonergic antidepressant; NDRI=norepinephrine-dopamine reuptake inhibitor; SARI=serotonin agonist and serotonin reuptake inhibitor; SSNRI=selective serotonin-norepinephrine reuptake inhibitor; SMS=serotonin modulator and stimulator.

between fluoxetine levels and efficacy or safety has been found (Blázquez et al. 2014; Koelch et al. 2012).

Adverse Effects Profile

Overall, fluoxetine is well tolerated, and side effects parallel other SSRIs. Fluoxetine has a high margin of safety in overdose. One patient ingested 8 g and survived. However, deaths have been reported in patients ingesting as little as 520 mg. The largest known pediatric ingestion is 3 g (patient recovered).

Fluoxetine should not be used in combination with any MAOI or within a minimum of 14 days of discontinuing an MAOI. Furthermore, fluoxetine should be discontinued for at least 5 weeks before starting an MAOI.

Efficacy

To date, three large RCTs in pediatric MDD have been conducted with fluoxetine, with all three demonstrating superiority over placebo (Emslie et al. 1997, 2002; March et al. 2004). It is the only antidepressant to demonstrate efficacy in more than one RCT in pediatric MDD. Only one small RCT of fluoxetine (n=40) has failed to demonstrate a positive response over placebo. However, the results of this study are difficult to interpret because of the small sample size and incompletely described methodology (Simeon et al. 1990).

Unlike some of the other SSRIs, fluoxetine appears to be equally effective in the younger age group (<12 years) as in adolescents. Random regression of the Children's Depression Rating Scale, Revised (CDRS-R) showed a treatment group by age group interaction ($f_{1,338}=4.10$, $P=.044$), indicating that the treatment effect was significantly more pronounced in children than adolescents (Mayes et al. 2007). Bridge et al. (2007) confirmed this in their meta-analysis, indicating that in children younger than age 12 with MDD, only fluoxetine showed benefit over placebo.

Fluoxetine has also been studied in three RCTs of children and adolescents with OCD, totaling 160 subjects (Geller et al. 2001; Liebowitz et al. 2002; Riddle et al. 1992). In the largest of the three studies (n=103), response was significantly greater with fluoxetine compared with placebo (49% vs. 25%; P=0.03) (Geller et al. 2001).

Three RCTs of other anxiety disorders have also demonstrated efficacy for fluoxetine in youth. In a small trial (n=15) of selective mutism plus social phobia in 6- to 11-year-olds, fluoxetine was more efficacious than placebo in improving anxiety and mutism (Black and Uhde 1994). In a larger study of generalized anxiety disorder (GAD), social phobia, and separation anxiety in 74 children and adolescents, fluoxetine led to greater response rates than placebo for GAD (67% vs. 36%; P=0.04) and social phobia (76% vs. 21%; P<0.001) but not for separation anxiety (54% vs. 41%; not significant). Across all disorders, fluoxetine was superior to placebo (61% vs. 35%; P=0.03) (Birmaher et al. 2003). In a study comparing fluoxetine (n=10), clomipramine (n=9), and placebo (n=11) in youth (ages 7–17 years) with GAD, separation anxiety, or social phobia, all three groups showed significant improvement after 12 weeks of treatment. Fluoxetine was superior to placebo but not to clomipramine, but no differences were seen between clomipramine and placebo (da Costa et al. 2013).

Finally, liquid fluoxetine was superior to placebo in reducing repetitive behaviors in 45 children and adolescents with autism in a double-blind, placebo-controlled crossover study (Hollander et al. 2005).

Thus, fluoxetine is the only antidepressant to have more than one positive RCT for MDD, OCD, and anxiety disorders. It is the only antidepressant with an FDA-approved indication for treatment of depression in both children and adolescents and is one of three antidepressants with an FDA indication for treatment of pediatric OCD. It may also be beneficial in improving OCD symptoms associated with other disorders (e.g., repetitive symptoms associated with autism).

Fluvoxamine

Chemical Structure and Pharmacology

Fluvoxamine maleate is a 2-aminoethyl oxime ether of aralkylketone with a structure that is unique among other SSRIs and TCAs. Fluvoxamine's mechanism of action is similar to that of other SSRIs. It inhibits the presynaptic reuptake of serotonin in brain neurons, thereby enhancing serotonergic transmission. Fluvoxamine has no clinically significant affinity for histaminergic, alpha- or beta-adrenergic, muscarinic, or dopaminergic receptors.

Pharmacokinetics

After oral ingestion, fluvoxamine is easily, and more than 90%, absorbed. Food does not affect its bioavailability, which is approximately 53% because of fast and extensive first-pass metabolism. Nearly 100% of orally administered fluvoxamine is excreted in the urine, but only minute amounts are unchanged. Gender differences in metabolism have been reported at dosages of 100 mg/day, with blood levels significantly higher in female subjects. This effect attenuates if the daily dose is doubled (Hiemke and Härtter 2000). Multiple-dose studies of children and adolescents indicate that steady-state plasma concentrations are significantly higher in children than adolescents. Peak plasma concentrations are significantly higher in female children compared with male children, but there are no gender differences in adolescents. Thus, female children may need lower doses, although this has not yet been studied. In adolescents, steady-state concentrations of fluvoxamine are similar to those in adults after 300 mg (Labellarte et al. 2004).

Fluvoxamine has multiple cytochrome P450 interactions. Clinicians should consult references for drug-drug interactions and maintain a high index of caution.

Adverse Effects Profile

The most common side effects of fluvoxamine are sleep disturbances (either somnolence or insomnia). Fluvoxamine is thought to have the lowest incidence of sexual side effects of all the SSRIs. Its cytochrome P450 inhibition should be considered when co-administering with other agents. Otherwise, its side effect profile is similar to other SSRIs. In overdoses, fluvoxamine appears to have a wide margin of safety, as patients ingesting up to 9 g have had mild symptoms and a complete recovery (Henry 1991).

Efficacy

Fluvoxamine has an FDA-approved indication for the treatment of childhood OCD. In a multicenter RCT, fluvoxamine-treated subjects showed statistically significant improvements compared with placebo on the primary outcome (CY-BOCS) at weeks 1, 4, 6, and 10. The active treatment group also displayed significantly greater improvement than placebo in secondary efficacy measures (National Institute of Mental Health Global Obsessive-Compulsive Scale and Clinical Global Impressions Scale) at all postrandomization visits (Riddle et al. 2001). Fluvoxamine has also demonstrated greater reduction in anxiety symptoms compared with placebo in a study of youth with social phobia, separation anxiety, or GAD (The Research Unit on Pediatric Psychopharmacology Anxiety Study Group 2001). However, a pilot trial of sequential treatment for 25 children with comorbid ADHD and anxiety showed no benefit in adding fluvoxamine for subjects on stimulants with stable ADHD symptoms but with ongoing anxiety (Abikoff et al. 2005).

Most studies of SSRIs in autism spectrum disorder in children have not been promising (McDougle et al. 2000). However, one study suggested that genetic polymorphisms of the serotonin transporter gene promoter region (5-HTTLPR) may affect response to fluvoxamine in young patients with autism (Sugie et al. 2005).

Fluvoxamine has not been studied in pediatric depression.

Paroxetine

Chemical Structure and Pharmacology

Paroxetine hydrochloride is a pure enantiomer salt of a phenylpiperidine compound and is structurally unrelated to other antidepressants. Among the SSRIs, it is the most potent serotonin and norepinephrine reuptake inhibitor. Its muscarinic acetylcholine antagonism also rivals that of TCAs and surpasses desipramine and maprotiline. However, it has minimal affinity for histamine; α_1-, α_2-, or α-adrenergic; dopamine (D_1 or D_2); and serotonin (5-HT_1 and 5-HT_2) receptors (Hiemke and Härtter 2000).

Pharmacokinetics

Paroxetine is easily and almost completely absorbed after oral administration. Calculations of bioavailability range from 50% to 100% in normal volunteers (DeVane 1992). Food does not affect absorption. Paroxetine is subject to first-pass metabolism. At least one-third of ingested paroxetine is excreted through feces, with less than 1% of this amount being unaffected drug. Paroxetine is highly lipophilic (at least 95% protein bound) and has a large volume of distribution (2–12 L/kg). Unlike fluoxetine and sertraline, paroxetine's metabolites have no activity related to monoamine reuptake (DeVane 1992; Hiemke and Härtter 2000).

Like other SSRIs, paroxetine's effects are thought to relate to its inhibition of the serotonin transporter leading to increased synaptic serotonin levels. It differs from other SSRIs in that it has the most potent serotonergic blockade and antagonistic activity at the norepinephrine transporter (DeVane 1992; Hiemke and Härtter 2000).

Paroxetine pharmacokinetics in children have been examined in two studies. The first was a single-dose (10 mg) study of 30 depressed subjects (ages 6–17). The average half-life was 11.1 hours, with a wide range. Investigators also found that metabolism correlated with CYP2D6 phenotype. Subsequently, blood levels were collected weekly during 8 weeks of treatment. Youth who had a dose increase had a nearly sevenfold increase in paroxetine blood levels (Findling et al. 1999, 2006b). Another study involved a 6-week trial of patients with MDD or OCD with 27 children (ages 7–11) and 35 adolescents (ages 12–17). This study also supported the idea that paroxetine has nonlinear kinetics and that optimal treatment for younger children may involve smaller doses (Findling et al. 2006b).

Adverse Effects Profile

Paroxetine's side effects are similar to other SSRIs. Because of its short half-life in children, its discontinuation symptoms are thought to be more severe than with other SSRIs. Thus, slow tapering is recommended to avoid psychological or somatic discontinuation symptoms. Paroxetine is relatively safe in large ingestions. Ingestions of 100–800 mg of paroxetine have been reported in children, with no resultant deaths or serious sequelae (Myers and Krenzelok 1997).

Efficacy

Three RCTs have been conducted in pediatric MDD with inconsistent findings. A study including only adolescents (N=275) demonstrated efficacy on some outcomes, although the primary outcome was negative (Keller et al. 2001). Two other RCTs of paroxetine, however, were negative on all outcome measures. In one of these studies, older adolescents (≥16 years) showed greater response to active treatment than placebo, suggesting that the older age group may be more responsive to this medication (Berard et al. 2006). In addition, in the study that included both children and adolescents, children had significantly higher dropout rates due to adverse events with paroxetine than with placebo. It is difficult to interpret efficacy outcomes for the younger age group because of the high dropout rates. It is possible that smaller doses may be beneficial in prepubertal children (Emslie et al. 2006).

One multicenter RCT of paroxetine has been conducted in pediatric OCD. The mean difference in decrease in scores on the CY-BOCS between paroxetine and placebo showed statistically significant superiority for paroxetine. Further, on three of six secondary efficacy measures paroxetine was statistically significantly better than placebo. However, similar to the pediatric MDD trial, 10% of the paroxetine-treated patients withdrew early because of adverse events (Geller et al. 2004). Unlike fluoxetine, fluvoxamine, and sertraline, which all received an FDA pediatric indication following one positive RCT, paroxetine does not have an FDA-approved indication for treatment of pediatric OCD.

One multicenter RCT examined paroxetine in children and adolescents with social anxiety disorder and reported greater improvement with paroxetine than placebo at all time points (Wagner et al. 2004a).

Sertraline

Chemical Structure and Pharmacology

Sertraline is the second most potent SSRI (second to paroxetine) and the only SSRI with affinity for dopamine receptors. It is similar to paroxetine in that it has two chiral centers. The marketed preparation of this drug contains only the more potent enantiomer (1S, 4S). It has no clinically relevant affinity for β-adrenergic, histaminergic, γ-aminobutyric acid (GABA), or benzodiazepine receptors. However, its α_1 antagonism is at least 10 times greater than that of other SSRIs. This antagonism apparently causes no significant cardiac effects such as hypotension or tachycardia (DeVane et al. 2002; Hiemke and Härtter 2000).

Pharmacokinetics

Unlike other SSRIs, food intake significantly increases sertraline's maximum plasma levels (by approximately 25%) and reduces time to peak plasma concentrations. Sertraline is 98% protein bound (DeVane et al. 2002; Hiemke and Härtter 2000).

One pharmacokinetic study of 29 children (ages 6–12) and 32 adolescents (ages 13–17) with OCD and MDD suggested that at daily doses of 200 mg, half-lives were similar to those for adults (26 hours for children and 27 hours for adolescents). Children appeared to have higher peak plasma concentrations, but this was likely due to body weight differences. Studies suggest that lower doses of sertraline will have decreased half-lives in adolescents. Hence, twice-daily dosing may be considered in doses less than 200 mg (Axelson et al. 2002; Findling et al. 2006a). In a naturalistic study of 90 children and adolescents treated with sertraline, serum concentrations were not associated with efficacy. However, youth with side effects had significantly greater sertraline serum concentrations than those without side effects (Taurines et al. 2013).

Adverse Effects Profile

Sertraline's side effects are similar to those of other SSRIs. Sertraline appears to be relatively safe in large overdoses, although death has been reported in some adult patients following large doses.

Efficacy

Two identical RCTs were conducted to compare sertraline and placebo in children and adolescents with MDD. Although the two studies individually did not demonstrate significant differences between sertraline and placebo, the combined studies found sertraline to be superior to placebo in improving MDD symptoms. Of interest is that greater differences were noted in adolescents than in children (Wagner et al. 2003).

In a large RCT involving 187 children and adolescents with OCD (ages 6–17 years), sertraline led to greater improvement in OCD symptoms than placebo at week 3, which persisted through the remaining 9 weeks of the study (March et al. 1998). On the basis of this study, sertraline received FDA approval for an indication in the treatment of pediatric OCD.

Sertraline has also been examined as part of the Pediatric Obsessive-Compulsive Disorder Treatment Study (POTS), which compared sertraline alone, cognitive-behavioral therapy (CBT) alone, combined sertraline and CBT, and pill placebo for 12 weeks in 112 children and adolescents. Combined treatment, CBT, and sertraline each displayed statistically meaningful benefit versus placebo, with combined treatment being superior to both of the individual modalities. Individual sertraline and CBT treatments did not display statistically significant differences compared with each other. The investigators concluded that initial treatment for children and adolescents with OCD should consist of sertraline plus CBT or CBT alone (Pediatric OCD Treatment Study Team 2004). In another study, 47 youth (ages 7–17 years) with OCD were randomly assigned to standard dosing of sertraline, slow dosing of sertraline, or placebo, with all youth receiving CBT. In this smaller study, there was no evidence of greater improvement with sertraline over placebo when added to CBT (Storch et al. 2013).

Other anxiety disorders have also been examined. Children and adolescents (n=488) with separation anxiety disorder, generalized anxiety disorder, or social phobia were randomly assigned to CBT, sertraline, combination CBT plus sertraline, or a placebo drug for 12 weeks. Combination treatment was more effective than both monotherapies and placebo, with 80.7% responding. Response rates were also higher for both CBT (59.7%) and sertraline alone (54.9%) than placebo (23.7%) (Walkup et al. 2008).

In contrast, sertraline in conjunction with trauma-focused CBT (TF-CBT) was no more effective than TF-CBT plus placebo in a pilot study of 24 female subjects (ages 10–17) with posttraumatic stress disorder (PTSD) related to a history of sexual abuse. Although the study was underpowered, the authors concluded that for children with PTSD, evidence suggests that an initial trial of an evidence-based psychotherapy is warranted prior to treatment with an SSRI (Cohen et al. 2007).

Finally, a small study of 22 children and adolescents with GAD demonstrated some superiority of sertraline over placebo, although this study warrants replication with a larger sample (Rynn et al. 2001).

Atypical Antidepressants

Atypical antidepressants, including bupropion, desvenlafaxine, duloxetine, mirtazapine, trazodone, and venlafaxine, have unique mechanisms. Although they are widely used in clinical practice and have FDA-approved indications for some adult disorders (Table 36–4), limited data are available regarding use in children and adolescents. In addition, three newer antidepressants (vilazodone, vortioxetine, and levomilnacipran) have FDA-approved indications for treatment of MDD in adults, although they have not been evaluated in youth and are less widely used. Table 36–5 describes the formulations and recommended dosing for the atypical antidepressants used in children and adolescents. Of note, nefazodone (a mixed serotonin antagonist and reuptake inhibitor) is also an atypical antidepressant; however, because Serzone has been taken off the market in the United States because of the risk of hepatotoxicity, nefazodone is not recommended for children and adolescents, and therefore it will not be reviewed in this chapter.

General Side Effects

Atypical antidepressants display a lower side effect profile than TCAs and MAOIs. Generally, these medications

TABLE 36–5. Formulations and dosing for atypical antidepressants

Medication	Formulations	Initial dose, mg	Target dose, mg		
			Children	Adolescents	Maximum dose
Bupropion, bupropion SR	Tablet: 75 mg, 100 mg Tablet ER: 100 mg, 150 mg, 200 mg	100	150–300	300	300
Bupropion XL	Tablet ER: 150 mg, 300 mg	150	150–300	450	450
Desvenlafaxine	Tablet ER: 50 mg, 100 mg	50	50	50–100	100
Duloxetine	Capsule: 20 mg, 30 mg, 60 mg	20 bid	40–60	40–60	60
Levomilnacipran	Capsule ER: 20 mg, 40 mg, 80 mg, 120 mg	20 bid for 2 days then 40	40–120	40–120	120
Mirtazapine	Tablet: 15 mg, 30 mg, 45 mg Tablet (dissolving): 15 mg, 30 mg, 45 mg	7.5–15	15–45	15–45	45
Trazodone	Tablet: 50 mg, 100 mg, 150 mg, 300 mg	25–50	100–150	100–150	150
Venlafaxine XR	Capsule: 37.5 mg, 75 mg, 150 mg	37.5	150–225	150–225	300
Vilazodone	Tablet: 10 mg, 20 mg, 40 mg	10	15–30	30–40	40
Vortioxetine	Tablet: 5 mg, 10 mg, 15 mg, 20 mg	10	20	20	20

Note. bid=twice a day; ER=extended release; SR=sustained release; XL=extended release; XR=extended release.

(except trazodone) have no sexual side effects but otherwise share similar untoward effects as the SSRIs. Most side effects manifest within the first few weeks of treatment, and while there is a great deal of individual variation, most resolve with time. Ideally, atypical antidepressants are tapered slowly to avoid discontinuation symptoms. These symptoms are most pronounced with venlafaxine. These novel antidepressants have a higher margin of safety in overdoses compared with TCAs and MAOIs. However, in some cases deaths have been reported with large ingestions.

Contraindications

Atypical antidepressants should not be taken with any of the MAOIs (or within 2 weeks of beginning or discontinuing MAOIs), as these combinations may lead to confusion, high blood pressure, tremor, hyperactivity, and death. In addition, tryptophan can cause headaches, nausea, sweating, and dizziness when taken concurrently with these antidepressants. Although rare, co-administration with tramadol hydrochloride can cause seizures. Bupropion should not be given to patients with eating disorders, epilepsy, or high risk for seizures. Given some evidence of potential increases in blood pressure with venlafaxine and duloxetine, blood pressure should be monitored at each visit during initiation of and dose changes with venlafaxine and duloxetine. If blood pressure remains stable within a few weeks of medication changes, periodic monitoring (e.g., every 6–12 months) is adequate if no other clinical indications warrant increased monitoring.

Efficacy

Each of these agents has an FDA-approved indication for the treatment of major depressive disorder in adults, and some have additional indications (Table 36–4). Currently, there are no approved indications for children and adolescents, and data supporting their pediatric efficacy are limited. However, on the basis of current guidelines from the Texas Children's Medication Algorithm Project for childhood MDD, bupropion, venlafaxine, mirtazapine, and duloxetine are stage 3 interventions. This means that depressed children should have failed at least two adequate trials of SSRIs prior to treatment with these novel agents (Hughes et al. 2007). In a meta-analysis of all newer antidepressants, Bridge and colleagues found that the pooled benefit-risk difference favored antidepressants (including SSRIs and atypical antidepressants) for MDD, OCD, and anxiety disorders. Of note, for depression this analysis included one trial of nefazodone and two trials each of mirtazapine and venlafaxine. The anxiety disorder analysis included two venlafaxine trials: one in GAD and one for social anxiety disorder (Bridge et al. 2007). Table 36–6 describes pharmacokinetics for atypical antidepressants. Further information on specific atypical antidepressants is provided in the following sections.

Bupropion

Chemical Structure and Pharmacology

Bupropion is a structurally novel antidepressant that resembles diethylpropion and is related to phenylethylamine. It is classified as a monocyclic phenylbutylamine aminoketone and is highly lipophilic. Bupropion was originally synthesized with the hopes of creating a compound with antidepressant activity but divergent pharmacology from TCAs and MAOIs. Bupropion is a norepinephrine and dopamine reuptake inhibitor. Its effects on serotonin are negligible. It

TABLE 36–6. Pharmacodynamics and pharmacokinetics of atypical antidepressants

Medication	Half-life	Time to steady state	CYP enzyme inhibited	Kinetics
Bupropion	Biphasic: 1.5 hours 14 hours	8 days	2D6 (potent)	Linear
Bupropion SR	21 hours	8 days	2D6 (potent)	Linear
Desvenlafaxine	11 hours	4–5 days	Primarily metabolized by UGT conjugation and CYP 3A4 (minor) No inhibition	Linear
Duloxetine	12.5 hours	3 days	1A2 (potent) 2D6 (potent)	Linear
Levomilnacipran	12 hours	Unknown	3A4	Linear
Mirtazapine	20–40 hours	4 days	No known inhibition substrate for 1A2, 2D6, 3A4	Linear
Trazodone	Biphasic: 3–6 hours 5–9 hours	Unknown	No known inhibition substrate for 3A4, 2D6	Nonlinear
Venlafaxine XR	10.3 hours	3 days	2D6 (weak) 3A4 (weak)	Linear
Vilazodone	25 hours	3 days	Minor induction CYP2C19 CYP2C8 inhibition	Linear
Vortioxetine	57–66 hours	2 weeks	2D6	Linear

Note. CYP=cytochrome P450; SR=sustained release; XR=extended release.

does not have cholinergic activity and is not sympathomimetic (DeVane 1998). It is marketed in immediate-, sustained-, and extended-release forms.

Pharmacokinetics

Bupropion has rapid absorption after oral administration. It is 80% protein bound and has a bioavailability of 90% and a volume of distribution of 27–60 L/kg. Administration with food has no clinically significant effects on absorption or metabolism. Hepatic impairment appears to extend the half-life of this drug. The effects of renal disease are unknown, but this could likely delay elimination as well (DeVane 1998).

Pharmacokinetic studies have been conducted with adolescent smokers. No differences were found between smoking and nonsmoking adolescents in a study of 75 subjects. However, female adolescents had significantly higher blood levels, a larger volume of distribution, and longer half-lives than males. Bupropion clearance normalized with body weight and did not differ with gender. Although the pharmacokinetics of bupropion in adolescents and adults are similar, studies involving its metabolite, hydroxybupropion, have shown significant differences in adults and adolescents (Daviss et al. 2006; Hsyu et al. 1997; Stewart et al. 2001).

Adverse Effects Profile

Seizures have occurred with bupropion and are thought to be dose related. At 300 mg/day, the risk for seizure is 0.1%. This increases to 0.4% at dosages of 400 mg/day. Bupropion is contraindicated in patients with epilepsy or eating disorders or other individuals at risk for seizures. In addition, co-administration with tramadol hydrochloride can cause seizures. This medication can also precipitate mania, but this may be less likely than with SSRIs. Large overdoses of bupropion appear to be nonlethal.

Efficacy

No double-blind, placebo-controlled RCTs of bupropion for anxiety disorders or depression have been conducted in pediatric psychiatry. Bupropion has been shown to have equal efficacy and safety to methylphenidate in a small study (n=40) of youth with ADHD, although no placebo control was used in this study (Jafarinia et al. 2012). For additional information on the use of bupropion for ADHD, see Chapter 35, "Medications Used for Attention-Deficit/Hyperactivity Disorder."

Bupropion has also been studied for smoking cessation in youth. Two placebo-controlled studies have been completed. The first included 312 adolescents who were randomly assigned to bupropion SR (150 mg or 300 mg) or placebo with all conditions, including weekly individual therapy. Youth treated with 300 mg showed greater abstinence at both 12 and 24 weeks. Despite the significant findings, only 14.5% of those receiving 300 mg of bupropion had abstained from smoking for the prior week (compared with only 5.6% receiving placebo; Muramoto et al. 2007). A second study examined 134 adolescents randomly assigned to receive bupropion or placebo, both conditions with or without contingency management (CM). Combination bupropion and CM was more effective than either treatment alone (Gray et al. 2011). Bupropion has also been studied as an augmenting treatment to a nicotine patch in 211 youth; however, addition of bupropion was no more effective than nicotine patch alone (Killen et al. 2004). Further research is needed, but it does appear that bupropion may improve abstinence in smoking cessation.

Desvenlafaxine

Chemical Structure and Pharmacology

Desvenlafaxine succinate (*O*-desmethylvenlafaxine [ODV]) is a novel salt form of the isolated major active metabolite of venlafaxine, and therefore it demonstrates some structural similarities, including two chemical rings that are not adjacent to each other. Similar to venlafaxine, desvenlafaxine inhibits presynaptic serotonin and norepinephrine reuptake. In vitro studies have demonstrated that desvenlafaxine has a tenfold higher selectivity for serotonin reuptake inhibition compared with norepinephrine reuptake inhibition (Deecher et al. 2006). Desvenlafaxine demonstrates a weak inhibitory effect on the reuptake of dopamine similar to that of venlafaxine. Desvenlafaxine lacks significant affinity for muscarinic-cholinergic, H_1-histaminergic, and α_1-adrenergic receptors in vitro (Wyeth Pharmaceuticals 2013). Desvenlafaxine also lacks monoamine oxidase (MAO) inhibitory activity. It is available only as extended release tablets (50 mg and 100 mg) and is dosed once daily.

Pharmacokinetics

Desvenlafaxine single-dose pharmacokinetics are linear and dose-proportional in a dose range of 50–600 mg/day. With recommended once-daily dosing, steady-state plasma concentrations are achieved within approximately 4–5 days with 80% oral bioavailability. Desvenlafaxine is primarily metabolized through conjugation and to a lesser extent through oxidative metabolism via the P-450 isoenzyme system (3A4; Sansone and Sansone 2014). The CYP2D6 metabolic pathway is not involved; 45% of the drug is excreted unchanged in the urine, and the conjugated metabolite is not pharmacologically active. Desvenlafaxine can be taken without regard to food.

Adverse Effects Profile

The most commonly observed adverse reactions (incidence ≥5% and at least twice the rate of placebo in premarketing adult studies) included nausea, dizziness, insomnia, hyperhidrosis, constipation, somnolence, decreased appetite, anxiety, and male sexual dysfunction. Discontinuation rates were as high as 12%. Treatment with desvenlafaxine has also resulted in sustained hypertension. Clinical trial experience with desvenlafaxine in overdose is limited, but it is reported to be similar to that of venlafaxine (it may be associated with an increased risk of fatal outcomes compared with that observed with SSRI antidepressant products but lower than that for tricyclic antidepressants).

Efficacy

No efficacy studies have been conducted in children and adolescents using desvenlafaxine. In an open-label safety study of 40 children and adolescents with MDD, 7 youth (4 children and 3 adolescents) withdrew because of adverse events. One adolescent with no suicidal ideation at baseline reported development of suicidal ideation after screening (Findling et al. 2014). The investigators concluded that desvenlafaxine is generally safe and well tolerated in youth, although RCTs are needed for further understanding of the role of desvenlafaxine in treating children and adolescents.

Duloxetine

Chemical Structure and Pharmacology

Duloxetine is a selective serotonin-norepinephrine reuptake inhibitor with comparatively high affinity for neurotransmitter systems. It has less potent dopaminergic reuptake inhibition and has minimal affinity for serotonergic, adrenergic, cholinergic, histaminergic, opioid, dopamine, glutamate, and GABA receptors. Duloxetine does not affect monoamine oxidase. These properties are thought to confer less risk for side effects compared with TCAs and MAOIs. Its multiple metabolites do not appear to have relevant pharmacological activity (Hunziker et al. 2005).

Pharmacokinetics

Duloxetine has extensive absorption after oral administration and reaches peak blood levels in approximately 6 hours. Food intake does not appear to have any effect on bioavailability. This drug is not recommended in patients with severe or end-stage renal disease, but mild to moderate renal insufficiency does not appear to affect its clearance. Duloxetine is not recommended for patients with hepatic failure, as metabolism and elimination are decreased (Hunziker et al. 2005). Only one study has been reported in youth treated with duloxetine. Seventy-two children and adolescents with MDD received duloxetine 20–200 mg for up to 32 weeks. Duloxetine clearance was 42%–60% higher than seen in adults. However, body weight and age did not affect other duloxetine pharmacokinetic parameters (Prakash et al. 2012).

Adverse Effects Profile

Slightly increased heart rate and blood pressure have been reported with duloxetine. In clinical trials, duloxetine increased transaminase levels in some patients. Small but significant weight gain (1.4–1.9 kg) has been reported in trials lasting 6 months. In the previously mentioned study of 72 youth, 50% of patients experienced transient blood pressure elevations (Prakash et al. 2012). Patients treated with duloxetine should have blood pressure monitored during treatment. Duloxetine should be given with caution in patients with epilepsy. At this time, there are limited data on safety in large dose ingestions.

Efficacy

Duloxetine was released in 2004, and there have been only two RCTs examining its efficacy. These were the first studies to use both a proven active comparator (fluoxetine) and placebo to examine safety and efficacy in youth with MDD. One was a fixed-dose study with 463 youth (Emslie et al. 2014), and the other was a flexible dose study of 337 youth (Atkinson et al. 2014). Both studies included a 10-week acute phase, followed by a 26-week continuation phase. In both studies, placebo response rates were quite high, and neither duloxetine nor fluoxetine was shown to be more effective than placebo, resulting in inconclusive findings. Safety outcomes, however, were consistent with results from adult studies (Atkinson et al. 2014; Emslie et al. 2014).

No RCTs of duloxetine have been reported for any other psychiatric disorders in youth. Two case reports have suggested that duloxetine may improve experience of pain and depressive symptoms in three cases of adolescent females with chronic or severe pain and depressive symptoms (Desarkar et al. 2006; Meighen 2007).

Mirtazapine

Chemical Structure and Pharmacology

Mirtazapine is a piperazino-azepine with a unique pharmacological profile in that it is a noradrenergic and specific serotonergic antidepressant. It is a racemic mixture with potent serotonergic antagonism at 5-HT_2 and 5-HT_3 receptors but has no affinity for 5-HT_{1A} and 5-HT_{1B} receptors. Mirtazapine is also a central α_2-adrenergic and peripheral α_1-adrenergic antagonist. Its 5-HT_2 and 5-HT_3 antagonism is thought to modulate serotonergic neurotransmission by an increase in 5-HT_{1A} activity. It is also a potent histamine (H_1) antagonist. Mirtazapine also has some antagonism for muscarinic receptors. It has no affinity for dopamine receptors and does not block serotonin reuptake (Kent 2000).

Pharmacokinetics

Mirtazapine absorption is rapid and complete after oral intake and food does not appear to affect its absorption. Of note, mirtazapine's pharmacokinetics appear to vary with enantiomers, with the *R*-enantiomer having higher plasma levels and a longer half-life. Females and elderly patients appear to have higher blood levels than males and young people. Liver and renal failure can decrease mirtazapine clearance by 30%–50% (Timmer et al. 2000).

Pharmacokinetic data in children and adolescents come from a study of one single 15-mg dose for 16 subjects (ages 7–17) with depression. Half-life increased significantly (ranging from 17.8 to 48.4 hours) with increased weight, and maximum plasma concentration decreased with increased age (Findling et al. 2006a).

Adverse Effects Profile

Mirtazapine has fewer side effects than other antidepressants and generally is well tolerated, although the substantial weight gain noted with mirtazapine should be considered when prescribing to youth. Mirtazapine can lead to hypotension, elevated liver enzymes, and leukopenia with a flulike syndrome. Mirtazapine appears to not have any untoward effects on the seizure threshold or cardiovascular system. It appears to have a high margin of safety in overdose. All reported deaths have involved polydrug ingestions. Nonfatal, single-dose ingestions of 900–1,500 mg have been reported (Kirkton and McIntyre 2006).

Efficacy

Two multicenter trials of children and adolescents (ages 7–17) with MDD were conducted to compare mirtazapine (15–45 mg/day) and placebo, with no significant differences on any of the outcome variables in either study (Cheung et al. 2005).

No RCTs of mirtazapine in other psychiatric disorders in youth have been reported. An open case series of eight children and adolescents with chronic or cyclic vomiting suggested some promise for mirtazapine in reducing vomiting (Coskun and Alyanak 2011).

Trazodone

Chemical Structure and Pharmacology

Trazodone is a triazolopyridine derivative with a unique structure. However, it does resemble side-chain groups of phenothiazines and TCAs. Its triazole moiety is thought to confer antidepressant properties. Trazodone blocks presynaptic reuptake of serotonin with lower potency than SSRIs. It is relatively specific and has negligible effects on dopamine or norepinephrine reuptake. Other serotonergic effects of this drug are complex and include serotonin receptor antagonism, particularly 5-HT_2. Its major active metabolite, *m*-chlorophenylpiperazine, is a potent serotonin agonist. Thus, trazodone is a serotonin reuptake inhibitor and a mixed serotonergic agonist and antagonist.

Pharmacokinetics

Trazodone is almost completely absorbed after oral administration and reaches peak plasma concentrations in approximately 1 hour on an empty stomach (2 hours if taken with food). Age and food do not appear to alter bioavailability. Trazodone is approximately 90%–95% protein bound. It has biphasic elimination with half-lives of 3–6 hours for the first phase and 5–9 hours for the second phase.

Adverse Effects Profile

Side effects with trazodone can be immediate but usually wane with time. Specific adverse events include dry mouth, sedation, dizziness, and fatigue. Like other α-adrenergic blocking agents, trazodone is associated with priapism. Priapism, defined as full or partial penile erection continuing 4 hours beyond sexual stimulation or in the absence of sexual stimulation, more commonly occurs in the first 28 days of treatment and with doses ≥150 mg/day (Warner et al. 1987). Ischemic priapism is an emergency and can be resolved without surgery in many cases if treatment is initiated promptly. Erectile dysfunction invariably results if it is left untreated. Parents and male patients should be forewarned about this risk and educated to seek emergency care if priapism occurs. Thompson et al. (1990) suggest screening for a past history of prolonged erection in male patients prior to the initiation of trazodone, as approximately half of males who develop this condition report a prior history of delayed detumescence. Trazodone can be lethal when combined with alcohol or other drugs. Other antidepressants, such as SSRIs, can increase trazodone's blood level.

Efficacy

No placebo-controlled RCTs have examined trazodone for treatment of pediatric depressive or anxiety disorders. One double-blind crossover trial evaluated trazodone for treatment of migraines in pediatric patients. Although both the active treatment and placebo groups improved initially, only those on trazodone during the second phase of the study continued to show improvement in migraines (Battistella et al. 1993).

Despite the frequent use of trazodone to improve sleep disturbance, no studies have been conducted to examine the effects of trazodone on sleep. One retrospective chart review suggested that trazodone treatment led to faster improvement in sleep disturbance compared with fluoxetine (2 days vs. 4 days). However, the difference, although statistically significant, was not considered clinically significant by the authors (Kallepalli et al. 1997). There is concern about the interaction effect between SSRIs and trazodone, with some suggestion that the combination may lead to worsening of depression (Shamseddeen et al. 2012).

Venlafaxine

Chemical Structure and Pharmacology

Venlafaxine is a novel bicyclic phenylethylamine derivative that inhibits presynaptic serotonin and norepinephrine reuptake. It is a weak inhibitor of dopamine. Venlafaxine's major active metabolite, ODV, has similar actions. Venlafaxine and ODV have no clinically meaningful affinity for cholinergic, histaminergic, or α-adrenergic receptors. This drug has one chiral center and is a racemic mixture. Its *R*-enantiomer confers dual inhibition of serotonin and norepinephrine reuptake. The *S*-enantiomer primarily inhibits serotonin. Other minor metabolites with lower potencies include *N*-demethylvenlafaxine and *N,O*-didemethylvenlafaxine. Venlafaxine is marketed in immediate- and extended-release formulations (Horst and Preskorn 1998).

Pharmacokinetics

Venlafaxine is easily absorbed with oral administration. It is subject to extensive hepatic metabolism to form ODV. Food can slow the rate of absorption but does not decrease its absolute bioavailability (which is 45%). Among antidepressants, venlafaxine has a favorable side effect profile with regard to the cytochrome P450 system.

There is one multiple-dose pharmacokinetic study of venlafaxine in children and adolescents. This involved six children and six adolescents on daily doses near 2 mg/kg. Investigators concluded that exposure to venlafaxine and ODV was lower in children and adolescents than was observed in adults with similar dosing regimens (Findling et al. 2006a).

Adverse Effects Profile

Dropout rates are high in clinical trials of this medication. Venlafaxine has caused electrocardiogram changes and blood pressure elevations, so blood pressure should be monitored regularly. Treatment-emergent suicidal thinking and agitation in children and adolescents may be more common with venlafaxine than with other antidepressants. In the safety analyses conducted by the FDA, venlafaxine was the only individual antidepressant to have significantly more suicide-related adverse events than placebo, which was primarily driven by increased suicidal ideation (Hammad et al. 2006). Patients require close monitoring when initiating and taking this medication. A fatal 30 g overdose of venlafaxine has been reported (Mazur et al. 2003).

Efficacy

Three double-blind controlled trials of venlafaxine have been conducted in children and adolescents with MDD, none of which demonstrated efficacy of venlafaxine over placebo (Emslie et al. 2007; Mandoki et al. 1997). Emslie et al. (2007) combined the two large studies. Although there was still no difference between active treatment and placebo in the overall sample, the subgroup of adolescents had greater improvement in depression with venlafaxine over placebo, suggesting that adolescents may show more response to venlafaxine treatment than younger children.

As a result of limited acute efficacy support and the increased risk of emergent suicidal thinking, venlafaxine is currently a third-line treatment option for youth with treatment-resistant MDD. Brent et al. (2008) reported from the Treatment of SSRI-Resistant Depression in Adolescents (TORDIA) trial on 334 adolescents with depression who had not responded to SSRI treatment and were subsequently randomly assigned to an alternative SSRI or venlafaxine (each medication with or without added CBT). No differences were found between the two medication options, although adding CBT improved outcomes. Thus, in youth who do not improve with initial SSRI treatment, switching to an alternative SSRI or venlafaxine is equally effective, although the group randomly assigned to receive venlafaxine reported more side effects.

Venlafaxine has also been examined for the treatment of GAD and social phobia. Two RCTs were combined to evaluate venlafaxine in 320 children and adolescents (ages 6–17 years) with GAD. Venlafaxine demonstrated greater reduction of anxiety symptoms than placebo. In the individual studies, one study was positive on the primary and secondary outcomes, while the second study was positive on only some secondary outcomes (Rynn et al. 2007). The RCT of venlafaxine for social phobia showed superiority of venlafaxine compared with placebo in reducing anxiety symptoms (March et al. 2007). Thus, venlafaxine appears to be more efficacious for pediatric anxiety disorders than depression.

Additional Atypical Antidepressants

Levomilnacipran, vilazodone, and vortioxetine are newer atypical antidepressants. All three have an FDA indication for treatment of MDD in adults but have no available data in the pediatric age group. A study of vilazodone is under way in adolescents ages 12–17 years with MDD. No dosing or safety data are available for any of these medications in youth.

Tricyclic Antidepressants

TCAs include tertiary amines (amitriptyline, clomipramine, and imipramine) and secondary amines (such as desipramine and nortriptyline). Tertiary amines are serotonin and norepinephrine reuptake inhibitors, while secondary amines (which are the metabolites of tertiary amines) primarily inhibit the norepinephrine transporter. The use of these agents in children has fallen out of favor with the advent of newer antidepressants and case reports of sudden death in children taking TCAs.

Adverse effects of TCAs involve anticholinergic side effects, such as dry mouth, blurred vision, and constipation. Long-term use may be associated with weight gain. Documented cardiovascular effects include tachycardia, hypertension, arrhythmias, and impaired conduction. Children younger than the age of 12 may be more susceptible to these effects, as they are presumed to have increased metabolism to the desmethyl forms of some TCAs, which are more cardiotoxic.

TCAs have been employed for the treatment of depression, ADHD, enuresis, OCD, separation anxiety disorder, and pervasive developmental disorders (autism spectrum disorder) in children and adolescents. Meta-analyses of TCAs have shown no significant differences from placebo in depressed youth (Maneeton and Srisurapanont 2000). However, TCAs may be efficacious for anxiety disorders. Three small controlled studies of clomipramine for OCD demonstrated benefit (DeVeaugh-Geiss et al. 1992; Flament et al. 1985; Leonard et al. 1989). However, clomipramine did not show better efficacy than placebo in an RCT for school refusal (Berney et al. 1981). Three RCTs of imipramine for school phobia have demonstrated efficacy (Bernstein et al. 1990, 2000; Gittelman-Klein and Klein 1973). One other study of imipramine for separation anxiety did not demonstrate efficacy (Klein et al. 1992).

Thus, the unfavorable side effect profile of TCAs and limited evidence of efficacy make it difficult to determine the role of TCAs in pediatric psychopharmacology. They might be considered in cases where multiple agents have failed or when other family members have had a positive response, but they are not considered a first-line treatment option for any disorder.

Monoamine Oxidase Inhibitors

MAOIs (such as phenelzine, isocarboxazid, tranylcypromine, selegiline, moclobemide, and brofaromine) modulate the concentration of monoamines in the central nervous system by inhibiting either MAO-A or MAO-B isoforms. These medications are seldom used in children and adolescents because of requisite dietary restrictions, multiple side effects, and multiple dangerous (possibly fatal) drug-drug interactions.

Selegiline is an irreversible inhibitor of monoamine oxidase with affinity for the MAO-B isoform when administered at low doses. It may have other pharmacological effects unrelated to MAO inhibition. In 2006, a transdermal selegiline system was approved by the FDA for treatment of MDD in adults. It appears to have efficacy similar to other antidepressants with no clinically relevant impact on weight or sexual functioning (Citrome et al. 2013). A recent multicenter trial with adolescents (N=308) failed to demonstrate statistically significant efficacy findings, although the selegiline transdermal system was safe and adequately tolerated in this sample of adolescents (DelBello et al. 2014).

Alternative Antidepressant Treatments

The use of alternative or complementary medicine is popular among pediatric patients despite little empirical evidence. The most commonly used remedies for depressive and anxiety disorders are St. John's wort, omega-3 fatty acid, and *S*-adenosylmethionine.

In open studies of St. John's wort, a daily dose between 300 mg and 1,800 mg was well tolerated by children. No RTCs of St. John's wort in pediatric depression or anxiety disorders have been published.

One small controlled study with pediatric depression has been done with omega-3 fish oil. Nemets et al. (2006) reported data on 20 Israeli children with depression randomly assigned to receive omega-3 fish oil or placebo for 16 weeks. Of children who received a 1,000 mg daily dose of omega-3 fish oil, 70% responded versus 0% in the placebo group. The omega-3 fish oil was well tolerated, and no significant side effects were reported. No studies of omega-3 fish oil have been reported in pediatric anxiety disorder.

No pediatric studies in pediatric depressive or anxiety disorders have been done for *S*-adenosyl-methionine.

Summary Points

- SSRIs are generally well tolerated in children and adolescents and have demonstrated efficacy in depression and anxiety disorders.
- SSRIs are considered the first-line pharmacological treatment for both MDD and anxiety disorders.
- Fluoxetine is the only antidepressant with an FDA indication for treatment of both children and adolescents with MDD. Escitalopram has an FDA indication for adolescents with MDD. Fluoxetine, sertraline, and fluvoxamine have an FDA indication for treatment of pediatric OCD.

- No non-SSRIs have demonstrated efficacy for acute MDD, but some appear to be efficacious in anxiety disorders. Non-SSRIs may be beneficial for youth who do not respond to SSRIs, although only one study of treatment-resistant MDD has been conducted to examine this strategy.
- Dose-finding studies are needed.

References

Abikoff H, McGough J, Vitiello B, et al: Sequential pharmacotherapy for children with comorbid attention-deficit/hyperactivity and anxiety disorders. J Am Acad Child Adolesc Psychiatry 44(5):418–427, 2005 15843763

Aronson S, Delgado P: Escitalopram. Drugs Today (Barc) 40(2):121–131, 2004 15045034

Atkinson SD, Prakash A, Zhang Q, et al: A double-blind efficacy and safety study of duloxetine flexible dosing in children and adolescents with major depressive disorder. J Child Adolesc Psychopharmacol 24(4):180–189, 2014 24813026

Axelson DA, Perel JM, Birmaher B, et al: Sertraline pharmacokinetics and dynamics in adolescents. J Am Acad Child Adolesc Psychiatry 41(9):1037–1044, 2002 12218424

Battistella PA, Ruffilli R, Cernetti R, et al: A placebo-controlled crossover trial using trazodone in pediatric migraine. Headache 33(1):36–39, 1993 8436497

Baumann P, Larsen F: The pharmacokinetics of citalopram. Reviews in Contemporary Pharmacotherapy 6:287–295, 1995

Berard R, Fong R, Carpenter DJ, et al: An international, multicenter, placebo-controlled trial of paroxetine in adolescents with major depressive disorder. J Child Adolesc Psychopharmacol 16(1–2):59–75, 2006 16553529

Berney T, Kolvin I, Bhate SR, et al: School phobia: a therapeutic trial with clomipramine and short-term outcome. Br J Psychiatry 138:110–118, 1981 7020816

Bernstein GA, Garfinkel BD, Borchardt CM: Comparative studies of pharmacotherapy for school refusal. J Am Acad Child Adolesc Psychiatry 29(5):773–781, 1990 2228932

Bernstein GA, Borchardt CM, Perwien AR, et al: Imipramine plus cognitive-behavioral therapy in the treatment of school refusal. J Am Acad Child Adolesc Psychiatry 39(3):276–283, 2000 10714046

Bezchlibnyk-Butler K, Aleksic I, Kennedy SH: Citalopram—a review of pharmacological and clinical effects. J Psychiatry Neurosci 25(3):241–254, 2000 10863884

Birmaher B, Axelson DA, Monk K, et al: Fluoxetine for the treatment of childhood anxiety disorders. J Am Acad Child Adolesc Psychiatry 42(4):415–423, 2003 12649628

Birmaher B, Brent D, Bernet W, et al: Practice parameter for the assessment and treatment of children and adolescents with depressive disorders. J Am Acad Child Adolesc Psychiatry 46(11):1503–1526, 2007 18049300

Black B, Uhde TW: Treatment of elective mutism with fluoxetine: a double-blind, placebo-controlled study. J Am Acad Child Adolesc Psychiatry 33(7):1000–1006, 1994 7961338

Blázquez A, Mas S, Plana MT, et al: Plasma fluoxetine concentrations and clinical improvement in an adolescent sample diagnosed with major depressive disorder, obsessive-compulsive disorder, or generalized anxiety disorder. J Clin Psychopharmacol 34(3):318–326, 2014 24743718

Brent D, Emslie G, Clarke G, et al: Switching to another SSRI or to venlafaxine with or without cognitive behavioral therapy for adolescents with SSRI-resistant depression: the TORDIA randomized controlled trial. JAMA 299(8):901–913, 2008 18314433

Bridge JA, Iyengar S, Salary CB, et al: Clinical response and risk for reported suicidal ideation and suicide attempts in pediatric antidepressant treatment: a meta-analysis of randomized controlled trials. JAMA 297(15):1683–1696, 2007 17440145

Cheung AH, Emslie GJ, Mayes TL: Review of the efficacy and safety of antidepressants in youth depression. J Child Psychol Psychiatry 46(7):735–754, 2005 15972068

Cheung AH, Zuckerbrot RA, Jensen PS, et al: Guidelines for Adolescent Depression in Primary Care (GLAD-PC), II: treatment and ongoing management. Pediatrics 120(5):e1313–e1326, 2007 17974724

Citrome L, Goldberg JF, Portland KB: Placing transdermal selegiline for major depressive disorder into clinical context: number needed to treat, number needed to harm, and likelihood to be helped or harmed. J Affect Disord 151(2):409–417, 2013 23890583

Cohen JA, Mannarino AP, Perel JM, et al: A pilot randomized controlled trial of combined trauma-focused CBT and sertraline for childhood PTSD symptoms. J Am Acad Child Adolesc Psychiatry 46(7):811–819, 2007 17581445

Connolly SD, Bernstein GA, Work Group on Quality Issues: Practice parameter for the assessment and treatment of children and adolescents with anxiety disorders. J Am Acad Child Adolesc Psychiatry 46(2):267–283, 2007 17242630

Coskun M, Alyanak B: Psychiatric co-morbidity and efficacy of mirtazapine treatment in young subjects with chronic or cyclic vomiting syndromes: a case series. J Neurogastroenterol Motil 17(3):305–311, 2011 21860824

da Costa CZ, de Morais RM, Zanetta DM, et al: Comparison among clomipramine, fluoxetine, and placebo for the treatment of anxiety disorders in children and adolescents. J Child Adolesc Psychopharmacol 23(10):687–692, 2013 24350814

Daviss WB, Perel JM, Birmaher B, et al: Steady-state clinical pharmacokinetics of bupropion extended-release in youths. J Am Acad Child Adolesc Psychiatry 45(12):1503–1509, 2006 17135996

Deecher DC, Beyer CE, Johnston G, et al: Desvenlafaxine succinate: a new serotonin and norepinephrine reuptake inhibitor. J Pharmacol Exp Ther 318(2):657–665, 2006 16675639

DelBello MP, Hochadel TJ, Portland KB, et al: A double-blind, placebo-controlled study of selegiline transdermal system in depressed adolescents. J Child Adolesc Psychopharmacol 24(6):311–317, 2014

Desarkar P, Das A, Sinha VK: Duloxetine for childhood depression with pain and dissociative symptoms. Eur Child Adolesc Psychiatry 15(8):496–499, 2006 16732464

DeVane CL: Pharmacokinetics of the selective serotonin reuptake inhibitors. J Clin Psychiatry 53(suppl):13–20, 1992 1531816

DeVane CL: Differential pharmacology of newer antidepressants. J Clin Psychiatry 59(suppl 20):85–93, 1998 9881541

DeVane CL, Liston HL, Markowitz JS: Clinical pharmacokinetics of sertraline. Clin Pharmacokinet 41(15):1247–1266, 2002 12452737

DeVeaugh-Geiss J, Moroz G, Biederman J, et al: Clomipramine hydrochloride in childhood and adolescent obsessive-compulsive disorder—a multicenter trial. J Am Acad Child Adolesc Psychiatry 31(1):45–49, 1992 1537780

Emslie GJ, Rush AJ, Weinberg WA, et al: A double-blind, randomized, placebo-controlled trial of fluoxetine in children and adolescents with depression. Arch Gen Psychiatry 54(11):1031–1037, 1997 9366660

Emslie GJ, Heiligenstein JH, Wagner KD, et al: Fluoxetine for acute treatment of depression in children and adolescents: a placebo-controlled, randomized clinical trial. J Am Acad Child Adolesc Psychiatry 41(10):1205–1215, 2002 12364842

Emslie GJ, Wagner KD, Kutcher S, et al: Paroxetine treatment in children and adolescents with major depressive disorder: a randomized, multicenter, double-blind, placebo-controlled trial. J Am Acad Child Adolesc Psychiatry 45(6):709–719, 2006 16721321

Emslie GJ, Findling RL, Yeung PP, et al: Venlafaxine ER for the treatment of pediatric subjects with depression: results of two placebo-controlled trials. J Am Acad Child Adolesc Psychiatry 46(4):479–488, 2007 17420682

Emslie GJ, Ventura D, Korotzer A, et al: Escitalopram in the treatment of adolescent depression: a randomized placebo-controlled multisite trial. J Am Acad Child Adolesc Psychiatry 48(7):721–729, 2009 19465881

Emslie GJ, Prakash A, Zhang Q, et al: A double-blind efficacy and safety study of duloxetine fixed doses in children and adolescents with major depressive disorder. J Child Adolesc Psychopharmacol 24(4):170–179, 2014 24815533

Findling RL, Reed MD, Myers C, et al: Paroxetine pharmacokinetics in depressed children and adolescents. J Am Acad Child Adolesc Psychiatry 38(8):952–959, 1999 10434486

Findling RL, McNamara NK, Stansbrey RJ, et al: The relevance of pharmacokinetic studies in designing efficacy trials in juvenile major depression. J Child Adolesc Psychopharmacol 16(1–2):131–145, 2006a 16553534

Findling RL, Nucci G, Piergies AA, et al: Multiple dose pharmacokinetics of paroxetine in children and adolescents with major depressive disorder or obsessive-compulsive disorder. Neuropsychopharmacology 31(6):1274–1285, 2006b 16319918

Findling RL, Robb A, Bose A: Escitalopram in the treatment of adolescent depression: a randomized, double-blind, placebo-controlled extension trial. J Child Adolesc Psychopharmacol 23(7):468–480, 2013 24041408

Findling RL, Groark J, Chiles D, et al: Safety and tolerability of desvenlafaxine in children and adolescents with major depressive disorder. J Child Adolesc Psychopharmacol 24(4):201–209, 2014 24611442

Flament MF, Rapoport JL, Berg CJ, et al: Clomipramine treatment of childhood obsessive-compulsive disorder. A double-blind controlled study. Arch Gen Psychiatry 42(10):977–983, 1985 3899048

Friedman RA, Leon AC: Expanding the black box—depression, antidepressants, and the risk of suicide. N Engl J Med 356(23):2343–2346, 2007 17485726

Geller DA, Hoog SL, Heiligenstein JH, et al: Fluoxetine treatment for obsessive-compulsive disorder in children and adolescents: a placebo-controlled clinical trial. J Am Acad Child Adolesc Psychiatry 40(7):773–779, 2001 11437015

Geller DA, Wagner KD, Emslie G, et al: Paroxetine treatment in children and adolescents with obsessive-compulsive disorder: a randomized, multicenter, double-blind, placebo-controlled trial. J Am Acad Child Adolesc Psychiatry 43(11):1387–1396, 2004 15502598

Gittelman-Klein R, Klein DF: School phobia: diagnostic considerations in the light of imipramine effects. J Nerv Ment Dis 156(3):199–215, 1973 4698665

Gray KM, Carpenter MJ, Baker NL, et al: Bupropion SR and contingency management for adolescent smoking cessation. J Subst Abuse Treat 40(1):77–86, 2011 20934835

Hammad TA, Laughren T, Racoosin J: Suicidality in pediatric patients treated with antidepressant drugs. Arch Gen Psychiatry 63(3):332–339, 2006 16520440

Henry JA: Overdose and safety with fluvoxamine. Int Clin Psychopharmacol 6(suppl 3):41–45, discussion 45–47, 1991 1806634

Hiemke C, Härtter S: Pharmacokinetics of selective serotonin reuptake inhibitors. Pharmacol Ther 85(1):11–28, 2000 10674711

Hollander E, Phillips A, Chaplin W, et al: A placebo controlled crossover trial of liquid fluoxetine on repetitive behaviors in childhood and adolescent autism. Neuropsychopharmacology 30(3):582–589, 2005 15602505

Horst WD, Preskorn SH: Mechanisms of action and clinical characteristics of three atypical antidepressants: venlafaxine, nefazodone, bupropion. J Affect Disord 51(3):237–254, 1998 10333980

Hsyu PH, Singh A, Giargiari TD, et al: Pharmacokinetics of bupropion and its metabolites in cigarette smokers versus nonsmokers. J Clin Pharmacol 37(8):737–743, 1997 9378846

Hughes CW, Emslie GJ, Crismon ML, et al: Texas Children's Medication Algorithm Project: update from Texas Consensus Conference Panel on Medication Treatment of Childhood Major Depressive Disorder. J Am Acad Child Adolesc Psychiatry 46(6):667–686, 2007 17513980

Hunziker ME, Suehs BT, Bettinger TL, et al: Duloxetine hydrochloride: a new dual-acting medication for the treatment of major depressive disorder. Clin Ther 27(8):1126–1143, 2005 16199241

Hyttel J, Arnt J, Sanchez C: The pharmacology of citalopram. Reviews in Contemporary Pharmacotherapy 6:271–285, 1995

Jafarinia M, Mohammadi MR, Modabbernia A, et al: Bupropion versus methylphenidate in the treatment of children with attention-deficit/hyperactivity disorder: randomized double-blind study. Hum Psychopharmacol 27(4):411–418, 2012 22806822

Kallepalli BR, Bhatara VS, Fogas BS, et al: Trazodone is only slightly faster than fluoxetine in relieving insomnia in adolescents with depressive disorders. J Child Adolesc Psychopharmacol 7(2):97–107, 1997 9334895

Keller MB, Ryan ND, Strober M, et al: Efficacy of paroxetine in the treatment of adolescent major depression: a randomized, controlled trial. J Am Acad Child Adolesc Psychiatry 40(7):762–772, 2001 11437014

Kent JM: SNaRIs, NaSSAs, and NaRIs: new agents for the treatment of depression. Lancet 355(9207):911–918, 2000 10752718

Killen JD, Robinson TN, Ammerman S, et al: Randomized clinical trial of the efficacy of bupropion combined with nicotine patch in the treatment of adolescent smokers. J Consult Clin Psychol 72(4):729–735, 2004 15301658

Kirkton C, McIntyre IM: Therapeutic and toxic concentrations of mirtazapine. J Anal Toxicol 30(9):687–691, 2006 17137530

Klein N, Sacher J, Geiss-Granadia T, et al: Higher serotonin transporter occupancy after multiple dose administration of escitalopram compared to citalopram: an [123I]ADAM SPECT study. Psychopharmacology (Berl) 191(2):333–339, 2007 17235610

Klein RG, Koplewicz HS, Kanner A: Imipramine treatment of children with separation anxiety disorder. J Am Acad Child Adolesc Psychiatry 31(1):21–28, 1992 1347039

Koelch M, Pfalzer AK, Kliegl K, et al: Therapeutic drug monitoring of children and adolescents treated with fluoxetine. Pharmacopsychiatry 45(2):72–76, 2012 22086744

Labellarte M, Biederman J, Emslie G, et al: Multiple-dose pharmacokinetics of fluvoxamine in children and adolescents. J Am Acad Child Adolesc Psychiatry 43(12):1497–1505, 2004 15564819

Leonard HL, Swedo SE, Rapoport JL, et al: Treatment of obsessive-compulsive disorder with clomipramine and desipramine in children and adolescents. A double-blind crossover comparison. Arch Gen Psychiatry 46(12):1088–1092, 1989 2686576

Liebowitz MR, Turner SM, Piacentini J, et al: Fluoxetine in children and adolescents with OCD: a placebo-controlled trial. J Am Acad Child Adolesc Psychiatry 41(12):1431–1438, 2002 12447029

LoVecchio F, Watts D, Winchell J, et al: Outcomes after supratherapeutic escitalopram ingestions. J Emerg Med 30(1):17–19, 2006 16434330

Luchini D, Morabito G, Centini F: Case report of a fatal intoxication by citalopram. Am J Forensic Med Pathol 26(4):352–354, 2005 16304470

Mandoki MW, Tapia MR, Tapia MA, et al: Venlafaxine in the treatment of children and adolescents with major depression. Psychopharmacol Bull 33(1):149–154, 1997 9133767

Maneeton N, Srisurapanont M: Tricyclic antidepressants for depressive disorders in children and adolescents: a meta-analysis of randomized-controlled trials. J Med Assoc Thai 83(11):1367–1374, 2000 11215868

March JS, Biederman J, Wolkow R, et al: Sertraline in children and adolescents with obsessive-compulsive disorder: a multicenter randomized controlled trial. JAMA 280(20):1752–1756, 1998 9842950

March J, Silva S, Petrycki S, et al: Fluoxetine, cognitive-behavioral therapy, and their combination for adolescents with depression: Treatment for Adolescents With Depression Study (TADS) randomized controlled trial. JAMA 292(7):807–820, 2004 15315995

March JS, Entusah AR, Rynn M, et al: A randomized controlled trial of venlafaxine ER versus placebo in pediatric social anxiety disorder. Biol Psychiatry 62(10):1149–1154, 2007 17553467

Mayes TL, Tao R, Rintelmann JW, et al: Do children and adolescents have differential response rates in placebo-controlled trials of fluoxetine? CNS Spectr 12(2):147–154, 2007 17277715

Mazur JE, Doty JD, Krygiel AS: Fatality related to a 30-g venlafaxine overdose. Pharmacotherapy 23(12):1668–1672, 2003 14695048

McDougle CJ, Kresch LE, Posey DJ: Repetitive thoughts and behavior in pervasive developmental disorders: treatment with serotonin reuptake inhibitors. J Autism Dev Disord 30(5):427–435, 2000 11098879

Meighen KG: Duloxetine treatment of pediatric chronic pain and co-morbid major depressive disorder. J Child Adolesc Psychopharmacol 17(1):121–127, 2007 17343560

Muramoto ML, Leischow SJ, Sherrill D, et al: Randomized, double-blind, placebo-controlled trial of 2 dosages of sustained-release bupropion for adolescent smoking cessation. Arch Pediatr Adolesc Med 161(11):1068–1074, 2007 17984409

Myers LB, Krenzelok EP: Paroxetine (Paxil) overdose: a pediatric focus. Vet Hum Toxicol 39(2):86–88, 1997 9080633

Nemets H, Nemets B, Apter A, et al: Omega-3 treatment of childhood depression: a controlled, double-blind pilot study. Am J Psychiatry 163(6):1098–1100, 2006 16741212

Pediatric OCD Treatment Study Team: Cognitive-behavior therapy, sertraline, and their combination for children and adolescents with obsessive-compulsive disorder: the Pediatric OCD Treatment Study (POTS) randomized controlled trial. JAMA 292(16):1969–1976, 2004 15507582

Personne M, Persson H, Sjöberg E: Citalopram toxicity. Lancet 350(9076):518–519, 1997 9274602

Prakash A, Lobo E, Kratochvil CJ, et al: An open-label safety and pharmacokinetics study of duloxetine in pediatric patients with major depression. J Child Adolesc Psychopharmacol 22(1):48–55, 2012 22251023

Rao N: The clinical pharmacokinetics of escitalopram. Clin Pharmacokinet 46(4):281–290, 2007 17375980

The Research Unit on Pediatric Psychopharmacology Anxiety Study Group: Fluvoxamine for the treatment of anxiety disorders in children and adolescents. N Engl J Med 344(17):1279–1285, 2001 11323729

Riddle MA, Scahill L, King RA, et al: Double-blind, crossover trial of fluoxetine and placebo in children and adolescents with obsessive-compulsive disorder. J Am Acad Child Adolesc Psychiatry 31(6):1062–1069, 1992 1429406

Riddle MA, Reeve EA, Yaryura-Tobias JA, et al: Fluvoxamine for children and adolescents with obsessive-compulsive disorder: a randomized, controlled, multicenter trial. J Am Acad Child Adolesc Psychiatry 40(2):222–229, 2001 11211371

Rynn MA, Siqueland L, Rickels K: Placebo-controlled trial of sertraline in the treatment of children with generalized anxiety disorder. Am J Psychiatry 158(12):2008–2014, 2001 11729017

Rynn MA, Riddle MA, Yeung PP, et al: Efficacy and safety of extended-release venlafaxine in the treatment of generalized anxiety disorder in children and adolescents: two placebo-controlled trials. Am J Psychiatry 164(2):290–300, 2007 17267793

Sansone RA, Sansone LA: Serotonin norepinephrine reuptake inhibitors: a pharmacological comparison. Innov Clin Neurosci 11(3–4):37–42, 2014 24800132

Shamseddeen W, Clarke G, Keller MB, et al: Adjunctive sleep medications and depression outcome in the treatment of serotonin-selective reuptake inhibitor resistant depression in adolescents study. J Child Adolesc Psychopharmacol 22(1):29–36, 2012 22251024

Simeon JG, Dinicola VF, Ferguson HB, et al: Adolescent depression: a placebo-controlled fluoxetine treatment study and follow-up. Prog Neuropsychopharmacol Biol Psychiatry 14(5):791–795, 1990 2293257

Stewart JJ, Berkel HJ, Parish RC, et al: Single-dose pharmacokinetics of bupropion in adolescents: effects of smoking status and gender. J Clin Pharmacol 41(7):770–778, 2001 11452710

Storch EA, Bussing R, Small BJ, et al: Randomized, placebo-controlled trial of cognitive-behavioral therapy alone or combined with sertraline in the treatment of pediatric obsessive-compulsive disorder. Behav Res Ther 51(12):823–829, 2013 24184429

Sugie Y, Sugie H, Fukuda T, et al: Clinical efficacy of fluvoxamine and functional polymorphism in a serotonin transporter gene on childhood autism. J Autism Dev Disord 35(3):377–385, 2005 16119478

Taurines R, Burger R, Wewetzer C, et al: The relation between dosage, serum concentrations, and clinical outcome in children and adolescents treated with sertraline: a naturalistic study. Ther Drug Monit 35(1):84–91, 2013 23318280

Thompson JW Jr, Ware MR, Blashfield RK: Psychotropic medication and priapism: a comprehensive review. J Clin Psychiatry 51(10):430–433, 1990 2211542

Timmer CJ, Sitsen JM, Delbressine LP: Clinical pharmacokinetics of mirtazapine.

Clin Pharmacokinet 38(6):461–474, 2000 10885584

Trivedi MH, Rush AJ, Gaynes BN, et al: Maximizing the adequacy of medication treatment in controlled trials and clinical practice: STAR(*)D measurement-based care. Neuropsychopharmacology 32(12):2479–2489, 2007 17406651

U.S. Food and Drug Administration: Guidance for Industry: Industry Supported Scientific and Educational Activities. Fed Regist 62(232):64093–64100, 1997

U.S. Food and Drug Administration: FDA drug safety communication: abnormal heart rhythms associated with high doses of Celexa (citalopram hydrobromide). Silver Spring, MD, U.S. Food and Drug Administration, 2012. Available at: http://www.fda.gov/Drugs/DrugSafety/ucm269086.htm. Accessed June 30, 2014.

von Knorring AL, Olsson GI, Thomsen PH, et al: A randomized, double-blind, placebo-controlled study of citalopram in adolescents with major depressive disorder. J Clin Psychopharmacol 26(3):311–315, 2006 16702897

Wagner KD, Ambrosini P, Rynn M, et al: Efficacy of sertraline in the treatment of children and adolescents with major depressive disorder: two randomized controlled trials. JAMA 290(8):1033–1041, 2003 12941675

Wagner KD, Berard R, Stein MB, et al: A multicenter, randomized, double-blind, placebo-controlled trial of paroxetine in children and adolescents with social anxiety disorder. Arch Gen Psychiatry 61(11):1153–1162, 2004a 15520363

Wagner KD, Robb AS, Findling RL, et al: A randomized, placebo-controlled trial of citalopram for the treatment of major depression in children and adolescents. Am J Psychiatry 161(6):1079–1083, 2004b 15169696

Wagner KD, Jonas J, Findling RL, et al: A double-blind, randomized, placebo-controlled trial of escitalopram in the treatment of pediatric depression. J Am Acad Child Adolesc Psychiatry 45(3):280–288, 2006 16540812

Walkup JT, Albano AM, Piacentini J, et al: Cognitive behavioral therapy, sertraline, or a combination in childhood anxiety. N Engl J Med 359(26):2753–2766, 2008 18974308

Warner MD, Peabody CA, Whiteford HA, et al: Trazodone and priapism. J Clin Psychiatry 48(6):244–245, 1987 3584080

Wyeth Pharmaceuticals: Pristiq Extended Release–Desvenlafaxine Succinate Tablet, Extended Release, 2013. Available at: http://labeling.pfizer.com/showlabeling.aspx?id=497. Accessed July 15, 2013.

CHAPTER 37

Mood Stabilizers

Barbara L. Gracious, M.D.
Arman Danielyan, M.D.
Robert A. Kowatch, M.D., Ph.D.

The mood stabilizers lithium and valproate have been used to treat children and adolescents with mood and seizure disorders for many years. Lithium was first used more than 40 years ago to treat "manic-depressive" illness in children (Annell 1969). Since then, a variety of potentially mood stabilizing agents have been used to treat psychiatric disorders in children and adolescents. *Mood stabilizers* can be divided into traditional agents lithium, valproate, and carbamazepine and newer or *novel* agents, including the anticonvulsants lamotrigine, oxcarbazepine, topiramate, and gabapentin (Weisler et al. 2006). The use of anticonvulsants migrated from pediatric neurology to child psychiatry after clinicians noticed their mood and behavioral effects. Now often used as second-line choices behind atypical antipsychotics for overall efficacy, they may still have cost or other advantages for specific youth, as monotherapy or together with an atypical antipsychotic. The evidence base for the long-term safety and efficacy of these two mood stabilizers as well as the newer antiepileptic agents in children and adolescents remains modest (Kowatch and DelBello 2006; Pavuluri et al. 2005). Table 37–1 provides mood stabilizer dosing and monitoring guidelines.

Lithium

Lithium carbonate is the best-studied classic mood stabilizer in children and adolescents and is the only one approved by the U.S. Food and Drug Administration (FDA) for the treatment of "manic episodes of manic-depressive illness" in patients ages 12 years and older. Lithium carbonate is a naturally occurring salt whose mood-stabilizing properties in adults with mania were first published by Australian John Frederick Joseph Cade (1912–1980) (Cade 1949). Lithium has multiple complex effects in the cen-

TABLE 37–1. Mood stabilizer dosing and monitoring guidelines

Generic name	U.S. trade name	How supplied (mg)	Starting dose	Target dose	Therapeutic serum level	Cautions
Carbamazepine Carbamazepine XR	Tegretol Tegretol XR Equetro Carbatrol	100, 200 100, 200, 400	Outpatients: 7 mg/kg/day 2–3 daily doses	Based on response and serum levels	8–11 mg/L	Monitor for P450 drug interactions
Gabapentin	Neurontin	100, 300, 400	100 mg bid or tid; hs only for sleep	Based on response and up to 1,800 mg/day	NA	Watch for behavioral disinhibition
Lamotrigine	Lamictal	5, 25, 100, 200	12.5 mg qd	Increase weekly on the basis of response	NA	Monitor carefully for rashes, serum sickness
Lithium carbonate Lithium carbonate Lithium citrate	Lithobid Eskalith Cibalith-S	300 (and 150 generic) 300 or 450 CR 5 cc=300 mg	Outpatients: 25 mg/kg/day 2–3 daily doses	30 mg/kg/day 2–3 daily doses	0.8–1.2 mEq/L	Monitor for hypothyroidism Avoid where possible in pregnancy
Oxcarbazepine	Trileptal	150, 300, 600	150 mg bid	20–29 kg: 900 mg/day 30–39 kg: 1,200 mg/day >39 kg: 1,800 mg/day	NA	Monitor for hyponatremia
Topiramate	Topamax	25, 100	25 mg qd	100–400 mg/day	NA	Monitor for memory problems, blurred vision, kidney stones
Valproic acid Divalproex sodium	Depakene Depakote	125, 250, 500	15 mg/kg/day 2 daily doses	20 mg/kg/day 2–3 daily doses	85–110 µg/mL	Monitor liver functions and for pancreatitis Monitor for polycystic ovary symptoms in females Contraindicated in pregnancy

Note. bid=twice a day; hs=at bedtime; CR=controlled release; qd=once a day; tid=three times a day; XR=extended release.

tral nervous system (CNS), particularly at the second messenger level. These effects include 1) blocking the activity of inositol polyphosphatase 1-phosphatase and inositol second messenger systems, 2) inhibiting adenyl cyclase by competing with magnesium in this second messenger system, 3) down-regulating hippocampal serotonin (5-HT_{1A}) receptors, 4) increasing low-affinity β-receptors, 5) inducing subsensitivity of α_2-receptors, and 6) increasing dopamine levels in tuberoinfundibular pathways (Alessi et al. 1994). In addition, lithium (and valproate) have neurotrophic effects via indirectly regulating cell survival pathways, including cyclic adenosine monophosphate response element-binding protein, brain-derived neurotrophic factor, apoptosis regulator protein B-cell lymphoma 2 (Bcl-2), and mitogen-activated protein kinases (Manji and Zarate 2002).

Disorders in Which Lithium May Be Useful

Lithium has been used for many years in children and adolescents to treat mania (Brumback and Weinberg 1977; Campbell et al. 1984; Dyson and Barcai 1970; Varanka et al. 1988), as well as bipolar depression (Patel et al. 2006), aggressive behavior in hospitalized children with conduct disorder (Campbell et al. 1972, 1995a, 1995b; Malone et al. 2000), adolescents with comorbid bipolar and substance use disorders (Geller et al. 1998a), and manic symptoms secondary to traumatic brain injury in children (Cohn et al. 1989).

Lithium may also be useful for preventing recurrent mood episodes in children and adolescents with bipolar disorder. Strober et al. (1990) followed the naturalistic course of 37 adolescents whose mood had been stabilized with lithium while hospitalized. After 18 months, of 35% who had discontinued lithium, 92% had relapsed compared with 38% who remained lithium compliant, suggesting lithium is useful for maintenance treatment in adolescents.

Evidence for Efficacy

Of six older controlled trials of lithium in bipolar children and adolescents, four (DeLong and Nieman 1983; Gram and Rafaelsen 1972; Lena 1979; McKnew et al. 1981) used a crossover design, not ideal for assessing outcome in an illness whose inherent nature is to wax and wane. The small number of subjects (average N=18) and variable response rates (33%–80%) reflect heterogeneity of the samples and differences among study designs. Several larger open-label studies reported that 40%–50% of manic children and adolescents with bipolar disorder improved with lithium monotherapy (Findling et al. 2003; Kowatch et al. 2000; Youngerman and Canino 1978).

In a small (n=25), prospective placebo-controlled trial of lithium in children and adolescents with bipolar disorder and comorbid substance abuse, those assigned to lithium for 6 weeks showed a significant improvement in global assessment of functioning (46% response rate vs. 8% response rate in the placebo group), as well as a statistically significant decrease in positive urine toxicology screens (Geller et al. 1998a). In an open prospective study of 100 adolescents treated with lithium for an acute manic episode, 63 responded and 26 remitted by week 4 (Kafantaris et al. 2003). Response was not predicted by prominent depressive features, age at first mood episode, severity of mania, or comorbidity with attention-deficit/hyperactivity disorder (ADHD). Kafantaris et al. (2004) subsequently reported results of a placebo-controlled discontinuation study of lithium in 40 adolescents with mania. After receiving open treatment with lithium at therapeutic serum levels (mean 0.99 mEq/L) for at least 4 weeks, responders were then randomly assigned to continue or discontinue lithium during a 2-week double-blind, placebo-controlled phase. The exacerbation rate in patients maintained on lithium (53%) was no different than that of patients changed to placebo (62%). It is possible that if the discontinuation period had been longer, a clear separation between groups would have been observed.

More recently, in the Collaborative Lithium Trials funded by the National Institute of Child Health and Human Development to develop evidence-based strategies for lithium use in youth with bipolar I disorder (manic or mixed), 58% of youth ages 7–17 years achieved response after 8 weeks of lithium. Effectiveness, safety, and tolerability did not differ among three different dosing strategies (Findling et al. 2011). A 16-week extension phase was then conducted in the 41 youth who had a partial or full response (Findling et al. 2013). With a mean weight-adjusted total daily dose of 27.8 (SD6.7) mg/kg/day and an average lithium level of 1.0 mEq/L, remitted youth remained in remission. Adjunctive medication was required in 61%, largely for refractory mania (32%) and for comorbid ADHD (37%). Partial responders did not improve further beyond the first 8 weeks of lithium.

Patel et al. (2006) evaluated the use of lithium for depressive episodes associated with bipolar I disorder in 27 adolescents. Open-label lithium dose was adjusted to achieve a therapeutic serum level of 1.0–1.2 mEq/L. Significant reduction in scores from baseline to endpoint on the Childhood Depression Rating Scale, Revised (CDRS-R) resulted in a large effect size of 1.7. These findings suggest that lithium is effective for treating acute depressive episodes in adolescents with bipolar disorder, although controlled trials are needed.

Several studies have demonstrated the usefulness of lithium for aggressive behaviors in the context of conduct disorder. Campbell et al. (1972) reported that lithium was effective in "hyperactive severely disturbed young children." Subsequent controlled studies by Campbell and others found lithium efficacious for children and adolescents with aggression and conduct disorder (Campbell et al. 1995a; Malone et al. 2000).

Baseline Assessments

Baseline studies prior to initiating treatment with lithium should include a general medical history and physical examination; serum electrolytes creatinine, blood urea nitrogen, and serum calcium levels; thyroid function tests; electrocardiogram (ECG); complete blood count with differential; urinalysis; and a pregnancy test for sexually active females (Danielyan and Kowatch 2005).

Contraindications

Lithium should be titrated cautiously and serum levels monitored carefully in patients with significant renal, cardiovascular, or thyroid disease or severe dehydration, in collaboration with pediatric subspecialists. Lithium has been associated with an increased rate of cardiac abnormalities in fetuses, and its use is typically avoided in pregnant or potentially pregnant females (Cohen et al. 1994).

Side Effects

Common side effects in children and adolescents include nausea, diarrhea, abdominal distress, sedation, tremor, polyuria, weight gain, enuresis, and acne. These side effects may affect adherence, especially in adolescents, who often find the possibility of weight gain and acne to be disincentives for continued treatment. Less common side effects requiring dose reduction or cessation include visual changes related to corneal swelling or persistent severe headaches and papilloedema from pseudotumor cerebri. Lithium can be difficult for pediatric patients to tolerate because of its very narrow therapeutic window (0.8–1.2 mEq/L). Patients may develop lithium toxicity when this window is exceeded. Signs of lithium toxicity include nausea, vomiting, slurred speech, and dyscoordination. With blood levels ≥3.0 mEq/L, seizures and coma can occur, resulting in potentially fatal outcomes (Gelenberg et al. 1989). Very young children (younger than 6 years) are more prone to developing neurological side effects, especially at the start of lithium treatment (Hagino et al. 1998).

Cardiac Side Effects

Lithium may occasionally affect cardiac conduction, causing first-degree atrioventricular block, irregular sinus rhythms, and increased premature ventricular contractions (Gelenberg et al. 1989). Reversible conduction abnormalities have been reported in children (Campbell et al. 1984). It is recommended that a baseline ECG be obtained, followed by another ECG once a therapeutic level has been reached.

Renal Side Effects

There are no studies of the effect of lithium use longer than 18 months on renal function in children and adolescents. Long-term lithium use in adults can result in clinically significant reduction in the glomerular filtration rate and in the maximum urinary concentrating capacity (Bendz et al. 1994). In addition, because of lithium's action on antidiuretic hormone in the distal tubules and collecting ducts, reversible cases of diabetes insipidus have been reported (Gelenberg et al. 1989). Focal glomerulosclerosis has occasionally been reported in children taking lithium, but it typically remits once lithium is discontinued (Sakarcan et al. 2002). Renal function should be tested every 2–3 months during the first 6 months of treatment (McClellan et al. 2007). Thereafter, renal function should be checked every 6 months or when clinically indicated. A newer serum renal test, cystatin-C, may be a more reasonable option for periodically evaluating glomerular filtration rates for those remaining on maintenance lithium, in place of the often difficult to obtain 24-hour urine for creatinine clearance. Chronic treatment with lithium can cause hyperparathyroidism; therefore, serum calcium levels should be checked once a year (Bendz et al. 1996a, 1996b).

Thyroid

There have been case reports of youth who developed hypothyroidism, goiter, and thyroid autoantibodies while taking lithium (Alessi et al. 1994; DeLong and Aldershof 1987). In one sample of children and adolescents treated with lithium and valproate for bipolar disorder, one-quarter showed thyroid-stimulating hormone (TSH) elevations of at least 10 mU/L with an average exposure to lithium of less than 3 months (Gracious et al. 2004). Factors associated with elevation in TSH in these lithium-treated subjects included a higher baseline TSH level and a higher lithium level. Close monitoring of thyroid function in children and adolescents taking lithium is recommended, as some may require supplemental thyroid hormone. Thyroid function should be tested during the first 6 months of treatment and then every 6 months or when clinically indicated.

Cognition

Another concern in children and adolescents treated with lithium is a potential for negative effects on cognitive functioning. In one double-blind, placebo-controlled study of lithium in 91 hospitalized children with conduct disorder, severe aggression, and explosiveness, some children appeared to develop cognitive impairment at low plasma levels (Campbell et al. 1991).

Teratogenicity

Adequate birth control measures must be followed in adolescent females taking lithium, as lithium has been associated with an increased rate of cardiac abnormalities following fetal exposure (Cohen et al. 1994). Although more recent prospective epidemiological studies have indicated bias in the initial reports and a lower rate of cardiac abnormalities that may not be elevated compared with control pregnancies, potential benefits for lithium treatment in those young women with severe illness must be balanced with a discussion of potential risk and appropriate fetal monitoring by high-level ultrasound (Yacobi and Ornoy 2008). Table 37–2 lists management tactics for the common side effects of lithium.

Drug Interactions

Medications that may increase lithium levels include several antibiotics (e.g., ampicillin, tetracycline), nonsteroidal anti-inflammatory agents (e.g., ibuprofen), angiotensin-converting enzyme inhibitors, calcium channel blockers, antipsychotic agents, propranolol, and serotonin-specific reuptake inhibitors.

Clinical Use

Lithium is a mood stabilizer with a moderate effect size that all child psychiatrists should be comfortable prescribing. Lithium is readily absorbed from the gastrointestinal system, with peak levels occurring 2–4 hours after each dose. Lithium is excreted by the kidneys, and the serum half-life in children and adolescents is estimated to be approximately 18 hours (Vitiello et al. 1988). Serum lithium levels in the range of 0.8–1.2 mEq/L are typically necessary for mood stabilization for bipolar I manic episodes. To obtain a therapeutic serum level of 0.8–1.2 mEq/L, lithium should typically be titrated to a dosage of 30 mg/kg/day in two to three divided doses.

Valproate

Valproate (valproate sodium) is a simple branched-chain fatty acid first introduced in the United States in 1978 as an antiseizure agent. It is currently approved by the FDA for the treatment of adults with partial complex seizures, migraines, or manic episodes of bipolar illness.

Disorders in Which Valproate May Be Useful

In children and adolescents, valproate may be effective in the treatment of mania, aggression, and migraine headaches.

Evidence for Efficacy

Valproate has been historically used to treat adults with mania. A review of five controlled studies of valproate for treatment of acute mania in adults showed an average response rate of 54%, demonstrating efficacy for valproate versus placebo (McElroy and Keck 2000). In most of these studies, positive results were

TABLE 37–2. Management of common lithium side effects

System	Side effects	Tactic
Central nervous system	Tremor, sedation, headache	Use a slow-release formulation; dose twice daily
Dermatological	Acne	Collaborate with primary care physician for management of acne; avoid retinoids
Endocrine	Hypothyroidism	Consult with endocrinologist; augment with triiodothyronine
Gastrointestinal	Nausea, diarrhea	Split into 2–3 daily doses; use a slow-release formulation
Metabolic	Weight gain	Encourage diet and exercise; consider a trial of metformin (Klein et al. 2006)
Renal	Polyuria, decreases in renal function	Write note to school that allows the patient to use the bathroom as needed during school; monitor serum creatinine or creatinine clearance, serum urea nitrogen, and urine osmolality every 6 months

obtained even though patients were selected from a population previously refractory to lithium treatment and were characterized by rapid cycling, mixed affective states, and irritability. Wagner et al. (2002) performed an open-label study of valproate in 40 children and adolescents (ages 7–19 years) with bipolar disorder. Subjects started at an initial dosage of 15 mg/kg/day of divalproex. The mean final dosage was 17 mg/kg/day. Twenty-two subjects (61%) showed ≥50% improvement in mania rating scores during the open-label phase of treatment.

Findling et al. (2005) conducted a discontinuation trial of lithium and divalproex to determine whether divalproex was superior to lithium in the maintenance monotherapy of 139 youth diagnosed with bipolar disorder I or II disorder. Participants (mean age 10.8±3.5 years) were initially treated with a combination of lithium and divalproex, for a mean duration of 10.7±5.4 weeks. Those meeting remission criteria for 4 consecutive weeks were then randomly assigned in a double-blind fashion to treatment with either lithium alone (n=30) or divalproex alone (n=30) for up to 76 weeks. At the end of the study, the lithium and divalproex treatment groups did not differ in either survival time (until emerging symptoms of relapse) or discontinuation for any reason. The authors concluded that lithium was not superior to divalproex as maintenance treatment in youth stabilized on combination lithium and divalproex pharmacotherapy. The mean survival time in this trial for both agents was about 16 weeks, demonstrating that monotherapy was not sufficient for overall maintenance treatment of children and adolescents with bipolar disorder.

A large, randomized, placebo-controlled, double-blind, multicenter study evaluated the safety and efficacy of Depakote ER (slow-release divalproex sodium) for bipolar I disorder, manic or mixed episode, in 150 outpatient children and adolescents ages 10–17 years across 20 sites (Wagner et al. 2009). Subjects had a Young Mania Rating Scale (YMRS) score ≥20 at screening and baseline. Subjects were randomly assigned in a 1:1 ratio to receive 4 weeks of Depakote ER (as 250 mg and/or 500 mg tablets) or matching placebo tablets, with an optional 1-week taper period. A 6-month open-label extension phase included 66 youth who elected to continue from the acute phase. There were no statistically significant differences between valproate and placebo on the primary or secondary outcome measures from either phase. Kowatch et al. (2007) published results of a large National Institute of Mental Health–funded, randomized, placebo-controlled, double-blind trial in 153 outpatients ages 7–17 years with bipolar I disorder. Participants (mean age 10.6±2.7; 86% male) were assigned to treatment with lithium, divalproex, or placebo for up to 24 weeks in a 2:2:1 ratio. Primary outcome measures were weekly YMRS and Clinical Global Impression–Improvement (CGI-I) scale ratings at the end of 8 weeks (Geller et al. 1998b). Divalproex demonstrated efficacy on both a priori outcome measures, whereas lithium did not. Response rates based on a CGI-I score of 1 or 2 (much or very much improved) were divalproex, 54%; lithium, 42%; and placebo, 29%. There was a trend toward efficacy for lithium, but it did not separate from placebo on the primary outcome measures.

Steiner et al. (2003) conducted the only randomized controlled trial (RCT) of divalproex sodium (Depakote) with 71 incarcerated youth with conduct disorder. Subjects were randomly assigned into high- and low-dose (subtherapeutic) conditions and were openly managed by a clinical team with subjects and independent outcome raters blind to the low-versus high-dose treatment condition assigned. Self-reported weekly impulse control was significantly better in the high-dose condition. Further controlled studies are needed in this population.

Baseline Assessments

Baseline studies prior to initiating treatment with valproate in children and adolescents should include general medical history and physical examination with height and weight, liver function tests, complete blood count with differential and platelets, and a pregnancy test for sexually active females. A complete blood count with differential, platelet count, and liver functions should be checked every 6 months or when clinically indicated, as divalproex can cause liver dysfunction and reduced platelet counts.

Contraindications

Caution must be used and serum level and liver functions monitored carefully if valproate is given to patients with significant liver dysfunction (Asconapé 2002) or patients with inborn errors of ammonia metabolism (König et al. 1994; Treem 1994). Valproate should be avoided in pregnancy.

Side Effects

Common side effects of valproate in children and adolescents include nausea, increased appetite, weight gain, sedation, thrombocytopenia, transient hair loss, tremor, and vomiting. Pancreatitis (Sinclair et al. 2004; Werlin and Fish 2006) and liver failure (Ee et al. 2003; König et al. 1994) are rare but have occurred in children treated with valproate. Fetal exposure to valproate is associated with an increased risk for neural tube defects.

Valproate-induced hyperammonemia has been observed in children and adolescents treated for psychiatric disorders (Carr and Shrewsbury 2007; Raskind and El-Chaar 2000; Treem 1994). It can present as lethargy, disorientation, and reversible cognitive deficits, which may progress to marked sedation, coma, and even death. It is often a transient and asymptomatic phenomenon but can become chronic if undetected.

There is an association between valproate and polycystic ovarian syndrome (PCOS), an endocrine disorder characterized by ovulatory dysfunction and hyperandrogenism, an autosomal dominant condition affecting more than 3%–5% of women overall (Rasgon 2004). The initial reports linked hyperandrogenism and adverse metabolic changes with divalproex exposure in women with epilepsy. The association was particularly strong if their exposure was during adolescence (Isojärvi et al. 1993). In adults with bipolar disorder, a sevenfold increased risk of new-onset oligomenorrhea with hyperandrogenism in women treated with valproate was found (Joffe et al. 2006). Common signs and symptoms of PCOS include irregular or absent menstruation, lack of ovulation, weight gain, adverse metabolic changes including hyperinsulinemia, hirsutism, and/or acne. Females treated with valproate should have a baseline assessment of menstrual cycle patterns and continued monitoring for menstrual irregularities, as well as for the above symptoms. If symptoms of PCOS develop, referral to an endocrinologist should be considered. Women with PCOS are often treated with hormonal contraceptives or metformin, in part because of the insulin resistance and risk for type 2 diabetes, a feature of the disorder. Of note, women already taking hormonal contraceptive agents are not susceptible to developing valproate-induced PCOS. Table 37–3 lists management tactics for the common side effects of valproate.

Drug Interactions

Valproate is metabolized in the liver by cytochrome P450 enzymes and has interactions with several medications that also are metabolized by this system. Medications that will increase valproate levels include erythromycin, selective serotonin reuptake inhibitors, cimetidine, and salicylates. Valproate may increase the levels of phenobarbital, primidone, carbamazepine, phenytoin, tricyclics, and lamotrigine.

Clinical Use

Valproate is readily absorbed from the gastrointestinal system; peak levels occur 2–4 hours after each dose. If given with meals to decrease nausea, peak levels may not be reached for 5–6 hours. Valproate is highly protein bound. It is metabolized in the liver and has a serum half-life of 8–16 hours in children and young adolescents (Cloyd et al. 1993). A starting dosage of divalproex sodium of 15 mg/kg/day in 2–3 divided doses in children and adolescents will produce serum valproate levels in the range of 50–60 μg/mL. Once this low serum level is attained, the dose is usually titrated upward depending on the subject's tolerance and response. It is best to measure serum valproate levels 12 hours after the last dose. Optimal serum levels for treating mania in adults are 85–110 μg/mL, and the same appears true in children and adolescents (Bowden et al. 1996).

Carbamazepine

Carbamazepine is an anticonvulsant structurally similar to imipramine, first introduced in the United States in 1968. It is metabolized by the P450 hepatic system to an active metabolite, carbamazepine-10,11-epoxide. Carbamazepine induces its own metabolism, and this "autoinduction" is complete 3–5 weeks after achieving a fixed dose, often requiring dose adjustment. Initial carbamazepine serum half-lives range from 25 to 65 hours and then decrease

TABLE 37–3. Management of common valproate side effects

System	Side effects	Tactic
Central nervous system	Tremor, headache, sedation	Use a slow-release formulation; split the dose
Endocrine	Polycystic ovary syndrome	Check for weight gain, abnormal menstrual periods, and hirsutism; consult with endocrinologist about management/laboratory work
Gastrointestinal	Nausea, stomach pains	Take with food; use a slow-release formulation
Hematological	Leukopenia, thrombocytopenia	Consult with hematologist; consider switching to a different mood stabilizer
Hepatic	Elevated liver function enzymes or pancreatic enzymes	Recheck lab values; consult with gastroenterologist

to 9–15 hours after autoinduction of the P450 enzymes (Wilder 1992).

Disorders in Which Carbamazepine May Be Useful

A long-acting form of carbamazepine has an FDA-approved indication for the treatment of acute manic or mixed episodes in adults with bipolar I disorder. In children and adolescents, carbamazepine may be useful for mania, mixed mania, bipolar depression, ADHD, and conduct disorder.

Evidence for Efficacy

Two controlled studies of a long-acting preparation of carbamazepine in adults with bipolar disorder demonstrated efficacy for carbamazepine as monotherapy for mania (Weisler et al. 2006). Joshi et al. (2010) performed a small prospective open-label trial of 8 weeks of extended-release carbamazepine monotherapy in 27 children, finding statistically significant, modest levels of improvement in mania, as well as in depressive, ADHD, and psychotic symptoms. Two subjects developed a skin rash. Findling and Ginsberg (2014) reported an industry-sponsored multisite study of open-label extended-release carbamazepine for acute manic or mixed bipolar I episodes in 60 children ages 10–12 and 97 adolescents. Doses were titrated over the initial 5 weeks and continued for up to 21 weeks. At study end, final dosages ranged from 200 to 1,200 mg/day; the most prevalent dosage was 1,200 mg/day, in about one-quarter of the adolescents and one-third of the children. The YMRS decreased significantly ($P<0.0001$), with just over half responding. The CDRS-R and CGI-I were also significantly decreased ($P<0.0001$). Concomitant mood-stabilizing medication was permitted if clinically necessary ($N=15$). Six children developed a rash, and five who had decreases in white blood cell counts were discontinued from the study. Serious adverse events considered related to the study drug included one case of thrombocytopenia and one case of erythema multiforme.

Pleak et al. (1988) found that 6 of 20 youth given carbamazepine for ADHD and conduct disorder worsened. Its chemical structure, in the tricyclic family, may contribute to its potential for worsening of mood in those children susceptible to this effect. A small negative double-blind placebo-controlled study for aggressive children with conduct disorder found no improvement over placebo (Cueva et al. 1996), but a smaller open trial found benefit in hospitalized aggressive children with conduct disorder (Kafantaris et al. 1992).

Randomized controlled trials are needed to assess efficacy of carbamazepine as a first-line agent for bipolar disorder in youth. Clinical use can be difficult because of the numerous P450 drug interactions (including with oral contraceptives), as well as relatively high rates of serious skin rashes and potential for worsening mood.

Baseline Assessments

Complete pretreatment blood counts, including platelets, should be obtained at baseline prior to treatment. If a patient in the course of treatment exhibits low or decreased white blood cell or platelet counts, the patient's counts should be monitored closely with pediatric consultation.

Serious and sometimes fatal dermatological reactions, including toxic epidermal necrolysis (TEN) and Stevens-Johnson syndrome (SJS), have been reported with carbamazepine treatment. The risk of these events is estimated to be about 1–6 per 10,000 new users in countries with mainly white populations. Retrospective case control studies have found that in patients of broad Asian ancestry there is a strong association between the risk of developing SJS or TEN with carbamazepine treatment and the presence of an inherited variant of the HLA-B gene, *HLA-B*1502. HLA-B*1502* is largely absent in individuals not of Asian origin (e.g., whites, African Americans, Hispanics, American Indians). Therefore, in patients of Asian ancestry, it is recommended that testing for *HLA-B*1502* be performed before starting carbamazepine.

Contraindications

Carbamazepine should not be used in patients positive for *HLA-B*1502* unless the benefits clearly outweigh the risks. Carbamazepine should not be used in patients with a history of previous bone marrow depression, hypersensitivity to the drug, or known sensitivity to any tricyclic compounds.

Side Effects

Common side effects of carbamazepine in children and adolescents include headache, sedation, ataxia, dizziness, blurred vision, nausea, and vomiting. Uncommon side effects include aplastic anemia, agranulocytosis, hyponatremia, TEN, and SJS (Devi et al. 2005; Keating and Blahunka 1995). The risk of agranulocytosis is 6 per million; aplastic anemia 2 per million, and SJS and TEN about 1–6 per 10,000 new users in countries with mainly white populations. Carbamazepine should be discontinued at the first sign of a serious rash unless the rash is clearly not drug-related. If signs or symptoms suggest SJS or TEN, carbamazepine should not be resumed. Carbamazepine can cause fetal harm and is therefore contraindicated during pregnancy.

Drug Interactions

Because of its stimulation of the hepatic P450 isoenzyme system, carbamazepine has many clinically significant drug interactions. Carbamazepine decreases lithium clearance, increasing the risk of lithium toxicity. Medications that will increase carbamazepine levels include erythromycin, cimetidine, fluoxetine, verapamil, and valproate. Carbamazepine may decrease the levels of the following medications: oral contraceptives, clonazepam, glucocorticoids, phenobarbital, primidone, phenytoin, tricyclics, valproate, and lamotrigine (Ciraulo et al. 1995). Carbamazepine can also decrease the serum levels of many of the atypical antipsychotics (Besag and Berry 2006), leading to symptomatic relapses in some patients.

Clinical Use

In patients ages 6–12 years, a reasonable starting dosage of carbamazepine is 100 mg twice daily and in patients ages 12 years and older, 100 mg three times daily. Carbamazepine serum levels 8–11 mg/mL are necessary for seizure control; however, the range of serum level for therapeutic effects in youth with bipolar disorder is unknown. The maximum daily dosage of carbamazepine should not exceed 1,000 mg/day in children ages 6–12 years and 1,200 mg/day in patients ages 13 years and older.

Oxcarbazepine

Oxcarbazepine is indicated for use as monotherapy or adjunctive therapy in the treatment of partial seizures in adults and as monotherapy in the treatment of partial seizures in children. It is the 10-keto analogue of carbamazepine that is biotransformed by hydroxylation to its active metabolite 10,11-dihydro-10-hydroxy carbamazepine (MHD). MHD is the primary active metabolite and accounts for the antiseizure properties of oxcarbazepine.

Wagner et al. (2006) reported the results of an industry-sponsored, multisite, randomized, double-blind, placebo-controlled study in children and adolescents with bipolar disorder. During this study, 116 youth with bipolar disorder (mean age 11.1±2.9 years) were randomly assigned to receive either oxcarbazepine or placebo. Between the treatment groups, the difference in the primary outcome variable—change in YMRS mean scores—was neither statistically nor clinically significant. This single negative trial does not support the use of oxcarbazepine as monotherapy in the treatment of mania in children and adolescents, but further controlled trials are needed. Whether this medication may be useful for the treatment of hypomania, bipolar depression, bipolar disorder not otherwise specified (NOS), or cyclothymia is unknown.

Lamotrigine

Lamotrigine is an antiseizure agent indicated as adjunct therapy for partial seizures, the generalized seizures of Lennox-Gastaut syndrome, and primary generalized tonic-clonic seizures in adults and children >2 years of age. It works by blocking voltage-sensitive sodium channels and inhibiting the release of excitatory neurotransmitters, particularly glutamate and aspartate (Ketter et al. 2003). Lamotrigine also inhibits serotonin reuptake, suggesting antidepressant properties. The FDA has approved lamotrigine for the maintenance treatment of bipolar I disorder in adults to delay the time to reoccurrence of mood episodes (e.g., depression, mania, hypomania, mixed episodes) in patients already treated for acute mood episodes with standard therapy.

Disorders in Which Lamotrigine May Be Useful

Lamotrigine is used to treat seizure disorders, and it may be useful for bipolar or unipolar depression.

Evidence for Efficacy

Several prospective studies in adults with bipolar disorder (bipolar I, bipolar II, and other specific/unspecified bipolar and related disorders) suggest that lamotrigine may be beneficial for the treatment of mood (especially depressive) symptoms in bipolar disorder (Bowden et al. 2003; Calabrese et al. 1999). Chang et al. (2006) published an 8-week, open-label trial of lamotrigine alone or as adjunctive therapy for the treatment of 20 adolescents with bipolar disorder (bipolar I, II, and not otherwise specified), who were experiencing a depressive or mixed episode. The mean final dosage was 131.6 mg/day. Of these subjects, 84% were rated on the CGI scale as much or very much improved. Shon et al. (2014) found a response rate of 46% in a retrospective chart review of 37 adolescents with unipolar and bipolar depression, with no difference in response between those with bipolar versus unipolar depression. The mean dosage was 65.4±37.5mg/day (range 12.5–181.7mg/day); rash occurred in 13.5% (n=5) and resolved after discontinuation of lamotrigine. Larger, placebo-controlled studies of lamotrigine in children and adolescents with bipolar disorder are needed.

Baseline Assessments

Prior to starting lamotrigine, a complete blood cell count, differential, platelet count, and liver function tests should be obtained.

Contraindications

Lamotrigine is contraindicated in patients who have demonstrated hypersensitivity to it.

Side Effects

The most common side effects of lamotrigine are dizziness, tremor, somnolence, nausea, asthenia, and headache. Blurred vision and cognitive difficulties, including word-finding problems, can occur and may respond to lowering the dose. Cases of lupus, leukopenia, agranulocytosis, hepatic failure, and multiorgan failure associated with lamotrigine treatment have been reported (Sabers and Gram 2000). However, lamotrigine has been well tolerated as long-term treatment in pediatric patients with epilepsy.

Benign rashes develop in 12% of adult patients, typically within the first 8 weeks of lamotrigine therapy (Calabrese et al. 2002). Rarely, severe cutaneous reactions such as SJS and TEN have been described. The risk of developing a serious rash is approximately three times greater in children and adolescents younger than age 16 years compared with adults. The FDA has issued a black box warning that states, "Lamictal is not indicated for use in patients below the age of 16 years." The frequency of serious rash associated with lamotrigine (rashes requiring hospitalization and discontinuation of treatment), including SJS, is approximately 1/100 (1%) in children ages younger than 16 years and 3/1,000 (0.3%) in adults (GlaxoSmithKline 2001).

Drug Interactions

Lamotrigine is primarily eliminated by hepatic metabolism through glucuronidation processes (Sabers and Gram 2000). Glucuronidation of lamotrigine is inhibited by valproic acid and induced by carbamazepine. Adding carbamazepine to lamotrigine decreases lamotrigine blood levels by 50%. Concomitant treatment with valproate increases lamotrigine blood levels; therefore, it is advisable to use lower lamotrigine doses and proceed very cautiously when coadministering these medications. Patients on oral contraceptives may require increased lamotrigine doses since estrogen induces the metabolism of lamotrigine. If contraceptives are discontinued or the patient is postpartum, the dose of lamotrigine should be decreased since lamotrigine levels may double (Reimers et al. 2005).

Clinical Use

The starting dosage of lamotrigine for an adolescent not on valproate is 25 mg/day for 2 weeks, with a gradual titration to up to 100–300 mg/day based on clinical response. If the patient is on valproate, then the starting dosage of lamotrigine is 25 mg every other day for 2 weeks. It is important to follow the current dosing guidelines recommended by GlaxoSmithKline for lamotrigine to avoid serious rashes. For patients <12 years, the dosing of lamotrigine is weight based, and these guidelines can be found within the package insert at https://www.gsksource.com/gskprm/htdocs/documents/LAMICTAL-PI-MG.PDF (accessed December 4, 2014).

Gabapentin

Gabapentin is an antiseizure agent approved for the treatment of partial seizures in patients older than age 12 years and postherpetic neuralgia in adults. It is structurally similar to γ-aminobutyric acid (GABA), increases GABA release from glia, and may modulate sodium channels. Gabapentin is eliminated from the systemic circulation by renal excretion, as it is not appreciably metabolized in humans. The half-life of gabapentin in children averages 4.7 hours.

Adult double-blind controlled studies of gabapentin as adjunctive therapy to lithium or valproate or as monotherapy have found it is no more effective than placebo for the treatment of mania (Pande et al. 2000); however, gabapentin may be useful in combination with other mood-stabilizing agents for the treatment of comorbid anxiety disorders in individuals with bipolar disorder (Keck et al. 2006). Vieta et al. (2006) found efficacy for sleep and manic symptoms in a very small 1-year double-blind placebo-controlled multicenter study. An open trial of its major metabolite, pregabalin, as an acute and maintenance adjunctive treatment for outpatient adults (N=58) with treatment-resistant bipolar disorder found that 41% were acute responders, with 42% of that group continuing adjunctive pregabalin for an average of 45 months, suggesting that double-blind controlled studies are needed (Schaffer et al. 2013).

In children and adolescents, gabapentin may be useful as a second- or third-line treatment, usually for anxiety or sleep disorders comorbid with bipolar disorder; however, there are no studies to date of gabapentin or pregabalin for youth with bipolar disorder. Laboratory tests are not necessary prior to starting gabapentin. It has a relatively benign side effect profile, with the most common side effects in bipolar disorder study participants including sedation, dizziness, tremor, headache, ataxia, fatigue, edema, and weight gain. Gabapentin has been reported to cause mania in adults and behavioral disinhibition in younger children (Lee et al. 1996; Tallian et al. 1996). Although drug-drug interactions are few because of lack of systemic metabolism or protein binding, gastrointestinal absorption of gabapentin is decreased by antacids, orlistat, and sodium citrate/citric acid and likely lithium citrate as well. Additionally, co-medication with CNS depressants should be minimized and monitored closely because of potential for additive effects. Multiorgan hypersensitivity has been reported. Gabapentin dosing in children and adolescents for seizures is 600–1,800 mg/day, starting at 50–100 mg. For anxiety it is commonly given in divided doses (three times a day) because of saturable absorption. Bioavailability of gabapentin is decreased by 20% with concomitant use of aluminum/magnesium hydroxide antacids.

Topiramate

Topiramate is indicated for monotherapy in patients ≥10 years of age with epilepsy and in adults for prophylaxis of migraine headache. It is a sulfamate-substituted monosaccharide, with several potential mechanisms of action, including blockade of voltage-gated sodium channels, antagonism of the kainate/α-amino-3-hydroxy-5-methyl-4-isoxazolepropionic acid subtype of glutamate receptor, enhancement of GABA activity, and carbonic anhydrase inhibition. Topiramate has been shown to be moderately effective in causing weight loss in adult and adolescent patients with psychotropic-induced obesity (McElroy et al. 2007; Tramontina et al. 2007). It has not been shown to be an effective mood stabilizer. DelBello et al. (2005) published results of an industry-funded, double-blind, placebo-controlled study of topiramate monotherapy for acute mania in children and adolescents with bipolar disorder type I. The trial was discontinued early by the pharmaceutical company after several adult mania trials with topiramate failed to show efficacy. During the pediatric trial, 56 children and adolescents (ages 6–17 years) with bipolar disorder type I were randomly assigned to receive topiramate or placebo. The mean final dosage of topiramate was 278±121 mg/day. Change in the primary outcome variable, the mean YMRS score from baseline to final visit, was not statistically different between the topiramate and the placebo groups. This is considered a negative trial, although results are largely inconclusive because of premature termination of the study.

Measurement of baseline and periodic serum bicarbonate during topiramate treatment is recommended. Topiramate is contraindicated in patients who have demonstrated hypersensitivity to it. The side effects of topiramate include sedation, fatigue, impaired concentration, visual changes (including acute closure glaucoma), and psychomotor slowing. In patients with epilepsy, there is a 1%–2% rate of nephrolithiasis because of carbonic anhydrase inhibition. Word-finding difficulties have been reported in up to one-third of adult patients treated with topiramate, and this also has been reported in children. Topiramate can be started at 25 mg twice daily and titrated to 100–200 mg/day over 3–4 weeks. A lower starting dose and slower titration may decrease some of the side effects of topiramate. Pediatric patients have a 50% higher clearance of topiramate and consequently a shorter elimination half-life than adults. Topiramate is a weak inducer of cytochrome P450 enzymes and therefore is potentially associated with a risk of oral contraceptive failure (particularly low-dose estrogen oral contraceptives). Topiramate is associated with limb agenesis in rodents and should be used with caution in females with childbearing potential.

Complementary and Alternative Medical Treatments

Omega-3 Fatty Acids

Long-chain polyunsaturated fatty acids (LC-PUFAs) include the omega n-3 and n-6 fatty acid subgroups, known by the position of the last double bond in their chemical structures. Omega-3 fatty acids are essential, meaning they are obtained only from naturally occurring diet sources. Mammals cannot synthesize them de novo, and can only elongate and desaturate, changing plant-based α-linolenic acid into eicosapentaenoic acid (EPA) and EPA into docosahexaenoic acid (DHA). Western diets are deficient in omega-3 fats because of relatively low seafood intake, high processed food consumption, and food industry changes over the last century resulting in greater corn and soy oil use, which are high in the omega-6 fatty acid linoleic acid (Hibbeln et al 2006). It has been speculated that insufficient dietary intake of LC-n-3 PUFAs may have contributed to the rise of mental disorders, including depression and bipolar disorder, during the twentieth century, as evidenced by epidemiological data showing lower rates of bipolar I, II, and NOS disorders in countries with higher seafood consumption (Noaghiul and Hibbeln 2003).

Disorders in Which LC-n-3 PUFAs May Be Helpful

Omega-3 fatty acids (O3Fas) may be helpful for bipolar depression, anxiety, ADHD, and comorbid metabolic conditions, including hypertriglyceridemia.

Evidence for Efficacy

Evidence from open-label and controlled trials is best summarized in the first meta-analysis of omega-3 fatty acids used specifically for bipolar disorder (Sarris et al. 2012). Six RCTs, including only one pediatric trial, had acceptable methodology for inclusion. The results support an effect for bipolar depression, but not manic symptoms, with small to moderate effect sizes. The authors concluded that omega-3 fish oils should now be recommended in the adjunctive treatment of bipolar disorder, especially for those with comorbid cardiovascular or metabolic conditions. They echo past calls for additional research to establish optimal formulations and doses for LC-n-3PUFA treatment in bipolar disorder.

There is strong biological plausibility to the theory that developing brains and bodies are more sensitive to or have differential results when given treatment doses of LCn-3 PUFAs (Kuratko et al. 2013; Montgomery et al. 2013). There are four published pediatric pilot studies of LCn-3 PUFAs for depressive and bipolar illness that document safety and tolerability, but sample sizes and methodological factors preclude definitive results. Analysis and submission for publication of several RCTs of fish oil for depression and bipolar disorder NOS in children are under way.

Omega-3 supplementation may improve concentration in youth with bipolar disorder who have comorbid ADHD. DHA supplementation in healthy boys has been found to increase activity in attention networks in the prefrontal cortex during sustained attention tasks (McNamara et al. 2010). Two recent meta-analyses concluded that omega-3 levels are reduced in children with ADHD and that dietary supplementation appears to improve symptoms, with effects perhaps greater for hyperactivity than attention (Hawkey and Nigg 2014).

Baseline Assessments

No specific studies are uniformly recommended. Periodic monitoring of lipids for increases in low-density lipoprotein and coagulation measures in those with a history of bleeding disorders is recommended.

Contraindications

Those youth with a history of hepatic impairment or bleeding disorders should be monitored closely, and omega-3 fatty acids should be discontinued if any worsening of the underlying disorder occurs. Fish oil is contraindicated in those with known hypersensitivity to fish or shellfish.

Side Effects

The most commonly reported side effects include stomach upset, "fish burps," and diarrhea. Changing dose timing or preparations or administering with or after food should eliminate most of these concerns.

Drug Interactions

In general, there are no expected drug interactions, but there may be additive effects with antiplatelet treatments and warfarin.

Clinical Use

Currently accepted dose recommendations are an EPA/DHA mix at a dosage of about 1,000 mg/day, which can be increased gradually, watching for emergence of increased cycling (Freeman et al. 2010). Several capsules per day of fish oil may be required to achieve this dose, depending on the product purchased. Families should be educated to examine the nutritional content label on the back of the bottles for EPA and DHA amounts to determine a suitable product; labels should also say that the product has been purified to exclude harmful heavy metals such as mercury. The presence of a U.S. Pharmacopeia Convention (USP) verified mark also indicates that the product has been voluntarily submitted to the USP Dietary Supplement Verification Program to meet federally recognized standards in quality, purity, and potency.

Broad-Spectrum Multinutrient Supplements

Clinicians may have families asking about or children presenting while taking broad-spectrum multinutrient supplements, possibly for bipolar disorder depression, ADHD, obsessive-compulsive disorder, autism spectrum disorder, substance use disorders, violent/antisocial behaviors, or acute stress disorder. There are no published RCTs examining the use of these supplements in youth, although an RCT of 80 adults with ADHD found nearly half reporting improvement in attention and hyperactivity. Post hoc analyses revealed improvement in depressive symptoms as well for those adults with comorbid moderate to severe depression. A 1-year naturalistic follow-up of 72 of the sample found ongoing perceived benefit of continuing micronutrients (Rucklidge et al. 2014). Secondary analyses of clinical reports describing broad-spectrum micronutrient use and effects in child and adolescent bipolar disorder, as well as theoretical mechanistic papers and a safety and tolerability review, have been published (Kaplan et al. 2007; Rucklidge et al. 2010; Simpson et al. 2011).

Side effects include nausea, vomiting, sleep disturbance, and headache. Anxiety, agitation, or impulsivity can occur if the dose is too high. Worsening of preexisting *Candida* (yeast) infections has been noted. Strict contraindications to multinutrient use include 1) Wilson disease (risk of copper overload), 2) hemochromatosis and hemosiderosis (risk of iron overload), 3) phenylketonuria (risk of phenylalanine overload), and 4) trimethylaminuria (risk of choline overload). Relative contraindications include 1) recreational drug dependence involving cannabis, caffeine, alcohol, and/or nicotine (reduced bioavailability or action of micronutrient supplements); 2) recent use of prescription drugs with potential withdrawal syndromes; 3) ongoing necessary medical treatment with CNS-active agents; 4) treatment-resistant

Candida infections; 5) autoimmune thyroid disease or nodular goiter (iodine); 6) high alcohol intake; 7) hyperlipidemia; and 8) severe protein malnutrition (associated with increased susceptibility to vitamin A toxicity).

Depending on ingredients, multinutrient supplements can interact with virtually all psychiatric drugs and other medications with CNS effects, especially medications associated with discontinuation syndromes. These interactions typically potentiate side effects of psychotropic medications. Antibiotics reduce gastrointestinal absorption of nutrients, so higher micronutrient dosages are necessary during antibiotic treatment.

Dosing is usually more than once a day; the total daily dose has been 8–15 capsules or tablets, depending on the product. Titration to the full dose has been generally performed quickly, within 1 week. Doses may need to be lowered to a level tolerated by each patient. Improvements have been reported as fairly quick for manic symptoms and by 4–6 weeks for depressive symptoms. Because of the large number and complexity of potential drug-nutrient interactions, it is recommended that clinicians monitor use of broad-spectrum micronutrient treatments in medication-naïve patients and only after familiarizing themselves with a specific product and related publications and consultation with clinicians with expertise with these treatments (Popper 2014).

Suicide and Mood Stabilizers

At a joint meeting in July 2008, members of the FDA peripheral and CNS and psychopharmacology advisory committees voted in favor of adding warnings and precautions about suicidality risk to the package inserts of all antiepileptic drugs—but not in the form of a black box warning. The FDA analyzed almost 200 studies of 11 antiseizure drugs, some of which have been on the market for decades. The studies tracked almost 28,000 people given the medications and another 16,000 given placebos. Suicidal thoughts or behavior were very rarely reported. Still, the FDA found that drug-treated patients had about twice the risk: 0.43% of drug-treated patients experienced suicidal thoughts or behavior, compared with 0.22% of placebo takers. Overall, four people in the drug-treated groups committed suicide and none in the placebo groups. The FDA concluded that for every 1,000 patients, about 2 more drug-treated patients experienced suicidal thoughts than those taking placebo. Antiseizure drugs are used for a variety of illnesses in addition to epilepsy, including migraines, certain nerve pain disorders, and psychiatric diseases such as bipolar disorder, which themselves carry a risk of suicide. The FDA found that drug-treated patients were at increased risk whatever their diagnosis, but the risk was highest for subjects with epilepsy. The 11 drugs included in the analysis were carbamazepine, divalproex sodium, felbamate, gabapentin, lamotrigine, levetiracetam, oxcarbazepine, pregabalin, tiagabine, topiramate, and zonisamide. Clinicians who prescribe any of these agents should take the following steps:

- Balance the risk with the patient's need for the drug
- Tell patients and their families about the risk so they will watch for changes in mood, thinking, or behavior
- Make sure patients and families know to contact a doctor in case of suicide warning signs such as talking or thinking about hurting oneself, becoming

preoccupied with death or socially withdrawn, becoming depressed or experiencing worsening depression, and giving away prized possessions

Maintenance Treatment

The question of how long to continue a mood stabilizer is difficult to answer because there have been few pediatric studies of these agents used for psychiatric indications that lasted longer than several months. It is reasonable to maintain a child or adolescent with bipolar disorder who has had a single manic episode on a mood-stabilizing agent for several years. If the patient is then euthymic and asymptomatic, the clinician may slowly taper the mood-stabilizing agent over several months. If mood symptoms recur, the mood-stabilizing agent(s) should be reintroduced. If a child or adolescent with bipolar disorder has been psychotic, he or she should be maintained on an antipsychotic (typical or atypical) for a minimum of 1 month, even if the psychosis has resolved (Kafantaris et al. 2001).

Future Directions

Both the traditional and novel mood stabilizers may be effective in the treatment of children and adolescents with mood and behavior disorders. The evidence is strongest for lithium, modest for valproate, and weaker for the other agents. What is clear is that the atypical antipsychotics are more powerful and generally work faster than mood stabilizers (DelBello et al. 2006). Risperidone and aripiprazole have FDA indications for the short-term (risperidone) and long-term (aripiprazole) treatment of acute manic or mixed episodes associated with bipolar I disorder in children and adolescents ages 10–17 years. Classical mood stabilizers may be relegated to second- or third-line treatment for child and adolescent psychiatric disorders because of the broad range and power of the atypical antipsychotics. However, the traditional mood stabilizers may remain more affordable for the uninsured. They may be useful as combination therapy with an atypical antipsychotic for those who do not fully remit on one alone as well as for acute and maintenance monotherapy in a lucky few who respond positively. Additional RCTs are needed to determine response in pediatric bipolar disorder for carbamazepine and some of the other anticonvulsants as well as for omega-3 fatty acids and multinutrient supplements before their use can be generally recommended.

Summary Points

- The traditional and novel mood stabilizers are widely used to treat pediatric patients with bipolar disorders, conduct disorders, seizure disorders, migraine headaches, and other disorders.
- Lithium is a good mood stabilizer with a moderate clinical effect size. In some patients, it may take as long as 6–8 weeks for a full response to lithium. The side effects of weight gain, enuresis, and exacerbation of acne may limit the use of lithium in some patients. There are still unanswered concerns about long-term effects on renal function.

- Valproate is usually better tolerated than lithium and works faster, generally in 4–6 weeks, in patients with bipolar disorder.
- Carbamazepine is considered a third-line agent after lithium and valproate because of its numerous P450 drug interactions.
- Fish oils with adequate EPA and DHA may be a useful adjunct for bipolar depression. There is emerging interest in the use of broad-spectrum multinutrient supplements, but randomized controlled pediatric trials are needed to assess safety and efficacy.

References

Alessi N, Naylor MW, Ghaziuddin M, et al: Update on lithium carbonate therapy in children and adolescents. J Am Acad Child Adolesc Psychiatry 33(3):291–304, 1994 8169173

Annell AL: Manic-depressive illness in children and effect of treatment with lithium carbonate. Acta Paedopsychiatr 36(8):292–301, 1969 4904303

Asconapé JJ: Some common issues in the use of antiepileptic drugs. Semin Neurol 22(1):27–39, 2002 12170391

Bendz H, Aurell M, Balldin J, et al: Kidney damage in long-term lithium patients: a cross-sectional study of patients with 15 years or more on lithium. Nephrol Dial Transplant 9(9):1250–1254, 1994 7816284

Bendz H, Sjödin I, Toss G, et al: Hyperparathyroidism and long-term lithium therapy—a cross-sectional study and the effect of lithium withdrawal. J Intern Med 240(6):357–365, 1996a 9010382

Bendz H, Sjödin I, Aurell M: Renal function on and off lithium in patients treated with lithium for 15 years or more. A controlled, prospective lithium-withdrawal study. Nephrol Dial Transplant 11(3):457–460, 1996b 8671815

Besag FM, Berry D: Interactions between antiepileptic and antipsychotic drugs. Drug Saf 29(2):95–118, 2006 16454538

Bowden CL, Janicak PG, Orsulak P, et al: Relation of serum valproate concentration to response in mania. Am J Psychiatry 153(6):765–770, 1996 8633687

Bowden CL, Calabrese JR, Sachs G, et al: A placebo-controlled 18-month trial of lamotrigine and lithium maintenance treatment in recently manic or hypomanic patients with bipolar I disorder. Arch Gen Psychiatry 60(4):392–400, 2003 12695317

Brumback RA, Weinberg WA: Mania in childhood. II. Therapeutic trial of lithium carbonate and further description of manic-depressive illness in children. Am J Dis Child 131(10):1122–1126, 1977 910765

Cade JF: Lithium salts in the treatment of psychotic excitement. Med J Aust 2(10):349–352, 1949 18142718

Calabrese JR, Bowden CL, Sachs GS, et al: A double-blind placebo-controlled study of lamotrigine monotherapy in outpatients with bipolar I depression. Lamictal 602 Study Group. J Clin Psychiatry 60(2):79–88, 1999 10084633

Calabrese JR, Sullivan JR, Bowden CL, et al: Rash in multicenter trials of lamotrigine in mood disorders: clinical relevance and management. J Clin Psychiatry 63(11):1012–1019, 2002 12444815

Campbell M, Fish B, Korein J, et al: Lithium and chlorpromazine: a controlled crossover study of hyperactive severely disturbed young children. J Autism Child Schizophr 2(3):234–263, 1972 4567547

Campbell M, Perry R, Green WH: Use of lithium in children and adolescents. Psychosomatics 25(2):95–101, 105–106, 1984

Campbell M, Silva RR, Kafantaris V, et al: Predictors of side effects associated with lithium administration in children. Psychopharmacol Bull 27(3):373–380, 1991 1775612

Campbell M, Adams PB, Small AM, et al: Lithium in hospitalized aggressive children with conduct disorder: a double-blind and placebo-controlled study. J Am Acad Child Adolesc Psychiatry 34(4):445–453, 1995a 7751258

Campbell M, Kafantaris V, Cueva JE: An update on the use of lithium carbonate in aggressive children and adolescents with conduct disorder. Psychopharmacol Bull 31(1):93–102, 1995b 7675995

Carr RB, Shrewsbury K: Hyperammonemia due to valproic acid in the psychiatric setting. Am J Psychiatry 164(7):1020–1027, 2007 17606652

Chang K, Saxena K, Howe M: An open-label study of lamotrigine adjunct or monotherapy for the treatment of adolescents with bipolar depression. J Am Acad Child Adolesc Psychiatry 45(3):298–304, 2006 16540814

Ciraulo DA, Shader RJ, Greenblatt DJ, et al (eds): Drug Interactions in Psychiatry. Baltimore, MD, Williams and Wilkins, 1995

Cloyd JC, Fischer JH, Kriel RL, et al: Valproic acid pharmacokinetics in children. IV. Effects of age and antiepileptic drugs on protein binding and intrinsic clearance. Clin Pharmacol Ther 53(1):22–29, 1993 8422737

Cohen LS, Friedman JM, Jefferson JW, et al: A reevaluation of risk of in utero exposure to lithium. JAMA 271(2):146–150, 1994 8031346

Cohn JB, Collins G, Ashbrook E, et al: A comparison of fluoxetine imipramine and placebo in patients with bipolar depressive disorder. Int Clin Psychopharmacol 4(4):313–322, 1989 2607128

Cueva JE, Overall JE, Small AM, et al: Carbamazepine in aggressive children with conduct disorder: a double-blind and placebo-controlled study. J Am Acad Child Adolesc Psychiatry 35(4):480–490, 1996 8919710

Danielyan A, Kowatch RA: Management options for bipolar disorder in children and adolescents. Paediatr Drugs 7(5):277–294, 2005 16220995

DelBello MP, Findling RL, Kushner S, et al: A pilot controlled trial of topiramate for mania in children and adolescents with bipolar disorder. J Am Acad Child Adolesc Psychiatry 44(6):539–547, 2005 15908836

DelBello MP, Kowatch RA, Adler CM, et al: A double-blind randomized pilot study comparing quetiapine and divalproex for adolescent mania. J Am Acad Child Adolesc Psychiatry 45(3):305–313, 2006 16540815

DeLong GR, Nieman GW: Lithium-induced behavior changes in children with symptoms suggesting manic-depressive illness. Psychopharmacol Bull 19(2):258–265, 1983 6867235

DeLong GR, Aldershof AL: Long-term experience with lithium treatment in childhood: correlation with clinical diagnosis. J Am Acad Child Adolesc Psychiatry 26(3):389–394, 1987 3597294

Devi K, George S, Criton S, et al: Carbamazepine—the commonest cause of toxic epidermal necrolysis and Stevens-Johnson syndrome: a study of 7 years. Indian J Dermatol Venereol Leprol 71(5):325–328, 2005 16394456

Dyson WL, Barcai A: Treatment of children of lithium-responding parents. Curr Ther Res Clin Exp 12(5):286–290, 1970 4986244

Ee LC, Shepherd RW, Cleghorn GJ, et al: Acute liver failure in children: A regional experience. J Paediatr Child Health 39(2):107–110, 2003 12603798

Findling RL, Ginsberg LD: The safety and effectiveness of open-label extended-release carbamazepine in the treatment of children and adolescents with bipolar I disorder suffering from a manic or mixed episode. Neuropsychiatr Dis Treat 10:1589–1597, 2014 25210452

Findling RL, McNamara NK, Gracious BL, et al: Combination lithium and divalproex sodium in pediatric bipolarity. J Am Acad Child Adolesc Psychiatry 42(8):895–901, 2003 12874490

Findling RL, McNamara NK, Youngstrom EA, et al: Double-blind 18-month trial of lithium versus divalproex maintenance treatment in pediatric bipolar disorder. J Am Acad Child Adolesc Psychiatry 44(5):409–417, 2005 15843762

Findling RL, Kafantaris V, Pavuluri M, et al: Dosing strategies for lithium monotherapy in children and adolescents with bipolar I disorder. J Child Adolesc Psychopharmacol 21(3):195–205, 2011 21663422

Findling RL, Kafantaris V, Pavuluri M, et al: Post-acute effectiveness of lithium in pediatric bipolar I disorder. J Child Adolesc Psychopharmacol 23(2):80–90, 2013 23510444

Freeman MP, Fava M, Lake J, et al: Complementary and alternative medicine in major depressive disorder: the American Psychiatric Association Task Force report. J Clin Psychiatry 71(6):669–681, 2010 20573326

Gelenberg AJ, Kane JM, Keller MB, et al: Comparison of standard and low serum levels of lithium for maintenance treatment of bipolar disorder. N Engl J Med 321(22):1489–1493, 1989 2811970

Geller B, Cooper TB, Sun K, et al: Double-blind and placebo-controlled study of lithium for adolescent bipolar disorders with secondary substance dependency. J Am Acad Child Adolesc Psychiatry 37(2):171–178, 1998a 9473913

Geller B, Warner K, Williams M, et al: Prepubertal and young adolescent bipolarity versus ADHD: assessment and validity using the WASH-U-KSADS, CBCL and TRF. J Affect Disord 51(2):93–100, 1998b 10743842

GlaxoSmithKline: Lamictal (lamotrigine) product information, in Physicians Desk Reference, 56th Edition. Research Triangle Park, NC, Thomson Healthcare, 2001. Available at: http://www.pdr.net/full-prescribing-information/lamictal-xr?druglabelid=207. Accessed March 29, 2015.

Gracious BL, Findling RL, Seman C, et al: Elevated thyrotropin in bipolar youths prescribed both lithium and divalproex sodium. J Am Acad Child Adolesc Psychiatry 43(2):215–220, 2004 14726729

Gram LF, Rafaelsen OJ: Lithium treatment of psychotic children and adolescents. A controlled clinical trial. Acta Psychiatr Scand 48(3):253–260, 1972 4617490

Hagino OR, Weller EB, Weller RA, et al: Comparison of lithium dosage methods for preschool- and early school-age children. J Am Acad Child Adolesc Psychiatry 37(1):60–65, 1998 9444901

Hawkey E, Nigg JT: Omega-3 fatty acid and ADHD: blood level analysis and meta-analytic extension of supplementation trials. Clin Psychol Rev 34(6):496–505, 2014 25181335

Hibbeln JR, Nieminen LR, Blasbalg TL, et al: Healthy intakes of n-3 and n-6 fatty acids: estimations considering worldwide diversity. Am J Clin Nutr 83(6 suppl):1483S–1493S, 2006 16841858

Isojärvi JI, Laatikainen TJ, Pakarinen AJ, et al: Polycystic ovaries and hyperandrogenism in women taking valproate for epilepsy. N Engl J Med 329(19):1383–1388, 1993 8413434

Joffe H, Cohen LS, Suppes T, et al: Valproate is associated with new-onset oligoamenorrhea with hyperandrogenism in women with bipolar disorder. Biol Psychiatry 59(11):1078–1086, 2006 16448626

Joshi G, Wozniak J, Mick E, et al: A prospective open-label trial of extended-release carbamazepine monotherapy in children with bipolar disorder. J Child Adolesc Psychopharmacol 20(1):7–14, 2010 20166791

Kafantaris V, Campbell M, Padron-Gayol MV, et al: Carbamazepine in hospitalized aggressive conduct disorder children: an open pilot study. Psychopharmacol Bull 28(2):193–199, 1992 1513924

Kafantaris V, Dicker R, Coletti DJ, et al: Adjunctive antipsychotic treatment is necessary for adolescents with psychotic mania. J Child Adolesc Psychopharmacol 11(4):409–413, 2001 11838823

Kafantaris V, Coletti D, Dicker R, et al: Lithium treatment of acute mania in adolescents: a large open trial. J Am Acad Child Adolesc Psychiatry 42(9):1038–1045, 2003 12960703

Kafantaris V, Coletti DJ, Dicker R, et al: Lithium treatment of acute mania in adolescents: a placebo-controlled discontinuation study. J Am Acad Child Adolesc Psychiatry 43(8):984–993, 2004 15266193

Kaplan BJ, Crawford SG, Field CJ, et al: Vitamins, minerals, and mood. Psychol Bull 133(5):747–760, 2007 17723028

Keating A, Blahunka P: Carbamazepine-induced Stevens-Johnson syndrome in a child. Ann Pharmacother 29(5):538–539, 1995 7655141

Keck PE Jr, Strawn JR, McElroy SL: Pharmacologic treatment considerations in co-occurring bipolar and anxiety disorders. J Clin Psychiatry 67(suppl 1):8–15, 2006 16426111

Ketter TA, Wang PW, Becker OV, et al: The diverse roles of anticonvulsants in bipolar disorders. Ann Clin Psychiatry 15(2):95–108, 2003 12938867

Klein DJ, Cottingham EM, Sorter M, et al: A randomized, double-blind, placebo-controlled trial of metformin treatment of weight gain associated with initiation of atypical antipsychotic therapy in children and adolescents. Am J Psychiatry 163(12):2072–2079, 2006 17151157

König SA, Siemes H, Bläker F, et al: Severe hepatotoxicity during valproate therapy: an update and report of eight new fatalities. Epilepsia 35(5):1005–1015, 1994 7925143

Kowatch RA, DelBello MP: Pediatric bipolar disorder: emerging diagnostic and treatment approaches. Child Adolesc Psychiatr Clin N Am 15(1):73–108, 2006 16321726

Kowatch RA, Suppes T, Carmody TJ, et al: Effect size of lithium, divalproex sodium, and carbamazepine in children and adolescents with bipolar disorder. J Am Acad Child Adolesc Psychiatry 39(6):713–720, 2000 10846305

Kowatch R, Findling R, Scheffer R, et al: Placebo controlled trial of divalproex versus lithium for bipolar disorder. Presented at the American Academy of Child and Adolescent Psychiatry 54th Annual Meeting, Boston, MA, October 2007

Kuratko CN, Barrett EC, Nelson EB, et al: The relationship of docosahexaenoic acid (DHA) with learning and behavior in healthy children: a review. Nutrients 5(7):2777–2810, 2013 23877090

Lee DO, Steingard RJ, Cesena M, et al: Behavioral side effects of gabapentin in children. Epilepsia 37(1):87–90, 1996 8603631

Lena B: Lithium in child and adolescent psychiatry. Arch Gen Psychiatry 36(8 Spec No):854–855, 1979 378162

Malone RP, Delaney MA, Luebbert JF, et al: A double-blind placebo-controlled study of lithium in hospitalized aggressive children and adolescents with conduct disorder. Arch Gen Psychiatry 57(7):649–654, 2000 10891035

Manji HK, Zarate CA: Molecular and cellular mechanisms underlying mood stabilization in bipolar disorder: implications for the development of improved therapeutics. Mol Psychiatry 7(suppl 1):S1–S7, 2002 11986989

McClellan J, Kowatch R, Findling RL, et al: Practice parameter for the assessment and treatment of children and adolescents with bipolar disorder. J Am Acad Child Adolesc Psychiatry 46(1):107–125, 2007 17195735

McElroy SL, Keck PE Jr: Pharmacologic agents for the treatment of acute bipolar mania. Biol Psychiatry 48(6):539–557, 2000 11018226

McElroy SL, Frye MA, Altshuler LL, et al: A 24-week, randomized, controlled trial of adjunctive sibutramine versus topiramate in the treatment of weight gain in overweight or obese patients with bipolar disorders. Bipolar Disord 9(4):426–434, 2007 17547588

McKnew DH, Cytryn L, Buchsbaum MS, et al: Lithium in children of lithium-responding parents. Psychiatry Res 4(2):171–180, 1981 6939008

McNamara RK, Able J, Jandacek R, et al: Docosahexaenoic acid supplementation increases prefrontal cortex activation during sustained attention in healthy boys: a placebo-controlled, dose-ranging, functional magnetic resonance imaging study. Am J Clin Nutr 91(4):1060–1067, 2010 20130094

Montgomery P, Burton JR, Sewell RP, et al: Low blood long chain omega-3 fatty acids in UK children are associated with poor cognitive performance and behavior: a cross-sectional analysis from the DOLAB study. PLoS ONE 8(6):e66697, 2013 23826114

Noaghiul S, Hibbeln JR: Cross-national comparisons of seafood consumption and rates of bipolar disorders. Am J Psychiatry 160(12):2222–2227, 2003 14638594

Pande AC, Crockatt JG, Janney CA, et al: Gabapentin in bipolar disorder: a placebo-controlled trial of adjunctive therapy. Bipolar Disord 2(3 Pt 2):249–255, 2000 11249802

Patel NC, DelBello MP, Bryan HS, et al: Open-label lithium for the treatment of adolescents with bipolar depression. J Am Acad Child Adolesc Psychiatry 45(3):289–297, 2006 16540813

Pavuluri MN, Birmaher B, Naylor MW: Pediatric bipolar disorder: a review of the past 10 years. J Am Acad Child Adolesc Psychiatry 44(9):846–871, 2005 16113615

Pleak RR, Birmaher B, Gavrilescu A, et al: Mania and neuropsychiatric excitation following carbamazepine. J Am Acad Child Adolesc Psychiatry 27(4):500–503, 1988 3182607

Popper CW: Single-micronutrient and broad-spectrum micronutrient approaches for treating mood disorders in youth and adults. Child Adolesc Psychiatr Clin N Am 23(3):591–672, 2014 24975626

Rasgon N: The relationship between polycystic ovary syndrome and antiepileptic drugs: a review of the evidence. J Clin Psychopharmacol 24(3):322–334, 2004 15118487

Raskind JY, El-Chaar GM: The role of carnitine supplementation during valproic acid therapy. Ann Pharmacother 34(5):630–638, 2000 10852092

Reimers A, Helde G, Brodtkorb E: Ethinyl estradiol, not progestogens, reduces lamotrigine serum concentrations. Epilepsia 46(9):1414–1417, 2005 16146436

Rucklidge JJ, Gately D, Kaplan BJ: Database analysis of children and adolescents with bipolar disorder consuming a micronutrient formula. BMC Psychiatry 10:74, 2010 20875144

Rucklidge JJ, Frampton CM, Gorman B, et al: Vitamin-mineral treatment of attention-deficit hyperactivity disorder in adults: double-blind randomised placebo-controlled trial. Br J Psychiatry 204:306–315, 2014 24482441

Sabers A, Gram L: Newer anticonvulsants: comparative review of drug interactions and adverse effects. Drugs 60(1):23–33, 2000 10929928

Sakarcan A, Thomas DB, O'Reilly KP, et al: Lithium-induced nephrotic syndrome in a young pediatric patient. Pediatr Nephrol 17(4):290–292, 2002 11956885

Sarris J, Mischoulon D, Schweitzer I: Omega-3 for bipolar disorder: meta-analyses of use in mania and bipolar depression. J Clin Psychiatry 73(1):81–86, 2012 21903025

Schaffer LC, Schaffer CB, Miller AR, et al: An open trial of pregabalin as an acute and maintenance adjunctive treatment for outpatients with treatment resistant bipolar disorder. J Affect Disord 147(1–3):407–410, 2013 23040739

Shon SH, Joo Y, Lee JS, et al: Lamotrigine treatment of adolescents with unipolar and bipolar depression: a retrospective chart review. J Child Adolesc Psychopharmacol 24(5):285–287, 2014 24813210

Simpson JS, Crawford SG, Goldstein ET, et al: Systematic review of safety and tolerability of a complex micronutrient formula used in mental health. BMC Psychiatry 11:62, 2011 21501484

Sinclair DB, Berg M, Breault R: Valproic acid-induced pancreatitis in childhood epilepsy: case series and review. J Child Neurol 19(7):498–502, 2004 15526953

Steiner H, Petersen ML, Saxena K, et al: Divalproex sodium for the treatment of conduct disorder: a randomized controlled clinical trial. J Clin Psychiatry 64(10):1183–1191, 2003 14658966

Strober M, Morrell W, Lampert C, et al: Relapse following discontinuation of lithium maintenance therapy in adolescents with bipolar I illness: a naturalistic study. Am J Psychiatry 147(4):457–461, 1990 2107763

Tallian KB, Nahata MC, Lo W, et al: Gabapentin associated with aggressive behavior in pediatric patients with seizures. Epilepsia 37(5):501–502, 1996 8617181

Tramontina S, Zeni CP, Pheula G, et al: Topiramate in adolescents with juvenile bipolar disorder presenting weight gain due to atypical antipsychotics or mood stabilizers: an open clinical trial. J Child Adolesc Psychopharmacol 17(1):129–134, 2007 17343561

Treem WR: Inherited and acquired syndromes of hyperammonemia and encephalopathy in children. Semin Liver Dis 14(3):236–258, 1994 7939785

Varanka TM, Weller RA, Weller EB, et al: Lithium treatment of manic episodes with psychotic features in prepubertal children. Am J Psychiatry 145(12):1557–1559, 1988 3195675

Vieta E, Manuel Goikolea J, Martínez-Arán A, et al: A double-blind, randomized, placebo-controlled, prophylaxis study of adjunctive gabapentin for bipolar disorder. J Clin Psychiatry 67(3):473–477, 2006 16649836

Vitiello B, Behar D, Malone R, et al: Pharmacokinetics of lithium carbonate in children. J Clin Psychopharmacol 8(5):355–359, 1988 3141484

Wagner KD, Weller EB, Carlson GA, et al: An open-label trial of divalproex in children and adolescents with bipolar disorder. J Am Acad Child Adolesc Psychiatry 41(10):1224–1230, 2002 12364844

Wagner KD, Kowatch RA, Emslie GJ, et al: A double-blind, randomized, placebo-controlled trial of oxcarbazepine in the treatment of bipolar disorder in children and adolescents. Am J Psychiatry 163(7):1179–1186, 2006 16816222

Wagner KD, Redden L, Kowatch RA, et al: A double-blind, randomized, placebo-controlled trial of divalproex extended-release in the treatment of bipolar disorder in children and adolescents. J Am Acad Child Adolesc Psychiatry 48(5):519–532, 2009 19325497

Weisler RH, Cutler AJ, Ballenger JC, et al: The use of antiepileptic drugs in bipolar disorders: a review based on evidence from controlled trials. CNS Spectr 11(10):788–799, 2006 17008822

Werlin SL, Fish DL: The spectrum of valproic acid-associated pancreatitis. Pediatrics 118(4):1660–1663, 2006 17015559

Wilder BJ: Pharmacokinetics of valproate and carbamazepine. J Clin Psychopharmacol 12(1 suppl):64S–68S, 1992 1541720

Yacobi S, Ornoy A: Is lithium a real teratogen? What can we conclude from the prospective versus retrospective studies? A review. Isr J Psychiatry Relat Sci 45(2):95–106, 2008 18982835

Youngerman J, Canino IA: Lithium carbonate use in children and adolescents. A survey of the literature. Arch Gen Psychiatry 35(2):216–224, 1978 623508

CHAPTER 38

Antipsychotic Medications

Christoph U. Correll, M.D.

Since their discovery in the 1950s, antipsychotics have become an important pharmacological treatment option for a number of severe mental disorders. In children and adolescents, antipsychotics are increasingly used for both psychotic and nonpsychotic disorders (Olfson et al. 2012). Data from randomized controlled trials (RCTs) indicate that antipsychotics have significantly greater efficacy than placebo for pediatric mania, schizophrenia, and irritability and aggression associated with autism spectrum disorder, disruptive behavior disorders, and Tourette's disorder. Because of physiological developmental differences between children and adults, higher antipsychotic doses per kilogram weight are generally required in pediatric patients to achieve similar serum levels and efficacy. More frequent dosing per day may be required in younger children. In addition, pediatric patients appear to be more sensitive than adults to several relevant antipsychotic adverse effects (Correll 2008), mandating careful treatment selection and adverse effect monitoring and management in this vulnerable group of patients.

Pharmacology

Pharmacokinetic Considerations

Table 38–1 shows the pharmacokinetic properties of second-generation antipsychotics (SGAs) and selected first-generation antipsychotics (FGAs). Knowledge about specific cytochrome P450 (CYP) enzymes that metabolize antipsychotics is important in predicting and managing potential drug-drug interactions. Six CYP enzymes located in the brain and the periphery are responsible for approximately 90% of all the CYP activity (Meyer 2007). Whenever medications are metabolized by the same liver enzyme, the competition can

This work was supported in part by the Zucker Hillside Hospital NIMH Advanced Center for Intervention and Services Research for the Study of Schizophrenia MH 074543-01.

TABLE 38–1. Pharmacokinetic information for first- and second-generation antipsychotics

Antipsychotic	Principal liver enzyme target	Protein binding	Bioavailability	Half-life	Time to peak level	CHLOR dose equivalent, mg[a]	Typical PED starting dose, mg[a,b]	Typical PED titration interval[b]	Typical PED dose range, mg[b,c]	Maximum regulatory approved adult dose, mg[a]	Dose strength, mg	Route of administration/formulation	Pediatric indication in the United States
Second-generation antipsychotics													
ARI	2D6>3A4	>99%	87%	po: 75 hours; im long: 30–47 days	po: 3–5 hours; im short: 1–3 hours; im long: 5–7 hours	7.5	2–5	SCZ, BD: 2 mg/d, 5 mg/d after 2 days, 10 mg/d after 2 days; increase by 5 mg/d Autism: 2 mg/d; increase at intervals ≥1 week to 5–15 mg/d TD: 2 mg/d, 5 mg/d after 2 days, 10 mg/d on day 8; dose adjustment ≥1 week	10–30	30	Tablets: 2, 5, 10, 15, 20, 30; Diss: 10, 15; Liquid: 1 mg/mL (except: 30 mg=25 mL); im short: 9.75/1.3 mL; im long: 300/.5 mL, 400/2.0 mL	po, diss, liquid, im short, im long	Irritability associated with autism spectrum disorder, ages 6–17 years Bipolar I disorder, manic or mixed, ages 10–17 years (acute monotherapy and adjunctive with lithium or valproate, maintenance) Schizophrenia ages 13–17 years (acute, maintenance) Tourette's disorder ages 6–17 years
ASE	1A2>3A4	98	35% (≤if swallowed)	First: 6 hours, terminal: 24 hours	0.5–1.5 hours	7.5	2.6 bid	2.5 bid, 5 mg bid on day 4	2.5–10	20	Tablets: 5, 10	Sublingual (avoid eating or drinking for 10 minutes after administration)	Bipolar I disorder, manic or mixed, ages 10-17 years (acute)

TABLE 38–1. Pharmacokinetic information for first- and second-generation antipsychotics *(continued)*

Antipsychotic	Principal liver enzyme target	Protein binding	Bioavailability	Half-life	Time to peak level	CHLOR dose equivalent, mg[a]	Typical PED starting dose, mg[a,b]	Typical PED titration interval[b]	Typical PED dose range, mg[b,c]	Maximum regulatory approved adult dose, mg[a]	Dose strength, mg	Route of administration/formulation	Pediatric indication in the United States
CLO	1A2 (30%) >2C19 (24%) >3A4 (22%) >2C9 (12%) >2D6 (6%)	97%	50%–60%	12 hours	1.5–2.5 hours	50	12.5	12.5–25	50–600	900	Tablets: 25, 50, 100, 200 Diss: 12.5, 25, 100, 150, 200 Liquid: 50 mg/mL	po	–
ILO	2D6>3A4>1A2	95%	96%	18 hours	2–4 hours	5	NA (adults: 1 mg bid)	NA (adults: 1 mg bid × 1 day, 2 mg × 1 day, then increase 2 mg/d daily to therapeutic dose	12–24	24	Tablets: 1, 2, 4, 6, 8, 10, 12	po	–
LUR	3A4	99%	9%–19%	18 hours	1–3 hours	25	SCZ: 40–80 BD depression, autism: 20	20–40	40–120	180	Tablets: 20, 40, 80, 120	po (with ≥350 kcal meal)	–
OLA	1A2, 2D6, 3A4	93%	60%	30 hours	po: 6 hours; im short: 15–45 minutes; im long: 7 days	5	2.5–5	2.5–5	10–20	20	Tablets: 2.5, 5, 7.5, 10, 15, 20; Diss: 5, 10, 15, 20 im short: 10/ mL; im long: 150/1.3 mL, 210/1.3 mL, 300/1.8 mL, 405/2.3 mL	po, diss, im short, im long	Bipolar I disorder, manic or mixed ages 13–17 years (acute) Schizophrenia ages 13–17 years (acute)

TABLE 38–1. Pharmacokinetic information for first- and second-generation antipsychotics *(continued)*

Antipsychotic	Principal liver enzyme target	Protein binding	Bioavailability	Half-life	Time to peak level	CHLOR dose equivalent, mg[a]	Typical PED starting dose, mg[a,b]	Typical PED titration interval[b]	Typical PED dose range, mg[b,c]	Maximum regulatory approved adult dose, mg[a]	Dose strength, mg	Route of administration/formulation	Pediatric indication in the United States
PAL	< 10% first-pass hepatic clearance	74%	28%	po: 23 hours; im long: 25–49 days	po: 24 hours; im long: 13 days	3	6	3 mg every ≤5 days	3–12	12	Tablets: 1.5, 3, 6, 9; im long: 39/0.25 mL, 78/0.5 mL, 117/0.75mL, 156/ mL, 234/1.5 mL	po (ER); im long	Schizophrenia ages 12–17 years (acute)
QUE	3A4	83%	100%	6–7 hours	IR: 1.5 hours, XR: 6 hours	75	IR 25 bid; ER: 50	IR 25–50 bid; XR: 50–100	SCZ: 400–800; BD: 400–600	800	Tablets: IR: 25, 50, 100, 200, 300, 400; XR: 50, 150, 200, 300, 400	po (IR, XR)	Bipolar I disorder, manic, ages 10–17 years (acute monotherapy and adjunctive with lithium or valproate) Schizophrenia ages 13–17 years (acute)
RIS	2D6>3A4	90%	70%	3 hours	3 hours	2	0.25 (<20 kg) to 0.5 (≥20 kg)	SCZ, BD: 0.5–1 at intervals ≥24 hours Autism: <20 kg/≥20 kg); 0.25/0.5 initially; may be increased after ≥4 to 0.5/1	1–6	16	Tablets: 0.5, 1, 2, 3, 4; Diss: 0.5, 1, 2, 3, 4; Liquid: 1 mg/mL; im long: 12.5/1 mL, 25/2 mL, 37.5/2 mL, 50/2 mL	po, diss, liquid, im long	Irritability associated with autism spectrum disorder ages 5–17 years Bipolar I disorder, manic or mixed, ages 10–17 years (acute) Schizophrenia ages 13–17 years (acute)
ZIP	Aldehyde oxidase (2/3) >3A4 (1/3)	>99%	60%	po: 7 hours; im short: 2–5 hours	po: 6–8 hours; im short: ≤60 minutes	60	20	20 mg every other day to every day	SCZ: 60–160; BD: 40–160	160	Tablets: 20, 40, 60, 80 im short: 20/1 mL	po (with im short ≥ 500 kcal meal); im short	-

TABLE 38–1. Pharmacokinetic information for first- and second-generation antipsychotics *(continued)*

Antipsychotic	Principal liver enzyme target	Protein binding	Bioavailability	Half-life	Time to peak level	CHLOR dose equivalent, mg[a]	Typical PED starting dose, mg[a,b]	Typical PED titration interval[b]	Typical PED dose range, mg[b,c]	Maximum regulatory approved adult dose, mg[a]	Dose strength, mg	Route of administration/formulation	Pediatric indication in the United States
First-generation antipsychotics													
CHLOR	2D6	>90	20%	30 hours	2–4 hours	100	25–100 mg	po: 25–100 mg; im short: 25 mg, followed by 25–50 mg as needed after 1–4 hours	50–300	2,000	Tablets: 10, 25, 50, 100, 200; Spansule: 30, 75, 150 Syrup: 5 mL=10 mg Liquid: 25 mg/5 mL; im short: 25/mL Supp: 25, 100	po, im short, im long	Severe behavioral problems and short-term treatment of hyperactive children showing excessive motor activity with accompanying conduct disorders ages 1–12 years (extrapolated from adults)
HAL	3A4	92%	60%–70%	po: 18 hours; im short: 10–20 hours; im long: 3 weeks	po: 2–6 hours; im short: 10–20 minutes; im long: 6–7 days	2	0.5–2	1–2	2–10	60	Tablets: 0.5, 1, 2, 5, 10, 20 Liquid: 2 or10 mg/mL im short: 5 im long: 50 mg/mL, 100 mg/mL	po, im short, im long	Psychotic disorders ages 3–17 years (extrapolated from adults) Nonpsychotic behavior disorders and Tourette's disorder 3–17 years (extrapolated from adults) Severely disturbed, nonpsychotic or hyperactive children with accompanying conduct disorders who failed to respond to psychotherapy or medications other than antipsychotics, ages 3–17 years (extrapolated from adults)

TABLE 38–1. Pharmacokinetic information for first- and second-generation antipsychotics *(continued)*

Antipsychotic	Principal liver enzyme target	Protein binding	Bioavailability	Half-life	Time to peak level	CHLOR dose equivalent, mg[a]	Typical PED starting dose, mg[a,b]	Typical PED titration interval[b]	Typical PED dose range, mg[b,c]	Maximum regulatory approved adult dose, mg[a]	Dose strength, mg	Route of administration/formulation	Pediatric indication in the United States
PER	2D6	>90%	40%	9–12 hours	1–3 hours	10	2–4	2–4	8–32	64	Tablets: 2, 4, 8, 16	po	Schizophrenia ages 12–17 years (extrapolated from adults)

Note. ARI=aripiprazole; ASE=asenapine; BD=bipolar disorder; CHLOR=chlorpromazine; CLO=clozapine; diss=dissolvable tablet; ER=extended release; HAL=haloperidol; ILO=iloperidone; im=intramuscularly; IR=immediate release; LUR=lurasidone; NA=not applicable; OLA=olanzapine; PAL=paliperidone; PED=pediatric; PER=perphenazine; po=by mouth; QUE=quetiapine; RIS=risperidone; SCZ=schizophrenia; supp=suppository; XR=extended release; ZIP=ziprasidone.
[a]CHLOR dose equivalents (i.e., dose given in the table is equivalent to 100 mg of CHLOR) (for references on which that conversion is based, see Correll 2008).[b]Doses need to be individualized on the basis of efficacy and tolerability.[c]Average dose range provided for adolescents with schizophrenia or bipolar disorder; for prepubertal patients or those with other diagnoses, average dose may be approximately 33%–50% lower.
[d]Grandfathered in, not based on studies meeting modern standards of regulatory approval.

Source. Correll et al. 2011; package insert information for each medication.

lead to increased serum levels of both drugs. Conversely, medications, nutraceuticals, and smoking can induce CYP enzyme production that may lower antipsychotic serum levels. The CYP enzymes 3A4, 2D6, and 1A2 are most important for antipsychotic clearance. CYP3A4 is a low-affinity, high-capacity enzyme, making it relatively immune to saturation unless very potent inhibitors are present. CYP3A4 is relevant mainly for haloperidol, lurasidone, quetiapine, and olanzapine clearance. CYP2D6 is a high-affinity, low-capacity enzyme. It is very efficient and not readily inducible, but it can be saturated more easily (Meyer 2007). Moreover, most known genetic polymorphisms affect CYP2D6. Aripiprazole, iloperidone, perphenazine, and risperidone are predominantly cleared by CYP2D6. The CYP1A2 enzyme is also a low-affinity, high-capacity enzyme and is relevant for the clearance of clozapine and, to some degree, olanzapine. CYP2C19 and 2C9 are relevant only for clozapine clearance. In addition, the aldehyde oxidase system, which is neither saturable nor inhibitable, is responsible for 67% of ziprasidone's metabolism. Since <10% of paliperidone and only 33% of ziprasidone undergo CYP first-pass metabolism, the likelihood of drug-drug interactions is lowest with these two antipsychotics. Updated CYP450 interactions are available at http://medicine.iupui.edu/flockhart/table.htm.

Knowledge about the half-life of antipsychotics can help predict how quickly steady state is achieved and how quickly the body eliminates the drug. In general, it takes about five times the half-life of a drug for both steady state and elimination. As shown in Table 38–1, the half-life differs considerably among antipsychotics. Titration can be faster (daily) with drugs that achieve almost full steady state within 24 hours (e.g., quetiapine, ziprasidone), particularly beyond the initial titration phase when peripheral receptors responsible for early side effects are saturated. Conversely, dose increase intervals may have to be as long as 5–7 days for asenapine, lurasidone, olanzapine, and risperidone/paliperidone. For aripiprazole, a rational dose increase interval (after steady state is reached) is 10–14 days. However, the initial titration of aripiprazole can be faster (e.g., every 3–5 days), as a lower starting dose seems to minimize early side effects that are likely due to partial D_2 agonism (i.e., nausea, vomiting, psychomotor restlessness). Such a titration schedule was used in two randomized, placebo-controlled trials in children and adolescents with schizophrenia (Findling et al. 2008) and bipolar disorder (Findling et al. 2009), where doses were increased every third day, escalating from 2 mg to 5 mg and 10 mg (reached by day 5) and further to 15 mg, 20 mg, 25 mg, and 30 mg (reached by day 11 or 13, respectively). Nevertheless, it is important to note that the half-life is measured via peripheral serum levels, not in cerebrospinal fluid or by functional regional receptor activity. Thus, it is possible that central nervous system (CNS) actions are more prolonged. Moreover, many antipsychotics have active metabolites about which less information is available and which may have a longer half-life than the parent drug.

The time until peak level can help to predict the rapidity of the onset of therapeutic action and side effects after a single dose. Again, antipsychotics differ considerably (see Table 38–1). Because antipsychotic peak levels are measured peripherally, time to maximum level and onset of action in the CNS may differ. Most likely, peripheral side effects are more closely related to time to peak levels. If the clinician wants to reduce peak level–related side effects during titration, splitting the dose or administration with fatty food (which slows down drug absorption) will reduce peak levels, leaving unaltered the total dose delivered (i.e., total area under the curve). Doses needed for sufficient dopamine blockade to reach antipsychotic, antimanic, anti-tic, and/or antiaggressive efficacy (see Table 38–1) depend in part on the affinity for the dopamine D_2 receptor that varies across antipsychotics. Table 38–1 provides the relative dose strengths expressed as chlorpromazine equivalents that allow estimating dose requirements during a switch from one antipsychotic to another. Dose equivalences are only approximations, however. Finally, dosing and titration strategies also depend on pharmacodynamics aspects (see the next subsection). For example, for iloperidone, a stepwise initial titration (starting with 1 mg bid and not increasing by more than 2 mg bid until the target dosage of 6–12 mg bid) is needed because of strong α-adrenergic blockade in order to avoid orthostatic hypotension.

Pharmacodynamic Considerations

The central feature of all antipsychotics is their ability to block the dopamine D_2 receptor. This activity seems to be associated with the antipsychotic, antimanic, anti-tic, and antiaggressive effects of antipsychotic medications. The overall goal of treatment is to reduce the hyperactivity of pathways that at least in part mediate psychosis, mania, tics, and aggression. Simultaneously, the pathways that regulate motor movements, prolactin secretion, and especially cognition and motivation need to be preserved. Most antipsychotic drugs also bind to serotonin and α-adrenergic, histaminic, or muscarinic receptors, which can in part predict the therapeutic and adverse effects during therapy with a particular drug (Correll et al. 2010). Antipsychotics that bind more tightly to receptors other than dopamine D_2 receptors contain these effects in addition to the antidopaminergic efficacy. In the case of antipsychotics with relatively weak dopamine binding (e.g., clozapine, quetiapine), non-antidopaminergic effects can predominate at low doses. The tighter binding at nondopaminergic receptors can be beneficial, as in the tighter binding of SGAs to 5-HT_2 receptors, which seems to be associated with less propensity for extrapyramidal symptoms (EPS). Conversely, the stronger binding to non-dopaminergic receptors can also lead to lasting adverse effects of an antihistaminergic or anticholinergic nature.

The dose, degree of receptor occupancy, and intrinsic activity at the receptor to which the antipsychotic binds are all important determinants of therapeutic and adverse effects. With a full antagonist, approximately 60%–70% dopamine receptor occupancy is needed for antipsychotic efficacy. With a partial agonist (e.g., aripiprazole), receptor occupancy is not equivalent to blockade, and a higher degree of occupancy (at least 80%–85%) is required to achieve the same level of blockade (Burris et al. 2002).

Pharmacokinetic and Pharmacodynamic Rebound Phenomena

Rebound effects that can diminish the initial therapeutic efficacy may occur during medication changes because of receptor level interactions between the previous medication and the new medication, particularly when the properties of the two antipsychotics vary greatly and when the change is too fast. Depending on the receptor system(s) involved, withdrawal or rebound symptoms can manifest as anxiety, insomnia, agitation, mania, psychosis, confusion, EPS, or akathisia, mimicking psychiatric worsening and primary inefficacy of the new agent (Correll et al. 2010). Pharmacokinetic rebound effects can be seen in the following circumstances:

- When a patient becomes nonadherent or when the new antipsychotic is relatively underdosed
- During switching (without adequate overlap) if the first antipsychotic has a relatively short half-life and is replaced by an antipsychotic with a much longer half-life that requires longer to achieve steady-state concentrations (e.g., aripiprazole)
- When the new antipsychotic
    a. Requires slower titration (e.g., clozapine)
    b. Is less absorbed, unless given with food (e.g., ziprasidone, lurasidone)
    c. Crosses the blood-brain barrier less readily, requiring higher doses to achieve equivalent levels (e.g., switching from risperidone to paliperidone)

Pharmacodynamic rebound effects are most likely when receptor binding profiles are very different between the first and second agent (Correll et al. 2010). This is especially likely when a patient discontinues a strongly antihistaminic or anticholinergic drug, such as chlorpromazine, clozapine, olanzapine, or quetiapine. Histamine blockade is associated with anxiolytic, calming, sleep-inducing, and EPS-reducing effects. Cholinergic blockade is associated with calming and anti-EPS effects. During a rapid switch from a potently antihistaminergic or anticholinergic antipsychotic to an agent with less sedation and less anticholinergic blockade (e.g., aripiprazole, ziprasidone, and less so, asenapine, iloperidone, lurasidone, risperidone, or paliperidone), upregulated, sensitized receptors can promote the transmission of histaminergic and muscarinic activity. This can result in (transient) rebound agitation, insomnia, anxiety, restlessness, EPS, and akathisia. Similarly, switching from a strongly antidopaminergic drug—such as a high- or medium-potency FGA or risperidone or paliperidone—to a less tightly binding antipsychotic (such as clozapine or quetiapine) or to a partial D_2 agonist (aripiprazole) can result transiently in a relative lack of dopamine blockade in the presence of hypersensitive and upregulated D_2 receptors (unless the new antipsychotic is dosed high enough). Clinically, this can manifest as rebound psychosis, mania, agitation, aggression, akathisia, or withdrawal dyskinesia.

Rebound phenomena may be avoided in many cases by using an overlapping or "plateau" cross-titration (Correll et al. 2010) or by treating withdrawal and rebound symptoms with time-limited, targeted use of benzodiazepines, antihistamines, anticholinergics, gabapentin, mirtazapine, or nonbenzodiazepine anxiolytics and sedatives.

Indications

Table 38–1 shows the U.S. Food and Drug Administration (FDA) regulatory pediatric indications for antipsychotics as of November 2014. As can be seen, antipsychotics are used clinically for far more indications than those for which they have FDA approval. Among antipsychotics, only the SGAs have trials that meet modern regulatory criteria for pediatric approval. FGAs that have regulatory or dosing language for pediatric patients in the package insert were grandfathered in on the basis of old studies. Pharmaceutical company trials for regulatory approval of some pediatric indications are currently ongoing for iloperidone, lurasidone, and ziprasidone.

Efficacy From Randomized Controlled Trials

Early Onset Schizophrenia

Twenty-four RCTs (*N*=2,394) in pediatric patients with schizophrenia have been published. Of these, 2 older trials (*n*=87) compared FGAs with placebo, 7 modern trials compared SGAs with placebo/pseudoplacebo in adolescents ages 13–17 (*N*=1,529), and 14 mostly small trials (*N*=724) compared different antipsychotics head-to-head. Only one maintenance trial (*N*=54) has been published. The study and patient characteristics and main efficacy outcomes, including study-defined response, are summarized in Table 38–2. In general, antipsychotics were superior to placebo, without greater efficacy in higher-dose arms in fixed-dose studies (Kendall et al. 2013). Conversely, in active controlled trials, antipsychotics did not differ significantly from each other on efficacy (Schimmelmann et al. 2013). An exception is clozapine, which even in relatively small active-controlled trials was superior in several efficacy measures (especially negative symptoms) at mean dosages of 176–403 mg/day compared with haloperidol, olanzapine, and "high-dose" olanzapine. A clinically useful measure for the difference between treatment groups is the number needed to treat (NNT), which is the number of patients who need to be exposed to a treatment until one additional positive event of interest occurs in excess of the rate in the comparator. NNTs of 10 or lower are considered clinically relevant. The NNTs for study-specific "response" in early onset schizophrenia ranged from 3 to 13 when nonclozapine antipsychotics were compared with placebo and from 3 to 6 for clozapine compared with olanzapine.

Confirming data in adults, two recent post hoc analyses in adolescents with schizophrenia spectrum disorders indicated that lack of at least minimal improvement after 3 weeks (Correll et al. 2013) or 4 weeks (Stentebjerg-Olesen et al. 2013) of adequately dosed antipsychotic treatment makes an adequate response (at least much improved) unlikely, so a switch to another antipsychotic should be considered.

Bipolar I Disorder

Fifteen RCTs (*N*=2,258) in pediatric patients with bipolar disorder have been published. The study and patient characteristics and main efficacy outcomes, including study-defined response and remission, are summarized in Table 38–3. Seven studies (*N*=1,213) demonstrated superior efficacy of SGAs compared with placebo in pediatric patients ages 10–17 years with bipolar mania (Correll et al. 2010). In bipolar depression, two studies of quetiapine were negative, while another study of olanzapine-fluoxetine combination was superior to placebo. Three active controlled studies (*N*=395) that compared quetiapine or risperidone with valproate and/or lithium demonstrated superior efficacy of the antipsychotic versus the mood stabilizer for bipolar mania, despite adequate mood stabilizer levels. In two placebo-controlled maintenance studies, aripiprazole was superior to placebo in main-

TABLE 38–2. Double-blind, randomized, placebo-controlled, and active-controlled trials of antipsychotics in children and adolescents with schizophrenia

Study	Design	Inclusion criteria	Drug	Mean dose, mg/day	*N*	Male, %	White, %	Age, mean (range)	Primary outcome	Response (as study defined), %	NNT response	≥7% weight gain,%	NNH ≥7% weight gain,%
Schizophrenia, placebo-controlled, acute													
First-generation antipsychotics													
Pool et al. 1976	4-week DB-RPCT	SCZ	Total		75				BPRS-C: ns (sign from baseline for all groups)				
			LOX	87.5	26	39		15.6		88	2		
			HAL	9.8	25	72		15.7		70	3		
			Pbo	5.4	24	63		15.3 (13–18)		36			
Spencer et al. 1992	8-week DB-RPCT	SCZ	Total		12	75		8.8 (5–12)	CGI-I and CGI-S: HAL>Pbo				
			HAL	2.0									
			Pbo										
Second-generation antipsychotics													
Findling et al. 2008	6-week DB-RPCT	SCZ	Total		302	57	59.9 (181)	15.5 (13–17)	PANSS: ARI 10 and ARI 30>Pbo				
			ARI	10 (9.5)	100					68	8	4	34
			ARI	30 (27.8)	102					71	6	5	25
			Pbo		100					54		1	
Kryzhanovskaya et al. 2009	6-week DB-RPCT	SCZ	Total		107				PANSS: OLA>Pbo				
			OLA	11.1	72	71	72	16.1		38	6	46	4
			Pbo		35	69	71	16.3 (13–17)		26		15	

TABLE 38–2. Double-blind, randomized, placebo-controlled, and active-controlled trials of antipsychotics in children and adolescents with schizophrenia *(continued)*

Study	Design	Inclusion criteria	Drug	Mean dose, mg/day	*N*	Male, %	White, %	Age, mean (range)	Primary outcome	Response (as study defined), %	NNT response	≥7% weight gain,%	NNH ≥7% weight gain,%
Singh et al. 2011	6-week DB-RPCT	SCZ	Total		200	59	68	15.4	PANSS: PAL 3 or 6>Pbo (nonweight group based: PAL 3, 6, and 12>Pbo)				
			PAL	1.5	54	56	65	15.1		39	20	6	25
			PAL	3 or 6	48	65	71	15.3		65	4	13	10
			PAL	6 or 12	47	70	68	15.5		51	6	13	10
			Pbo		51	45	69	15.7 (13–17)		33		2	
Findling et al. 2012b	6-week DB-RPCT	SCZ	Total		220	41	61	15.4	PANSS: QUE 400 and Que 800>Pbo				
			QUE	400	73	57	62	15.4		28 (38.4)	13	23	7
			QUE	800	74	60	60	15.4		27 (36.5)	11	18	10
			Pbo		73	58	63	15.3 (13–17)		19 (26)		7	
Haas et al. 2009b	6-week DB-RPCT	SCZ	Total		160	36	53	15.6	PANSS: RIS 1–3 and RIS 4–6>Pbo				
			RIS	1–3 (2.6)	55	46	60	15.7		65	4	15	8
			RIS	4–6 (5.3)	51	28	47	15.7		72	3	16	8
			Pbo		54	65	50	15.5 (13–17)		35		2	
Haas et al. 2009c	8-week DB-RPCT	SCZ	Total		257				PANSS: RIS 1.5–6>RIS 0.15–0.6				
			RIS	1.5–6 (4.0)	125	44	85	15.6		73	5	39	5
			RIS	0.15–0.6	132	48	85						
			(pseudo-Pbo)	(0.5)		39	85	15.6 (13–17)		50		16	

TABLE 38–2. Double-blind, randomized, placebo-controlled, and active-controlled trials of antipsychotics in children and adolescents with schizophrenia *(continued)*

Study	Design	Inclusion criteria	Drug	Mean dose, mg/day	*N*	Male, %	White, %	Age, mean (range)	Primary outcome	Response (as study defined), %	NNT response	≥7% weight gain,%	NNH ≥7% weight gain,%
Findling et al. 2013b	6-week DB-RPCT	SCZ	Total		283	60	62		BPRS-A: ns (p=0.15; per protocol: ZIP>Pbo)				
			ZIP	80–160 (≥45 kg)	193	57	60	15.2					
			Pbo	40–80 (<45 kg)	90	69	67	15.4 (13–17)					
Wolpert et al. 1967	8-week DB-RCT	SCZ	Total	Range:	16				Not specified, Central Islip Nurses Rating Scale of Autistic Children, Global Impression				
			THIX	6–30	8			11.4		50	8		
			TRIFL	6–30	8			11.5 (8–15)		38 ("improved")			
Engelhardt et al. 1973	12-week DB-RCT	SCZ	Total		30		27	9.2	Not specified, CGI, Children's Psychiatric Rating Scale				
			FLU	10.4	15	80		8.9		93	16		
			HAL	10.4	15	93		9.5 (6–12)		87			
Paprocki and Versiani 1977	4-week DB-RCT	SCZ	Total		50				Not specified, BPRS, Nurses Observation Scale for Inpatient Evaluation, CGI				
			LOX	70.4	25	92	44	16.0		64			
			HAL	7.6	25	100	48	16.2 (13–18)		79 ("good improvement")	7		

TABLE 38–2. Double-blind, randomized, placebo-controlled, and active-controlled trials of antipsychotics in children and adolescents with schizophrenia *(continued)*

Study	Design	Inclusion criteria	Drug	Mean dose, mg/day	*N*	Male, %	White, %	Age, mean (range)	Primary outcome	Response (as study defined), %	NNT response	≥7% weight gain,%	NNH ≥7% weight gain,%
Realmuto et al. 1984	4–6 week SBRCT	SCZ	Total		21				BPRS-C and CGI-S: ns between groups				
			THIX	16.2	13			15.1					
			THIO	178	8			16.1 (11–18)					
Mozes et al. 2006	12-week OL- RCT	SCZ	Total		25				PANSS: ns (from baseline for all groups)				
			RIS	1.62	13	39		10.7		46			
			OLA	8.18	12	42		11.5 (9–14)		67	5		
Sikich et al. 2004	8-week DB-RCT	SCZ spectrum: 52%; mood d/o with psychosis: 48%	Total		50	60	60	14.8	BPRS-C: ns (from baseline for all groups)				
			RIS	4.0	19	68	47	14.6		74	5		
			OLA	12.3	16	56	63	14.6		88	3, 8		
			HAL	5.0	15	53	73	15.4 (8–19)		53			
Kumra et al. 1996	6-week DB-RCT	SCZ, resistant to ≥2 APs	Total	176	21	50		14.4	BPRS-C: CLO>HAL (P=.04)				
			CLO	16	10	54		13.73					
			HAL		11								
Shaw et al. 2006	8-wk DB-RCT	SCZ, resistant to ≥2 APs	Total		25				SAPS, SANS, CGI-S: ns (from baseline for both groups)				
			CLO	327	12	67	58	11.7		33	6		
			OLA	18.1	13	54	54	12.8 (7–16)		15			

TABLE 38–2. Double-blind, randomized, placebo-controlled, and active-controlled trials of antipsychotics in children and adolescents with schizophrenia *(continued)*

Study	Design	Inclusion criteria	Drug	Mean dose, mg/day	*N*	Male, %	White, %	Age, mean (range)	Primary outcome	Response (as study defined), %	NNT response	≥7% weight gain,%	NNH ≥7% weight gain,%
Kumra et al. 2008	12-week DB-RCT	SCZ, resistant to ≥2 APs	Total		39				BPRS-C: ns (from baseline for both groups)				
			CLO	403.1	18	44	13	15.8		67	3		
			OLA	26.2	21	62	29	15.5 (10–18)		33			
Sikich et al. 2008	8-week DB-RCT	SCZ spectrum	Total		119				BPRS-C: ns (from baseline for all groups)				
			OLA	11.4	35					49	34		
			RIS	2.8	41					46			
			MOL	59.9	40					60	8, 10		
Jensen et al. 2008	12-week OL-RCT	SCZ spectrum	Total		30	67	60	15.2	PANSS: ns (post hoc: RIS>QUE)				
			OLA	14.0	10	50	50	15.3		50	5	60	5
			QUE	611	10	70	60	14.8		30		50	
			RIS	3.4	10	80	70	15.6 (10–18)		70	3, 5	80	4
Arango et al. 2009	24-week OL-RCT	SCZ spectrum: 80%; mood d/o with psychosis: 20%	Total		50			16.0	PANSS: ns (from baseline for all groups)				
			OLA	9.7	26	76	77	15.7					
			QUE	533	24	79	88	16.3 (12–18)					

TABLE 38–2. Double-blind, randomized, placebo-controlled, and active-controlled trials of antipsychotics in children and adolescents with schizophrenia *(continued)*

Study	Design	Inclusion criteria	Drug	Mean dose, mg/day	*N*	Male, %	White, %	Age, mean (range)	Primary outcome	Response (as study defined), %	NNT response	≥7% weight gain,%	NNH ≥7% weight gain,%
Swadi et al. 2010	6-week OL-RCT (blind ratings)	SCZ spectrum 68%; mood d/o with psychosis: 32%	Total		22	55		<19 yrs old	Not specified, PANSS: ns	64	4	55	10
			QUE	607	11	64				91		46	
			RIS	2.9	11								
Savitz et al. 2015	8-week DB-RPCT	SCZ	Total		226	66	76	15.3	PANSS: ns (from baseline for all groups)				
			ARI	11.6	114	67	75	15.4		82	21	18	
			PAL	6.75	112	65	77	15.3 (12–17)		77		26	13
Findling et al. 2010	44-week DB extension phase	SCZ spectrum	Total		54	69	69		BPRS-C: ns (from baseline for all groups)				
			RIS	3.9	21	76	62						
			OLA	9.6	13	92	69						
			MOL	76.5	20	45	75						

Note. APs=antipsychotics; ARI=aripiprazole; BPRS-C=Brief Psychiatric Rating Scale for Children; CGI-I=Clinical Global Impressions–Improvement Scale; CGI-S=Clinical Global Impressions Severity of Symptoms Scale; CLO=clozapine; DB-RCPT=double-blind, randomized, placebo-controlled trial; d/o=disorder; FLU=fluphenazine; HAL=haloperidol; LOX=loxapine; MOL=molindone; NNH=number needed to harm; NNT=number needed to treat; ns=not significant; OLA=olanzapine; PAL=paliperidone; PANSS=Positive and Negative Syndrome Scale; Pbo=placebo; RIS=risperidone; SANS=Schedule for the Assessment of Negative Symptoms; SAPS=Schedule for the Assessment of Positive Symptoms; SBRCT=single-blind, randomized controlled trial; SCZ=schizophrenia; THIO=thioridazine; THIX=thiothixene; TRIFL=trifluoperazine.

TABLE 38–3. Double-blind, randomized, placebo-controlled trials of antipsychotics in children and adolescents with bipolar disorders

Study	Design	Inclusion criteria	Drug	Mean dose, mg/day	*N*	Male, %	White, %	Age, mean (range)	Primary outcome	Response (as study-defined), %	NNT response	Remission (study defined), %	NNT remission	≥7% weight gain,%	NNH 7% weight gain,%
Bipolar disorder, manic or manic/mixed, placebo controlled, acute															
Findling et al. 2009	4-week DB-RPCT	Bipolar I	Total		296	54	65	13.4 (10–17)	YMRS: ARI 10 and ARI 30>Pbo						
			ARI	10 (9.5)	98					45	6	25	5	4	–100
			ARI	30 (28.5)	99					64	3	48	3	12	15
			Pbo		99					26		5		5	
Tramontina et al. 2009	6-week DB-RPCT	Bipolar I or II disorder, with ADHD	Total		43	47	91	11.94	YMRS: ARI>Pbo						
			ARI	13.61	18	33	83	11.72		89	3	72	3		
			Pbo		25	56	96	12.16		52		32			
Tohen et al. 2007	3-week DB-RPCT	Bipolar I disorder	Total		161				YMRS: OLA>Pbo						
			OLA	8.9	107	57	66	15.1		49	4	35		42	3
			Pbo		54	44	76	15.4 (13–17)		22		11		2	
DelBello et al. 2002	6-week DB-RPCT	Bipolar I disorder	Total		30			14.3 (12–18)	YMRS: QUE+VPA >Pbo+VPA (p=0.05)						
			QUE+DVP	432+102 g/mL	15					87	3				
			Pbo+DVP		15					53					

TABLE 38–3. Double-blind, randomized, placebo-controlled trials of antipsychotics in children and adolescents with bipolar disorders *(continued)*

Study	Design	Inclusion criteria	Drug	Mean dose, mg/day	*N*	Male, %	White, %	Age, mean (range)	Primary outcome	Response (as study-defined), %	NNT response	Remission (study defined), %	NNT remission	≥7% weight gain,%	NNH 7% weight gain,%
Pathak et al. 2013	3-week DB-RPCT	Bipolar I mania	Total		277	56	77	13.2	YMRS: QUE 400 and QUE 600>Pbo						
			QUE	400	93	56	79	13.1		64	5	53	5	15	7
			QUE	600	95	58	77	13.1		58	4	54	5	10	10
			Pbo		99	61	74	13.3 (10–17)		37		30		0	
Haas et al. 2009c	3-week DB-RPCT	Bipolar I disorder	Total		169	49	77	13.0 (10–17)	YMRS: RIS 0.5–2.5 and RIS 3–6>Pbo						
			RIS	0.5–2.5	50	56	70			59	3	43	4	14	12
			RIS	3–6	61	43	82			63	3	43	4	10	20
			Pbo		58	48	78			26		16		5	
Findling et al. 2008, 2013b	4-week DB-RPCT	Bipolar I disorder	Total		237	55			YMRS: ZIP>Pbo						
			ZIP	40–160	149	56	79	13.6		62	4			7	34
			Pbo		88	53	81	13.7 (10–17)		35				4	
Bipolar disorder, depressed, placebo-controlled, acute															
DelBello et al. 2009	8-week DB-RPCT	Bipolar I disorder	Total		32	10	81		CDRS: ns						
			QUE	403	17	29	82	16		71	26	35			
			Pbo		15	33	80	15		67		40	20		

TABLE 38–3. Double-blind, randomized, placebo-controlled trials of antipsychotics in children and adolescents with bipolar disorders *(continued)*

Study	Design	Inclusion criteria	Drug	Mean dose, mg/day	*N*	Male, %	White, %	Age, mean (range)	Primary outcome	Response (as study-defined), %	NNT response	Remission (study defined), %	NNT remission	≥7% weight gain,%	NNH 7% weight gain,%
Findling et al. 2014a	8-week DB-RPCT	Bipolar I disorder	Total		193	51	65	14.0	CDRS: ns						
			QUE	150–300	93	49	71	13.9		63	13	46	9	13	16
			XR		100	52	60	14.0		55		34		6	
			Pbo												
Detke et al. 2012	8-week DB-RPCT	Bipolar I disorder	Total		255	51	71	14.7	CDRS: OLA+FLU >Pbo						
			OLA+FLU	12/50	170	49.4	70	14.6		78	6	59	7		
			Pbo		85	54.1	72	15 (10–17)		78		59			
Bipolar disorder, placebo controlled, maintenance															
Findling et al. 2012a	72-week DB-RPC with-drawal trial	Bipolar disorder	Total		60	70		6.9	Time to all-cause discontinuation: ARI>Pbo	Mood relapse					
			APZ	0.26 mg/kg	30	63		7.1		73	5				
			Pbo		30	77		6.7		97					
Findling et al. 2013a	28-week DB extension phase	Bipolar I disorder	Total		210				YMRS: ARI>Pbo						
			ARI	10	75		60	13.6		58.7%	4				
			ARI	30	71		66	13.1		64.8%	3				
			Pbo		64		66	13.3 (10–17)		29.7%					

TABLE 38–3. Double-blind, randomized, placebo-controlled trials of antipsychotics in children and adolescents with bipolar disorders *(continued)*

Study	Design	Inclusion criteria	Drug	Mean dose, mg/day	*N*	Male, %	White, %	Age, mean (range)	Primary outcome	Response (as study-defined), %	NNT response	Remission (study defined), %	NNT remission	≥7% weight gain,%	NNH 7% weight gain,%
Bipolar disorder, active controlled, acute															
DelBello et al. 2006	4-week DB-RPCT	Bipolar I disorder	Total		50	42	26	15.0 (12–18)	YMRS: ns (but faster onset with QUE, *P*=0.01)						
			QUE	412	25					60	4	55	3		
			DVP	101 µg/mL	25					28		17			
Pavuluri et al. 2010	6-week DB-RPCT	Bipolar I disorder	Total		66	61	57	10.9	YMRS: RIS>DVP						
			RIS	1.4	33	63	63	10.5		78	4	63	4		
			DVP	96 µg/dL	33	58	52	11.2 (8–18)		46		33			
Geller et al. 2012	6-week DB-RPCT	Bipolar I disorder	Total		279	50	73	10.1	CGI-I: RIS>LITH, RIS>VPA						
			RIS	2.6	89	47	67	11		69	3, 3				
			LITH	1.1 mEq/L	90	59	73	9.7		36	9				
			DVP	114 µg/mL	100	44	77	9.7 6–15)		24					

Note. ARI=aripiprazole; DBD=disruptive behavior disorder; CDRS=Child Depression Rating Scale; CGI-I=Clinical Global Impressions–Improvement Scale; DVP=divalproex; d/o=disorder; FLU=fluoxetine; LITH=lithium; NNH=number needed to harm; NNT=number needed to treat; OLA=olanzapine; Pbo=placebo; QUE=quetiapine; RIS=risperidone; VPA=valproate; YMRS=Young Mania Rating Scale; ZIP=ziprasidone.

taining efficacy. In pediatric mania, NNTs of an SGA compared with placebo for response (defined as at least a 50% reduction in the Young Mania Rating Scale [YMRS] total score) and for remission (defined by a YMRS total score ≤12) ranged from 3 to 6 (Correll et al. 2010). In the active controlled trials of SGAs versus mood stabilizers, the NNTs for response and remission were 3–4.

Irritability and Aggressive Behaviors Associated With Autism Spectrum Disorder

Fourteen RCTs (*N*=907) in pediatric patients with autism spectrum disorder have been published. The study and patient characteristics and main efficacy outcomes, including study-defined response, are summarized in Table 38–4. Eight studies (*N*=665) demonstrated superior efficacy of aripiprazole, olanzapine (*N*=11 only), and risperidone compared with placebo in patients ages 5–17 years. In three small active-controlled trials (*N*=101), antipsychotics did not differ from each other. In three relapse prevention studies (*N*=141), aripiprazole and risperidone were superior to placebo. NNTs for study-defined response in autism spectrum disorder ranged from 2 to 7 for the acute response and 2 to 6 for relapse prevention.

Irritability and Aggressive Behaviors Associated With Disruptive Behavior Disorders, ADHD, and Subaverage IQ/Intellectual Disability

Eleven RCTs (*N*=1,068) in pediatric patients with disruptive behavior disorders have been published. The study and patient characteristics and main efficacy outcomes, including study-defined response, are summarized in Table 38–5. Nine studies (*N*=702) demonstrated superiority chiefly of risperidone compared with placebo for aggressive behaviors associated with conduct disorder, disruptive behavior disorders, attention-deficit/hyperactivity disorder (ADHD), and/or subaverage IQ. In one additional, active-controlled trial (*N*=31), molindone was found to be superior to thioridazine for conduct disorder in youth. Molindone is currently unavailable, having been discontinued by the manufacturer. However, on the basis of results from a phase 2a study, the FDA "fast tracked" the further development of molindone for the treatment of impulsive aggression in youth with ADHD, and phase 3 trials are expected to start in 2015.

NNTs for study-defined "response" in studies without concurrent psychosocial treatment ranged from 2 to 5 for risperidone in patients with aggression due to disruptive behavior spectrum disorders. NNT in one relapse prevention study (*N*=335) was 7 for risperidone. Although efficacy data exist for risperidone in disruptive behavior disorders, use of antipsychotics for aggression or impulsivity is recommended only after treatments for underlying disorders and nonpharmacological interventions and have been exhausted (Knapp et al. 2012; Scotto Rosato et al. 2012; toolkit: http://www.chainonline.org/CHAINOnline/assets/File/TMAY%20final_120926.pdf).

Tourette's Disorder

Five parallel-group RCTs (*N*=199) in pediatric patients with Tourette's or tic disorder have been published. The study and patient characteristics and main efficacy outcomes, including study-defined response, are summarized in Table 38–5. Three studies (*N*=115) demonstrated superiority of aripiprazole, risperidone, and ziprasidone compared with placebo

TABLE 38–4. Double-blind, randomized, placebo-controlled, and active-controlled trials of antipsychotics in children and adolescents with autism spectrum disorders

Study	Design	Inclusion criteria	Drug	Mean dose, mg/day	*N*	Male, %	White, %	Age, mean (range)	Primary outcome	Response (as study-defined), %	NNT response	≥7% weight gain, %	NNT ≥7% weight gain, %
Autism spectrum disorders, placebo controlled, acute													
Owen et al. 2009	8-week DB-RPCT	Autistic disorder	Total		98	88	75		ABC-I and CGI-I				
			ARI	2–15	47	89	68	9.7		52	3	29	5
			Pbo		51	86	80	8.8 (6–17)		14		6	
Marcus et al. 2009	8-week DB-RPCT	Autistic disorder	Total		218	89			ABC-I and CGI-I				
			ARI	5	53	89	70	9.0		56	5	33	4
			ARI	10	59	85	70	10.0		49	7	15	15
			ARI	15	54	93	78	9.5		53	6	30	5
			Pbo		52	92	67	10.2		35		8	
Hollander et al. 2006	8-week DB-RPCT	PDD	Total		11	82	64	9.0	OASS and CGI-S: ns				
			OLA	10	6	100	50	9.3		50	4	67	2
			Pbo		5	60	80	8.9 (6–14)		20		20	
McCracken et al. 2002	8-week DB-RPCT	Autistic disorder	Total		101	81	66	8.8 (5–17)	ABC: RIS>Pbo				
			RIS	1.8	49					69	2		
			Pbo		52					12			
Luby et al. 2006	6-month DB-RPCT	Autistic disorder	Total		23				CARS: ns				
			RIS	1.14	11	82	91	4.1					
			Pbo		12	67	92	4 (2–6)					

TABLE 38–4. Double-blind, randomized, placebo-controlled, and active-controlled trials of antipsychotics in children and adolescents with autism spectrum disorders *(continued)*

Study	Design	Inclusion criteria	Drug	Mean dose, mg/day	*N*	Male, %	White, %	Age, mean (range)	Primary outcome	Response (as study-defined), %	NNT response	≥7% weight gain, %	NNT ≥7% weight gain, %
Shea et al. 2004	8-week DB-RPCT	Autistic disorder, PDD	Total		79				ABC and N-CBRF: RIS > Pbo				
			RIS	1.48	40	73	67	7.6		54	4		
			Pbo		39	82	72	7.3 (5–12)		18			
Nagaraj et al. 2006	6-month DB-RPCT	Autistic disorder	Total		39	87			CARS: RIS>Pbo				
			RIS	1	19	84		4.8		95	2		
			Pbo		20	90		5.3 (2–9)		30			
Kent et al. 2013	6-week DB-RPCT	Autistic disorder	Total		96	88	70	9	ABC-I: high-dose RIS (1.25 mg/day [20 to < 45 kg], 1.75 mg/day [> 45 kg])>Pbo				
			RIS	1.25–1.75	31	90	81	9		83	3		
			RIS	0.125–0.175	30	83	70	10		52	10		
			Pbo		35	89	60	9 (5–17)		41			
Autism spectrum disorder, placebo controlled, relapse prevention													
Research Units on Pediatric Psychopharmacology Autism Network 2005	8-week DB-RPCT	Autistic disorder	Total		32	49	44	8.6	Relapse: RIS< Pbo	Relapse:			
			Risp	2.0	16					13	2		
			Pbo		16					63			

TABLE 38–4. Double-blind, randomized, placebo-controlled, and active-controlled trials of antipsychotics in children and adolescents with autism spectrum disorders *(continued)*

Study	Design	Inclusion criteria	Drug	Mean dose, mg/day	*N*	Male, %	White, %	Age, mean (range)	Primary outcome	Response (as study-defined), %	NNT response	≥7% weight gain, %	NNT ≥7% weight gain, %
Troost et al. 2005	8-week DB-RPCT	Autism spectrum (PDD: 67%)	Total		24	92	92	9.0	Relapse: RIS<PBo	Relapse:			
			Risp	1.9	12		100	9.4		25	3		
			Pbo		12		83	8.7 (5–17)		7			
Findling et al. 2014b	16-week DB-RPCT	Autistic disorder	Total		85	80	69	10.4	Relapse: ns (0.097)	Relapse:			
			APZ	2–15	41	73	76	10.1		35	6		
			Pbo		44	86	64	10.8 (6–17)		52			
Autism spectrum disorder, active controlled, acute													
Ghanizadeh et al. 2014	8-week DB-RCT	Autism spectrum (autistic disorder: 65%)	Total		59			9.6	ABC: ns (from baseline for both groups)		7		
			ARI	5.5	27	86		9.5 (4–18)		33	7		
			RIS	1.1	29	77				17			
Malone et al. 2002	6-week ROT	Autistic disorder	Total		12	67	58	7.8	CGI-I, CGI-S, and CPRS: ns				
			OLA	7.9	6	67	50	8.5		83	3		
			HAL	1.4	6	67	68	7.3 (4–12)		50			

TABLE 38–4. Double-blind, randomized, placebo-controlled, and active-controlled trials of antipsychotics in children and adolescents with autism spectrum disorders *(continued)*

Study	Design	Inclusion criteria	Drug	Mean dose, mg/day	*N*	Male, %	White, %	Age, mean (range)	Primary outcome	Response (as study-defined), %	NNT response	≥7% weight gain, %	NNT ≥7% weight gain, %
Miral et al. 2008	12-week DB-RCT	Autistic disorder	Total		30				ABC and Turgay DSM-IV PDD: RIS>HAL				
			RIS	2.6	15	87		10.9		60	4		
			HAL	2.6	15	73		10.0 (7–17)		85			

Note. ABC=Aberrant Behavior Checklist; ADHD=attention-deficit/hyperactivity disorder; CARS=Childhood Autism Rating Scale; CD=conduct disorder; CGI-I=Clinical Global Impressions–Improvement Scale; CGI-S=Clinical Global Impressions Severity of Symptoms Scale; DBD-NOS=disruptive behavior disorder not otherwise specified; DB-RPCT=double-blind, randomized, placebo-controlled trial; HAL=haloperidol; N-CBRF=Nisonger Child Behavior Rating Form; NNH=number needed to harm; NNT=number needed to treat; OASS=Overt Agitation Severity Scale; ODD=oppositional defiant disorder; OLA=olanzapine; Pbo=placebo; PDD=pervasive developmental disorder; RIS=risperidone; ROT=randomized open trial; RUPP=Research Units on Pediatric Psychopharmacology; Turgay DSM-IV PDD=Turgay DSM-IV Pervasive Developmental Disorder Scale.

TABLE 38–5. Double-blind, randomized, placebo-controlled trials of antipsychotics in children and adolescents with disruptive behavior disorders and Tourette's disorder

Study	Design	Inclusion criteria	Drug	Mean dose, mg/day	*N*	Male, %	White, %	Age, mean (range)	Primary outcome	Response (as study-defined), %	NNT response	≥7% weight gain, %	NNT ≥7% weight gain, %
Disruptive behavior disorders, placebo-controlled, acute													
Campbell et al. 1984	4-week DB-RPCT	CD	Total		61	93	16	8.9 (5–12)	CPRS, hyperactivity, hostility, aggression: HAL and lithium>Pbo				
			HAL		20	90							
			Lithium	3.0	21	100							
			Pbo	1.2	20	90							
Findling et al. 2000	10-week DB-RPCT	CD	Total		20	95	50		ABC and RAAPP: RIS>Pbo				
			RIS	1.3	10			10.7					
			Pbo		10			8.2 (5–15)					
Aman et al. 2002	6-wk DB-RPCT	Disruptive behavior, subaverage IQ	Total	1.2	118	85	51	8.7	ABC: RIS>Pbo				
			RIS		55	79	62	8.1		54	3		
			Pbo		63					8			
Van Bellinghen and De Troch 2001	4-week DB-RPCT	Behavioral disturbances, subaverage IQ	Total		13	39			ABC: RIS>Pbo	83	2		
			RIS	1.2	6	33		10.5		0			
			Pbo		7	43		11.0 (6–14)					
Buitelaar et al. 2001	6-week DB-RPCT	Aggression, subaverage IQ	Total		38				ABC: RIS>Pbo				
			RIS	2.9	19	90		14.0					
			Pbo		19	84		13.7					

TABLE 38–5. Double-blind, randomized, placebo-controlled trials of antipsychotics in children and adolescents with disruptive behavior disorders and Tourette's disorder *(continued)*

Study	Design	Inclusion criteria	Drug	Mean dose, mg/day	*N*	Male, %	White, %	Age, mean (range)	Primary outcome	Response (as study-defined), %	NNT response	≥7% weight gain, %	NNT ≥7% weight gain, %
Snyder et al. 2002	6-week DB-RPCT	CD, DBD, subaverage IQ	Total	1.0	110				ABC: RIS>Pbo	38	3		
			RIS		53	77	77	8.6		16			
			Pbo		57	74	74	8.8					
Aman et al. 2005	6-week DB-RPCT	CD, ODD, or DBD-NOS with comorbid ADHD	Total		155				ABC and N-CBRF: RIS>Pbo				
			RIS+Stim		35	86	66	9.0					
			RIS		43	81	56	8.6					
			Pbo+Stim		38	92	74	8.9					
			Pbo		39	74	56	8.3 (5–12)					
Armenteros et al. 2007	4-week DB-RPCT	ADHD+aggressive behavior	Total		25				CAS-P and CAS-T: ns	100	5		
			RIS	1.1	12	83	50	7.3		77			
			Pbo		13	92	46	8.8 (7–12)					
Connor et al. 2008	7-week DB-RPCT	CD	Total		19	74	74	14.1	CGI-I, CGI-S: QUE>Pbo				
			QUE	294	9	78	78	13.1		89	2		
			Pbo		10	70	70	15.0 (12–17)		10			
Aman et al. 2014	9-week DB-RPCT	ADHD with comorbid CD (26%) or ODD (74%)	Total		168	77	53	9	NCBRF disruptive Total subscale: RIS>Pbo				
			RIS	1.7	84	77	57	9		79	11		
			Pbo		84	76	49	8.8 (6–12)		70			

TABLE 38–5. Double-blind, randomized, placebo-controlled trials of antipsychotics in children and adolescents with disruptive behavior disorders and Tourette's disorder *(continued)*

Study	Design	Inclusion criteria	Drug	Mean dose, mg/day	*N*	Male, %	White, %	Age, mean (range)	Primary outcome	Response (as study-defined), %	NNT response	≥7% weight gain, %	NNT ≥7% weight gain, %
Disruptive behavior disorders, placebo controlled, relapse prevention													
Reyes et al. 2006	6-month DB-RPCT	Disruptive behavior disorders	Total	0.81<50 kg	335	87		10.8	Relapse	Relapse			
			RIS		172	82		10.9		27	7		
			Pbo	1.22≥50 kg	163	91		10.8 (5–17)		42			
Disruptive behavior disorders, active controlled, acute													
Greenhill et al. 1985	8-week DB-RCT	CD	Total		31	100	19		CGI-S: MOL>THIO				
			MOL	26.8	15			9.8					
			THIO	170	16			10.3 (6–11)					
Tourette's and other tic disorders, placebo controlled, acute													
Scahill et al. 2003	8-week DB-RPCT	Tourette's disorder	Total		26	96		11.1	YGTSS: RIS>Pbo				
			RIS	2.5	12					75	2		
			Pbo		14					7			
Sallee et al. 2000	8-week DB-RPCT	Tourette's disorder	Total		28	79			YGTSS: ZIP>Pbo				
			ZIP	28.2	16	88		11.3					
			Pbo		12	67		11.8 (7–17)					
Yoo et al. 2013	10-week DB-RPCT	Tourette's disorder	Total		61		0		TS-CGI-I				
			ARI	11.0	31	94	0	11	APZ>Pb	66	5		
			Pbo		29	79	0	10.9 (6–18)		45			

TABLE 38–5. Double-blind, randomized, placebo-controlled trials of antipsychotics in children and adolescents with disruptive behavior disorders and Tourette's disorder *(continued)*

Study	Design	Inclusion criteria	Drug	Mean dose, mg/day	*N*	Male, %	White, %	Age, mean (range)	Primary outcome	Response (as study-defined), %	NNT response	≥7% weight gain, %	NNT ≥7% weight gain, %
Tourette's and other tic disorders, active controlled, acute													
Bruggeman et al. 2001	12-week DB-RCT	Tourette's disorder	Total		24			<20	TSSS: ns (from baseline for both groups)				
			PIM	2.9	11					38		18	
			RIS	3.8	13					54	7	62	3
Ghanizadeh and Haghighi 2014	8-week DB-RCT	Tic disorder	Total		60			11.1	YGTSS: ns (from baseline for both groups)				
			ARI	3.2	31	82		10.2 (6–18)		90	9		
			RIS	0.6	29	86				79			

Note. ABC=Aberrant Behavior Checklist; ADHD=attention-deficit/hyperactivity disorder; CAS-P=Children's Aggression Scale—Parent; CAS-T=Children's Aggression Scale—Teacher; CD=conduct disorder; CGI-I: Clinical Global Impression–Improvement scale; CGI-S=Clinical Global Impression Severity scale; CPRS=Conners' Parent Rating Scale; DBD=disruptive behavior disorder; DB-RPCT=double-blind, randomized, placebo-controlled trial; d/o=disorder; HAL=haloperidol; IQ=intelligence quotient; MOL=molindone; NCBRF: Nysonger Child Behavior Rating Form; NNH=number needed to harm; NNT=number needed to treat; PDD=pervasive developmental disorder; PIM=pimozide; RAAPP=Rating of Aggression Against People and/or Property Scale; RIS=risperidone; THIO=thioridazine; TSSS=Tourette Symptom Severity Scale; YGTSS=Yale Global Tic Severity Scale; ZIP=ziprasidone.

in youth with Tourette's disorder. In two small, active controlled trials (N=84), risperidone differed from neither aripiprazole nor pimozide regarding efficacy for tic severity. NNTs for study-defined efficacy ranged from 2 (risperidone) to 5 (aripiprazole).

Adverse Effects

Children and adolescents seem to be more sensitive to most antipsychotic adverse effects, including sedation, EPS (except for akathisia), withdrawal dyskinesia, prolactin abnormalities, weight gain, and metabolic abnormalities (Correll et al. 2006). On the other hand, adverse effects that require a longer time to develop (e.g., diabetes mellitus) and that are related to greater medication dose and lifetime exposure (e.g., tardive dyskinesia [TD]) are less prevalent in youth than in adults. However, there is concern that these later-onset adverse effects are not seen because of short follow-up periods and that they may emerge in vulnerable patients prematurely in adulthood the earlier antipsychotics are started in childhood. Table 38–6 summarizes general side effect propensities across 10 SGAs available in the United States and 3 selected FGAs.

Neuromotor Adverse Effects

Extrapyramidal Side Effects

In general, children and adolescents are more sensitive than adults to EPS associated with FGAs and SGAs (Correll et al. 2006). An RCT of 40 youth with psychotic disorders comparing haloperidol (mean dosage 5 mg/day), risperidone (mean dosage 4 mg/day), and olanzapine (mean dosage 12 mg/day) found substantial EPS not only with haloperidol (67%) but also with olanzapine (56%) and risperidone (53%), although haloperidol-treated patients reported more severe EPS (Sikich et al. 2004). In another study of 119 pediatric patients with schizophrenia, molindone (mean dosage 60 mg/day) was associated with greater benztropine use (48%) compared with risperidone (37%, mean dosage 2.8 mg/day) and olanzapine (26%, mean dosage 11 mg/day), even though patients randomly assigned to receive molindone received 0.5 mg benztropine bid prophylactically (Sikich et al. 2008). Clozapine and quetiapine appear to be associated with relatively low rates of EPS in pediatric patients (as in adults). For aripiprazole and ziprasidone, rates of EPS appear to increase with increasing dose.

Since reported incidence of EPS is highly dependent on dose and elicitation method, results have to be interpreted within these limitations, especially as most of the risperidone trials were conducted in prepubertal boys with aggressive spectrum disorders in whom low doses of risperidone (only around 1 mg/day) were used. Moreover, noticeable rates of EPS in the placebo arms of placebo-controlled trials suggest that some rates could be inflated by carryover effects of prior antipsychotic treatment.

Akathisia

In youth, less is known regarding the risk for akathisia, which is substantial with FGAs across age groups and which seems to be similar across antipsychotics in pediatric compared with adult patients. Incidence of akathisia from placebo-controlled RCTs in pediatric schizophrenia has been reported for aripiprazole (5% for placebo, 5% in the 10 mg/day group, 11.8% in the 30 mg/day group) and risperidone (6% for pla-

TABLE 38–6. Adverse effect profiles of antipsychotics in children and adolescents

Adverse effect	Suspected mechanism	Dose/titration dependent	Second-generation antipsychotics										First-generation antipsychotics		
			ARI	ASE	CLO	ILO	LUR	OLA	PALI	QUE	RIS	ZIP	CHLOR	HAL	PER
Anticholinergic effect	M1–4 blockade	++	0	0	+++	0	0	++	0	+/++	0	0	++	0	0/+
Acute parkinsonism	D_2 blockade	+++	+	++	0	0/+	+ /++	0/+	++	0	++	+	+	+++	++
Akathisia	? D_2 blockade and alpha, 5-HT interaction	+++	++	++	+	0/+	+/++	+	+	+	+	+/++	+	+++	++
Cerebrovascular events	? D_2 mediated hypercoagulability	0 ?	+[a,b]	+?[a,b]	+?[a,b]	+?[a,b]	+?[a,b]	+[a,b]	+?[a,b]	+[a,b]	+[a,b]	+?[a,b]	+?[a,b]	+?[a,b]	+?[a,b]
Diabetes	Weight gain, ?direct effects	0 ?	0/+	0/+	+++	+	0/+	+++	+	++	+	0/+	+++	0/+	+
↑ Lipids	Weight gain, ?direct effects	0/+	0/+	0/+	+++	+	0/+	+++	+	++	+	0/+	+++	0/+	+
Hypersalivation (due to overproduction)	M4 agonism	+	0	0	++	0	0	0	0	0	0	0	0	0	0
Neutropenia	?	+?	0/+	0/+	++	0/+	0/+	0/+	0/+	0/+	0/+	0/+	0/+	0/+	0/+
Orthostasis	Alpha 1 blockade	+++	0/+	+	+++	+++	0/+	++	+	++[c]	+	0	++	0	+
↑ Prolactin/sexual dysfunction	D_2 blockade	+++	0	+	0	0/+	+	+	+++	0	+++	+	+	++ / +++	++
↓ Prolactin	D_2 agonism	+ ?	+	0	0	0	0	0	0	0	0	0	0	0	0
↑ QTc interval	Cardiac ion channel effects	+	0/+[d]	+[d]	+[d]	++[d]	0/+[d]	0/+[d]	+[d]	+[d]	+[d]	++[d]	0/+[d]	0+[d]	+[d]
Sedation	H_1 blockade	+++	0/+	+	+++	0/+	+/++	+/++	0/+	++c	+	+	++	+	+
Seizures	? dopamine blockade	+++	0/+	0/+	++	0/+	0/+	0/+	0/+	0/+	0/+	0/+	0/+	0/+	0/+
Tardive dyskinesia	? D_2 receptor desensitization	++	0/+	0/+	0	0/+	0/+	0/+	0/+	0/+	0/+	0/+	++	++	++
Withdrawal dyskinesia	D_2 blockade rebound	+++	+/++	+	0	+	+	0/+	+	0/+	+	+	0/+	++	+/++
Weight gain[a]	?H_1, D_2, 5-HT_{2c} blockade	+	0/+	+	+++	+/++	0/+	+++	++	++	++	0/+	+++	+	++

Note. A large part of the data information is extrapolated from adult populations. Therefore, information contained in this table may change as more data from large pediatric populations become available.

[a]Insufficient long-term data to fully determine the risk.

[b]Unlikely to be due to low risk factors in childhood and adolescents and long lag time for cerebrovascular disease to develop disease.

[c]Less at higher doses than lower doses (potential threshold≥300 mg/day).

[d]Relevance for the development of torsades de pointes not established.

0=none; 0/+=minimal; +=mild; ++=moderate; +++=severe; ?=unclear/questionable; ↑=increased; ↓=decreased; ARI=aripiprazole; ASE=asenapine; CLO=clozapine; CHLOR=chlorpromazine; HAL=haloperidol; ILO=iloperidone; LUR=lurasidone; OLA=olanzapine; PAL=paliperidone; PER=perphenazine; QUE=quetiapine; RIS=risperidone.

cebo, 6% in the 1–3 mg/day group, 10% in the 4–6 mg/day group), corresponding to the number needed to harm (NNH) of 14.7 to no risk for aripiprazole 30 mg/day and 5 mg/day, respectively, and NNH of 25 to no risk for risperidone 4–6 mg/day and 1–3 mg/day, respectively (Correll 2008). In an RCT in pediatric bipolar disorder, akathisia rates were 2.1% for placebo, 8.2% for aripiprazole 10 mg/day, and 11.8% for aripiprazole 30 mg/day, with corresponding NNTs of 9.1–14.1, respectively (Correll 2008). The relatively high akathisia rates for placebo, especially in the pediatric schizophrenia trials, suggest the potential presence of a relevant carryover effect from prior antipsychotic treatment, miscoding agitation-restlessness as akathisia, or the possibility of withdrawal phenomena after a brief washout from antipsychotics and/or medications that can mitigate akathisia. In the Treatment of Early Onset Schizophrenia Spectrum Disorders (TEOSS) study, molindone, but not olanzapine or risperidone, was associated with a significant increase in the Barnes Akathisia Scale score (Sikich et al. 2008). However, in interpreting these results, the clinician needs to remember that the occurrence of akathisia may depend on dose and speed of titration and that the identification and differentiation of akathisia from agitation, restlessness, or anxiety can be quite difficult.

Withdrawal Dyskinesia

During FGA treatment, youth are at risk of developing withdrawal dyskinesias. However, unlike in adults, the dyskinesias are frequently reversible (Campbell et al. 1997). Withdrawal dyskinesia rates appear to be lower with SGAs compared with FGAs (Connor et al. 2001), although a switch from an antipsychotic with strong D_2 affinity (risperidone, aripiprazole) to one with less potent affinity (quetiapine, clozapine) may predispose to withdrawal dyskinesia.

Tardive Dyskinesia

A meta-analysis of 10 studies lasting at least 11 months reported on TD rates in 783 patients ages 4–18 years (weighted mean 10 years). Most patients were prepubertal (80%), male (82%), and white (79%). Across these studies, only three cases of TD were reported, resulting in an annualized incidence rate of 0.4% (Correll and Kane 2007). While this pediatric rate is approximately half of the risk found in a meta-analysis that included 1,964 nonelderly adults (Correll et al. 2004), firm conclusions are precluded by the fact that none of the pediatric studies was designed specifically to detect TD, antipsychotic doses were low, and lifetime exposure was relatively short.

Neuroleptic Malignant Syndrome

Neuroleptic malignant syndrome (NMS) is a rare but potentially fatal complication of antipsychotic treatment. It has been suggested that SGAs may be associated less with NMS than FGAs and that SGAs are associated with a more benign course of NMS (Ananth et al. 2004), but this is unclear. In children and adolescents, cases of SGA-associated NMS have been reported. Thus, clinicians should be vigilant for NMS in youth treated with antipsychotics who present with fever, tachycardia, and marked motor rigidity and measure white cell count and creatine kinase levels, which would both be elevated in NMS. Creatine kinase levels are typically found to be 1,000 or higher in cases of true NMS. Notably, in case reports of five adults, clozapine rechallenge with slower titration avoided recurrence of NMS (Manu et al. 2012).

Weight Gain and Metabolic Adverse Effects

Weight Gain

In general, youth with psychiatric disorders seem to be at increased risk for being overweight or obese, especially when exposed to antipsychotics (Maayan and Correll 2011). Age-inappropriate weight gain is of particular concern in pediatric patients because of its association with glucose and lipid abnormalities and cardiovascular morbidity/mortality (American Diabetes Association et al. 2004; Correll et al. 2009). Reasons for weight gain are complex and include psychiatric illness, unhealthy lifestyle, and treatment effects. The weight gain potential of SGAs follows roughly the same rank order as found in adults (see Table 38–6), but the magnitude is greater (De Hert et al. 2011; Maayan and Correll 2011). Exceptions may be a greater relative weight gain propensity of risperidone and a greater likelihood of aripiprazole and ziprasidone to not be weight neutral in subgroups of pediatric patients (De Hert et al. 2011). Of note, combined treatment with an SGA and a stimulant does not seem to attenuate SGA-induced weight gain, whereas combined SGA plus mood stabilizer treatment seems associated with more weight gain than mood stabilizer monotherapy and even combined mood stabilizer treatment (Maayan and Correll 2011).

In a meta-analysis of 24 placebo-controlled studies of antipsychotics in 3,048 youth across diagnosis, ziprasidone (–0.04 kg; 95% confidence interval [CI]: –0.38 to +0.30) was associated with the lowest weight gain, followed by aripiprazole (0.79 kg; CI: 0.54–1.04), quetiapine (1.43 kg; CI: 1.17–1.69) and risperidone (1.76 kg; CI: 1.27–2.25), with olanzapine being associated with the most weight gain (3.45 kg; CI: 2.93–3.97). Using ≥7% weight gain as a threshold for clinically significant weight gain in these short-term trials, NNTs ranged from 36 (CI: –1 to +7, not significant) with ziprasidone to 12 (CI: 9–17) with aripiprazole, 9 (CI: 7–14) with quetiapine, 6 (CI: 5–7) with risperidone, and 3 (CI: 3–4) with olanzapine (with lower NNHs indicating greater weight gain) (De Hert et al. 2011). However, significant weight gain was more prevalent in youth with autism spectrum disorder, for which no data were available with quetiapine and ziprasidone. The greater observed weight gain in youth with autism spectrum disorder is likely due to their being younger and more antipsychotic-naïve than those with schizophrenia or bipolar disorder. Less prior antipsychotic treatment is a major risk factor for greater observed weight gain (Correll et al. 2009; Maayan and Correll 2011). Thus, in more comparable samples that exclude patients with autism spectrum disorder, the respective NNHs for weight gain of ≥7% were 39 (CI: –1 to +6, not significant) for aripiprazole, 36 (CI: –1 to +7, not significant) for ziprasidone, 9 (CI: 7–14) for quetiapine, 6 (CI: 5–8) for risperidone, and 3 (CI: 3–4) for olanzapine. NNHs for ≥7% with specific antipsychotics in each diagnostic category are provided in Tables 38–3, 38–4, and 38–5.

Metabolic Adverse Effects

The magnitude of adverse metabolic changes in fasting glucose and insulin and, especially, in total cholesterol, low-density lipoprotein (LDL) cholesterol, and triglycerides, generally follows the magnitude of weight gain (Pringsheim et al. 2011; Maayan and Correll 2011). However, clozapine and olanzapine appear to have additional direct, dose-dependent adverse effects on glucose and lipid metabolism, and quetiapine appears to have additional direct, dose-dependent adverse effects on lipid metabolism (Maayan and Correll 2011). The risk for type 2 diabetes mellitus, one of the most feared consequences of antipsychotic-related metabolic abnormalities, is relatively low, at least during 2 years of observation, but does appear to be elevated in youth treated with antipsychotics, compared with both healthy pediatric samples and psychiatric control subjects (Galling and Correll 2015).

Prolactin-Related Side Effects

Both FGAs and SGAs can elevate prolactin levels. Hyperprolactinemia can result in sexual side effects, although prolactin levels are not tightly correlated with symptoms including amenorrhea or oligomenorrhea, erectile dysfunction, decreased libido, hirsutism, and breast symptoms such as enlargement, engorgement, pain, or galactorrhea (Correll 2008). Data also suggest that hyperprolactinemia is dose dependent, reduces over time, and resolves after antipsychotic discontinuation. The relative potency of antipsychotic drugs in increasing prolactin levels is higher in adolescents than in adults but follows roughly the same pattern: paliperidone≥risperidone>haloperidol>olanzapine>ziprasidone>quetiapine≥clozapine>aripiprazole (Correll 2008). To date, adequate long-term data are lacking to determine if hyperprolactinemia at levels found during antipsychotic therapy alters bone density, sexual maturation, or the risk for benign prolactinomas. Because aripiprazole is a partial agonist at the D_2 receptor, prolactin levels can decrease below baseline. To date, no adverse effects have been described that might be related to low prolactin. Complicating the interpretation of available studies in youth is the fact that sexual side effects may not be present or expressed in prepubertal or sexually inactive youth. Also, these symptoms are infrequently asked about. More research is needed to determine long-term effects of prolactin-level changes during development.

Cardiac Side Effects

QTc Prolongation

Antipsychotics can differentially prolong the heart rate–corrected QT interval of the electrocardiogram (ECG), which may be associated with torsades de pointes, a potentially fatal arrhythmia. In adults, QTc prolongation is usually minimal compared with placebo, except for thioridazine. A meta-analysis evaluated QTc data from 55 prospective studies, including 108 treatment arms, 9 antipsychotics, and 5,423 youth (age 12.8±3.6 years, 32.1% female) (Jensen et al. 2014). Treatments included aripiprazole: 14 studies, n=814; haloperidol: 1 study, n=15; molindone: 3 studies, n=125; olanzapine: 5 studies, n=212; paliperidone: 3 studies, n=177; pimozide: 1 study, n=25; quetiapine: 5 studies, n=336; risperidone: 23 studies, n=2,234; ziprasidone: 10 studies, n=523; and placebo: 19 studies, n=962. From baseline to endpoint, aripiprazole significantly decreased the QTc interval (–1.44 milliseconds, CI: –2.63 to –0.26, P=0.017), while risperidone (+1.68, CI: +0.67 to +2.70, P=0.001) and, especially, ziprasidone (+8.74, CI: +5.19 to +12.30, P<0.001) significantly increased QTc. Compared with placebo, none of the investigated antipsychotics caused a significant increase in the incidence of QTc prolongation measures (i.e., >440–470 milliseconds, QTc >500 milliseconds, QTc change >60 milliseconds), but few studies reported these outcomes. Although clinically relevant QTc prolongation seems to be rare in youth, ECGs may need to be obtained if there is a family history of early sudden death or prolonged QT syndrome or a personal history of irregular heartbeat, unexplained tachycardia or shortness of breath at rest, dizziness on exertion, or syncope.

Myocarditis

Only clozapine has been associated with a myocarditis risk, which is greatest early in treatment. Clinical signs of acute myocarditis include palpitations, chest pain, shortness of breath, and syncope. Characteristic ECG changes include ectopic beats, atrioventricular block, atrial fibrillation or flutter, intraventricular conduction disturbance, ventricular tachycardia or fibrillation, and low QRS voltages. In youth, the incidence seems relatively low (Wehmeier et al. 2004).

Miscellaneous Adverse Effects

Sedation or Somnolence

Sedation is a frequent and often impairing antipsychotic side effect that usually is dose dependent, although tolerance may develop. An exception to the dose-dependent nature of sedation may be quetiapine, which seems to be less sedating at dosages above 200–300 mg/day, where α_2 blockade sets in, increasing noradrenergic tone. Although limited by different methodologies, a comparison of adult FDA labeling trials with pediatric data suggested a similar rank order of sedation but increased rates in youth (Correll et al. 2006). Sedation rates were 0%–33% for aripiprazole, 42%–69% for ziprasidone, 25%–80% for quetiapine, 29%–89% for risperidone, 44%–94% for olanzapine, and 46%–90% for clozapine. These rates are of particular concern in youth because of the potential interference with learning and school performance.

Liver Enzyme Abnormality or Toxicity

Abnormal liver enzymes have been reported with pediatric antipsychotic use (Kumra et al. 1997; Sikich et al. 2004, 2008). In two RCTs of olanzapine (Kryzhanovskaya et al. 2009; Tohen et al. 2007), significantly more patients had abnormal liver function tests of greater than three times the norm than patients on placebo. Abnormal aspartate transaminase (AST) was present in 35% versus 7% and 22% versus 2% of patients with schizophrenia and bipolar disorder, respectively. Abnormal alanine transaminase was present in 48% versus 3% and 34% versus 2% of patients with schizophrenia and bipolar disorder, respectively. These frequencies translate into an NNH of 3–5 for abnormal liver function with olanzapine compared with placebo. In the TEOSS study, olanzapine, but not risperidone or molindone, increased transaminases, with a significant baseline to endpoint increase for AST (Sikich et al. 2008). Although the extent and significance of liver enzyme abnormalities are unclear, the combination of divalproex with antipsychotics, particularly olanzapine, may increase the risk of abnormal liver function (Gonzalez-Heydrich et al. 2003).

Neutropenia and Agranulocytosis

With the exception of clozapine, the antipsychotic-associated decrease in white blood cell counts is generally not clinically significant. In a chart review of 172 clozapine-treated pediatric patients (Gerbino-Rosen et al. 2005), the cumulative 1-year probability of an initial adverse hematological event was 16% (13% for neutropenia, 0.6% for agranulocytosis). However, 48% of the 24 children and adolescents with newly emerging neutropenia were successfully rechallenged, and only 8 patients discontinued clozapine because of neutropenia (n=7) or agranulocytosis (n=1).

Adverse Effect Assessment and Monitoring

Adverse effect assessment and monitoring should be proactive, taking into consideration developmental norms and thresholds. Suggested baseline and follow-up assessments and intervals (Correll 2008; Pringsheim et al. 2011) are detailed in Table 38–7.

Healthy Lifestyle

Healthy (or unhealthy) lifestyle behaviors related to diet, activity, sleep, and substance use should be inquired about and compared with recommendations in the pediatric (American Medical Association 2007) or psychiatric (Correll 2008) population. These recommendations are summarized as follows.

1. Allow child to self-regulate meals; encourage authoritative parenting style supporting increased physical activity and reduced sedentary behavior; provide tangible and motivational support; discourage overly restrictive parenting
2. No sugar- or sugar replacement–sweetened beverages; assess for excessive consumption of 100% fruit juice; replace with water or moderate amounts of unsweetened tea or milk
3. Four to five separate meals per day, with two meals or less in the evening or at night
4. Daily breakfast
5. Promote serving small meal portions and slow eating, considering second helpings only after a delay
6. Preferentially eat food with a low glycemic index (i.e., 55 or less; http://www.glycemicindex.com)
7. At least 25–30 g of soluble fiber per day; five or more servings of fruits and vegetables per day
8. Avoid snacking in a satiety state, replace high-fat, high-calorie snacks with fruits and vegetables
9. Limit meals outside the home, especially in fast-food restaurants; family meals at least 5–6 times/week
10. Two or fewer hours of screen time per day, and no television in the room where the child sleeps
11. One hour or more of daily physical activity

Neuromotor Adverse Effects

Parkinsonian side effects and akathisia should be monitored at baseline, during titration, at 3 months, and annually (more often if abnormalities are noted). Dyskinetic movements should be assessed at least at baseline, at 3 months, and annually (more often if abnormalities are noted). It can be useful to measure these adverse effects with widely available rating scales, such as the Simpson-Angus Scale for parkinsonian side effects, the Barnes Akathisia Rating Scale for akathisia, and the Abnormal Involuntary Movement Scale for TD.

Body Weight and Composition

Ideally, weight should be monitored at each clinical visit (see Table 38–7). Clinically, the most commonly used measures to monitor weight include absolute weight change, percentage weight

TABLE 38–7. Suggested monitoring strategies in children and adolescents treated with antipsychotic agents[a]

Assessment	Baseline	Each visit	During titration and at target dose	At 3 months	Every 3 months	Every 6 months	Annually
Lifestyle behaviors[b]	✓	✓	-	-	-	-	-
Sedation/somnolence	✓	✓	-	-	-	-	-
Height, weight (calculate BMI percentile, BMI z score[c])	✓	✓	-	-	-	-	-
Sexual/reproductive dysfunction	✓	-	✓	✓	✓	-	-
Fasting blood glucose (or hemoglobin A1C) and lipids	✓	-	-	✓	-	✓	-
Parkinsonism (SAS or ESRS), akathisia (AIMS or ESRS)	✓	-	✓	✓	-	-	✓
Tardive dyskinesia	✓	-	-	✓	-	-	✓
Blood pressure (calculate sex- and age-adjusted percentiles[c]) and pulse	✓	-	-	✓	-	-	✓
Personal and family medical history[d]	✓	-	-	-	-	-	✓
Liver function tests	If symptomatic or significant weight gain	-	-	✓	-	-	If symptomatic or significant weight gain
Electrolytes, full blood count, renal function	If symptomatic; regular blood counts if on clozapine	-	-	-	-	-	If symptomatic; regular blood counts if on clozapine
Electrocardiogram	If on ziprasidone or clozapine	-	✓ If on ziprasidone; if on clozapine only if symptomatic	-	-	-	-
Prolactin[e]	If symptomatic	-	If symptomatic	If symptomatic	If symptomatic	If symptomatic	If symptomatic

Note. AIMS=Abnormal Involuntary Movement Scale (Guy 1976); BMI=body mass index; ESRS=Extrapyramidal Symptom Rating Scale (Chouinard et al. 1980); SAS=Simpson Angus Rating Scale (Simpson and Angus 1970).

[a]More frequent assessments of abnormalities occur or patient is at very high risk for specific adverse effects by personal or family history.

[b]Lifestyle behaviors=diet, exercise, smoking, substance use, sleep hygiene.

[c]Use, for example, the following online calculator based on data from the U.S. Centers for Disease Control and Prevention: http://www.quesgen.com/BMIPedsCalc.php.

[d]Include components of the metabolic syndrome (obesity, arterial hypertension, diabetes, dyslipidemia), past medical history for coronary heart disease or coronary heart disease equivalent disorders (e.g., diabetes mellitus, peripheral arterial disease, abdominal aortic aneurysm, symptomatic carotid artery disease), history of premature coronary heart disease in first-degree relatives (males <55 years and females <65 years), and past efficacy and adverse effect experiences in patients and/or family members.

[e]In case of abnormal sexual symptoms or signs; draw fasting in the morning and approximately 12 hours after the last antipsychotic dose.

change (weight change/baseline weight), and change in body mass index (BMI). Although easily obtained and valid in adults, these measures are useful only for periods of ≤3 months in pediatric patients, as they do not account for normal growth. Therefore, age- and sex-adjusted BMI percentiles (used to determine weight category; Table 38–8) and BMI z scores (used for change over time) need to be calculated, using growth charts (www.cdc.gov/growthcharts/) or calculators based on data from the U.S. Centers for Disease Control and Prevention (e.g., http://www.quesgen.com/BMIPedsCalc.php). A score (standard deviation) of zero and the 50th BMI percentile represent the population mean. Continuation on the same BMI *z* score or percentile represents stable relative weight over time. Although in adults waist circumference is preferred over BMI as a metabolic syndrome criterion, it is not recommended as a routine assessment in youth because of difficulty in accurate measurements and uncertainty of age-dependent cutoffs (American Medical Association 2007).

Blood Sugar and Insulin

To assess the risk for hyperglycemia and emerging diabetes (see Table 38–8), fasting blood glucose should be measured at baseline, at 3 months, and every 6 months (see Table 38–7) (Correll 2008). Families should be instructed that the patient must consume nothing but water for ≥8 hours prior to the blood draw. High-risk patients (e.g., family history of diabetes, nonwhite, BMI ≥95th percentile, weight gain >0.5 BMI *z* score) may require more frequent assessments. Patients should be asked at each visit about unintended weight loss, polyuria, and polydipsia to rule out emerging diabetes. Developing insulin resistance (i.e., increased insulin secretion) is more likely than diabetes in the context of weight gain as long as pancreatic β cells are able to compensate for the decreased insulin sensitivity. A simple measure of insulin resistance is the homeostatic model assessment (HOMA-IR): insulin (μU/mL) × fasting glucose (mmol/L)/22.5. HOMA-IR of ≥4.4 represents insulin resistance in adolescents (Lee et al. 2006). Nevertheless, insulin levels are not currently recommended in clinical practice, as they are expensive and not subject to standardized assays in the United States. Moreover, HOMA-IR predominantly reflects hepatic insulin sensitivity, which determines fasting levels of glucose and insulin, whereas insulin resistance also occurs in skeletal muscle, particularly early on. The ratio of fasting triglycerides to high-density lipoprotein (HDL) cholesterol has also been proposed as a widely applicable and sensitive measure of insulin resistance, with 3.5 being discussed as the threshold predicting insulin resistance, but this marker has not been evaluated in youth. While nonfasting or postprandial glucose levels are not recommended as screening tests for hyperglycemia or diabetes (Correll 2008), hemoglobin A1C levels (which are not affected by nonfasting status) are now recommended for identifying prediabetes or diabetes and tracking glucose homeostasis over time (see Table 38–8).

Blood Lipids

Like blood sugar, fasting serum lipids should be obtained at baseline, at 3 months, and every 6 months (see Table 38–7), with shorter intervals in case of abnormal lipids or significant weight gain (Correll 2008). The panel should include total cholesterol, HDL cholesterol, LDL cholesterol, and triglycerides. Table 38–8

TABLE 38–8. Clinically relevant thresholds for body weight and metabolic parameters in children and adolescents

Parameter	Threshold
Body weight	
Underweight	**BMI <5th percentile for sex and age[a]**
Normal weight	**BMI 5th to <85th percentile for sex and age[a]**
Overweight (previously "at-risk for overweight" in pediatric patients)	**BMI 85th to <95th percentile for sex and age[a]**
Obese (previously "overweight" in pediatric patients)	**BMI ≥95th percentile for sex and age[a]**
Blood glucose or hemoglobin A1C (hbA1C)	
Fasting hyperglycemia ("prediabetes")	Glucose: 100–125 mg/dL or HbA1C 5.7%–6.4%
2-hour postglucose load hyperglycemia ("impaired glucose tolerance")	140–199 mg/dL
Fasting diabetes (needs to be repeated)	Glucose: ≥126 mg/dL or HbA1C >6.4%
2-hour postglucose load diabetes	≥200 mg/dL
Insulin and insulin resistance	
Fasting hyperinsulinemia	**>20 µmol/L**
Homeostatic model assessment (HOMA)[b]	**≥4.4**
Triglycerides: HDL-cholesterol ratio	**>3.5 (exact cutoff in youth is still unclear and may be age-dependent)**
Blood lipids	
Total cholesterol	**≥170 mg/dL**
LDL cholesterol	**≥130 mg/dL**
HDL cholesterol	**<40 mg/dL in males and females**
Triglycerides	**≥110 mg/dL**
Metabolic syndrome (more than three out of five criteria required)	
Abdominal obesity criterion	**Waist circumference ≥90th percentile or BMI ≥95th percentile for sex and age[c]**
Fasting triglycerides criterion	**≥110 mg/dL**
Fasting HDL cholesterol criterion	**<40 mg/dL in males and females**
Blood pressure criterion	**≥90th percentile for sex and age[d]**
Fasting glucose criterion	≥110 mg/dL
Adjusted fasting glucose criterion	≥100 mg/dL

Note. Thresholds shown in bold are specific for children and adolescents.

BMI=body mass index; HDL=high-density lipoprotein; LDL=low-density lipoprotein.

[a]Sex- and age-adjusted BMI expressed in percentile (population norm: 50th BMI percentile) or BMI z scores (population norm: 0 BMI *z* score); growth charts (www.cdc.gov/growthcharts/) or Web-based calculators (e.g., http://www.quesgen.com/BMIPedsCalc.php). Stable age- and sex-adjusted weight is indicated by absence of any change in BMI percentile and BMI *z* score over time.

[b]HOMA: homeostatic model assessment=fasting insulin (µmol/L)×glucose (mmol/L)/22.5; glucose mmol/L=glucose m/dL/17.979797 or fasting insulin (mg/dL)×glucose (mg/dL)/405.

[c]Sex- and age-adjusted waist circumference percentile tables (Fernández et al. 2004).

[d]Sex- and age-adjusted blood pressure percentile tables (National High Blood Pressure Education Program Working Group on High Blood Pressure in Children and Adolescents 2004) or Web-based calculator (e.g., http://www.quesgen.com/BMIPedsCalc.php).

summarizes pediatric-specific blood lipid thresholds.

Blood Pressure

Blood pressure should be measured with a cuff large enough that 80% of the upper arm is covered. To assess for hypertension, the patient's height percentile has to be calculated (http://reference.medscape.com/calculator/height-age-percentile-boys; http://reference.medscape.com/calculator/height-age-percentile-girls). The measured blood pressure is compared with population norms from children of the same age, sex, and height (hypertension: ≥90th percentile for sex and age; see Table 38–8) (National High Blood Pressure Education Program Working Group on High Blood Pressure in Children and Adolescents 2004). To simplify the process, online calculators can be used to determine the systolic and diastolic percentiles for sex and age (e.g., http://www.quesgen.com/BMIPedsCalc.php).

Prolactin and Sexual/Reproductive System Side Effects

In case of hyperprolactinemia, common causes such as hormonal contraception or pregnancy, hypothyroidism, or renal failure need to be ruled out by measuring serum human chorionic gonadotropin, thyroid-stimulating hormone, or creatinine, respectively. To identify hyperprolactinemia-related hypogonadism, the clinician should inquire at baseline, during drug titration, and quarterly about menstruation, nipple discharge, breast enlargement, sexual functioning, and (if appropriate) pubertal development. Since the effects of subclinical prolactin elevations are unclear, current thinking dictates that prolactin levels be measured only if clinical symptoms develop. Because prolactin undergoes diurnal variations and increases with exercise, stress, and food intake, it should be measured in the morning, after fasting, and 8–12 hours after the last medication dose. Prolactin thresholds are laboratory dependent and higher for postpubertal youth and females (upper level ~20–30 ng/mL) than in males (upper level ~11–15 ng/mL) or age in years up until age 18.

Liver Enzymes

Liver enzyme testing to check for potential signs of fatty liver infiltration should be considered in patients who 1) have abdominal/gastrointestinal symptoms, 2) gain ≥7% of their baseline body weight over 3 months, or 3) have ≥0.5 BMI z scores when treated for >3 months. In patients with AST, alanine aminotransferase, or γ-glutamyl transferase levels three times the norm and without other medical causes, discontinuation of the antipsychotic or of possibly responsible co-medications should be considered.

White Cell and Granulocyte Counts

The increased risk of agranulocytosis associated with clozapine requires enrollment in a central national database. Guidelines mandate weekly monitoring of the white blood cell count (WBC) and absolute neutrophil count (ANC) for the first 6 months. If the counts are normal (WBC >3,500 and ANC >2,000), intervals change to biweekly for the next 6 months and monthly thereafter. If there is a single drop or cumulative drop within 3 weeks of WBC ≥3,000/mm^3 or of ANC ≥1,500/mm^3, or if WBC is <3,500/mm^3 and ≥3,000/mm^3 or ANC is <2,000/mm^3 and ≥1,500/mm^3 (mild leukopenia/granulocytopenia), twice-weekly blood monitoring is to be initiated until WBC >3,500/mm^3 and ANC >2,000/mm^3, at which point the clinician may return to previous monitoring frequency. In case of moderate leukopenia/granulocytopenia (WBC <3,000/mm^3 and ≥2,000/mm^3 and/or ANC <1,500/mm^3 and ≥1,000/mm^3), clozapine is to be stopped and daily blood tests are required until WBC >3,000/mm^3 and ANC >1,500/mm^3, followed by twice-weekly blood tests until WBC >3,500/mm^3 and ANC >2,000/mm^3. Clozapine rechallenge is permitted when WBC >3,500/mm^3 and ANC >2,000/mm^3. However, if clozapine rechallenge is initiated, weekly monitoring is required for 1 year before returning to the usual monitoring schedule of every 2 weeks for 6 months and then every 4 weeks as long as results are normal. In case of WBC <2,000/mm^3 and/or ANC <1,000/mm^3, clozapine is to be discontinued and a rechallenge is not permitted.

Of note, the thresholds for discontinuing clozapine do not take into account ethnic variations. Considering ethnic variations is important, as a subgroup of patients with African descent (25%–50%) and some people of Middle Eastern origin have habitually low white counts in the absence of any infections—also called benign ethnic (or cyclic) neutropenia (Rajagopal 2005). African Americans have lower WBCs and ANCs than whites, and people of African descent have lower values than people of African American descent. Men have lower values than women, independent of ethnicity (Hsieh et al. 2007). On the basis of these findings and successful clozapine treatment in patients with benign ethnic neutropenia (Whiskey and Taylor 2007), adjusted thresholds for patients with habitually low white counts have been proposed (Rajagopal 2005) that are 500/mm^3 lower than in the general population for normal white cell/neutrophil count (≥3,000/≥1,500/mm^3 instead of ≥3,500/≥2,000/mm^3), mild leukopenia/neutropenia (≥2,500–3,000/≥1,000–1,500 mm^3 instead of ≥3,000–3,500/≥1,500–2,000/mm^3), and moderate leukopenia/neutropenia (<2,500 to >2,000/<1,000 to >500/mm^3 instead of <3,000 to >2,000/<1,500 to >1,000/mm^3).

Cardiac Conduction and Repolarization

Although a very uncommon complication of antipsychotic treatment, any QTc value of ≥500 ms, confirmed by manual reading, should lead to a discontinuation of the antipsychotic, unless other QT-prolonging agents can be discontinued instead or hypomagnesemia or hypokalemia is present that can be corrected.

Managing Adverse Effects

In addition to discussion in this section, Table 38–9 lists some suggested adverse effect management strategies in children and adolescents treated with antipsychotic agents.

Neuromotor Adverse Effects

Extrapyramidal adverse effects are dose and titration dependent. In milder cases, a dose reduction or slowing of the titration can bring relief. In cases of more severe parkinsonian side effects, oral or (especially for acute dystonia) intramuscular anticholinergics, antihistamines, or adjunctive benzodiazepines can be used. Once the patient is stabilized and on maintenance therapy, gradual with-

TABLE 38–9. Suggested adverse effect management strategies in children and adolescents treated with antipsychotic agents

Assessment	Selected interventions for relevant abnormality
Unhealthy lifestyle behaviors[a]	Provide healthy lifestyle instruction or intervention program
Sedation/somnolence	Wait first for potential tolerance to develop; decrease dose (increase if on low-dose quetiapine, which may lead to less sedation at doses ≥300 mg/day); switch to lower-risk drug; modafinil coadministration
Postural hypotension/dizziness/syncope	Slow down titration, reduce dose (increase if on low-dose quetiapine, which may lead to less orthostasis at doses >300 mg/day); increase fluid intake; switch to lower-risk drug
Parkinsonism	Slow down titration, reduce dose; switch to lower-risk drug; add anticholinergic agent,[b] antihistamine,[b] or benzodiazepine[a,b]
Akathisia	Slow down titration, reduce dose; switch to lower-risk drug; add benzodiazepine,[a,b,c] β-blocker,[c] antihistamine,[b] or anticholinergic agent
Tardive dyskinesia	Reduce dose; increase dose (masking); if possible, replace with non-antipsychotic; switch to clozapine; possibly add vitamin E
Developmentally inappropriate weight gain	Switch to lower-risk drug; healthy lifestyle intervention; add weight-loss agents (e.g., metformin [best evidence],[d] topiramate [second best evidence],[b] orlistat,[e] amantadine,[f,g] bupropion[g])
Arterial hypertension/tachycardia	Switch to lower-risk drug; healthy lifestyle intervention; add weight-loss agents (e.g., metformin,[d] orlistat,[e] amantadine,[f,g] topiramate,[b] bupropion[g]); add antihypertensive
Hyperglycemia/diabetes	Switch to lower-risk drug; healthy lifestyle intervention; add weight-loss agents (e.g., metformin,[d] orlistat,[e] topiramate,[b] bupropion[g]); add antihyperglycemic agent
Dyslipidemia	Switch to lower-risk drug; healthy lifestyle intervention; add weight-loss agents (e.g., metformin,[d] topiramate,[b] orlistat,[e] bupropion[g]); add lipid-lowering agent
Clinically relevant abnormal electrolytes, full blood count, renal function	Switch to lower-risk drug; address specific abnormality as needed
Abnormally elevated liver enzymes (>2 upper limit)	Reassess need for medication; consider switch
Hyperprolactinemia	If asymptomatic, may wait if values normalize with time; reduce dose; switch to lower-risk drug if symptomatic Only if symptomatic hyperprolactinemia continues despite switch to a low-risk antipsychotic: obtain MRI of the sella turcica or bone density scan or add a full (e.g., bromocriptine,[f,g] amantadine[f,g]) or partial (e.g., aripiprazole) dopamine agonist
Sexual/reproductive dysfunction	Reduce dose; switch to lower-risk drug; for performance: add bupropion,[g] sildenafil
Clinically relevant ECG abnormalities	Reassess need for medication; consider switch

Note. ECG=electrocardiogram; MRI=magnetic resonance imaging.
[a]Can impair coordination.
[b]Can impair cognitive abilities.
[c]Can cause bradycardia, dizziness, and syncope.
[d]Lactic acidosis and hypoglycemia no real risk in children; nausea, stomachache, flatulence, and diarrhea can occur.
[e]Unless low-fat diet is observed, flatulence, diarrhea, and involuntary encopresis can occur.
[f]Potential risk for exacerbation of psychosis.
[g]Potential risk for exacerbation of mania.

drawal of the adjunctive treatments for the neuromotor adverse effects can be tried to reduce the potential cognitive burden that anticholinergics especially may have. Often, patients adapt to the dopamine blockade over time and do not require sustained anticholinergic treatment. For akathisia, β-blockers, benzodiazepines, dopamine agonists, or mirtazapine can be helpful. Unfortunately, unless the patient can be maintained without antipsychotic therapy, no evidence-based therapy for TD exists, but dose reduction (or dose increase to mask the movements) or a switch from an FGA to an SGA or to clozapine can be tried.

Weight and Metabolic Dysfunction

Medical health strategies for youth treated with antipsychotics have been summarized (Correll 2008). *Primary preventive strategies* include 1) educating about and maximizing adherence to healthy lifestyle behaviors and 2) choosing an agent with the lowest likelihood of adverse effects on body composition and metabolic status. *Secondary preventive strategies* in overweight patients and those with mild baseline metabolic abnormalities, significant weight gain, or beginning metabolic abnormalities (see Table 38–9) during therapy include 1) intensification of healthy lifestyle instructions, 2) consideration of switching to a lower-risk agent, and 3) a nonpharmacological weight-loss treatment or adjunctive pharmacological intervention that targets normalization or reversal of weight abnormalities (see Table 38–9). *Tertiary preventive* strategies in patients who are obese or have clinically defined related abnormalities (e.g., hyperglycemia, diabetes, dyslipidemia, hypertension; see Table 38–8) require intensified weight reduction interventions, attempts at changing to or initiating lower-risk medications for the underlying psychiatric condition, and targeted treatments of these suprathreshold metabolic or endocrine abnormalities, often in conjunction with a subspecialist.

Despite concern about age-inappropriate weight gain in pediatric patients, no consensus exists regarding the cutoff for clinically meaningful weight change. Rather, BMI≥85th percentile (i.e., overweight or obese) is the accepted threshold for intervention (American Medical Association 2007) (see Table 38–8). However, in psychiatric practice, where the underlying illness in conjunction with adverse treatment effects can lead to significant and often rapid weight gain, clinicians require guidance regarding at what point to consider changing therapy or using adjunctive treatments. Operational criteria for clinically significant weight gain or abnormal weight status in psychiatrically ill patients that requires reconsideration of the current treatment plan include (Correll 2008):

1. Greater than 5% weight gain during 3 months or
2. Any of the following three conditions at any time during treatment:
   a. Greater than 0.5 increase in BMI z score
   b. BMI percentile ≥85–94.9 plus one adverse health consequence (hyperglycemia; dyslipidemia; hyperinsulinemia; hypertension; orthopedic, gallbladder, or sleep disorder)
   c. BMI ≥95th percentile or abdominal obesity (>90th percentile).

As outlined earlier, the treatment of choice for abnormalities in body weight or metabolic health includes healthy lifestyle education and modification strategies. While such strategies have been tested and shown to be successful to a certain degree in adults (Caemmerer et al. 2012), the effects of healthy lifestyle programs have not yet been reported in youth treated with an antipsychotic. The American Medical Association (2007) Expert Committee stage 1 recommendations for healthy lifestyle behaviors in pediatric patients that can be implemented widely without significant training are summarized in the subsection "Healthy Lifestyle." Progression to the *structured* stage 2 weight management protocol is indicated if after 3–6 months no improvement in weight status has occurred and if the patient and family show readiness for change. Stage 2 interventions can be implemented by a primary care physician or allied health care provider highly trained in weight management and include the following:

1. Structured dietary and physical activity behaviors
   a. Plan development for a balanced macronutrient diet containing few energy-dense foods
   b. Structured daily meals and snacks
   c. Supervised active play of ≥60 minutes daily
   d. Screen time of ≤1 hour daily
2. Increased monitoring (e.g., of screen time, physical activity, dietary intake, restaurant logs) by provider, patient, or family
3. Goal setting of weight maintenance resulting in a decreasing BMI percentile as age and height increase

If no improvement in BMI percentile or weight occurs after 3–6 months, the patient should be advanced to stage 3, consisting of a comprehensive protocol implemented by a multidisciplinary obesity care team and aiming at weight maintenance or gradual weight loss until BMI <85th percentile (American Medical Association 2007).

If behavioral measures alone are insufficient, pharmacological weight loss interventions may be added. Foremost therapies that have had some success in producing weight loss in pediatric patients receiving antipsychotics include metformin (e.g., 250 mg/day tid if <50 kg or 500 mg/day tid to 1,000 mg/day bid if ≥50 kg titrated over 3–4 weeks) and topiramate (e.g., 25–400 mg/day) (Maayan et al. 2010). Dyslipidemia should be treated initially with dietary measures; if this is not sufficient, drug therapy may be given using a fibric acid derivative (e.g., gemfibrozil, fenofibrate), a statin, fish oil, or niacin, if appropriate. Diabetes may be treated with diet, oral hypoglycemic agents, or insulin as needed, but diabetes induced by atypical antipsychotic agents sometimes disappears when the drug is stopped or changed to a lower-risk agent (Correll 2008). While medications used to mitigate or reverse antipsychotic-induced weight gain may be prescribed by psychiatric health care providers, medications used to treat dyslipidemia or hyperglycemia are likely managed by pediatricians or pediatric endocrinologists.

Hyperprolactinemia and Sexual/Reproductive System Side Effects

If serum prolactin is <200 ng/mL, management strategies include antipsychotic dose reduction or change to a prolactin-sparing drug, such as aripiprazole, quetiapine, or in treatment-resistant patients, clozapine (Correll 2008). If serum prolactin is >200 ng/mL or is persistently elevated despite change to a prolactin-sparing drug, the clinician should obtain a magnetic resonance imaging (MRI) scan of the sella turcica to look for a pituitary adenoma or parasellar tumor. If the MRI scan is normal, sex steroid replacement therapy (e.g., oral contraceptives for women of menstrual age, testosterone for men) may be used to treat the hypogonadism, or drugs such as bisphosphonates (e.g., alendronate, risedronate) can be given to treat and prevent osteoporosis. Prolactin levels can also be lowered by adding a dopamine agonist (e.g., amantadine, bromocriptine) or by adding a partial dopamine agonist (e.g., aripiprazole 5–15 mg/day), which can be effective without worsening psychosis or mania (Shim et al. 2007). The beneficial effects on prolactin levels after a switch to a lower-risk agent or addition of a full or partial dopamine agonist can be evaluated at least five times the half-life after the offending drug is stopped and the new agent has been titrated to the target dose.

Neutropenia

Since neutropenia may follow a diurnal variation pattern, afternoon levels in patients with habitually low white blood counts should be obtained to reconsider clozapine initiation in such patients (Esposito et al. 2006). Moreover, lithium at low to medium dosages (300–600 mg/day) may be used to increase white blood counts, which increase because of both a shedding of white cells from the vascular walls and bone marrow stimulation (Sporn et al. 2003; Whiskey and Taylor 2007). In cases where agranulocytosis has developed, treatment with granulocyte colony–stimulating factor can be lifesaving (Whiskey and Taylor 2007).

Summary Points

- RCTs in youth have demonstrated efficacy of antipsychotics for schizophrenia, bipolar mania, irritability/aggressive behaviors associated with autism spectrum and disruptive behavior disorders, and Tourette's disorder.
- Various antipsychotics have FDA-approved indications for use in youth with schizophrenia, bipolar mania, and irritability associated with autism spectrum and tic disorders. Although efficacy data exist for risperidone in disruptive behavior disorders, use of antipsychotics for aggression or impulsivity is recommended only after treatments for underlying disorders and nonpharmacological interventions have been exhausted.
- While differences in antipsychotic efficacy (except for clozapine in refractory patients) are likely relatively small and difficult to predict, differences in adverse effects between antipsychotic agents are clinically relevant and easier to predict.
- Pharmacokinetic and pharmacodynamic profiles of antipsychotics can be used to predict the likelihood of adverse effects and drug-drug interactions that can manifest as overdose or rebound and withdrawal phenomena.
- Children and adolescents are at risk to develop antipsychotic-induced sedation, acute extrapyramidal side effects (except for akathisia), withdrawal dyskinesia, hyperprolactinemia, age-inappropriate weight gain, and lipid abnormalities.

- Safety assessments need to use developmentally adjusted measures and thresholds.
- Treatment selection should be guided by individual patient factors (e.g., age, development, illness phase, target symptoms, past response, side effect pattern) and by medication factors, choosing first to use medications with the lowest likelihood of causing relevant adverse effects.
- Education of patients and families about and proactive assessment of antipsychotic adverse effects in youth should be routine clinical practice.
- While adverse effects need to be balanced against efficacy gains, clinicians should be prepared to carefully change antipsychotic treatment or initiate interventions to reduce bothersome as well as physically problematic adverse effects to improve overall psychiatric and physical outcomes.

References

Aman MG, De Smedt G, Derivan A, et al: Double-blind, placebo-controlled study of risperidone for the treatment of disruptive behaviors in children with subaverage intelligence. Am J Psychiatry 159(8):1337–1346, 2002 12153826

Aman MG, Arnold LE, McDougle CJ, et al: Acute and long-term safety and tolerability of risperidone in children with autism. J Child Adolesc Psychopharmacol 15(6):869–884, 2005 16379507

Aman MG, Bukstein OG, Gadow KD, et al: What does risperidone add to parent training and stimulant for severe aggression in child attention-deficit/hyperactivity disorder? J Am Acad Child Adolesc Psychiatry 53(1):47–60, e1, 2014 24342385

American Diabetes Association, American Psychiatric Association, American Association of Clinical Endocrinologists, et al: Consensus development conference on antipsychotic drugs and obesity and diabetes. J Clin Psychiatry 65(2):267–272, 2004 15003083

American Medical Association: Expert Committee Recommendations on the Assessment, Prevention, and Treatment of Child and Adolescent Overweight and Obesity: Recommendations for Treatment of Pediatric Obesity. Chicago, IL, American Medical Association, January 25, 2007. Available at: http://www.ama-assn.org/ama1/pub/upload/mm/433/ped_obesity_recs.pdf. Accessed March 18, 2008.

Ananth J, Parameswaran S, Gunatilake S, et al: Neuroleptic malignant syndrome and atypical antipsychotic drugs. J Clin Psychiatry 65(4):464–470, 2004 15119907

Arango C, Robles O, Parellada M, et al: Olanzapine compared to quetiapine in adolescents with a first psychotic episode. Eur Child Adolesc Psychiatry 18(7):418–428, 2009 19198920

Armenteros JL, Lewis JE, Davalos M: Risperidone augmentation for treatment-resistant aggression in attention-deficit/hyperactivity disorder: a placebo-controlled pilot study. J Am Acad Child Adolesc Psychiatry 46(5):558–565, 2007 17450046

Bruggeman R, van der Linden C, Buitelaar JK, et al: Risperidone versus pimozide in Tourette's disorder: a comparative double-blind parallel-group study. J Clin Psychiatry 62(1):50–56, 2001 11235929

Buitelaar JK, van der Gaag RJ, Cohen-Kettenis P, et al: A randomized controlled trial of risperidone in the treatment of aggression in hospitalized adolescents with subaverage cognitive abilities. J Clin Psychiatry 62(4):239–248, 2001 11379837

Burris KD, Molski TF, Xu C, et al: Aripiprazole, a novel antipsychotic, is a high-affinity partial agonist at human dopamine D2 receptors. J Pharmacol Exp Ther 302(1):381–389, 2002 12065741

Caemmerer J, Correll CU, Maayan L: Acute and maintenance effects of non-pharmacologic interventions for antipsychotic associated weight gain and metabolic abnormalities: A meta-analytic comparison of randomized controlled trials. Schizophr Res 140(1–3):159–168, 2012 22763424

Campbell M, Small AM, Green WH, et al: Behavioral efficacy of haloperidol and lithium carbonate. A comparison in hospitalized aggressive children with conduct disorder. Arch Gen Psychiatry 41(7):650–656, 1984 6428371

Campbell M, Armenteros JL, Malone RP, et al: Neuroleptic-related dyskinesias in autistic children: a prospective, longitudinal study. J Am Acad Child Adolesc Psychiatry 36(6):835–843, 1997 9183140

Chouinard G, Ross-Chouinard A, Annabel L, et al: The Extrapyramidal Symptom Rating Scale. Can J Neurol Sci 7(3):233, 1980

Connor DF, Fletcher KE, Wood JS: Neuroleptic-related dyskinesias in children and adolescents. J Clin Psychiatry 62(12):967–974, 2001 11780878

Connor DF, McLaughlin TJ, Jeffers-Terry M: Randomized controlled pilot study of quetiapine in the treatment of adolescent conduct disorder. J Child Adolesc Psychopharmacol 18(2):140–156, 2008 18439112

Correll CU: Antipsychotic use in children and adolescents: minimizing adverse effects to maximize outcomes. J Am Acad Child Adolesc Psychiatry 47(1):9–20, 2008 18174821

Correll CU, Kane JM: One-year incidence rates of tardive dyskinesia in children and adolescents treated with second-generation antipsychotics: a systematic review. J Child Adolesc Psychopharmacol 17(5):647–655, 2007 17979584

Correll CU, Leucht S, Kane JM: Lower risk for tardive dyskinesia associated with second-generation antipsychotics: a systematic review of 1-year studies. Am J Psychiatry 161(3):414–425, 2004 14992963

Correll CU, Penzner JB, Parikh UH, et al: Recognizing and monitoring adverse events of second-generation antipsychotics in children and adolescents. J Child Adolesc Psychiatr Clin N Am 15(1):177–206, 2006 16321730

Correll CU, Manu P, Olshanskiy V, et al: Cardiometabolic risk of atypical antipsychotics during first-time use in children and adolescents. JAMA 302(16):1765–1773, 2009 PMC3055794

Correll CU, Schenk EM, DelBello MP: Antipsychotic and mood stabilizer efficacy and tolerability in adult and pediatric patients with bipolar I mania: a comparative analysis of acute, randomized, placebo-controlled trials. Bipolar Disord 12(2):116–141, 2010 20402706

Correll CU, Kratochvil CJ, March J: Developments in pediatric psychopharmacology: focus on stimulants, antidepressants and antipsychotics. J Clin Psychiatry 72(5):655–670, 2011 21658348

Correll CU, Zhao Q, Carson WH, et al: Validity of early antipsychotic response to aripiprazole in adolescents with schizophrenia and its predictive value for clinical outcomes. J Am Acad Child Adolesc Psychiatry 52(7):689–698, 2013

De Hert M, Dobbelaere M, Sheridan EM, et al: Metabolic and endocrine adverse effects of second-generation antipsychotics in children and adolescents: A systematic review of randomized, placebo controlled trials and guidelines for clinical practice. Eur Psychiatry 26(3):144–158, 2011 21295450

DelBello MP, Schwiers ML, Rosenberg HL, et al: A double-blind, randomized, placebo-controlled study of quetiapine as adjunctive treatment for adolescent mania. J Am Acad Child Adolesc Psychiatry 41(10):1216–1223, 2002 12364843

DelBello MP, Kowatch RA, Adler CM, et al: A double-blind randomized pilot study comparing quetiapine and divalproex for adolescent mania. J Am Acad Child Adolesc Psychiatry 45(3):305–313, 2006 16540815

DelBello MP, Chang K, Welge JA, et al: A double-blind, placebo-controlled pilot study of quetiapine for depressed adolescents with bipolar disorder. Bipolar Disord 11(5):483–493, 2009 19624387

Detke HC, DelBello M, Landry J, et al: Safety and efficacy of olanzapine/fluoxetine combination vs. placebo in patients ages 10 to 17 in the acute treatment of major depressive episodes associated with bipolar I disorder. Presented at the American College of Neuropsychopharmacology 51st Annual Meeting, Hollywood, FL, December 2–8, 2012

Engelhardt DM, Polizos P, Waizer J, et al: A double-blind comparison of fluphenazine and haloperidol in outpatient schizophrenic children. J Autism Child Schizophr 3(2):128–137, 1973 4583792

Esposito D, Chouinard G, Hardy P, et al: Successful initiation of clozapine treatment despite morning pseudoneutropenia. Int J Neuropsychopharmacol 9(4):489–491, 2006 16191206

Expert Panel on Detection, Evaluation, and Treatment of High Blood Cholesterol in Adults: Executive Summary of The Third Report of The National Cholesterol Education Program (NCEP) Expert Panel on Detection, Evaluation, And Treatment of High Blood Cholesterol In Adults (Adult Treatment Panel III). JAMA 285(19):2486–2497, 2001 11368702

Fernández JR, Redden DT, Pietrobelli A, et al: Waist circumference percentiles in nationally representative samples of African-American, European-American, and Mexican-American children and adolescents. J Pediatr 145(4):439–444, 2004 15480363

Findling RL, McNamara NK, Branicky LA, et al: A double-blind pilot study of risperidone in the treatment of conduct disorder. J Am Acad Child Adolesc Psychiatry 39(4):509–516, 2000 10761354

Findling RL, Robb A, Nyilas M, et al: A multiple-center, randomized, double-blind, placebo-controlled study of oral aripiprazole for treatment of adolescents with schizophrenia. Am J Psychiatry 165(11):1432–1441, 2008 18765484

Findling RL, Nyilas M, Forbes RA, et al: Acute treatment of pediatric bipolar I disorder, manic or mixed episode, with aripiprazole: a randomized, double-blind, placebo-controlled study. J Clin Psychiatry 70(10):1441–1451, 2009 19906348

Findling RL, Johnson JL, McClellan J, et al: Double-blind maintenance safety and effectiveness findings from the Treatment of Early Onset Schizophrenia Spectrum (TEOSS) study. J Am Acad Child Adolesc Psychiatry 49(6):583–594, quiz 632, 2010 20494268

Findling RL, Youngstrom EA, McNamara NK, et al: Double-blind, randomized, placebo-controlled long-term maintenance study of aripiprazole in children with bipolar disorder. J Clin Psychiatry 73(1):57–63, 2012a 22152402

Findling RL, McKenna K, Earley WR, et al: Efficacy and safety of quetiapine in adolescents with schizophrenia investigated in a 6-week, double-blind, placebo-controlled trial. J Child Adolesc Psychopharmacol 22(5):327–342, 2012b 23083020

Findling RL, Correll CU, Nyilas M, et al: Aripiprazole for the treatment of pediatric bipolar I disorder: a 30-week, randomized, placebo-controlled study. Bipolar Disord 15(2):138–149, 2013a 23437959

Findling RL, Cavuş I, Pappadopulos E, et al: Efficacy, long-term safety, and tolerability of ziprasidone in children and adolescents with bipolar disorder. J Child Adolesc Psychopharmacol 23(8):545–557, 2013b 24111980

Findling RL, Pathak S, Earley WR, et al: Efficacy and safety of extended-release quetiapine fumarate in youth with bipolar depression: an 8 week, double-blind, placebo-controlled trial. J Child Adolesc Psychopharmacol 24(6):325–335, 2014a 24956042

Findling RL, Mankoski R, Timko K, et al: A randomized controlled trial investigating the safety and efficacy of aripiprazole in the long-term maintenance treatment of pediatric patients with irritability associated with autistic disorder. J Clin Psychiatry 75(1):22–30, 2014b 24502859

Galling B, Correll CU: Do antipsychotics increase diabetes risk in children and adolescents? Expert Opin Drug Saf 14(2):219–241, 2015 25480466

Geller B, Luby JL, Joshi P, et al: A randomized controlled trial of risperidone, lithium, or divalproex sodium for initial treatment of bipolar I disorder, manic or mixed phase, in children and adolescents. Arch Gen Psychiatry 69(5):515–528, 2012 22213771

Gerbino-Rosen G, Roofeh D, Tompkins DA, et al: Hematological adverse events in clozapine-treated children and adolescents. J Am Acad Child Adolesc Psychiatry 44(10):1024–1031, 2005 16175107

Ghanizadeh A, Haghighi A: Aripiprazole versus risperidone for treating children and adolescents with tic disorder: a randomized double blind clinical trial. Child Psychiatry Hum Dev 45(5):596–603, 2014 24343476

Ghanizadeh A, Sahraeizadeh A, Berk M: A head-to-head comparison of aripiprazole and risperidone for safety and treating autistic disorders, a randomized double blind clinical trial. Child Psychiatry Hum Dev 45(2):185–192, 2014 23801256

Gonzalez-Heydrich J, Raches D, Wilens TE, et al: Retrospective study of hepatic enzyme elevations in children treated with olanzapine, divalproex, and their combination. J Am Acad Child Adolesc Psychiatry 42(10):1227–1233, 2003 14560173

Greenhill LL, Solomon M, Pleak R, et al: Molindone hydrochloride treatment of hospitalized children with conduct disorder. J Clin Psychiatry 46(8 Pt 2):20–25, 1985 3894338

Guy W (ed): ECDEU Assessment Manual for Psychopharmacology (Publ ABM 76-338). Washington, DC, U.S. Department of Health, Education, and Welfare, 1976, pp 534–537

Haas M, Unis AS, Armenteros J, et al: A 6-week, randomized, double-blind, placebo-controlled study of the efficacy and safety of risperidone in adolescents with schizophrenia. J Child Adolsc Psychopharmacol 19(6):622–632, 2009a 20035579

Haas M, Eerdekens M, Kushner S, et al: Efficacy, safety and tolerability of two dosing regimens in adolescent schizophrenia: double-blind study. Br J Psychiatry 194(2):158–164, 2009b 19182179

Haas M, Delbello MP, Pandina G, et al: Risperidone for the treatment of acute mania in children and adolescents with bipolar disorder: a randomized, double-blind, placebo-controlled study. Bipolar Disord 11(7):687–700, 2009c

Hollander E, Wasserman S, Swanson EN, et al: A double-blind placebo-controlled pilot study of olanzapine in childhood/adolescent pervasive developmental disorder. J Child Adolesc Psychopharmacol 16(5):541–548, 2006 17069543

Hsieh MM, Everhart JE, Byrd-Holt DD, et al: Prevalence of neutropenia in the U.S. population: age, sex, smoking status, and ethnic differences. Ann Intern Med 146(7):486–492, 2007 17404350

Jensen JB, Kumra S, Leitten W, et al: A comparative pilot study of second-generation antipsychotics in children and adolescents with schizophrenia-spectrum disorders. J Child Adolesc Psychopharmacol 18(4):317–326, 2008 18759641

Jensen KG, Juul K, Fink-Jensen A, et al: Corrected QT changes during antipsychotic treatment of children and adolescents: A systematic review and meta-analysis of clinical trials. J Am Acad Child Adolesc Psychiatry 54(1):25–36, 2014 25524787

Kendall T, Hollis C, Stafford M, et al: Recognition and management of psychosis and schizophrenia in children and young people: summary of NICE guidance. BMJ 346:f150, 2013 23344308

Kent JM, Kushner S, Ning X, et al: Risperidone dosing in children and adolescents with autistic disorder: a double-blind, placebo-controlled study. J Autism Dev Disord 43(8):1773–1783, 2013 23212807

Knapp P, Chait A, Pappadopulos E, et al: Treatment of maladaptive aggression in youth: CERT guidelines I. Engagement, assessment, and management. Pediatrics 129(6):e1562–e1576, 2012 22641762

Kryzhanovskaya L, Schulz SC, McDougle C, et al: Olanzapine versus placebo in adolescents with schizophrenia: a 6-week, randomized, double-blind, placebo-controlled trial. J Am Acad Child Adolesc Psychiatry 48(1):60–70, 2009 19057413

Kumra S, Frazier JA, Jacobsen LK, et al: Childhood-onset schizophrenia. A double-blind clozapine-haloperidol comparison. Arch Gen Psychiatry 53(12):1090–1097, 1996 8956674

Kumra S, Herion D, Jacobsen LK, et al: Case study: risperidone-induced hepatotoxicity in pediatric patients. J Am Acad Child Adolesc Psychiatry 36(5):701–705, 1997 9136506

Kumra S, Kranzler H, Gerbino-Rosen G, et al: Clozapine and "high-dose" olanzapine in refractory early onset schizophrenia: a 12-week randomized and double-blind comparison. Biol Psychiatry 63(5):524–529, 2008 17651705

Lee JM, Okumura MJ, Davis MM, et al: Prevalence and determinants of insulin resistance among U.S. adolescents: a population-based study. Diabetes Care 29(11):2427–2432, 2006 17065679

Luby J, Mrakotsky C, Stalets MM, et al: Risperidone in preschool children with autistic spectrum disorders: an investigation of safety and efficacy. J Child Adolesc Psychopharmacol 16(5):575–587, 2006 17069546

Maayan L, Correll CU: Weight gain and metabolic risks associated with antipsychotic medications in children and adolescents.

J Child Adolesc Psychopharmacol 21(6):517–535, 2011 22166172

Maayan L, Vakhrusheva J, Correll CU: Effectiveness of medications used to attenuate antipsychotic-related weight gain and metabolic abnormalities: a systematic review and meta-analysis. Neuropsychopharmacology 35(7):1520–1530, 2010 20336059

Malone RP, Maislin G, Choudhury MS, et al: Risperidone treatment in children and adolescents with autism: short- and long-term safety and effectiveness. J Am Acad Child Adolesc Psychiatry 41(2):140–147, 2002 11837403

Manu P, Sarpal D, Muir O, et al: When can patients with potentially life-threatening adverse effects be rechallenged with clozapine? A systematic review of the published literature. Schizophr Res 134(2–3):180–186, 2012 22113154

Marcus RN, Owen R, Kamen L, et al: A placebo-controlled, fixed-dose study of aripiprazole in children and adolescents with irritability associated with autistic disorder. J Am Acad Child Adolesc Psychiatry 48(11):1110–1119, 2009 19797985

McCracken JT, McGough J, Shah B, et al: Risperidone in children with autism and serious behavioral problems. N Engl J Med 347(5):314–321, 2002 12151468

Meyer J: Drug-drug interactions with antipsychotics. CNS Spectr 12(12 suppl 21):6–9, 2007 18389925

Miral S, Gencer O, Inal-Emiroglu FN, et al: Risperidone versus haloperidol in children and adolescents with AD: a randomized, controlled, double-blind trial. Eur Child Adolesc Psychiatry 17(1):1–8, 2008 18080171

Mozes T, Ebert T, Michal SE, et al: An open-label randomized comparison of olanzapine versus risperidone in the treatment of childhood-onset schizophrenia. J Child Adolesc Psychopharmacol 16(4):393–403, 2006 16958565

Nagaraj R, Singhi P, Malhi P: Risperidone in children with autism: randomized, placebo-controlled, double-blind study. J Child Neurol 21(6):450–455, 2006 16948927

National High Blood Pressure Education Program Working Group on High Blood Pressure in Children and Adolescents: The fourth report on the diagnosis, evaluation, and treatment of high blood pressure in children and adolescents. Pediatrics 114(2 suppl 4th rep):555–576, 2004 15286277

Olfson M, Blanco C, Liu SM, et al: National trends in the office-based treatment of children, adolescents, and adults with antipsychotics. Arch Gen Psychiatry 69(12):1247–1256, 2012 22868273

Owen R, Sikich L, Marcus RN, et al: Aripiprazole in the treatment of irritability in children and adolescents with autistic disorder. Pediatrics 124(6):1533–1540, 2009 19948625

Paprocki J, Versiani M: A double-blind comparison between loxapine and haloperidol by parenteral route in acute schizophrenia. Curr Ther Res Clin Exp 21(1):80–100, 1977 12922

Pathak S, Findling RL, Earley WR, et al: Efficacy and safety of quetiapine in children and adolescents with mania associated with bipolar I disorder: a 3-week, double-blind, placebo-controlled trial. J Clin Psychiatry 74(1):e100–e109, 2013 23419231

Pavuluri MN, Henry DB, Findling RL, et al: Double-blind randomized trial of risperidone versus divalproex in pediatric bipolar disorder. Bipolar Disord 12(6):593–605, 2010

Pool D, Bloom W, Mielke DH, et al: A controlled evaluation of loxitane in seventy-five adolescent schizophrenic patients. Curr Ther Res Clin Exp 19(1):99–104, 1976 812671

Pringsheim T, Panagiotopoulos C, Davidson J, et al: Evidence-based recommendations for monitoring safety of second-generation antipsychotics in children and youth. Paediatr Child Health 16(9):581–589, 2011 PMC3223902

Rajagopal S: Clozapine, agranulocytosis, and benign ethnic neutropenia. Postgrad Med J 81(959):545–546, 2005 16143678

Realmuto GM, Erickson WD, Yellin AM, et al: Clinical comparison of thiothixene and thioridazine in schizophrenic adolescents. Am J Psychiatry 141(3):440–442, 1984 6367494

Research Units on Pediatric Psychopharmacology Autism Network: Risperidone treatment of autistic disorder: longer-term benefits and blinded discontinuation after 6 months. Am J Psychiatry 162(7):1361–1369, 2005 15994720

Reyes M, Buitelaar J, Toren P, et al: A randomized, double-blind, placebo-controlled study of risperidone maintenance treatment in children and adolescents with disruptive behavior disorders. Am J Psychiatry 163(3):402–410, 2006 16513860

Sallee FR, Kurlan R, Goetz CG, et al: Ziprasidone treatment of children and adolescents with Tourette's syndrome: a pilot study. J Am Acad Child Adolesc Psychiatry 39(3):292–299, 2000 10714048

Savitz AJ, Lane R, Nuamah I, et al: Efficacy and safety of paliperidone extended release in adolescents with schizophrenia: a randomized, double-blind study. J Am Acad Child Adolesc Psychiatry 54(2):126–137, 2015

Scahill L, Leckman JF, Schultz RT, et al: A placebo-controlled trial of risperidone in Tourette syndrome. Neurology 60(7):1130–1135, 2003 12682319

Schimmelmann BG, Schmidt SJ, Carbon M, et al: Treatment of adolescents with early onset schizophrenia spectrum disorders: in search of a rational, evidence-informed approach. Curr Opin Psychiatry 26(2):219–230, 2013 23364281

Scotto Rosato N, Correll CU, Pappadopulos E, et al: Treatment of maladaptive aggression in youth: CERT guidelines II. Treatments and ongoing management. Pediatrics 129(6):e1577–e1586, 2012 22641763

Shaw P, Sporn A, Gogtay N, et al: Childhood-onset schizophrenia: A double-blind, randomized clozapine-olanzapine comparison. Arch Gen Psychiatry 63(7):721–730, 2006 16818861

Shea S, Turgay A, Carroll A, et al: Risperidone in the treatment of disruptive behavioral symptoms in children with autistic and other pervasive developmental disorders. Pediatrics 114(5):e634–e641, 2004 15492353

Shim JC, Shin JG, Kelly DL, et al: Adjunctive treatment with a dopamine partial agonist, aripiprazole, for antipsychotic-induced hyperprolactinemia: a placebo-controlled trial. Am J Psychiatry 164(9):1404–1410, 2007 17728426

Sikich L, Hamer RM, Bashford RA, et al: A pilot study of risperidone, olanzapine, and haloperidol in psychotic youth: a double-blind, randomized, 8-week trial. Neuropsychopharmacology 29(1):133–145, 2004 14583740

Sikich L, Frazier JA, McClellan J, et al: Double-blind comparison of first- and second-generation antipsychotics in early onset schizophrenia and schizo-affective disorder: findings from the treatment of early onset schizophrenia spectrum disorders (TEOSS) study. Am J Psychiatry 165(11):1420–1431, 2008 18794207

Simpson GM, Angus JW: A rating scale for extrapyramidal side effects. Acta Psychiatr Scand Suppl 212:11–19, 1970 4917967

Singh J, Robb A, Vijapurkar U, et al: A randomized, double-blind study of paliperidone extended-release in treatment of acute schizophrenia in adolescents. Biol Psychiatry 70(12):1179–1187, 2011 21831359

Snyder R, Turgay A, Aman M, et al: Effects of risperidone on conduct and disruptive behavior disorders in children with subaverage IQs. J Am Acad Child Adolesc Psychiatry 41(9):1026–1036, 2002 12218423

Spencer EK, Kafantaris V, Padron-Gayol MV, et al: Haloperidol in schizophrenic children: early findings from a study in progress. Psychopharmacol Bull 28(2):183–186, 1992 1513922

Sporn A, Gogtay N, Ortiz-Aguayo R, et al: Clozapine-induced neutropenia in children: management with lithium carbonate. J Child Adolesc Psychopharmacol 13(3):401–404, 2003 14642024

Stentebjerg-Olesen M, Jeppesen P, Pagsberg AK, et al: Early nonresponse determined by the clinical global impressions scale predicts poorer outcomes in youth with schizophrenia spectrum disorders naturalistically treated with second-generation antipsychotics. J Child Adolesc Psychopharmacol 23(10):665–675, 2013 24266529

Swadi HS, Craig BJ, Pirwani NZ, et al: A trial of quetiapine compared with risperidone in the treatment of first onset psychosis among 15- to 18-year-old adolescents. Int Clin Psychopharmacol 25(1):1–6, 2010 19809337

Tohen M, Kryzhanovskaya L, Carlson G, et al: Olanzapine versus placebo in the treatment of adolescents with bipolar mania. Am J Psychiatry 164(10):1547–1556, 2007 17898346

Tramontina S, Zeni CP, Ketzer CR, et al: Aripiprazole in children and adolescents with bipolar disorder comorbid with attention-deficit/hyperactivity disorder: a pilot randomized clinical trial. J Clin Psychiatry 70(5):756–764, 2009 19389329

Troost PW, Lahuis BE, Steenhuis MP, et al: Long-term effects of risperidone in children with autism spectrum disorders: a placebo discontinuation study. J Am Acad Child Adolesc Psychiatry 44(11):1137–1144, 2005

Van Bellinghen M, De Troch C: Risperidone in the treatment of behavioral disturbances in children and adolescents with borderline intellectual functioning: a double-blind, placebo-controlled pilot trial. J Child Adolesc Psychopharmacol 11(1):5–13, 2001 11322745

Wehmeier PM, Schüler-Springorum M, Heiser P, et al: Chart review for potential features of myocarditis, pericarditis, and cardiomyopathy in children and adolescents treated with clozapine. J Child Adolesc Psychopharmacol 14(2):267–271, 2004 15319023

Whiskey E, Taylor D: Restarting clozapine after neutropenia: evaluating the possibilities and practicalities. CNS Drugs 21(1):25–35, 2007 17190527

Wolpert A, Hagamen MB, Merlis S: A comparative study of thiothixene and trifluoperazine in childhood schizophrenia. Curr Ther Res Clin Exp 9(9):482–485, 1967

Yoo HK, Joung YS, Lee JS, et al: A multicenter, randomized, double-blind, placebo-controlled study of aripiprazole in children and adolescents with Tourette's disorder. J Clin Psychiatry 74(8):e772–e780, 2013 24021518

PART VI

Psychosocial Treatments

CHAPTER 39

Individual Psychotherapy

Lenore Terr, M.D.

Individual psychotherapy is important for every child and adolescent psychiatrist to know and understand. Its associated techniques are also crucial to supervision, conferences, meetings with educators, community gatherings, and policy-setting agendas. One hundred years' worth of clinical case reports in the professional literature attest to the usefulness of child psychotherapy.

Several factors have delayed the conduct of the kind of research that might enable nonmanualized individual psychotherapy to reach the current criteria for being *evidence based.* It is difficult to follow control subjects for as long as some individual cases actually take in psychotherapy. It is even more difficult to locate the proper comparison groups and to offer the young people in them a good alternative to psychotherapy. *Blinding* is challenging, and *double blinding* is virtually impossible. Furthermore, interventional research on children is often difficult to have funded or institutionally approved. The proper parental and child consents (and/or assents) may be problematic to obtain (Group for the Advancement of Psychiatry Committee on Child Psychiatry 1989). All of this leads to just a few clinical case series and a handful of controlled research projects in a field that has existed for years (Gerber et al. 2011; Midgley and Kennedy 2011).

Despite the dearth of contemporary research on psychotherapy, the well-trained mental health professional dealing with children should understand how to use psychotherapy and how to collaborate with a psychotherapist. In this chapter I present and summarize psychotherapy, both as an idea and as a set of techniques.

Throughout the chapter, words given in bold are defined in Table 39–1.

Today's child and adolescent psychotherapy is eclectic, combining a number of Freudian principles (**psychodynamic psychotherapy**) with other ideas coming from the medical, educational, and non-Freudian psychological fields. Current individual psychotherapy consists of 30–45 minutes spent between clinician and young patient, conversing and using play, art, word games, metaphor,

TABLE 39–1. Glossary of terms

Term or phrase (in order of presentation)	Definition
Psychodynamic psychotherapy	Psychological treatment of a child, based on such Freudian principles as internal conflict, the unconscious, repetition compulsion, and transference
Uncovering psychotherapy	A type of treatment primarily using exploration of defenses, conscience, secret wishes, and transference in order to resolve internal unconscious conflict
Supportive psychotherapy	A type of treatment using the real relationship with the therapist, education, suggestions, and reinforcements to help a patient cope with the external world
Displacement	Defense mechanism in which the object of a conflict is moved over to someone else, an animal, or even a thing or idea
Oedipal	The conscious or unconscious wish to marry the parent of the opposite sex and rid the self of the same-sex parent
Id	The psychological space (and energies) occupied by primitive, raw sexual and aggressive drives, most of which are unconscious
Ego	The psychological space (and energies) occupied by ways of coping, defending against the drives, thinking things through, and dealing with loved ones and the world—both conscious and unconscious
Interpretation	The therapist's bringing together of ideas about the patient's defenses, wishes, conscience, and/or dealings with the world that makes unconscious mechanisms visible and therefore workable
Superego	The particular ways "conscience," ethics, ideals, morals, and role models operate in mentality—both conscious and unconscious
Clarification	The therapist's putting new words to something the patient already knows in a different way
Transference	The patient's particular defensive displacement toward the therapist, based on old attitudes and feelings about important others in the patient's life
Education	Teaching something to the patient
Suggestion	Guiding the patient to a conclusion the patient eventually makes, which can be unconscious on the patient's part or entirely conscious
Modeling	Showing the patient—in the therapist's actions—how to act or be
Reinforcement	Responding to the patient's actions or story positively or negatively and thereby demonstrating how the therapist wants the patient to behave
Real therapist	Either being actual or telling the patient who the actual person treating him or her is
Mentalization	The ability to reflect on and hold in mind the mental states (feelings, thoughts, beliefs) of oneself and others

TABLE 39–1. Glossary of terms *(continued)*

Term or phrase (in order of presentation)	Definition
Diagnosis	The synthesis of history, observation, and tests, leading to the indication of a certain medical condition that is treated in a prescribed way
Formulation	The working psychological explanation for a patient's feelings, behavior, and thinking
Abreaction	The expression of emotion relating to a problem, particularly psychic trauma
Context	The perspective and understanding, particularly of a psychic trauma, in terms of history, geography, science, peer group, criminology, and so forth
Correction	The imaginary or real solution to a traumatic event, even if it is an old one and/or virtually unsolvable
Denial in fantasy	Defense mechanism in which a painful reality is overlooked or forgotten by constructing a situation in one's imagination that negates or obscures the reality
Family therapy	Treating a dysfunctional unit (siblings, parent(s), step- or half-siblings, originally targeted child, other key figures)
Filial therapy	Treating a child through the parent (who takes the doctor's ideas home and tries them out on the young person)
Collaborative therapy	Treating a child while having one or more other clinicians treat the parent(s) or sibling(s)
Countertransference	The clinician's unreasonable, personally based responses to a patient
Repetition compulsion	The need to refeel, retell, redream, or reenact (in conflicted or traumatized people)
Reenactment	Repetitive behavior (often related to past trauma) that replays a thought, a fear, or an original behavior from the event(s)
Ego ideal	Who and what a person wishes to become, or a person's better self

and other forms of interaction. Sometimes a parent is present for the entire session. Frequently, a parent is seen for the first 5–15 minutes (or, less frequently, for the last few minutes). Most of the time, however, a parent is not in the room as the youngster is working with the practitioner.

Not only is contemporary psychotherapy used both for *uncovering* and for *supportive* purposes, but it is also used in more severe cases of pathology (e.g., character problems, psychic trauma) than it was first conceived to treat. For example, when Sigmund Freud, in 1909, indirectly treated his first modern-day child psychotherapy patient through the 5-year-old boy's father (who carefully implemented Freud's suggestions), the child, "Little Hans," was cured of his newly developed and mild problem, phobia of horses. Within a few sessions of working with the boy's major defense pattern (**displacement**) and his hidden fears and wishes (his fright of his father and his desire for an **Oedipal** victory), the phobia cleared. It took just a few good talks between the doctor and the parent and then between the parent and the little boy. The problem was acute and mild. The psychotherapeutic answer was *Freudian,* including an analysis of **id** (the boy's secret sexual and aggressive wishes) and **ego** (his displacement defense). The solution was ultimately simple (Freud 1909/1955). Today, however, when psychotherapy is used with a child or adolescent, it may occur in much harsher settings than Freud's—and in much more confrontational situations (Terr 2008). Still, the technique can work dramatically—as it did with Little Hans. And it may take no more time.

Anna Freud, Sigmund Freud's daughter, observed and commented on children's play, especially at her Hampstead, England, housing facility and school for children evacuated from the London blitz of World War II (Freud and Burlingham 1943). Before the war, Miss Freud expanded on her father's ideas about the defenses, especially those developing in childhood (Freud 1928). She thus helped child psychotherapy switch its emphasis from id to ego (Freud 1936/1946). She consistently preferred watching and listening to a child and carefully making remarks about the child's conflicts afterward. These spoken verbal interventions by the therapist are called **interpretations.**

In the several years following the war, child psychotherapy adopted the concepts of ego, **superego,** and id. It followed adult psychiatry in separating the idea of uncovering (Freudian-minded psychotherapy) from support (ego building, conscience building, community-related help, education). Child psychiatry eventually came to incorporate both forms—uncovering and support—into its general approach to psychotherapy. To uncover with an adult, the therapist needed interpretation and **clarification.** The therapist also needed to maintain a neutral and relatively passive stance. This rather distant approach was intended to encourage **transference,** the displacement of old attitudes, especially about the patient's family of origin, to the therapist. To support a child, on the other hand, the therapist was taught to employ more **education, suggestion, modeling,** and positive or negative **reinforcement** (largely in the therapist's attitude toward the patient). The psychotherapist was also encouraged to be *real* with the patient in order to avoid potentially dangerous transference in seriously disordered children and to help very disturbed young people learn how to act in society.

There is still discussion in the field of child and adolescent psychiatry as to what persona to adopt with which child. Over the years, child psychotherapists have recognized that transference is not as important a phenomenon in the treatment of young children as it is in adults. This happens because children are still primarily involved in their families of origin and therefore do not consistently displace these feelings to their treating physician or counselor. Therapists do not have to be as passive or neutral as Sigmund Freud might have suggested. The corollary to this observation is the important idea that while knowing and understanding himself or herself well, the psychiatrist might remain *real* and inspire a good therapeutic relationship with the child (Harrison et al. 1970; Terr et al. 2005; Weiner and King 1977). No one rule, however, applies to all youngsters. In fact, not all child psychology is universal—various cultures offer different ways of raising children and, thus, of building young personalities. To keep these important cultural differences in mind, the treating psychotherapist must understand the child's racial, ethnic, and religious background and adjust his or her treatment of the young person to that understanding (Erikson 1950). Any child and adolescent psychotherapist, in fact, needs to be cautioned about the use of pure Freudian-derived psychotherapy. The clinician must be careful to include education, clarification, and other "supports" in any psychotherapy with children (Hartmann 1956). In other words, a contemporary child psychotherapist does not choose between uncovering or supportive treatment with young people—he or she combines the two. The clinician does not automatically assume a single type of therapeutic persona with all children. The clinician must be flexible.

Winnicott (1971b) taught that the spirit of play must infuse psychotherapy. Not only must the therapist be playful, but the patient may need to be shown how to play. Play reveals the inner world of the child, and it also releases considerable emotional energy (Levy 1939). Play also enables the therapist to interact entirely inside the pretend or the game (Kline 1932) and to insert new corrective ideas into the more hidden, playful life of the child.

Today's child psychotherapy applies to a broader age range of childhood than may have traditionally been considered. There are contemporary psychotherapeutic techniques geared to adolescents (Mishne 1986), as well as techniques specific to infants and toddlers (Fraiberg 1977). In fact, a recently developed psychoanalytic principle, **mentalization** (Fonagy and Bateman 2008), has been applied in both adolescent (Bleiberg 2013; Rossouw and Fonagy 2012) and infant psychotherapy (Schechter and Willheim 2009). A wider variety of disorders have fallen under the aegis of child psychotherapy, such as the (acute and chronic) posttraumatic conditions (see Terr 1991, 2003), problems of childhood personality (Kernberg et al. 2000; Thomas et al. 1968), physical and psychosomatic illness (Lewis and King 1994), congenital and hereditary differences and/or anomalies (Green and Solnit 1964), and disorders of attention and/or neurological integration (Silver 2003). Cognitive-behavioral techniques are frequently used in the individual psychodynamic psychotherapies (Terr 2008). It would not be uncommon, for example, for a therapist exploring the inner reasons for an obsession to also work out a behavioral program to extinguish the accompanying compulsions in a child.

For an excellent reference on child psychotherapy through most of the twentieth century, see *The Process of Child Therapy* (Group for the Advancement of Psychiatry 1982). Table 39–2 illustrates the major historical changes in the practice of child psychotherapy over the past 100 years. For recent approaches to psychodynamic psychotherapy, see Kernberg et al. (2012) and Ritvo and Henderson (2013).

In summary, contemporary child and adolescent psychotherapy is increasingly eclectic, flexible, and able to treat (in many cases, along with medication treatment) all ages and most conditions of childhood.

Which Child Needs Individual Psychotherapy?

In conducting a diagnostic evaluation of a child—and in initially interviewing parents and sometimes siblings—two important opinions are reached by the psychiatrist. One is the **diagnosis.** The second is the **formulation.** Each opinion is equally meaningful in deciding what to do with a mentally disordered or

TABLE 39–2. One hundred years of child psychotherapy

Early twentieth-century child psychotherapy	Early twenty-first-century child psychotherapy
Prekindergarten through late latency ages	All ages from birth into young adulthood
Children of the same culture as therapist	Children of all cultures
Talk emphasized	Talk plus all modes of play and art
Uncovering	Uncovering and supportive
Geared toward neurosis and problems of development	Potentially useful in any disorder or problem of development, as well as in prevention
Dealing with imagination	Dealing with imagination and reality
Therapist is entirely objective and distant	Therapist assumes various ways of relating to the child and/or is real
Parents are primary and must be engaged in therapy themselves	Parents are important but are given advice, counseling, modeling—not necessarily therapy
Rules for administering therapy strict, largely Freudian	Rules for administering therapy loose and eclectic
Interpretation of internal id-ego conflicts and of transference	Interpretation of child's relationship to the real world, as well as id, ego, and/or transference
Insight is a goal	Insight is not necessarily a goal
Ethics: "first do no harm"	Ethics: "first do no harm"

developmentally disturbed young person (Jellinek and McDermott 2004; Shapiro 1989; Terr et al. 2006c). Because the formulation consists of a working psychological explanation of the patient's feelings, behaviors, and thinking, it expresses the "art" of the medical and mental health evaluation, as opposed to the "science," or the diagnosis. Both are essential to setting up a treatment program for a child. (See Chapter 1, "The Process of Assessment and Diagnosis," for more detailed discussion of diagnosis and formulation.)

For any proposed treatment, the child will need an understandable explanation, careful education about the condition, a coordinated treatment program to be carried out by the family, and meaningful follow-up over a long enough time to see if the program works. In other words, at least minimal individual supportive psychotherapy is necessary whenever the clinician treats a child. The child must know who the therapist is and how he or she will be working with the therapist.

Some cases clearly signal the need for individual nonmanualized psychotherapy. The use of maladaptive defenses defines a likely case for individual psychotherapy. Also, if a stress or series of stressors or, even worse, a traumatic event is affecting a child, this often requires psychotherapy. Trauma psychotherapy usually involves **abreaction:** helping the child define and express all the emotions inherent in what is taking or has taken place. It also involves understanding the event(s) in **context** and finding **corrections**—even fantasized or historical ones—for such situations (Terr 2003, 2009). For a summary of the types of cases for which psychotherapy is often warranted, see Table 39–3.

An example in which psychotherapy is the preferred method of treatment is a child who behaves well and is accomplished at school but appears angry much of the time at home. For several years, his mother and sisters have been the continuous objects of his rage. Neither oppositional defiant disorder nor conduct disorder encompass his strengths as well as his symptoms. Now the preadolescent boy is serving as president of his all-boys' sixth grade class. In school, he is easy to get along with and popular. His father is "too busy" to participate in the psychiatric evaluation. When asked about his activities with his dad, the boy lies: "He jogged with me lots of times last summer," he says. "In the winter, we played hockey." The boy's mother reports that there were no such games, play, or practice. In fact, the boy's father prefers the company of men his own age and hardly participates in family life. A divorce is being contemplated. At whom is the boy really angry—his mother who loves and protects him or his father who usually doesn't give him "the time of day?" The boy is defending himself with **denial in fantasy** and displacement. He is developing attitudes about women that will not serve him well in the future. His phenomenological diagnosis does not suggest a type of treatment. His formulation, however, leads directly to the consideration of individual psychotherapy. What moves the choice away from treatment with mood stabilizing drugs and a course of family therapy or anger management training? It is the psychological meaning of the preadolescent's behaviors. This meaning will direct the subsequent individual psychotherapy.

Another situation often calling for psychotherapy (again, considering the formulation but bearing in mind, too, the diagnosis) is slowdown, misdirection, or even an omission in social or emotional development (Gilmore and

TABLE 39–3. Cases for which individual psychotherapy may be warranted

Situations in the child	Situations affecting the family
Use of maladaptive defenses	Response to the child
Stressors	Stressors
Traumatic event	Response to child Traumatic event to the family Familial perpetration of trauma and/or neglect
Emotional or social development Slowdown Misdirection Omission Conflicts around a developmental issue	Response to the child Parental naiveté or mistakes in rearing Mentalization problems in a parent
Child psychiatric disorders Mood Attention Anxiety	Response to the child Medication management Health management
Pediatric disorders Congenital defects and disorders Pre- or postsurgery Dying child Chronic illness (e.g., diabetes, neurological disorder, asthma)	Parental guilt and/or grief Response to the child Health management
The child wants a therapist and/or therapy	Parents think therapy will help Parents will not allow medications for their child
Early personality problems	Response to the child Parent has personality disorder Parent has "superego lacunae" (Johnson 1949) Parental naiveté or mistakes Family perpetration of trauma and/or neglect

Meersand 2014). Babies who cannot feed properly, toddlers who cannot be toilet trained, smart youngsters who do not talk—all of this calls for close collaboration among parents, child, and clinician. In many such situations, the child will require some psychotherapy sessions by himself—or with a parent there to observe and/or participate (Fraiberg 1977; Gaensbauer as cited by Terr et al. 2006b; Lieberman and Van Horn 2008).

If a child's problems are related to a conflict around a developmental issue, such as attachment, autonomy, gender, self-esteem, getting older, sexuality, or identity, this kind of conflict usually requires treatment with psychotherapy. In addition, if a young person appears to be experimenting with a new line of behavior and in this way has come to a "fork in the road" (Schulman et al. 1977), he or she may require a brief course of individual therapy. Furthermore, if a child shows personality quirks that have impaired peer or family relationships or diminished the youngster's ability to concentrate and work or to experience joy, that child may need psychotherapy. In other words, even when a child does not meet the criteria for a full disease or disorder, the clinician may consider psychotherapy as an option. Similar to the pediatrician's efforts, a good deal of the child mental health professional's work centers on prevention.

Many common childhood psychiatric disorders (e.g., mood, attention, and anxiety disorders) often require first-line treatments with medication and/or cognitive-behavioral therapy. A number of children with these conditions, however, also need considerable attention, education, help with "Why me?" questions, observation for suicidality, and a deeper understanding of the interior conflicts and family difficulties that are associated with these conditions. Individual psychotherapy is often prescribed as an important addition to drugs and/or brief manualized treatments in these kinds of cases. Along the same line, children with conditions along the autism spectrum need a great deal of educational and parental support. If the child is able to form a meaningful relationship with a psychotherapeutic clinician, long-term individualized treatment may greatly improve his or her prognosis.

The psychiatrist gathers clues from the child during the evaluation process that may lead to a decision in favor of psychotherapy. The child "gets" something the evaluator says, for instance, and responds with appropriate words and/or emotion. Or the child drops a huge "clue" for the psychiatrist that no one else has picked up before. Or the psychiatrist tries a simple interpretation and the child "sees" what is meant and offers feedback or an evident emotional response. Or the youngster actually asks the clinician to treat her. Or the clinician notices that a bond with the child is forming. In these situations, the relationship serves as a cue to strongly consider individual therapy.

Parents, guardians, or institutions are often reluctant to medicate youngsters. Many adults fear unknown long-term effects and possible complications from giving drugs to children. In such situations, individual psychotherapy may be the child's only option. If it is appropriate for the child in terms of both the diagnosis and formulation, psychotherapy may be tried and may indeed be successful.

How Does a Child's Treatment Begin?

Once the decision to treat a child with psychotherapy is made, a time schedule is selected. Often this corresponds to the parents' or caregivers' ability to transport the child to the office, the youngster's schedule at home and school, and life circumstances. The clinician must consider these realities carefully, alongside what might be therapeutically optimal. Typically, once-weekly psychotherapy is about right for a school-age child. On the other hand, if the child or adolescent is entering treatment during a crisis period (serious illness of a parent, early in the wake of a trauma, suicidal thoughts), the clinician might consider two (or sometimes three) times a week to start and then cut back to once weekly within a month or two. Also, when emergencies arise during the course of psychotherapy, stepping up the frequency of sessions is often helpful.

Child patients should be given a developmentally tailored explanation so that they know what to expect. For example: "I'm a worry doctor." "I talk to children and play with them." "I help kids get along better at school." "I want to help you figure out how to make friends." "I've heard you're sad a lot, and I'd like to help you feel less depressed." For most children, it is important to let them know that this kind of doctor will not be undressing them, examining them, or giving them shots. The psychotherapist gears what is said at the beginning of therapy to what the child has expressed during the evaluation, as well as the child's stage of development. "I'm a talking doctor" is about all the clinician might say to a toddler. But with an adolescent, the clinician would have to offer a fuller explanation. When a psychiatrist will be prescribing medicine as well as psychotherapy, this must be discussed.

If the psychotherapist is also working with the child's parents, a sentence or two about confidentiality should be shared with the young patient. How much will the therapist say? Will the therapist listen to parents? Teachers? Who else? Why? If the therapist may also have to testify in court on a child patient's behalf, the therapist must fully explain that his or her notes will go to "a judge who decides things" or that the therapist may have to go to court and testify as well.

In beginning therapy with a child, the psychiatrist must make sure that the youngster has enough opportunity to ask questions and make statements about the treatment. Most young people do not have much to say at these early stages, however, and it is often a good idea to launch into play and/or talk about the child's life soon after the beginning of the first hour. A child patient must find out quickly in the early course of treatment that psychotherapy is often fun and funny, even though there will be painful moments as well.

Where Do Parents Fit Into Child and Adolescent Psychotherapy?

Parents need to understand—in an ongoing fashion—what the individual psychotherapy with their child is attempting to accomplish and where that accomplishment presently stands. They must know, therefore, the general outlines of the treatment as it is being carried out. The child patient should give a form of oral assent for the parents being told by the therapist why the child is being treated and what is currently happening in therapy. With an adolescent, it is often wise to tell the young patient what will be said to parents. Adolescents also benefit from an idea of what their parents think about their general progress. This therapist-patient understanding about conveying general information back and forth should be established at the onset of psychotherapy and repeated as treatment proceeds. Child patients need to believe that the therapist will not give away the details of their secret lives and thoughts. Otherwise, it will be difficult to either establish or maintain a trusting relationship.

It is best for both parents to be engaged in facilitating their youngster's psychotherapy. Even if one parent is busier than the other—or has moved out of the area or has established a new, separate family—it is still important to enlist that parent's support and, from time to time, see that parent in the office. What does the more-or-less absent parent think of the child's progress? What has that parent observed over summers, on vacations, or when the child is with the new family? On the other hand, if there has been a total break between an absent parent and a child, there is no set rule about trying to reestablish the child-parent relationship. Often, trauma and/or neglect demand a continuation of such separations. Each case is considered individually. Any past legal decisions to permanently terminate parental rights must be honored by the clinician until, at least, a time when the child has achieved legal adulthood and can decide how to proceed.

There are several ways to engage parents in the child's psychotherapy. In addition to occasionally giving a "temperature reading" on their youngster's progress, the clinician can ask parents about aspects of their child's life that the youngster currently does not understand, perceive, or choose to tell. The clinician can actually have parents in the same room with the young patient, reflecting on the realities of what their child is saying. This may be helpful for children with severe personality or social problems. Ordinarily, however, this approach will not work for more than a few sessions with school-age children and adolescents. If, on the other hand, the clinician routinely schedules the first several minutes of each of the child's sessions for one or more parents alone, then the child is less likely to perceive this information sharing as tattling, refuting, or blaming.

Sometimes parents have a poor understanding or almost total naiveté regarding how to be a parent. How does one play with a child? How does one talk? What does one say? In such instances, the clinician may include the parents in all of the child's sessions, from beginning to end, as a form of **family therapy.** Or the clinician may proceed as if the child were alone in individual therapy while the parent(s) watch, both for modeling from the therapist and for new ideas about the child's thinking and experience directly from the young patient. This kind of session often needs active psychiatric "translation" of the child's behaviors for the parents, as well as a steady flow of comments and/or play between the psychiatrist and the child.

The Little Hans method of child treatment—working only with a parent and then having the parent make the suggested therapeutic interventions and commentaries—has been elaborated by Erna Furman into what is known as **filial therapy.** This treatment can be especially useful in preschoolers or with crisis management situations, such as coping with a seriously ill adolescent or a health emergency in a latency-age child (Furman 1957).

Finally, **collaborative therapy** on behalf of children—based on the American child guidance system model, in which the child is assigned to one professional while the parents are assigned to another (Group for the Advancement of Psychiatry 1982)—has become less and less common with changes in the economics and practicalities of delivering services. Collaborative therapy can work, but it is expensive, and it also carries the potential to stir up conflict or competition among professionals, especially if there is a discrepancy in their status or their treatment philosophies (Group for the Advancement of Psychiatry 1982). For collaborative treatment to succeed it is essential for all involved to communicate frequently. If the collaborators steadily keep the child in mind, complicated collaborative treatments may proceed smoothly. There must be a spoken or tacit understanding, however, about who will be the leader.

Even the best individual psychotherapy with a child may fail if the parents or other treating professionals are not on board. Because the rest of this chapter will deal with what happens inside the clinician's office with the child patient alone, the author refers the reader to other chapters in Part V, "Somatic Treatments," that cover other psychosocial interventions.

The Therapist's Persona

Forming a therapeutic alliance with a child is essential to performing effective individual psychotherapy. This alliance, however, is not necessarily easy to attain with the young and immature. At times, the relationship depends on what kind of person—in the child's eyes—the therapist appears to be. All clinicians have options as to what traits in themselves they choose to emphasize with a specific child or adolescent patient in psychotherapy. Certainly, the clinician must be professional. This would include being calm, unhurried, willing to listen, nonjudgmental, relatively objective, focused on the patient, and committed to the basic principle behind the Hippocratic oath, "First do no harm." Beyond this professionalism, the child and adolescent mental health clinician must also consider how to "be" when with a specific child (Bugental 1964).

Sometimes a very calm, noncommenting, unemotional approach is exactly what is needed. A child going through a heated divorce, for instance, may respond well to this typically "psychoanalytic" persona in the clinician. It serves as a good foil to the overemotionality at home. A child with a life-threatening disease may also respond at his or her best to this impassive stance. Others around the child are showing their agony—perhaps crying, shrieking in frustration, being irritable. The unflappable clinician in situations such as these can become a stabilizing force in a childhood world falling apart.

Another choice for the psychotherapist, however, is to emphasize the positive in his or her personality (Allen 1962). Never failing to notice something good about a child or the world outside the child can become an important foil to years of neglect or negative criticism. This positive approach may work well for violent children, for children with histories of poor attachments, and for adolescents residing in institutions geared to delinquency. The psychiatric director of a California childhood residential care institution for latency-age children, for instance, set up a plan whereby his entire program could present a consistently positive persona to its young patients (Rosenfeld and Wasserman 1990). Many children achieved success through experiencing this institutional approach.

Another approach is to become a "player"—with commentary, of course—in the child's life. Play is usually similar—not opposite—to a child's previous life experience. Play and humor considerably lighten the load of the youngster's psychotherapy and make it more palatable (Terr 2003). Play also aids the therapeutic alliance (Terr et al. 2006b). The player is close to the actual persona of many child and adolescent clinicians. It works well in helping young patients express their deeper feelings and secret imaginings.

Although for adult patients, the classic psychodynamic psychotherapeutic persona is that of passive listener and occasional commentator, the child and adolescent psychotherapeutic persona is often more active, serving as "tutor" or "coach." Most cognitive-behavioral therapists are seen by children as a kind of teacher as they educate and support and send their young patients off to do homework assignments until the next scheduled session. In most cases, this does not destroy the therapist-patient relationship. Instead, it furthers the idea that the therapist is there to help the child. When a combination of individual work and behavioral modification is being attempted in nonmanualized individual therapy, the therapist frequently takes this same kind of tutorial approach. Habit disturbances, obsessive-compulsive symptoms, phobias, and some personality trait problems require that the psychotherapist employ a two-pronged technique: 1) uncovering (How did this particular problem arise? What basically is bothering the patient?) while simultaneously 2) coaching (How can the patient begin to extinguish his or her maladaptive habits, starting with the easiest?). Here, the therapist performs as both investigator and educator.

For example, a latency-age boy with encopresis, whose peer-given nickname was "Stink Bomb," was taken for short periods by his male psychiatrist into side-by-side stalls in a large public men's room at the hospital clinic where the psychiatrist worked. They spoke out loud so anyone could hear. While training the youngster to push hard to defecate, the psychiatrist simultaneously uncovered the boy's rage at his divorced father who lived in a distant city and the boy's paralyzing fear that to defecate meant to personally "explode." It took just a few months of this combination of uncovering and teaching to eradicate the symptom while strengthening the boy's adaptive abilities (see reference by McDermott cited by Terr et al. 2005). Interestingly, at the end of his treatment, the patient voiced regret that his doctor would not be available to coach him at T-ball.

Taking a detective-like stance with a young patient is an interesting behavioral option for the child and adolescent psychotherapist. Not nosy or overly intrusive in these instances, the therapist allows the young patient to join in the work of investigation: "How can we find out what happened?" "Do you have any old friends from that neighborhood who knew you before?" The "mystery game" is a fascinating one for children making a difficult life transition, recovering from trauma, getting over a terrible illness, or trying to understand placement in foster care. Comprehending trauma puts the child's life stress into context. Understanding gives the trauma boundaries and, in fact, a possible solution. For instance, one child who could not sleep after watching the film *A Nightmare on Elm Street* worked as a "detective" on the problem along with his therapist (see reference by Dodson cited by Terr 2008). Therapist and patient first tried a number of behavioral techniques for the boy's intractable insomnia. None worked. But the therapist—willing to investigate further—decided, with the boy's permission, to write to the film's conceiver and director, Wes Craven. Mr. Craven answered the letter. The boy, who had recently moved to a new home, new school, and new state, suddenly gained a new perspective on his problem. What had made Mr. Craven dream up the monster Freddy Krueger for the movies, in fact, had been entirely different and separate from what had been bothering the young patient. No longer did the boy have to fear Freddy Krueger. Freddy belonged to somebody else's imagination. This individual course of therapy was very brief, taking only a month or two. It is clear from these instances that individual, nonmanualized therapy does not have to be long term, intensively insightful, or enormously expensive.

Although there are other possible personas for practicing clinicians, the "real doctor" is often the most useful, the most positive, and also the most potent role for a psychotherapist to take. For example, an adolescent spots the therapist's sports car out on the road. The therapist was speeding, the patient says. Was he? The truth is the best answer, whatever it is. "Are you pregnant?" a child asks her therapist. This calls for truth. "I saw you coming out of a synagogue last Saturday. Are you Jewish?" An honest response is best. These realities about the therapist play into the treatment alliance and must be discussed with unvarnished truth and dignity. Their meaning to the child must be taken up as well.

Children may see their therapists on television. They can view their therapists' Web sites and follow discussions about them or even pictures of them on the Internet. Sometimes a child's peer at school is also visiting the same therapist, and an appointment is inadvertently scheduled back to back. Sometimes, the cultural chasm is so vast between therapist and young patient that the therapist must admit to ignorance or ask questions that point to his or her naiveté. If the therapist's country of origin (even from generations ago) is at war with that of the patient (across the ocean and also removed by time), it may still require an open talk and an indication that the psychiatrist is willing to accept further discussion.

Of course, **countertransference** (the therapist's feelings, often based on old unresolved conflicts that the patient's attitudes may bring to the surface) occasionally must be dealt with in order to save the therapeutic alliance with the child (Marshall 1979; Tsiantis et al. 1996). This, too, requires dealing with reality—often in small bits, but sometimes in one fell swoop (see reference by Blos and Metcalf cited by Terr 2008). A thorough acquaintance with the concepts of transference and countertransference is important in doing psychotherapy with children (see Winnicott 1958). It is also important to be able to talk with a supervisor or with colleagues about these types of very personal responses to children.

Truthfulness and openness are important because the therapist-patient relationship in child psychotherapy is one of the main avenues to a child's improvement. Children change when they sense that their therapist cares enough about them to be real. They change when they believe that people can be honest with one another, no matter how painful that straight talk might be. They come to trust an adult who levels with them. They come to see that their intimate dialogues with others might safely be open and nonsecretive as well.

A good example of a statement from psychotherapy of a therapist's reality comes from a psychiatrist who was allergic to eggs (see reference by Deeney cited by Terr et al. 2005). The psychiatrist noticed himself becoming sick in his office as a rebellious and sad adolescent patient with a Mohawk haircut repeatedly ran his fingers through his upright hair. Then, the boy spontaneously complained that the egg whites he had used to stiffen his "do" were not effectively doing their job. Realizing that the boy's egg whites were leading him toward anaphylaxis, the psychiatrist told his patient that he needed to excuse himself to take some medicine. When he returned, the psychiatrist explained what had happened, and the boy—for the first time in his treatment—expressed sincere empathy and offered to end the session early. From then on, the therapist-patient relationship turned around. The boy's psychotherapy became productive. As a matter of fact, the boy, now a young man, chose his life's work among the "helping" professions. The therapist's realistic and truthful explanation was given without hesitation or defensiveness. Briefly painful as it was for both therapist and patient, the "real" moment between them became an anchor for the boy's treatment and eventual cure.

Atmosphere of the Therapy Sessions

Individual child and adolescent psychotherapy requires a room in which to be alone with the young patient that is as appealing as possible. In certain instances, psychotherapy may also be conducted on walks with a young person (see reference by Stewart or Zrull cited by Terr 2008), or it might occur in a child's hospital room (see reference by Fine or Livingston cited by Terr 2008). In general, however, it usually takes place in an office furnished with enough shelves and drawers to house attractive and easy-to-use art supplies as well as a collection of toys. With these objects, a child patient will be able to express a multiplicity of feelings, problems, impulses, conflicts, and fantasies. This happens because children's play and art represent miniaturizations of life-size situations.

A youngster's conflicts and concerns are often expressed in terms of animals (hence, animal puppets and small dinosaurs are important office equipment); vehicles (a set of cars, fire and rescue equipment, pickup and tow trucks, police cars—and perhaps even a bus to the local prison—are helpful); a baby doll; older girl dolls and, if possible, a boy doll; a deck of cards; checkers; a doll house with miniature furniture and a small doll family; an army including men (and women) and their equipment; and some popular culture items (e.g., a *Frozen* toy or two, *Star Wars* figures, princesses, and Batman or Spider-Man). Other kinds of objects, including some larger dolls and some movable ones—such as circus figures—and some simple games for two—such as cards or checkers—are also useful.

A toy (or choice of toys) may be purchased to suit a specific child's problem. All items should be kept clean, in good repair, and easily reachable by the child patient. Keeping glue on hand is helpful. If a child breaks something, the clinician should consider fixing it in front of the patient—this shows that situations (and people) can be made "right"—or at least put into working order. If a toy is irreparable, the therapist should try to buy another similar one in time for the child to see its replacement. If this is impossible, however, the therapist would be well advised to discuss with the young patient the reality of what happened.

It is helpful for a well-equipped therapy office to be furnished with easily opening and closing toy cupboards and shelves so that adult patients, children's parents, and older adolescents can speak to the therapist without focusing on an office full of playthings. This does not mean that adults do not enjoy playing, too, or fiddling as they speak with something smoothly movable—such as small magnetic acrobats, tile puzzles, or tiny-ball-bearings-in-the-hole games. These things can be kept on open tables or a desktop. A nesting set of tables is a good furnishing for the psychotherapy office because children can pull these tables out and use them to arrange their play or artwork. Clay and finger paints, which have the capacity to ruin walls and carpeting, are best avoided. Attractive, washable baby rattles, blocks, and animals, on the other hand, are very useful, either for babies who accompany their parents to the office or in observing and assessing the infants themselves.

In thinking about establishing a playful atmosphere, the therapist must also consider the needs and tastes of adolescents. For example: A therapist who had previously spent an unproductive, silent hour with a rebellious teenage girl, the daughter of an army sergeant deployed in Iraq, decided to suggest a game of pickup sticks at the beginning of the girl's second appointment. By the time the girl had won the game (which was new to her and therefore of considerable interest), she exposed her entire problem in a running monologue that accompanied her play (see reference by Massie cited by Terr et al. 2006b). Suggesting play had broken the girl's initial negative transference. Without a handy game for teenagers in the office, this breakthrough might not have happened.

Children sometimes fantasize with toys in unique fashions far from the original intent of the toy (Waelder 1933). This often conveys meaning to the therapist. For instance, one angry boy used erasers to kick up chalk dust rather than to clean the clinician's chalkboard. The therapist turned to the boy, showing him how to bring the erasers together gently. They immediately created a mutually enjoyable, albeit dusty, game for two. In so doing, the psychotherapist was able to help the boy modify his violent behaviors in a larger world outside the office (see reference by Teal cited by Terr 2008). The clinician can glean from this example that in individual psychotherapy, toys may be used to condense a child's problems into a nutshell, making them small enough to deal with.

Play does not happen only with toys and art. It happens with words. Words can be used playfully—as in word games like Pig Latin or William Steig's (1968) CDB language; codes or metaphors, especially ones that last for a while in treatment; rhymes; and little scenarios, set up and acted out by the child or adolescent patient. All of these plays on words charge the atmosphere with the spirit of fun and of mutual discovery. For instance, a convicted juvenile rapist was treated during his 6-month sentence of psychotherapy by initially agreeing to call his crime—and his other serious problems with peers and authorities—"massive misunderstandings" (Terr et al. 2006b). Many years later, he contacted the psychiatrist for advice about helping his children through an impending divorce. "Don't worry," he said as if he had been in the office the day before, "[My divorce] was *not* a 'massive misunderstanding'!"

Not only should the psychotherapeutic office atmosphere reflect playfulness through the toys it contains and the words spoken there, but it also should reflect a willingness to wait, if needed. The clinician may have to patiently "hold the fort" until a particular child responds—or to explain the next step in treatment and then accept a break in therapy while the patient thinks. Many a child psychotherapist has to patiently sit through a child's screaming tantrum, a refusal to talk, or even an avoidance of looking at the therapist. Sometimes monotonous games go on until the therapist fully appreciates the meaning of a young patient's behavior. Calmness and patience on the part of the psychotherapist are important characteristics to be developed in child and adolescent psychiatrists and other child mental health clinicians (see reference by Sack cited by Terr 2008). They also become part of the therapist's atmosphere. Sooner or later, skilled therapists—and their patients—find their way out of such impasses (see reference by Jetmalani cited by Terr 2008). The therapist thinks of something new, remembers something old, attends a conference, has a good talk with a colleague, or reads a book or a chapter. With effort and creativity, many of the "waiting games" played out in psychotherapy eventually benefit the patient.

The Clinician's Reading of the Child

Clinicians develop formulations about a youngster's problems during the evaluation phase. Later, clinicians may make shifts in the way they view the child's psychology (Group for the Advancement of Psychiatry 1982). Flexibility is required as any treatment moves along. As psychotherapy progresses, the therapist follows the child's leads, takes the child's "tests," and enters the young person's fields of interest, seeking answers for the patient's dilemma. All of these methods of joining children on their personal journeys can work. Therapeutic collaboration works best when the clinician is finally able to "read" the child.

Children are likely to repeat a symptom in one form or another as long as that conflict or problem continues to exist. This **repetition compulsion,** one of Freud's most important observations of human behavior (Freud 1920/1955), gives the psychotherapist an opportunity to really "see" the child, even if other clues have previously been ignored or misunderstood. In other words, if the clinician misses what the child was conveying one time, he or she will have a second chance to catch on later. One of the beauties of doing play therapy in this context is that a child may repeat a certain theme endlessly in office play (Webb 2007). Not only does a child's play disclose these themes, but they are evident in drawings, poetry, songs, and other creative endeavors. They show up in dreams. And they show up in behaviors—both in the small, repeated habits children develop and in their large-scale **reenactments.**

When a clinician "gets" something about a child, he or she has a number of choices. For instance, he or she may choose to continue to play it out with the child without leaving the arena of play. The therapeutic understanding may be interpreted directly to one of the characters in the child's play scenario, for instance. Or, as if the child were a screenwriter, the solution may be offered as an addition to the plot. Here, the treating clinician stays completely inside the play, the child's drawing, or the rhyming couplets. All help is offered to the fictional characters inside the child's creation.

On the other hand, the therapist also has the option of moving outside the play and interpreting the child to himself. "You feel this way or that, but you can't express it because you're afraid of this or that," she might say, for instance. An interpretation is most often given, as in the previous example. But a confrontation may be offered instead. "You actually *like* having a ghost in your life" (see Beitchman cited by Terr et al. 2006a) or "You'd rather have a *boy* therapist" (see reference by Winters cited by Terr et al. 2006b).

Some children prefer being talked to inside of their play. Others prefer being directly approached as themselves. It may boil down to experiments of trial and error. But because of the repetition compulsion, the practitioner will get more than one chance to discover what works for a specific child. Sometimes, in fact, both techniques work for the same individual.

"Getting" the child may come in a flash. Or it may come from careful listening and study. One clinician suddenly understood what his selectively mute boy patient was trying to express to him when he accompanied his own children to the Disney film *The Little Mermaid* (see reference by Jetmalani cited by Terr et al. 2006c). Another clinician watched her small Iranian patient, who was also selectively mute, search and search for the "right" doll to play with (see reference by Rogers cited by Terr et al. 2005). Realizing that the little boy could not find the right doll, this psychiatrist fashioned a small, nondescript doll from a rag—on which the child quickly placed a head scarf. He named the doll "Grandma," eventually revealing his story of a wrenching removal from Iran, along with a total cutoff from his beloved grandmother. Once the boy was allowed to telephone his grandmother, he began speaking with everyone else. None of this would have happened without a therapist who could bridge the cultural gap. The practitioner did so with a piece of clean white cloth and some profound understanding.

Occasionally, a child patient leads the psychotherapist into a test that he or she must take (Terr 2008). Testing, like play, requires a sincere attempt on the psychiatrist's part to "get" the youngster. Like play, it also requires a technical decision—to stay inside or move outside the test. Adolescents are the most likely group to deliver such tests. Why? Because they can. And because psychotherapy so often feels to them like a deprivation. It takes away from "their" time. It chips away at their developing selves—their defenses, deviant actions, and fears. In other words, therapists practicing psychotherapy are doing slow surgery, cutting out dysfunctional parts while their young patients are fully awake, without anesthetic. No wonder tests are administered by the patient in the hope that the therapist will fail.

Although most of these child-given tests come early in the course of evaluation or therapy, they may occur later as well. This is one of the main places where a clinician sees—and can interpret—transference. It also becomes an opportunity for the therapist to massively improve the relationship by playing along. As in the case of psychotherapeutic play, the clinician can sit apart, watch, and then comment on the test. Or the clinician can enter in and then correct the situation from inside the test itself. The important thing about a child-initiated test is to "get" the fact that an examination is taking place. Children may use a "bad" response as a quick way to achieve an exit from psychotherapy. They may decide to tell their parents, guardian, or school that their therapist is stupid. If the authorities in the child's life insist that the youngster wait it out, however, there is a high probability that the psychiatrist will be tested again. Because of the repetition compulsion, the therapist will receive a second chance.

Two case examples will be presented here: the first, a severely neglected teenager (see reference by Powers cited by

Terr et al. 2006c), and the second, an ignored little boy (see reference by Stewart cited by Terr 2008).

Case Example 1

An adolescent girl, Taylor—who had lived in succession with a drug-abusing mother; an unseeing, neglectful older sister; a middle sister who existed in chaos; and, finally, a more stable paternal cousin—was undergoing psychotherapy with a male psychotherapist whom her grandmother had chosen. They had worked together briefly (on Taylor's "conduct disorder") while she lived with her middle sister, but the chaos that drove her from her sister's home also disguised her silent dropout from psychotherapy. When she was forced to return 2 years later, and after about 3 months of grudging compliance, Taylor suggested that she come to the therapist's office only twice a month (he had prescribed once a week). The psychotherapist considered this an unpassable "test." If he went along with Taylor's request, he would be seen by her as neglectful, like her mother and sisters (Silberschatz 2005). If he said no, on the other hand, Taylor would consider him one of the unthinking authorities who regularly stimulated rebellious feelings in her. The therapist refused to take the test. Musing aloud about both no-win options, he would not choose one side or the other. Taylor argued, persuaded, cajoled, and finally left the office—for 2 weeks off. But when Taylor came back, she announced that she had settled on a course of weekly psychotherapy. Her attitude turned positive for the first time. She plunged into treatment. The test had been enunciated, interpreted, and passed by the therapist. As a result, Taylor developed a meaningful relationship with him.

The second case illustrates a test given and taken without interpretation. It comes from a much younger child, a boy of 5.

Case Example 2

A kindergartener, Danny, had a slightly older brother on whom his parents doted. The patient himself was virtually ignored. At school Danny hid under desks and curled into a fetal position. He feared bodily injury, saying that all his fluids might flow out of him. Two years of steady once-a-week psychotherapy led to some positive changes, but Danny still felt afraid of carnivorous animals and his school classmates. Then one day, he claimed he needed to interrupt his psychotherapeutic session to go to the bathroom. When the psychiatrist went looking for him, he found the boy gripping his erect penis and smiling expectantly. The psychiatrist instructed Danny to return to the office at once. Over the next few months, this happened four or five more times. The psychiatrist knew he was being tested, but the only response he could think of was to ask his patient to come back to the office. Then one day—during the same routine—the psychiatrist found Danny standing atop a clinic bathroom sink, pants down, erect penis in hand, and a huge smile on his face. A new thought suddenly came to the psychiatrist. "That's a great one," the psychiatrist said. Danny beamed at his therapist, put his pants back on, climbed down from the sink, and never interrupted a session again. He improved afterward, so quickly in fact that his treatment was terminated in a few months' time. This is a situation in which the therapist—after thinking about this case for months—found a good solution in an instant. It was a "Eureka!" moment. The little boy's test was passed. Nor was any interpretation necessary. The child's masculinity had been confirmed for the very first time by, of all people, his psychiatrist.

Another way to show children that their therapists "get" them is to follow their interests. If a child in psychotherapy loves Harry Potter, for example, it helps if the therapist reads some of the books, too. If an adolescent girl is talking about vampire romances or avatars, it certainly helps her to learn that her therapist has some ideas about such things as well. Superheroes may be used to enhance children's treatments (Brody 2012; Rubin 2007). For instance, considering what a character like Spider-Man or Batman might do in the child's personal situation gives the child a new way of seeing himself. Not only can popular culture and movie heroes be used in individual therapy, but, depending on the particular child, nonfictional athletes, cancer survivors, and historical figures may also be used. For example, one late-latency boy, whom the writer of this chapter treated for apathy, learning delays, and depression, became briefly interested in Julius Caesar (Terr 2008). How would Caesar have handled the politics of this young man's seventh-grade classroom? How would Caesar have planned to become friends with the boys he admired—or the girls? This patient gained 2 years' worth of academic reading skills during the 2 months he talked (and read) about Caesar. His grades went up dramatically. Despite years of receiving a number of diagnoses at a well-known clinic, taking several potent medications, and receiving tutoring in special classes, the idea of being like a great historical figure whom he admired was what finally turned this particular adolescent around.

Individual child psychotherapy gears itself to the psychological needs of a specific youngster. Instead of aiming at a particular disorder, individualized therapy gives special attention to one particular child's ways of coping, internalized meanings, defensive choices, understandings of the world, and loves.

The Psychotherapeutic Response

In days past, psychotherapists felt the need to interpret a child's conflicts in terms of the youngster's secret wishes, defenses, past experiences, here-and-now behaviors, and/or transference. It was felt that the interpretation would be the most effective whenever most of these elements could be brought together in a single comment or group of comments. The defenses were stressed as being more acceptable to children than the "naughty" desires. Therefore, if a psychotherapist could make an interpretation as an ego explanation (about coping and defense) rather than a comment about badness or mischief (the id), the child would handle it better (see Group for the Advancement of Psychiatry 1982).

Currently, however, therapeutic statements to children cover a far wider gamut of issues than those noted in the previous paragraph. Past realities in the child's life—the death of a peer's parent, an illness, a broken arm—loom larger in the twenty-first century than they used to. Present realities—trouble at school, problems with classmates, joblessness at home, bullies, gangs in the neighborhood—are given far more room for exploration and discussion than they were in the past.

What a child envisions in the future and whom a child might wish to emulate as an **ego ideal** are extremely important in contemporary psychotherapy (Terr 2003). How does the youngster imagine what will happen before his or her next birthday? Later in adulthood? How will he or she die? When? What about marriage, children, career? Discussing the future in terms of the youngster's present coping skills or behaviors often offers a new perspective to the child and thus a new way to combat old conflicts. It also sets up goals for the young patient. These issues must be taken into account right along with the classic issues—defenses and coping, secret unattainable desires, transference, and countertransference.

In current child psychotherapy, many of the therapist's responses to a youngster come as play rather than as speech. They come in the form of metaphor rather than as a direct hit. Some responses are conveyed as stories, supposedly about others but really about the young patient. All psychotherapeutic responses, however, carry one element in common: They try to help the child make sense of his inner self or her external world. And in so doing, they allow the child to reassess, consciously or unconsciously, how he or she wishes to be.

Psychotherapeutic commentary can be calculated—as in the instance of a psychiatric resident watching a nonpsychotic hospitalized boy (with a psychotic identical twin brother) playing with "broken elevators" made up of blocks. After a consultation with his supervisor, the trainee came up with a carefully premeditated response—that elevator repairmen can fix certain elevators but have a much tougher time with others (see reference by Zrull cited by Terr et al. 2005). This calculated response came about a week after the boy's play was first observed. It impressively relieved the young patient. However, a psychiatrist's quickly blurted-out or counterintuitive commentary can be just as effective. For example, a very angry boy seemed ready to destroy his psychiatrist's office. The psychiatrist knew that both the boy's teacher and his babysitter had quit their jobs that week. The psychiatrist caught a similarity between how the boy responded to her and her symbolic stand-ins, the teacher and the babysitter. "Despite what may have happened with them," she unhesitatingly told her angry patient, "I'm not leaving!" The patient settled down, and for the first time ever, he verbally expressed his ever-present sense of ambivalence about people, including his therapist. This was the key to the boy's psychology—and the crucial interpretation actually came from his own mouth, not from the psychiatrist's. But first, the psychiatrist said what immediately came to mind, putting the key into a door that the boy could now open by himself (see reference by Donner cited by Terr 2008).

At times a verbal response to a child offers the youngster a solution to his own personal mystery. Louis Fine, for instance, wondered for years why so many children with congenital anomalies did poorly—especially in terms of depression—after rehabilitative surgeries aimed at giving them better functioning. He solved the mystery by asking a number of youngsters about their postsurgical depressions. They were used to their congenital problems, they told him. Their problems had been with them forever. They liked their heavy shoes, with which they could kick their tormentors, or their wheelchairs and canes, with which they had always felt comfortable. Once Dr. Fine solved the mystery for one child (with his pointed commentary), he began solving the same mystery for others (with back and forth dialogue about these children's perceived dangers regarding their physical improvements). This consulting psychiatrist was thus able to solve similar dilemmas for many children by using very brief individual psychotherapies during their postsurgical hospitalizations (see reference by Fine cited by Terr 2008).

With children it is sometimes appropriate to create a dramatic moment, a grand gesture that conveys to the child almost the entire meaning of the child's psychotherapeutic experience. Sometimes the therapist confronts the young child with exactly what he or she is doing or is wishing for (see reference by Beitchman or Winters cited by Terr 2008). On the right occasion, on the other hand, it may be possible to say a poem, tell a story, or draw a picture that almost perfectly conveys to the young patient a sense of the therapist's understanding. Sometimes, using an established method of working in psychotherapy, such as Winnicott's squiggle game (in which the therapist starts a doodle and the child finishes it [Winnicott 1971a]) or Gardner's mutual storytelling technique (in which the therapist and patient work out the beginnings of a story to which the therapist—or better yet, the patient—affixes a corrective ending [Gardner 1971]), creates just what was needed. Shapiro (1983), for instance, worked with a 5-year-old girl for only two sessions, using Winnicott's squiggle game. This psychotherapeutic approach completely relieved the young child's previously intractable insomnia. With children suffering from terrible experiences (Terr 2003), a story resembling the trauma can be started with the patient, and the child is then asked to find a correction.

Letters to a person who the child feels needs to receive this kind of communication is another dramatic way for a young psychotherapeutic patient to find comfort and self-awareness. Letters do not necessarily have to be actually sent. Letters to Santa, even letters to God, for instance, have long been a childhood tradition. When this tradition is used on behalf of the individual youngster in psychotherapy, it may bring with it a sense of control and relief (Terr 2008).

Some gifted psychotherapists improvise just the right drama for the specific child. In fact, some of these little dramas are produced on the spur of the moment. One kindergarten-age girl, for instance, was brought to a Montreal emergency room because she had become afraid to eat. For a couple of days, she had refused all food, claiming she might inadvertently kill a living being, like a fly. "What is the worst thing that would happen," the psychiatrist asked her, "if you *did* swallow a fly?" The youngster could not answer. The psychiatrist responded, "It would come out in your poo" (see reference by Minde cited by Terr et al. 2006b). Entranced, the little girl's 2-year-old sister chanted, "Fly in the poo! Ha! Ha!" The psychiatrist began to sing and dance, on the basis of the toddler's chant. The entire family eventually joined in. The kindergartener left the emergency room that night, no longer afraid to eat.

If a child will not talk, the gifted psychotherapist might try a *soliloquy for two,* another dramatic gesture. In a soliloquy for two, the therapist tells a story about an imaginary child who, of course, is just like the patient herself (see reference by Robson cited by Terr 2008). In a different context, if a child happens to give away something intimate about himself, the gifted therapist might say something so dramatic it requires ongoing discussion. Consider, for instance, the phrase "Your secret will be safe with me" (from the 1942 film *Casablanca*). An institutionalized teenager, who was spotted feigning psychosis, heard this phrase coming from his psychiatrist, and the patient wished to discuss it. This adolescent was eventually able to leave the residential center, where he was incarcerated because of the ongoing psychotherapeutic talks that followed from his psychiatrist's provocative remark (see reference by Livingston cited by Terr 2008). Many dramatic circumstances are so unique that they cannot be duplicated. Studying good books and research reports, watching others, and talking to peers can lead to calculated or instinctive solutions, where the impetus to create memorable moments for children can safely be followed.

Ending Treatment

If the clinician has the option of deciding when to end psychotherapy (and many times he or she does not), the clinician considers the original goals—have they been met?—and any secondary goals that arose during treatment—have they been met as well? After thinking these goals through, the clinician suggests an end date and may taper the frequency of sessions in order to assess how the young patient does without as much access to psychotherapy. Clinician and child talk about their relationship, what they each believe the treatment meant and accomplished, and what the child will do if a problem arises in the future.

Often the clinician makes sure that the child knows how to reach another good practitioner—or the same therapist—in the future, if one is needed. The clinician might also suggest yearly checkups for a while, if that option seems appropriate. Furthermore, the clinician might make it clear that "booster shots" or briefer treatment periods may be necessary when the youngster enters a new phase of life. This is particularly common in cases of psychic trauma, in which the old trauma is experienced differently as new developmental challenges arise (Terr 2003).

Frequently, psychotherapy ends prematurely by the therapist's standards. For example, the young patient moves to a new city. The patient goes to a boarding school or college. The parents divorce. The family can no longer afford the therapy. Insurance plans change. Insurance carriers decide "No more." The trainee therapist completes his or her educational program. Even improvement is sometimes cause for a premature termination, at least in the therapist's opinion. The family sees the child's improvement as sufficient to stop the treatment, while the therapist still wishes to help strengthen and mature some of the child's underlying coping and defensive strategies.

In such cases, it is best to provide the young patient with two or three termination sessions, perhaps at increasing time intervals. If the clinician can obtain agreement from the family for a few therapy hours to wrap up, it is usually the most helpful way to end a child's therapeutic work.

Some parents decide that summer vacation from school is the time for ending treatment. If a child fails to reappear in the fall, it is worthwhile to make a phone inquiry and to ask for further in-person conversation with the family. Often, from the child's point of view, summer is a natural time to stop. School stops, as do certain sports and music lessons. In the case of therapy, however, missing the chance to say good-bye may lead to later confusion as to what those visits to the therapist were all about. Unfortunately, even when termination with a child is handled with the greatest of skill, youngsters often still fail to understand why they went through a course of psychotherapy. Insight is, in fact, an almost-adult trait and a very difficult one for any young patient to develop.

Future Directions

One interesting aspect of psychotherapy open for future study is the "turning point." What accounts for almost instantaneous meetings of the mind between therapists and young patients? Daniel Stern (2004) and his associates have watched and discussed this phenomenon, as have the author and her colleagues. Interest in the instantaneous gesture and intuitive move by the well-trained and experienced clinician may eventually lead in new and fruitful directions.

Most importantly, let us hope that innovative new studies allow us—with vigor and enthusiasm—to eventually supply an evidence base to this crucial field.

Summary Points

- Make a full diagnosis and formulation, suggesting psychotherapy where appropriate and potentially helpful.
- Find a way for the child's parents or guardians to participate.
- Pick a persona in yourself that will enhance the child's chances of therapeutic success.
- Be willing to show your "realness" when called for.
- Outfit an office that can be adapted to be comfortable for children, adolescents, and adults.
- Use a variety of techniques tailored to the particular child, such as conversation, play, art, and storytelling.
- Watch and listen, following the child's leads.
- Nurture the relationship with appropriate gestures and comments.
- Make therapeutic responses geared to the youngster's inner problems, problems with the real world, and/or problems in the relationship itself.
- Think and talk about the child's future.
- Stay flexible.

References

Allen F: Positive Aspects of Child Psychiatry. New York, Basic Books, 1962

Bleiberg E: Mentalizing-based treatment with adolescents and families. Child Adolesc Psychiatr Clin N Am 22(2):295–330, 2013 23538015

Brody M: Seductive Screens: Children's Media—Past, Present, and Future. Cambridge, UK, Cambridge Scholars Publishing, 2012

Bugental JF: The person who is the psychotherapist. J Consult Psychol 28:272–277, 1964 14174915

Erikson E: Childhood and Society. New York, WW Norton, 1950

Fonagy P, Bateman A: The development of borderline personality disorder—a mentalizing model. J Pers Disord 22(1):4–21, 2008 18312120

Fraiberg S: Insights From the Blind. New York, Basic Books, 1977

Freud A: Introduction to the Technique of Child Analysis. Washington, DC, Nervous and Mental Disease Publishing Company, 1928

Freud A: The Ego and the Mechanisms of Defense (1936). New York, International Universities Press, 1946

Freud A, Burlingham D: War and Children (Report 12). New York, Medical War Books, 1943

Freud S: Analysis of a phobia in a five-year old boy (1909), in The Standard Edition of the Complete Psychological Works of Sigmund Freud, Vol 10. Translated and edited by Strachey J. London, Hogarth, 1955, pp 3–147

Freud S: Beyond the Pleasure Principle (1920), in The Standard Edition of The Complete Psychological Works of Sigmund Freud, Vol 18. Translated and edited by Strachey J. London, Hogarth, 1955, pp 7–64

Furman E: Treatment of under-fives by way of parents. Psychoanal Study Child 12:250–262, 1957

Gardner R: Therapeutic Communications With Children: The Mutual Storytelling Technique. New York, Science House, 1971

Gerber AJ, Kocsis JH, Milrod BL, et al: A quality-based review of randomized controlled trials of psychodynamic psychotherapy. Am J Psychiatry 168(1):19–28, 2011 20843868

Gilmore K, Meersand P: Normal Child and Adolescent Development: A Psychoanalytic Primer. Washington, DC, American Psychiatric Publishing, 2014

Green M, Solnit AJ: Reactions to the threatened loss of a child: the vulnerable child syndrome. Pediatric management of the dying child, part III. Pediatrics 34:58–66, 1964 14181986

Group for the Advancement of Psychiatry: The Process of Child Therapy. New York, Brunner/Mazel, 1982

Group for the Advancement of Psychiatry Committee on Child Psychiatry: How old is old enough? The ages of rights and responsibilities. Rep Group Adv Psychiatry 126:1–124, 1989 2813874

Harrison SI, McDermott JF Jr, Schrager J, et al: Social status and child psychiatric practice: the influence of the clinician's socioeconomic origin. Am J Psychiatry 127(5):652–658, 1970 5491541

Hartmann H: Notes on the reality principle. Psychoanal Study Child 11:31–53, 1956

Jellinek MS, McDermott JF: Formulation: putting the diagnosis into a therapeutic context and treatment plan. J Am Acad Child Adolesc Psychiatry 43(7):913–916, 2004 15213593

Johnson A: Sanctions for superego lacunae of adolescents, in Searchlights on Delinquency. Edited by Eissler K. Oxford, UK, International Universities Press, 1949, pp 225–254

Kernberg PF, Weiner AS, Bardenstein K: Personality Disorders in Children and Adolescents. New York, Basic Books, 2000

Kernberg PF, Ritvo R, Keable H, et al: Practice Parameter for psychodynamic psychotherapy with children. J Am Acad Child Adolesc Psychiatry 51(5):541–557, 2012 22525961

Kline M: The Psychoanalysis of Children. London, Hogarth, 1932

Levy D: Release therapy. Am J Orthopsychiatry 9:713–736, 1939

Lewis M, King R (eds): Consultation-Liaison in Pediatrics (Child and Adolescent Psychiatric Clinics of North America, Vol 3, Pt 3). Philadelphia, PA, WB Saunders, 1994

Lieberman A, Van Horn P: Psychotherapy With Infants and Young Children. New York, Guilford, 2008

Marshall R: Countertransference in the psychotherapy of children and adolescents. Contemp Psychoanal 15(4):599–629, 1979

Midgley N, Kennedy E: Psychodynamic psychotherapy for children and adolescents: a critical review of the evidence base. Journal of Child Psychotherapy 37:232–260, 2011

Mishne JM: Clinical Work With Adolescents. New York, Free Press, 1986

Ritvo R, Henderson S (eds): Psychodynamic Treatment Approaches to Psychopathology (special issue). Child and Adolescent Psychiatric Clinics of North America 22(2):149–374, 2013

Rosenfeld AR, Wasserman S: Healing the Heart: A Therapeutic Approach to Disturbed Children in Group Care. Washington, DC, Child Welfare League of America, 1990

Rossouw TI, Fonagy P: Mentalization-based treatment for self-harm in adolescents: a randomized controlled trial. J Am Acad Child Adolesc Psychiatry 51(12):1304–1313, e3, 2012 23200287

Rubin LC (ed): Using Superheroes in Counseling and Play Therapy. New York, Springer, 2007

Schechter DS, Willheim E: When parenting becomes unthinkable: intervening with traumatized parents and their toddlers. J Am Acad Child Adolesc Psychiatry 48(3):249–253, 2009 19242290

Schulman JL, de la Fuente ME, Suran B: An indication for brief psychotherapy. The fork in the road phenomenon. Bull Menninger Clin 41(6):553–562, 1977 588787

Shapiro T: The unconscious still occupies us. Psychoanal Study Child 38:547–567, 1983 6647668

Shapiro T: The psychodynamic formulation in child and adolescent psychiatry. J Am Acad Child Adolesc Psychiatry 28(5):675–680, 1989 2793795

Silberschatz G: The control mastery theory, in Transformative Relationships. Edited by Silberschatz G. New York, Routledge, 2005, pp 3–24

Silver L: Attention-deficit/Hyperactivity Disorder: A Clinical Guide to Diagnosis and Treatment for Health and Mental Health Professionals. Washington, DC, American Psychiatric Publishing, 2003

Steig W: CDB! New York, Aladdin, 1968

Stern D: The Present Moment in Psychotherapy and Everyday Life. New York, WW Norton, 2004

Terr LC: Childhood traumas: an outline and overview. Am J Psychiatry 148(1):10–20, 1991 1824611

Terr LC: "Wild Child": how three principles of healing organized 12 years of psychotherapy. J Am Acad Child Adolesc Psychiatry 42(12):1401–1409, 2003 14627874

Terr L: Magical Moments of Change: How Psychotherapy Turns Kids Around. New York, WW Norton, 2008

Terr LC: Using context to treat traumatized children. Psychoanal Study Child 64:275–298, 2009 20578442

Terr LC, McDermott JF, Benson RM, et al: Moments in psychotherapy. J Am Acad Child Adolesc Psychiatry 44(2):191–197, 2005 15689733

Terr LC, Beitchman JH, Braslow K, et al: Children's turn-arounds in psychotherapy: the doctor's gesture. Psychoanal Study Child 61:56–81, 2006a 17370455

Terr LC, Deeney JM, Drell M, et al: Playful "moments" in psychotherapy. J Am Acad Child Adolesc Psychiatry 45(5):604–613, 2006b 16670655

Terr LC, Abright AR, Brody M, et al: When formulation outweighs diagnosis: 13 "moments" in psychotherapy. J Am Acad Child Adolesc Psychiatry 45(10):1252–1263, 2006c 17003671

Thomas A, Chess S, Birch HG: Temperament and Behavior Disorders in Children. New York, New York University Press, 1968

Tsiantis J, Sandler A-M, Anastasopoulos D, et al: Countertransference in Psychoanalytic Psychotherapy With Children and Adolescents. London, Karnac, 1996

Waelder R: The psychoanalytic theory of play. Psychoanal Q 2:208–224, 1933

Webb NB (ed): Play Therapy With Children in Crisis, 3rd Edition. New York, Guilford, 2007

Weiner MF, King JW: Self-disclosure by the therapist to the adolescent patient, in Adolescent Psychiatry, Vol 5. Edited by Feinstein S, Giovacchini P. New York, Jason Aronson, 1977, pp 449–459

Winnicott DW: Clinical varieties of transference, in Collected Papers: Through Pediatrics to Psychoanalysis. New York, Basic Books, 1958, pp 295–299

Winnicott DW: Playing and Reality. New York, Basic Books, 1971a

Winnicott DW: Therapeutic Consultations in Child Psychiatry. New York, Basic Books, 1971b

CHAPTER 40

Parent Counseling, Psychoeducation, and Parent Support Groups

Amy N. Mendenhall, Ph.D., M.S.W.
L. Eugene Arnold, M.D., M.Ed.
Mary A. Fristad, Ph.D., ABPP

Mental illness in children affects the entire family. Children are dependent on their parents to help recognize and meet their needs, so education and support for both the child and the caregivers about disorders and treatment are essential. Various parent and family interventions have been developed for families with a child with a serious emotional or behavioral disorder. Table 40–1 lists the distinguishing features of some of these programs.

In this chapter we describe three interventions that provide support and education to parents of children with serious emotional and behavioral disturbances: parent counseling, psychoeducation, and parent support groups. *Parent counseling* is a broad category of parent-focused work that combines a mixture of education and psychotherapy based on the needs of each parent. As a specific subset of parent counseling, *psychoeducation* is an explicit manualized intervention that focuses on education and skill building for both parents and children. *Parent support groups* are less formal than parent counseling and psychoeducation. They gather together parents experiencing similar situations to create a network of support. Despite these differences, the interventions have a common focus—to help parents of children with emotional and behavioral disorders in order to aid the children indirectly.

TABLE 40–1. Parent and family interventions

Intervention	Definition and distinguishing features	Relative importance of trained professional
Family assessment	Assesses child diagnosis, family needs, and necessary services and treatment	++++
Family therapy	Psychotherapeutic approach focusing on family interactions and relationships to promote change Classically based on a "systems" framework: may also include interventions from other theoretical models (e.g., behavioral)	++++
Multifamily psychoeducation groups[a]	Psychoeducation in context of multifamily group, providing knowledge, support, and skill building to families with a common problem	++++
Parent counseling[a]	Continuum of interventions to help parents understand their child and the mental illness; targets parent attitudes and behavior; includes advice, supportive therapy	++++
Parent training in behavior management ("parent management training")	Teaches and coaches parents how to manage their child's problem behaviors, mainly using behavior modification strategies and techniques	+++
Parent support groups[a]	Create a support network of parents experiencing similar situations; focus on self-help, identification, and guilt reduction	+
Psychoeducation[a]	Manualized approach focusing on education about the disorder; its treatment; accessing of services; and skill building in communication, problem solving, and symptom management	++++
Wraparound services	Creation of a network of community services and natural supports individualized to the needs of the child and family	++
Treatment of parent's own mental disorder	Parent is treated directly for a diagnosed mental disorder that impairs parenting	++++
Counseling in context of parent's treatment	Parent in treatment for own problem brings up difficulty with child during treatment	++++

Note. [a]Interventions described in the current chapter.

Parent Counseling and Psychoeducation

What Is Parent Counseling?

Parent counseling or parent guidance has been used more generally to describe parent education and therapy separate from work with the child. It refers to a continuum of interventions aimed to help parents understand their children and their moods and behaviors. It sometimes targets parent attitudes and behaviors that may contribute to overall difficulties in the family. Interventions range from basic education to psychotherapy and can include clarification, advice, persuasion, facilitation, and exploration of feelings (Arnold 1978). The decision of which intervention to use is based on the nature of the problem, family personality and strengths, obstacles to effective parenting, and type of help the parents are willing to accept.

Regardless of the specific intervention, it should be accompanied by the sincere valuing of parents for their experience in caring for their children and their expertise in understanding their children and their needs (Arnold 1978). Recognizing parental expertise and beliefs can lead to better personalization of treatment, a stronger therapeutic relationship, and more positive outcomes. Table 40–2 lists basic principles of parent counseling, and Table 40–3 lists some strategies to use while working with parents in this modality. In this chapter we focus on one specific type of parent counseling, psychoeducation, which refers to manualized educational programs for parents and children. Parent training, also an educational parent counseling approach, is covered in Chapter 41, "Behavioral Parent Training."

What Is Psychoeducation?

The term psychoeducation has been applied to a wide range of interventions of varying intensities from simple, short-term educational efforts to integration of education with therapy. In this chapter, the focus is on psychoeducation that integrates psychotherapeutic and educational methods with the intention of educating both the patient and the family to reach better outcomes for all (Lukens and McFarlane 2004). Psychoeducation covers topics such as diagnoses, course of illness, medications, other treatments, and symptom management. This form of psychoeducation has been termed *psychoeducational psychotherapy* by some to differentiate it from short-term psychoeducation such as books, films, and Web sites (Mendenhall and Fristad 2010). Psychoeducation is designed as an adjunctive treatment to medications or other treatment already in progress. It has been applied to many different areas within the health and mental health fields. Growing literature on the effectiveness of psychoeducation led to national and international recommendations to use psychoeducation for the treatment of schizophrenia and other mental illnesses.

History of Psychoeducation

Psychoeducation emerged from efforts to improve the prognosis of schizophrenia. Goldstein et al. (1978) gave recently discharged adults with schizophrenia and their families a program designed to help them understand the illness and its treatment and plan for future crises. The program was the first to combine medi-

TABLE 40–2. Basic characteristics and principles of parent counseling

1. Education and therapy are provided to parents rather than directly to the child
2. Parents are essential to treatment because they spend the most time with their child
3. The experience and expertise parents have from caring for their children should be valued and used in treatment
4. The appropriate choice of intervention depends on the problem, the circumstances, and the family
5. The professional acts as a consultant to help parents identify problems and learn skills needed to manage their child's illness successfully on their own
6. Counseling helps parents understand normal child development, their own child, and their child's needs and problems
7. Counseling helps parents modify their own attitudes, behaviors, and parenting that may be unwittingly contributing to the problem
8. Efficiency, effectiveness, and practicality are emphasized to the exclusion of moral judgment or blame
9. It is assumed that parent-child conflicts are two-way vicious cycles

Source. Adapted from Arnold (1978).

TABLE 40–3. Strategies for working with parents in parent counseling

Help parents reframe the problem in a way that seems manageable and does not place responsibility solely on them

Model appropriate parent-child behavior for parents to observe

In cases where punishment has been excessively frequent or severe (which usually means it has been ineffective), guide parents in understanding the purpose of consequences and finding a humane consequence that works for their child

Help parents understand the importance of counterbalancing punishment with rewards (both carrot and stick)

Provide parents with supplemental reading to reinforce topics discussed in sessions

Refer parents to other services that cannot be provided in counseling

Encourage parents to seek therapy for themselves, not just for their child

Encourage parents to be patient and to expect small increments of change rather than a quick cure

Source. Adapted from Arnold (1978).

cation and family intervention, and the combined program was found to be more effective than either separate intervention. Also during this time period, Carol Anderson and Gerald Hogarty (Anderson et al. 1980) developed the family psychoeducation approach, combining psychoeducation and social skills training for families of individuals with schizophrenia. Miklowitz and Goldstein (1995) also successfully adapted the psychoeducation model to address bipolar disorder in adults. Success of these programs spurred a series of studies on the use of psychoeducation for schizophrenia, bipolar disorder, and other adult mental health disorders, followed by adaptations and studies examining its use with children and adolescents, with some positive outcomes.

Theoretical Background of Parent Counseling and Psychoeducation

Parents are the primary caregivers and decision makers in their children's lives. Parents of a child with mental illness have the added responsibility of managing their child's symptoms and treatment. Educated parents are better positioned to help their child manage symptoms and to access services appropriate to their child's needs.

Psychoeducation combines several clinical approaches, including cognitive-behavioral, learning, narrative, systems, client-centered, stress and coping, and social support theories (Lukens and McFarlane 2004). Techniques such as role-playing encourage parents to practice applying new information and skills learned. Systems theory provides a framework to understand mental illness in relation to all relevant systems, including family, school or work, and social network. Group psychoeducation provides an atmosphere for social learning and support among group members. A biopsychosocial approach presents mental illness as a "no fault illness." Psychoeducation participants are specifically told they are not to blame for the illness; rather, they are taught how to separate themselves from the symptoms (Fristad et al. 1999).

Description of Parent Counseling and Psychoeducation

Parent counseling and psychoeducation can have very different structures, depending on the problem being addressed and the setting in which the interventions are being provided. The interventions can be delivered to individual families or in multifamily groups (Fristad 2006). Individual family psychoeducation consists of one family working one on one with the clinician to learn more about their child's diagnosis and treatment. Multifamily psychoeducation groups consist of multiple families in similar situations following a standardized format of education. A group of researchers at Ohio State University have developed and tested both individual family and multifamily psychoeducation interventions (Fristad 2006). Different strengths were found for each format, as listed in Table 40–4. McFarlane et al. (1995) found that multifamily group psychoeducation was even more effective in reducing relapse rates and increasing functioning in adults than individual or family psychoeducation; however, this has not been tested in families of children and adolescents.

Psychoeducation interventions usually consist of a set of sessions focused on providing information about mental illness and its treatment. These sessions are typically the same for every individual or group, with each session's topic area described in detail in a treatment manual. Information can be presented through lecture, discussions, video, and role-playing. Areas commonly covered are diagnosis, symptom management, communication, medication, other treatment, and skill building. Session length and duration may vary among different programs, but typically, sessions last 1–2 hours and 1–20 sessions are planned. Some psychoeducation treatments have one or more built in "flex" sessions to be used as needed for specific parent and family concerns.

Psychoeducation is easily adapted to a variety of settings including hospitals, schools, mental health centers, jails or detention centers, and online Web sites. Format, length, duration, and treatment

TABLE 40–4. Relative advantages of the two psychoeducation formats

Individual family psychoeducation	Multifamily psychoeducation groups
Easy for private practice clinician to implement	Cost-effective way to deliver services within a large clinic
Privacy	Opportunity to talk and share with both professionals and other families
Flexibility in scheduling	
Flexibility to tailor topics to individualized needs	Development of support network
	Identifying with and learning from other families' successes

focus may vary on the basis of the setting. The professionals leading the intervention may include psychiatrists or other physicians, psychologists, social workers, teachers, and nurses. Regardless of their profession, psychoeducation leaders serve as facilitators and teachers. They are responsible for developing the intervention to meet the needs, motivations, strengths, and weaknesses of the patients.

Adaptation of psychoeducation for children and adolescents requires several changes in the content and format of the intervention. Fristad et al. (1996) suggest six adaptations to psychoeducational approaches based on children's developmental needs (Table 40–5).

Benefits of Parent Counseling and Psychoeducation

Education about specific disorders helps parents to understand their child's experiences and how to help their child. Education about types of available treatments, classes of medications, side effects, and building a treatment team can promote treatment adherence and efficiency. Increased knowledge about the problem allows parents to react more appropriately.

Another benefit is a focus on the parents, their feelings, and their stress, which often have been neglected in pursuit of the child's treatment. The impact of mental illness on caregivers and families can be enormous, and psychoeducation tries to alleviate some of the difficulties of caring for a child with mental illness. Psychoeducation addresses these stresses not only by empowering parents with knowledge about their child's illness and treatment but also by promoting healthy communication, symptom management, and parent health and mental health and by addressing parental needs. Parents are offered support, validation, and recognition of their own struggles (Fristad et al. 2003b).

Additionally, psychoeducation targets expressed emotion (EE), which may be a factor contributing to perpetuation of symptoms. EE refers to the type and quality of interactions and attitudes regarding a person who is mentally ill. The term emerged from a series of studies that found high familial EE associated with relapse rates in adults with schizophrenia (Brown et al. 1972). High EE has been identified as a risk factor for depression onset (Burkhouse et al. 2012) and has been found to relate to poor outcomes in mood disorders in youth (Asarnow et al. 1993). Psychoeducation provides parent support and education that can help families adapt a strategy of problem-focused coping rather than emotion-focused coping, leading to better family communication and symptom

TABLE 40–5. Age adjustments needed for psychoeducation with children and adolescents with mental illness, compared with programs for adults

Psychoeducational adjustments for children and adolescents	Reason for the adjustment
Clarification for the child and family about what the disorder is and what the child's traits are: distinction between personality and symptoms	With a much earlier age of onset than adults, children may not have had an opportunity to develop a healthy identity separate from symptoms
Emphasis on social skills training	Children may not have had the opportunity to develop age-appropriate social skills because of early onset
Assistance in adjusting environmental expectations	Education and intervention are often needed at school to help adjust the environment to one in which the child can succeed despite symptoms
Emphasis on the importance of the home environment and how to improve it	Children are still dependent on their parents and thus are particularly vulnerable to unhealthy home environments
Greater intensity of treatment and longer follow-up	Earlier onset often leads to a more pernicious course and greater treatment resistance
Developmentally appropriate group content	Children and adolescents differ in their developmental level, so separate content or groups are needed for the two ages

Source. Adapted from Fristad et al. (1996).

management (Sloper 1999). Lowering negative EE through psychoeducation may lead to an improved environment for the child suffering from an emotional or behavioral disorder.

Research on Psychoeducation for Children's Mental Health

Family psychoeducation is an evidence-based practice in adult mental health. The application of psychoeducation has spread to children's mental health, and research on psychoeducation for various children's mental health disorders is ongoing. Table 40–6 lists examples of family psychoeducation as it has been applied to various mental disorders in children and adolescents. The table excludes psychoeducation interventions designed only for the child and not the parents or family.

As shown in Table 40–6, family or parent psychoeducation interventions have been designed for attention-deficit/hyperactivity disorder (ADHD), depressive disorders, bipolar disorders, disruptive behavior disorders, eating disorders, and trauma- and stressor-related disorders. Programs have also been designed for general emotional and behavioral disturbances rather than for specific disorders. Across diagnoses, the active treatment components of these family psychoeducation interventions were all very similar and included medications, other forms of treatment, symptom management, parenting, and coping and communication skills. Some mood disorder interventions had pharmacotherapy and psychoeducation offered as a treatment package. Interventions followed structured formats, most commonly led by a mental health professional and typically outlined in a treatment manual. Material was taught through a variety of

TABLE 40–6. Studies of the use of psychoeducation in children's mental health

Study	Population	Design and sample	Active treatment protocol	Structure and duration	Outcomes
Attention-deficit/hyperactivity disorder (ADHD)					
Ferrin et al. 2014	Children ages 5–18 years with ADHD and their families	Blind RCT Control group received parent counseling and support intervention N=81 (20% female)	Manualized psychoeducation	12 sessions, 90 minutes in length	Treatment group had significantly reduced ADHD symptoms after intervention compared with control group ($P<0.01$).
Lopez et al. 2005	Children ages 6–17 years with ADHD and their families	Open study N=90 (mean age=9.9; 29% female)	Psychoeducation through written materials and physicians and clinical assistants	Varied for each family	Parents used available education materials; they indicated satisfaction with intervention at the end of treatment.
Disruptive behavior disorders					
Bradley et al. 2003	Parents of children ages 3–4 years who have trouble managing their child's behavior	RCT Wait list control N=222 (mean age=3.8; 35% female)	Immediate multifamily psychoeducation based on the 1-2-3 Magic video vs. wait list control	2-hour group meeting weekly for 3 weeks with booster session 4 weeks later	Parenting practices improved ($P<0.001$), and child behavior improved from pretest to posttest compared with control group ($P<0.05$).
Smith et al. 2006	93 parents and 102 adolescents with substance abuse and behavior disorders	Open study N=93 parents and 102 adolescents	Psychoeducation vs. control group	2-hour meeting weekly for 3 weeks with a booster session 4 weeks after	Substance abuse declined ($P<0.001$); 85% did not relapse over the course of an entire year posttreatment.
Eating disorders					
Geist et al. 2000	Females ages 12–17 years with anorexia nervosa and their families	RCT Alternative treatment control N=25 (mean age=14.3; 100% female)	Family therapy vs. multifamily psychoeducation	8 total sessions every 2 weeks over 4 months	No significant differences between groups were found. Significant time effect was found for both treatment groups for restoration of body weight ($P<0.001$).

TABLE 40–6. Studies of the use of psychoeducation in children's mental health *(continued)*

Study	Population	Design and sample	Active treatment protocol	Structure and duration	Outcomes
Holtkamp et al. 2005	Parents of adolescents in treatment for eating disorders	Open study N=153 (mean age=15.3)	Multifamily psychoeducation	Five 90-minute group sessions	Parents rated psychoeducation as helpful in coping with child's disorder and would recommend to others.
Mood disorders					
Fristad et al. 2009	Children ages 8–11 years with major mood disorders and their families	RCT Wait list control N=165 (30% depressive spectrum, 70% bipolar spectrum)	Adjunctive multifamily psychoeducational psychotherapy	8 sessions, 90 minutes in length, with separate parent and child groups	Immediate treatment group had less severe mood symptoms at follow-up compared with wait list group (P=0.03). Wait list group showed similar improvements in mood severity after they also received treatment.
Miklowitz et al. 2008	Adolescents with bipolar disorder ages 12–17 years and family members	RCT Enhanced care (3 family sessions) and pharmacotherapy control N=58 (mean age=14.5; 57% female)	Family-focused psychoeducation and pharmacotherapy	21 sessions over 9 months	Youth in treatment group recovered from baseline depressive symptoms compared with comparison group (P<0.05). These youth also spent fewer weeks in depressive episodes and had more favorable trajectory of depressive symptoms for 2 years.
Miklowitz et al. 2013	Adolescents ages 9–17 years with mood disorder symptoms at high risk for bipolar disorder	RCT Family education control N= 40 (mean age=12.3; 42.5% female)	Brief early family-focused psychoeducational intervention	12 sessions, 60 minutes in length, over 4 months	Youth in treatment group had more rapid recovery from their initial mood symptoms (P=0.47), more weeks in remission, and a more favorable trajectory of mania symptoms over 1 year than youth in the control group.

TABLE 40–6. Studies of the use of psychoeducation in children's mental health *(continued)*

Study	Population	Design and sample	Active treatment protocol	Structure and duration	Outcomes
Pavuluri et al. 2004	Youth with early onset bipolar spectrum disorder	Open study N=34 (mean age=11.3; 29% female)	Combination of psychoeducation, family-focused therapy, and CBT with pharmacotherapy	12 family sessions 1 hour in length	From pretest to posttest, children displayed reductions in symptom severity ($P<0.001$) and increases in overall global functioning ($P<0.001$). High levels of treatment adherence and satisfaction were also noted.
Sanford et al. 2006	Adolescents ages 13–18 years with major depressive disorder and their families	RCT Usual treatment control N=41 (mean age=15.9; 65% female)	Family psychoeducation and treatment as usual	Twelve 90-minute family sessions in the home and 1 booster session at 3-month follow-up	Treatment group showed greater improvement in social functioning and adolescent-parent relationships from pretest to posttest than control subjects ($P<0.05$, effect size >0.5). Parents reported greater treatment satisfaction than control subjects posttest ($P<0.01$).
Psychosis					
O'Brien et al. 2014	Youth or young adults at clinical high risk for psychosis	RCT Enhanced care control (3 sessions over 1 month) N=103 (mean age=17; 39% female)	Family-focused psychoeducation	18 sessions over 6 months, 50 minutes in length	Treatment group had greater improvement in constructive communication ($P<0.01$) and decreases in conflictual behaviors ($P<0.01$) during family interactions compared with the control group.

TABLE 40–6. Studies of the use of psychoeducation in children's mental health *(continued)*

Study	Population	Design and sample	Active treatment protocol	Structure and duration	Outcomes
Serious emotional and behavioral disturbances in general					
Davidson and Fristad 2004	Families of children with mental illness	Open study $N=46$	Multifamily psychoeducation	8-week class led by other family members	Parents reported lower stress in relationships ($P=0.02$), improved mental health ($P=0.04$), more compliance with child's chores ($P=0.04$), fewer self-harming acts by the child ($P<0.01$), and fewer public rages ($P=0.01$) from pretest to posttest.
Ruffolo et al. 2005	Parents of children with serious emotional disturbance	RCT Usual treatment control $N=94$ (mean age=11.5; 25% female)	Multifamily psychoeducation and intensive case management vs. intensive case management	Open group format, 2-hour meetings twice a month	No statistically significant differences were found between groups in social support; behavior improved in both groups.
Pollio et al. 2005	Families of children receiving school social work services or related services	Open study $N=15$	Multifamily psychoeducation	Eight 90-minute sessions twice monthly or twelve 90-minute sessions weekly	There was a high level of participation and satisfaction with the group experience.
Trauma- and stressor-related disorders					
Copping et al. 2001	Children ages 3–17 years who had experienced trauma and their caregivers	Open study $N=27$ (mean age=9.8; 48% female)	Psychoeducation and CBT	21 sessions of varying length, including 6 group psychoeducation sessions, 7 individualized CBT sessions, and 4 assessment sessions, followed by 4 treatment sessions	There was a reduction in conduct disorder ($P=0.001$), problems in social relations ($P=0.039$), and caregiver depression ($P=0.006$) from pretest to posttest.

Note. CBT=cognitive-behavioral therapy; RCT=randomized controlled trial.

methods, including lecture, video, role-playing, reading, and discussion. Most psychoeducation programs included both children and parents. Program length ranged from 1 session to 21 sessions. Most had 90-minute sessions. Study designs included case studies, open trials, and a few randomized controlled studies. Outcomes relate to level of knowledge and beliefs about mental illness, symptom severity, social and family functioning, and satisfaction with the intervention. Overall, the findings are supportive in several disorders for inclusion of psychoeducation as part of the treatment package for families of children with serious mental illness.

More research on psychoeducation interventions for children with psychiatric disorders is needed before their effectiveness is as well established as psychoeducation for families of adults with schizophrenia and bipolar disorder. However, ongoing research is testing various interventions with larger samples, more stringent research methods (randomized clinical trials), and a variety of disorders and populations. The following subsection provides a more detailed description of one of these psychoeducation interventions.

Example of a Psychoeducation Intervention: Multifamily Psychoeducational Psychotherapy for Children With Mood Disorders

Multifamily psychoeducational psychotherapy (MF-PEP) was developed as an adjunctive intervention for families of children ages 8–12 years with mood disorders (Fristad et al. 2003a). The guiding principle of MF-PEP is that education, support, and skill building will lead to a better understanding of the illness, which in turn will lead to better treatment adherence, less conflict, and better outcomes for all. Eight 90-minute sessions are manualized with a nonblaming biopsychosocial model using systems and cognitive-behavioral techniques. Table 40–7 lists the weekly session topics for the parents and children.

Sessions start with children and parents together for a discussion of the day's content area, issues brought up in previous sessions, unanswered questions, and reports on the previous week's homework projects. Then the parents and youth separate into groups for their separate lessons. They rejoin for a wrap-up at the end of the session. Parents and children are assigned projects to complete between sessions to practice skills learned in the group. The child group is led by two co-therapists, and the parent group is led by one therapist. Goals for the parent group are social support, information, and skill building (Goldberg-Arnold et al. 1999). Goals for the child group are meeting and interacting with other children who struggle with similar issues, increased awareness of symptoms and symptom management, increased affect regulation skills, and social skills building.

A National Institute of Mental Health–funded randomized controlled trial ($N=165$) found that youth who received MF-PEP had a significantly greater decrease in mood symptom severity at follow-up compared with wait list control with improvement maintained through an 18-month follow-up period (Fristad et al. 2009). The strongest treatment effect was seen in severely impaired children (MacPherson et al. 2014b). MF-PEP was also associated with decreases in symptoms of ADHD, oppositional defiant disorder,

TABLE 40–7. Weekly topic schedule for multifamily psychoeducational psychotherapy

Parents	Children
1. Welcome and overview of group and mood disorders	1. Welcome and overview of group and mood disorders
2. Medications	2. Medications
3. Systems of care	3. Symptom management techniques
4. Mood disorders and family life	4. Connection of thoughts, feelings, actions
5. Problem-solving skills	5. Problem-solving skills
6. Communication	6. Nonverbal communication
7. Symptom management techniques	7. Verbal communication
8. Review and graduation	8. Review and graduation

Source. Adapted from Fristad et al. (2003b).

and overall disruptive behavior (Boylan et al. 2013). Results suggest that MF-PEP helps parents become better consumers of mental health services by increasing their knowledge about mood disorders and treatment, which then leads them to access higher-quality services. Consequently, when children receive services appropriate for meeting their needs, the severity of their symptoms decreases (Mendenhall et al. 2009). Preliminary results also support the implementation of MF-PEP in community settings and suggest associated improvement in clinical outcomes (MacPherson et al. 2014a).

Starting a Multifamily Psychoeducation Group

Establishing a curriculum is the first step. Regardless of type of disorder, a curriculum for a new psychoeducation program should address several main content areas (Table 40–8). Addressing these areas provides families with a well-rounded education and skill development to help them successfully manage symptoms and access appropriate care. However, aspects of the programs should be specialized for the disorder being targeted. Table 40–9 lists suggested disorder-specific adaptations to psychoeducation based on the studies summarized in the subsection "Research on Psychoeducation for Children's Mental Health." Integrated into the curriculum should be techniques for practicing and monitoring newly learned knowledge and skills. Techniques are often adapted from therapeutic approaches such as cognitive-behavioral therapy, narrative therapy, or learning theory. Table 40–10 describes some commonly used psychoeducational techniques.

When developing a group, logistical decisions—such as location, whether to include the youth, optimal group size, length of program, and duration of sessions—must be made on the basis of the setting and targeted disorder. Possible complications in implementing psychoeducation groups and how to address them should also be considered before starting the group. Table 40–11 lists some complications and options for possible solutions or responses.

For those seeking further guidance, many psychoeducation programs have developed treatment manuals or other literature on their programs. Additionally, the Substance Abuse and Mental Health Services Administration devel-

TABLE 40–8. Core psychoeducation content areas

Types of disorders and symptoms
Medication and side effects
Cognitive restructuring
Behavioral skills and techniques
Problem-solving skills
Relapse prevention
Daily routines and healthy habits
Communication skills
Social functioning
Treatment and services (traditional and non-traditional)

oped an extensive toolkit for implementing family psychoeducation based on the adult literature and research. The toolkit is available at http://store.samhsa.gov/product/Family Psychoeducation-Evidence-Based-Practices-EBP-KIT/SMA09-4423. Although not based specifically on psychoeducation with families of children with mental illness, information from the site may be helpful in starting a group for this population.

Parent Support Groups

What Are Parent Support Groups?

Parent support groups bring together parents of children with similar symptoms or diagnoses in an environment designed to be safe for mutual sharing and learning. These groups can be started in any setting or for any diagnosis and can be led by professionals or consumers. Such groups can alleviate parent burden by providing essential information, peer support, coping skills, and respite from the strain of life with a chronically ill child (Hellander et al. 2003). These goals match well with the three basic needs for which individuals join self-help groups: social support, practical information, and a sense of shared purpose or advocacy (Bennett et al. 1996; Koroloff and Friesen 1991). A national survey of parents of children with emotional or behavioral disorders showed that 72% of respondents found emotional support to be the most helpful aspect of family support services (Friesen and Koroloff 1990). Approximately 70% of Americans suffering from mental disorders rely solely on self- and mutual-help options rather than specialized mental health care (Norcross 2000).

History of Parent Support Groups

During the 1970s and 1980s, the mental health recovery movement led to a boom in support groups and other consumer-led efforts to help individuals with mental illness and to promote change in the whole mental health system. The recovery movement emerged as former patients and other advocates gathered together to protest issues such as involuntary hospitalization and the state of mental health treatment. The central philosophy was that individuals with mental illness can and do recover. A key component in the recovery process is being around other people who offer hope, understanding, and support and who encourage self-determination and self-actualization. This emphasis on the importance of mutual help led to a growth in support groups and self-help programs. Now support groups exist for almost every problem or illness that has been identified in adults and children. Groups are held for individuals experiencing mental illness themselves and for family members and caregivers of adults or children with serious emotional or behavioral disorders.

TABLE 40–9. Potential psychoeducation adaptations by disorder

Disorder	Adaptation	Rationale for adaptations
ADHD	Share information with the school	Much impairment occurs at school
	Include tips to improve organizational skills, time management, and study skills	These skills are most often lacking
	Include information about medications	Pharmacotherapy is an important part of decreasing symptoms
Disruptive behavior disorders	Train parents in discipline strategies	Parents often use inadequate methods to discipline these children
	Discuss and develop behavior contracts	Discuss and implement limits on behavior to help youth understand what is acceptable
Eating disorders	Include nutrition education and monitoring	Help youth and parents understand healthy eating patterns
	Include weight monitoring	Help monitor progress in weight normalization and potential relapses
Mood disorders	Encourage assessment and treatment of parents for mood disorders	Parents of youth with mood disorders frequently have mood disorders as well, which makes parenting more challenging
	Use mood charts to monitor mood changes	Mood charts help to clarify the circumstances associated with mood changes
	Include pharmacotherapy as treatment component	Pharmacotherapy is an important part of decreasing symptoms
Trauma- and stressor-related disorders	Assess and treat parents for their own trauma response	Parents have often experienced the same trauma
	When appropriate, redefine acting-out behavior as a response to the trauma	Correct attributions may assist the parents to empathically address difficult behavior

TABLE 40–10. Examples of techniques used in psychoeducation

Psychoeducational techniques	Description of technique
Bibliotherapy	Using written materials, video, or Web sites to further educate families about mental illness
Daily routine tracking	Tracking daily routines such as sleep-wake cycles, eating, and other daily activities to determine their effect on mood and behavior
Mood chart	Tracking changes in mood, when they occur, and the circumstances that happen around the time of the changes
Naming the enemy[a]	Helping the child and parents determine the difference between the child's symptoms and his or her own personality
Thinking, feeling, doing[a]	Increasing insight of parents and child into the connections among their thoughts, feelings, and behavior
Toolkit[a]	Developing a variety of pleasant or relaxing activities for the child to use in affect regulation

Note. [a]Techniques used in multifamily psychoeducational psychotherapy.

Theoretical Background of Parent Support Groups

The theoretical assumption behind parent support groups is that parents need the opportunity to discuss their situation with other parents who have had similar experiences and therefore can understand what they are going through. These groups provide members with knowledge, support, and an outlet for their feelings. Two basic helping processes occur among support group members: giving help and support and receiving help and support (Roberts et al. 1999). Providing help to other group members allows participants to feel they have strengths to offer others, thus enhancing feelings of competence and usefulness. Help received can be in the form of knowledge and support, helping parents to be better prepared to manage their child's illness. Key components include information, group cohesiveness, universality of the problem, identification with others, altruism, catharsis, instillation of hope, interpersonal learning, self-understanding, adoption of an ideological framework, and advocacy (Citron et al. 1999). Of course, these components may not occur within every support group or for every member.

The impact of a support group is determined by the specific group environment and the process the group goes through together. The process may differ slightly depending on whether the group is time limited or open-ended. Time-limited groups occur for a set number of sessions and typically have the same members for the duration. Revolving open-ended groups are continuous, with members joining and leaving the group freely. In professionally led support groups, four phases of group process have been identified: exchanging information, developing intimacy, solidifying relationships, and terminating (Shulman 1992). Groups begin by superficially exchanging information; slowly, they become more intimate as more personal information and experiences are shared. As members become more intimate, the relationships between members become stronger, so that sharing and advice become more

TABLE 40–11. Complications frequently faced by parent group and support group leaders

Complications	Possible responses, solutions, and alternatives
Arguing among members	Restate ground rules Comment on strong feelings behind the opinions and point out potential learning experience for group if the reasons can be shared Invite members to share why they have such strong feelings on the topic
Crying	Empathize and encourage others to empathize Offer tissues Reflect their pain Remind the group that one purpose of the group is to share such experiences
Discussion of inappropriate topics	Change the topic Remind group of its purpose and the ground rules Ask if everyone feels comfortable with topic
Discussion shifts away from scheduled topic	Restate topic Ask group if they want to continue with diversionary topic or return to scheduled topic Find connection between diversionary topic and scheduled topic
Incomplete homework	Reassign Complete as a group Explore reasons not completed
Late arrival	If the late arrival is a member already familiar with the group or is a member who frequently causes disruptions, ignore and continue discussion If the late arrival is a new member, reintroduce everyone, recap what has been discussed, and restate topic of discussion
Nonparticipation	Invite the nonparticipant to comment on another member's comment Suggest each parent share his or her story for 2 minutes
Not enough time to cover topic	Ask if group wants to stay longer Finish at following meeting Adapt homework assignment if topic not finished
Only one family attends group	Proceed the same way, following the manual Adapt to individual family psychoeducation for one session Explore family's feelings about being the only family
One parent dominates discussion	Set limits Take turns for a set amount of time Remind group of time Thank parent for sharing and ask if others would also like to share
Silence	Empathize with difficulty talking about the problems Provide anecdote to start discussion Use humor to break the ice Suggest each parent share his or her story for 2 minutes
Technology disruptions (e.g., ringing phones, text messaging)	Ask members to silence their phones at the beginning of the group. Require members to leave the room if they need to take a call or use their phone for texting or other purposes

profound. In revolving open-ended groups, individual group members episodically terminate and new members join and the process repeats itself. In contrast to traditional group therapy, in which contact between group members outside the group setting is often discouraged, in support groups relationships beyond the group are often encouraged.

Description of Parent Support Groups

Support groups are typically affiliated or linked with social agencies, larger formal organizations, or consumer organizations (e.g., community mental health agencies, a local National Alliance on Mental Illness chapter, a hospital, a residential facility). The affiliation often provides the groups with financial and professional support, resources, recognition, and legitimacy, as well as referral of new members. Mental health professionals or agencies are the most common referral sources for family support groups (Heller et al. 1997).

Support groups for parents of children with emotional disorders can vary greatly in membership, format, and longevity (Koroloff and Friesen 1991). Groups can be professionally led and sponsored by a specific agency or can be completely consumer driven. Regardless of who leads the group, the support group facilitator has several roles to fulfill for the group to be successful, which are outlined in Table 40–12. Common issues the facilitator must handle during a support group include most of those listed in Table 40–11 for psychoeducation groups. One of the most difficult tasks is moderating parental sharing during discussion, especially making sure that other group members are not overwhelmed. In regard to such sharing, problems could arise in several ways: 1) members feeling reluctant to share enough to allow an appropriate response or to fit in as one of the group (playing the observer role too long), 2) members sharing too much and scaring others or inducing guilt that they "do not have it so bad," 3) members developing a "more unfortunate than thou" contest, and 4) members sharing successes to the extent that others feel inferior. Note that these are problems of quantity, not quality, and can be moderated or titrated by an astute group leader. For example, in the first situation, the leader could comment that it seems difficult for that parent to talk about family problems and ask a more forthcoming group member to describe how hard it was to begin sharing. Additional group members could then be encouraged to comment on the topic of how hard it is to begin opening up.

Regardless of the type of support group, facilitators generally follow the same meeting format. The facilitator starts the meeting by introducing himself or herself and describing the purpose and expectations of the group. Group guidelines are then outlined and include confidentiality, accepting other members, and being nonjudgmental. Then all present may introduce themselves for the benefit of new members. Next, the meeting core begins with either open discussion or individual extended turns. The meeting's discussion topic may be decided by the members, or there may be a predetermined topic for the session. The meeting is concluded with a summary of the discussion and a reminder of the next meeting date.

Internet support groups have recently emerged as another option for parents in need of support and information. They are often available on the Web sites of disorder-specific organizations (Table 40–13). A survey of caregivers of chil-

TABLE 40–12. Role and tasks of a support group facilitator

Manage logistics	Secure meeting location, set meeting date, arrange for refreshments, remind members of dates
Promote the group	Raise awareness in the community about the group; increase membership
Moderate member sharing during the meeting	Ensure all members have an opportunity to share and no one monopolizes the discussion
Listen	Be an attentive and empathic listener for all members
Assess when members may need more help	Recognize members who need more help than the group can provide
Create a safe environment	Ensure members do not feel threatened or uncomfortable sharing; stress confidentiality
Refer members to resources	Have knowledge about local resources to which to refer members

TABLE 40–13. Support groups and Internet resources

Organizations

- American Self-Help Group Clearinghouse: Self-Help Group Sourcebook Online, http://mentalhelp.net/selfhelp
- Anxiety and Depression Association of America (ADAA), www.adaa.org
- Autism Society, www.autism-society.org
- Children and Adults With Attention-Deficit/Hyperactivity Disorder (CHADD), www.chadd.org
- Depression and Bipolar Support Alliance (DBSA), www.dbsalliance.org
- Learning Disabilities Association of America (LDA), www.ldaamerica.org
- Mental Health America (MHA), www.mentalhealthamerica.net
- National Alliance on Mental Illness (NAMI), www.nami.org
- National Institute of Mental Health (NIMH), www.nimh.nih.gov
- Substance Abuse and Mental Health Services Administration (SAMHSA), www.samhsa.gov

Publications

- Carlson H: *The Courage to Lead: Start Your Own Support Group—Mental Illnesses and Addictions.* Branford, CT, Bick Publishing House, 2001
- Kurtz LF: *Self-Help and Support Groups: A Handbook for Practitioners.* Thousand Oaks, CA, Sage, 1997
- Nichols K, Jenkinson J: *Leading a Support Group: A Practical Guide.* New York, Open University Press, 2006
- Schiff HS: *The Support Group Manual: A Session-by-Session Guide.* New York, Penguin, 1996

dren with early onset bipolar disorder reported that the main advantage of online support groups is convenience (Hellander et al. 2003). Groups are always available; parents can go online in their homes and receive immediate information and support. Additionally, some parents indicated that the anonymity of online interaction was more comfortable than face-to-face interaction. However, one small study found no significant differences in child mood or anxiety symptoms, parenting stress, or positive perceptions in parents of children with autism spectrum disorders who participated in an online support group compared with a no-treatment comparison group (Clifford and Minnes 2013), although parents in the support group reported that the group was helpful and were satisfied with support from the group.

Regardless of format, common problems with parent support groups are frequent dropouts and low membership, which can threaten the group's longevity. Common reasons for dropouts include child care issues, not having enough time to attend, no longer finding the group helpful, having problems with transportation and parking, experiencing inadequate leadership, and lacking comfort with other members (Heller et al. 1997). Ironically, children in crisis can also prevent parents from attending support groups when they need it most. These challenges must all be considered and addressed by group facilitators in order for a parent support group to thrive.

Benefits of Parent Support Groups

Parent support groups can lead to positive outcomes in three ways. First, interaction with other parents of children with mental illness can be informative, relieving, and therapeutic. Through this interactive process, friendships and social connections form that can help improve parental mental health. Connecting with other parents in a similar situation helps parents feel less isolated and allows them to share and compare experiences, which is often a type of support that other family and friends cannot provide (Kerr and McIntosh 2000).

Second, the interaction of parents with differing levels of knowledge and experience with their child's mental illness provides a forum for knowledge and skill building. Parents can learn from each other's experiences with managing their children's symptoms, seeking services, and juggling responsibilities. One study found that parents who were involved in support groups reported more use of information and services than did parents who were not involved in support groups (Koroloff and Friesen 1991).

Third, parent support groups can help families develop effective advocacy skills and become more active in advocacy efforts. Besides advocating for their own child, parents often become involved in advocating for better overall services at the community, state, or national level for all children with mental illness. As a result of these three benefits of support groups, parents are likely to be more comfortable in their roles as caregiver and case manager for their mentally ill child.

Research on Parent Support Groups for Children's Mental Health

Little research has been conducted on the effects of support group membership on parents of children with serious emotional or behavioral disturbances. Research on these parent support groups is difficult because of continually changing membership, inability to assign members in an experimental design, and difficulty accessing groups (King et al. 2000). Below are summaries of a few studies.

- One study explored the experience of implementing a parent support group in a children's inpatient psychiatric hospitalization setting (Slowik et al. 2004). This open group met for 1 hour every 2 weeks for 9 months during the family visiting time. Each group meeting had three to seven members in attendance. Many discussion themes emerged in the groups, including the effects of the hospitalization on parents and siblings, relationships with and attitudes toward professionals, positive coping strategies, and the effects and usefulness of the group. As a result of attending the group, parents felt less isolated and began to support each other and not rely exclusively on the experts. Parents also felt the doctors were more approachable at the group meetings. Doctors found it beneficial to interact with family members in a less formal setting and often learned more about the parents' experiences. Unit staff had to address several difficulties in setting up and running the group, including opposition from other staff, timing of the group, and engaging and maintaining a sufficient number of parents.

- As part of an outpatient treatment program, another study evaluated the benefits gained from parent participation in a support group for adolescents with eating disorders (Pasold et al. 2010). The open-ended parent support group was held weekly at the same time as the patient psychotherapy group and was co-facilitated by two professionals. The groups included discussion of personal experiences in addition to psychoeducation provided by the facilitators. Evaluation surveys were completed by 261 parents or guardians, and results indicated high parent satisfaction with the group. Parents reported that the group was a source of emotional support and that it helped them understand eating disorder symptoms and treatment and how to support their child.
- Focusing on structure and organization rather than outcomes, a qualitative study conducted interviews and observed support groups to learn more about support groups for parents of children with special needs (King et al. 2000). Interviews were conducted with 20 parents, and six group meetings were observed. The study found that challenges for groups include encouraging new leaders, attracting new members, obtaining funds or assistance to support their activities, and meeting the changing needs of members. Characteristics associated with group longevity included committed and effective leadership, community connections providing needed funds and practical assistance, and group members' willingness to change the group to meet changing needs.

Research has been conducted primarily in restrictive settings such as hospitals and residential placements, as groups in these settings are more readily accessible. Little research is available on support groups with a self-help format run by members, most likely because of the difficulty in accessing these groups. However, the studies described here do reveal that parents felt more knowledgeable and supported and less stressed following participation in parent support groups. Several studies examined support groups that incorporated education into their programs; therefore, it is difficult to separate out the unique benefit of the support, per se. Overall, the combination of support and education can be a powerful tool to help parents of children with mental illness.

Conclusion

Parent counseling, psychoeducation, and parent support groups all provide parents with support from professionals or from other parents in similar situations. These interventions aim to educate parents about their children's mental illness and how to manage and treat it. All these approaches view parents as essential to child outcomes and recognize parents as experts on their own family. They also encourage parents to take care of their own health to better help their child. Overall, these parent interventions focus on improving the mental health of children by focusing on the knowledge, beliefs, and behaviors of the parents. Together, these parent approaches paired with other treatment such as medication, psychotherapy, and school services can help to decrease the negative impact of symptoms and improve the quality of life for children and adolescents suffering from mental illness.

Summary Points

- Parent intervention is as important as child intervention because parents are responsible for recognizing and addressing their child's needs.
- Parent counseling and psychoeducation are adjunctive educational interventions aimed at providing parents with the knowledge and skills needed to be effective caregivers and case managers for their child with emotional or behavioral disorders.
- Research on parent psychoeducation has been promising, with positive parent and child outcomes, but more randomized controlled studies are needed.
- Parent support groups provide parents the opportunity to interact with and receive informational and emotional support from other parents in similar situations.
- Most research on parent support groups has occurred in restrictive placements such as hospitals and residential care. Studies have tentatively demonstrated that a combination of support and education can lead to positive outcomes for children in these settings. More research is needed on support groups in other settings.
- Parent interventions should be combined with other family or child-focused interventions—such as family therapy, individual therapy, medication, and school services—to systemically address the symptoms and impairment caused by the child's disorder.

References

Anderson CM, Hogarty GE, Reiss DJ: Family treatment of adult schizophrenic patients: a psycho-educational approach. Schizophr Bull 6(3):490–505, 1980 7403810

Arnold LE (ed): Helping Parents Help Their Children. New York, Brunner/Mazel, 1978

Asarnow JR, Goldstein MJ, Tompson M, et al: One-year outcomes of depressive disorders in child psychiatric in-patients: evaluation of the prognostic power of a brief measure of expressed emotion. J Child Psychol Psychiatry 34(2):129–137, 1993 8444988

Bennett T, DeLuca DA, Allen RW: Families of children with disabilities: positive adaptation across the life cycle. Children & Schools 18:31–44, 1996

Boylan K, Macpherson HA, Fristad MA: Examination of disruptive behavior outcomes and moderation in a randomized psychotherapy trial for mood disorders. J Am Acad Child Adolesc Psychiatry 52(7):699–708, 2013 23800483

Bradley SJ, Jadaa DA, Brody J, et al: Brief psychoeducational parenting program: an evaluation and 1-year follow-up. J Am Acad Child Adolesc Psychiatry 42(10):1171–1178, 2003 14560166

Brown GW, Birley JL, Wing JK: Influence of family life on the course of schizophrenic disorders: a replication. Br J Psychiatry 121(562):241–258, 1972 5073778

Burkhouse KL, Uhrlass DJ, Stone LB, et al: Expressed emotion-criticism and risk of depression onset in children. J Clin Child Adolesc Psychol 41(6):771–777, 2012 22838507

Citron M, Solomon P, Draine J: Self-help groups for families of persons with mental illness: perceived benefits of helpfulness. Community Ment Health J 35(1):15–30, 1999 10094507

Clifford T, Minnes P: Logging on: evaluating an online support group for parents of children with autism spectrum disorders. J Autism Dev Disord 43(7):1662–1675, 2013 23143075

Copping VE, Warling DL, Benner DG, et al: A child trauma treatment pilot study. J Child Fam Stud 10(4):467–475, 2001

Davidson KH, Fristad MA: The Hand-to-Family Education Program: a means of reducing parental stress and increasing support in families of children with brain disorders. Child Adolesc Psychopharmacol News 9(2):7–9, 2004

Ferrin M, Moreno-Granados JM, Salcedo-Marin MD, et al: Evaluation of a psychoeducation programme for parents of children and adolescents with ADHD: immediate and long-term effects using a blind randomized controlled trial. Eur Child Adolesc Psychiatry 23(8):637–647, 2014 24292412

Friesen BJ, Koroloff NM: Family centered services: implications for mental health administration and research. J Ment Health Adm 17(1):13–25, 1990 10104410

Fristad MA: Psychoeducational treatment for school-aged children with bipolar disorder. Dev Psychopathol 18(4):1289–1306, 2006 17064439

Fristad MA, Gavazzi SM, Centolella DM, et al: Psychoeducation: a promising intervention strategy for families of children and adolescents with mood disorders. Contemp Fam Ther 18(3):371–384, 1996

Fristad MA, Gavazzi SM, Soldano KW: Naming the enemy: Learning to differentiate mood disorder "symptoms" from the "self" that experiences them. J Fam Psychother 10(1):81–88, 1999

Fristad MA, Gavazzi SM, Mackinaw-Koons B: Family psychoeducation: an adjunctive intervention for children with bipolar disorder. Biol Psychiatry 53(11):1000–1008, 2003a 12788245

Fristad MA, Goldberg-Arnold JS, Gavazzi SM: Multi-family psychoeducation groups in the treatment of children with mood disorders. J Marital Fam Ther 29(4):491–504, 2003b 14593691

Fristad MA, Verducci JS, Walters K, et al: Impact of multifamily psychoeducational psychotherapy in treating children aged 8 to 12 years with mood disorders. Arch Gen Psychiatry 66(9):1013–1021, 2009 19736358

Geist R, Heinmaa M, Stephens D, et al: Comparison of family therapy and family group psychoeducation in adolescents with anorexia nervosa. Can J Psychiatry 45(2):173–178, 2000 10742877

Goldberg-Arnold JS, Fristad MA, Gavazzi SM: Family psychoeducation: giving caregivers what they want and need. Fam Relat 48(4):411–417, 1999

Goldstein MJ, Rodnick EH, Evans JR, et al: Drug and family therapy in the aftercare of acute schizophrenics. Arch Gen Psychiatry 35(10):1169–1177, 1978 211983

Hellander M, Sisson DP, Fristad MA: Internet support for parents of children with early onset bipolar disorder, in Bipolar Disorder in Childhood and Early Adolescence. Edited by Geller B, DelBello M. New York, Guilford, 2003, pp 314–329

Heller T, Roccoforte JA, Hsieh KF, et al: Benefits of support groups for families of adults with severe mental illness. Am J Orthopsychiatry 67(2):187–198, 1997 9142352

Holtkamp K, Herpertz-Dahlmann B, Vloet T, et al: Group psychoeducation for parents of adolescents with eating disorders: the Aachen program. Eat Disord 13(4):381–390, 2005 16864352

Kerr SM, McIntosh JB: Coping when a child has a disability: exploring the impact of parent-to-parent support. Child Care Health Dev 26(4):309–322, 2000 10931070

King G, Stewart D, King S, et al: Organizational characteristics and issues affecting the longevity of self-help groups for parents of children with special needs. Qual Health Res 10(2):225–241, 2000 10788285

Koroloff NM, Friesen BJ: Support groups for parents of children with emotional disorders: a comparison of members and non-members. Community Ment Health J 27(4):265–279, 1991 1864076

Lopez MA, Toprac MG, Crismon ML, et al: A psychoeducational program for children with ADHD or depression and their families: results from the CMAP feasibility study. Community Ment Health J 41(1):51–66, 2005 15932052

Lukens EP, McFarlane WR: Psychoeducation as evidence-based practice: considerations for practice, research, and policy. Brief Treatment and Crisis Intervention 4:205–225, 2004

MacPherson HA, Fristad MA, Leffler JM: Implementation of Multi-Family Psychoeducational Psychotherapy for childhood mood disorders in an outpatient community setting. J Marital Fam Ther 40(2):193–211, 2014a

MacPherson HA, Algorta GP, Mendenhall AN, et al: Predictors and moderators in the randomized trial of multifamily psychoeducational psychotherapy for childhood mood disorders. J Clin Child Adolesc Psychol 43(3):459–472, 2014b 23795823

McFarlane WR, Link B, Dushay R, et al: Psychoeducational multiple family groups: four-year relapse outcome in schizophrenia. Fam Process 34:127–144, 1995 7589414

Mendenhall AN, Fristad MA: Psychoeducational approaches to children with bipolar disorder, in Bipolar Disorder: A Developmental Psychopathology Approach. Edited by Miklowitz DJ, Cicchetti D. New York, Guilford, 2010, pp 494–521

Mendenhall AN, Fristad MA, Early TJ: Factors influencing service utilization and mood symptom severity in children with mood disorders: effects of multifamily psychoeducation groups (MFPGs). J Consult Clin Psychol 77(3):463–473, 2009 19485588

Miklowitz DJ, Goldstein MJ: The effectiveness of psychoeducation family therapy in the treatment of schizophrenic disorders. J Marital Fam Ther 21(4):361–376, 1995

Miklowitz DJ, Axelson DA, Birmaher B, et al: Family focused treatment for adolescents with bipolar disorder: results of a 2-year randomized trial. Arch Gen Psychiatry 65(9):1053–1061, 2008 18762591

Miklowitz DJ, Schneck CD, Singh MK, et al: Early intervention for symptomatic youth at risk for bipolar disorder: a randomized trial of family focused therapy. J Am Acad Child Adolesc Psychiatry 52(2):121–131, 2013 23357439

Norcross JC: Here comes the self-help revolution in mental health. Psychotherapy 37(4):370–377, 2000

O'Brien MP, Miklowitz DJ, Candan KA, et al: A randomized trial of family focused therapy with populations at clinical high risk for psychosis: effects on interactional behavior. J Consult Clin Psychol 82(1):90–101, 2014 24188511

Pasold TL, Boateng BA, Portilla MG: The use of a parent support group in the outpatient treatment of children and adolescents with eating disorders. Eat Disord 18(4):318–332, 2010 20603732

Pavuluri MN, Graczyk PA, Henry DB, et al: Child- and family-focused cognitive-behavioral therapy for pediatric bipolar disorder: development and preliminary results. J Am Acad Child Adolesc Psychiatry 43(5):528–537, 2004 15100559

Pollio DE, McClendon JB, North CS, et al: The promise of school-based psychoeducation for parents of children with emotional disorders. Children & Schools 27:111–115, 2005

Roberts LJ, Salem D, Rappaport J, et al: Giving and receiving help: interpersonal transactions in mutual-help meetings and psychosocial adjustment of members. Am J Community Psychol 27(6):841–868, 1999 10723537

Ruffolo MC, Kuhn MT, Evans ME: Support, empowerment, and education: a study of multifamily group psychoeducation. J Emot Behav Disord 13(4):200–212, 2005

Sanford M, Boyle M, McCleary L, et al: A pilot study of adjunctive family psychoeducation in adolescent major depression: feasibility and treatment effect. J Am Acad Child Adolesc Psychiatry 45(4):386–495, 2006 16601642

Shulman L: The Skills of Helping: Individuals, Families, and Groups. Itasca, IL, FE Peacock, 1992

Sloper P: Models of service support for parents of disabled children. What do we know? What do we need to know? Child Care Health Dev 25(2):85–99, 1999 10188064

Slowik M, Willson SW, Loh EC, et al: Service innovations: developing a parent/carer support group in an in-patient adolescent setting. Psychiatr Bull 28:177–179, 2004

Smith TE, Sells SP, Rodman J, et al: Reducing adolescent substance abuse and delinquency: pilot research of a family orientated psychoeducation curriculum. J Child Adolesc Subst Abuse 15(4):105–115, 2006

CHAPTER 41

Behavioral Parent Training

Linda J. Pfiffner, Ph.D.
Nina M. Kaiser, Ph.D.

Theoretical Underpinnings and Key Concepts

Behavior therapy has a long history of success in treating childhood problems. This approach is based on several core assumptions that highlight methodological rigor, empirical evaluation, a focus on observable behaviors as the most beneficial targets of intervention, and the importance of behavioral assessment in both design and ongoing evaluation of treatment plans. Behavior therapy approaches emphasize the importance of environmental and social contingencies in fostering and maintaining problem behavior—that is, *contingency theory* (Patterson 1982). Contingency-based behavioral interventions involve one or more of four key concepts: behavior is increased either by following it with something desirable (*positive reinforcement*) or by removing something undesirable (*negative reinforcement*); behavior is decreased either by following it with something undesirable (*punishment*) or by removing something desirable (*extinction*). Current behavioral treatments also draw from social learning theory (Bandura 1977), which incorporates contingency theory into a more general model that also includes modeling and imitation and cognitive factors (e.g., cognitive appraisals and attributions).

Behavioral interventions usually begin with a *functional behavior analysis,* which involves specifying behaviors (positive behaviors to increase or negative behaviors to decrease) and then identifying each behavior's antecedents (variables setting the stage for or preceding the behavior) and consequences (variables maintaining the behavior). On the basis of this analysis, specific strategies for modifying antecedents and consequences are selected for a behavioral intervention plan with the goal of reducing problem behavior and promoting desired behavior. Maximally effective behavioral interventions consider the function of the problem behavior when attempting to reduce it. For example, if a child exhibits disruptive behavior in order to gain parental attention, a behavioral intervention might teach the child to gain attention through more appropriate behavior and reinforce this appropriate behavior when it occurs. Generally, the behavioral approach to intervention selects target behaviors for treatment that cause impairment in daily living (e.g., academic, social behavior) rather than targeting diagnostic symptoms per se, although it is important to note that these interventions often do have powerful direct and indirect effects on diagnostic symptoms. A behavioral approach can be very effective in modifying behavior and improving overall adjustment, whatever the underlying disorder.

Behavior therapy has been applied to a wide variety of childhood problems and within multiple different settings. Our main focus in this chapter will be on behavioral parent training (BPT), one of the most widely used forms of behavior therapy for disruptive behavior problems (also variously referred to as parent management training, parent training, or behavioral family therapy). In this approach, the therapist teaches parents skills to improve the quality of family relationships, promote positive child behaviors, and decrease child deviant behaviors. We include information about core components of parent training as well as adjunctive interventions used to address problems at school, with peers, and in the family system.

Rationale for Using Parent Training With Disruptive Behavior Disorders

Parent training programs are based largely on theory and data showing that families with a child displaying behavior problems tend to exhibit dysfunctional parent-child interaction patterns. One prominent pattern, described by Patterson (1982), is referred to as the *coercive process* and specifies that families with children having behavior problems learn to control one another through negative reinforcement. More specifically, children exhibit negative behaviors to the parent and the parent responds aversively to this behavior; this type of response from the parent in turn leads to an escalation of the child's negative behavior and so on until either the parent or the child gives in to the demands of the other, thereby reinforcing the other's negative behavior. One example of this type of pattern might be a child learning that unwanted parental demands (e.g., to do chores or homework) might be withdrawn if he or she provides a counterattack (e.g., arguing, refusing, exhibiting high levels of negative affect). Alternatively, a parent who discovers that the child complies when the parent engages in yelling or other extremely aversive behavior is more likely to employ this type of behavior in the future. Observational studies of family interaction (Dishion et al. 1991; Patterson et al. 1992) show that disrupted family management skills, most notably parent discipline and monitoring, appear to be key factors in antisocial behavior development. Subsequent studies consistently have found that problematic parenting practices (e.g., overly negative and controlling, lacking in warmth and positive involvement) are strongly related to disruptive behavior disorders (Johnston and Mash 2001). The importance of maladaptive parenting practices in perpetuating disruptive behavior problems is underscored by findings that the adverse effects of contextual factors on children such as stress, social disadvantage, divorce, and/or parent depression are mediated largely by these practices (Patterson et al. 1992).

Child behavior problems most commonly addressed by parent training map onto the DSM-5 diagnoses of attention-deficit hyperactivity disorder (ADHD; classified under neurodevelopmental disorders) and oppositional defiant disorder and/or conduct disorder (classified under disruptive, impulse-control, and conduct disorders). For this chapter, we refer to this triad of disorders as disruptive behavior disorders (DBDs). Parent training for DBDs is supported by extensive data that children with these problems show dysfunctional responses to usual contingencies that disrupt these children's ability to regulate behavior according to typical consequences (for a review, see Luman et al. 2005). More specifically, because of a weak inhibition system, children with DBDs display a lack of sensitivity to partial reinforcement, elevated reward thresholds, a marked aversion to delays in reinforcement, and less avoidance of or caution toward cues of punishment or nonreward. Children with conduct disorder have a reward-dominant style, in which their behavior is motivated more by the possibility of gaining a reward than avoiding punishment. Together, these findings suggest that the families of children with DBDs are likely to benefit from parent training precisely because of this approach's focus on modification of external contingencies, such as use of consistent, salient, and immediate rewards; well-delivered negative consequences; clear rules and directions; and predictable routines.

Parent training programs also can address attachment deficiencies between children and their parents. Lower levels of attachment are theorized to lead to emotional dysregulation and a lack of mutual responsiveness between parent and child (Harwood and Eyberg 2004; Herschell et al. 2002). Parent training addresses these emotional factors by fostering responsiveness, communication, and nurturance between parent and child. These processes in turn enable the child to develop secure attachments with others and improved emotional regulation.

Models of Parent Training

Models for delivering parent training involve a therapist working with parents to teach a variety of behavioral strategies; the parents then apply these strategies at home. Troubleshooting the use of each strategy occurs within the context of each individual family during each therapy session. Parent training may be offered in combination with behavioral school consultation and/or with child-focused interventions, such as skill-building groups or cognitive-behavioral interventions.

Parent training can be administered individually with parents, with families (parents and children together), or in groups of parents. The group format may be especially useful for parents who would benefit from receiving support from and/or sharing ideas with other parents. Reluctant parents often become more open to using a strategy after hearing firsthand about the success another parent has had with that particular strategy. However, not all parents benefit equally from a group experience. Groups seem to be most useful when members share very similar problems. Working with the individual family is indicated when more intensive and tailored interventions are needed; this may be the case when there are very severe child problems, for parents who have interpersonal styles that would be difficult for a group, or when a slower pace is desirable. In some cases, individual sessions interspersed with the group meetings are helpful.

Parent training is intended to be time limited. The number of sessions typically varies from 6 to 12, with some programs lasting as long as 20–25 weeks; duration generally depends on the severity of the problems and developmental level of the child (Kazdin 1997; McMahon and Forehand 2005; Webster-Stratton et al. 2004). During sessions, the therapist presents specific strategies, discusses their rationale, has parents practice the skills (e.g., via role-plays), and instructs parents to implement the skills at home with their child between sessions. If therapists opt to have parents practice skills in vivo with their child(ren), parents can be observed and coached by having the parents wear a "bug-in-the-ear" (wireless ear piece with radio transmission) while the therapist is behind a one-way mirror; alternatively, in-room coaching can be effective with young children. Programs in which parents observe videotaped examples of effective and ineffective parenting strategies with opportunity for discussion of the strategies also have substantial research support for efficacy (Webster-Stratton et al. 2004). Parent training has been successfully delivered remotely via weekly telephone coaching sessions (McGrath et al. 2011) and videoconferencing (Reese et al. 2012).

Recent innovations in smartphone technology also have been applied to parent training. For example, Jones et al. (2014) developed a technology-enhanced version of Helping the Noncompliant Child (McMahon and Forehand 2005) that incorporated videos of parenting skills, tracking of daily skill use, video call check-ins, videotaped home practice for review and feedback, and text message reminders of home practice. Enhancements like these appear to improve the parent's engagement in treatment and, as a result, improve child outcomes.

Baseline Assessments Prior to Starting Treatment

Initial assessments typically include the usual diagnostic work-up and gathering of information about functional impairment at home, at school, and with peers. This information ideally is obtained from the child's parents and teachers using a combination of empirically based and standardized rating scales, as well as more qualitative measures, including direct observation of the family interactions or school functioning (if possible). However, it is important to emphasize that behavioral forms of treatment are guided more by functional analysis of behavior and less by a diagnosis or symptoms per se. Therefore, parents typically are asked questions at the initiation of parent training about the frequency and specific types of behaviors of concern, as well as the antecedents (e.g., when they occur) and consequences (e.g., what happens after they occur) of each problem behavior. Parents often keep a chart of these behaviors during the first week or two prior to starting a behavior plan. This chart can then serve as a baseline for comparison after specific strategies are implemented in order to determine if the program is having its intended effect. Assessment of target behaviors continues throughout behavioral treatment as an important guide to decision making about which strategies are most effective for each family.

Setting Treatment Goals

In behavioral approaches, setting goals for treatment is an individualized and collaborative process between parent and therapist. Usually, the parents' initial goal simply involves modifying the child's behavior. However, in parent training, treatment goals include the parents changing their own behavior. Although this goal does not always need to be explicitly stated, some discussion of this issue usually is helpful. It is important that the therapist communicates to the parents that they are not being blamed for their child's difficulties. Instead, parents are told that children's difficulties are multiply determined (including biological and environmental factors) and that children with behavioral challenges are more difficult to parent. The goal is to find the best "fit" between their child's personality and their parenting practices. We often tell parents of children having behavioral concerns that there is a need to become "superparents," providing a structured "superenvironment" that is more demanding than what average parents need to manage their children.

Initial treatment goals are set at levels that ensure that both the child and the parent experience some success at the outset (and consequently are motivated to continue). Thus, initial target behaviors and parenting strategies taught are relatively simple and easy to change (e.g., positive attention during nonconfrontational situations, compliance with nonprovocative commands). At treatment onset, parents typically are encouraged to target only one or two behaviors for change. A shaping process is then used so that as initial goals are reached, more difficult or complex behaviors and skills are added. Behaviors important to the child's family, social, and academic functioning generally are included as primary goals (e.g., following directions the first time asked, completing chores, completing homework, playing well with siblings), and both prosocial and antisocial behaviors are included. After parents have obtained some success with home-based targets, treatment goals may be expanded to incorporate problem behavior outside the home or with other adults.

Core Session Topics

Although a number of different approaches to parent training exist, all approaches generally involve some combination of the core topics we describe in Appendix 41–1 at the end of this chapter. Different approaches vary somewhat in the session time that is allocated to each topic, the order in which topics are presented, and/or supplemental topics that are also covered by the treatment package. In addition, we note that clinicians may pick and choose specific topics to be covered on the basis of differences in the problems with which a given child and family present. For example, we have found that parents of children who are particularly impulsive or oppositional tend to need more instruction on effective discipline than do parents of children with mostly attentional problems. For each topic, we discuss and troubleshoot common parental concerns and questions.

Please note that we intend our descriptions of session topics to serve as an educational overview of each topic rather than step-by-step instructions. We reference a variety of excellent treatment manuals throughout this chapter that provide more explicit information on conducting BPT, and we encourage those interested in implementing this type of intervention to consult these manuals for further guidance.

Psychoeducation and Background Information

Overview

The first session of BPT generally involves providing parents with background information and psychoeducation regarding childhood behavior problems, family interactions, and behavior therapy (see Appendix 41–1). In addition, parents are introduced to the antecedent-behavior-consequence (ABC) model of behavior that sets the framework for all topics presented in this chapter.

Troubleshooting

As mentioned in the subsection "Setting Treatment Goals," one question that often arises relates to why parents (as opposed to the child) participate in treatment, as the child is the identified patient. In response to these concerns, therapists typically acknowledge that the temperaments of children with externalizing problems make these children more difficult to parent; consequently, parent training is presented as a way for parents to obtain additional strategies for their parenting toolboxes that will help them more effectively manage their child's behavior. In addition, it may be helpful to briefly describe research literature suggesting that parent-focused intervention is more effective than are child-focused treatments alone, likely at least in part as a result of core skill deficits underlying child behavior problems.

Attending and Ignoring

Overview

The focus of this session is on improving the parent-child relationship, under the assumption that 1) this relationship has been impaired by negative parent-child interaction cycles and 2) children are more likely to comply with parental instructions in the context of a positive parent-child relationship. Parents thus are taught to spend "special time" with their child during which they actively attend to their child's behavior (see Appendix 41–1). After parents master this skill, they learn to generalize the attending skill and differentially attend to positive behaviors they would like to see increase and ignore negative behaviors that they aim to decrease.

Troubleshooting

During discussion of attending and ignoring, parents may raise the following concerns:

- *Why shouldn't I ask questions, praise my child, or be directive during special time?*

  Parents are encouraged to let the child direct the activity to the greatest extent possible in order for the child to feel that the activity is most pleasant and validating. Asking questions, praising, and redirecting the child all are subtle ways of controlling the situation and consequently are to be avoided during the attending/special time exercise.
- *How should I deal with misbehavior?*

  Parents are encouraged to ignore mild misbehavior during special time. Obviously, however, it is inappropriate to ignore behaviors that are unsafe, and parents should employ their usual system of consequences to cope with any such behaviors that occur.
- *How will I find time? What about my other kids?*

  Parents are encouraged to practice attending even if the special time lasts only for brief periods of time (5–10 minutes) or in the context of an activity that the child already is doing. Often, looking for opportunities to practice attending (rather than scheduling attending as a separate event) feels more manageable to parents. Parents with multiple children may find that all children are eager to have parents do attending with them; if this is the case, parents may choose to do special time with one child on one day and another child the next day.

- *I'm ignoring, but my child's behavior is getting worse!*

  It is important to warn parents that with ignoring, behaviors generally get worse before they get better; because the child often escalates in an attempt to obtain the parents' attention, the most unbearable behavior often occurs immediately before the child gives up. Once the child begins to behave appropriately, the parent is directed to resume attending.

Praise and Positive Reinforcement

Overview

As negative behavior generally is much more salient to parents than positive behavior, parents often unintentionally ignore positive behaviors when these behaviors do occur. Session content consequently focuses on reinforcing and rewarding positive behavior with praise and tangible reinforcers such as activities or token prizes (see Appendix 41–1).

Troubleshooting

The following issues or concerns may come up during a discussion of praise and positive reinforcement:

- *Giving rewards feels like bribing my child for things that he or she should be doing anyway.*

  Therapists may wish to point out that the child is not doing the task at the moment and that use of positive reinforcement can be helpful in getting the child to complete the task (and can consequently be faded out over time). It also may be useful to draw a parallel between this type of positive reinforcement and that experienced by parents in the workforce, few of whom likely would go to work if they were not paid.

- *My child is upping the ante and saying things like "I'll do it if you get me...."*

  Parents are encouraged to provide rewards only in the context of structured reward programs, as opposed to spontaneous rewards (particularly in situations in which the child is trying to manipulate the situation in order to obtain a reward). Giving in to this kind of request makes it more likely to happen in the future.

Token Economy or Point System

Overview

A crucial component of parent training programs for parents of school-age children involves working with parents to establish a home reward system in which the child earns tokens, points, or privileges for positive behavior; the child then can cash in earned tokens or points for activities or token reinforcers (see Appendix 41–1 and Figure 41–1).

Case Example 1: Token Economy/Shaping and Fading/Integrating Home Challenge and Classroom Challenge

Melissa, a 7-year-old girl, was brought in to the clinic by her parents, Mr. and Mrs. Smith. The Smiths' primary concern was Melissa's need

NAME: Melissa S.

DATE:____________

	DAY				
TARGET BEHAVIORS	**Monday**	**Tuesday**	**Wednesday**	**Thursday**	**Friday**
Home Target Behavior Getting ready in the morning: (5 points each) 1. Out of bed by 7:00 2. Dressed by 7:15 3. Breakfast by 7:45 4. Brush teeth by 7:55 5. Get backpack and ready to leave for school by 8:05					
Daily Report Card Points					
TOTAL Points					
WEEKLY TOTAL	____ **points**				

Possible Daily Earnings = 40 points

Daily Rewards:	***Game with parent**	**10 points/15 minutes**
	***8:30 bedtime**	**15 points**
	***TV Time**	**20 points/30 minutes**
Weekly Rewards:	***Dinner out**	**60 points**
	***Trip to park**	**40 points/1 hour**
	***Go to movie**	**80 points**

FIGURE 41–1. Sample token economy for Melissa.

for excessive supervision when completing morning routine tasks, which made the entire family late to school and work on almost a daily basis; the Smiths indicated that they currently were giving Melissa four or more reminders for each task she needed to accomplish in the morning. In addition, Melissa's teacher reported that Melissa had difficulty completing her work independently in the classroom and that she required reminders to stay seated appropriately during class time. Mr. and Mrs. Smith set up a token economy system with five specific target behaviors for Melissa to accomplish during morning routine (see Figure 41–1). Melissa could earn 5 points for each behavior that she completed with two or fewer reminders from her parents, for a total of 25 points per day. In addition, Melissa's teacher agreed to implement a daily behavior report card (Figure 41–2) in the classroom to help Melissa complete her work independently, remain seated during class time, turn in completed homework, and remember to bring the report card to the teacher each day (awarded with a bonus point). Melissa could earn an additional 15 points for successfully performing these behaviors.

Before beginning the program, the Smiths developed a reward menu with Melissa's assistance; as Melissa could earn up to 40 points each school day (for a total of 200 points per week), the Smiths assigned point values to each reward accordingly (see Figure 41–1). After posting the morning routine checklist and implementing the token economy, Mr. and Mrs. Smith reported an immediate improvement in Melissa's compliance with the morning routine. After 2 weeks, Melissa needed only one to two reminders for each morning routine behavior and consequently was regularly earning all 25 possible points every morning. At this point, Mr. and Mrs. Smith decided that because Melissa now was doing so well, they would change the criterion; now, Melissa would need to complete each task with one or fewer reminders in order to earn her points. After Melissa met this goal regularly, the Smiths then required Melissa to complete each morning routine behavior without any reminders in order to earn her points. The Smiths were able to phase out the token economy once Melissa was regularly completing the morning routine checklist independently, although they continued to praise her every morning for getting the checklist done on her own. Melissa's teacher continued to implement the daily behavior report card in the classroom throughout the remainder of the school year.

Troubleshooting

For clinicians, it is important to be aware that token economies are somewhat sensitive interventions, with minor differences in intervention structure often resulting in vastly different outcomes and efficacy (Table 41–1). Consequently, if a token economy is not initially effective, it is important to troubleshoot the intervention rather than to deem it ineffective and discontinue it. One frequent challenge is that parents often want to address a large number of behaviors and end up developing complicated programs that are difficult for the child to understand and for the parents to implement consistently (Table 41–1). It is best for parents to start with a simple system that focuses on increasing three or four positive behaviors and then revise the system as the child responds to the initial demands.

In addition, parents must set the criteria for earning the tokens or rewards low enough that the child is able to regularly obtain rewards; if the behaviors are too difficult relative to the child's current functioning, the child likely will become discouraged and the system will not work.

Name: Melissa S. **Date:** ______

MY CHALLENGE

	TIME		
TARGET BEHAVIORS			
Completed classwork independently	0 1 2	0 1 2	0 1 2
Followed class rules	0 1 2	0 1 2	0 1 2
Turned in completed homework		0 1 2	
Gave challenge to teacher		1 bonus point	
DAILY TOTAL		= _____ **POINTS**	

Point Scale 0 = Needs Improvement
1 = Okay
2 = Super Job

Teacher signature: ____________________

FIGURE 41–2. Sample daily report card for Melissa.

Giving Effective Instructions

Overview

Discussion of effective instructions shifts the focus from the consequences of behaviors to the antecedents of those behaviors. More specifically, parents discuss how to give instructions in a manner that maximizes the chance that the child will comply (see Appendix 41–1).

Troubleshooting

- *What do I do when my child does not comply?*

  Parents often want to jump ahead to a discussion of punishment, particularly in the context of this module, but it is important for them to master giving instructions in a maximally effective manner prior to implementing a punishment for noncompliance. To this end, parents are encouraged simply to practice giving effective instructions and to praise compliance without implementing any particular consequences for noncompliance.

Time-Out

Overview

Time-out, or time away from positive reinforcement (e.g., parental attention, another enjoyable activity) can be a powerful consequence for negative behavior. This session involves reviewing parents' past experiences with time-out, as well as discussion of mechanical and logistical issues of the time-out procedure (see Appendix 41–1 and Figure 41–3).

Case Example 2: Time-Out/Integrating Strategies

Kyle is a 10-year-old boy whose parents, Mr. and Mrs. Miller, reported concerns including aggressive behavior toward his younger sister and noncompliance with parental commands. The Millers decided to employ a time-out procedure to address both of these problem behaviors. They selected a time-out location (in the living room on the sofa, away from any distractions such as

TABLE 41–1. Troubleshooting token economies

Question	Solution
Is the target behavior defined very clearly?	Define target behavior in observable, positive terms.
Is the goal set too high?	Set goal at a level that allows the child to be successful immediately.
Is the child motivated by the reinforcer and not able to have it without earning it?	Make sure the child wants the reinforcer and can get it only when earned.
Does the child understand the program?	Have the child repeat all steps of the program, including goals and reinforcers.
Is the child overly anxious about the program or complaining that it is too hard?	Make sure goals are within the child's reach and ignore the child's complaining if it is intended to get the parents to stop the program.
Is the child interested in the reinforcer?	Make sure the child wants the reinforcer.
Is the reinforcer given immediately and frequently?	Reinforcement needs to occur as often as necessary to ensure goals are met and soon after the behavior.
Are there other factors maintaining the problem behavior (e.g., getting peer attention, getting out of doing work, getting someone else to do it for him or her)?	Address any competing factors directly.
Did the child do well for a while and then start to backslide?	Encourage parents to consider changing consequences to something more meaningful but to be consistent in keeping the program in place.
Are all caretakers supporting the program?	Communicate with caretakers in addition to the parents (e.g., grandparents, babysitters) so that everyone understands the program and can support it.
Did the child start having more problems when the reward program was being faded?	Successfully fading a program is a gradual process (e.g., via gradual increases in requirements for rewards) and should be presented to the child as a positive accomplishment. Expect that some contingencies may always need to be in place for optimal outcomes.

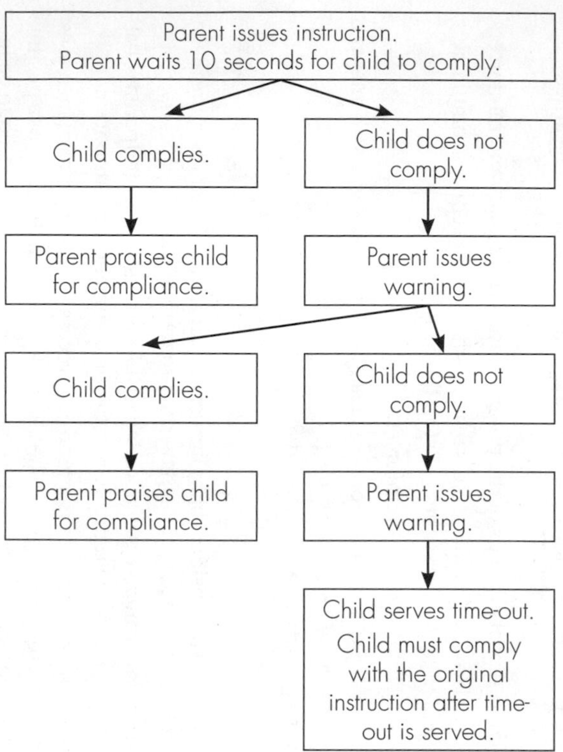

FIGURE 41–3. Time-out flowchart.

TV or toys) and decided that Kyle's time-outs would be 10 minutes long (1 minute for each year of his age). The Millers sat down with Kyle and explained that from now on, every time he displayed aggressive behavior toward his sister (e.g., hitting, kicking, pinching), he would earn an automatic time-out. In addition, Kyle now would be expected to follow parental instructions with only one reminder; if he did not follow the instructions after a warning was provided, he would earn a time-out. If Kyle chose not to serve this time-out, he would not be able to play video games or watch TV for the remainder of the day. Mr. and Mrs. Miller posted these rules on the refrigerator.

Later that day, Kyle was playing video games when Mr. Miller instructed him to pick up his shoes and put them away. Kyle ignored the instruction. After waiting 10 seconds for Kyle to comply, Mr. Miller stated, "I've asked you to pick up your shoes and put them away. If you do not pick up your shoes now, you will earn a 10-minute time-out." Kyle continued to ignore his father. Mr. Miller then informed Kyle that he had earned a 10-minute time-out and should proceed directly to the living room sofa to serve his time-out. When Kyle refused to do so, Mr. Miller calmly reminded Kyle that if he did not serve his time-out, he would be choosing to lose video games and TV for the remainder of the day. Although Kyle grumbled under his breath on his way to time-out, he served the time-out appropriately. At the end of the 10 minutes, Mr. Miller allowed Kyle to leave time-out and instructed him to pick up his shoes. Kyle complied, and then he was able to return to playing video games.

Troubleshooting

The following concerns often come up during a discussion of time-out.

- *I've tried time-out before and it did not work.*

  Discussion about the mechanics of time-out used in the past and how the time-out being recommended may differ from the procedure employed in the past likely will address these concerns. However, therapists should be prepared to troubleshoot the time-out procedure with parents as they implement this strategy at home.
- *What if my child refuses to go to time-out?*

  Parents may handle time-out refusal in one of two ways. First, parents can modify the time-out procedure and use either an escalating or escalating-reducible time-out. In an escalating time-out, the child earns additional time in time-out for each refusal to go to time-out. In an escalating-reducible time-out, the duration of the child's time-out increases each time that he or she refuses to go to time-out, but the child has the chance to earn half off his or her time-out by proceeding to time-out and serving the time-out appropriately. An alternative way to handle time-out refusal involves implementing a back-up consequence, such as removal of a favorite activity, should the child choose not to go to time-out.

Response-Cost Procedures

Overview

Parents also are taught punishment strategies that involve removing tokens, points, or privileges after the child demonstrates target negative behaviors; these strategies can be implemented either within the existing home reward system or separately (see Appendix 41–1).

Troubleshooting

Again, parents may get carried away with the number of behaviors that they want to address. Parents who employ response-cost procedures within the token economy must be cautioned to monitor the reward system in order to ensure that the child continues to earn rewards and remains motivated.

Parents also must be warned about punishment spirals that result in the child losing all of his or her tokens or points or losing activities or toys for unreasonably long periods of time. If a child continues to misbehave after the initial response-cost fine, the parent should implement a back-up consequence instead of continuing to fine the child tokens or points. Further, it may be helpful to discuss children's difficulty estimating time (as well as the fact that if parents take away toys or activities for extended periods of time, they are limiting their future response-cost options should the behavior recur).

Developing a Plan for Homework

Overview

Some programs include one or more sessions that specifically address homework time in the home environment (see Power et al. 2001). Key points of this session generally are related to the development of a plan to increase the structure of the time set aside for homework by making rules for this time explicit, thinking ahead about potential problems, and instituting consequences for specific homework target behaviors (see Appendix 41–1).

Troubleshooting

Children may not clearly record school homework assignments or may not bring home the needed materials. Using a homework assignment notebook containing daily assignments, materials, and due dates is advisable. Children and parents should be made aware of the teacher's procedure for assigning homework, and children should be reinforced for using the homework notebook. The teacher may also sign the notebook each day to ensure accuracy.

Parents also may be somewhat resistant to setting a specific and consistent time for homework in the context of other family activities. Although this is a valid concern, parents should be cautioned that children are likely to be most compliant with a homework hour that occurs at a routine time.

Home-School Report Cards

Overview

Many parent training intervention programs include a session teaching families to develop a daily behavior report card (DRC) targeting between one and four problem behaviors that the teacher fills out and sends home with the child each day (Kelley 1990) (see Appendix 41–1 and Figure 41–2). The child can earn daily rewards at home based on his or her behavior at school. This type of program encourages better communication between parents and teachers and provides the child with incentives for positive behavior in the classroom. Degree of therapist involvement in developing these programs depends on the particular intervention model, as well as the type of service (i.e., group vs. individual treatment) being provided. Some programs include regular school consultation meetings for the duration of treatment, while other programs teach parents how to set up a classroom intervention with limited or no therapist contact with the school. The latter approach is more efficient in use of therapist time and is likely to be successful with reasonably skilled parents and with teachers who already are familiar with the approach.

Troubleshooting

Children may forget to bring home the DRC or fail to bring it home on days with negative ratings. Usually this can be addressed successfully by treating that day as if the target goals were not achieved, and therefore the daily home reward is not earned.

Parents and teachers may select too many behaviors on which to focus or set the bar for rewards too high. As with home-based interventions, home-school report cards must have a manageable number of behaviors (typically between two and four) and permit the child some success.

Finally, teachers may informally expand target behaviors to address more general misbehavior over the course of the intervention rather than adhering to the originally specified operational definitions of DRC goals. Should this be the case, the child may not understand exactly what he or she needs to do in order to be considered successful. Specific, concrete expectations should be set and then consistently adhered to, with any modification or expansion of goals formalized and explicitly explained to the child.

Managing Behavior in Public Places

Overview

Parents often report child misbehavior in public places outside the home setting in which the strategies that they have learned to use at home are not immediately available. Parents are encouraged to anticipate problem behavior by employing the ABC model before entering the public place in order to alter antecedents and minimize the chance that the child will engage in problem behavior (see Appendix 41–1).

Troubleshooting

Parents often raise concerns about feeling embarrassed about their child's misbehavior or about implementing punishment techniques in public; discussion of these concerns often may help parents to be more comfortable and less self-conscious about using available strategies. In the end, however, parents must realistically select strategies that they are willing and able to implement consistently.

When-Then

Overview

In addition to the formal rewards that parents have learned to use in their token economy systems, there are many activities that parents permit children to have for free that also can be used as rewards. During discussion of "Grandma's rule" or Premack contingencies, parents learn to use more desirable activities as reinforcers for the completion of less desirable activities (see Appendix 41–1). For example, a parent might say, "If you do your homework, then you can watch TV." For families struggling to implement a more structured token economy system, a less complex when-then contingency implemented consistently can serve as a more easily administered alternative to a token or point system (e.g., "If you are ready to leave for school by 7:45 A.M., then you can play the iPad in the car on the way to school.").

Troubleshooting

Parents occasionally will attempt to use this strategy with desirable activities that they are not willing to withhold (e.g., family vacations or other outings); it is important to remind parents that they should employ this strategy only when the desired activity is one that they are willing and able to withhold if the child fails to complete the less desirable task.

Planning Ahead

During the final session, parents review the strategies that they have learned over the course of treatment and discuss ways to apply these strategies to future situations (see Appendix 41–1).

Supplemental Topics

Child Skills

BPT can be combined with child-focused skill training treatments, such as social skills training, anger management, or organizational and study skills training, that permit direct skill instruction and practice for children (e.g., Abikoff et al. 2013; Kazdin et al. 1992; Pfiffner et al. 2007, 2014). Parents also can be taught strategies, as part of BPT, for helping their child's skills develop in these domains (e.g., Parental Friendship Coaching developed by Mikami et al. 2010). (Table 41–2 contains details on addressing social and organizational

TABLE 41–2. Teaching parents about child skills

Social skills	Organizational skills
Discussing importance of providing children with opportunities to practice their social skills (e.g., one-on-one playdates and participation in activities)	Addressing antecedents of organized vs. disorganized behavior
Structuring playdates in a manner that minimizes antecedents of problem behavior and makes playdates successful experiences for the child:	Establishing an organizational structure at home that will encourage the child to be more organized:
Selecting an easygoing or mild-mannered peer the child likes	Modeling organizational skills
Keeping the playdate brief	Organizing the home environment (perhaps by implementing a system using boxes, labels, shelves, and visual cues such as colors and pictures)
Planning an activity that both children will enjoy	Teaching parents to serve as skill coaches:
Setting up a plan before the playdate to reward positive behavior	Explaining the organizational process to the parent
Teaching parents to serve as skill coaches:	Demonstrating organizational skills for the child in a specific area (e.g., a backpack or desk) and then disorganizing the area and asking the child to reorganize it
Discussing each skill and what it means with the child	This strategy requires a time investment on the part of the parent that can be reduced over time, but any organization system established will continue to require monitoring and reinforcement on the part of the parent.
Cuing the child about when to use each skill	
Rewarding the child for using each skill successfully	

Note. For additional information please see Abikoff et al. 2013; Frankel and Myatt 2003; Pfiffner and McBurnett 1997; Pfiffner et al. 2014.

problems.) Session content generally includes two primary components. The first component involves working with the parents to address antecedents of skilled versus unskilled behavior on the part of the child and to structure the environment and provide the child with opportunities to be successful. Second, the parents also are taught to serve as skill coaches for their child by working with the child to focus on specific skills (e.g., engaging in discussion with the child about what a specific skill may mean, cuing the child about when to use the skill, rewarding the child for successfully demonstrating the skill).

Parent Stress Management

Parents usually are receptive to the idea that their own stress levels affect their child's behavior and that higher levels of parental stress are related to increased behavior problems on the part of the child (as well as increased relational stress between the child and the parent). Likewise, parents usually agree that when they are able to manage their own stress levels, they are better able to meet their child's needs. Parents may be engaged in discussion about their values and priorities and how these correspond to the manner in which they allocate their time. Further, parents also may be taught specific coping strategies to use when they are feeling pressured; these strategies may include relaxation, participating in pleasurable leisure activities, taking a time-out when they can feel themselves getting upset or angry, engaging in good sleep hygiene and other healthy habits, and finding additional sources of support (e.g., see Sanders et al. 2000; Webster-Stratton 1994).

Parent Cognitions and Emotion Management

Chronis et al. (2004) note that parental psychopathology and/or emotional dysregulation is one major moderator of treatment response for those participating in parent training. Clinicians recently have given more weight to the discussion of parents' own cognitions and emotions, particularly as they pertain to the child. These interventions may include teaching parents cognitive restructuring techniques to help them differentiate between unhelpful and helpful thoughts about the child or situation (e.g., see Bloomquist 1996). Therapists generally make the point that some thoughts may cause the parents either to become angry with the child and escalate the situation (e.g., age-inappropriate expectations or thoughts that the child is misbehaving intentionally) or to become discouraged and give up (e.g., thoughts that attempts to exert control over the child are hopeless or that the parents themselves are ineffective or inadequate parents), whereas other thoughts are more likely to help the parents remain calm and to deal with the child's behavior in a more rational manner. Parents are taught to identify the first type of thought as well as ways to respond to this kind of thinking that will be most effective in promoting calm and rational interactions with their child. These strategies may be especially useful adjuncts for depressed and/or multiply stressed parents (e.g., Chacko et al. 2009; Chronis-Tuscano et al. 2013)

In addition, teaching parents mindfulness strategies also may help in addressing parent cognitions and emotions. More specifically, advocates of mindfulness in parent training argue that parents and children become enmeshed in automatic cycles and that being mindful of these interactions serves as a step toward altering them. Dumas (2005) describes the following key components of a mindfulness approach: 1) teaching parents to accept where the child and they themselves are in the moment without judging; 2) teaching parents to distance themselves from situations that could induce negative emotion; and 3) collaborating with the parents to rationally develop and implement a plan to meet goals relevant to both parents and child.

Monitoring Treatment Progress

In behavior therapy, treatment progress is monitored each session by reviewing the data, such as the child's progress on behavior charts and DRCs (if used). Written documents (e.g., charts or graphs of point totals) can facilitate a more objective appraisal of gains over time (although we note that gathering and constructing charts of such data can be time intensive for the parents and/or therapist). Objective data can be supplemented with more qualitative parent impressions regarding treatment progress (as well as teacher impressions regarding school-based interventions). To effectively monitor progress, parents should be asked specific questions about how they are implementing the programs (e.g., Which behaviors did you praise this week? How often did you do special time? How often did you catch yourself giving effective vs. ineffective instructions? Did you use the point system? How calm were you when you gave the time-out?) and about how their child is responding (e.g., How much did your child seem to enjoy special time? How often did your child complete his or her target behaviors? What rewards did your child earn and how often? How often did he or she earn a time-out? How well did he or she take the time-out?). Brief behavior rating scales also can be used to track progress, as can questionnaires regarding parents' understanding of social learning principles and effective parenting practices. Consumer satisfaction ratings also can be very helpful for assessing parents' understanding of and perceptions about the usefulness of content covered during each session. When such ratings are gathered each session, these data can alert the therapist to potential dissatisfaction that might lead to premature termination or failure to follow through on programs at home. In addition, observations of parent-child interactions can be extremely useful in determining whether parents are able to successfully implement the procedures and also in evaluating the child's response.

Potential Adverse Effects or Complications

In general, this approach to treatment is associated with a very low risk for any serious adverse effects, making the risk-benefit ratio quite small. Instead, unwanted effects usually are mild and transient and result from parents using skills taught in an inappropriate manner. These effects can be addressed by making modifications to the program. We discuss typical pitfalls in the earlier subsections on troubleshooting session content (see "Core Session Topics") and in Table 41–1. The most serious complications may occur around the topic of punishment, as overly critical or potentially violent parents may overuse these approaches to the exclusion of the more positive ones. In these cases, an errorless learning approach may be particularly helpful (Ducharme et al. 2000). *Errorless learning* is a success-based noncoercive intervention that involves the gradual introduction of more demanding requests so that child noncompliance and associated consequences for non-compliance are minimized throughout treatment. Another potential complication is that children presenting with aggressive behavior may become aggressive toward parents or other authority figures when punishment is used. In these cases, reward-only programs may be best, or there may be a need for additional intervention, such as collaborative family problem solving (Greene 2014) or medication.

Misuse of rewards may also lead to untoward effects. Studies show that rewarding behaviors that already have intrinsic value will decrease their intrinsic value (Deci et al. 1999). Also, rewarding the termination of a problem behavior may inadvertently increase that behavior through negative reinforcement (e.g., "If you stop the tantrum, you can have dessert" or in the case of children demanding rewards to complete tasks). In addition, studies show that children who receive ability-focused praise are more likely to become discouraged and give up during challenging tasks, whereas effort-focused praise is best for improving motivation and persistence on challenging tasks (see Dweck 2006). These studies highlight the need to carefully design and judiciously use praise and other reward-based programs.

A common problem in behavior therapy (as in other forms of psychotherapy) is noncompliance or resistance to treatment, as indicated by failure to complete homework between sessions, poor attendance, or other resistance to using recommended strategies. In these cases, it is important to determine the contributing factors (e.g., the parent did not understand homework; he or she was too busy; it was too difficult). Research shows that the relationship between the therapist and parents greatly influences parental compliance with behavioral treatment in the same manner in which this type of relationship is important to the success of other forms of psychotherapy. Thus, even though a behavioral approach tends to be inherently directive, it is most effective in the context of a collaborative parent-therapist relationship (see Webster-Stratton and Herbert 1993). The therapist's warmth, humor, support, optimism, and knowledge are key factors in establishing this type of relationship. A Socratic style of interaction in which the therapist asks parents questions to facilitate their reaching desired conclusions often improves parent-therapist collaboration and can increase parents' motivation to change. It also is incumbent on the therapist to use the same reinforcement principles with parents that they are teaching parents to use with their children (e.g., praise their efforts). Other procedures that also can improve adherence to treatment include making reminder phone calls, holding sessions only after the parent has completed the homework, scheduling sessions at convenient times, offering child care, and addressing transportation needs.

When to Expect Response

Children typically respond to initial strategies within the first few weeks of the time that parents put these strategies into practice (i.e., within the first several sessions of treatment). Some parents are surprised by how much change occurs with their use of contingent positive attention. More serious problems usually are not resolved until stronger reward-based and/or punishment programs are used. With a well-conceived behavior plan, initial improvement in specific target behaviors is expected within 1 week of starting the program. Continued improvement toward long-term treatment goals is achieved via a gradual shaping process of both child and parent behavior. For example, when the child successfully earns a reward for initial target behaviors (e.g., brushes teeth with only one reminder), the requirements for earning the reward are gradually increased (e.g., dresses and brushes teeth with no reminders) until the final goal is achieved (e.g., completes entire morning routine with no reminders; see Case Example 1). However, it is common for children (and parents) to backslide about half-way through the program. Troubleshooting usually can revamp a faltering program, and parents who had stopped using the program, thinking the child's gains were going to be durable without it, often see the importance of maintaining consistency.

When to Change to or Add a Different Treatment

In some cases, the ongoing weekly assessment of progress shows that desired effects are not being achieved. There are two critical areas to assess: 1) adherence to treatment (are the parents implementing the program consistently, or are the procedures only partially implemented, explaining the poor response to treatment?) and 2) what exactly is the child's response, and how unsuccessful is the progress? In some cases, the treatment goals or behavioral criteria initially may have been too high and the child may display more success if the criteria are reduced to a more realistic level. Goals then can be increased more gradually via a shaping process. In other cases, unsuccessful programs may be helped by adding other strategies (e.g., adding response cost to a reward program) or adding a behavioral program in another setting for problems specific to that setting (e.g., school, peers). Parents may wish to consider adding medication if either severe behavior problems make it difficult to implement the program consistently or milder problems do not respond to tweaking of the behavioral program or cross-site implementation of the program. The combination of medication and behavioral treatments is considered the most potent intervention for many cases of ADHD, improving symptoms and functioning across domains (Subcommittee on Attention-Deficit/Hyperactivity Disorder et al. 2011). Other forms of treatment also may be needed in order to address problems with the family system (marital therapy, cognitive-behavioral therapy for parental depression, treatment for parental ADHD); these adjunctive treatments can occur concurrently with BPT, or parent training can be paused temporarily until gains in alternative treatments are achieved.

How Long to Continue Successful Treatment

Fading and termination of treatment usually are a collaborative decision between therapist and family. Many programs involve a set number of sessions, after which time a decision is made about whether additional treatment is needed. When most treatment goals are met, the frequency of individual sessions typically is reduced gradually in order to best maintain treatment gains (e.g., from once per week to once every other week and then once per month). Parents often become less motivated to come to sessions when their child is having success; termination thus is often initiated by the parents. After termination, booster sessions may be provided (and often are encouraged) during predictable transitional periods (start or change of school) or at times of high stress. For more severe or chronic problems, a continued-care model may be necessary. For example, given that ADHD is considered a chronic disorder, it is likely that some sort of intervention may be needed throughout childhood, adolescence, and into adulthood. The precise nature and intensity of these interventions may vary somewhat depending on environmental circumstances and developmental stage, but it seems reasonable to expect that maintenance of improvements following initial successful treatment will require continued intervention and troubleshooting from time to time.

Indications

BPT is strongly indicated for oppositional and conduct problems and ADHD on the basis of numerous empirical studies and is recommended by the major professional organizations in psychiatry, pediatrics, and psychology (American Psychological Association Working Group on Psychoactive Medications for Children and Adolescents 2006; Steiner et al. 2007; Subcommittee on Attention-Deficit/Hyperactivity Disorder et al. 2011). Both boys and girls spanning the full age range (toddler to adolescent) can benefit from this approach, although developmental considerations may require modifications (see the section "Developmental Issues"). BPT also can be helpful for youth with comorbid internalizing problems such as anxiety or depression, although minor modifications may be made for children presenting primarily with these types of problems.

Contraindications

The demands of parent training can be substantial, as parents are required to learn specific procedures and complete homework each week to practice skills taught during group. As a result, the primary contraindications are parent psychopathology (ADHD, depression), marital discord, or some other type of family dysfunction that is sufficiently severe that it prevents parents from participating or making the necessary time investment. Alternatives would be to teach the skills in a more gradual manner, have the parents receive individual or couples counseling prior to parent training, or provide these interventions concurrently.

Developmental Issues

Parent training can be applied across developmental levels with various modifications. For the preschool and early elementary school ages, parents and other caretakers assume dominant roles in socialization, and young children typically are very responsive to parental and caretaker attention. Several behavioral programs have been developed for this age group. These interventions include The Incredible Years (Webster-Stratton and Reid 2010), Parent Child Interaction Training (Menting et al.

2013), and Helping the Noncompliant Child (McMahon and Forehand 2005). Each of these programs follows a similar two-stage process. In the first, child-directed stage, parents are taught skills to foster a close, secure relationship with their child through use of traditional play therapy skills such as using attending and praising without questions, commands, and criticisms. In the second, parent-directed stage, parents are taught specific techniques for giving effective commands, labeled (or specific) praise, selective attention (ignoring), and time-out for more serious problems (e.g., hitting, tantrums).

At the elementary school level, there are greater expectations placed on children for independent functioning, and children develop the ability to delay gratification for longer periods of time, to work toward specific goals over time, and to understand the relationship between their behavior and contingencies. As exemplified by programs developed by Barkley (2013), Cunningham et al. (1995), Kazdin (2005), Sanders et al. (2000), and Webster-Stratton and Reid (2010; Webster-Stratton et al. 2004), interventions for this age group focus on daily and weekly reward programs or contracts as well as discipline techniques such as response cost (taking away privileges) and time-out. Treatment also often includes contact with schools and a focus on homework for the purpose of addressing academic problems.

Parent training without the direct involvement of the child may be less effective during adolescence because of teens' greater need for autonomy, increased risk-taking behaviors, reduced responsiveness to direct parent control, and greater influence of peer groups on values and behavior (relative to the influences of family or authority figures). For adolescents, contingency management and discipline (response cost and restitution through chores rather than time-out) continue to be part of the treatment, but there is a need for greater involvement of the adolescent in the problem-solving process. Treatment focuses on teaching teens and their parents effective skills for communication, negotiation, and family problem solving (Barkley and Robin 2014; Dishion and Kavanagh 2003). Formal behavioral contracts typically are used. Treatment for adolescents also focuses on improving parental monitoring and oversight of their teen's behavior. As with younger youth, treatment often includes consulting with the school to address academic and/or social problems in that setting.

Research Evidence for Efficacy and Effectiveness

Numerous outcome studies and meta-analyses show strong and clinically meaningful effects of BPT for the disruptive behavior disorders during preschool and elementary school (Evans et al. 2013; Fabiano et al. 2009; Menting et al. 2013; Pfiffner and Haack, in press). Gains occur in child compliance and reduction of problem behaviors, moving many children into the nonclinical range of functioning relative to their peers (Kazdin 1997). BPT also improves parenting skills, including use of effective commands, praise, attending, ignoring, and monitoring, and decreases controlling and negative parenting. The extent of changes in parenting usually predicts the extent of improvement in child behavior (Chronis-Tuscano et al. 2011; Dishion et al. 2003; Hinshaw et al. 2000). Gains made in parent training can be maintained several years posttreatment (Nock 2003). During adolescence, family-centered behavioral interventions (including the teen in the treatment sessions) show positive effects (Barkley and Robin 2014; Dishion and Kavanagh 2003).

BPT also has positive effects on parent functioning. Parents who participate in parent training often show reductions in parenting stress (Anastopoulos et al. 1993; Gerdes et al. 2012) and depression and greater confidence in their ability to manage their child's behavior (Herschell et al. 2002). Treatment effects can extend to untreated siblings (Herschell et al. 2002). Parent training also can be effective in alleviating marital distress that is caused by disagreements over childrearing, by unifying the parents' approach (Beauchaine et al. 2005). Parent satisfaction for this form of intervention tends to be high (Herschell et al. 2002). The addition of components to address parents' problem solving, stress, depression, and marital discord increases effects of BPT on overall parent, child, and family functioning (Nock 2003).

Multicomponent Behavioral Interventions

BPT is likely to be most potent when combined with school- and/or child-focused interventions, as together these interventions can target the range of risk factors and settings contributing to child problems and synergize the effects of the individual components. The combination of parent training with school-based interventions, such as those reviewed in Chapter 48, "School-Based Interventions" (see also Pfiffner et al. 2006), and/or child-focused interventions, such as anger management training, problem solving, and social skills, has been found to be effective in improving attention and externalizing problem behavior, parent-child interactions, homework problems, and social skills in a number of studies across age groups (Kern et al. 2007; Langberg et al. 2010; Nock 2003; Pfiffner and McBurnett 1997; Pfiffner et al. 2007, 2014; Power et al. 2012; Webster-Stratton et al. 2011). Including a child component can reduce premature termination in BPT (Miller and Prinz 1990), suggesting that these adjunctive interventions exert a positive effect on parents' motivation for treatment. In addition, when medication is needed, there is evidence that combining behavioral and medication treatments may permit a lower dose of medication (Fabiano et al. 2007; Pelham et al. 2014).

Factors Affecting Outcome

A number of studies have evaluated under which conditions and for whom behavioral interventions work best. Generally, the more difficult the living conditions and the more impaired the child functioning and parent functioning, the less favorable the outcome is. In particular, past research suggests that low socioeconomic status (SES) predicts poorer outcome (Eamon and Venkataraman 2003). It is likely that the limited resources of families from lower levels of SES contribute to these families' greater likelihood of early termination from treatment. For example, transportation issues, need for daytime attendance (i.e., during working hours), lack of child care for siblings, and other such issues may present greater treatment barriers for these families relative to more affluent families. For families facing financial disadvantage, an individual approach to BPT that allows for more tailoring of treatment to individual family circumstances may be significantly more effective than group-based approaches (Harwood and Eyberg 2004; Lundahl et al. 2006). There is no evidence that low SES increases dropout differentially for behavior therapy versus other psychosocial treatments. There has been some question as to whether fathers need to attend parent training; outcome studies tend to show that having both parents attend may not affect posttreatment outcome but may improve maintenance of treatment gains (Fabiano et al. 2012; Miller and Prinz 1990). Recently, BPT has been adapted for fathers of children with ADHD (Fabiano et al. 2012). The adapted intervention integrates standard BPT with a recreational sports activity (e.g., soccer game) for fathers to practice newly learned parenting skills with their children. This approach has been shown to improve fathers' engagement in the treatment. Generally, we advise that all caretakers attend sessions but require only the primary caretaker to attend every week.

A number of other parent and family factors may affect outcomes. Single-parent families, high parent stress, and a lack of parent social support all predict less favorable outcomes (Harwood and Eyberg 2006; Nock 2003; Schneider et al. 2013). Parents' beliefs about their child and his or her capacity to change can also affect outcome. Parents who think that their child is behaving badly on purpose or that their child is destined to display negative behavior ("There is nothing I can do") often are less likely to feel motivated to implement new behavioral strategies. Further, perceived stigma about receiving mental health services may prevent parents from continuing to receive services or from accessing them at all.

A number of child factors also predict response to parent training. The severity and nature of symptoms and problems likely are the strongest predictors of whether or not (or to what degree) treatment produces desired change. For example, children with conduct disorder who are high on callous-unemotional traits show a poorer response to parent training in general than do children low on these traits, and these children show an especially poor response to time-out as compared with reward programs (Hawes and Dadds 2005). Children with very severe oppositional defiant disorder or explosive behavior also may respond less well to traditional parent training approaches and require a more collaborative family problem-solving model (Greene 2014) relative to children presenting without these problems. For child-focused treatments, level of motivation and cognitive ability on the part of the child also are likely to be positively related to response.

Cultural and racial backgrounds affect treatment-seeking behavior, in that members of minority groups are less likely to seek or obtain services, and therefore much of the existing treatment outcome research is based largely on white samples (Forehand and Kotchick 1996). For families completing treatment, past research typically shows few differences in response to interventions after controlling for SES (Butler and Eyberg 2006), and recently several culturally modified treatments for children have been developed with positive results (McCabe and Yeh 2009). In light of differences in parenting across cultures, it seems important to take cultural factors into consideration. For example, in cultures involving the extended family in child care and emphasizing communal parenting, it may be important for nonparent providers to take part in or observe the training. In order to address cultural conceptions regarding behavior and psychological functioning (and particularly the increased stigma that may be associated with psychological disorders or participation in mental health services), the language used to describe the treatment may require modification (e.g., "understanding your child and resolving conflicts" or "parent coaching" instead of "parent training" [see Butler and Eyberg 2006]). Similarly, the types of reinforcers, activities, and privileges may need to be adapted depending on family and cultural values. Response to treatment also may benefit from a cultural match between therapist and family.

As noted earlier, there are a variety of process factors associated with implementation of parent training that also can affect outcome. As with any intervention, the therapist-client relationship influences outcome in behavior therapy (Webster-Stratton and Herbert 1993). Therapist warmth, knowledge of social learning principles and disruptive behavior disorders, likability, and communication skills all are likely to contribute to more positive outcomes. Helpful therapist behaviors include active listening skills to guide and maintain parents' responses to open-ended questions, whereas overly supportive statements early in therapy may reinforce feelings of client helplessness, which might contribute to dropout (Harwood and Eyberg 2004). Compliance with treatment also can be enhanced using motivational strategies (Dishion et al. 2003; Nock and Kazdin 2005) and specific prompts (e.g., reminder phone calls between sessions that prompt parents to complete homework or to come to the next session). Active parental engagement and compliance with treatment as measured by parental adherence to between-session assignments (e.g., the extent to which they implement the strategies they are taught) and to a lesser extent attendance at sessions are important predictors of child outcomes (Clarke et al. 2013).

Cost-Benefit Issues

Relative to long-term "traditional" individual therapy, behavior therapy is very cost-effective. The substantial gains of BPT can result from as few as 8–12 parent training sessions. The cost-benefit of parent training may be especially favorable when it is administered in a group setting, which for many families is as effective as individual approaches (Chronis et al. 2004). Large community-based group parent training programs held in the child's neighborhood also provide a cost-effective and perhaps less stigmatizing approach than clinic-based services (Cunningham et al. 1995). Self-administered parent training (e.g., via workbooks, videos) does not appear to be sufficient for most families (Sanders et al. 2000; Webster-Stratton 1990).

Summary Points

- Behavioral parent training (BPT) is a well-established and evidence-based treatment for a wide variety of child and adolescent behavior problems that can be adapted across developmental levels and is also useful for prevention of behavior problems. The positive effects of BPT include reductions in children's deviant behavior and symptoms; improvement in child compliance, parenting skills, and the quality of parent-child interactions; and improvement in parents' stress, self-confidence, and well-being.
- BPT interventions employ functional behavior analysis—the antecedent-behavior-consequence (ABC) model of behavior—in order to examine problem behaviors and identify potential antecedents and/or consequences of maintaining those behaviors. BPT programs then include some combination of core topics that teach parents to alter either antecedents (attending, giving effective instructions, managing behavior in public places, planning ahead) or consequences (praise and positive reinforcement, time-out, token economy, when-then, response cost) to improve the behavior.
- Behavioral interventions designed to target school-based problems such as homework completion or school behavior can be taught during BPT sessions and therapist consultation with the child's teacher.
- Additional child problems, such as social or organizational skills deficits, can be addressed in additional parent sessions (often including the child) and in parallel skills-training group treatment for the child.
- Sessions also can be added to address concurrent parent stress management or maladaptive cognitions or emotions on the part of the parents; these sessions typically employ combinations of behavioral, cognitive-behavioral, and/or mindfulness techniques.
- Parent factors that often reduce positive outcomes include low SES, single-parent status, severe marital discord, and parent psychopathology (depression, ADHD, substance abuse). These issues may be addressed through adjunctive treatments or (in the case of limited resources) some alteration of the parent training protocol.
- Combinations of BPT with other cognitive-behavioral treatments and/or medication likely produce the most potent outcomes for children and families having the most impairment. In some cases of ADHD, behavioral treatments add benefit to medication and may permit decreased medication use and dose.

References

Abikoff H, Gallagher R, Wells KC, et al: Remediating organizational functioning in children with ADHD: immediate and long-term effects from a randomized controlled trial. J Consult Clin Psychol 81(1):113–128, 2013 22889336

American Psychological Association Working Group on Psychoactive Medications for Children and Adolescents: Psychopharmacological, Psychosocial, and Combined Interventions for Childhood Disorders: Evidence Base, Contextual Factors, and Future Directions. Report of the Working Group on Psychoactive Medications for Children and Adolescents. Washington, DC, American Psychological Association, 2006

Anastopoulos AD, Shelton TL, DuPaul GJ, et al: Parent training for attention-deficit hyperactivity disorder: its impact on parent functioning. J Abnorm Child Psychol 21(5):581–596, 1993 8294653

Anastopoulos AD, Rhoads LH, Farley SE: Counseling and training parents, in Attention Deficit Hyperactivity Disorder: A Handbook for Diagnosis and Treatment. Edited by Barkley RA. New York, Guilford, 2006, pp 453–479

Bandura A: Social Learning Theory. Englewood Cliffs, NJ, Prentice-Hall, 1977

Barkley RA: Defiant Children, 3rd Edition: A Clinician's Manual for Assessment and Parent Training. New York, Guilford, 2013

Barkley RA, Robin A: Defiant Teens, 2nd Edition: A Clinician's Manual for Assessment and Family Intervention. New York, Guilford, 2014

Beauchaine TP, Webster-Stratton C, Reid MJ: Mediators, moderators, and predictors of 1-year outcomes among children treated for early onset conduct problems: a latent growth curve analysis. J Consult Clin Psychol 73(3):371–388, 2005 15982136

Bloomquist ML: Skills Training for Children With Behavior Disorders: A Parent and Therapist Guidebook. New York, Guilford, 1996

Butler AM, Eyberg SM: Parent-child interaction therapy and ethnic minority children. Vulnerable Child Youth Stud 1(3):246–255, 2006

Chacko A, Wymbs B, Wymbs F, et al: Enhancing traditional behavioral parent training for single mothers of children with ADHD. J Clin Child Adolesc Psychol 38(2):206–218, 2009 19283599

Chronis AM, Chacko A, Fabiano GA, et al: Enhancements to the behavioral parent training paradigm for families of children with ADHD: review and future directions. Clin Child Fam Psychol Rev 7(1):1–27, 2004 15119686

Chronis-Tuscano A, O'Brien KA, Johnston C, et al: The relation between maternal ADHD symptoms and improvement in child behavior following brief behavioral parent training is mediated by change in negative parenting. J Abnorm Child Psychol 39(7):1047–1057, 2011 21537894

Chronis-Tuscano A, Clarke TL, O'Brien KA, et al: Development and preliminary evaluation of an integrated treatment targeting parenting and depressive symptoms in mothers of children with attention-deficit/hyperactivity disorder. J Consult Clin Psychol 81(5):918–925, 2013 23477479

Clarke AT, Marshall SA, Mautone JA, et al: Parent attendance and homework adherence predict response to a family school intervention for children with ADHD. J Clin Child Adolesc Psychol 2013 23688140 Epub ahead of print

Cunningham CE, Bremner R, Boyle M: Large group community-based parenting programs for families of preschoolers at risk for disruptive behaviour disorders: utilization, cost effectiveness, and outcome. J Child Psychol Psychiatry 36(7):1141–1159, 1995 8847377

Deci EL, Koestner R, Ryan MM: A meta-analytic review of experiments examining the effects of extrinsic rewards on intrinsic motivation. Psychol Bull 125(6):627–668, 1999 10589297

Dishion TJ, Kavanagh KK: Intervening in Adolescent Problem Behavior: A Family Centered Approach. New York, Guilford, 2003

Dishion TJ, Patterson GR, Kavanagh KK: An experimental test of the coercion model: linking theory, measurement, and intervention, in Preventing Antisocial Behavior. Edited by McCord J, Tremblay RE. New York, Guilford, 1991, pp 253–282

Dishion TJ, Nelson SE, Kavanagh KK: The family check-up with high risk young adolescents: preventing early onset substance use by parent monitoring. Behav Ther 34(4):553–571, 2003

Ducharme JM, Atkinson L, Poulton L: Success-based, noncoercive treatment of oppositional behavior in children from violent homes. J Am Acad Child Adolesc Psychiatry 39(8):995–1004, 2000 10939227

Dumas JE: Mindfulness-based parent training: strategies to lessen the grip of automaticity in families with disruptive children. J Clin Child Adolesc Psychol 34(4):779–791, 2005 16232075

Dweck C: Mindset: The New Psychology of Success. New York, Random House, 2006

Eamon MK, Venkataraman M: Implementing parent management training in the context of poverty. Am J Fam Ther 31(4):281–293, 2003

Evans S, Owens J, Bunford N: Evidence-based psychosocial treatments for children and adolescents with attention-deficit/hyperactivity disorder. J Clin Child Adolesc Psychol 43(4):527–551, 2013 24245813

Fabiano G, Pelham W, Gnagy E, et al: The single and combined effects of multiple intensities of behavior modification and methylphenidate for children with attention deficit hyperactivity disorder in a classroom setting. School Psych Rev 36(2):195–216, 2007

Fabiano GA, Pelham WE Jr, Coles EK, et al: A meta-analysis of behavioral treatments for attention-deficit/hyperactivity disorder. Clin Psychol Rev 29(2):129–140, 2009 19131150

Fabiano GA, Pelham WE, Cunningham CE, et al: A waitlist-controlled trial of behavioral parent training for fathers of children with ADHD. J Clin Child Adolesc Psychol 41(3):337–345, 2012 22397639

Forehand R, Kotchick BA: Cultural diversity: a wake-up call for parent training. Behav Ther 27:187–206, 1996

Frankel F, Myatt R: Children's Friendship Training. New York, Brunner-Routledge, 2003

Gerdes AC, Haack LM, Schneider BW: Parental functioning in families of children with ADHD: evidence for behavioral parent training and importance of clinically meaningful change. J Atten Disord 16(2):147–156, 2012 20837977

Greene RW: The Explosive Child: A New Approach for Understanding and Parenting Easily Frustrated, "Chronically Inflexible" Children, Revised 5th Edition. New York, HarperCollins, 2014

Harwood MD, Eyberg SM: Therapist verbal behavior early in treatment: relation to successful completion of parent-child interaction therapy. J Clin Child Adolesc Psychol 33(3):601–612, 2004 15271617

Harwood MD, Eyberg SM: Child-directed interaction: prediction of change in impaired mother-child functioning. J Abnorm Child Psychol 34(3):335–347, 2006 16708275

Hawes DJ, Dadds MR: The treatment of conduct problems in children with callous-unemotional traits. J Consult Clin Psychol 73(4):737–741, 2005 16173862

Herschell AD, Calzada EJ, Eyberg SM, et al: Parent-child interaction therapy: new directions in research. Cogn Behav Pract 9:9–16, 2002

Hinshaw SP, Owens EB, Wells KC, et al: Family processes and treatment outcome in the MTA: negative/ineffective parenting practices in relation to multimodal treatment. J Abnorm Child Psychol 28(6):555–568, 2000 11104317

Johnston C, Mash EJ: Families of children with attention-deficit/hyperactivity disorder: review and recommendations for future research. Clin Child Fam Psychol Rev 4(3):183–207, 2001 11783738

Jones DJ, Forehand R, Cuellar J, et al: Technology-enhanced program for child disruptive behavior disorders: development and pilot randomized control trial. J Clin Child Adolesc Psychol 43(1):88–101, 2014 23924046

Kazdin AE: Parent management training: evidence, outcomes, and issues. J Am Acad Child Adolesc Psychiatry 36(10):1349–1356, 1997 9334547

Kazdin A: Parent Management Training: Treatment for Oppositional, Aggressive, and Antisocial Behavior in Children and Adolescents. New York, Oxford University Press, 2005

Kazdin AE, Siegel TC, Bass D: Cognitive problem-solving skills training and parent management training in the treatment of antisocial behavior in children. J Consult Clin Psychol 60(5):733–747, 1992 1401389

Kelley ML: School-Home Notes: Promoting Children's Classroom Success. New York, Guilford, 1990

Kern L, DuPaul GJ, Volpe RJ, et al: Multisetting assessment-based intervention for young children at risk for attention deficit hyperactivity disorder: initial effects on academic and behavioral functioning. School Psych Rev 36(2):237–255, 2007

Langberg JM, Arnold LE, Flowers AM, et al: Parent-reported homework problems in the MTA study: evidence for sustained improvement with behavioral treatment. J Clin Child Adolesc Psychol 39(2):220–233, 2010 20390813

Luman M, Oosterlaan J, Sergeant JA: The impact of reinforcement contingencies on AD/HD: a review and theoretical appraisal. Clin Psychol Rev 25(2):183–213, 2005 15642646

Lundahl B, Risser HJ, Lovejoy MC: A meta-analysis of parent training: moderators and follow-up effects. Clin Psychol Rev 26(1):86–104, 2006 16280191

McCabe K, Yeh M: Parent-child interaction therapy for Mexican Americans: a randomized clinical trial. J Clin Child Adolesc Psychol 38(5):753–759, 2009 20183659

McGrath PJ, Lingley-Pottie P, Thurston C, et al: Telephone-based mental health interventions for child disruptive behavior or anxiety disorders: randomized trials and overall analysis. J Am Acad Child Adolesc Psychiatry 50(11):1162–1172, 2011 22024004

McMahon R, Forehand R: Helping the Noncompliant Child: Family Based Treatment for Oppositional Behavior, 2nd Edition. New York, Guilford, 2005

Menting AT, Orobio de Castro B, Matthys W: Effectiveness of the Incredible Years parent training to modify disruptive and prosocial child behavior: a meta-analytic review. Clin Psychol Rev 33(8):901–913, 2013 23994367

Mikami AY, Lerner MD, Griggs MS, et al: Parental influence on children with attention-deficit/hyperactivity disorder: II. Results of a pilot intervention training parents as friendship coaches for children. J Abnorm Child Psychol 38(6):737–749, 2010 20339911

Miller GE, Prinz RJ: Enhancement of social learning family interventions for childhood conduct disorder. Psychol Bull 108(2):291–307, 1990 2236385

Nock MK: Progress review of the psychosocial treatment of child conduct problems. Clinical Psychology: Science and Practice 10(1):1–28, 2003

Nock MK, Kazdin AE: Randomized controlled trial of a brief intervention for increasing participation in parent management training. J Consult Clin Psychol 73(5):872–879, 2005 16287387

Patterson GR: Coercive Family Process. Eugene, OR, Castalia, 1982

Patterson GR, Reid JB, Dishion TJ: Antisocial Boys. Eugene, OR, Castalia, 1992

Pelham WE, Burrows-MacLean L, Gnagy EM, et al: A dose-ranging study of behavioral and pharmacological treatment in social settings for children with ADHD. J Abnorm Child Psychol 42(6):1019–1031, 2014 24429997

Pfiffner L, Haack L: Nonpharmacological treatments for childhood ADHD and their combination with medication, in A Guide to Treatments That Work, 4th Edition. Edited by Nathan P, Gordon J. New York, Oxford University Press, in press

Pfiffner LJ, McBurnett K: Social skills training with parent generalization: treatment effects for children with attention deficit disorder. J Consult Clin Psychol 65(5):749–757, 1997 9337494

Pfiffner L, Barkley RA, DuPaul GJ: Treatment of ADHD in school settings, in Attention Deficit Hyperactivity Disorder: A Handbook for Diagnosis and Treatment. Edited by Barkley RA. New York, Guilford, 2006, pp 547–589

Pfiffner LJ, Yee Mikami A, Huang-Pollock C, et al: A randomized, controlled trial of integrated home-school behavioral treatment for ADHD, predominantly inattentive type. J Am Acad Child Adolesc Psychiatry 46(8):1041–1050, 2007 17667482

Pfiffner L, Hinshaw S, Owens E, et al: A two-site randomized clinical trial of integrated psychosocial treatment for ADHD-inattentive type. J Consult Clin Psychol 2014, 24865871 Epub ahead of print

Power TJ, Karustis JL, Habboushe DF: Homework Success for Children With ADHD: A Family School Intervention Program. New York, Guilford, 2001

Power TJ, Mautone JA, Soffer SL, et al: A family school intervention for children with ADHD: results of a randomized clinical trial. J Consult Clin Psychol 80(4):611–623, 2012 22506793

Reese RJ, Slone NC, Soares N, et al: Telehealth for underserved families: an evidence-based parenting program. Psychol Serv 9(3):320–322, 2012 22867126

Sanders MR, Markie-Dadds C, Tully LA, et al: The triple P-positive parenting program: a comparison of enhanced, standard, and self-directed behavioral family intervention for parents of children with early onset conduct problems. J Consult Clin Psychol 68(4):624–640, 2000 10965638

Schneider B, Gerdes A, Haack L, et al: Predicting treatment drop-out in parent training intervention in families of school-age children with ADHD. Child Fam Behav Ther 35(2):144–169, 2013

Steiner H, Remsing L, American Academy of Child and Adolescent Psychiatry Work Group on Quality Issues: Practice parameter for the assessment and treatment of children and adolescents with oppositional defiant disorder. J Am Acad Child Adolesc Psychiatry 46(1):126–141, 2007 17195736

Subcommittee on Attention-Deficit/Hyperactivity Disorder et al: ADHD: clinical practice guideline for the diagnosis, evaluation and treatment of attention deficit/hyperactivity disorder in children and adolescents. Pediatrics 128(5):1007–1022, 2011 22003063

Webster-Stratton C: Enhancing the effectiveness of self-administered videotape parent training for families with conduct-problem children. J Abnorm Child Psychol 18(5):479–492, 1990 2266221

Webster-Stratton C: Advancing videotape parent training: a comparison study. J Consult Clin Psychol 62(3):583–593, 1994 8063985

Webster-Stratton C, Herbert M: Behav Modif 17(4):407–456, 1993 8216181

Webster-Stratton C, Reid J: The Incredible Years Parents, Teachers, and Children Training Series: A Multifaceted Treatment Approach by Young Children With Conduct Disorders. New York, Guilford, 2010

Webster-Stratton C, Reid MJ, Hammond M: Treating children with early onset conduct problems: intervention outcomes for parent, child, and teacher training. J Clin Child Adolesc Psychol 33(1):105–124, 2004 15028546

Webster-Stratton CH, Reid MJ, Beauchaine T: Combining parent and child training for young children with ADHD. J Clin Child Adolesc Psychol 40(2):191–203, 2011 21391017

APPENDIX 41–1. Core parent training topics

Topic	Key elements
Psychoeducation/background information	What is behavior therapy/parent training? Why is this the treatment of choice for childhood behavior problems? If treatment is targeted toward parents of children with a specific disorder (e.g., attention-deficit/hyperactivity disorder, conduct disorder), provide information regarding core symptoms, diagnostic criteria, etiology, and empirically supported treatments. Parent-child coercive interaction cycles: negative behaviors on the part of both parent and child are accidentally reinforced and perpetuated. Antecedent-behavior-consequence (ABC) model: modifying behavior by altering either the *antecedents* (i.e., the way in which the situation is set up) or *consequences* (i.e., rewards or punishments) of any given behavior.
Attending and ignoring	Use attending skills during child-directed special time, with goal of improving parent-child relationship: Child directs the activity. Parent actively attends to child's behavior by narrating activity in a nondirective, noncoercive, and neutral manner (without interrupting or making suggestions). Expand on attending during special time by differentially attending to positive and negative behaviors in other parent-child interactions: Attend to and praise positive behavior. Ignore mild negative behavior.
Praise/positive reinforcement	Deliver praise, rewards, or other positive reinforcement for positive behaviors that often are ignored, as they are less salient to parents than are negative behaviors. Effective vs. ineffective praise; examples of important aspects of effective praise include the following: Praise is specific: "I like the way you followed my instruction" rather than "Nice job." Praise immediately follows positive target behavior each and every time it occurs. Praise is not contaminated by negative affect on the part of the parent. There is a need for consistency (and immediacy) in delivering praise or positive reinforcement. Develop a reward menu with child's assistance that provides multiple options, such as token prizes or activities that can be paired with verbal praise.

APPENDIX 41–1. Core parent training topics *(continued)*

Topic	Key elements
Token economy/point system	Child earns tokens, points, or privileges for positive behavior at home that then can be cashed in for rewards such as small toys, stickers, or valued activities.
	Generate lists of daily and weekly rewards.
	Select clearly observable and specific target behaviors that include both difficult and relatively easy tasks in order to ensure that the child earns rewards and remains motivated.
	Assign points or token values to each behavior (behaviors can all earn the same number of points or can be weighted by importance or difficulty level).
	Set point or token costs for each reward on the basis of the total number of points or tokens that the child can earn in any given day and week.
	Use reward menu from list of daily and weekly rewards.
Giving effective instructions	Effective vs. ineffective instructions; effective instructions involve the following:
	Getting the child's attention
	Keeping the command brief, specific, and framed as what the child should do (vs. what he or she should *not* do)
	Phrasing commands as statements rather than questions or "let's" statements
	Using a neutral voice
	Giving the child time (up to 10 seconds) to respond
	Giving praise if the child complies or implementing a consequence if the child does not comply
	Attention to phrasing and consistency is needed.
Time-out	Time-out from positive reinforcement or enjoyable activity as a consequence of two or three specific target negative behaviors (e.g., noncompliance with commands or rule violations such as physical aggression or destruction of property)
	Discussion and troubleshooting of parents' past experience with time-out
	Mechanics of three-step procedure (see Figure 55–3), including the following:
	Give an instruction.
	Wait 5–10 seconds for the child to comply (counting aloud can improve compliance).

Appendix 41–1. Core parent training topics *(continued)*

Topic	Key elements
	If the child does not comply, issue a warning (e.g., "I've asked you to pick up your shoes. If you do not pick up your shoes now, you will earn a 5-minute time-out.").
	If the child does not comply, inform the child that he or she has earned a time-out and should proceed directly to the prespecified time-out location.
	The child must serve minimum time in time-out and is permitted to leave time-out only if he or she has served the last moment or two of the time-out appropriately; avoid reinforcing negative behavior by approaching or engaging with the child in time-out when he or she is displaying disruptive behavior.
	For noncompliance, child must complete original instruction following release from time-out; if child resists, time-out cycle should be repeated until child follows through on instruction in order to ensure that he or she does not use time-out to avoid following parental directions.
	For rule violations, no warning is necessary prior to assigning time-out (as long as parent has discussed this with child in advance).
	Specific logistical issues:
	Location for time-out: safe, easily monitored, no potential for positive reinforcement
	Duration of time-out may vary according to child's age (e.g., 1 minute for each year) or type of time-out procedure parents have chosen
	Behaviors that earn time-out
Response-cost procedures	Removal of tokens, points, or privileges when child displays target negative behaviors
	Can be done in several ways:
	Within token economy system
	Can provide prespecified number of tokens/points at the beginning of day or week and then assess a fine each time the behavior occurs (i.e., subtract fined tokens from the initial amount)
	Can directly fine child tokens or points he or she has already earned
	Can add a separate line to the token economy for rule infractions and then total points earned minus points lost at the end of the week
	Separate from token economy system: parents can take away privileges, activities, or toys

APPENDIX 41–1. Core parent training topics *(continued)*

Topic	Key elements
	Parents should continue to frame the token economy system in a positive manner to the child even after adding a response-cost component and also ensure that the child continues to earn rewards even if tokens are being subtracted for negative behavior.
Developing a plan for homework	Increase structure for homework time by making rules explicit and planning ahead for potential problems:
	Ensure necessary materials are available.
	Use an assignment system so that parents are aware of work needing to be completed.
	Prespecify a location for homework that is free of distractions.
	Set a consistent time for homework (or designate a "homework hour," during which time child must engage in quiet activities even if schoolwork is completed).
	Discuss with parents what their role or level of involvement in homework should be.
	Extend the token economy to the homework time, with tokens earned and lost for specific homework-related behaviors.
Home-school report cards	Parents learn to work collaboratively with teachers in developing and implementing a daily behavior report card that targets between one and four specific school-based problem behaviors.
	Parents provide the child with rewards at home for positive behavior at school.
	Teacher involvement can vary in time commitment or intensity; teachers may track the precise number of times a problem behavior occurs or provide a Likert rating of how well the child is doing on each target over the course of the school day.
Managing behavior in public places	Employ the ABC model before entering the public place in order to minimize possible problem behavior.
	Anticipate potential problems and restructure antecedents accordingly.
	Have preplanned consequences in place and communicate these to the child in advance.
	Reward positive behavior.
	Assign consequences (e.g., modified time-out) for negative behavior.
When-then/if-then/ "Grandma's rule" (Premack contingencies)	Use more desirable activities as reinforcers for completion of less desirable activities: "When/if you do what I want you to do, *then* you do what you want to do"; for example, parents using this strategy might tell their child, "When you finish your homework, then you can watch TV."

APPENDIX 41–1. Core parent training topics *(continued)*

Topic	Key elements
Planning ahead/anticipating future behavior problems	Review strategies learned to date. Apply the ABC model to new problems. Troubleshoot existing interventions: make sure rewards are motivating for the child, interventions are manageable in size for both child and parents, and reward and punishment (e.g., time-out, response cost) procedures are being implemented consistently.

Note. For additional information please see Anastopoulos et al. 2006; Barkley 2013; Bloomquist 1996; Kazdin 2005; McMahon and Forehand 2005; Pfiffner et al. 2014.

CHAPTER 42

Family-Based Assessment and Treatment

Richard Wendel, Ph.D.
Karen R. Gouze, Ph.D.

Unlike adults, children do not walk into a therapy office asking for help. Rather, children and adolescents typically find themselves in a therapist's consultation room when they have exceeded the limits of their environment to care for them (as in externalizing disorders) or have raised the concerns of significant others in their lives (as with internalizing disorders). Given this reality, the therapist must ask himself or herself, "Does it really make sense for me to leave these 'others' in the waiting room while I treat this child individually as I would an adult?" The role of the family in the treatment of child and adolescent mental health has evolved greatly. During the early to mid twentieth century, largely as a function of the influence of psychoanalysis, it was believed that parents should not be involved in child treatment because they were regarded as the cause of their child's psychological or psychiatric problems. This attitude was replaced during the 1950s and 1970s as research and practice revealed the enormous impact parents and other family members have on the well-being of children. It was during this era that family therapy established itself as a legitimate treatment modality, although still separate from mainstream child and adolescent psychiatry. Later, in the 1980s, families became more actively engaged as "partners in treatment." Today, best practices in all child and adolescent mental health disciplines accept that for optimal outcomes and to ensure engagement and therapeutic progress families need to be active participants in their children's mental health treatment (American Psychological Association Presidential Task Force on Evidence-Based Practice 2006; Diamond and Josephson 2005).

Research has established that family functioning and involvement powerfully affect treatment engagement and dropout rates in child mental health (Brookman-Frazee et al. 2008). Specific family factors found to affect engagement in services include family poverty, stress levels, single parent status, effectiveness of parent management strategies, and family cohesion (Gopalan et al. 2010). Family-reported empowerment and engagement also correlate with improvements in child adjustment (Taub et al. 2001). In a meta-analysis of published studies involving family support in children's mental health, Hoagwood et al. (2010) found that when parent support was integrated into child treatment, overall results were positive for child symptom reduction, parental satisfaction with the treatment, improved parenting skills, parental knowledge of the child's illness, and perceived social support. Treating children in their familial context makes sense from both the biopsychosocial and the developmental psychopathology perspectives. Thus, the American Academy of Child and Adolescent Psychiatry has consistently maintained that family assessment and treatment are indispensable for child and adolescent mental health practice (Josephson and American Academy of Child and Adolescent Psychiatry Work Group on Quality Issues 2007).

In spite of these findings and public policy initiatives, family therapy has begun only recently to develop a significant literature on empirically supported interventions. In this chapter we provide a framework for this work by first introducing the reader to the evolution of the field and key concepts, which is followed by a discussion of common factors and mechanisms of change that influence child and family outcomes. A discussion of the contributions made by developmental psychopathology research to family therapy follows. Finally, the reader is introduced to the Integrative Module-Based Family Therapy (IMBFT) approach, an integrative model consistent with current mandates in the field (see Lebow 2014) that provides a road map for assessing families and identifying appropriate empirically supported treatments for intervention.

The Evolution of Family Therapy

During the early decades of the twentieth century several forces came together to create family therapy. The Child Guidance Movement turned our attention to the psychosocial needs of children and the importance of early intervention. Growth in the practice of psychology and psychiatry led to robust theory development and clinical experimentation. The first generation of practitioners found working directly with couples and families to be thought provoking and clinically beneficial. Schools of thought developed around these pioneers. In this period, clinical practice was far ahead of empirical support. However, 20 years of empirical studies now provide strong confirmation that family therapy and family-based practices are effective and necessary for good patient care. Nevertheless, today we are in the unusual position of having abundant evidence that "family work" is efficacious for a variety of disorders, while many clinicians and clinical training programs pay insufficient attention to it. One of the difficulties in learning family-based treatments is that there are many manualized treatments for specific disorders, too many for clinicians to learn. These treatments often originate in the purity of the laboratory and address narrow and specific needs. Although these empirically supported treatments (ESTs) demonstrate the utility and benefits of family therapies, they were not designed for real world practice and multiproblem patients and families. Thus, the rollout from research protocol (efficacy) to everyday clinical treatment (effectiveness) has been uneven. Real life clinical settings require greater treatment flexibility and guidelines for adjusting to the needs of specific patients and families. When one balances the value of specific ESTs with the common factors (see subsection "Key Concepts") of all successful treatments, one is able to translate the scientifically established benefits of ESTs to typical patients in tailored and effective ways.

Key Concepts

Family therapy has developed its own descriptive vocabulary that aids the clinician in maintaining the dual focus on the patient and the relevant social forces. The *identified patient* is the person (the child or adolescent) originally presenting for treatment. Family therapy uses this term to remind clinicians that other family members and the family as a whole, in some sense, are also "patients" requiring assessment and intervention. For instance, there are strong associations between the emergence of conduct problems in young people and parents who are inconsistent or use overly harsh punishment (Kazdin 2005). It is quite difficult to attend to the primary problems of the identified patient without addressing the family and/or parental dysfunction.

From the beginning, family therapists have assessed and intervened on multiple levels. Thinking in terms of an interactive *sequence* allows clinicians to trace the critical moments and decisions of each dyad or family interaction. For example, if we are dealing with "last night's fight" or behavioral dysregulation, we can ask those involved to begin with a time before things got out of hand. Then the family therapist can trace the interaction from a calm moment through the fight. This way provocations, inappropriate communications, and amplified and dysregulated affects can be identified and the participants can be asked to think through their emotional and behavioral reactions so that in the future a conflict is less likely to occur.

Family therapy has long been associated with the notion of "system" or "systemic." When family therapists use the word *system* they are recognizing that psychosocial influences can come from multiple sources. The interlocking nature of family interactions is well captured in the term *circular causality.* Linear causality seeks to identify, in a sequential fashion, when and how a certain problem began. For instance, the child's behavior problems increased when a parent moved out of the household. However, many human difficulties arise within a social or interactional context, and a specific moment when the problem emerged cannot be identified. In this regard, trying to find a first cause to a family argument often fails because each participant can cite a previous grievance (in some cases, going back years). Employing circular causality frees the clinician from evaluating who (or what) started the problem. Family therapists often describe this in terms of a *nag-withdrawal pattern.* A parent may say, "Yes, I nag you (try to get you to talk) because you are so withdrawn," and the young person may say, "I tune you out because you nag me all the time." Seeing the circularity of the interaction prevents the useless search for a first cause or someone to blame and allows for interventions that address how both individuals may be a little right and a little wrong—but participants can change the cycle if they choose. Over the years the term "system" and its variants have been used so broadly that today it is better to think in terms of *interactive, bidirectional,* or *transactional processes.* For example, the escalation of *negative affective reciprocity* (perceiving negative emotion from someone and amplifying one's in-kind response) has been found to be frequently associated with lower levels of attachment and relational stability (Gottman 1994). Helping dyads understand this interactive process and teaching them to resist increasing their retaliatory responses helps them create and sustain a stable and satisfying bond. Because families are made up of interconnected dyads, helping patients construct stable and beneficial relationships is an important focus for clinical intervention.

From the beginning, family therapy has thought in terms of several parallel and sometimes intertwined *developmental trajectories.* Besides the developmental needs of the identified patient, family therapists consider the developmental processes of couple and family formation and how parent-child interactions are affected by them and how interactional styles of parents and children must change with maturation. For instance, one child may become symptomatic when the youngest sibling enters school and the mother returns to work. Helping the family and the identified patient to adapt to the change is an important clinical consideration.

Since the 1990s, family therapists have focused on the kinds of stories or *narratives* families tell. These stories identify family cultures and often reflect the kinds of images, roles, and cognitive constructions family members have of one another. For example, if parents see a child as troublesome, this child may often be blamed for things he or she did not do. This assigned role may also discourage him or her from trying to change. Helping the family shift the narrative to more constructive images (Freeman et al. 1997; White and Epston 1990) is important. Within the last decade, we have seen cross-fertilization between cognitive-behavioral therapy (CBT) and narrative (family) therapies in theory formation and intervention. This is a fruitful area of exploration and practice.

The Social Environment for Children and Adolescents

D.W. Winnicott, an early major figure in child psychiatry, emphasized the significance of the social environment for the child in terms of two interlocking processes. The first is the developmental process from *absolute dependence* through *relative dependence* to *independence* (Winnicott 1965). The second process is the profoundly beneficial influence of an *emotionally facilitating environment.* Winnicott posited that the adequacy of this social environment is essential for normal human development and psychological growth. Perhaps more than anything else, it is the dependence of infants, children, and adolescents and the sensitivity and reactivity of young people to their environment that distinguish working with children and adolescents from the treatment of adults. Winnicott's theory is now firmly established in the literature. There are a variety of regulatory processes, biologically based and environmentally shaped, that influence emotional outcomes, from health and vitality to the manifestation of behavioral disorders. A central component of Winnicott's theory is the *holding environment:* that is, the provision of a safe and need-fulfilling social context within which the infant and young child can develop. The creation of this holding environment requires an early and primary *parental preoccupation* in order to facilitate the growth of children, which gradually recedes as the child matures. This is one reason why the family is so important to child and adolescent mental health practice. Adults may be able to be treated without reference to their family (although many rightly question the wisdom of this), but the dependency of children requires the assessment and involvement of the family.

Similarly, John Bowlby's (1988) work on attachment posits the importance of the transactional relationship between parent and infant in promoting a sense of "felt security" that allows the infant or child to explore the environment and seek out independence in a manner that contributes to ongoing healthy development. Attachment theorists have long argued that context is critical to the development of resilience throughout childhood and that an ongoing secure attachment is foundational for creating the frame within which healthy development takes place (Bowlby 1988; Davies and Cicchetti 2004). From an attachment perspective, treating a child independently of the context of his or her primary relationships, specifically caregiving relationships, is unlikely to promote resilience or alter current patterns of psychopathology.

Finally, developmental psychopathology, the field of study devoted to the understanding of risk and protective factors in child development, emphasizes the importance of both a systems principle and a multilevel principle. The *systems principle* states that "psychopathology arises from complex interactions…between the individual and the multiple systems in which the life of the individual is embedded (Masten 2006, p. 48), while the *multilevel principle* argues that "processes involved in psychopathology occur within and across multiple levels of functioning, from the molecular or genetic to cultural or societal systems" (Masten 2006, p. 48). Clearly, from the perspective of researchers in child development and developmental psychopathology it is impossible either to understand or to alter patterns of psychopathology without attending to the context of children's lives. In this regard, the family is the most powerful system within which these lives are embedded.

The formative role played by families in promoting or attenuating mental health in children has been well documented in the developmental psychopathology literature. For example, a strong relationship is found between externalizing behavior in school-age children and family conflict, parental hostility and warmth, and parental scaffolding (Grant et al. 2006; Hipwell et al. 2008; Zimet and Jacob 2001). Morris et al. (2007) argued that family context is critical to the development of emotion control in children and adolescents and operates through three processes: observation/modeling, parenting practices, and the emotional climate of the family. Still others have demonstrated clear relationships between high levels of family stress and conflict and internalizing disorders in toddlers and preschoolers (Côté et al. 2009) and in older children and adolescents (Hammen et al. 2004). Parental support and hostility have also been linked to internalizing disorders in preschoolers (Lovejoy et al. 2000) and in older children and adolescents (Ge et al. 1996). In response to findings such as these, clinicians have worked to develop empirically supported interventions that target family risk factors including poor attachment (Diamond et al. 2014), family conflict (Szapocznik et al. 2012), poor family emotional control (Keiley 2002), and poor parenting practices (Webster-Stratton and Reid 2010; Zisser and Eyberg 2010). Our primary goal in this chapter is to present a model for assessing family functioning that allows for careful selection of appropriate empirically supported treatments that address the familial risk and protective factors ameliorating, maintaining, or exacerbating individual child and adolescent psychopathology.

Common Factors and Mechanisms of Change

In addition to specific treatments that have demonstrated positive therapeutic effects, there are widely shared aspects of all therapies that positively influence outcomes. Common factors are those broad elements of good clinical care that contribute to desired outcomes (Sprenkle et al. 2009). For example, clinicians who create and maintain a strong alliance, including making adjustments to fit the patient's temperament and needs, have more successful treatments. The expression of respect for patients and the creation of hope contribute to good care. Regulating the therapeutic climate and improving emotional regulation in persons and relationships is known to contribute to positive outcomes. Clinicians are more successful when they strive for workable strategies for desired change, redefining behaviors and problems toward more constructive viewpoints and helping patients to engage in new and beneficial behaviors. In dyadic and family-based treatments the following have been identified as enhancing positive outcome: involving others in treatment, creating good alliances with pertinent family members, conceptualizing problems in terms of social interaction, disrupting harmful relational cycles, ensuring agreement on tasks and treatment goals, helping all members see their part in negative patterns, slowing down and softening the interactive and emotional processes, and encouraging personal responsibility for negative and positive processes (Sprenkle et al. 2009).

An important and interesting debate has centered on this question: What accounts for clinical change in psychotherapy, factors common to all established treatments or the specific protocols of ESTs (Asay and Lambert 1999; Lambert and Barley 2001; Sprenkle et al. 2009)? The discussion has evolved and now can be posed in a different way. First, we know that when therapists follow a manualized protocol, clinicians differ in their outcomes (Anderson et al. 2009; Blatt et al. 1996; Podell et al. 2013). These differences are attributable to some clinicians possessing a higher level of the skills common within good clinical care as discussed. These studies examine the relative impact of therapist and patient characteristics and specific treatment effects. Most often, the therapist's and patient's contributions to outcomes are greater than specific treatment effects (Lambert and Barley 2001; Luborsky et al. 1986).

Researchers have also examined the impact of specific elements of ESTs on outcomes. Treatment effects that moderate pathology serve as specific mechanisms of change in therapy (Kazdin 2007). Findings from this research can influence model development and intervention planning. For instance, Jacobson et al. (1996) have shown that behavioral activation (BA), a component of CBT for depression, is as effective alone as the full version of CBT. BA is now used as a stand-alone treatment for depression (Jacobson et al. 2001; Martell et al. 2010). Lipsitz and Markowitz (2013) argued that Interpersonal Psychotherapy (IPT) contains at least three important mechanisms of change: improving social support, decreasing interpersonal stress, and improving the processing of emotions. Gallagher et al. (2013) argued that increasing a sense of self-efficacy and decreasing anxiety sensitivity are central change mechanisms in the treatment of panic disorder using CBT. Dietz et al. (2014) found that improving adolescent social problem solving significantly contributes to outcome, whether it occurs in CBT or family-based treatments. Henggeler et al. (2009) found that decreases in antisocial behavior are associated with improved caregiver discipline, disengagement from deviant peers, and improved family functioning. Shahar et al. (2010) found that reducing brooding (an aspect of rumination) and increasing mindfulness serve as mechanisms of change in the treatment of depression.

There are many ESTs for specific disorders. Since we now possess evidence of shared mechanisms of change, do we need to follow the manualized form of these ESTs? Is treatment outcome lessened or improved when components of these ESTs are used? Chorpita, Weisz, and colleagues provide an answer and a treatment planning road map to these questions. These researchers have established that a tailored and modular approach, using aspects of empirically supported treatments, is actually more effective in real world settings than the manualized treatments for anxiety, depression, and conduct problems (Chorpita and Weisz 2009; Weisz et al. 2012).

With this information in mind one can see that establishing ESTs is not the end-point of outcome research. Rather, our ESTs require the next step in the process, which is teasing out the mechanism(s) of change. These mechanisms, when executed within sound common factors practice, are the actual agency of change in clinical care. When both the positive impact of the common factors of therapies and the core mechanisms of change within ESTs are considered, one is left with the conclusion that it is not an either/or distinction but both/and. That is, the skills found in the common factors serve as the vehicle or atmosphere through which the empirically supported techniques (as mechanisms of change) have potency. This is all the more convincing when modular approaches demonstrate superiority over fixed treatment protocols and are flexibly tailored to each patient. IMBFT is a modular family-based therapy that uses ESTs within an overarching clinical approach that strives to benefit from specific skills identified within the common factors. Lebow et al. (2012, p. 159) have argued that integrative practices that rely on evidence-based methods "may be taken to have support by proxy."

General Principles

Successful family-based treatments share specific characteristics. In therapies for individuals, when the patient enters the consultation room, it is reasonable for the clinician to ask, in a variety of ways, "What is the problem?," whereas working with dyads and families requires different tactics. Families, by definition, involve multiple people, often with different experiences and perspectives on the "problem." So clinicians who ask "What is the problem?" are likely to hear the most verbal and most frustrated person, probably a parent, launch into a *problem-saturated description* (White and Epston 1990), such as that portrayed in the case example in the section "Implementing Integrative Module-Based Family Therapy." The neediness and frustrations of family members are often overwhelming, and beginning therapists find themselves unable to redirect the speaker, quickly losing control of the session. At the same time, the child who is the identified patient is likely to become flooded with negative emotion and either fight back or shut down. Either way, therapists with an individual therapy orientation find themselves in an alienating situation. Family therapists actively use a technique known as *joining* to do three things. First, they avoid the "What's wrong?" question. Second, family therapists begin with relationship-building small talk with each person in the room. Third, they postpone (interrupting if necessary) the serious issues until everyone in attendance has had a chance to enter the process (in as low stress an atmosphere as possible). Following this joining with the family, the therapist solicits each person's view of the problem in turn. Only after everyone's story has been heard is it wise to move on to the next stage.

Family therapists listen to the description of the problem from each family member and note points of agreement and disagreement. Discrepancies are expected, and family therapists begin to construct in their own minds a view of the problem that is clinically workable and most likely to be shared by all. This may be done in one session or several sessions. When family therapists together with the family and identified patient have generated a shared explanation of the problem (*shaping a workable presenting problem*), then and only then can they begin to think in terms of solutions and interventions. It should be noted that family therapists routinely delay formal assessment until they have built a working alliance with each pertinent family member. This may be difficult in many clinical settings and may work better if diagnostic assessment and treatment are separated. This relational style models good relationship formation and has been found to be one of the most powerful "common factors" (Bachelor and Horvath 1999; Blatt et al. 1996; Sprenkle et al. 2009) in effective psychotherapeutic practice. This working relationship with all family members also enhances assessment cooperation. As assessment comes to a close, family therapists move to *create a shared tenable treatment plan.* This requires, in most cases, agreement among all family members present; otherwise, a misalliance may be created, leading to treatment dropout or nonadherence.

Indications

In the last two decades family therapy and family-based treatments have moved from theory-guided practice to the application of more empirically supported interventions. Several reviews highlight that family therapy and family-based approaches are effective and beneficial for a wide variety of disorders (Baldwin et al. 2012; Bond et al. 2013; Carr 2014; Couturier et al. 2013; Henggeler and Sheidow 2012; Kaslow et al. 2012; Lucksted et al. 2012; Rowe 2012; Shields et al. 2012). Family assessment is called for in all child and adolescent patient contacts since families can activate a host of risk and protective factors. Furthermore, family intervention can be used either as a stand-alone treatment or as a treatment augmentation. See Table 42–1 for examples of applicable family-

TABLE 42–1. Examples of empirically supported treatments and best practices per domain

Psychiatric and related medical conditions domain, possible modular interventions
- Somatizing patients: Medical Family Therapy
- Autism spectrum disorders: Pivotal Response Treatment
- Substance abuse: substance abuse treatment and family therapy (CSAT); Multidimensional Family Therapy; Brief Strategic Family Therapy
- Eating disorders: Maudsley family-based treatment
- Parent Management Training
- Other chapters in this text
- Practice parameters of the American Academy of Child and Adolescent Psychiatry

Attachment/relationship domain, possible modular interventions
- Attachment/relationship-based therapies: Attachment-Based Family Therapy
- Attachment therapy for depressed and/or suicidal adolescents: Attachment-Based Family Therapy
- Attachment therapy for trauma: Child-Parent Psychotherapy

Family structure domain, possible modular interventions
- Family structure interventions: Brief Strategic Family Therapy; techniques from Structural Family Therapy

Family communication domain, possible modular interventions
- Communication and problem solving: problem-solving communication training; Collaborative Problem-Solving Therapy
- Working with intense affect: Emotion Focused Therapy

Developmental domain, possible modular interventions
- Normal family processes
- Developmental psychopathology: Holmbeck et al. 2010; Masten and Cicchetti 2010
- Addressing developmental needs of families: Attachment-Based Family Therapy; Child-Parent Psychotherapy; Narrative Therapy

Affect regulation domain, possible modular interventions
- Reducing intensity of expressed emotion in families: family treatment of expressed emotion; Emotion Focused Therapy; contextual emotion-regulation therapy; multifamily psychoeducation groups
- Mood disorders: Family-Focused Treatment; Narrative Family Therapy; MATCH-ADTC
- Adolescent depression: Interpersonal Psychotherapy for Adolescents
- Anxiety disorders: Exposure-Based Cognitive-Behavioral Therapy
- Bipolar disorder: Family-Focused Treatment; multifamily psychoeducation groups

Behavior regulation domain, possible modular interventions
- Reducing behavior problems in young children: Parent Management Therapy; Parent-Child Interaction Therapy; The Incredible Years training program
- Family intervention to improve limit setting and reduce coercive cycles of discipline: Functional Family Therapy; Multisystemic Therapy: The Defiant Teens Program; MATCH-ADTC

Cognitive/narrative domain, possible modular interventions
- Use of narrative structure to rewrite the family story: Narrative Family Therapy
- Use of externalization to understand a problem-saturated story: Narrative Family Therapy
- Extension of CBT techniques from individual to family: Cognitive-Behavioral Family Treatment; CBT

TABLE 42–1. Examples of empirically supported treatments and best practices per domain *(continued)*

Mastery domain, possible modular interventions
Academic skill encouragement
Skills training for externalizing children: skills training
Family resilience interventions
Community domain (e.g., social context, gender, culture, race, sexual orientation)
Sensitivity to culture, race, gender, and sexual orientation: Boyd-Franklin 2008; McGoldrick and Hardy 2008
Sensitivity to gender: Haddock et al. 2000
Sensitivity to sexual orientation: Bepko and Johnson 2000
Sensitivity to religion: Josephson and Peteet 2004

Source. Adapted from Gouze and Wendel 2008; Wendel and Gouze 2010.

Note. CBT=cognitive-behavioral therapy; CSAT=Center for Substance Abuse Treatment; MATCH-ADTC=Modular Approach to Therapy for Children with Anxiety, Depression, Trauma, or Conduct Problems.

based treatments. See other chapters in this text for more details on treatment of specific disorders.

Integrative Module-Based Family Therapy

Jay Lebow's (1997) influential article identified a dramatic change in family therapy practice, which he described as an "integrative revolution in couple and family therapy" (p. 1). He called attention to empirically supported treatments, evidence-based practice, and best practice standards that have led clinicians to "do what works" rather than be loyal to and practice within one of the older theoretical models. Since the late 1990s, integrative empirically supported practice has superseded the classic models. Treatments today commonly employ a multimodal approach and draw from a variety of pertinent ESTs.

The IMBFT approach (Gouze and Wendel 2008; Wendel and Gouze 2010) combines previous integrative family therapy models with empirically supported and best practice approaches to family treatment and theoretical and empirical knowledge from the fields of developmental psychology and psychopathology, family studies, and psychiatry to provide a road map for assessment and treatment of families.

IMBFT describes 10 areas referred to as *domains* in which there are empirically established or reasonably assumed mechanisms of change. By employing 10 domains, IMBFT is more comprehensive than other forms of family therapy, whether they are the classical models or more narrowly defined family-based ESTs. The 10 domains are as follows:

1. *Psychiatric/biological domain* (intervention here includes psychopharmacology)—This domain entails assessing the psychiatric status of the identified patient (i.e., the child or adolescent) initially presenting for treatment using standard criteria from DSM-5 (American Psychiatric Association 2013). The assumption is that successful family intervention requires a complete understanding of the child or adolescent's more biologically based difficulties. For exam-

ple, a child with moderate to severe attention-deficit/hyperactivity disorder (ADHD) might require pharmacological intervention before significant progress can be made through family therapy. Similarly, identifying the biological basis of disorders in participating family members, particularly parents, may be a prerequisite for improvement through family therapy. A depressed or substance abusing parent, for example, may require adjunctive individual treatment before progress can be made with the identified patient through family intervention.

2. *Attachment/relationship domain*—This domain is derived from a large body of literature (see Table 42–1) that demonstrates the relationship between secure parent-child attachments and healthy child development. This attachment relationship provides a secure base from which children can explore the environment and functions as a template for future relationships. As children and adolescents grow, their relationships with their parents serve as a fundamental source of self-esteem. When family relationships are fractured, it is difficult to move past the negative aspects of these relationships unless this domain is addressed first.
3. *Family structure domain*—Since the early days of family therapy, family structure has been seen as an important contributor to the formation and maintenance of individual pathology within families. A family with a child with oppositional defiant disorder, for example, often has a poorly functioning parenting dyad. Assessment of and intervention in this domain require attention to roles, family rules, hierarchies, family alliances, and boundaries.
4. *Family communication domain*—From the inception of family therapy, every model, in its own way, has dealt with the type, method, and content of communication in families. Healthy families communicate clearly, express and respond to emotional content, are attuned to nonverbal messages, and are able to problem solve without avoidance or escalating into conflict. The questions within the IMBFT assessment instrument help the clinician to identify strengths and problems of communication in families.
5. *Developmental domain*—Since the beginning of modern psychiatry, the formation and maintenance of pathology have been viewed as a hierarchical integration of chronological and interactive processes (developmental psychopathology). Assessment and intervention within this domain necessitate an understanding of normal family processes (see Chapter 31, "Family Transitions: Challenges and Resilience") and child development. An example of the need for treatment within this domain is the emergence of symptoms as a child and his or her family begin to negotiate the demands of adolescence.
6. *Affect regulation domain*—Poor affect regulation is, almost by definition, indicative of poor psychological functioning. Note, for example, the number of diagnoses that have irritability as a core symptom. The ability to regulate affect has been shown to be critical to the mental health of individual members of the family (see Table 42–1). Not only do individual family members who themselves affectively dysregulate contribute to high levels of negative emotionality, but the reverse is also true. Families

that are successful in helping one another regulate affect contribute to greater stability in psychiatrically impaired members (see Table 42–1). Children and adolescents learn to regulate their own affect within the context of their families, making this a central area of intervention for children and adolescents who present with affective disturbances.

7. *Behavior regulation domain*—Behavior dysregulation is a core feature of externalizing disorders. This area draws on the array of empirically supported treatments in the parenting literature, including Parent Management Training, The Incredible Years, Multisystemic Therapy, and Functional Family Therapy (see Table 42–1), that demonstrate that treatment of externalizing disorders often requires behavioral intervention at the family level. Parental monitoring of behavior programs, providing structure for accomplishing tasks (e.g., homework), and the setting of household rules are examples of interventions that fall within this domain.
8. *Cognitive/narrative domain*—This domain draws on literature in two areas: the Narrative Family Therapy tradition and cognitive-behavioral therapies that make mental and descriptive activity cornerstones of treatment. This domain is addressed first if family stories or myths continue to support maladaptive behavior in an individual child or adolescent (e.g., "He's the lazy one in the family."). Or it might be the first domain engaged in intervention if cognitive restructuring is required to shift a family's focus from a problem-focused view of a child to the things he or she does right. *Reframing*—a time-honored technique in family therapy, in which a more positive perspective is placed on what is otherwise seen as a maladaptive behavior—falls in this category. An example might be when a parent complains that an anxious child is driving her crazy with her clingy behavior and the therapist reframes this as the child's need to be close to her mother.
9. *Mastery domain*—Mastery is a core concept in developmental psychology and psychopathology. Winnicott, Freud, and Erikson all identify mastery as central to the growing child's development of self-esteem and a core self. The mastery domain is important to address in families in which individual members' failures of mastery (e.g., inability to hold a job, poor school performance, inability to make friends) are contributing to or serving to maintain mental health problems.
10. *Community domain*—This broad domain encompasses the need for family therapists to be sensitive to the role that culture, socioeconomic level, immigration status, religion, race, gender, and sexual orientation play in creating conditions that produce or maintain psychopathology. Even when this domain is not the prime focus of intervention, it is important that it be considered as a frame for working within all the other domains.

Implementing Integrative Module-Based Family Therapy

A step-by-step assessment instrument and sample assessment questions for each domain can be found in Tables 42–2 and 42–3. Assessment of the family across all 10 domains provides the clinician with a starting point for intervention. The clinician's initial intervention should be based on two criteria. The first concern is to focus on the most acute problem area. Second, the therapist must assess whether leaving a particular problem area unresolved will interfere with progress in another domain and thereby block therapeutic progress. For example, if familial relationships are badly fractured and there is poor behavior regulation, it is likely that some repair of the attachments will have to precede the behavioral intervention or the efforts will fail. This is why most parenting programs begin with instructing parents how to engage in descriptive play with their children before teaching discipline techniques such as time-out. Once a domain is selected as the focus for beginning intervention, the clinician is encouraged to search the literature (e.g., Medline and PsycINFO) or practice guidelines to determine the best applicable therapies or empirically supported treatments (see also Chapter 24, "Evidence-Based Practice"). Table 42–1 provides a sample of empirically based and best practice interventions to guide treatment for each of the domains. Following the choice of domain and subsequent modular intervention, it is important that the clinician assess progress using standard outcome measures such as ratings of symptoms, standard checklists, or regular discussions with the family concerning movement toward shared therapeutic goals. When treating children and adolescents, depending on the presenting problems, it is often important for the clinician to get measures from outside the family (e.g., teachers). IMBFT was designed to be flexible and, therefore, responsive to changing clinical presentations or new challenges that affect treatment. As the clinician proceeds, ongoing evaluation of outcomes and barriers guides the clinician toward new domains and modules for intervention. As the therapist moves to address new symptoms or overcome barriers, she or he can easily return to using the assessment instrument for the family's current state and choose new domains as points of intervention. This systematic approach provides a heuristic frame for treatment that is readily accessible even to less experienced family therapists.

Case Example

You welcome a plainly dressed mother with a serious and distressed look on her face and a teenage male, Michael, who is wearing clothes that look slept in, with his underwear showing atop his low-slung pants. He does not make eye contact, avoids a handshake, drops into your consultation chair, and begins to stare out the window. His mother turns to you and says, "See, he has no respect for others. You gotta straighten him out." That is only the beginning, as the mother launches into a 10-minute monologue about how Michael will not talk "normally" to his parents. He yells and "starts a fight if you say anything to him." He is not doing well in school. He has been caught with cheap whiskey in his room, and "last week he was arrested for driving without a license." Michael's mother enacts a dramatic pause and exclaims, "And he's only 14." As you realize that the teenager is actually in the room, you notice that his mood is sullen and he has been shaking his head in disgust. When you try to ask him what he makes of what his mother has just said, he replies, "Yeah whatever," as his mother begins to yell at him. Michael interrupts her and shouts, "I was just going to see Brandy." Even though it is unpleasant, you decide to let the two of them argue, just so you can hear something from Michael and watch how they relate. After about 5 minutes you

TABLE 42–2. Integrative Module-Based Family Therapy: step-by-step assessment

1. Patient identification
   a. Age and gender
   b. Cultural and/or social variables
   c. Family composition (members of household, pertinent extended family)
2. Diagnostic assessment and indicators
   a. DSM-5 symptoms in the identified patient
   b. Diagnostically unanswered questions
   c. Current or tentative diagnosis
   d. Medications (if any)

   Until the patient is psychiatrically stable, supportive and psychoeducational interventions are indicated.
3. Diagnostic assessment of psychosocial indicators
   a. *Attachment/relationship:* How strained or conflicted are the relationships within the family? It is difficult to form a viable treatment plan until there is an understanding that improving relationships and managing conflict are priorities. Rate from high concern (7) to low concern (1). List strengths and weaknesses in the family relationships.

      Strengths Weaknesses
   b. *Family structure:* Are there indications that structural issues (e.g., excessive discipline, inconsistent discipline, poor parental leadership) are exacerbating the presenting problem? Rate from high concern (7) to low concern (1). List strengths and weaknesses in the family.

      Strengths Weaknesses
   c. *Family communication:* Do family members speak directly to one another? Are the messages clear? Do family members feel heard? Do family members hear and respond to one another's feelings? Do family members interrupt one another? Do family members use feeling words, and is the emotion vocabulary sufficiently broad? Is parenting done through imperatives with no explanation? Do family members speak with "I" statements? Can family members discuss emotionally charged issues without avoidance or conflict? Can family members perceive and respond to nonverbal cues? Rate from high concern (7) to low concern (1). List strengths and weaknesses in the family.

      Strengths Weaknesses
   d. *Developmental issues:* How pertinent are individual and/or family developmental issues to the presenting problem? Are there foundational issues (e.g., maternal role dissatisfaction, depression) that cause negative cascading effects and need to be addressed? Rate from high concern (7) to low concern (1). List strengths and weaknesses in the family.

      Strengths Weaknesses
   e. *Affect regulation:* Are individuals able to regulate affects? Are there relationships within the family that are prone to dysregulation? What are the triggers that cause family members to become dysregulated? Rate from high concern (7) to low concern (1). List strengths and weaknesses in the family.

      Strengths Weaknesses

TABLE 42–2. Integrative Module-Based Family Therapy: step-by-step assessment *(continued)*

f. *Behavior regulation:* Are there individuals in the family who are prone to behavioral dysregulation? Are there specific relationships where this is more common? Who in the family is best able to regulate the behavior of the ones who lose control? How do parents maintain structure and behavioral control in the family? Are there power coercive cycles that must be addressed? Rate from high concern (7) to low concern (1). List strengths and weaknesses in the family.

Strengths Weaknesses

g. *Cognitive/narrative concerns* (family narratives): Is there evidence of cognitive distortions, exaggerated thoughts, or opinions about one another based more on emotion than facts? Are there family myths or negative role assignments that contribute to or maintain symptoms? Rate from high concern (7) to low concern (1). List strengths and weaknesses in the family.

Strengths Weaknesses

h. *Mastery:* Is the family successful in helping members achieve mastery, self-efficacy, and self-esteem? Is this related to the presenting problem? Rate from high concern (7) to low concern (1). List strengths and weaknesses in the family.

Strengths Weaknesses

i. *Community* (e.g., race, gender, worldview, religion, culture, sexual orientation): Are there relevant community issues that make achieving therapeutic goals difficult? Rate from high concern (7) to low concern (1). List strengths and weaknesses in the family's community context.

Strengths Weaknesses

4. Formulation

In light of the psychiatric diagnosis and the assessment of relevant psychosocial dimensions, describe how the presenting problem has become difficult for this particular patient and his or her family to manage. Or, how is the primary psychiatric diagnosis embedded within the familial context? What strengths within the family may be used to further clinical goals? What weaknesses complicate treatment?

5. Treatment plan

a. Domains of high concern generally require initial attention. Evidence-based therapies and best practice standards aid treatment planning. If treatment is not progressing, consider ways to strengthen the alliance with important family members in order to aid treatment adherence. Describe the (proposed or to-date) treatment plan.

b. Assess how well the patient and the family agree with the treatment plan.

Source. Adapted from Gouze and Wendel 2008; Wendel and Gouze 2010.

learn that he isn't the only one shouting at home. Apparently, mom and dad fight regularly because dad goes out and no one knows where he is. Michael's older brother left for college earlier in the year and has not come home for a visit.

How and where does one begin? First of all, it is generally best not to allow the problem-saturated description to take over the therapeutic process. The clinician will have to interrupt the mother and state that the problems will be fully addressed later, but at this point it is more important for the therapist to get to know both the mother and her son. This would begin the three-step joining process described earlier in the section "General Principles." As the therapist builds a relationship and rapport with both the mother and Michael, several questions emerge: Assess for substance

TABLE 42–3. Sample assessment questions for Integrative Module-Based Family Therapy domains

Psychiatric and related medical conditions domain

Standard psychiatric diagnostic questions guided by DSM-5, such as "Does your child have difficulty completing tasks?" "Does he or she get easily distracted?" "Does he or she seem sad most days?" "Does he or she have difficulty being left with a babysitter?"

Describe your child's medical history—any hospitalizations, medical conditions, current or past medications?

Attachment/relationship domain

Who in the family has the closest relationship with your child?

What is your relationship with your parents? Are you close?

Whom do you go to for support with your parenting?

Who is the best listener in the family?

Whom does the child trust with his or her distressing challenges?

Family structure domain

Who is most likely to enforce the rules in your family?

How are chores assigned to the children? Who assigns them? Who makes sure they are done?

Do you (parents) usually agree about how things should be done? If you disagree, how do you decide?

If you are planning a family outing, how do you decide where to go?

Family communication domain

Do family members feel heard?

Can family members tell what others are feeling?

How do you (parents) present and explain your directives?

Do family members engage in reflective listening?

Do family members talk over one another?

Developmental domain

Your child is starting school in the fall. How do you feel about this transition?

What was school like for you? (Ask other children in the family, "How do you guys feel about school?" "Do you do well?")

What are your hopes and dreams for your child?

How will having all your children in school all day change your life? What will you do with your free time during the day?

Affect regulation domain

Who has the worst temper in your family? Anyone else with a bad temper? What does that person do when he or she is angry?

How do people in your family calm down after an argument? How long does it take to restore positive relationships? How is that accomplished?

Do you think of your family as a pretty calm family or a very emotional one? Tell me more about that.

Behavior regulation domain

What are the rules about acceptable and unacceptable behavior in your family?

What kinds of rewards and consequences do you use?

Do the adults in your family follow rules and model good behavior, or do the adults push the limits (e.g., ignore parking regulations, lie about children's ages to get them into the movies for less money)?

TABLE 42–3. Sample assessment questions for Integrative Module-Based Family Therapy domains *(continued)*

Cognitive/narrative domain
Do you have favorite family stories or traditions that would help me understand your family?
Do you think of different members of the family in particular ways? If they were characters in a novel, how would you describe each of them?
How do different family members react to your child when he or she is nervous? Do you all seem to follow the same script when this happens?
Mastery domain
Are you pleased with your performance in school? Who else in your family has opinions about how you do in school?
What other things are you good at? Do you do sports or music or art?
Do you feel effective as a parent? What kinds of things make you feel more or less effective?
Community domain
What were gender roles like in your own family of origin? How have you worked these out in your current family?
Are you involved with a religious or community group of any type?
What has it been like for you to immigrate to this country? How do you feel that this affects your relationship with your children?

Source. Adapted from Gouze and Wendel 2008.

abuse? Depression? ADHD? Conduct disorder? Individual sessions with the teen or conjoint clinical hours with the teen and mom? What about dad? Clearly, there is no simple algorithm. By applying the 10 domains of IMBFT (Tables 42–2 and 42–3), the clinician begins to form a road map for intervention. Step 1 (Table 42–2) involves soliciting descriptive information from the identified patient and his family. It is important to see the "problem" within the larger familial context. Asking questions like "Please describe a typical day for the family from rising until bedtime" or "Are there times when the 'problem' isn't a problem?" can be quite informative. The clinician should be attuned to family transitions known to be times of increased vulnerability. Accounts from more than one person can be compared for differences and similarities. This type of discussion helps the clinician do two things. First, it provides important information without stimulating a problem-saturated description and helps the family therapist begin to form a view of overall family life and functioning. Second, it allows the clinician to indirectly consider DSM symptoms.

As the atmosphere calms, the therapist can seek more specific information related to pathology (step 2). In the case example, conduct disorder, ADHD, depression with agitation, and drug abuse need to be considered and viewed within overall family function. Table 42–3 provides sample questions the clinician can ask to determine the primacy of the other nine domains: attachments, family structure, communication, development, affect regulation, behavior regulation, cognitive/narrative concerns, mastery, and community. Ranking from low concern (1) to high concern (7) helps set priorities. In reviewing these scales, the therapist notes that modulating affect and behavior regulation are areas of concern. Also, the strained attachments suggest that cooperation and treatment adherence are unlikely until the familial relationships improve. Why are mom and dad fighting? Are they modeling hostile and impulsive interactional styles? Where does the dad go? Whom is he with? Is the teen doing what dad does? Do mom and dad exhibit positive and consistent parental structure focusing more on rewards than punishments, or the reverse? Why are the family attachments strained? Did this happen recently or is it longstanding? Who in the family is best able to help regulate Michael's affects, and what are the differences between the one who is best and the one who is worst at regulating his emotional response? Why hasn't the older brother come home from college? Questions such as these help the clinician construct a formulation in which the problem is seen in the context of overall family functioning.

Before the family therapist moves toward a treatment plan, session configuration needs to be considered. In this case, family or dyadic sessions are more appropriate, but the marital and familial climates are significant complicating factors. The clinician must guard against allowing the parents to prematurely focus on the teen's problems, which would be likely to stimulate an outburst confirming the parents' views and agenda but alienating the identified patient. The clinician could meet separately with each and compare accounts. Perhaps a better plan would be to invite other family members so viewpoints can be verified or dismissed. The clinician would have to exert more session management so as not to let the emotional level escalate. As the clinician formulates the case and considers treatment foci and options, the next step is entering into a discussion with the family and seeking agreement. In this example, Emotionally Focused Therapy may be applied in order to down regulate negative affective interaction and promote more empathic familial communication. After there is some improvement in the family's affective and behavioral regulation and their relationships with one another, the therapist might shift to delays in developmental success and achievement of mastery for the teen. It is hard to focus and apply oneself within an emotionally labile and hostile atmosphere. As a clinician identifies the priority domains (Table 42–2) and intervenes accordingly, he or she is able to engage in a cycle of reassessment that will lead to a new focus until treatment is complete.

Summary Points

- Clinicians are encouraged to do the following.
    1. Build a relationship with all family members and encourage each one to tell his or her story.
    2. Assess through 10 domains (psychiatric/biological, attachment/relationship, family structure, family communication, developmental, affect regulation, behavior regulation, cognitive/narrative, mastery, and community).
    3. Choose an initial focus.
    4. Form a feasible shared treatment plan.
    5. Learn (know) what empirically supported treatments or best practice standards are available after comprehensive family assessment.
    6. Tailor interventions to the needs and temperaments of the patient and family.
    7. Assess progress toward goals and make treatment shifts when necessary.

References

American Psychiatric Association: Diagnostic and Statistical Manual of Mental Disorders, 5th Edition. Arlington, VA, American Psychiatric Association, 2013

American Psychological Association Presidential Task Force on Evidence-Based Practice: Evidence-based practice in psychology. Am Psychol 61(4):271–285, 2006 16719673

Anderson T, Ogles BM, Patterson CL, et al: Therapist effects: facilitative interpersonal skills as a predictor of therapist success. J Clin Psychol 65(7):755–768, 2009 19437509

Asay TP, Lambert MJ: The empirical case for the common factors in therapy: quantitative findings, in The Heart and Soul of Change: What Works in Therapy. Edited by Hubble MA, Duncan BL, Miller SD. Washington, DC, American Psychological Association, 1999, pp 23–55

Bachelor A, Horvath A: The therapeutic relationship, in The Heart and Soul of Change: What Works in Therapy. Edited by Miller SD. Washington, DC, American Psychological Association, 1999, pp 133–178

Baldwin SA, Christian S, Berkeljon A, et al: The effects of family therapies for adolescent delinquency and substance abuse: a meta-analysis. J Marital Fam Ther 38(1):281–304, 2012 22283391

Bepko C, Johnson T: Gay and lesbian couples in therapy: perspectives for the contemporary family therapist. J Marital Fam Ther 26(4):409–419, 2000 11042835

Blatt SJ, Sanislow CA 3rd, Zuroff DC, et al: Characteristics of effective therapists: further analyses of data from the national institute of mental health treatment of depression collaborative research program. J Consult Clin Psychol 64(6):1276–1284, 1996 8991314

Bond C, Woods K, Humphrey N, et al: Practitioner Review: The effectiveness of solution focused brief therapy with children and families: a systematic and critical evaluation of the literature from 1990–2010. J Child Psychol Psychiatry 54(7):707–723, 2013 23452301

Bowlby J: A Secure Base: Parent-Child Attachment and Healthy Human Development. New York, Basic Books, 1988

Boyd-Franklin N: Black Families in Therapy: Understanding the African America Experience, 2nd Edition. New York, Guilford, 2008

Brookman-Frazee L, Haine RA, Gabayan EN, et al: Predicting frequency of treatment visits in community-based youth psychotherapy. Psychol Serv 5(2):126–138, 2008 20396643

Carr A: The evidence base for family therapy and systemic interventions for child-focused problems. J Fam Ther 36(2):107–157, 2014

Chorpita B, Weisz JR: Modular Approach to Therapy for Children with Anxiety, Depression, Trauma, or Conduct Problems (MATCH-ADTC). Satellite Beach, FL, PracticeWise, 2009

Côté AS, Boivin M, Liu X, et al: Depression and anxiety symptoms: onset, developmental course and risk factors during early childhood. J Child Psychol Psychiatry 50(10):1201–1208, 2009 19519755

Couturier J, Kimber M, Szatmari P: Efficacy of family based treatment for adolescents with eating disorders: a systematic review and meta-analysis. Int J Eat Disord 46(1):3–11, 2013 22821753

Davies PT, Cicchetti D: Toward an integration of family systems and developmental psychopathology approaches. Dev Psychopathol 16(3):477–481, 2004 15605621

Diamond G, Josephson A: Family based treatment research: a 10-year update. J Am Acad Child Adolesc Psychiatry 44(9):872–887, 2005 16113616

Diamond GS, Diamond GM, Levy SA: Attachment-Based Family Therapy for Depressed Adolescents. Washington, DC, American Psychological Association, 2014

Dietz LJ, Marshal MP, Burton CM, et al: Social problem solving among depressed adolescents is enhanced by structured psychotherapies. J Consult Clin Psychol 82(2):202–211, 2014 24491077

Freeman J, Epston D, Lobovits D: Playful Approaches to Serious Problems: Narrative Therapy With Children and Their Families. New York, W.W. Norton, 1997

Gallagher MW, Payne LA, White KS, et al: Mechanisms of change in cognitive behavioral therapy for panic disorder: the unique effects of self-efficacy and anxiety sensitivity. Behav Res Ther 51(11):767–777, 2013 24095901

Ge X, Best KM, Conger RD, et al: Parenting behaviors and the occurrence and co-occurrence of adolescent depressive symptoms and conduct problems. Dev Psychol 32(4):717–731, 1996

Gopalan G, Goldstein L, Klingenstein K, et al: Engaging families into child mental health treatment: updates and special considerations. J Can Acad Child Adolesc Psychiatry 19(3):182–196, 2010 20842273

Gottman JM: What Predicts Divorce? The Relationship Between Marital Processes and Marital Outcomes. Hillsdale, NJ, Lawrence Erlbaum Associates, 1994

Gouze KR, Wendel R: Integrative module-based family therapy: application and training. J Marital Fam Ther 34(3):269–286, 2008 18717919

Grant KE, Compas BE, Thurm AE, et al: Stressors and child and adolescent psychopathology: evidence of moderating and mediating effects. Clin Psychol Rev 26(3):257–283, 2006 16364522

Haddock SA, Zimmerman TS, MacPhee D: The Power Equity Guide: attending to gender in family therapy. J Marital Fam Ther 26(2):153–170, 2000 10776603

Hammen C, Brennan PA, Shih JH: Family discord and stress predictors of depression and other disorders in adolescent children of depressed and nondepressed women. J Am Acad Child Adolesc Psychiatry 43(8):994–1002, 2004 15266194

Henggeler SW, Sheidow AJ: Empirically supported family based treatments for conduct disorder and delinquency in adolescents. J Marital Fam Ther 38(1):30–58, 2012 22283380

Henggeler SW, Letourneau EJ, Chapman JE, et al: Mediators of change for multisystemic therapy with juvenile sexual offenders. J Consult Clin Psychol 77(3):451–462, 2009 19485587

Hipwell A, Keenan K, Kasza K, et al: Reciprocal influences between girls' conduct problems and depression, and parental punishment and warmth: a six year prospective analysis. J Abnorm Child Psychol 36(5):663–677, 2008 18172753

Hoagwood KE, Cavaleri MA, Serene Olin S, et al: Family support in children's mental health: a review and synthesis. Clin Child Fam Psychol Rev 13(1):1–45, 2010 20012893

Holmbeck GN, Devine KA, Bruno EF: Developmental issues and considerations in research and practice, in Evidence-Based Psychotherapies for Children and Adolescents. Edited by Kazdin AE, Weisz JR. New York, Guilford, 2010, pp 28–39

Jacobson NS, Dobson KS, Truax PA, et al: A component analysis of cognitive-behavioral treatment for depression. J Consult Clin Psychol 64(2):295–304, 1996 8871414

Jacobson NS, Martell CR, Dimidjian S: Behavioral activation treatment for depression: returning to contextual roots. Clin Psychol Sci Pract 8:255–270, 2001

Josephson AM, American Academy of Child and Adolescent Psychiatry Work Group on Quality Issues: Practice parameter for the assessment of the family. J Am Acad Child Adolesc Psychiatry 46(7):922–937, 2007 17581454

Josephson AM, Peteet JR (eds): Handbook of Spirituality and Worldview in Clinical Practice. Washington, DC, American Psychiatric Publishing, 2004

Kaslow NJ, Broth MR, Smith CO, et al: Family based interventions for child and adolescent disorders. J Marital Fam Ther 38(1):82–100, 2012 22283382

Kazdin AE: Parent Management Training: Treatment for Oppositional, Aggressive, and Antisocial Behavior in Children and Adolescents. New York, Oxford University Press, 2005

Kazdin AE: Mediators and mechanisms of change in psychotherapy research. Annu Rev Clin Psychol 3:1–27, 2007 17716046

Keiley MK: Attachment and affect regulation: a framework for family treatment of conduct disorder. Fam Process 41(3):477–493, 2002 12395570

Lambert MJ, Barley DE: Research summary on the therapeutic relationship and psychotherapy outcome. Psychotherapy 38(4):357–361, 2001

Lebow J: The integrative revolution in couple and family therapy. Fam Process 36(1):1–17, discussion 19–24, 1997 9189750

Lebow JL: Couple and Family Therapy: An Integrative Map of the Territory. Washington, DC, American Psychological Association, 2014

Lebow JL, Chambers AL, Christensen A, et al: Research on the treatment of couple distress. J Marital Fam Ther 38(1):145–168, 2012 22283385

Lipsitz JD, Markowitz JC: Mechanisms of change in interpersonal therapy (IPT). Clin Psychol Rev 33(8):1134–1147, 2013 24100081

Lovejoy MC, Graczyk PA, O'Hare E, et al: Maternal depression and parenting behavior: a meta-analytic review. Clin Psychol Rev 20(5):561–592, 2000 10860167

Luborsky L, Crits-Christoph P, McLellan AT, et al: Do therapists vary much in their success? Findings from four outcome studies. Am J Orthopsychiatry 56(4):501–512, 1986 3789096

Lucksted A, McFarlane W, Downing D, et al: Recent developments in family psychoeducation as an evidence-based practice. J Marital Fam Ther 38(1):101–121, 2012 22283383

Martell CR, Dimidjian S, Herman-Dunn R: Behavioral Activation for Depression: A Clinician's Guide. New York, Guilford, 2010

Masten AS: Developmental psychopathology: pathways to the future. Int J Behav Dev 30(1):47–54, 2006

Masten AS, Cicchetti D: Developmental cascades. Dev Psychopathol 22(3):491–495, 2010 20576173

McGoldrick M, Hardy KV (eds): Re-Visioning Family Therapy: Race, Culture, and Gender in Clinical Practice. New York, Guilford, 2008

Morris AS, Silk JS, Steinberg L, et al: The role of the family context in the development of emotion regulation. Soc Dev 16(2):361–388, 2007 19756175

Podell JL, Kendall PC, Gosch EA, et al: Therapist factors and outcomes in CBT for anxiety in youth. Prof Psychol Res Pr 44(2):89–98, 2013

Rowe CL: Family therapy for drug abuse: review and updates 2003–2010. J Marital Fam Ther 38(1):59–81, 2012 22283381

Shahar B, Britton WB, Sbarra DA, et al: Mechanisms of change in mindfulness-based cognitive therapy for depression: preliminary evidence from a randomized controlled trial. Int J Cogn Ther 3:402–418, 2010

Shields CG, Finley MA, Chawla N, et al: Couple and family interventions in health problems. J Marital Fam Ther 38(1):265–280, 2012 22283390

Sprenkle DH, Davis SD, Lebow JL: Common Factors in Couple and Family Therapy: The Overlooked Foundation for Effective Practice. New York, Guilford, 2009

Szapocznik J, Schwartz SJ, Muir JA, et al: Brief strategic family therapy: an intervention to reduce adolescent risk behavior. Couple Family Psychol 1(2):134–145, 2012 23936750

Taub J, Tighe TA, Burchard J: The effects of parent empowerment on adjustment for children receiving comprehensive mental health services. Children's Services: Social Policy, Research, and Practice 4(3):103–122, 2001

Webster-Stratton C, Reid MJ: The Incredible Years parents, teachers, and children: a multifaceted treatment approach for young children with conduct disorders, in Evidence-Based Psychotherapies for Children and Adolescents. Edited by Weisz JR, Kazdin AE. New York, Guilford, 2010, pp 194–210

Weisz JR, Chorpita BF, Palinkas LA, et al: Testing standard and modular designs for psychotherapy treating depression, anxiety, and conduct problems in youth: a randomized effectiveness trial. Arch Gen Psychiatry 69(3):274–282, 2012 22065252

Wendel R, Gouze KR: Family therapy: assessment and intervention, in Dulcan's Textbook of Child and Adolescent Psychiatry. Edited by Dulcan MK. Washington, DC, American Psychiatric Publishing, 2010, pp 869–886

White M, Epston D: Narrative Means to Therapeutic Ends. New York, W.W. Norton, 1990

Winnicott DW: The Maturational Processes and the Facilitating Environment: Studies in the Theory of Emotional Development. Oxford, UK, International Universities Press, 1965

Zimet DM, Jacob T: Influences of marital conflict on child adjustment: review of theory and research. Clin Child Fam Psychol Rev 4(4):319–335, 2001 11837462

Zisser A, Eyberg SM: Parent-child interaction therapy and the treatment of disruptive behavior disorders, in Evidence-Based Psychotherapies for Children and Adolescents. Edited by Kazdin AE, Weisz JR. New York, Guilford, 2010, pp 179–193

CHAPTER 43

Interpersonal Psychotherapy for Depressed Adolescents

Meredith L. Gunlicks-Stoessel, Ph.D.
Laura Mufson, Ph.D.

Interpersonal psychotherapy for depressed adolescents (IPT-A; Mufson et al. 2004b) is a time-limited, manualized psychotherapeutic intervention adapted from interpersonal psychotherapy for adults (IPT; Weissman et al. 2000). IPT is based on the principle that regardless of the underlying cause, depression occurs within an interpersonal context. The goal of treatment, therefore, is to decrease depressive symptoms by focusing on current interpersonal difficulties and helping the individual improve his or her relationships and communication patterns.

The theoretical basis for IPT comes from the work of Adolf Meyer, Harry Stack Sullivan, and other interpersonal theorists, who have stated that interpersonal interactions form the basis of personality and functioning and that psychopathology develops out of and is perpetuated by problems in these interactions (Meyer 1957; Sullivan 1953). Consistent with these principles, IPT focuses on helping patients become aware of their current communication patterns and the types of responses these patterns elicit from others. They can then observe that by altering their communication patterns, the nature of their relationships is changed, and this, in turn, can lead to improvements in mood. Attachment theory is also relevant for IPT. Bowlby (1978) proposed that people have a tendency and need to develop strong bonds to significant others. When these bonds are disrupted in some way, the individual experiences emotional distress, including symptoms of depression. IPT addresses the role of attachment in depression by targeting interpersonal conflicts, transitions, and grief in relationships that may affect the patient's attachment experiences and contribute to the development of depression.

IPT was originally designed as an intervention for nonpsychotic depressed adults treated as outpatients, and there is strong empirical support for its use (Weissman et al. 2000). IPT-A is a developmental adaptation that is designed to treat adolescents, ages 12–18 years, with nonpsychotic, unipolar depression. Depressed adolescents with comorbid anxiety disorders, attention-deficit/hyperactivity disorder, and oppositional defiant disorder have been successfully treated with IPT-A, although IPT-A is most effective when depression is the primary diagnosis. IPT-A is not recommended for adolescents who have intellectual disability, active suicidal or homicidal thoughts with a plan and/or intent, psychosis, or bipolar disorder or are actively abusing substances.

Course of Treatment

IPT-A is designed to be delivered once a week for 12 weeks, although the treatment schedule can be more flexible, if necessary. If a crisis occurs or supplementary sessions are needed for other reasons, the treatment duration can be extended or sessions can be temporarily scheduled for more frequently than once a week. The school-based model allows for 12 sessions in 16 weeks to accommodate the school calendar. However, it is crucial to keep the treatment time limited, even when negotiating additional sessions, by restating the treatment contract with those modifications.

IPT-A is an individual treatment that recommends, but does not require, parental participation. Parental session attendance can range from none to several sessions, although nonattendance is strongly discouraged. Parental absence from sessions is sometimes necessary, however, depending on the family's circumstances. It is recommended that parents attend at least one session in the beginning of treatment in order to be educated about depression and the IPT-A treatment and at least one session at the end of treatment in order to learn about the adolescent's warning signs of depression and strategies for managing potential recurrence. Parental participation can also be helpful in the middle phase of treatment, as parental participation provides adolescents with opportunities to practice learned skills with their parents.

IPT-A is divided into three treatment phases: initial, middle, and termination. Each session begins with the therapist assessing the adolescent's depressive symptoms and asking the adolescent to rate his or her mood using a 1–10 scale (10 most depressed). Any changes in depressive symptoms that occurred since the last session are noted and linked to interpersonal events that happened during the week. The symptom review and mood ratings are useful ways for both the therapist and the adolescent to monitor treatment progress. Following the review of symptoms, the therapist and adolescent focus on tasks that are specific to the adolescent's current phase of treatment.

Initial Phase (Sessions 1–4)

Confirm the Depression Diagnosis and Suitability of IPT-A

Prior to entering IPT-A, the adolescent should have already completed a full psychiatric evaluation to assess current symptoms and diagnoses, as well as psychiatric, family, developmental, medical, social, and academic history

(Mufson et al. 2004b). However, it is important to confirm the depression diagnosis in the first session, using a clinical interview.

Provide Psychoeducation About Depression

The therapist should provide the adolescent and his or her family with information about depression, including its associated symptoms and behaviors. For example, many families do not realize that irritability is a symptom of depression. They also may not realize that a decline in academic performance may be a function of reduced concentration, anhedonia, fatigue, and other symptoms of depression, rather than an indication that the adolescent is being oppositional or lazy. It is also useful to place depression in the context of a medical illness that can be treated. This can decrease the stigma often associated with depression, take the blame off of the adolescent for causing the depression, and provide an optimistic prognosis that the depression will improve with treatment.

Psychoeducation also includes assigning the adolescent the *limited sick role.* This involves explaining that like someone with a medical illness, adolescents who have symptoms of depression may not be able to do as many things or do things as well as they did before the depression developed. The goal of the limited sick role is for the adolescent to try to do as many of his or her usual activities as possible, with the awareness and acceptance that he or she might not do these things as often or as well as before the depression developed. It is important for the family to understand the limited sick role so that they can be more supportive of the adolescent's efforts in these activities and less critical of the outcomes.

Explain the Theory and Goals of IPT-A

The therapist should explain the theory and structure of IPT-A to the adolescent and family so that they know what to expect. This includes educating the family about the premise that depression occurs within an interpersonal context. Specifically, regardless of what initially caused the depression, depression affects people's relationships, and relationships affect people's moods. Thus, the treatment will focus on improving the adolescent's relationships by teaching communication and interpersonal problem-solving skills that can lead to a reduction in the adolescent's depressive symptoms.

Conduct the Interpersonal Inventory

The interpersonal inventory is used to identify the interpersonal issues that are most closely related to the adolescent's depression. First, the adolescent identifies the significant relationships in his or her life by completing a *closeness circle.* A closeness circle is a series of four concentric circles that resembles a bull's-eye. The therapist writes the adolescent's name in the innermost circle and places the names of the people in the adolescent's life in the other circles according to the closeness of their relationship. People to whom the adolescent feels closest, even if the relationship is not always positive, are put in the circle closest to the adolescent, with other people placed in the middle or outer circle. Once the closeness circle has been completed, the therapist and adolescent discuss each relationship in more depth, placing particular emphasis on the relationships that the adolescent feels are most related to his or her mood in either positive or negative ways. The therapist typically asks the adolescent to identify four to five people from the circle who are important to discuss to understand their role in the adolescent's depression. For each relationship, the therapist should ask about the frequency and content of their interactions, terms and expectations for the relationship, positive and negative aspects of the relationship, ways in which the relationship is associated with the adolescent's depression, and changes the adolescent would like to make in the relationship (Mufson et al. 2004b).

Identify the Interpersonal Problem Area(s)

On the basis of the interpersonal inventory, the therapist helps the adolescent link the status and quality of his or her relationships to his or her depressive symptoms. The therapist identifies common themes or problems in the adolescent's relationships, and together with the adolescent identifies one of four interpersonal problem areas that will be the focus of treatment: grief due to death, interpersonal role disputes, interpersonal role transitions, or interpersonal deficits. Generally, only one interpersonal problem area is identified, but it is also possible to identify a secondary problem area.

Grief Due to Death

Grief is selected as the problem area when an adolescent experiences the death of a loved one and the loss is associated with normal bereavement or prolonged grief, significant depressive symptoms, and impairment in functioning. The goal of IPT-A for adolescents with this problem area is to facilitate the resolution of the delayed normal mourning process and to develop or improve other relationships that can provide the support, nurturance, companionship, or guidance that has been lost (Mufson et al. 2004b).

Interpersonal Role Disputes

An interpersonal role dispute involves the adolescent and at least one significant other having different expectations about the terms and/or guidelines for behavior within their relationship (Weissman et al. 2000). Interpersonal role dispute is selected as the problem area if the adolescent's depressive episode coincides with a relationship conflict. The goal of treatment is to help the adolescent develop skills to attempt to resolve the dispute. If resolution is not possible, the goal is to help the adolescent develop strategies for coping with the relationship (Mufson et al. 2004b).

Interpersonal Role Transitions

A role transition occurs when a life change requires an alteration of behavior from an old role to a new role (Weissman et al. 2000). Role transitions may be biologically determined (transitioning from childhood to puberty) or a result of social and cultural practices (transitioning from middle school to high school). In addition to these more normative transitions, adolescents may also experience unexpected changes that require them to take on new social roles, such as a change in family structure due to parents' separation or divorce. An adolescent may develop symptoms of depression in response to a role transition if the role is unexpected or undesired, the adolescent is not psychologically or emotionally prepared for the new role, or the adolescent preferred the old role. Depression may also exacerbate the adolescent's ability to successfully negotiate a transition. For adolescents experiencing a role transition, the goal of IPT-A is to help them mourn the loss of the old role and develop the skills they need to manage the new role more successfully (Mufson et al. 2004b).

Interpersonal Deficits

Interpersonal deficits refer to underdeveloped social and communication skills that impair the adolescent's ability to have positive relationships (Weissman et al. 2000). Deficits may include difficulty initiating or maintaining relationships, verbally expressing one's feelings or needs, or eliciting information from others to establish communication. The goal of treatment is to develop the interpersonal skills needed to have more satisfying relationships and reduce social isolation (Mufson et al. 2004b). Adolescents whose interpersonal deficits may be due to severe social skills deficits or autism spectrum disorder diagnoses are not well suited to IPT-A because the treatment aims to build on existing skills in a short period of time and assumes that at least some of the skill deficits are due to the depression and are considered transient.

Make the Treatment Contract

Once the problem areas have been identified, the adolescent and therapist make a verbal treatment contract regarding the adolescent's and therapist's roles in treatment, the interpersonal problem area(s) that will be the focus of treatment, and the practical details of the treatment. This includes explaining to the adolescent that for the treatment to be most helpful, the adolescent will need to bring in information about relationships and interpersonal interactions each week for the therapist and adolescent to discuss and problem solve. The therapist also informs the adolescent that his or her parent(s) may be invited to attend a treatment session to work on the identified problem area(s).

Middle Phase (Sessions 5–9)

During the middle phase of treatment, the therapist and adolescent begin to work directly on the identified interpersonal problem area(s). This is accomplished by identifying effective strategies for managing the problem and practicing and implementing the strategies. Some of the therapeutic techniques used during this phase of treatment are specific to the identified problem area(s), and others are used across problem areas. It is best to start with an interpersonal issue that is relatively simple and has a high likelihood of success. This generates hope that the strategies learned can help facilitate change in relationships and improve mood.

General Techniques

Encouragement of Affect and Linkage With Interpersonal Events

These techniques are used to help the adolescent become aware of, acknowledge, and accept negative emotions about events and relationships and understand how emotions affect relationships (Weissman et al. 2000). It is our experience that adolescents tend to present in one of two ways. Some adolescents experience their emotions intensely and can readily express them but do not seem to be aware of how the emotions are related to the events in their lives. Other adolescents can easily describe events in their lives but do so without any mention of emotion. For both types, it is important to help them link interpersonal events with their mood. If the adolescent describes a change in mood without an awareness of the cause, the therapist and adolescent may review the week in great detail to unearth an event or relationship that may have led to the change in mood. If the adolescent describes a difficult interaction with a significant other without awareness of the feelings associated with it, the therapist may ask the adolescent how the event made the adolescent feel and how it affected his or her depressive symptoms. This educates the adolescent about the link between interpersonal events and mood and helps the adolescent become more comfortable and skilled in identifying, understanding, and communicating his or her feelings.

Communication Analysis

Communication analysis is used to explore the adolescent's patterns of interacting with others in order to identify ways in which his or her communication is problematic and skills the adolescent needs to master to have more satisfying relationships. Communication analysis involves asking the adolescent to describe a recent interpersonal event in great detail. The therapist may ask the adolescent questions, such as the following (Mufson et al. 2004b): "How did the discussion start?" "When and where did it take place?" "What exactly did you say?" "What did the other person say back?" "Then what happened?" "How did that make you feel?" "How do you think it made the other person feel?" "Is that the outcome you wanted?" Through this process, the therapist helps the adolescent recognize the impact of his or her words on others, the feelings that arose during the interactions, and the feelings he or she conveys verbally and nonverbally.

Once the therapist and adolescent have an understanding of the interaction, they discuss how doing things differently at various points might have led to a different outcome and different emotional experience. Some common communication techniques to be taught and modeled include 1) selecting an optimal time to initiate a conversation, 2) communicating feelings and opinions directly ("I" statements), 3) attempting to see the problem from the other person's perspective, 4) being specific when talking about a problem and focusing on the present problem at hand (avoid "you always" or "you never"), and 5) generating some solutions prior to the conversation and being willing to compromise (Mufson et al. 2004b).

Decision Analysis

Decision analysis is similar to problem-solving techniques that are used in other models of therapy but is focused more specifically on addressing interpersonal problems. It involves selecting an interpersonal situation that is causing the adolescent problems, determining the goal, generating a list of alternative strategies (some of these may come out of the communication analysis), evaluating the pros and cons of each potential solution or strategy, and selecting a strategy to try first in session and then, if it looks promising, outside of the session (Mufson et al. 2004b). Once the adolescent has tried the strategy, the therapist and adolescent should evaluate the outcome and determine if there is a need to select an alternative strategy.

Role-Playing

Role-playing is a way for adolescents to practice the communication and interpersonal problem-solving skills that they have learned in order to feel more comfortable using them in real life. To be most helpful, the therapist and adolescent should not simply talk about what it would be like to have the conversation using the new strategies; they should actually act it out. It can be useful to give the adolescent the opportunity to play both roles, in turn, so the adolescent can better understand the other person's perspective. This also helps the therapist understand the adolescent's experience of the other person. It is also useful to try the role-play more than once, with different outcomes to the interactions, both positive and negative, so that the adolescent can become more skilled in handling different kinds of situations that might develop. Once the adolescent is able to role-play the interaction effectively, the therapist should encourage the adolescent to try having the conversation with the other person prior to the next therapy session. The therapist and adolescent can then use communication analysis in the next therapy session to process how the conversation went and determine if further action is needed.

Problem Area–Specific Techniques

Grief Due to Death

The treatment goal for adolescents with the identified problem area of grief is to facilitate the delayed normal grieving process. This involves detailed discussions of the adolescent's relationship with the deceased, including both positive and negative aspects of the relationship and conflicts in the relationship. The therapist should also gently encourage expression of affect about the relationship and its loss and help the adolescent to connect current depressive symptoms and behaviors to feelings surrounding the death. As the treatment progresses, the therapist helps the adolescent develop skills for communicating thoughts and feelings about the loss with other people in the adolescent's life. The idea is to help the adolescent develop new relationships or further develop existing relationships to fill in the support that was lost with the death of the loved one.

Interpersonal Role Disputes

An adolescent may present with interpersonal role disputes that may be in one of three stages: renegotiation, impasse, or dissolution (Weissman et al. 2000). An adolescent and significant other are in the *renegotiation stage* if they are still communicating with one another and are attempting to resolve the conflict. They are in the *impasse stage* if they are no longer attempting to negotiate the conflict and social distancing (or "the silent treatment") has occurred. In the *dissolution stage,* the adolescent and significant other have already decided that the dispute cannot be resolved, and they have chosen to end the relationship. For adolescents whose disputes are in the renegotiation or impasse stages, the goal of treatment is to help the adolescent define and resolve the dispute. This involves working with the adolescent and the other person, if possible, to describe the dispute, identify existing patterns of communication, teach new communication skills, and generate solutions to the dispute (Mufson et al. 2004b). If complete resolution of the problem does not appear to be possible, the therapist works with the adolescent to develop strategies for coping with a relationship that cannot be changed. This may include developing other relationships that the adolescent can use as a means of support. It is often helpful to point out that although a relationship may not be changeable, simply decreasing the frequency or intensity of conflict can lead to improved mood. If the dispute is in the dissolution stage, treatment focuses on mourning the loss of the relationship. This involves discussing the dispute and lost relationship, developing an understanding of what occurred, and helping the adolescent establish new relationships.

Interpersonal Role Transitions

For adolescents experiencing an interpersonal role transition, treatment involves identifying and defining the transition, helping the adolescent give up the old role and accept the new one, and helping the adolescent develop a sense of competence in the new role (Mufson et al. 2004b). The therapist should provide the adolescent and parents, when possible, with information about the effect that transitions can have on functioning. The therapist then explores with the adolescent the meaning of the transition, feelings and expectations about the old and new roles, and gains and losses associated with the transition. The therapist also helps the adolescent learn and practice new communication and interpersonal problem-solving skills that can be used to manage the new role and develop relationships that can provide ongoing support during the transition.

Interpersonal Deficits

For adolescents with interpersonal deficits, treatment begins with helping the adolescent identify and label repetitive interpersonal problems and connect these problems with his or her depressive symptoms (Mufson et al. 2004b). If the adolescent does not have many current relationships, the therapist can review past relationships to look for patterns of difficulty as well as strengths on which to build. The therapist can also use his or her own relationship with the adolescent to explore the adolescent's interpersonal deficits. The therapist then helps the adolescent learn and practice new skills for developing and maintaining relationships, such as how to initiate and sustain a conversation, ask a peer to join in an activity, or share feelings with someone. The therapist works with the adolescent to identify existing relationships that he or she would like to build on and/or new relationships that the adolescent would like to develop. It is important with these adolescents to focus on strengths as much as on deficits. The therapist should draw attention to skills the adolescent has used in other relationships or in the therapy session to help the adolescent build a sense of confidence and competence and to reinforce positive communication patterns.

Termination Phase (Sessions 10–12)

The termination phase of IPT-A is similar to the termination phases of other therapy models. This phase involves reviewing the course of the adolescent's depressive symptoms and how these symptoms have changed. The therapist and adolescent should also review the changes that occurred in the adolescent's communication style and relationship functioning, link these changes to the improvement in the adolescent's mood, and highlight the skills and strategies the adolescent found particularly useful. It is also helpful to discuss anticipated future difficult situations and review strategies that the adolescent can use to negotiate those situations. As part of termination, it is also important to discuss the adolescent's feelings about ending treatment and the relationship with the therapist. Finally, the therapist and adolescent should discuss the possibility of recurrence of depression, the warning symptoms of depression that are particular to that adolescent, and strategies for managing a recurrence (Mufson et al. 2004b). It is recommended that parents attend a session during the termination phase in order to review the adolescent's progress, plans for managing future interpersonal difficulties, warning signs for recurrence of depression, and strategies for managing the depression, should it recur.

The following case example illustrates the IPT-A techniques and course of treatment.

Case Example

Tianna is a 14-year-old African American girl who had recently begun ninth grade in a new high school. She was referred for treatment by her school counselor for possible depression after three incidents in which other students reported finding Tianna crying in the bathroom. Tianna lives with her mother, older sister, and younger brother. Her depressive symptoms reportedly began approximately 6 months prior to the evaluation and included irritability, reduced interest in spending time with peers, insomnia, fatigue, and decreased appetite. Her mother also described her as more quiet and isolative around the house. Tianna had consistently been a strong student, and this had not changed with the onset of her depressive symptoms. On the basis of the clinical evaluation, she was diagnosed with major depressive disorder.

Initial Phase

During the first session, the therapist met with Tianna and her mother to hear their perspectives on Tianna's depressive symptoms and to confirm the depression diagnosis. The therapist provided them with information about depression, including describing depression as a medical illness that can be treated. The therapist assigned the limited sick role, which for Tianna meant trying to continue socializing with peers and communicating with her family, despite her reduced interest in doing so—but also not being too critical of herself at times when she does not feel able to socialize. The session ended with the therapist explaining the theory and structure of IPT-A and addressing Tianna's and her mother's questions.

The next three sessions were spent completing the interpersonal inventory. In the closeness circle, Tianna identified her mother, sister, brother, two aunts who lived close by, and one friend from middle school as the important people in her life. With respect to her mother and siblings, Tianna described their relationships as distant. Tianna noticed that her mother and siblings were more talkative than she was. She felt that she spent a lot of time listening to them talk about the events of the day and their problems, but they did not reciprocate. Whenever she tried to talk, one of her family members would interrupt her or talk over her. Consequently, Tianna kept her problems to herself. She felt overlooked by her family, and this left her feeling depressed. She spent increasing amounts of time in her room to avoid her family.

Tianna also talked about her two aunts who lived close by. She reported seeing them a few times a week and stated that she had fun with them, but she had never used them as a means of support in coping with problems at home or elsewhere. In terms of peers, Tianna continued to see and talk regularly with one friend from middle school who did not go to her high school. Tianna stated that most of the kids at her new school seemed nice, but she had not developed friendships with any of them.

After the interpersonal inventory, Tianna and the therapist developed an interpersonal formulation of Tianna's depression. Tianna's primary interpersonal problem area appeared to be interpersonal deficits. She was having difficulty expressing her feelings, problems, and needs with her immediate and extended family; she had only one existing friendship; and she was having difficulty developing new social connections at her high school. The therapist and Tianna discussed how Tianna's difficulty talking about her feelings and problems with her family left her feeling depressed. Her depression caused her to withdraw even more, and her withdrawal then prevented her from getting support from family and friends. The therapist and Tianna made a treatment contract to work on communication skills that would help Tianna better express her feelings and needs so that she could have more satisfying relationships.

Middle Phase

During the middle phase of treatment, the therapist and Tianna worked to develop a better understanding of Tianna's difficulty expressing herself and soliciting support from others. This involved conducting communication analysis on several interactions Tianna had with her mother and siblings to examine how and what Tianna communicated to her family and how these interactions made her feel. Through these analyses, the therapist and Tianna became aware that Tianna tended to wait for one of her family members to ask her how she was doing rather than initiating a conversation when she needed support. In addition, if Tianna's mother or siblings interrupted her when she was talking, Tianna tended to just let the other person talk. These interactions left Tianna feeling depressed and angry. The therapist and Tianna discussed how Tianna could initiate a conversation with her mother or siblings when she needed some support, at a time when her mother or siblings seemed like they might be particularly receptive to listening to her (e.g., letting mom relax a bit after she gets home from work before trying to talk to her). Tianna practiced initiating a conversation and expressing her feelings using a role-play, and she was asked to try the conversation at home. Tianna attempted the conversation and reported back to the therapist that when she tried to talk to her mother, her sister came in and interrupted the conversation. Tianna and the therapist discussed and practiced having Tianna explain to her sister that when she interrupts it makes Tianna feel ignored and unimportant. Tianna also had the idea of telling her sister that she would like to hear what her sister has to say and proposing that her sister have a turn to talk when Tianna is finished.

The therapist also worked with Tianna to help her enhance her relationships with her aunts and develop friendships at her new high school. This included having Tianna talk to her aunts about her depression and the difficulties she had been having communicating with her mother and siblings. The therapist and Tianna also conducted communication analysis regarding interactions Tianna had with her friend. Through the course of these analyses, the therapist was able to highlight the communication skills Tianna used in this relationship that could be applied toward developing relationships at her new school. Tianna identified two girls with whom she would like to initiate friendships, and Tianna and the therapist role-played having conversations with them. As changes in Tianna's relationships began to occur, Tianna's depressive symptoms began to improve. The therapist pointed out the link between the improvements in Tianna's relationships and her improved mood.

Termination Phase

During the termination phase, the therapist and Tianna reviewed the course of Tianna's depressive symptoms, noting that Tianna felt better when she was able to talk more to her family members and friends about her problems and needs. They discussed the interpersonal strategies that Tianna found most helpful, including directly expressing her feelings and needs and selecting an appropriate time to initiate a conversation. During this discussion, Tianna and the therapist also discussed the strategies that Tianna could continue to use after treatment had ended. Tianna also discussed her feelings about ending treatment. Tianna's mother joined Tianna and the therapist for the last session. Together they reviewed Tianna's progress in treatment, discussed Tianna's warning signs for recurrence of depression, and discussed how to seek help should the depression recur.

Group Psychotherapy

IPT-A has been adapted to be delivered in a group format (Mufson et al. 2004a). Group IPT-A consists of a combination of individual and group therapy sessions delivered over the course of 14 weeks. Two to three individual pregroup sessions are conducted with each adolescent and his or her parent(s) to collect information about the adolescent's depressive symptoms and significant relationships and to identify the interpersonal problem area(s). There are 12 group sessions. Adolescents participate in group exercises in which they coach each other to use better communication and problem-solving skills. In addition, they report to each other on their experiences trying the new techniques outside of the group, which provides opportunities for adolescents to learn from each other's successes and mistakes. Parents are also invited to participate in a single family session midtreatment and posttreatment. The midtreatment session provides the adolescent with an opportunity to practice newly learned communication skills with his or her parents. The posttreatment session is used to review with parents the adolescent's progress and to discuss strategies for managing potential recurrence of depression.

Empirical Support

The efficacy and effectiveness of IPT-A for reducing adolescents' depressive symptoms have been examined in four randomized controlled clinical trials (Mufson et al. 1999, 2004c; Rosselló and Bernal 1999; Rosselló et al. 2008). Depressed adolescents treated with IPT-A demonstrated fewer depressive symptoms, better social functioning, and better global functioning at the completion of treatment than adolescents in control conditions, although in one study by Rosselló et al. (2008), IPT did not show as much improvement as CBT. The Rosselló and Bernal (1999) and Rosselló et al. (2008) studies used their own adaptation of IPT for use with adolescents, and in the Rosselló et al. (2008) study, there was low fidelity adherence to the IPT treatment, which may explain their weaker results for IPT. IPT-A has been shown to be particularly effective for adolescents with high levels of parent-adolescent conflict (Gunlicks-Stoessel et al. 2010; Young et al. 2009). On the basis of the empirical support for treatment efficacy, IPT-A meets the American Psychological Association Division 12 criteria for a "well-established" psychotherapy for depression in youth.

A modified version of group IPT-A, titled Interpersonal Psychotherapy–Adolescent Skills Training (IPT-AST), has also been developed as a prevention intervention for adolescents with elevated symptoms of depression (Young et al. 2006, 2010). In a clinical trial, adolescents who received IPT-AST had significantly fewer depressive symptoms and depressive diagnoses and had better overall functioning posttreatment than adolescents who received school counseling (Young et al. 2006, 2010).

Summary Points

- Interpersonal psychotherapy for depressed adolescents (IPT-A) is based on the observation that depression occurs within an interpersonal context. The goal of treatment is to decrease depressive symptoms by helping the adolescent improve his or her relationships and communication patterns.
- As part of the psychoeducation about depression, the therapist should assign the adolescent the limited sick role. This involves encouraging the adolescent to try to do as many of his or her usual activities as possible, with the understanding that he or she might not do these things as often or as well as before the depression developed.
- To identify the interpersonal issues that are most closely related to the adolescent's depression, the therapist conducts an interpersonal inventory. The adolescent identifies the significant relationships in his or her life by completing a closeness circle, and the therapist probes each relationship in depth.
- On the basis of the interpersonal inventory, the therapist identifies one of four interpersonal problem areas that will be the focus of treatment: grief due to death, interpersonal role disputes, interpersonal role transitions, or interpersonal deficits.
- During the middle phase of treatment, adolescents learn to use exploration of affect, communication analysis, decision analysis, and role-plays to acquire and practice skills for managing their interpersonal problems.
- Adolescents are encouraged to try the interpersonal skills they have learned outside of the therapy setting. This "work at home" is not predetermined by the therapist but rather grows out of each therapy session's specific focus and content.
- During the termination phase of treatment, the therapist should highlight interpersonal skills gained, promote generalization of specific strategies, and help the adolescent identify warning signs of depression that might indicate that he or she should seek treatment again.

References

Bowlby J: Attachment theory and its therapeutic implications. Adolesc Psychiatry 6:5–33, 1978 742687

Gunlicks-Stoessel M, Mufson L, Jekal A, et al: The impact of perceived interpersonal functioning on treatment for adolescent depression: IPT-A versus treatment as usual in school-based health clinics. J Consult Clin Psychol 78(2):260–267, 2010 20350036

Meyer A: Psychobiology: A Science of Man. Springfield, IL, Charles C Thomas, 1957

Mufson L, Weissman MM, Moreau D, et al: Efficacy of interpersonal psychotherapy for depressed adolescents. Arch Gen Psychiatry 56(6):573–579, 1999 10359475

Mufson L, Gallagher T, Dorta KP, et al: A group adaptation of interpersonal psychotherapy for depressed adolescents. Am J Psychother 58(2):220–237, 2004a 15373283

Mufson L, Dorta KP, Moreau D, et al: Interpersonal Psychotherapy for Depressed Adolescents, 2nd Edition. New York, Guilford, 2004b

Mufson L, Dorta KP, Wickramaratne P, et al: Arch Gen Psychiatry 61(6):577–584, 2004c

Rosselló J, Bernal G: The efficacy of cognitive-behavioral and interpersonal treatments for depression in Puerto Rican adolescents. J Consult Clin Psychol 67(5):734–745, 1999 10535240

Rosselló J, Bernal G, Rivera-Medina C: Individual and group CBT and IPT for Puerto Rican adolescents with depressive symptoms. Cultur Divers Ethnic Minor Psychol 14(3):234–245, 2008 18624588

Sullivan HS: The Interpersonal Theory of Psychiatry. New York, WW Norton, 1953

Weissman MM, Markowitz JC, Klerman GL: Comprehensive Guide to Interpersonal Psychotherapy. New York, Basic Books, 2000

Young JF, Mufson L, Davies M: Efficacy of interpersonal psychotherapy–adolescent skills training: an indicated preventive intervention for depression. J Child Psychol Psychiatry 47(12):1254–1262, 2006 17176380

Young JF, Gallop R, Mufson L: Mother-child conflict and its moderating effects on depression outcomes in a preventive intervention for adolescent depression. J Clin Child Adolesc Psychol 38(5):696–704, 2009 20183654

Young JF, Mufson L, Gallop R: Preventing depression: a randomized trial of interpersonal psychotherapy-adolescent skills training. Depress Anxiety 27(5):426–433, 2010 20112246

CHAPTER 44

Cognitive-Behavioral Treatment for Anxiety and Depression

Deborah C. Beidel, Ph.D., ABPP
Mark A. Reinecke, Ph.D., ABPP, ACT

Anxiety and depressive disorders are among the most prevalent childhood psychiatric conditions. Despite their initial dismissal as not serious (see Beidel and Alfano 2011), there is now sufficient evidence that childhood anxiety symptoms are serious, chronic, distressing, and functionally impairing. Similarly, depressive disorders in children can be associated with severe functional impairment, including suicidal ideation. Thus, the need for efficacious interventions that can eliminate symptoms and enhance overall functioning is now firmly established. Over the past 30 years, a robust literature has developed, consisting of rigorous randomized controlled trials (RCTs) that confirm the efficacy of cognitive-behavioral treatment (CBT) for youth with anxiety or depressive disorders (Chu and Harrison 2007), suggesting that CBT not only decreases symptoms but improves general functioning. For anxiety disorders, CBT is considered the first-line treatment approach. In this chapter, we review CBT for anxiety and depressive disorders.

General Characteristics of Cognitive-Behavioral Treatment

CBT is formulation based and prescriptive. Interventions are selected on the basis of understanding the cognitive, behavioral, social, and environmental variables contributing to the child's distress. Thus, the specific interventions used in CBT are individually tailored and strategically directed toward changing maladaptive beliefs and attitudes, eliminating emotional distress, and alleviating social skill deficits and avoidance behaviors. An essential characteristic of CBT is its time-limited nature. Active and focused treatment is organized according to an agenda and begins with thorough psychoeducation regarding the nature of CBT and its goals and procedures. Outside of the clinic, homework assignments provide practice opportunities for skill reinforcement and generalization to the natural environment. The therapeutic relationship is characterized by collaboration among patient, family, and therapist, and in some cases will include school personnel. Treatment is not typically open-ended or long term. CBT attempts to bring about meaningful symptomatic improvement within 12–16 sessions. In community practice, however, comorbidities and the particular strengths and weaknesses of the family may require longer interventions. In the next subsections, we list the general characteristics of CBT for anxiety disorders and depressive disorders, followed by the relevant treatment outcome data.

Anxiety Disorders

Anxiety is best conceptualized as a multidimensional construct, consisting of physiological arousal, subjective (cognitive) distress, and behavioral avoidance. Depending on the therapist's specific theoretical orientation, intervention may initially target any one of these three components. However, successful outcome depends on change across all three dimensions.

There are several different theoretical models that are considered to play a role in the etiology of anxiety disorders. Vicarious conditioning (observational learning) is the process whereby a child may acquire a fear by observing another person behaving fearfully—if a parent behaves fearfully during a thunderstorm, a child may acquire a fear of thunderstorms. One of the most influential explanations for the etiology and maintenance of anxiety disorders is Mowrer's (1947) two-factor theory. Mowrer hypothesized that fears may be acquired by classical conditioning but are maintained by operant conditioning, where escape or avoidance behaviors eliminate physical and psychological distress. For example, Jackie has a fear of dogs, which developed because a dog once suddenly jumped on her, creating a startle reaction (her heart began to race, she could not catch her breath, and so forth). Her fear developed because of classical conditioning. Now, when playing outside, Jackie sees a dog and becomes anxious. If Jackie runs away, her anxiety dissipates. In turn, the feeling of relief increases the likelihood that in the future, Jackie will run away when she sees a dog. Therefore, her fear is maintained by operant conditioning—she acts on her environment, and by her actions, she maintains her fear. These same theoretical models—classical conditioning, operant conditioning, and vicarious conditioning—form the underpinnings of CBT.

There is uniform agreement that the key ingredient in CBT for anxiety disorders is exposure, a procedure whereby the individual is placed in contact with the object or situation that elicits fear or distress. Graduated exposure is based on a classical conditioning paradigm whereby situations that elicit a low level of fear are introduced first, followed over time by situations that elicit more intense fear. As the number of times that the child confronts the situation increases, even former "high fear" items no longer elicit distress. An example of a successful graduated exposure hierarchy for a child with selective mutism, an anxiety disorder found in children, is presented in Table 44–1. In many

TABLE 44–1. Hierarchy for a child with selective mutism

1. Whisper aloud to mom and dad so a friend can hear.
2. Talk aloud to mom and dad so a friend can hear.
3. Whisper aloud to a friend.
4. Talk aloud to a friend.
5. Talk aloud to two friends.
6. With mom present, say one word aloud to an unfamiliar adult.
7. With mom present, say one sentence aloud to an unfamiliar adult.
8. Say "hello" to next-door neighbor when parents are not present.
9. Say "hello" to teacher at school.
10. Say "hello" to a classmate.

instances, graduated exposure is combined with cognitive strategies such as *cognitive restructuring* (discussed later in this subsection) in an attempt to elicit and change negative thoughts that may be part of the fear complex.

In the case of children or adolescents with social anxiety disorder, an additional consideration is that their social anxiety is often accompanied by social skills deficits (Beidel and Alfano 2011). When present, deficits must be addressed during the course of treatment, typically through a procedure called *social skills training.* Using modeling, role-play, and corrective feedback, children practice conversational skills such as starting a conversation, asking questions, and being assertive. Nonverbal skills such as eye contact and vocal tone and volume are also taught when necessary. In some programs (Beidel et al. 2000, 2007; Spence et al. 2000) multicomponent interventions including social skills training, peer generalization, and graduated exposure effectively treat children and adolescents with social anxiety disorder.

Another behavioral intervention is *relaxation training,* a procedure in which children learn to decrease their physiological and subjective arousal by engaging in either muscle tension-relaxation sequences or cognitive meditation. Relaxation training is often used as part of multicomponent treatments for anxiety disorders but is rarely used as the sole intervention.

Cognitive conceptualizations of anxiety begin with the premise that emotional disorders result from maladaptive thought patterns, such as misperceiving neutral objects or situations as dangerous. *Cognitive restructuring* is based on the theory that negative thoughts can affect the emotional and behavioral response to the anxiety-provoking situations. The goal of treatment is to restructure faulty cognitions, which in turn should decrease subjective distress and eliminate avoidance behavior. The first step of cognitive restructuring is to help youth become aware of these maladaptive thoughts. On the basis of Socratic questioning, therapists help youth recognize errors in logic and see how particular beliefs may be maladaptive. In some cases, alternative (e.g., coping) statements may be used to counteract the negative thoughts. To promote skill generalization, homework is assigned so that youth learn to apply these cognitive skills to the events or situations that produce anxiety. Many cognitive programs also include exposure therapy so that youth have the opportunity to practice their cognitive restructuring skills in anxiety-provoking situations.

Depressive Disorders

From a CBT perspective, depressive disorders are based on faulty thinking patterns. Depressed youth report negative thoughts about themselves, the world, and their future; they may view themselves as unlovable, undesirable, or flawed and others as unreliable, unsupportive, and uncaring. They anticipate rejection and ruminate about their problems. Deficits in rational problem solving and problem-solving motivation also are present. All of these vulnerabilities are conceptualized via a cognitive diathesis-stress model (e.g., Abramson et al. 1989; Beck 1967). In this model, depression is precipitated by a cognitive vulnerability that interacts with a negative life event. Cognitive vulnerabilities are organized as *schemas:* stable cognitive structures that include representations of the self and others. These structures are latent until activated by stress (Beck 1963, 1983). These CBT targets and their corresponding interventions are illustrated in Tables 44–2 and 44–3 and discussed later in this subsection. We refer the interested reader to Friedberg and McClure (2002), Reinecke and Curry (2008), Reinecke et al. (2003), and Stallard (2002) for more detailed descriptions of CBT with children and adolescents with depressive disorders.

With respect to specific interventions, *mood monitoring* (via a mood diary) increases the child's awareness and understanding of emotions. *Activity scheduling* begins with the generation of activities identified as safe, active, inexpensive, readily available, legal, and genuinely enjoyable. Adolescents use self-reward for trying new activities, whereas the parents of younger children use tangible rewards such as stickers or activities enjoyed together. Developing mastery/accomplishment and pleasure/fun activity lists that are social in nature can enhance social interaction and social reward.

Social skills (described in the previous subsection) are another focus of treatment, as depressed youth are often withdrawn and behave in ways that alienate peers and family. *Problem solving* is a critical treatment component. Youth with depression often demonstrate poor problem-solving skills and low motivation. A formal model of problem solving uses the acronym RIBEYE: **R**elax, **I**dentify the problem, **B**rainstorm possible solutions, **E**valuate their strengths and weaknesses, say **Y**es to one (or two), and **E**ncourage yourself for success (Curry et al. 2005). Therapists provide youth with graduated experiences with clinic and in vivo (real life) practice.

Affect regulation and distress tolerance strategies help modulate negative moods. Youth identify thoughts, physiological sensations, and behavioral cues that occur immediately before mood escalation and then develop a list of cognitive, behavioral, and social strategies to prevent emotional outbursts. Changing automatic thoughts and relaxation training, described in the previous subsection, are also core strategies for treating depression in youth.

Adaptive counterthoughts allow the patient to "talk back" to negative cognitions. After learning to identify automatic thoughts, the adolescent learns specific strategies for rectifying these maladaptive cognitions. Upsetting thoughts are seen as questions or hypotheses to be tested, and evidence is sought to ascertain their validity and utility. Specifically, patients are taught to ask 1) What is the evidence that supports the thought? 2) Is there any contra-

TABLE 44–2. Common targets of cognitive-behavioral interventions with youth

	Targets
Cognitive interventions	Automatic thoughts (self, world, future) and images
	Perceptions
	Cognitive distortions
	Memories
	Schemata, assumptions
	Goals, wishes, plans, standards (e.g., perfectionism)
	Problem solving (rational skills and motivation)
	Attributions
	Ruminative style
Social and behavioral interventions	Social skills
	Communication skills
	Conflict resolution/negotiation
	Maladaptive coping
	Attachment difficulties (insecure, disorganized, fearful)
	Supports (peers, family, adults)
Environmental interventions	Stressors (major and minor)
	Cues and reinforcers

TABLE 44–3. Specific interventions commonly used in cognitive-behavioral therapy (CBT)

1. Introducing CBT model and treatment rationale
2. Goal setting
3. Mood monitoring
4. Activity scheduling (pleasant/social/mastery)
5. Rational problem solving and problem-solving motivation
6. Rationally disputing automatic thoughts, replacing with adaptive self-statements
7. Cognitive distortions
8. Affect regulation
9. Social skills
10. Assertiveness
11. Communication and compromise
12. Attachment security
13. Parent training
14. Booster sessions and relapse prevention

dictory evidence? Is there any evidence I have overlooked or anything that might lead me to think the thought may not be true? 3) Is there another way of looking at the situation? 4) If the negative thought is true, is it really so big a deal? 5) What's the solution? What can be done to handle this?

Empirical Support

To date, most RCTs demonstrate that CBT is superior to wait list and no-treatment control conditions, and CBT is considered an efficacious treatment for anxiety and depressive disorders. More recent RCTs using active treatment control conditions and meta-analyses confirm these initial positive findings.

Anxiety Disorders

To illustrate recent advances in establishing the efficacy of CBT, a comprehensive review published in 2008 found that no treatment for childhood anxiety disorders was considered "well-established" at that time (Silverman et al. 2008). Only four interventions (two for multiple anxiety disorders and two specifically for social anxiety disorder) met the criteria for "probably efficacious," meaning that there was at least one rigorous RCT demonstrating its efficacy. Since that time, a number of additional RCTs have been published and have established the efficacy of CBT for anxiety disorders. One well-known intervention (Coping Cat) has been replicated several times in individual and group formats (e.g., Kendall et al. 1997) and has been repeatedly demonstrated to be efficacious, with treatment gains maintained at least 7 years later. Other interventions, such as Silverman's individual and group CBT programs, have also been demonstrated to be efficacious in RCTs, with treatment gains maintained at follow-up (Silverman et al. 1999a, 1999b). These three interventions begin with the theoretical rationale that children with separation anxiety disorder, social anxiety disorder, specific phobia, or generalized anxiety disorder share basic clinical characteristics and that in many cases, children often meet diagnostic criteria for more than one anxiety disorder. Because of the similarity in symptom presentation, the therapeutic rationale is that an intervention that is multicomponent in nature will be efficacious across diagnostic groups. Coping Cat includes relaxation therapy, cognitive restructuring, and in vivo exposure to anxiety-producing situations. Individual CBT and group CBT include contingency management, self-control, cognitive restructuring, and in vivo exposure. Overall, these interventions, among others that are similar in content, were found to be efficacious for children with anxiety disorders (Hudson et al. 2009), although final sample sizes often precluded examination of outcome by primary diagnostic group.

Continuing with the idea that children with various anxiety disorders share enough characteristics to benefit from a multicomponent intervention, the Child/Adolescent Anxiety Multimodal Study (CAMS) examined the efficacy of CBT (Coping Cat), sertraline, the combination of CBT and sertraline, or placebo in a six-site RCT consisting of 488 children and adolescents. After 12 weeks of treatment, 80.7% of children treated with combination therapy were judged to be much or very much improved, as were 59.7% of the CBT group, 59.4% of the sertraline group, and 23.7% of the placebo group (Walkup et al. 2008). In effect, all interventions were superior to pill placebo, and the combination group was superior to either of the monotherapies. However, remission rates after 12 weeks of treatment (defined as no longer meeting diagnostic criteria for an anxiety disorder) were lower: 68% of the combination group, 46% of the sertraline group, 46% of the CBT group, and 24% of the placebo group (Ginsburg et al. 2011). Predictors of remission rate included younger age, nonminority status, lower baseline anxiety, the absence of other internalizing disorders, and the absence of a social anxiety disorder diagnosis. At 24- and 36-week follow-up, more than 80% of responders maintained treatment gains, although 15.7% of the combination group, 36.4% of the sertraline group, and 29.9% of the CBT group received additional treatment during these follow-up periods (Piacentini et al. 2014).

The smaller treatment response for youth with social anxiety disorder in the CAMS trial is not an isolated finding. An independent sample of youth with a social anxiety disorder diagnosis or symptoms treated with CBT (Coping Cat) demonstrated initial symptom improvement but were significantly less improved than children with other anxiety disorders at 7.4 years follow-up (Kerns et al. 2013). The outcome of these two investigations, among several others, suggests that social anxiety disorder may present unique treatment challenges and may not be most efficaciously treated with a generic or transdiagnostic intervention strategy.

This conclusion is consistent with the work of other investigators (e.g., Albano et al. 1995; Beidel et al. 2000; Spence et al. 2000) who developed and evaluated interventions specifically for youth with social anxiety disorder. Although each intervention has some unique elements, they all include social skills training. Social Effectiveness Therapy for Children (SET-C; Beidel et al. 2000, 2007), for example, combines social skills training, in vivo exposure, and peer generalization sessions. It has been demonstrated to be more efficacious than an active, nonspecific psychological treatment, pill placebo, or fluoxetine. Across both investigations, 53%–67% of youth achieve remission (no longer have a diagnosis), and the results are maintained at least 5 years posttreatment, with a relapse rate of less than 10% (Beidel et al. 2006). In one investigation (Beidel et al. 2007), both SET-C and fluoxetine decreased anxiety in social situations, but only SET-C produced an improvement in social skills, which are necessary for effective social interaction. These data suggest that there may be something unique about social anxiety disorder and that attention to improving social interaction/communication skills, as well as decreasing anxiety, may be the most efficacious strategy for youth with this disorder.

Depressive Disorders

There are fewer RCTs examining the efficacy of CBT for depressive disorders than for the anxiety disorders. Furthermore, data from two meta-analyses (Chu and Harrison 2007; Watanabe et al. 2007) suggest that the effectiveness of CBT for childhood depressive disorders is less than that of CBT for anxiety disorders. When compared with a variety of control conditions (no treatment, wait list, attention placebo, or treatment as usual), at posttreatment CBT was more efficacious than control for adolescents with moderate to severe depression, but the differences disappeared at 6-month follow-up (Watanabe et al. 2007). Another meta-analysis conducted at the same time reported that whereas CBT for anxiety produces moderate to large effects on behavioral, cognitive, physiological, and coping variables, CBT for depression produces only small effects for cognitive processes and no impact on behavioral or coping variables (Chu and Harrison 2007). Below we present several specific intervention packages developed for youth with depressive disorders. Following this description, we review other empirical data related to treating depression in youth.

The Adolescent Coping With Depression Course (CWD-A; Clarke et al. 1990) is a group treatment designed to have a classroom rather than clinical feel. Each participant has a student workbook. A leader's manual guides the therapists through lectures, discussions, role-plays, and homework. Major topics include social skills, relaxation, changing unpleasant cognitions, resolving conflicts, and planning for the future. The CWD-A can be adapted for use in individual therapy, although the authors stress that much can be gained from a group of adolescents learning together and from one another. A parallel course has been developed for the parents of depressed adolescents (Lewinsohn et al. 1991), allowing families to join sessions and practice their communication skills. The first study evaluating the program's efficacy (Lewinsohn et al. 1990) compared three conditions: the treatment of adolescents alone, the treatment of adolescents with a parallel parent group, and a wait list control. Adolescents treated with CWD-A demonstrated significant reductions in depressive symptoms relative to those in the control condition. These gains were maintained at 2-year follow-up. The parent training component did not appear to enhance clinical improvement. The CWD-A has been refined over the past 15 years, and it can be quite effective for treating mild to moderate depression in some teens.

The ACTION treatment and workbook (Stark et al. 2004) outline a gender-specific, developmentally sensitive program for depressed girls. The treatment program is based on a self-control model in which youth use coping, problem solving, and/or cognitive restructuring strategies to address their depression. Strengths of the ACTION program include its engaging activities as well as use of ACTION kits that help the child remember the central therapeutic concepts. Earlier iterations of ACTION (Stark and Kendall 1996) outlined a protocol for both girls and boys. Research with earlier versions of the treatment protocol suggests that it may be efficacious for alleviating depression among prepubertal youth (Stark 1990; Stark et al. 1987).

The Primary and Secondary Control Enhancement Training (PASCET; Weisz 1990; Weisz et al. 1993) is based on a two-process model of control, wherein primary control involves enhancing reward and reducing punishment by adjusting objective conditions, while secondary control involves adjusting oneself to more adaptively deal with situations that are more difficult to change. Core CBT techniques are delivered through group meetings, with additional individual meetings to fit the specific treatment elements to the individual child's situation. In one study, subjects receiving the PASCET program showed greater posttreatment reductions in depressive symptoms than the no-treatment control group (Weisz et al. 1997).

The multisite Treatment for Adolescents With Depression Study (TADS) was an RCT funded by the National Institute of Mental Health (NIMH) that examined the effectiveness of individual CBT in comparison with fluoxetine, placebo, and the combination of fluoxetine and CBT (March et al. 2004; Treatment for Adolescents With Depression Study Team 2003). The CBT protocol included eight skills considered essential (introduction to treatment rationale, mood monitoring, goal setting, pleasant activities, problem solving, automatic thoughts and cognitive distortions, realistic counterthoughts, and taking stock) and an additional five optional skills (social interaction, assertion, communication and compromise, relaxation, and affect regulation). Treatment was conducted with individual teens with optional family sessions. After 12 weeks, TADS CBT did not lead to more improvement in depression than the other TADS treatments (March et al. 2004). Youth who received any of the active treatments maintained their gains over 36 weeks. Although all active interventions yielded similar levels of clinical improvement (March et al. 2007), overall, the combination of CBT and fluoxetine resulted in more rapid alleviation of depressive symptoms than fluoxetine or CBT alone (March et al. 2004). The combination of CBT and fluoxetine was also more effective in improving global functioning, global health, and quality of life (Vitiello et al. 2006). As noted in the subsection on anxiety disorders, improvement and remission represent different outcomes, and these different outcomes are reflected in the TADS data as well. After 12 or 18 weeks, the combination treatment resulted in statistically significantly higher remission rates compared with CBT or fluoxetine alone (Kennard et al. 2009b). However, after 36 weeks of acute and maintenance treatment, remission rates were equal across all three groups (combination 60%, CBT 64%, and fluoxetine 55%). As noted by the investigators, selecting a single treatment may delay remission for a subset of adolescents with depression. However, even with the combination treatment, 40% of adolescents still failed to achieve remission 9 months later.

As a result of the TADS data that concomitant CBT produced better outcome and more rapid improvement for adolescents with suicidal ideation, the National Institute for Health and Care Excellence in the United Kingdom advised practitioners that selective serotonin reuptake inhibitors (SSRIs) should not be prescribed without a specific concomitant psychological treatment (Dubicka et al. 2010). A recent meta-analysis examined the validity of this recommendation, examining change in depressive symptoms, suicidality, impairment, and global improvement for adolescents with depressive disorder. The results indicated that adding CBT to an SSRI did *not* lead to additional benefit with regard to reduction in depressive symptoms, suicidality, or global improvement (Dubicka et al. 2010), but there was a statistically significant advantage for the combination on a clinician rating of overall impairment at immediate posttreatment. Another NIMH multicenter trial, the Treatment of SSRI-Resistant Depression in Adolescents (TORDIA), compared the outcomes of switching medication, adding another medication, or adding CBT to any medication class when adolescents with depression did not respond to initial treatment with an SSRI. Adding CBT plus switching medications yielded a higher response rate (54.8%) than a medication switch alone (40.5%) (Brent et al. 2008). In the TORDIA study, CBT consisted of cognitive restructuring, behavioral activation, emotion regulation, social skills, problem-solving family-oriented components, motivational interviewing, and relapse prevention. Subsequent to the initial study findings, in an effort to enhance CBT's efficacy, data analyses determined specific CBT elements that contributed to the positive outcome (Kennard et al. 2009a). The results indicated that adolescents were 2.5 times more likely to benefit from CBT if they attended at least 9 out of 12 sessions. As with medication, participating in the treatment as prescribed is necessary for the intervention to be successful. Furthermore, even when controlling for number of sessions, the adolescents were

2.3 times more likely to have a positive benefit if they had received problem-solving training and 2.6 times more likely to have a positive benefit if they had participated in social skills training. Thus, as discussed with CBT for anxiety disorders, specific elements in the CBT armamentarium may be more essential, or at least more critical, for certain disorders.

Transportability and Dissemination

Effective psychotherapeutic treatments for anxiety and depressive disorders are available. A continuing challenge, however, is how to transport and disseminate these treatments to nonresearch settings where the population may be different and there are fewer resources. One alternative is to use computer- and Web-based technology, where interventions available over the Internet could provide uniformity, standardization, ease of delivery, and cost-effectiveness (March 2009, p. 174). As computers and Web access technology now permeate the environment, researchers are beginning to examine how to harness this technology for transportability, dissemination, and positive treatment outcome. BRAVE-ONLINE is a CBT program developed for delivery to children (ages 8–12) or adolescents (ages 13–17) with anxiety disorders (Spence et al. 2008). The program includes relaxation strategies, coping self-talk and cognitive restructuring, graduated exposure, problem solving, and self-reinforcement of brave behavior. In a sample of adolescents, BRAVE delivered in the clinic or online was equally effective in decreasing anxiety symptoms and anxiety disorders. At 12-month follow-up, 78% of adolescents treated with the online version no longer met criteria for their principal diagnosis compared with 80% treated in the clinic (Spence et al. 2011). It should be noted, however, that children whose anxiety disorder was rated as "severe" by diagnostic clinicians were excluded from this treatment trial because one of the randomized groups would not be seen in the clinic. Therefore, the efficacy of this computer-based intervention for youth with the most severe anxiety disorders is not known. Additionally, an RCT with 7- to 12-year-old children with anxiety disorders resulted in small positive changes after the BRAVE-ONLINE program (March et al. 2009) but less than for the adolescent sample (Spence et al. 2011).

Camp Cope-A-Lot (CCAL) is a computer-based program for youth with anxiety disorders that uses multimedia, text, and interactive games to teach the components of Coping Cat: psychoeducation, cognitive restructuring, relaxation training, principles of exposure, and homework. Goals of CCAL are to eliminate the need for practitioners to have specific CBT training and to allow experiential learning rather than reading text online. In an initial effectiveness trial (Khanna and Kendall 2010) CCAL was compared with clinician-delivered individual CBT and a computer-assisted education support and attention program. All interventions were delivered by doctoral level clinicians with no prior experience in CBT. On clinician ratings, CCAL and CBT both produced equivalent symptom reduction when compared with the control condition, and both were superior to the control condition (81%, 70%, and 19%, respectively, no longer met diagnostic criteria for their principal anxiety disorder at posttreatment). However, all conditions (including the control condition) produced similar improvement on child ratings of anxiety. Therapist adherence to the treatment protocol was greater for CCAL than the other conditions, indicating that novice therapists could successfully use CCAL and produce positive treatment outcome with CBT.

Internet-based depression intervention/prevention programs have also been developed, and one, Competent Adulthood Transition with Cognitive-Behavioral, Humanistic and Interpersonal Training (CATCH-IT), has been effectively implemented in primary care settings (Van Voorhees et al. 2009). CATCH-IT includes three modules: behavioral activation, cognitive-behavioral therapy (Clarke et al. 1990), and interpersonal psychotherapy. The program has been reported to be effective in reducing the percentage of participants with clinically significant depressive symptoms as well as decreasing thoughts of self-harm and hopelessness and decreasing the likelihood of a subsequent depressive episode when compared with a brief advice condition.

Virtual reality (VR) and virtual environments (VEs) are becoming commonplace in exposure-based treatment of adults with anxiety disorders. Their use with adolescents and children is just beginning. In addition to presenting anxiety-eliciting stimuli for exposure therapy, VEs are being developed and used to assist in aspects of manualized interventions that are difficult to translate to traditional clinical practice. Pegasys-VR (D.C. Beidel and J. Spitalnick, "Pegasys VR: Integrating Virtual Humans in the Treatment of Child Social Anxiety," unpublished manuscript, University of Central Florida, 2014) is a VE that is designed to assist in the acquisition of social skills and to replace the peer generalization and homework components of SET-C (Beidel et al. 2007). These two treatment components were the targets of the VE development because feedback from clinicians indicated that SET-C implementation would be difficult in community settings because of the time and resources necessary to conduct and supervise the peer generalization sessions. Even in clinical research settings, homework compliance was often less than optimal when parents did not assist children in completing their homework (e.g., parent did not take child places to initiate conversations). The initial VE consisted of an elementary school with eight avatars (four adults and four children) typically found in a school setting (principal, teachers, children) and used multiple school locations (classrooms, hallways, gymnasium). The Pegasys school prototype included four social skill elements (greetings, asking questions, compliments, assertion). The therapist uses a computer interface that contains various verbal responses, which are keyed to each of the avatars. Using this program, the clinician controls the avatar's verbal communication, allowing the avatars to initiate and respond to the child's attempts at social interaction. As the children become more proficient, the avatar's responses can become more challenging, allowing the child to experience a variety of different responses and engage in challenging interactions. In addition, there is a computerized homework program that allows practice and reinforcement. The results of an initial development and feasibility study (Sarver et al. 2014) support the use of this VE in clinical and home settings for preadolescent children with social anxiety disorder. Parents and children rated the quality of the VE as very good to excellent, and children found the characters to be real and reported being comfortable talking to the virtual characters. Treatment credibility ratings were high—children and parents believed that the VE elements were logical and would be helpful in treating social anxiety disorder in children. Finally, although homework compliance was less than optimal (children completed only two-thirds of their homework assignments), compliance was still higher than in the traditional SET-C program, where only 50.3% of the children completed all of their homework assignments, 38.4% completed some assignments, and 11.2% did not complete any assignments (Beidel and Spitalnick, unpublished manuscript, 2014). On the basis of these positive prototype results, the development of the full Pegasys-VR system, including a revised homework strategy and additional VEs, is under way.

Developmental and Gender Considerations

CBT requires consideration of the child's developmental stage. Although chronological age is a useful starting point, clinicians also need to consider social aptitude, cognitive ability, emotional maturity, and idiosyncratic needs when implementing CBT with children and adolescents.

Research has not yet supported the use of CBT with very young children with depression (e.g., ages 3–5 years) or among youth with a severe learning disability or developmental delay. Some young children may not have the mental ability necessary to engage in metacognition (thinking about thinking), which is a necessary element of cognitive restructuring (Alfano et al. 2002). Fortunately, the elimination of this component from some CBT programs for anxiety disorders does not reduce the efficacy of the overall program (Spence et al. 2000). When cognitive restructuring is included in the treatment program, its implementation will vary as a function of developmental level. With younger children, tasks such as filling in cartoon thought bubbles or completing sentence prompts are often used to identify thoughts. Using child-friendly terms instead of psychological jargon is also recommended (e.g., *thinking traps* instead of *cognitive distortions* and *clues* as opposed to *evidence*). Using some of these modifications, CBT appears to be efficacious for children between ages 4 and 8 (Hirshfeld-Becker et al. 2010; Schneider et al. 2011; Waters et al. 2009), although more parental participation is required than for older youth.

When youth are treated for anxiety or depression, completion of homework assignments such as exposure, behavioral activation, or testing of cognitions is essential for successful outcome. These tasks must be developmentally appropriate. Younger patients may require parental involvement to complete homework assignments, whereas adolescents may need to be given more autonomy. Similarly, the use and type of reinforcers require consideration of developmental stage and individual preferences (e.g., stickers, toys, and other tangible items for preadolescents vs. extra time allowed on the phone or allowing a friend to visit for adolescents).

Gender may also influence treatment. Boys have a greater tendency to underreport symptoms (Ollendick et al. 1985), perhaps as a result of gender role expectations. Boys may also deny fear, minimizing fear intensity and its impact on functioning.

Positive Outcomes That May Be Expected

Efficacious CBT decreases physical and cognitive symptoms and improves behavioral functioning. Improvement in primary symptoms often leads to improvement in comorbid conditions and improved academic and family functioning. In the case of anxiety-based school refusal, the child returns to the school environment. For social anxiety disorder and depressive disorders, expected outcomes include increased socialization and improved peer relationships.

Factors Affecting Outcome

Several factors likely influence the efficacy of CBT for anxiety and depressive disorders. Chronological age may be a factor, but findings regarding the nature of this effect have been inconsistent. An early meta-analysis of the efficacy of CBT on different childhood disorders revealed that age, as an indicator of cognitive development, had a positive impact on treatment outcome; that is, older children were generally more responsive to CBT (Durlak et al. 1991). However, a subsequent investigation of treatment of anxiety disorders (Southam-Gerow et al. 2001) found that older age predicted *less* favorable treatment outcome. Among depressed youth, younger adolescents who were less chronically depressed and demonstrated higher functioning were more likely to benefit from 12 weeks of CBT treatment (March et al. 2007). These disparities may have more to do with the nature of the specific treatment program than the composition of the treated sample. CBT programs developed for preadolescents may need substantial modification for use with adolescents.

Baseline psychopathology also may affect treatment outcome. For children with primary anxiety disorders, comorbid symptoms of depression, and trait anxiety in particular or higher levels of childhood internalizing disorders in general were negatively associated with treatment efficacy (Berman et al. 2000; Southam-Gerow et al. 2001). Predictors of poor response for children with primary depressive disorders include greater severity of depression, higher levels of cognitive distortion (Brent et al. 1998; Clarke et al. 1992), and greater hopelessness (Brent et al. 1998; Curry et al. 2006), whereas lower levels of suicidal ideation and higher expectancies for treatment were predictive of 12-week positive outcomes. There is mixed evidence regarding the effect of comorbidity on depression outcomes, with some studies finding no effect (e.g., Weersing and Weisz 2002) and some finding that comorbidity predicts poor treatment response (e.g., Clarke et al. 1995; Curry et al. 2006).

Few data are available that specifically examine the number of treatment sessions necessary for optimal response. Outcome data from controlled trials indicate that many children demonstrate significant improvement after 12–16 weeks of treatment. In a trial comparing behavioral and pharmacological treatments for youth with social anxiety disorder (Beidel et al. 2007), fluoxetine appeared to achieve its maximum effectiveness by week 8, whereas behavior therapy (SET-C) continued to exert an effect through week 12, suggesting that 3 months of treatment may allow for consolidation of gains. Findings from TADS indicate that 12 weeks of CBT may be insufficient for many adolescents with depressive disorders. If treatment is continued for 36 weeks, however, approximately 80% of youth will demonstrate significant improvement. In anxiety disorders, frequency of the treatment sessions also affects response. Specifically, massed treatment sessions (frequent applications of the intervention, perhaps occurring two to three times per week) achieve superior outcome in a shorter period of time than once weekly sessions.

Parental psychopathology also may affect successful treatment of the child. Symptoms of depression, fear, hostility, psychoticism, and paranoia and obsessive-compulsive tendencies have all been negatively associated with treatment outcome for children with anxiety disorders (Berman et al. 2000). Family income may also moderate the effect of CBT for adolescents with depression (Curry et al. 2006). In contrast, sociodemographic variables do not seem to significantly affect treatment outcome for youth with anxiety disorders. Efficacy appears consistent across ethnicity, gender, and socioeconomic status (Berman et al. 2000; Ferrell et al. 2004; Pina et al. 2003).

Economic Cost-Benefit Issues

When taking into account both direct and indirect expenses, the annual cost of anxiety disorders (for all ages) is estimated to range between $42 and $47 billion (DuPont et al. 1996; Greenberg et al. 1999). Annual costs for depression (for all ages) have been estimated to be between $44 and $53 billion (Greenberg et al. 1993, 1996). The current cost would likely be significantly higher. This burden could be mitigated considerably by early detection, accurate diagnosis, and effective intervention.

Given the chronicity of these disorders, early effective intervention may offset later costs to society and to the individual. In comparison with combined or eclectic interventions, CBT tends to be less expensive and to require a shorter treatment period. Among children, group CBT appears to be less expensive than and equally as effective as individual CBT (Manassis et al. 2002), indicating that it may be a high-quality cost-effective alternative.

If CBT for any disorder is to be effective, it must be adopted for use by community therapists in community settings. In an initial test of transportability, community clinicians were trained and supervised in CBT (Weisz et al. 2009). Youth with depressive disorders were randomly assigned to CBT or usual care and were treated until "normal termination." Usual care therapists were more likely to use psychodynamic and family approaches than CBT. At posttreatment 75% of youth no longer had a depressive disorder, suggesting that both interventions were equally efficacious. However, compared with usual care, intervention with CBT was shorter (24 weeks vs. 39 weeks), resulted in a better therapeutic alliance with parents, was less likely to need adjunctive therapies, and was less costly. As models of heath care continue to evolve, less expense in terms of time and health care dollars may be particularly advantageous. Transportability and dissemination using technology may be useful in addressing these challenges.

Adverse Effects and Complications

Clinicians often make mistakes when learning to implement CBT. Although CBT protocols tend to be straightforward, attention must be given to individual, familial, and developmental factors. Maladaptive beliefs, attitudes, and behaviors are learned and function in a social context. Although CBT emphasizes rectifying intrapsychic cognitive processes that maintain pathological behavior, care should be taken to address ways in which parents, teachers, and peers may inadvertently be modeling or reinforcing these maladaptive patterns. Attention should be given to environmental factors, such as parental participation in treatment, parental mood, parenting practices (including cultural practices), parental attitudes and beliefs, and parental motivation for treatment. Consideration of cultural factors and ethnic minority status will enhance treatment. In treating depressed children, it is helpful to discuss low motivation as part of the disorder. Activity scheduling is helpful in alleviating some mood symptoms, which then may increase motivation. Last, the family as well as the clinician must be patient with the change process.

Nonspecific factors, including therapeutic warmth, responsiveness, and empathy, go a long way in forging an effective treatment alliance. Consistency in completing homework assignments is a strong predictor of outcome. The completion of homework encourages both the child and the family to generalize interventions "out of the office" and apply them in day-to-day life. It is vital to continue practicing each cognitive and behavioral skill until it is learned well, rather than exposing the child to multiple techniques all at once. The old adage "less is more" applies here. Progress must be assessed systematically. Objective assessment can help the clinician step back and reformulate the case if current interventions are not leading to clinical improvement. Attention to these common pitfalls will aid the clinician in effective CBT implementation.

Parental assumptions or negative biases may reinforce caution and behavioral avoidance and discourage risk-taking behaviors. These actions are counterproductive to CBT's goals and method of intervention, which encourage the child (in a controlled fashion) to approach situations or objects. In many instances, one of the therapist's first objectives is to correct misperceptions and educate the parent about the crucial role of exposure for effective intervention. Similarly, parents may fail to understand that anticipatory anxiety is often more severe than the distress experienced when actually contacting the feared stimulus or that anxiety during exposure sessions is actually less than what the child (and parent) imagined would occur, particularly in the case of gradual exposure. Without this understanding, parents often work at cross-purposes with the therapist, inadvertently reinforcing the child for anxious and avoidant behaviors rather than for positive approach behaviors.

Another complication for the implementation of CBT for anxiety disorders occurs when exposure sessions are too short to allow habituation to occur. Depending on the type of exposure selected (graduated or intensive) and the age of the patient (child or adolescent), sessions may need to last from 30 to 90 minutes. If exposure is discontinued prior to habituation, sensitization to the feared stimulus and an increase in fear may occur, thereby leading to a worsening of the child's condition.

Summary Points

- Cognitive-behavioral therapy (CBT) is a term for a group of interventions that share a commitment to empiricism and focus on behavior change.
- CBT is an efficacious treatment approach for children and adolescents with anxiety disorders and probably depressive disorders.
- Whereas developmental factors play a role in the manner in which CBT is implemented, the intervention appears efficacious across age, gender, race and ethnicity, and socioeconomic status.
- The presence of comorbid conditions may attenuate the efficacy of CBT.
- Parental biases, assumptions, or unwillingness to participate in the therapeutic process can hinder progress and must be addressed.
- Implementation of CBT procedures must be adapted to the individual patient and family.

References

Abramson L, Metalsky G, Alloy L: Hopelessness depression: a theory based subtype of depression. Psychol Rev 96(2):358–372, 1989

Albano AM, Marten PA, Holt CS, et al: Cognitive-behavioral group treatment for social phobia in adolescents. A preliminary study. J Nerv Ment Dis 183(10):649–656, 1995 7561811

Alfano CA, Beidel DC, Turner SM: Cognition in childhood anxiety: conceptual, methodological, and developmental issues. Clin Psychol Rev 22(8):1209–1238, 2002 12436811

Beck AT: Thinking and depression, I: idiosyncratic content and cognitive distortions. Arch Gen Psychiatry 9:324–333, 1963 14045261

Beck AT: Depression: Causes and Treatment. Philadelphia, University of Pennsylvania Press, 1967

Beck AT: Cognitive therapy of depression: new perspectives, in Treatment of Depression: Old Controversies and New Approaches. Edited by Clayton P, Barrett J. New York, Raven, 1983, pp 265–284

Beidel DC, Alfano CA: Childhood Anxiety Disorders: A Guide to Research and Treatment. New York, Routledge/Taylor and Francis Group, 2011

Beidel DC, Turner SM, Morris TL: Behavioral treatment of childhood social phobia. J Consult Clin Psychol 68(6):1072–1080, 2000 11142541

Beidel DC, Turner SM, Young BJ: Social effectiveness therapy for children: five years later. Behav Ther 37(4):416–425, 2006 17071218

Beidel DC, Turner SM, Sallee FR, et al: SET-C versus fluoxetine in the treatment of childhood social phobia. J Am Acad Child Adolesc Psychiatry 46(12):1622–1632, 2007 18030084

Berman SL, Weems CF, Silverman WK, et al: Predictors of outcome in exposure-based cognitive and behavioral treatments for phobic and anxiety disorders in children. Behav Ther 31(4):713–731, 2000

Brent D, Emslie G, Clarke G, et al: Switching to another SSRI or to venlafaxine with or without cognitive behavioral therapy for adolescents with SSRI-resistant depression: the TORDIA randomized controlled trial. JAMA 299(8):901–913, 2008 18314433

Brent DA, Kolko DJ, Birmaher B, et al: Predictors of treatment efficacy in a clinical trial of three psychosocial treatments for adolescent depression. J Am Acad Child Adolesc Psychiatry 37(9):906–914, 1998 9735610

Chu BC, Harrison TL: Disorder-specific effects of CBT for anxious and depressed youth: a meta-analysis of candidate mediators of change. Clin Child Fam Psychol Rev 10(4):352–372, 2007 17985239

Clarke G, Lewinsohn P, Hops H: Leader's Manual for Adolescent Groups: Adolescent Coping With Depression Course. Portland, OR, Kaiser Permanente Center for Health Research, 1990. Available at: http://www.kpchr.org/public/acwd/CWDA_manual.pdf. Accessed June 16, 2009.

Clarke G, Hops H, Lewinsohn PM, et al: Cognitive-behavioral group treatment of adolescent depression: prediction of outcome. Behav Ther 23(3):341–354, 1992

Clarke GN, Hawkins W, Murphy M, et al: Targeted prevention of unipolar depressive disorder in an at-risk sample of high school adolescents: a randomized trial of a group cognitive intervention. J Am Acad Child Adolesc Psychiatry 34(3):312–321, 1995 7896672

Curry J, Wells KC, Brent DA, et al: Treatment for Adolescents With Depression Study (TADS) Cognitive Behavior Therapy Manual. Durham, NC, Duke University, 2005. Available at: https://trialweb.dcri.duke.edu/tads/manuals.html. Accessed July 7, 2014.

Curry J, Rohde P, Simons A, et al: Predictors and moderators of acute outcome in the Treatment for Adolescents With Depression Study (TADS). J Am Acad Child Adolesc Psychiatry 45(12):1427–1439, 2006 17135988

Dubicka B, Elvins R, Roberts C, et al: Combined treatment with cognitive-behavioural therapy in adolescent depression: meta-analysis. Br J Psychiatry 197(6):433–440, 2010 21119148

DuPont RL, Rice DP, Miller LS, et al: Economic costs of anxiety disorders. Anxiety 2(4):167–172, 1996 9160618

Durlak JA, Fuhrman T, Lampman C: Effectiveness of cognitive-behavior therapy for maladapting children: a meta-analysis. Psychol Bull 110(2):204–214, 1991 1835106

Ferrell CB, Beidel DC, Turner SM: Assessment and treatment of socially phobic children: a cross cultural comparison. J Clin Child Adolesc Psychol 33(2):260–268, 2004 15136189

Friedberg RD, McClure JM: Clinical Practice of Cognitive Therapy With Children and Adolescents: The Nuts and Bolts. New York, Guilford, 2002

Ginsburg GS, Kendall PC, Sakolsky D, et al: Remission after acute treatment in children and adolescents with anxiety disorders: findings from the CAMS. J Consult Clin Psychol 79(6):806–813, 2011 22122292

Greenberg PE, Sisitsky T, Kessler RC, et al: The economic burden of anxiety disorders in the 1990s. J Clin Psychiatry 60(7):427–435, 1999 10453795

Greenberg PE, Stiglin LE, Finkelstein SN, et al: The economic burden of depression in 1990. J Clin Psychiatry 54(11):405–418, 1993 8270583

Greenberg PE, Kessler RC, Nells TL, et al: Depression in the workplace: an economic perspective, in Selective Serotonin Re-Uptake Inhibitors: Advances in Basic Research and Clinical Practice. Edited by Feighner JP, Boyer WF. New York, Wiley, 1996, pp 327–363

Hirshfeld-Becker DR, Masek B, Henin A, et al: Cognitive behavioral therapy for 4- to 7-year-old children with anxiety disorders: a randomized clinical trial. J Consult Clin Psychol 78(4):498–510, 2010 20658807

Hudson JL, Rapee RM, Deveney C, et al: Cognitive-behavioral treatment versus an active control for children and adolescents with anxiety disorders: a randomized trial. J Am Acad Child Adolesc Psychiatry 48(5):533–544, 2009

Kendall PC, Flannery-Schroeder E, Panichelli-Mindel SM, et al: Therapy for youths with anxiety disorders: a second randomized clinical trial. J Consult Clin Psychol 65(3):366–380, 1997 9170760

Kennard BD, Clarke GN, Weersing VR, et al: Effective components of TORDIA cognitive-behavioral therapy for adolescent depression: preliminary findings. J Consult Clin Psychol 77(6):1033–1041, 2009a 19968380

Kennard BD, Silva SG, Tonev S, et al: Remission and recovery in the Treatment for Adolescents with Depression Study (TADS): acute and long-term outcomes. J Am Acad Child Adolesc Psychiatry 48(2):186–195, 2009b 19127172

Kerns CM, Read KL, Klugman J, et al: Cognitive behavioral therapy for youth with social anxiety: differential short and long-term treatment outcomes. J Anxiety Disord 27(2):210–215, 2013 23474911

Khanna MS, Kendall PC: Computer-assisted cognitive behavioral therapy for child anxiety: results of a randomized clinical trial. J Consult Clin Psychol 78(5):737–745, 2010 20873909

Lewinsohn P, Clarke G, Hops H, et al: Cognitive-behavioral treatment for depressed adolescents. Behav Ther 21(4):385–401, 1990

Lewinsohn PM, Rohde P, Hops H, et al: Leader's Manual for Parent Groups: Adolescent Coping With Depression Course. Portland, OR, Kaiser Permanente Center for Health Research, 1991. Available at: http://www.kpchr.org/public/acwd/CWDA_parent_manual.pdf. Accessed June 16, 2009.

Manassis K, Mendlowitz SL, Scapillato D, et al: Group and individual cognitive-behavioral therapy for childhood anxiety disorders: a randomized trial. J Am Acad Child Adolesc Psychiatry 41(12):1423–1430, 2002 12447028

March JS: The future of psychotherapy for mentally ill children and adolescents. J Child Psychol Psychiatry 50(1–2):170–179, 2009 19220600

March J, Silva S, Petrycki S, et al: Fluoxetine, cognitive-behavioral therapy, and their combination for adolescents with depression: Treatment for Adolescents With Depression Study (TADS) randomized controlled trial. JAMA 292(7):807–820, 2004 15315995

March JS, Silva S, Petrycki S, et al: The Treatment for Adolescents With Depression Study (TADS): long-term effectiveness and safety outcomes. Arch Gen Psychiatry 64(10):1132–1143, 2007 17909125

March S, Spence SH, Donovan CL: The efficacy of an Internet-based cognitive-behavioral therapy intervention for child anxiety disorders. J Pediatr Psychol 34(5):474–487, 2009 18794187

Mowrer OH: On the dual nature of learning: a reinterpretation of "conditioning" and "problem solving." Harv Educ Rev 17:102–148, 1947

Ollendick TH, Matson JL, Helsel WJ: Fears in children and adolescents: normative data. Behav Res Ther 23(4):465–467, 1985 4026774

Piacentini J, Bennett S, Compton SN, et al: 24- and 36-week outcomes for the Child/Adolescent Anxiety Multimodal Study (CAMS). J Am Acad Child Adolesc Psychiatry 53(3):297–310, 2014 24565357

Pina AA, Silverman WK, Fuentes RM, et al: Exposure-based cognitive-behavioral treatment for phobic and anxiety disorders: treatment effects and maintenance for Hispanic/Latino relative to European-American youths. J Am Acad Child Adolesc Psychiatry 42(10):1179–1187, 2003 14560167

Reinecke MA, Curry JF: Adolescents, in Adapting Cognitive Therapy for Depression: Managing Complexity and Comorbidity. Edited by Whisman M. New York, Guilford, 2008, pp 394–416

Reinecke MA, Dattilio FM, Freeman A (eds): Cognitive Therapy With Children and Adolescents: A Casebook for Clinical Practice, 2nd Edition. New York, Guilford, 2003

Sarver NW, Beidel DC, Spitalnick JS: The feasibility and acceptability of virtual environments in the treatment of childhood social anxiety disorder. J Clin Child Adolesc Psychol 43(1):63–73, 2014 24144182

Schneider S, Blatter-Meunier J, Herren C, et al: Disorder-specific cognitive-behavioral therapy for separation anxiety disorder in young children: a randomized waiting-list-controlled trial. Psychother Psychosom 80(4):206–215, 2011 21494062

Silverman WK, Kurtines WM, Ginsburg GS, et al: Contingency management, self-control, and education support in the treatment of childhood phobic disorders: a randomized clinical trial. J Consult Clin Psychol 67(5):675–687, 1999a 10535234

Silverman WK, Kurtines WM, Ginsburg GS, et al: Treating anxiety disorders in children with group cognitive-behaviorial therapy: a randomized clinical trial. J Consult Clin Psychol 67(6):995–1003, 1999b 10596522

Silverman WK, Pina AA, Viswesvaran C: Evidence-based psychosocial treatments for phobic and anxiety disorders in children and adolescents. J Clin Child Adolesc Psychol 37(1):105–130, 2008 18444055

Southam-Gerow MA, Kendall PC, Weersing VR: Examining outcome variability: correlates of treatment response in a child and adolescent anxiety clinic. J Clin Child Psychol 30(3):422–436, 2001 11501258

Spence SH, Donovan C, Brechman-Toussaint M: The treatment of childhood social phobia: the effectiveness of a social skills training-based, cognitive-behavioural intervention, with and without parental involvement. J Child Psychol Psychiatry 41(6):713–726, 2000 11039684

Spence SH, Donovan CL, March S, et al: Online CBT in the treatment of child and adolescent anxiety disorders: Issues in the development of BRAVE-ONLINE and two case illustrations. Behav Cogn Psychother 36(special issue 4):411–430, 2008

Spence SH, Donovan CL, March S, et al: A randomized controlled trial of online versus clinic-based CBT for adolescent anxiety. J Consult Clin Psychol 79(5):629–642, 2011 21744945

Stallard P: Think Good, Feel Good: A Cognitive Behaviour Therapy Workbook for Children and Young People. New York, Wiley, 2002

Stark KD: Childhood Depression: School-Based Intervention. New York, Guilford, 1990

Stark KD, Kendall PC: Treating Depressed Children: Therapist Manual for ACTION. Ardmore, PA, Workbook Publishing, 1996

Stark KD, Reynolds WM, Kaslow NJ: A comparison of the relative efficacy of self-control therapy and a behavioral problem-solving therapy for depression in children. J Abnorm Child Psychol 15(1):91–113, 1987 3571741

Stark KD, Schnoebelen S, Simpson J, et al: Treating Depressed Children: Therapist Manual for ACTION. Ardmore, PA, Workbook Publishing, 2004

Treatment for Adolescents With Depression Study Team: Treatment for Adolescents With Depression Study (TADS): rationale, design, and methods. J Am Acad Child Adolesc Psychiatry 42(5):531–542, 2003 12707557

Van Voorhees BW, Fogel J, Reinecke MA, et al: Randomized clinical trial of an Internet-based depression prevention program for adolescents (Project CATCH-IT) in primary care: 12-week outcomes. J Dev Behav Pediatr 30(1):23–37, 2009 19194326

Vitiello B, Rohde P, Silva S, et al: Functioning and quality of life in the Treatment for Adolescents with Depression Study (TADS). J Am Acad Child Adolesc Psychiatry 45(12):1419–1426, 2006 17135987

Walkup JT, Albano AM, Piacentini J, et al: Cognitive behavioral therapy, sertraline, or a combination in childhood anxiety. N Engl J Med 359(26):2753–2766, 2008 18974308

Watanabe N, Hunot V, Omori IM, et al: Psychotherapy for depression among children and adolescents: a systematic review. Acta Psychiatr Scand 116(2):84–95, 2007 17650269

Waters AM, Ford LA, Wharton TA, et al: Cognitive-behavioural therapy for young children with anxiety disorders: Comparison of a Child + Parent condition versus a Parent Only condition. Behav Res Ther 47(8):654–662, 2009 19457471

Weersing VR, Weisz JR: Mechanisms of action in youth psychotherapy. J Child Psychol Psychiatry 43(1):3–29, 2002 11848335

Weisz JR: Development of control-related beliefs, goals, and styles in childhood and adolescence: a clinical perspective, in Self-Directedness and Efficacy: Causes and Effects Throughout the Life Course. Edited by Schaie KW, Rodin J, Schooler C. New York, Erlbaum, 1990, pp 103–145

Weisz JR, Sweeney L, Proffitt V, et al: Control-related beliefs and self-reported depressive symptoms in late childhood. J Abnorm Psychol 102(3):411–418, 1993 8408953

Weisz JR, Thurber CA, Sweeney L, et al: Brief treatment of mild-to-moderate child depression using primary and secondary control enhancement training. J Consult Clin Psychol 65(4):703–707, 1997 9256573

Weisz JR, Southam-Gerow MA, Gordis EB, et al: Cognitive-behavioral therapy versus usual clinical care for youth depression: an initial test of transportability to community clinics and clinicians. J Consult Clin Psychol 77(3):383–396, 2009 19485581

CHAPTER 45

Motivational Interviewing

Paul Nagy, M.S., LPC, LCAS, CCS
Sarah Armstrong, M.D., FAAP

Engaging parents and youth in discussions regarding behavior change can be a special challenge. It may be particularly difficult to motivate change when the young patient is engaged in behaviors, such as substance abuse, sexual risk taking, or speeding, that are positively reinforced by social, developmental, or biological conditions. The usual ways of delivering lifestyle and behavioral counseling, which typically focus on education delivery and provider-centered ideas for change, are generally known to be ineffective. Motivational interviewing (MI) is an alternative approach for raising problem awareness and facilitating change exploration with individuals who may be reluctant, stuck, or not yet ready to make behavioral changes. MI uses a patient-centered, collaborative approach that follows a particular set of principles and uses specific skills and techniques (Miller and Rollnick 1991). While MI has been studied primarily with adults, it is now being used with children and adolescents in a variety of settings, including pediatric practice, schools, juvenile justice settings, and emergency departments (Feldstein and Ginsburg 2006).

In this chapter we provide a brief description of MI and how it is done, a summary of the research and experience supporting the use and effectiveness of MI with children and adolescents, and an overview of several practical applications for implementing MI. The MI counselor should note that this technique is effective when used with children ages 10 and older; for children younger than age 10 (or the developmental equivalent), MI should be directed at the parent or guardian as the agent of change.

Motivational Interviewing Described

MI is "a collaborative conversation style for strengthening a person's own motivation and commitment to change" (Miller and Rollnick 2013, p. 12). The theoretical base for MI is self-determination theory, and it is further supported by Truax and

Carkaff (1967) and Gordon (1970). The core of MI instructs the counselor not to confuse *outcome* with *strategy.* For example, telling a patient he or she needs to lose weight to lower blood pressure (outcome) is less effective than helping a patient understand personal motivators to lose weight and collaboratively develop a plan. While MI adopts a traditional patient-centered style, it is intended to be more deliberate, directional, and goal oriented (Miller and Rollnick 2013) than traditional person-centered approaches.

Principles of Motivational Interviewing

The original concepts of the MI model are consistent with the trans-theoretical model (Prochaska and DiClemente 1982) that described change as a process and ambivalence toward change as normal. Resolving ambivalence, expressing commitment, and developing self-efficacy are considered to be the keys to change (Miller and Rollnick 1991). Motivation is viewed as a dynamic state, rather than a personality trait, because it can be modified and influenced by the provider's style (Miller and Rollnick 1991). It endorses the perspective that change is more likely to happen when the provider elicits a person's own reasons for change than when a provider argues for change through persuasive or directive methods. The persuasive method is often referred to as the *righting reflex,* or the tendency of a provider to "correct" a behavior that is detrimental to the patient by telling the patient to stop one behavior and adopt another, without consideration of the patient's knowledge, values, or opinions. The MI therapist's communication style is based on a "spirit" that emphasizes collaboration, evocations, and respect for patient autonomy (Miller and Rollnick 2002). The MI therapist is directive, exercising skills and techniques that address the patient's choices in relation to his or her own personal goals.

Does Motivational Interviewing Work? Evidence for Efficacy

MI has been studied in a variety of medical and therapeutic settings in which behavior change is the desired outcome. This includes adult and pediatric studies relevant to substance abuse, smoking cessation, medication adherence, and obesity counseling. Among adolescents, the literature shows that MI holds significant promise for addressing these concerns. MI counseling has demonstrated efficacy in reducing risky sexual behavior among inner-city teens, leading to reduced incidence of teen pregnancy and HIV exposure (Danielson et al. 2013; Williams et al. 2013). Teens are more likely to seek needed emergency contraception if their providers discuss options using MI (American Academy of Pediatrics Committee on Adolescence 2005). Sample findings related to substance abuse include those from the Cannabis Youth Treatment study. This study compared a variety of standardized treatments and found that a five-session motivational therapy intervention combined with cognitive-behavioral therapy had results comparable to those of longer-term interventions for the treatment of cannabis abuse (Dennis et al. 2004). Also, a series of studies (Barnett et al. 2001; Colby et al. 1998; Monti et al. 1999; Spirito et al. 2004) evaluated the effectiveness of MI in changing alcohol use behavior in adolescents and young adults treated in emergency settings. While postdischarge behaviors were similar in both conditions, those receiving the MI intervention demonstrated a greater decrease in drinking and driving episodes, alcohol-related injuries, and alcohol-related problems. Young adolescents whose providers use MI to discuss tobacco use demonstrate lower rates of smoking initiation (Winickoff et al. 2013). Adolescents prefer that their providers talk to them in a manner consistent with MI (Latham et al. 2012). The evidence in childhood is less clear. With children younger than age 12 years, it has been shown that a counseling focus on the parent's choices and behaviors is more effective than focus on the child. MI has been shown to be effective when aimed at parents of young children diagnosed with obesity. In this case, use of MI with the parent is associated with greater reductions in the child's BMI than traditional counseling, even when matched for the amount of time spent in the room with the family (Resnicow et al. 2006). MI seems to be a particularly good fit for adolescents because of normal developmental pulls toward identity formation, independence, acceptance, and connection (Berg-Smith et al. 1999; Channon et al. 2003) as well as the fact that MI is typically brief, focused, and personalized. Additional advantages in using MI with children and adolescents include a targeted approach for dealing with low motivation, avoidance of labels and judgment, recognition of personal autonomy and choices, validating versus discounting of patient desires and choices, and attention to strengths and accomplishments.

How Does Motivational Interviewing Work?

Motivational Interviewing Spirit

The MI model recognizes that change is more likely to be influenced when the provider adopts the *spirit* of MI in addition to *doing* MI. This spirit embodies the perspective, approach, and style of the provider. The effectiveness of MI is enhanced by being *with* and *for* patients through partnership, acceptance, compassion, and evocation (Miller and Rollnick 2013). When a patient experiences an interested, understanding, and nonjudgmental provider who views the patient as an "expert" partner, the patient is more likely to be comfortable; to engage; and to be open, honest, and receptive to feedback, information, and advice. Providers who genuinely recognize, honor, and express an individual's worth, potential, and autonomy through the skillful expression of empathy and affirmation have been shown to evoke hope and confidence and empower action.

Eliciting Change Talk

Change talk is language used by the patient that suggests that he or she is at least thinking about possible alternatives to current behavior (e.g., "If I didn't smoke, I could use the money for music"). *Sustain talk* is language reflecting commitment to the status quo (e.g., "I love smoking; there's nothing you or anyone else can say or do to get me to quit"). Both change talk and sustain talk are facilitated by the conversational dynamic between the provider and the patient, and both predict behavior change. Conversely, resistance to change is also influenced by provider style, which may explain why confrontational approaches are ineffective. A provider elicits and reflects change talk by asking questions that allow individuals to talk about behavior in the context of their interests, concerns, and values. In MI a provider adopts a curious, guiding style of communication consisting of open-ended questions and reflective statements. This *change conversation* also serves to identify any ambivalence that might exist because of circumstances such as competing desires (e.g., "I want to give up smoking marijuana, but I don't want to lose my friends"), assessed importance ("Will it matter?") or confidence ("Can I do it?"). In MI, ambivalence is viewed as a normal part of the change process. A principal focus of MI is to identify, explore, and resolve ambivalence when it is in the way of change (Miller and Rollnick 1991). This discovery clarifies what needs to happen for change to occur.

Mobilizing Commitment to Action

A primary goal of MI is to build motivation and consolidate commitment by facilitating recognition of a problem, eliciting statements of personal concern about that problem, and then *drawing out* motivation statements related to intention to change and being optimistic about change (Miller and Rollnick 2002). MI is also a directive approach for guiding and implementing change. Through the adoption of the four processes of MI described in the section "Structure of the MI Interview: The Four Processes," the provider assists the patient in targeting and planning a particular change (Miller and Rollnick 2013).

Skills of the Interview: OARS

MI uses a cluster of counseling skills referred to as OARS—open-ended questions, affirmations, reflective listening, and summaries. These core skills are used both to get to know the patient and also to guide and motivate change. Use of these skills depends on the nature of the interview, the presentation of the patient, and the stage of the conversational process. Skills such as open-ended questions and reflective listening would be used to help with patient engagement and to promote awareness and understanding. Affirmations can be helpful to build motivation and inform possibilities by focusing on strengths and accomplishments. Summaries can assist people in hearing their own change talk and for collecting and clarifying information, as well as for transitioning to other topics. Information sharing and advice giving can be a very useful way of guiding change. In MI, this skill is typically exercised with permission and readiness of the patient.

Structure of the MI Interview: The Four Processes

A useful guide for using MI skills and techniques are the four processes: engaging, focusing, evoking, and planning (Miller and Rollnick 2013). These processes reflect the flow and focus of the MI conversation with the intention of "meeting the person where they are" and guiding the flow of effort and focus of conversation. While these processes typically emerge in sequence, there is often an overlapping and recursive nature to the four processes in MI conversations. In some cases, the conversation may be anchored in one process until the patient is ready to move forward. For example, adolescents may require a fair amount of time engaging with the provider to build rapport and trust. The provider is likely to be more successful guiding a patient through change when engaging ahead of focusing, focusing ahead of evoking, and evoking ahead of planning. In addition to the core interviewing skills (OARS), the provider can use particular skills and techniques to focus the conversation in alignment with the processes.

Engaging

Engagement serves as the foundation for all that follows. During this process the provider's focus is developing a connection, engendering patient "buy in" and getting to know the patient. In particular, it is useful to attempt to discover the things in the patient's life that matter, motivate, and marvel. A goal of engagement is coming to a mutual awareness of the patient's hopes, wishes, and dreams and the things that offer the patient meaning, purpose, and value. When assessing patient needs or progress, taking a more conversational approach versus a question and answer approach will enhance the opportunity to fit the assessment into the interview rather than fitting the interview into the assessment.

Engagement techniques include the following:

- Agenda setting: Review of roles, purpose, and relevance of the visit and agreement about topics for discussion

  Example: "Robert, I am a counselor who helps parents and teens work on having better control of their diabetes. We have about 30 minutes set aside for our meeting today, and while I would like to review your recent lab results and discuss some ways of managing your diabetes, I am also interested to see if there is anything in particular you would like to discuss or accomplish during our visit today."
- Assessing readiness for change: Discuss the change process and assess change readiness (e.g., review the wheel of change [stages of change] and ask the patient to stage his assessed level of readiness to work on a specific change)

  Example: "I've explained the different stages of readiness with regard to making changes in behavior. Where would you say you are on this wheel?"
- Assessment with feedback

  Example: "From what you describe, relative to your peers, you have experienced some real hardship related to your drinking."
- Exploring values and goals and identifying behavioral discrepancies
- Accurate and empathetic validation of experiences and feelings
- Use of restraint by avoiding communication traps such as the question and answer and premature traps and resisting the righting reflex

Focusing

The goal of focusing is to identify achievable goals to determine the direction of working together. While goals can come from the patient, a referring provider, a parent, or the provider, prioritizing the patient's agenda is the intention of this process. Focusing is an ongoing process and assumes that a person's interests and priorities might change. The counseling style and particular techniques used in this process depend on the scenario. Patients may be clear, unclear, or confused about the direction in which they would like to go. The goal during this process is to identify a goal even if it is a goal to decide whether or not to have a goal. Some useful responses to the various states would be the following:

- Clear focus: Move to evoking
- Unclear focus or undecided: Review menu of options (agenda mapping), provide assessment with feedback,

share information (elicit-provide-elicit), and offer suggestions with permission (informing choices)

Example of agenda mapping and informing choices: "Dennis, at this time it seems as though you are not clear about what you would like to work on in counseling. I would be happy to review some of the choices or to discuss what others do in your situation and see what you think."

Example of information sharing:

Elicit—"Would you like to hear some of the things you could do to better control the way you express your anger?"

Provide—"One choice would be to work on how you talk to yourself about the things that make you angry to see if there are ways of changing your thoughts."

Elicit—"Do you think this is something that might be helpful?"

Evoking

Supported by the belief that individuals know best what they want and what they are willing to do to work for what they want, the provider engages with the patient in this process to determine readiness and ideas for change. It is also helpful during this process to identify those impediments to change to help the patient better recognize what needs to be out of the way in order to get on the way. Because strength of commitment matters when people decide on a goal, during this process the provider evokes, reflects, and builds on change talk as well as explores and assists the patient in working through any identified ambivalence. If a patient is clearly focused and motivated, this process is oriented to eliciting the patient's ideas about how he or she sees himself or herself changing and then transitioning to planning accordingly. A key to successfully working through this process is to avoid the righting reflex by avoiding telling the patient *your* reasons for why he should change and instead expressing the patient's autonomy.

Evoking techniques include the following:

- Elicit self-motivational statements by asking "DARN CAT" questions:

  Desire: How much do you want to make this change?

  Ability: How successful do you think you can be in making this change?

  Reason: What is a good reason for you to make this change?

  Need: Why is it important for you to make this change?

  Commitment: When will you know it is time to close the deal with yourself?

  Activation: What are you ready or willing to do? When might you get started?

  Taking steps: What have you done or how will you get started?
- Measure the importance of, commitment to, and confidence in the ability to change (see Figure 45–1). Key: elicit self-motivational statements by asking the patient's reasons for higher-scale answers (e.g., "How come you answered a 4 and not a 3 on seeing this change as important to make?")
- Review pros and cons of making or not making a change; weigh the answer according to expressed goals and values

  Example: "As you have outlined all the things you would gain and lose by quitting alcohol, which of your answers relates the best to the things that are most important to you?"
- Develop discrepancies (with permission); identify the distance between

On a scale of 0 to 10, how IMPORTANT is it for you right now to change?

0 ____ 1 ____ 2 ____ 3 ____ 4 ____ 5 ____ 6 ____ 7 ____ 8 ____ 9 ____ 10

Not at all Important — Extremely Important

On a scale of 0 to 10, how CONFIDENT are you that you could make this change?

0 ____ 1 ____ 2 ____ 3 ____ 4 ____ 5 ____ 6 ____ 7 ____ 8 ____ 9 ____ 10

Not at all Confident — Extremely Confident

FIGURE 45–1. Readiness scale.

the patient's expressed intentions and his or her choices

Example: "Would you be willing to help me understand your current motivation for quitting smoking? At our last visit you said you were highly motivated to stop smoking and would start by not buying cigarettes. Today you're carrying a carton of cigarettes with you, so I'm wondering whether your motivation has changed, or should we work on another approach to helping you quit?"

- Query extremes

  Example: "What is the worst thing that can happen if you continue to drink this way?"
- Explore others' concerns

  Example: "Why do you think your parents are worried about you?"
- Look forward

  Example: "How would you like things to be a month from now?" or "If you were to have made this change, how do you think you would have succeeded?"
- Evoke hope and confidence by affirming strengths and reviewing past successes

  Example: "Is there anything that you learned about yourself or about how to be successful when you passed your GED test?"
- Reflect change talk heard in ambivalent statements

  Example: "While I hear that you don't like having your parents have so much control over your life, you certainly are clear that you would like to have a better chance of having your driving privileges reinstated if you choose to honor your curfew."

Planning

During planning the goal is to move the patient from intention to action by helping with the development of an effective change plan (Table 45–1). During this process there is less discussion about whether and why to change and more about how. Some indicators for assessing patient readiness for change planning include clear and consistent desire and commitment statements ("I'm really serious about wanting to fit in my clothes"), queries about how to get to change ("How do others lose weight?"), and any activation or movement toward change ("I've started drinking only one soda a day"). A strong change plan is one that is motivated by expressed intrinsic reasons and includes elements that are specific, measurable, attainable, realistic, and timely. Identifying supports and anticipating setbacks or detours can offset potential implementa-

TABLE 45–1. Sample change plan

1. The change I want to make is ____________________ by this time: ________________
2. The expected benefit of making this change will be ______________________________
3. This is how and when I will get started: _____________________________________
4. The people who can help me are ____
5. The way they can help me will be ____
6. I will monitor my progress by ____
7. Things that could interfere with my plan would be _______________________________
8. The ways I will plan to deal with these challenges will be __________________________
9. This is how I will celebrate my success: ______________________________________

tion challenges. This process is also facilitated by applying the spirit and skills of MI (Table 45–2). Because change is rarely neat and linear, planning also includes opportunities for reassessing motivation, reevaluating the plan, and refocusing on new goals. Change sampling can be a useful way for the patient to try out new behaviors without further commitment ("One option you have identified for improving your grades is to not use marijuana the night before you have an exam. You can always try that to see if it makes a difference. It's up to you.").

Specific Applications

The pediatric and adolescent provider faces challenges, of which we describe a few commonly encountered situations and strategies.

Children

Primary Focus

Who should be the primary focus: the parent or the child? Adolescents (ages 12 years and older) should be the primary focus of the MI interview and often enjoy the opportunity to explore their emerging autonomy. Children younger than age 8 years are concrete in their cognitive developmental abilities and are less able to discuss causality, link current behavior with future goals, or respond to inferential questions. For these children, the focus should be on factors within the parent's control. For example, if a provider is meeting with an obese 6-year-old child, he might first *engage* and *focus* on the topic of weight-related health concerns, then *elicit* any long-term concerns the parent might have if the child's weight were to remain an issue. After understanding and reflecting the parent's long-term hopes for the child's health, the practitioner may explore any *plans* the parent may have to improve the child's weight (e.g., not buying soda, taking the child to the playground more often) and help the parent solidify commitment to this plan. For children ages 8–12 years, the focus necessarily is on both the child and the parent. A provider can help frame the discussion by reminding the parent-child pair that they may have different concerns about the issue (the parent wants to avoid diabetes in the child; the child wants to feel comfortable wearing a bathing suit) and still set a shared plan (mom agrees to buy some new vegetables to try; child agrees to try at least one bite).

Managing Blame

Often, a situation that requires change makes all members of a family feel

TABLE 45–2. Readiness and MI process–based interventions

Stage of change	MI process	Intervention	Technique
Precontemplation			
Not yet thinking about change	Engaging	Rapport building	Icebreakers
		Discovery and awareness	Client education
		Emphasizing personal choice	Assessment with personal feedback
			Exploring others' concerns
			Values clarification and identification of discrepancies
			Accurate empathy
			Resisting the righting reflex
Contemplation			
Thinking about change	Focusing	Identifying personal motivation and goals	Wheel of change
		Reviewing of behaviors in situational context	Agenda mapping
			Informing choices
			Elicit-provide-elicit
			Pros and cons/decisional balance
			Querying extremes
Preparation			
Preparing for change	Evoking	Assessing readiness to change	Scaling
		Identifying pathways to change	DARN CAT
		Strengthening commitment to change	Information and advice giving with permission
		Evoking hope and confidence	Use of hypotheticals
			Looking forward
			Querying extremes
			Affirmations
			Exploring successes
Action			
Implementing change	Planning	Mobilizing commitment to action	Change sampling
			Change planning

uncomfortable. A natural tendency to relieve discomfort is to place the blame elsewhere, and in a family there may be many people on whom to spread the blame. MI does not require the provider to address this issue. Rather, the provider should treat blame as any other resistance to change and "roll" with the resistance while listening for change talk. For example, the parents of an overweight child may blame the child for eating too much or too quickly or eating the "forbidden foods" in the home. The child may blame the parents for buying these foods. The MI approach would acknowledge these challenges and use open-ended questions to explore ideas for change (or successful strategies that have been used in the past). This *forward-looking* approach does not seek to resolve the conflict; rather, it aligns the child and parent in pursuit of a common goal.

Separate Households

Providers commonly care for children who live in more than one household. In some cases, the conditions for and commitment to behavior change vary drastically between these households. In some extreme examples, one household may actively "sabotage" the other's efforts to change (e.g., mom tries to get the child to eat only healthy foods; dad thinks mom is being overly strict and takes the child out for fast food to compensate). Unfortunately, in these situations, the child is usually the one to suffer the most. If the child is developmentally mature, a provider can conduct the four processes with the child and ask the child to write his or her evoked values and plan in the form of a letter to his or her parents (e.g., "Dear mom and dad, it is important for me to eat healthier because I can't run as fast as the other kids at school and it makes me feel bad. I want to try to stop drinking soda but this is hard for me because I like it so much. You can help me by not buying it at home and not drinking it in front of me when we go out. Can I count on you to help me?"). Younger children can often complete this activity with the help of the provider (not the parent) to do the writing.

Adolescents

Choices Inconsistent With Intentions

The developing brain does not always cooperate with motivation and intention. Because of the gradual maturation of the prefrontal cortex, there are limitations to the adolescent's capacity for reasoning, decision making, and impulse control (Galvan et al. 2006; Giedd 2004). Adolescents have an enhanced drive toward reward seeking and risk taking (Galvan et al. 2006). The immature prefrontal system cannot be expected to reliably mediate emotional drive and reward-seeking behaviors. Adolescents are naturally at risk for alcohol and drug use, risky sexual activity, and other forms of risk-taking behaviors. High emotional needs for peer acceptance, stimulation, or excitement may lead to increased vulnerability for risk taking, pending full brain maturation. Sole reliance on cognitive-behavioral strategies that instruct on ways to "think through behavior" may not work unless coupled with a strategy for enhancing motivation and resisting temptation by helping the adolescent emotionally connect with the target behavior change. Also, the capacity for awareness and insight is more limited in young patients who are not adequately equipped with the cognitive and reasoning abilities for effective decision making. When there are known discrepancies between a patient's actions and his or her expressed intentions, taking a curious, concerned, and validating approach can open the discussion. Assuming there is always a "good reason" or logic for every behavioral decision and focusing on understanding rather than "fixing" can be a useful approach. Example: "Frank, is it okay if I share an observation with you? Last week you mentioned you were highly motivated to quit smoking and today you are carrying a pack of cigarettes and a lighter. I'm wondering whether your motivation changed since last week, or is there something that is getting in the way of you quitting?" Also, highly valued behavior is more likely to be sustained. Discovering and focusing on core rather than superficial reasons for change is a key to building motivation and developing discrepancy. Example: "Having heard you say last week that your primary reason for staying off drugs is that your little brother told you he is worried you will be arrested again, I'm wondering whether you have any concern about this recent choice you made to buy drugs?"

Unrecognized Discrepancies

Adolescents often do not recognize how their choices work against their interests. Even when risk can be acknowledged, adolescents may view themselves as invincible and therefore immune from harm. For example, a young heroin user was encouraged by his therapist to learn from a friend's fatal overdose and was advised on a plan to avert a similar fate. He responded by saying that he was "smarter" than his friend and therefore not vulnerable to any such risk. In our experience, adolescents can easily view a provider who takes a "meet them where they are" approach as tacitly approving negative behaviors. The provider must be prepared to intervene as needed with regard to the health and safety of the patient. MI can be used even when the provider acknowledges that he or she is not neutral about the patient's choices. Most adolescents will accept that the provider has the responsibility to protect patients. An MI-informed approach can be taken even when communicating intention to influence a particular outcome. For example:

> You think I do not trust your ability to handle yourself when you drink and drive. You certainly have reasons to believe this, since, as you say, you have not yet had anything bad happen to you when you have done this. I care about you a great deal, and as your counselor I need to know that I am doing everything I can to keep you from hurting yourself or anyone else. I have choices about how I do that. Would you be willing to look at these choices with me and work together on a solution?

Also, depending on the seriousness of the situation, negotiating a change can be an appropriate strategy. For example:

> Susan, I want to be honest with you that I am worried about you having unprotected sex. I care about you and don't want you to suffer any serious consequences. I accept that you're not as worried as I am about you getting pregnant or contracting a sexually transmitted disease. Given that you are clear that you are not going to stop having sex, I'm wondering if you are willing to discuss some options for preventing pregnancy or catching a disease.

Planting seeds or attempting to move the patient from precontemplation to contemplation is another useful MI approach. For example: "Of all the things that could happen if you continue to have unprotected sex, is there anything that you would not like to happen? Is there something that you believe might have to happen first to change your mind?"

Change Is Not "Worth It"

One of the principal challenges in promoting behavior change with adolescents is that a positive change may not seem to be worth it. Adolescents may in fact experience negative consequences when making positive choices. For example, if an adolescent's substance use is reinforced by an important peer group, he or she may experience rejection or feelings of isolation and loss if choosing to not use drugs with his or her friends. Ideally, sharing factual information with permission about the benefits of change might be helpful. However, in the absence of any identified intrinsic motivators or with unwelcome tradeoffs, motivation will be affected. In these instances looking forward can be a helpful technique for guiding patients to an awareness of the benefits of change (e.g., "In what way might you imagine life could be better or that you would be closer to your goal of finishing high school if you were to stop using drugs?"). Another practical approach is to explore ways to work in partnership with the patient to assist with making the change worth it. For example:

> Debbie, as you continue to do your part to work on your goal of regaining your parents' trust, I certainly will do all I can to help your parents see you in a more trusting light if you continue on the path of remaining alcohol and drug free. If you would like, I can increase the number of drug screens we do and work with you and your parents on having your privileges reinstated in response to negative drug screens.

Additional Applications

There are a range of other application scenarios specific to the practice of MI with children, adolescents, and parents. These include doing MI in groups and with families as well as MI-informed strategies for addressing the needs of special populations such as those involved in juvenile justice or hospital- or school-based settings and those with specific mental health, behavioral, or health conditions. As MI is a complex skill set, those interested are encouraged to pursue available training. In particular, feedback and coaching of observed practice and participation in MI learning communities are demonstrated ways of learning MI and integrating it into practice (Miller and Rollnick 2013).

In summary, building the helping relationship through empathy and collaboration and attending to readiness of the patient and the flow of conversation through use of the four processes (engaging, focusing, evoking, planning) along with the five communication skills of MI (OARS and providing information with permission) facilitate a positive and outcome-driven working partnership.

Summary Points

- Motivational interviewing (MI) is a patient-centered, collaborative approach for strengthening a person's own motivation and commitment to change.
- MI works through a spirit of partnership, acceptance, evocation, and compassion and by eliciting change talk and mobilizing commitment to action.
- MI is done by working with individuals through the four processes: engaging, focusing, evoking, and planning.

- MI uses specific counseling skills such as open-ended questions, affirmations, reflective listening, summaries, and giving information and advice with permission.
- MI has been shown to improve client engagement and self-efficacy and improve behavioral outcomes in children and adolescents. It is a good fit with youth given its use of empathy, validation, and acceptance and its recognition of personal autonomy and attention to strengths and accomplishments.
- Motivating change in children and adolescents is a unique challenge given a range of developmental and practical issues. Catalyzing change requires that MI be skillfully applied in recognition of the limits of child and adolescent insight, judgment, and control. The spirit of MI can be expressed to positive effect even when the provider is not neutral about the adolescent's choices.

References

American Academy of Pediatrics Committee on Adolescence: Emergency contraception. Pediatrics 116(4):1026–1035, 2005 16147972

Barnett NP, Monti PM, Wood MD: Motivational interviewing for alcohol-involved adolescents in the emergency room, in Innovations in Adolescent Substance Abuse Interventions. Edited by Wagner EF, Waldron, HB. Amsterdam, Pergamon, 2001, pp 143–168

Berg-Smith SM, Stevens VJ, Brown KM, et al: A brief motivational intervention to improve dietary adherence in adolescents. Health Educ Res 14(3):399–410, 1999 10539230

Channon S, Smith VJ, Gregory JW: A pilot study of motivational interviewing in adolescents with diabetes. Arch Dis Child 88(8):680–683, 2003 12876161

Colby SM, Monti PM, Barnett NP, et al: Brief motivational interviewing in a hospital setting for adolescent smoking: a preliminary study. J Consult Clin Psychol 66(3):574–578, 1998 9642898

Danielson CK, McCauley JL, Jones AM, et al: Feasibility of delivering evidence-based HIV/STI prevention programming to a community sample of African American teen girls via the internet. AIDS Educ Prev 25(5):394–404, 2013 24059877

Dennis M, Godley SH, Diamond G, et al: The Cannabis Youth Treatment (CYT) study: main findings from two randomized trials. J Subst Abuse Treat 27(3):197–213, 2004 15501373

Feldstein SW, Ginsburg JID: Motivational interviewing with dually diagnosed adolescents in juvenile justice settings. Brief Treatment and Crisis Intervention 6(3):218–233, 2006

Galvan A, Hare TA, Parra CE, et al: Earlier development of the accumbens relative to orbitofrontal cortex might underlie risk-taking behavior in adolescents. J Neurosci 26(25):6885–6892, 2006 16793895

Giedd JN: Structural magnetic resonance imaging of the adolescent brain. Ann N Y Acad Sci 1021:77–85, 2004 15251877

Gordon T: Parent Effectiveness Training. New York, Wyden, 1970

Latham TP, Sales JM, Renfro TL, et al: Employing a teen advisory board to adapt an evidence-based HIV/STD intervention for incarcerated African-American adolescent women. Health Educ Res 27(5):895–903, 2012 21368023

Miller WR, Rollnick S: Motivational Interviewing: Preparing People to Change Addictive Behavior. New York, Guilford, 1991

Miller WR, Rollnick S: Motivational Interviewing: Preparing People for Change, 2nd Edition. New York, Guilford, 2002

Miller WR, Rollnick S: Motivational Interviewing, 3rd Edition. New York, Guilford, 2013

Monti PM, Colby SM, Barnett NP, et al: Brief intervention for harm reduction with alcohol-positive older adolescents in a hospital emergency department. J Consult Clin Psychol 67(6):989–994, 1999 10596521

Prochaska JO, DiClemente CC: Transtheoretical Therapy: Toward a more integrative model of change. Psychotherapy 19(3):276–288, 1982

Resnicow K, Davis R, Rollnick S: Motivational interviewing for pediatric obesity: conceptual issues and evidence review. J Am Diet Assoc 106(12):2024–2033, 2006 17126634

Spirito A, Monti PM, Barnett NP, et al: A randomized clinical trial of a brief motivational intervention for alcohol-positive adolescents treated in an emergency department. J Pediatr 145(3):396–402, 2004 15343198

Truax CB, Carkaff RR: Toward Effective Counseling and Psychotherapy. Chicago, IL, Aldine, 1967

Williams TH, Dumas BP, Edlund BJ: An evidence-based parenting intervention with inner-city teen mothers. J Natl Black Nurses Assoc 24(1):24–30, 2013 24218870

Winickoff JP, Nabi-Burza E, Chang Y, et al: Implementation of a parental tobacco control intervention in pediatric practice. Pediatrics 132(1):109–117, 2013 23796741

CHAPTER 46

Systems of Care, Wraparound Services, and Home-Based Services

Yann Poncin, M.D.
Joseph Woolston, M.D.

Systems of care (SOCs) and wraparound services represent philosophies of care rather than programs with clearly specified elements of treatment. An SOC recognizes the importance of family, school, and the community at large in a child's overall health. The SOC comprises the informal and formal supports and services available in a given community and their linkage, and coordinating access to services within the larger community is an integral part of an SOC. Wraparound services are one approach to working with families using an SOC philosophy. Wraparound "wraps" services in the community around a child and family, according to the needs of the individual family. Wraparound has a specifically defined clinical and theoretical orientation and is concerned with the process of how a child and family are engaged to create a service plan that accesses or creates the relevant services in the community. Core features of wraparound and SOCs include engagement with the family from a strength-based and culturally competent perspective and respecting the family's own perception of their needs and goals, along with helping them to obtain services to meet those goals (Walker and Bruns 2006). When SOC programs first emerged, the wraparound process became the favored approach to implementing the SOC philosophy; therefore, the two terms are closely linked.

Historical Roots: Emergence of SOCs and Wraparound

A predecessor of SOCs is the child guidance movement, which emerged at the turn of the nineteenth century and led a shift from a punishment model to a corrective model ("guiding" children) that emphasized advocacy in multiple life domains (Jones 1999). The U.S. Congress passed the Mental Retardation Facilities and Community Mental Health Centers (CMHCs) Construction Act in 1963 in order to create a national network of community mental health centers. As the act did not specifically address children, only half of the centers had children's services. The indirect costs of child services, such as consultation with schools, were poorly reimbursed, if at all. Once the planned transition of the responsibility for managing CMHCs moved to the states, few states had a child mental health system or expertise (Lourie 2003).

The book *Unclaimed Children* (Knitzer 1982), which described the inadequacies of the national response to children with serious emotional disturbances and their families, served as a rallying point for advocates. This concern, coupled with philosophical and financial concerns about the excessive use of institutional care, ultimately facilitated Congressional funding of the Child and Adolescent Service System Program (CASSP) in 1984 and later the Comprehensive Community Mental Health Services for Children and Their Families Program. These new programs, along with state and foundation funding, led to the development of community-based services for youth with significant emotional disturbance.

At the time CASSP was funded, children who had the most significant difficulties were also those least likely to obtain the range of services they might need. Mental health, education, child welfare, and juvenile justice each had elements of mental health service or had children with mental health needs within their purview but were largely disconnected from one another (Lourie 2003). CMHCs had the ability to manage children with mild to moderate problems, but services were inadequate for children with more severe or multiple needs. At times, families had to forego their parental rights to be able to access child welfare's financial resources for services. A goal of CASSP was to enable children with special needs to access services without resorting to the juvenile justice or child protective service systems (Lourie 2003). Improved communication and collaboration among agencies was another goal. The guiding principle of CASSP was the SOC, a multiagency approach to the delivery of services. The three core values of an SOC (see Table 46–1) are the child and family's needs, community-based services, and care that is culturally competent (Stroul 2003). CASSP included expectations of interagency efforts to meet children's needs, using state-level discussions among existing disconnected agencies. Another goal of CASSP was to develop and strengthen mental health resources for children, given that half of the states had no budget dedicated to children's mental health. With the focus on empowering families in forging individualized care plans, wraparound services and intensive home-based services also became common features of an SOC approach (Burns et al. 2000). Table 46–2 highlights the key features of an SOC.

SOCs and community-based services developed as the result of the interaction of social, legal, cultural, therapeutic, political, and economic changes. In providing wraparound care, a team is organized around a child and family, and interventions are determined collaboratively to access and link a range of community services and agencies. Advocacy for both children and families is essential. The term *wraparound*

TABLE 46–1. Systems of care: core values

Core values	Core values in action
Child and family centered	The family determines the mix of services
Community based	Management and decision making are at the community level
Culturally competent	Agencies and individuals are responsive to cultural and ethnic differences

Source. Adapted from Stroul 2003.

TABLE 46–2. Systems of care: guiding principles

Children with emotional disturbances should receive services that address their emotional, social, educational, and physical needs
Services should be individualized for the child and family
Services should be developmentally appropriate and least restrictive
Caregivers should be fully integrated into the planning and treatment process
Services should be integrated and linked to one another
Case management should be provided to coordinate care as needed
Early identification and intervention should be promoted to ameliorate outcomes
A smooth transition to adult services should be ensured
The rights of children with emotional disturbances should be protected and efforts at advocacy promoted
All children with emotional disturbances should receive services regardless of race, sex, physical disability, religion, or other characteristics

Source. Adapted from Stroul 2003.

was reportedly first used by Lenore Behar in North Carolina in the early 1980s (VanDenBerg 1999), following a lawsuit that resulted in the state's requirement to provide less restrictive services in the community (Behar 2003). The Individuals with Disabilities Education Act (P.L. 94-142), for example, which was passed in 1975, reinforced emerging ideas of inclusion and "least restriction" (see Chapter 48, "School-Based Interventions").

The U.S. Supreme Court's *Olmstead* decision (*Olmstead v. L.C.*, 527 U.S. 581, affirmed in part, vacated in part, and remanded [1999]) found that the institutionalization of individuals with disabilities could be a form of discrimination that is prohibited by the Americans with Disabilities Act. Cost is another factor increasing interest in community-based care. Although it has proved difficult to compare long-term outcomes or collateral or consequential costs, monies required for institution-based care (hospital or residential treatment) are much greater than those required for community-based care (Brown and Hill 1996; Urdapilleta et al. 2013).

Wraparound Services

Wraparound services are helpful when children and families have significant emotional and behavioral difficulties and have experienced treatment failures. The wraparound model has been particularly aimed at maintaining youth in their communities or with their families. Children and their families who are served by wraparound may be involved in foster care, child protective services, juvenile justice, residential treatment facilities, special education, and other agencies. Approximately 1,000 wraparound programs serve 100,000 children yearly in the United States (Bruns et al. 2011).

A consensus group of experts in 1998 defined the key elements of wraparound services. As can be seen in Table 46–3, many aspects of wraparound involve developing the appropriate perspective and attitude, rather than determining specific components of care. Three key characteristics of wraparound are 1) strength-based orientation, 2) the value placed on cultural competence, and 3) integration of the family as an active participant in building a treatment plan. Traditional mental health treatment uses a deficit model that identifies a problem and focuses on ameliorating the problem. A strength-based approach, one that identifies positive coping mechanisms and resiliency factors, can be especially helpful in engaging with and helping families who come to receive or are referred to wraparound or SOC services, as these families have significant needs and are often accustomed to working from the perspective of failure with multiple, often poorly coordinated, agencies and services.

Wraparound Services in Practice

Examples of well-known early wraparound services and those programs serving specific populations are listed in Table 46–4. Wraparound Milwaukee was a recent recipient of the Annie E. Casey Innovations Award in Children and Family System Reform bestowed by the John F. Kennedy School of Government at Harvard University, reflecting the increasing recognition of services that address youth and their families from a collaborative and community perspective. The characteristics of wraparound programming and SOCs depend on local ecologies and other factors. Some of the key elements for the process used by wraparound services are described in Table 46–5. Examples of informal and formal community supports are provided in Table 46–6. Implementing a wraparound approach presents challenges. Development of cultural competence requires team or individualized training and ongoing supervision. Enhancement of coordination among agencies and services requires systems change at the policy and leadership levels that must filter down to (or up from) the individual workers in the agencies and systems to be linked.

Wraparound Services and Research Considerations

Studies have examined qualitative and quantitative outcomes and have shown positive results. At times, lack of clarity in how adherent these were to the core elements of wraparound services and which exact approaches were used makes conclusive interpretations difficult. From a research perspective, there are several challenges. Wraparound services are highly individualized, applied to a variety of populations, and generally reserved for families who present with a complex range of function and psychosocial distress. Moreover, those elements that make up the so-called core elements of wraparound services remain somewhat unsettled. The key elements of wraparound services as determined by experts set the founda-

TABLE 46–3. Key elements in the wraparound process

The youth and family must be full and active partners at every level and in every activity of the wraparound process. They must have a voice.
The wraparound approach must be a team-driven process involving the family, the child, natural supports, agencies, and community services working together to develop, implement, and evaluate the individualized plan.
Wraparound services must be located in the community, with all efforts toward serving the identified youth in community, residential, and school settings.
The process must be culturally competent, building on the unique values, preferences, and strengths of children and families and their communities.
Services and supports must be individualized and built on strengths and must meet the needs of children and families across life domains to promote success, safety, and permanence in home, school, and community.
Wraparound plans must include a balance of formal services and informal community and family supports.
There must be an unconditional commitment to serve children and their families.
Plans of care should be developed and implemented on the basis of an interagency, community-based collaborative process.
Wraparound child and family teams must have flexible approaches and adequate and flexible funding.
Outcomes must be determined and measured for the system, for the program, and for the individual child and family.

Source. Adapted from Goldman and Faw 1999.

tion on which measures of model fidelity were developed, such as the Wraparound Observation Form (Epstein et al. 1998) and the Wraparound Fidelity Index (Bruns et al. 2004).

Evidence Base in SOCs and Wraparound Services

Randomized controlled studies by Clark et al. (1996, 1998) and Evans et al. (1996, 1998) have found benefits to wraparound services. Other less methodologically rigorous studies also support the wraparound approach (Eber et al. 1996; Hyde et al. 1996; Pullmann et al. 2006; Yoe et al. 1996).

Evidence on wraparound services also points in a negative direction (Bickman et al. 2003; Carney and Buttell 2003; Toffalo 2000). The Fort Bragg study (Bickman et al. 2003) found that outcomes for subjects receiving wraparound services did not differ in a number of domains compared with those receiving treatment as usual. The treatment as usual in this sample, however, was more intensive than that available in many communities. Even with adequate methodological rigor, studies involving wraparound can be difficult to generalize to other populations and localities. Overall, wraparound, if delivered with full fidelity, is considered an evidence-based treatment for children with serious emotional disturbance (Washington State Institute for Public Policy [WSIPP] 2014).

Home-Based Services

Home-based services are often an integral part of a system of care. Because of the resources, staffing, funding, and intensity of treatment required, home-

TABLE 46–4. Examples of wraparound services and systems of care

Program	Location	Features
Alaska Youth Initiative (AYI)	Alaska	Early wraparound system Alaska was a CASSP-designated state and had received funds from NIMH to implement systems of care for children Based on Kaleidoscope programs in Chicago, which used the principles of unconditional care and individualized services in the community Initially served returnees from out-of-state residential treatment centers
Washington Youth Initiative	Washington	Replication of AYI For children in or returning from long-term residential treatment centers
Project Wraparound	Vermont	Replication of AYI For children at risk of out-of-home placement
Project Milwaukee	Milwaukee	Example of Medicaid managed care behavioral health carve-out For children under court order in juvenile justice or child protective services
La Grange school district	Illinois	Example of school-based wraparound program with the goal of maintaining children in less restrictive school settings by improving collaboration between schools and families
Program UPLIFT (Uniting Partners to Link and Invest in Families Today)	Santa Clara County, California	Example of wraparound provided through private agency Serves children in the community in lieu of residential placement
Fostering Individualized Assistance Program	Florida	Designed to improve permanency outcomes of children placed in foster care

Note. CASSP=Child and Adolescent Service System Program; NIMH=National Institute of Mental Health.

Source. Adapted from Goldman and Faw 1999; VanDenBerg 1999.

TABLE 46–5. Implementation of a wraparound approach

What	Who	Role
Community team (informal and formal stakeholders)	Leaders of Agencies, public and private Schools Parent groups Advocacy groups Business Higher education Clergy	Provide services or support to the family according to the care plan
Identification and referral	"Subcommittee" of a community team	Determine which families will receive services, often decided by consensus vote; various test scores have been used
Referral sources	Vary by wraparound system May include a large referral pool or only those children who are in state custody or at risk of out-of-home placement	Work collaboratively with wraparound teams and help identify children suited for the wraparound process
Resource coordinator (or case manager or individualized service coordinator)	An agency brokers the services and is responsible for hiring resource coordinators who have bachelor's level or higher education	Identify key individuals in child and family's life
	The agency oversees the wraparound process and manages flexible funds	Perform strength-based assessment Conduct child and family team meetings Help family team create individualized service plan Evaluate helpfulness of current services Develop crisis plan Arrange services not currently being used or available Manage flexible funds Provide direct services Evaluate progress Arrange for transition

TABLE 46–5. Implementation of a wraparound approach *(continued)*

What	Who	Role
Family	Parent and child	Parent and child must be actively engaged and listened to, and once a plan is co-constructed with them, the parent and child agree to the plan and commit to it
Strengths discovery	Resource coordinator with family	Informal or formal assessment of strengths to determine which services will be tailored
Child and family team	Child, family, extended family, friends, professionals, neighbors (usually consisting of 4–10 members)	No more than half the team should be professionals to encourage family ownership of the process
Team meetings	Child and family team	Review strengths and develop individualized service plan
Review of major life domains	Child and family team Child may or may not be present, depending on developmental and emotional considerations	Examination of the following areas: Living arrangements Family—structure, needs, function Social Emotional and psychological Educational Legal Financial Spiritual Medical Cultural Safety
Creating a service plan	Resource coordinator with child and family team	Life domains are prioritized according to the most need; these are often voted on, and the family has ultimate say in deciding what these are Brainstorming of ideas to meet the needs Ideal plan focuses on informal supports as these are longer lasting than formal supports, which will end Detailed crisis plan with action steps for each team member is established

TABLE 46–5. Implementation of a wraparound approach *(continued)*

What	Who	Role
Review of plan	Community team	Review plan for consistency with individual and community values and consider safety issues
		Review budget to determine how needs can be met
		If team disagrees with plan, the plan is not stopped, but it is sent back for revision to the child and family team
Implementation of plan	Coordinator and child and family team	Coordinator implements the plan and meets with the child and family team every few weeks initially and then at least every quarter thereafter
		Major changes are undertaken only with the input of the child and family team
Outcomes	Resource coordinator and others	Typically, quantitative measures of behavioral change, reduction in drug use, school attendance, and out-of-home placement are used along with qualitative feedback from families

Source. Adapted from VanDenBerg and Grealish 1996.

TABLE 46–6. Potential sources of community support

Home life	Family, friends, family friends, grandparents, extended family, foster care agency, independent living center, group home, respite care
School	Teacher, special education teacher, paraprofessional aide, guidance counselor, school social worker, school psychologist, principal, peer groups, parent-teacher organization and other parent groups, sports activities, school programs and groups, student mentors, student tutors, alternative education, therapeutic day schools, general equivalency diploma programs
After-school programs	Community centers, recreation centers, sports leagues, any organized leisure activities
Mental health and allied services	Social worker, psychologist, psychiatrist, nurse, art therapist, recreation therapist, therapeutic mentor, social skills training, individual therapy, group therapy, family therapy, in-home services, intensive outpatient services, partial hospital treatment, speech and language therapist, occupational therapist
Legal sources	Probation officer, attorney, guardian ad litem, case manager
Employment	Vocational and job training agencies, job internships, employment
Spiritual sources	Church, mosque, pastors, ministers, imams, meditation, members of the congregation
Complementary sources	Complementary alternative medicine and other approaches
Economic sources	Flexible funding support

based services are typically reserved for families who have children at risk of being placed out of home, whether in a hospital, residential treatment center, correctional facility, foster care, or other location. The intent of the Adoption Assistance and Child Welfare Act of 1980 (P.L. 96-272) was to strengthen permanency planning for children. States were required to make reasonable efforts to prevent removal of youth from their family or to return them to their family, or, if attempts to have the child remain with the family are unsuccessful, to accomplish permanency planning within a reasonable amount of time. In 1993, Congress passed legislation establishing Title IV, Part B-2, of the Social Security Act, creating funding for family preservation and family support programs.

The first program with which the term *family preservation* became associated was the Homebuilders program in Tacoma, Washington, developed in 1974 to avert foster care placement. Homebuilders worked with the entire family using a treatment approach based on crisis intervention theory (Kinney and Dittmar 1995). Nowadays, intensive home-based family preservation refers to a wide array of treatment services and interventions with significantly different treatment models and implementation strategies. They differ from traditional treatment approaches in a number of ways. Services are provided in the home and community, at a time of day that more flexibly meets the family's schedule. Treatment is often time limited, usually lasting 1–6 months, although longer periods are common. Caseloads for therapists are small (two to eight families). Therapists have frequent in-home or in-community contact with families and care providers, or their proxies, are available to families on a 24-hour basis to respond to crises and treatment needs.

Home-Based Services and Mental Health

Home-based services generally serve children who are involved with child welfare, juvenile justice, and/or mental health. The specific home-based service provided and its focus will depend on the primary problem and the population served. The examples of home-based services in the following subsections are those that have been used to help children with mental health needs that are well known and systematically evaluated and/or widely disseminated.

Multisystemic Therapy

Multisystemic therapy (MST) is a home-based, family-focused program, meant to treat youth who have serious behavioral problems. It was developed and refined serving the juvenile justice population and has been available for more than two decades. An adapted model, applied to populations with primarily mental health needs, is called MST-Psychiatric and is considered an evidence-based program by the Substance Abuse and Mental Health Services Administration.

MST uses an ecological model as a guiding principle that places a child in the inner circle of expanding concentric circles that include child, family, peers, school, neighborhood, community, and culture. MST teams consist of two to four therapists. A therapist works with two to four families at a time. A supervisor conducts weekly clinical team supervision and individual supervision for cases in crisis. The duration of treatment ranges from 3 to 5 months. Discharge criteria are outcome based and must show that there has been an improvement in the problem behavior. MST has a rigorous quality assurance program, and for agencies to provide MST services, they must adhere to this program (Multisystemic Therapy Services 2007).

MST has a robust evidence base from randomized clinical trials for use with juvenile offenders and substance-abusing youth at risk for out-of-home placement. The evidence for populations with psychiatric problems as a primary concern is less established. In one large controlled trial, MST was associated with a reduced number of days of inpatient psychiatric hospitalization, improvement in externalizing symptoms, improved family relationships, and increased school attendance (Schoenwald et al. 2000). However, longer-term follow-up revealed few differences over time compared with the control group (Henggeler et al. 2003). Another controlled study, comparing MST with existing continuum of care services (the latter ranging from outpatient to home-based to out-of-home placement), showed a short-term decrease in out-of-home placements and externalizing symptoms (Rowland et al. 2005).

Intensive In-Home Child and Adolescent Psychiatric Services

The Intensive In-Home Child and Adolescent Psychiatric Services (IICAPS; Woolston et al. 2007), developed at Yale in 1997, is a home-based intervention for children and adolescents with serious emotional and behavioral problems. IICAPS is a Medicaid-funded service delivered throughout Connecticut and part of New York and is considered a promising practice. It is undergoing a randomized controlled trial but is not conclusively established as an evidence-based model of care (Cannata and Williams 2012). It is included here for review, as it conforms to the theme of this chapter, delivering care in the community to those youth who are at risk of requiring institutional care or have exhausted traditional outpatient services. Moreover, unlike in other models, the child and adolescent psychiatrist is an integral part of IICAPS, without which the model would not exist. The in-home, or family, component of IICAPS represents the view that the family is essential to and has the power to make and sustain change in a child's life. Families agree to participate voluntarily in treatment, to be partners in the work, and to co-lead treatment planning. Families are more likely to feel comfortable and empowered if services are provided in their own home. This also circumvents obstacles for families who have difficulty attending clinic-based care. In the home, the IICAPS team can see firsthand the multiple social and interaction factors—both strengths and vulnerabilities—that influence the vicious cycle of significant emotional disturbance for the child and family. Teams can provide direct psychiatric evaluation and treatment, parenting skills training, family management skills training, problem-solving skills training, 24/7 mobile crisis emergency services, and intensive case management.

IICAPS teams consist of a senior clinician with a master's level degree, usually in social work, and a mental health counselor with a bachelor's degree. Teams with two master's level clinicians are often used. All individual clinicians receive 15 hours of initial training. A more senior mental health clinician supervises the teams weekly. A child and adolescent psychiatrist serves as the medical director and co-leads interdisciplinary treatment rounds. Clinicians each treat 6–8 families for 4–6 months or longer, depending on need. The team is available 24/7 for mobile crisis interventions. Programmatically, IICAPS has a nested structure: 6–8 cases to a team, 4 teams to a rounds group, 1–4 rounds groups to a program, 15 programs to a network. The model is manualized, and adherence to the model at the team level is assured by clinician fidelity to the IICAPS tools and structures of treatment. At the program level, each site must demonstrate the use of specified tools for engagement, assessment, treatment, and quality assurance. IICAPS uses a Web-based system to collect data, with the goal of determining the effectiveness of IICAPS in both improving function and reducing out-of-home placement. IICAPS has yet to be evaluated empirically. A controlled trial is currently under way that randomly assigns children and families referred to IICAPS to one of two arms: treatment in the community as usual supplemented with the assistance of a case manager to broker services or IICAPS services.

As detailed in the following case example, IICAPS is an in-home service and reflects a system of care philosophy. IICAPS provides direct treatment and not coordination of care per se. Additional therapeutic and community supports are determined according to the child's and family's needs and are enlisted in the service of treatment.

Case Example: Stages of IICAPS Treatment

Julia is a 12-year-old girl referred to IICAPS after her second psychiatric hospital admission. She lives with her maternal grandmother, her grandmother's fiancé, a 21-year-old half-sister, and a 2-year-old niece. Child protective services had placed Julia in her grandmother's care at age 4 because of neglect. Julia entered outpatient treatment at age 6 after an aggressive outburst at school resulted in Julia being sent to the emergency room. Over the years, Julia and her family have had general outpatient services, parent management training, intensive outpatient services, partial hospital treatment, medication management, and inpatient psychiatric hospitalization. She has carried a number of diagnoses, including bipolar disorder, intermittent explosive disorder, attention-deficit/hyperactivity disorder, mood disorder not otherwise specified, posttraumatic stress disorder, psychotic disorder not otherwise specified, and borderline intellectual functioning. Although she has been suspended from school a number of times, she has not been identified for special education. Her institutional care to date has helped with acute behaviors and maintaining safety, but it has not addressed the domains in Julia's social ecology that promote the symptoms that lead to her hospitalization. In some aspects, hospitalization has even worsened Julia's function by exacerbating symptoms of trauma and abandonment.

After a referral from the hospital to IICAPS was accepted, the senior clinician (MSW) and the mental health counselor (BA) set up an appointment within the week and reviewed the tools and processes they would use to engage the family and co-construct a treatment plan for the *assessment and engagement phase* of treatment. The tools and objectives of this phase include developing the immediate action plan, defining and rating the initial main problem, creating a genogram, cataloging strengths and vulnerabilities in four domains, and reviewing the "cycle of the main problem."

At the first meeting, the family and team developed an *immediate action plan,* which included safety planning—that is, identifying what behaviors were considered an emergency for Julia and how the family would access help in a crisis. At the first visit, the team learned that the electricity had been turned off and that the grandmother's fiancé, the main breadwinner, had relapsed into substance use and was working only sporadically. The team and family decided that the mental health counselor would meet with Julia individually while the senior clinician would meet with Julia's grandmother and the fiancé. All would meet together for family work, which would include Julia's sister. The team and family arranged a schedule for three home visits per week. The team first helped the family get the electricity turned on (for reasons of medical necessity) and establish a payment plan with the company. The grandmother, however, remained guarded with the team and often confused their role with the role of child protective services, with which the family was involved. On several occasions, no one answered the door at the appointed visit times. Three weeks into treatment, Julia was rehospitalized after an aggressive outburst toward her 21-year-old half-sister, whom she threatened to kill. The team attended team rounds on the inpatient unit, met with Julia, and continued to meet with her grandmother at home. After Julia's discharge, the team renewed their home visits as scheduled. After continuous and ongoing efforts at engagement with the family, the grandmother warmed up to the team, appreciating their demonstration of commitment and support.

With Julia home, the family and team began to co-construct the treatment plan. Co-construction is a key philosophical element of IICAPS. The family takes the lead in establishing main problems and goals, and the IICAPS team, through their increasing familiarity with the family's psychosocial function, contributes as well. The team helped the family discuss and discover their *strengths and vulnerabilities in each of four domains*—child, family, school, and physical environment—and to review the impact of these on the main problem. The IICAPS model defines the main problem as the behavior that leads to a higher level of care, such as hospitalization. The strengths and vulnerabilities in each domain were mapped out on paper as the *cycle of the main problem.* This is a graphical representation of the cycle or pattern leading to manifestation of the main problem. The team and family then cocreated goals and action steps in each of the four domains to address the main problem. Goals and action steps were limited to one or two per domain and were phrased in the family's own words. Often families list too many goals and action steps, which dilutes efforts to address the very serious behaviors related to the main problem.

Julia's main problem was that "she gets angry and hits people." One child domain goal was that "Julia will not hit others," with one of the action steps being "Julia will go to her room when she is becoming upset." In the family domain, one goal was that "family members will respect each other and not yell." The action step included "Grandmother will spend nice, alone time with Julia." For the school domain, the goal was "Julia will attend school." The action steps included "Team and family will meet with school to get more information about Julia's function and abilities at school." In the physical environment domain, which highlights therapeutic and natural supports in the community, the family identified their minister as helpful and concerned. He, along with other church members, was enlisted as support. The team and grandmother also thought that Julia would benefit from a therapeutic mentor, someone who could provide individual support to Julia while taking her out into the community. The grandmother also mentioned needing help with day-to-day household chores; the team agreed to help the grandmother look into free day care services for the 2-year-old through another community organization. The team and family also decided that a meeting bringing together all the services involved in the family's life—child protective services, outpatient treatment team, and school, among others—would be helpful. The team wrote the treatment plan, and all members—the family, Julia, clinical team, team supervisor, and medical director—reviewed and signed the plan.

During treatment, the team met weekly with their supervisor and presented Julia's case in multidisciplinary team rounds every 3 weeks. In rounds, the team, supervisors, and the child psychiatrist contributed to the biopsychosocial formulation and the team's conceptualization of the case.

The next phase after assessment and engagement, which may take weeks or months, is the *work and action phase,* in which the main problem and goals are established, as described previously, and a treatment plan is signed. These are regularly reevaluated and rated by the family and team. The focus remains on developing problem-solving skills, parent management skills, and family management skills as they relate to the main problem. The purpose is to help the child stay out of institutional care, to function better in all aspects of the social ecology, and to improve the developmental trajectory.

The last phase of treatment is the *ending and wrap-up phase,* in which the course of treatment and goals are rereviewed and therapeutic and community supports are consolidated prior to discharge.

Functional Family Therapy

Functional Family Therapy (FFT) uses principles of systems theory and behavior modification to improve the interactions, communication, and problem solving within a family. FFT has existed for close to 40 years and targets youth between ages 11 and 18 years. It focuses on youth with disruptive behaviors, conduct disorder, and substance use, who may have a number of additional psychiatric diagnoses. It is often used in juvenile justice populations and as an alternative to out-of-home placement or incarceration (Alexander et al. 2002; Sexton and Alexander 2000). FFT is provided in 8–12 sessions over 3 months, including up to 30 direct service hours. FFT therapists have a master's degree in a human services field. FFT also examines the multiple systems involved in a child and family's life. FFT first discovers the family's strengths and then helps empower the family to be self-sufficient as they interact with or access multiple systems in the community (Alexander et al. 2002; Sexton and Alexander 2000).

Brief Strategic Family Therapy

Brief strategic family therapy (BSFT) is a 12- to 15-session problem-focused intervention delivered over 3 months. Its target population is school-age children and adolescents who have behavioral problems. Generally, it has been delivered in the office but has also been used as an in-home service. BSFT focuses on the family system and the patterns of interaction that influence each member. The therapist's goal is to help identify which family interactions lead to the child's problem behaviors. BSFT is manualized and has been empirically validated for the treatment of substance abuse and conduct problems and has also been modified to serve the cultural needs of Hispanic youth (Szapocznik et al. 2002).

Multidimensional Treatment Foster Care

Multidimensional treatment foster care (MTFC) is a program designed for youth who require out-of-home care. Children are placed in a foster family setting for 6–9 months. The MTFC team consists of a program supervisor, a family therapist, an individual therapist, a child skills trainer, and a daily telephone contact person. The foster parents undergo training and become part of the team. They attend a weekly meeting and provide a daily phone report, Monday through Friday. Foster parents have access to staff 24/7. The MTFC team meets weekly to review the child's progress, including the daily reports, and to adjust the treatment plan as indicated. The birth parents receive parent training and family therapy in preparation for their child's return home. The skills they learn resemble the approach to the child in the foster home. The goal of treatment is to have the child return home. MTFC has been shown to reduce out-of-home placements and juvenile delinquency (Chamberlain et al. 2007a, 2007b).

Nurse-Family Partnership

The nurse-family service is delivered in the home as both treatment for the parent and prevention for the child. In this program, nurses visit low-income, first-time mothers weekly or biweekly from the prenatal period until the child reaches age 2 years. Nurses focus on the mother's health and the environment, and they educate mothers about developmental expectations and caregiving issues. Family members are engaged, and access to services in the community is facilitated as needed. Senior nurses supervise the home visitors, each of whom carries a caseload of approximately 25. A 15-year follow-up study demonstrated a reduction in maternal behavior problems, maternal arrests, running away by children, arrests of children, and alcohol use by children. A reduction of child abuse and neglect also occurred, but the reduction was limited if high rates of domestic violence were present (Olds 2007).

The Affordable Care Act and Wraparound

The Affordable Care Act (ACA) was passed by Congress and signed into law by the president on March 23, 2010 and was upheld by the Supreme Court on June 28, 2012. The ACA has a number of provisions and legal mandates related to health care, many of which are not germane to wraparound or systems of care. However, one provision of the ACA allows states the option of implementing health homes (not to be confused with medical homes) under their Medicaid state plans, with matching federal funds as an incentive. The purpose of this option is to encourage states to implement models of health delivery that enhance access to and coordination of physical and behavioral health, both mental health and substance use, and community services for children and adults with chronic conditions. The definition of chronic condition includes serious emotional disturbance in children. The elements identified as being key to a health home approach are similar to or often the same as those elements found in wraparound, even if the exact terminology may differ. The health home elements include care coordination and health promotion, individual and family support, comprehensive care management, referral to community and support providers, and comprehensive transitional care from inpatient to other settings, among other elements, all of which lend themselves well to wraparound models (Pires 2013). Care coordination or wraparound for children differs from that of adults. For adult patients with chronic mental illness, it is their physical health that requires high-intensity services, and it is costly. For children, behavioral health treatments account for most of the cost of caring for such children. Moreover, care coordination for adults may be effective, with relatively high caseloads, up to 250 clients per care manager, whereas care coordination for children, which uses high-fidelity wraparound, requires a much lower case to care manager ratio, on the order of 10:1. Children have families and are involved with mental health, schools, juvenile justice, and child welfare, among others, which leads to complexity of management and a need for more in-person coordination. Such a ratio presents a significant cost to the payer, but data suggest, according to demonstration projects, such coordination reduces per-beneficiary costs by avoiding institutional care, such as residential care (Urdapilleta et al. 2013). Given the ACA provision, the option to receive matching funds, the potential benefit of reducing high utilizer costs, and the availability of an evidence-based model that aligns itself well with the health home intention, the increased implementation of wraparound models is likely over the next years.

Summary Points

- The system of care (SOC) philosophy recognizes the importance of family, school, and the community at large in a child's overall health and functioning.
- An important goal of SOCs is for the various agencies and treatment providers involved in a child's life to be linked to one another.
- Wraparound is a community-based service that implements an SOC philosophy. Wraparound services help provide and obtain services in the community by working with and advocating for a child and family.
- The wraparound process includes a focus on the child's and family's strengths, cultural competence, and co-construction with the family of a treatment plan. A case manager is assigned to and works with the family to help negotiate community services.
- Wraparound services have been used with youth in foster care, juvenile justice, schools, and mental health settings. Wraparound services are often used to work with families who have children at risk for out-of-home placement.
- Home-based services are delivered to the family in the community and usually include 24/7 team availability, small caseload, and intense short-term treatment lasting 6 weeks to 9 months.
- Multisystemic therapy is a specific well-known home-based service that has robust evidence of efficacy for youth who are in juvenile justice or who use substances and, to a lesser degree, youth who have mental illness.
- Mental health services programs for youth such as intensive In-Home Child and Adolescent Psychiatric Services, Brief Strategic Family Therapy, Functional Family Therapy, Multidimensional Treatment Foster Care, and Nurse-Family Partnerships are programs that have elements of a system of care philosophy and are promising for the treatment or prevention of mental illness.
- The Affordable Care Act provides for implementation of health homes to manage serious emotional disturbances. Wraparound services lend themselves well to implementation of such health homes.

References

Alexander J, Barton C, Gordon D, et al: Book Three: Functional Family Therapy. Boulder, Center for the Study and Prevention of Violence, Institute of Behavioral Science, University of Colorado, 2002

Behar LB: Using litigation to improve child mental health services: promises and pitfalls. Adm Policy Ment Health 30(3):199–218, 2003 12854676

Bickman L, Smith CM, Lambert EW, et al: Evaluation of a congressionally mandated wraparound demonstration. J Child Fam Stud 12(2):135–156, 2003

Brown RA, Hill BA: Opportunity for change: exploring an alternative to residential treatment. Child Welfare 75(1):35–57, 1996

Bruns EJ, Burchard JD, Suter JC, et al: Assessing fidelity to a community-based treatment for youth: the Wraparound Fidelity Index. J Emot Behav Disord 12(2):79–89, 2004

Bruns EJ, Sather A, Pullman MD, et al: National trends in implementing Wraparound: results from the state Wraparound survey. J Child Fam Stud 20(6):726–735, 2011

Burns BJ, Schoenwald SK, Burchard JD, et al: Comprehensive community-based interventions for youth with severe emotional disorders: multisystemic therapy and the wraparound process. J Child Fam Stud 9(3):283–314, 2000

Burns BK, Goldman SK: Executive summary, in Promising Practices in Wraparound for Children With Severe Emotional Disorders and Their Families (Systems of Care: Promising Practices in Children's Mental Health, Vol IV). Edited by Burns BK, Goldman SK. Washington, DC, Center for Effective Collaboration and Practice, 1999, pp 11–18

Cannata E, Williams M: Evidence Based and Promising Practices, 2012. Available at: www.ctkeepthepromise.org/uploads/EBPPpresentation.ppt. Accessed July 20, 2014.

Carney MM, Buttell F: Reducing juvenile recidivism: evaluating the wraparound services model. Res Soc Work Pract 13(5):551–568, 2003

Chamberlain P, Reid J, Fisher PA, et al: Multidimensional Treatment Foster Care, 2007a. Available at: http://www.mtfc.com. Accessed September 25, 2007a.

Chamberlain P, Leve LD, Degarmo DS: Multidimensional treatment foster care for girls in the juvenile justice system: 2-year follow-up of a randomized clinical trial. J Consult Clin Psychol 75(1):187–193, 2007b 17295579

Clark HB, Lee B, Prange ME, et al: Children lost within the foster care system: can wraparound service strategies improve placement outcomes? J Child Fam Stud 5(1):39–54, 1996

Clark HB, Prange ME, Lee B, et al: An individualized wraparound process for children in foster care with emotional/behavioral disturbances: follow-up findings and implications from a controlled study, in Outcomes for Children and Youth With Emotional and Behavioral Disorders and Their Families: Programs and Evaluation Best Practices. Edited by Epstein MH, Kutash K, Duchnowski A. Austin, TX, Pro-Ed, 1998, pp 513–542

Eber L, Osuch R, Redditt CA: School-based applications of the wraparound process: early results on service provision and student outcomes. J Child Fam Stud 5(1):83–99, 1996

Epstein MH, Jayanthi M, McKelvey J, et al: Reliability of the Wraparound Observation Form: an instrument to measure the wraparound process. J Child Fam Stud 7(2):161–170, 1998

Evans ME, Armstrong MI, Kuppinger AD: Family centered intensive case management: a step toward understanding individualized care. J Child Fam Stud 5(1):55–65, 1996

Evans ME, Armstrong MI, Kuppinger AD, et al: Preliminary outcomes of an experimental study comparing treatment foster care and family centered intensive case management, in Outcomes for Children and Youth With Emotional and Behavioral Disorders and Their Families: Programs and Evaluation Best Practices. Edited by Epstein MH, Kutash K, Duchnowski A. Austin, TX, Pro-Ed, 1998, pp 543–580

Goldman SK, Faw L: Three wraparound models as promising approaches, in Promising Practices in Wraparound for Children With Severe Emotional Disorders and Their Families (Systems of Care: Promising Practices in Children's Mental Health, Vol IV). Edited by Burns BK, Goldman SK. Washington, DC, Center for Effective Collaboration and Practice, 1999, pp 35–78

Henggeler SW, Rowland MD, Halliday-Boykins C, et al: One-year follow-up of multisystemic therapy as an alternative to the hospitalization of youths in psychiatric crisis. J Am Acad Child Adolesc Psychiatry 42(5):543–551, 2003 12707558

Hyde KL, Burchard JD, Woodworth K: Wrapping services in an urban setting. J Child Fam Stud 5(1):67–82, 1996

Jones K: Taming the Troublesome Child: American Families, Child Guidance, and the Limits of Psychiatric Authority. Cambridge, MA, Harvard University Press, 1999

Kinney J, Dittmar K: Homebuilders: helping families help themselves, in Home-Based Services for Troubled Children. Edited by Schwartz IM, AuClaire P. Lincoln, University of Nebraska Press, 1995, pp 29–54

Knitzer J: Unclaimed Children: The Failure of Public Responsibility to Children and Adolescents in Need of Mental Health Services. Washington, DC, The Children's Defense Fund, 1982

Lourie IS: A history of community child mental health, in The Handbook of Child and Adolescent Systems of Care: The New Community Psychiatry. Edited by Pumariega AJ, Winters NC. San Francisco, CA, Jossey-Bass, 2003, pp 1–16

Multisystemic Therapy Services: Complete Overview: Research on Effectiveness. Mt. Pleasant, SC, Multi-Systemic Therapy Services, 2007. Available at: http://www.mstservices.com/complete_overview.php. Accessed September 23, 2007.

Olds DL: Preventing crime with prenatal and infancy support of parents: the nurse-family partnership. Victims & Offenders 2(2):205–225, 2007

Pires S: Customizing Health Homes for Children with Serious Behavioral Health Challenges, March 2013. Available at: http://www.nwi.pdx.edu/pdf/CustomizingHealthHomes.pdf. Accessed July 19, 2014.

Pullmann MD, Kerbs J, Koroloff N, et al: Juvenile offenders with mental health needs: reducing recidivism using wraparound. Crime Delinq 52(3):375–397, 2006

Rowland MD, Halliday-Boykins CA, Henggeler SW, et al: A randomized trial of multisystemic therapy with Hawaii's felix class youths. J Emot Behav Disord 13(1):13–23, 2005

Schoenwald SK, Ward DM, Henggeler SW, et al: Multisystemic therapy versus hospitalization for crisis stabilization of youth: placement outcomes 4 months postreferral. Ment Health Serv Res 2(1):3–12, 2000 11254068

Sexton TL, Alexander JF: Functional Family Therapy. Washington, DC, U.S. Department of Justice, Office of Juvenile Justice and Delinquency Prevention, 2000. Available at: http://www.ncjrs.gov/pdffiles1/ojjdp/184743.pdf. Accessed October 1, 2007.

Stroul BA: Systems of care: a framework for children's mental health care, in The Handbook of Child and Adolescent Systems of Care: The New Community Psychiatry. Edited by Pumariega AJ, Winters NC. San Francisco, CA, Jossey-Bass, 2003, pp 17–34

Szapocznik J, Robbins MS, Mitrani VB, et al: Brief strategic family therapy, in Comprehensive Handbook of Psychotherapy: Integrative/Eclectic, Vol 4. Edited by Kaslow FW. Hoboken, NJ, Wiley, 2002, pp 83–109

Toffalo DAD: An investigation of treatment integrity and outcomes in wraparound services. J Child Fam Stud 9(3):351–361, 2000

Urdapilleta O, Geena K, Ying W, et al: National Evaluation of the Medicaid Demonstration Waiver Home- and Community-Based Alternatives to Psychiatric Residential Treatment Facilities, 2013. Available at http://www.medicaid.gov/Medicaid-CHIP-Program-Information/By-Topics/Delivery-Systems/Downloads/CBA-Evaluation-Final.pdf. Accessed July 19, 2014.

VanDenBerg JE: History of the wraparound process, in Promising Practices in Wraparound for Children With Severe Emotional Disorders and Their Families (Systems of Care: Promising Practices in Children's Mental Health, Vol IV). Edited by Burns BK, Goldman SK. Washington, DC, Center for Effective Collaboration and Practice, American Institutes for Research, 1999, pp 19–26

VanDenBerg JE, Grealish EM: Individualized services and supports through the wraparound process: philosophy and procedures. J Child Fam Stud 5(1):7–21, 1996

Walker JS, Bruns EJ: The wraparound process: Individualized, community-based care for children and adolescents with intensive needs, in Community Mental Health: Challenges for the 21st Century. Edited by Rosenberg J, Rosenberg S. New York, Routledge, 2006, pp 47–57

Washington State Institute for Public Policy (WSIPP): Inventory of Evidence-Based, Research-Based, and Promising Practices For Prevention and Intervention Services for Children and Juveniles in Child Welfare, Juvenile Justice, and Mental Health Systems, January 2014. Available at: http://www.wsipp.wa.gov/ReportFile/1552/Wsipp_Updated-Inventory-of-Evidence-based-Research-based-and-Promising-Practices-for-Prevention-and-Intervention-Services-for-Children-

and-Juveniles-in-the-Child-Welfare-Juvenile-Justice-and-Mental-Health-Systems_Inventory.pdf. Accessed July 19, 2014.

Woolston JL, Adnopoz J, Berkowitz SJ: IICAPS: A Home-Based Psychiatric Treatment for Children and Adolescents. New Haven, CT, Yale University Press, 2007

Yoe JT, Santarcangelo S, Atkins M, et al: Wraparound care in Vermont: program development, implementation, and evaluation of a statewide system of individualized services. J Child Fam Stud 5(1):23–37, 1996

CHAPTER 47

Milieu Treatment

Inpatient, Partial Hospitalization, and Residential Programs

Theodore A. Petti, M.D., M.P.H.

Inpatient hospital units (IUs), partial hospital (PH) or day treatment (DT) programs, and residential treatment centers (RTCs; sometimes grouped as *restrictive* or *intensive* services) play a critical role for children and adolescents (youth) with severe and/or persistent mental illness requiring extensive or intensive health and psychiatric services. Federal reports sometimes combine residential and inpatient statistics, while PH/DT programs are now pooled with outpatient treatments. A common set of values and expectations allows these programs to be considered together. A therapeutic milieu is central to each. In this chapter I describe common features across these milieu treatments (MTs) and consider each modality by defining the intervention and describing its structure, clinical role, and related issues.

Historical Context

Therapeutic milieus began as orphanages and boarding schools for youngsters with mental disabilities and psychiatric illness and evolved into child care institutions and group foster homes to assist emotionally disturbed and socially deviant children. Behavior problems were the predominant focus of IUs that began in the early 1920s. Ascendancy of a managed mental health care model and other forces led to their decreased use in the 1990s. Closing of mostly for-profit programs and publicly funded state and county units has resulted (Parmelee and Nierman 2006). Managed care has not lessened problems of access to and appropriate use of IU care across geographical areas but has resulted in decreased use and shortened length of stay (LOS; Case et al. 2007; Cuellar et al. 2001). PH/DT programs began after 1963 as a movement against the perceived antitherapeutic effects of institutional care and for cost-effective treatments and greater family and community roles. Blader and Foley (2007) provide a more detailed historical perspective of MTs.

Common Issues

The current political, fiscal, and clinical environments require a sufficiently flexible organizational structure to allow accommodation and adaptation to rapid regulatory and funding changes while being stable enough to provide predictability for all involved staff.

Parent or Sponsoring Body, Structure, and Administrative Issues

Programs offering MTs have various types of governing bodies and range from simple to multiple hierarchical layers. Administrative links to the governing body serve to define how a program functions. The administrative structure must deal with regulatory and certifying body authorities and demands by funders of care (Whitted 2004). With the impact of managed care, funders appear to exert a disproportionate influence (Cuellar et al. 2001). Expectations of accountability should facilitate use of evidence-based practice (EBP).

For many programs, full census determines solvency and viability; fluctuations represent threats to consistent staffing levels and sustaining morale. Professional staff members must devote time to justifying initial admission, continued stay, and level of treatment, thus raising expenses and lowering staff availability for direct clinical work. Requirements by regulatory and certifying bodies to evaluate outcome are particularly difficult for most milieu programs, in part because of the heterogeneous nature of populations served, diversity of programs, and the difficulties in developing operational definitions and measurement of delivered services. Epstein (2004) systematically reviewed studies measuring treatment effects. Basic methods suggested for studying MT service outcomes are change analysis, decision analysis, and outcome prediction (Lyons et al. 2001). Most studies employ change analysis (i.e., the differences between measures before and after service delivery) with standardized measures.

Outcome reviews are available for each type of program, but few generalizations can be made beyond concluding that some youth can benefit from such intensive treatments. Unfortunately, return to a dysfunctional or abusive family with high expressed emotion or failure to comply with agreed-on aftercare recommendations can easily eradicate any benefits from even a highly effective MT. In addition, long-term positive benefit is unlikely when aftercare services are limited, unavailable, or inaccessible or not culturally sensitive to family needs. Conclusive evidence demonstrating MT's effectiveness is lacking (Tse 2006; Whittaker 2004). To summarize multiple outcome studies, most RTC- and IU-treated children and adolescents improve, but studies are limited by admitting the most disturbed youth, with practical and ethical questions making controlled studies difficult to design and implement (Epstein 2004).

Table 47–1 lists factors essential for providing effective MT care. Community resources have expanded significantly, but in most geographical areas there are inadequate MT or alternative

TABLE 47–1. Essential milieu factors for patient assessment, safety monitoring and assurance, and transition to community

Patient assessment
Estimation of ability to form therapeutic alliance
Determination of critical factors existing prior to admission
Child and family functioning
Consistency of discipline within family
Family-perceived stress
Contact with delinquent peers (for those with disruptive disorders)
Extent of drug and/or alcohol use or abuse
Consideration of multiple domains in the life of the mentally ill child and the family
Safety monitoring and assurance
Protection of vulnerable populations of youth (e.g., autism spectrum, developmentally delayed, prior abuse or neglect)
Monitoring extent of the following:
Contact with delinquent peers
Potential harm to self or others
Adherence of patient and family to program rules and recommendations
Appropriate assessment of biopsychosocial risk factors (i.e., predisposing, precipitating, perpetuating, preventive factors)
Transition to community
Interdisciplinary functioning, coordination, and communication
Availability of aftercare by other services in the continuum of care
Transitional psychosocial services for step-down processes within the mental health system
Physicians and related professionals for medication management

services to address the needs of youth (Lieberman 2004). With increasing emphasis on crisis stabilization and reliance on medication and shorter LOS, concern about recycling youth among the types of acute and intermediate MT care settings and related disruption of care has been voiced (Case et al. 2007).

Clinical Issues

Quality assurance and continuing quality improvement efforts represent links between administrative and clinical issues. Maintaining well-trained and motivated staff, meeting fiscal goals, and nurturing constructive relationships with referral sources are common objectives. Surprisingly, admission criteria (illness severity, consideration of dangerousness and safety, need for separation from the family) of MT program types appear to differentiate poorly among residential programs, IU, and PH/DT programs. Criteria for MT care have been widely described and are compared in Table 47–2.

Formal education occurs in most programs. Exceptions are PH/DT programs provided after school or on weekends that focus on social skills and relationships or eating disorder symptoms. Education components vary from structured, certified school programs offering academic credit to certified teachers working with school books and assignments that families bring for the few hours a day the child spends in the school setting. Many

TABLE 47–2. Comparative criteria for milieu treatment programs

Criteria	Acute inpatient	Partial hospital	Day treatment	Residential treatment center
Danger to self and/or others				
High risk	2	2	1	0
Low risk	0	2	2	2
Moderate to severe psychopathology	2	2	2	1
Need for constant observation	2	0	0	0
Need for 24-hour care	2	0	0	1
Unstable home environment	2	1	1	2
Unstable home environment but manageable most of the time and patient not dangerous to self and/or others	0	2	2	1
Dangerous when nonadherent to treatment	2	2	1	2
Comprehensive evaluation required	1	1	1	1

Note. 2=generally applicable; 1=sometimes applicable; 0=not applicable.

children and adolescents admitted for MT are certified as requiring special education (Carman et al. 2004). Legal requirements for an individualized education program must be heeded when the youngster is expected to be in a program for an extended duration and requires special services. Youth in MT may have language delays, other developmental disabilities, and psychiatric disorders that impair learning and academic achievement (Pogge et al. 2014). These issues represent significant challenges to assessment and treatment during acute psychiatric admissions and are more likely to be addressed during intermediate to long-term IU, PH/DT, and RTC stays. Funding sources for such services vary. Programs depend increasingly on local public school systems to fund and/or provide school personnel to meet educational requirements. Flexibility and collaboration are necessary (Carman et al. 2004; Kiser et al. 2006). Coordinating the program-based school with other milieu components remains a challenge. Educating the child and family about the illness and its treatment is a basic component of care. Social skills and self-control training are present in virtually all programs, though labels and emphasis may differ. Health care concerns may differ among programs, with some devoted to comorbid medical and mental health problems (or poor adherence), psychosomatic illness, or eating disorders. Pediatrician or nurse practitioner involvement ranges from ongoing for all patients to as-needed consultations. Nursing staff to varying extents play a critical role in health and mental health care for youth receiving MT. The participation of milieu, recreation, physical, occupational, art, and music therapists varies depending on the facility and populations served.

Managing highly aggressive, violent, destructive youth is an expectation for all MT staff and relates directly to concerns about staff morale, regulations, and fiscal and regulatory issues. Aggressive youth influence everyone's perception of providing, working in, or residing in a safe environment. An extensive literature on seclusion and restraint regarding how to address violent and agitated behavior provides multiple perspectives on these interventions, from therapeutic to dangerous (Day 2007; Masters 2007). Regulatory agencies and advocacy groups are extensively involved in this critical area because of highly publicized adverse effects associated with mechanical and other forms of restraint (Nunno et al. 2007). Stricter federal policy is the result (Centers for Medicare and Medicaid Services 2006). Multiple approaches have reduced the incidence of aggression and agitation that often precede seclusion and/or restraint, lowered the incidence of seclusion, and eliminated mechanical restraint in some settings, often through organizational and cultural change (Greene et al. 2006; Nunno et al. 2007; Petti et al. 2005).

Perceptions vary about interventions that are widely accepted and employed across MT programs, such as seclusion and restraint, time-out, level systems, and as-needed (prn) medications (Mohr et al. 2009). Contrary to earlier studies advocating time-out, hospitalized children often prefer medication to time-outs or seclusion (Petti et al. 2003). The terms *chemical restraint* and *prn sedation* describing psychotropic use targeted for reduction in MT settings (Dean et al. 2006) deserve further thoughtful consideration before they are accepted as valid. Various types of aggression, especially those involving intellectual disability and developmental delay, are highly correlated with oppositional defiant or noncompliant behavior, which are frequent reasons for MT admission and are germane to the functioning of the milieu. In one study, although aggression was significantly associated with use of seclusion and restraint, noncompliant behavior was significantly associated with number of psychiatric medications at discharge and hospital LOS (Sukhodolsky et al. 2005). A challenge is to adapt the extensive options for treating disruptive and defiant behavior and to modify the milieu, especially for youth with autism spectrum disorder and other developmental and intellectual disabilities, in order to reduce aggression and improve outcome. Aggression and violence will continue to demand considerable attention until more effective interventions are found to lessen or eliminate agitation in impulsive youngsters with severe mental illness. To decrease agitation and aggression in MT settings, psychotropic medications within a framework of 14 recommendations have been suggested (Pappadopulos et al. 2003) and updated (Rosato et al. 2012).

Sexual perpetrators are a subset of aggressive youngsters referred for intensive, restrictive care. Of equal concern are referrals of youngsters who, having been sexually or physically abused, represent potential victims of peers or, very rarely, of deviant staff (Milne and Collin-Vézina 2014).

Risk of elopement (escape from the program space) has lessened as a safety concern following increased program security. Dynamics related to elopement from treatment programs are similar to those found in youth who exhibit self-injurious behavior (e.g., self-cutting, head banging, and ingesting foreign objects) (Petti et al. 2005). Effective communication among staff and between staff and patients is the best way to prevent elopement and other risky behaviors. Suicidal youth present an additional critical safety risk factor for MTs (Ash and Nurcombe 2007). Safety factors for consideration when admitting or discharging youngsters who are potentially dangerous to self and others are described in Table 47–3. Measures of depression severity remain significant predictors of suicidality (Sanislow et al. 2003).

Dialectical behavior therapy (DBT) is increasingly being employed in MT programs and is especially useful for suicidal and self-injurious youth by targeting impulsive aggression, noncompliance, and engagement in therapy. DBT has been demonstrated to be feasible in outpatient and acute and intermediate hospital settings (Katz et al. 2004; Petti et al. 2005) and is a valuable addition to the therapeutic program. It can be conducted in 2 weeks with follow-up in community settings. A DBT focus is expected to work best on a unit with staff trained in its principles and capable of assisting the youth in using and developing the ability to generalize the skills to other settings (Katz et al. 2004).

Repeated seclusion and restraint, sexualized behavior, and issues concerning safety are all threats to a program's integrity as related to licensure and certification. MT programs for mentally ill or developmentally delayed children and teens are under the observation of multiple entities. These range from the Center for Medicare and Medicaid Services to The Joint Commission (formerly known as the Joint Commission on the Accreditation of Healthcare Organizations), various state agencies, and related oversight bodies (Teich and Ireys 2007). Safety and outcome evaluation issues are raised by these regulatory and certifying bodies with demands for a structure and process to assure safety and demonstrate effectiveness of the MT program. National accrediting bodies for nonpsychiatric programs providing

TABLE 47–3. Risk factors for suicidal behavior warranting admission and conditions for safe discharge

Admission risk factors
Clearly abnormal mental state of a suicide attempter or someone with suicidal ideation
Stated persistent wish to die
Adequate supervision and support not possible outside therapeutic milieu
Unresolved biopsychosocial risk factors unlikely to change sufficiently to allow safe return home
Discharge safety factors
Crisis issue resolved to acceptable extent
Potential for suicide deemed minimal
Secured home environment
No access to firearms
Medication locked safely
Family-related issues addressed
Parental psychiatric illness
Dysfunctional family patterns
Aftercare in place
Appropriate education of family and patient
Realistic transition plan agreed on by all concerned
Psychosocial interventions
Medication monitoring

MTs are also developing standards (Friedman et al. 2006).

Required master treatment plans are expected to reflect the multidisciplinary and interdisciplinary nature of staff and programming and vary depending on program type and populations served. Critical elements include targeted psychiatric symptoms, medical issues, education and psychoeducation, and disposition. Accrediting, certifying, and other bodies have differing expectations and criteria for an acceptable plan; programs frequently struggle to develop plans that balance such competing interests.

The Milieu

Therapeutic milieus are generally characterized by their predominant environment, social organization, or culture, with a multidisciplinary professional and paraprofessional team devoted to diagnosis and treatment of children with major mental illness (Bellonci 2010). The milieu and its operation are based on program philosophy, leadership, history, culture, staff, and average LOS. The physical environment may determine the manner in which the milieu functions, as safety and aesthetic issues can affect morale and outcomes. Recognized as interventions able to lead to change by their ability to contain the child in a structured environment, MTs provide opportunities to comprehensively assess complex child- and family-related issues (Bellonci 2010; Tse 2006).

The Child or Adolescent Requiring Milieu Treatment

Youngsters admitted to MT programs differ from other children with emotional illness by the degree of stress they place on the home, school, and community. They have not benefited from, or had access to, individualized community services (Bellonci 2010; Friedman et al. 2006). More than 20% of IU patients are diagnosed with comorbid medical conditions (Case et al. 2007), and most have complex comorbid psychiatric disorders and difficult family dynamics. The out-of-home facilities where they are admitted range from small group homes for disruptive youth to comprehensive RTCs and highly sophisticated acute university hospital units.

The Family

The opportunity for contact between hospitalized youngsters or those in residential care and their family or others is inconsistent across programs. In the absence of research, The Joint Commission, the Child Welfare League, and other interested bodies have clearly defined expectations about residents' rights to have visits and/or contact with parents or family members. Restrictions need to be reasonable, detailed in the treatment plan, explained to the child and family, and reviewed at least monthly. Parents are expected to be integral to treatment planning and ongoing care for all MT programs, although this is not universal. Often parent management training or other EBPs are absent (Furniss et al. 2013; Tse 2006).

Role in a System of Care

The MTs play a critical role in the array of services necessary to provide effective care. The provision of service with long-term involvement by some MT programs can differentiate successful from unsuccessful responses to treatment (Whittaker 2004). Recommendations for the most effective MT are detailed in Table 47–4 (Leichtman et al. 2001; Lyons and Schaefer 2000; Whittaker 2004).

Family involvement, vitally needed in treatment plan development and implementation, is a problem for those without adequate transportation and child care for other children, poor and rural families, and those living a distance from the facility. Audio and video teleconferencing have been used in some programs. MT programs depend on other aftercare services to provide appropriate transition services to the general community (e.g., even in a program with significant resources allotted to discharge planning, one-third of adolescents consecutively discharged from a comprehensive RTC became homeless within 5 years, more than one-sixth in the first year) (Embry et al. 2000).

Residential Treatment Centers

RTCs provide 24-hour mental health and related care for youth who are often indistinguishable from those served in hospitals or PH/DT programs and who often transition among these settings. The federal government defines RTCs as "psychiatric organizations (exclusive of psychiatric hospitals) that provide residential services primarily to persons under age 18 who have been diagnosed as exhibiting moderate or severe emotional illness or psychiatric disorders" (Stroup et al. 1988, p. 2). Teich and Ireys (2007) found inconsistent definitions among states, noting that diverse state agencies share responsibility for handling complaints, licensing, and oversight. They categorized 71 facility types from the 3,628 facilities described by informants from 38 reporting states. Burgeoning private, largely unlicensed or unaccredited residential programs

TABLE 47–4. Recommendations for assuring effective milieu treatment

Optimize safety for patients, peers, and staff
Encourage family and patient collaboration in treatment plan development
Encourage ongoing family involvement
Ensure that transportation is available
Ensure adequate funding
Ensure that the treatment plan addresses factors identified in case formulation
Provide financial support for duration of required treatment
Discharge when lesser level of care will suffice and is appropriate

have generated critical media attention concerning lack of community contact, serious abuses, and inadequate mental health treatment (Teich and Ireys 2007). Accurate statistics do not exist for such programs and the youth being served—benefited or harmed—at these facilities (Friedman et al. 2006).

Presenting problems often include various combinations of family conflict or dysfunction, aggression, inability to succeed in school, depression, anxiety disorders, and delinquent behavior (Pottick et al. 2004). In some states, only youth with psychosis are eligible for publicly funded residential treatment. Residential treatment accounts for only 8% of total youth mental health services in the United States but almost 25% of child mental health expense (Teich and Ireys 2007). This does not include the cost of the private, largely unregulated programs described as programs, camps, or schools for behavior disordered youth (Friedman et al. 2006).

The increased number of facilities providing residential care and number of mentally ill children using RTCs are considered secondary to decreased LOS in acute IUs and fewer long-term state and other psychiatric hospital beds (Manderscheid et al. 2004). Data from 16 randomly selected New York State RTCs show a significant increase in children formerly served by the juvenile justice and mental health systems (Dale et al. 2007). To meet the changing needs, some RTCs have become integral components within systems of care and partner with managed care organizations (MCOs) to develop innovative strategies linking all the positive features of a system of care with family involvement and sophisticated technology. They have changed and modified their programs to provide increasingly shorter LOS and greater flexibility in keeping parents actively involved (Petti 2006).

Residential Care

Some RTCs provide more comprehensive services than hospital units, while others resemble group homes or halfway houses. These 24-hour facilities are not considered hospitals because nursing and medical care is not available around the clock. Some operate for only 5 days a week or have prolonged closures during which services are not provided. Some operate with two or three shifts of staff, while others have live-in house parents or counselors.

RTCs may be differentiated from psychiatric IUs by their group living and individual treatment focus. RTC youth view themselves as being a "resident" of the facility as contrasted to a hospitalized sick person. Less regression has been expected in residential compared with hospital treatment where total care, safety, and meeting dependency needs are paramount. RTCs expect "healthy" behavior as contrasted to the "sick" behavior allowed and expected during a hospital stay by parents, the court, advocates, community workers, and staff. These differences may diminish with the shortened LOS allowed for inpatient programs but may hold for intermediate and longer-term IUs. RTCs offer services for the resident to become self-sufficient. Located in communities, traditional RTCs are better able to facilitate the transition back to the residents' home communities and local schools since they frequently are integrated with community public schools and their residents often spend time in the community schools.

Per diem RTC costs, except for the most specialized units, are significantly less than comparable IU costs but more than most community programs. Some private residential facilities require families to make nonrefundable payments in advance (Friedman et al. 2006). Because some of these residential programs have been accused of maltreatment and even death of their charges, greater scrutiny has been given to them (Friedman et al. 2006). In the late 1990s, youth were often placed in RTCs for nonpsychiatric reasons (Lyons et al. 1998). More than one-third of residents in randomly selected Illinois RTCs had risk profiles suggesting that those youth might be better served in community placements since they represented no danger to themselves or others and had limited overall dysfunction and psychopathology. Older teens were the most likely to inappropriately remain. However, experts do not agree that danger to self or others is the only criterion for RTC placement. Some youngsters need long-term placement for a variety of reasons, including the need and opportunity for stability in their lives. This needy subpopulation of youth may be defined by absence of a supportive discharge environment and the child or adolescent's inability to benefit from prior community-based intensive treatment (Leichtman et al. 2001). After changes in the Illinois child welfare system (Parmelee and Nierman 2006), youth remaining in residential care were those who had not responded to the range of community-based services and had no viable placement alternatives because of their higher levels of required mental health interventions (Lyons and McCulloch 2006). Contrary to assertions that mental health services are disproportionately provided to white mentally ill juveniles compared with those of minority races (who are purported to be relegated to juvenile justice facilities), data indicate that admission rates for African Americans to mental health RTCs exceeded those for whites overall and for both males and females (Milazzo-Sayre et al. 2000). The racial balance among RTC residents in the organized mental health sector are similar to those of youth in child welfare (Pottick et al. 2004).

RTCs have often been classified by their functional orientation (e.g., therapeutic communities, token economies, chemical dependency programs, psychoeducational services, community-based residential group care). Some are behaviorally oriented; others are psychodynamic/psychoanalytic or cognitive-behaviorally based. A limited number serve youth with eating disorders, co-occurring medical illness, or chemical dependency, while others serve dually diagnosed mental illness and intellectual disability or related developmental issues. Some are built around the facility's education program with schools on site, some have their residents attend school in the community, and others have both. Many offer both outpatient and PH/DT programs (Milazzo-Sayre et al. 2000). Practical aspects of working or consulting in residential programs have been detailed (Cohen 2006; Fujita and Arnold 2006).

Outcome and Quality Assessment

Outcome studies of RTCs continue to suggest factors associated with poor outcomes including presence of psychosis, organic etiology for the psychiatric disorder, below-average level of intelligence, antisocial and bizarre behavior, dysfunctional family, insufficient duration of residential treatment to allow for consolidation of gains, and adequate aftercare services (Kutash and Rivera 1995). Defining an adequate residential care LOS is difficult and may relate to the overall difficulty in evaluating the cost and benefits of RTC care, including the absence of data on the extent to which children are helped or harmed and the number actually served (Friedman et al. 2006).

Although controlled and randomized studies are problematic to implement, there are some naturalistic comparative evaluations (Curry 2004; Epstein 2004). Curry (2004) suggested employing research designs that compare between-treatment, within-program, and across-program designs. Noting that residential treatment is not an isolated event in the life and treatment of a youth, he considers comparative outcome studies, emphasizes the need to control for the postdischarge environment, and suggests that EBP methods can be and have been adapted for RTCs, with special adaptations made for facility factors and for patients with histories of abuse or neglect or substance abuse.

Lyons and Schaefer (2000) found that the most dangerous youth were the most severely ill, and they benefited most from residential care. Lyons and McCulloch (2006) described a model for using outcomes research as an effective means to monitor residential treatment by identifying RTC site strengths, weaknesses, treatment progress trajectories, and trends. Use of the Child Functional Assessment Rating Scale, a major tool for a Residential Treatment Outcomes System evaluation, allows system-wide assessment with generated data that administrators and providers can report via a Web-based system efficiently and quickly. It allows comparison within and between providers and monitoring of individual patient progress or deterioration compared with a reference group.

Subramaniam et al. (2007), in a prospective study of adolescents following stays in an RTC for substance abuse treatment, reported that a Beck Depression Inventory baseline score of ≥11 predicted significantly poorer substance use outcome as measured by the mean percentage of days of nonnicotine substance use after discharge in 90-day blocks for 1 year. The authors' conclusions suggested the need to treat the comorbid depression for improved outcomes. More recently, youth at 12-month follow-up after discharge from an "integrated residential continuum of care" exiting at the lowest level of restrictiveness compared with those at higher levels of restrictiveness had more positive outcomes (i.e., they were most likely to be living at home or in a homelike setting and experiencing fewer postdeparture out-of-home placements) but no differences in substance use, arrests, school attendance, or graduation rate (Ringle et al. 2012).

Inpatient Hospitalization

Psychiatric IU care is the most restrictive and expensive MT. Usually reserved for the severely ill who require round-the-clock medical and nursing supervision, IUs may exist within psychiatric, pediatric, general, or freestanding child and adolescent psychiatric hospitals and may be obligated to serve within a system of care, be selective in caring for special populations, or be available to all within a certain age range or residential area. In 1997, 286,176 U.S. youth younger than age 18 were admitted for organized mental health IU care. More than two-thirds were ages 13–17, and 30% were ages 6–12 years (Pottick et al. 2004). Age ratios in IU community hospital discharges between 1999 and 2000 (N=29,590) were similar to the 1997 figures, as were primary payer sources: 43%–37% public insurer, 48%–55% private insurance, and 9% other. More white (78%–67%) and fewer black (14%–16%) and Hispanic (4%–14%) youth were seen in community hospitals (Case et al. 2007; Pottick et al. 2004). The number of discharges and population-based discharge rates with a mental health diagnosis from community hospitals between 1990 and 2000 for children 17 years and younger remained relatively stable. By 2007, for youth with a primary psychiatric diagnosis, the number of discharges from and hospital days in "short-stay facilities" markedly increased; public funding bore an increased share of the cost (Blader 2011).

Mean charges per stay and total LOS decreased by half, and median LOS decreased 63% from 12.2 to 4.5 days (Case et al. 2007). Nonclinical variables may best predict LOS for youth, contributing between 22% and 30% to the variance. Leon et al. (2006) reported that the most consistent, largest LOS predictor was the hospital itself. Clinical predictors accounted for only 7% of variance, with suicide risk predicting lower LOS; longer LOS was predicted by danger to others and consistency of symptoms across multiple contexts. Snowden et al. (2007) reported that although factors influencing IU admission decisions in a large foster care population were due to illness level related to safety and were clinically appropriate, multiple context issues (e.g., family problems) also played a significant role.

Inpatient Care

Acute IU care, the most common form of hospital-based care, now comprises several functions as listed in Table 47–5. Intermediate- and long-term IUs are becoming uncommon. Comprehensive assessment using resources of larger pediatric, psychiatric, or general hospitals is ideal. Intermediate-term facilities offer patients and families opportunities for more extensive assessment and consolidation of gains needed for successful transition to less restrictive settings. Requirement for "medical clearance" prior to IU admission has been questioned (Donofrio et al. 2014).

Conduct disturbance, broadly defined, most frequently precipitates preadolescent admission (Blader 2006). Table 47–6 lists frequency of presenting problems to acute IUs. Coded severity of psychiatric illness has continued to increase. Contemporary issues include potential undertreatment of minority youth, "diagnostic upcoding" (i.e., coding more serious psychiatric disorders or self-harm to justify admission or greater reimbursement), discrepancies in admissions between publicly and pri-

TABLE 47–5. Frequency of presenting problems to acute specialty mental health inpatient programs

Problem	Frequency
Depressed or anxious mood (including self-harm)	65%
Suicidality	55%
Aggression	49%
Family problems	47%
Alcohol or drug use	26%
Delinquent behavior	25%

Source. Pottick et al. 2004.

TABLE 47–6. Acute inpatient psychiatric unit functions

Assessment
Minimizing potential for harm
Separation from family and community
Monitoring behavior
Case formulation and diagnosis
Treatment plan development and brief implementation
Stabilization of symptoms and crisis
Disposition planning
Transition to less restrictive setting

vately insured youth, the highly significant increase in disposition to home rather than out-of-home placement, and significant decreases in both referral to another facility (12%–7%) and discharges against medical advice (5%–2%) (Case et al. 2007).

Providing therapy in acute IUs beyond resolving the precipitating crisis is challenging. Emphasis on therapeutic intervention is expected in longer-term facilities, although youth so hospitalized are seldom candidates for traditional therapies. Altering negative cognitions and training in social skills through cognitive, behavioral, and psychodynamic approaches within the milieu are standard in most treatment plans. DBT was equally effective in significantly reducing suicidal ideation, depressive symptoms, and parasuicidal behavior at 1-year follow-up when administered to suicidal adolescents in 10 daily sessions on one acute hospital unit compared with treatment as usual (psychodynamically oriented crisis assessment and treatment) on a matched unit. For both groups, mean LOS was 18 days, as-needed medications were employed, and symptom improvement was evident at discharge. The DBT group had significantly fewer behavioral incidents during hospitalization (Katz et al. 2004). Thus, positive therapeutic interactions employing traditional as well as innovative means can occur with lasting benefit, given sufficient time. Mentalizing approaches are also being added (Sharp et al. 2009).

Efforts devoted to family work depend on family availability, motivation for positive change, and complex family factors (Blader 2006). Aftercare is often difficult to implement. Concern about "institutionalizing" the patients in intermediate or longer-term care is real, particularly when patients feel more comfortable in the protective and nurturing environment than in the community environment. Aggression and violence are common foci of attention. Current quandaries for acute IU psychiatrists involve prescribing psychotropics and readmissions when aftercare is unavailable, as shown in the following case example.

Case Example

Thirteen-year-old Jennie's hospitalization following a suicide attempt was prolonged. On the basis of a case formulation of her mild to moderate depression, her treatment team concluded that intensive family work and social skills training were needed to prevent recurrence of her hopelessness; antidepressant medication demanded by the MCO to justify continued stay beyond 3 days for crisis stabilization was deemed clinically unwarranted. Sertraline was prescribed in part to secure additional approved days. Hospital discharge was delayed because a physician to monitor medication and an experienced therapist within reasonable distance from her home could not be located.

The aftercare problem—given the shortage of child and adolescent psychiatrists, the reluctance of many primary care physicians to prescribe psychotropic medications in light of U.S. Food and Drug Administration warnings, and the pressure by MCOs to prescribe medication and discharge once danger or other immediate precipitants for hospital justification are lessened—makes EBP difficult to implement and the likelihood for readmission higher than previously experienced. Attention to parental attitudes toward aftercare treatment and specific aspects of psychopathology may improve aftercare adherence to discharge recommendations (Burns et al. 2008).

Outcome and Quality Assessment

Readmissions to acute IUs are a potential measure of outcome. Defining outcomes and factors specific to IU care has been difficult. Blader (2004) followed 109 school-age children for 1 year after IU discharge. Predictors for readmission, 81% occurring within 90 days, included more severe conduct problems, disengaged parent-child relations, and harsh parental discipline. He concluded that readmissions might best be prevented by attention to the immediate postdischarge period, with efforts directed to family factors and severe conduct symptoms. The findings are consistent with those reported by Kolko (1992) for symptom abatement in formerly hospitalized elementary school– and middle school–age children at 2, 4, and 6 months after discharge. He suggested attending to factors improved in the higher-functioning youngsters: internalizing and externalizing symptom decreases, parental disciplinary effectiveness, adaptive involvement in recreation and leisure activities, positive peer interaction, and improved satisfaction with relationships. Interventions most likely to improve functioning were parent management training; exposure to group activities fostering prosocial behavior; cognitive-behavioral skills training; aftercare planning; and clarifying parent versus child variables, diagnoses, and other factors that contribute to outcome. Masters (2005) reports using cognitive-behavioral therapy components that can be effectively implemented within 5 hospital days.

Studies of multisystemic therapy (MST) suggest that intermediate- or long-term IU care can be dramatically decreased. However, for adolescents in psychiatric crisis (average age of 13 years, 64% African American, 65% male), acute hospitalization was subsequently required in 44% of MST-assigned cases (Henggeler et al. 1999), thus supporting the role of IUs in a total system of care. A similarly designed study of youth presenting for psychiatric hospitalization for dangerous behavior toward self or others found both standard IU care and MST effective, with MST superior to IU care in reducing suicide attempts but no difference in related symptoms (Huey et al. 2004).

Partial Hospitalization and Day Treatment

Multiple variations of PH or DT have been described. PH and DT are defined as less than 24-hour hospital-level daily care targeted to diagnosing and treating psychiatric disorders for which preventing relapse or hospitalization and improvement in the condition could be expected (Daily and Reddick 1993). The American Association for Partial Hospitalization has defined partial hospitalization as clinical services offering active ambulatory treatment within a stable therapeutic milieu that is time limited, therapeutically intensive, coordinated, and structured. Broadly defined, partial hospitalization refers to less than 24-hour care provided in a hospital setting, while DT is care provided as school based for at least 5 hours a day and involves integrated education, counseling, and family services.

PH/DT programs have been underutilized for children and teens with severe psychiatric disorders, often because of lack of insurance coverage, residence in rural areas, or poor access to programs not located in schools. Additional problems include the absence of admission criteria and clear definitions of outcome and reluctance to maintain seriously ill youngsters in the community. It is difficult to engage many parents in regular family therapy. With the emergence of MCOs and PH and DT programs, the expected growth and prominence in the pediatric mental health service system failed to materialize.

Partial Hospital and Day Treatment Care

Many PH and DT programs offer the intensive MT of an IU or RTC setting while maintaining the youngster in home and community. DT programs are the most common, including evening and after-school programs. They may be freestanding or within a hospital clinic or IU, a school, or an RTC. Most are highly structured, attend to their patients' educational needs, and provide multimodal treatments. They attempt to avoid the regression frequently found when psychiatrically ill children and adolescents enter other MTs. Patients are expected to have sufficient self-control to avert dangerous behavior and live safely in the community. However, quick access to the IU or RTC if needed is facilitated when the PH/DT unit is integrated with or a component of a more restrictive program. Care more intensive than multiple outpatient visits per week (as in an intensive outpatient program) is provided in PH on a variable but short-term crisis focus as an IU alternative. PH often serves as a step-down from an IU or RTC setting. Therapeutic school DTs often are of longer duration (e.g., one or more school years) and are funded by school systems.

Specialized MTs employing the PH model of care are available in some locales for patients with substance abuse and chemical dependency or eating disorders, victims of abuse, children under age 5 years (Furniss et al. 2013), and those with medical disorders and comorbid psychiatric difficulties. Tse (2006) suggests that DT programs may be the only place where disruptive children and their families find acceptance. Disruptive, attention-deficit/hyperactivity, and mood disorders are common diagnoses in referred children. Parents or caretakers must be able to regularly participate in family counseling, training, and therapy and adequately provide support of and control over their children during evenings and weekends. Reliable transportation must be available. PH restrictive practice (i.e., seclusion and restraint) depends on the hospital configuration; DT restrictive practice is generally limited to those methods acceptable and available in most school or home environments. Personal ("therapeutic") holding of young children and quiet rooms are used in some DT programs; chemical and manual restraints are not. Medication use on an as-needed basis is available in some settings, particularly PHs.

Understanding the interplay among family, environment, and the child is central to successful PH/DT program operation. Programs strive to provide the MT structure of IUs and RTCs while maintaining active, community, and family functional links. The academic domain is secondary to the social-emotional domain in many PH/DT programs, even when they are in educational settings; the school experience serves as a core for therapeutic interactions. Physician involvement depends on PH/DT type and psychiatric functions. Those settings serving as alternatives to or step-downs from IU care require more medical input and greater psychiatrist involvement; other settings employ the psychiatrist primarily as a consultant to provide diagnostic assessment and medication monitoring. Practical aspects of work in and consulting to PH and DT programs are detailed by Kiser et al. (2006).

Outcome and Quality Assessment

Studies of PH/DT programs suffer from similar problems to those faced by the other MTs. Studies measuring successful reintegration into regular school settings report effectiveness in 65%–70% of DT cases successfully discharged (Kutash and Rivera 1995). A comparison of PH programs to each other and to other forms of MT results in fair evidence for efficacy and effectiveness. Outcome studies suggest the following: a portion of children can benefit from this service or be reintegrated into school settings, individual and family functioning improves, gains are not generalized to the school setting, and families play critical roles posttreatment as measured by standardized scales (Grizenko 1997; Kutash and Rivera 1995). A randomized, multicenter, open trial comparing DT following short IU care with full IU treatment in 172 adolescents with anorexia nervosa found DT was not inferior to IU with regard to the body mass index at 12-month follow-up, with superior mental status and psychosexual adjustment. Thus, DT may be safe and cost-effective when combined with a short IU stay (Herpertz-Dahlmann et al. 2014).

Although DT programs for preschoolers (sometimes called "therapeutic nurseries") have been used extensively since the 1950s, Tse (2006) commented on the paucity of related literature. Her review of research reports (published between 1974 and 2004) on psychosocial intervention outcome data with preschool children identified one published controlled study reporting no long-term benefits and five studies reporting quantitative outcomes. She offered a list of prevention and efficacy studies that should improve DT for disruptive preschoolers that apply as well to all youngsters.

Moving Forward

Clinical questions and controversies regarding MTs that should be addressed in the next 5 years include the following:

1. Overcoming barriers to developing and translating EBP into MT settings and incorporating systematic evaluation
2. Improving aftercare services so that gains made in MT settings will be maintained
3. Determining modifiable factors related to failed return to home or other placements
4. Decreasing readmission rates
5. Expanding and evaluating use of standardized measures for MTs
6. Increasing manualized, time-limited treatments for families and patients in MTs
7. Regulating non–mental health residential facilities
8. Reducing impulsive aggression and violence
9. Decreasing injuries from seclusion and restraint in mental health MTs

Summary Points

- Milieu treatments (MTs) are critical components of a mental health system of care.
- The evidence base for MT effectiveness needs continued attention.
- Mental health MTs are heavily regulated, monitored, and affected by managed care.
- Aftercare following discharge must be enhanced.
- Standardized instruments can be effectively used for assessment, monitoring, and outcome.
- Alternatives to seclusion and restraint must be developed and evaluated.

References

Ash P, Nurcombe B: Malpractice and professional liability, in Lewis's Child and Adolescent Psychiatry: A Comprehensive Textbook, 4th Edition. Edited by Andres M, Volkmar FR. Philadelphia, PA, Lippincott Williams and Wilkins, 2007, pp 1018–1032

Bellonci C: Physician leadership in residential treatment for children and adolescents. Child Adolesc Psychiatr Clin N Am 19(1):21–30, 2010 19951804

Blader JC: Symptom, family, and service predictors of children's psychiatric rehospitalization within one year of discharge. J Am Acad Child Adolesc Psychiatry 43(4):440–451, 2004 15187804

Blader JC: Which family factors predict children's externalizing behaviors following discharge from psychiatric inpatient treatment? J Child Psychol Psychiatry 47(11):1133–1142, 2006 17076752

Blader JC: Acute inpatient care for psychiatric disorders in the United States, 1996 through 2007. Arch Gen Psychiatry 68(12):1276–1283, 2011 21810629

Blader JC, Foley CA: Milieu-based treatment: Inpatient and partial hospitalization, residential treatment, in Lewis's Child and Adolescent Psychiatry: A Comprehensive Textbook, 4th Edition. Edited by Andres M, Volkmar FR. Philadelphia, PA, Lippincott Williams and Wilkins, 2007, pp 865–878

Burns CD, Cortell R, Wagner BM: Treatment compliance in adolescents after attempted suicide: a 2-year follow-up study. J Am Acad Child Adolesc Psychiatry 47(8):948–957, 2008 18596554

Carman GO, Dorta N, Kon D, et al: Special education in residential treatment. Child Adolesc Psychiatr Clin N Am 13(2):381–394, 2004 15062352

Case BG, Olfson M, Marcus SC, et al: Trends in the inpatient mental health treatment of children and adolescents in US community hospitals between 1990 and 2000. Arch Gen Psychiatry 64(1):89–96, 2007 17199058

Centers for Medicare and Medicaid Services: Medicare and Medicaid Programs; Hospital Conditions of Participation: Patients' Rights; Final Rule. Fed Regist 42 CFR Part 482, 2006, pp 71377–71428

Cohen P: Chemical dependency program, in Community Child and Adolescent Psychiatry: A Manual of Clinical Practice and Consultation. Edited by Petti TA, Salguero C. Washington, DC, American Psychiatric Publishing, 2006, pp 205–218

Cuellar AE, Libby AM, Snowden LR: How capitated mental health care affects utilization by youth in the juvenile justice and child welfare systems. Ment Health Serv Res 3(2):61–72, 2001 12109839

Curry JF: Future directions in residential treatment outcome research. Child Adolesc Psychiatr Clin N Am 13(2):429–440, 2004 15062355

Daily S, Reddick C: Adolescent day treatment: an alternative for the future. Adolesc Psychiatry 19:523–540, 1993 8296995

Dale N, Baker AJL, Anastasio E, et al: Characteristics of children in residential treatment in New York State. Child Welfare 86(1):5–27, 2007 17408008

Day DD: A review of the literature on the therapeutic effectiveness of physical restraints with children and youth, in For Our Own Safety: Examining the Safety of High-Risk Interventions for Children and Young People. Edited by Nunno MA, Day DM, Bullard LB. Washington, DC, Child Welfare League of America, 2007, pp 27–44

Dean AJ, McDermott BM, Marshall RT: PRN sedation-patterns of prescribing and administration in a child and adolescent mental health inpatient service. Eur Child Adolesc Psychiatry 15(5):277–281, 2006 16583125

Donofrio JJ, Santillanes G, McCammack BD, et al: Clinical utility of screening laboratory tests in pediatric psychiatric patients presenting to the emergency department for medical clearance. Ann Emerg Med 63(6):666–675, 2014 24219903

Embry LE, Vander Stoep AV, Evens C, et al: Risk factors for homelessness in adolescents released from psychiatric residential treatment. J Am Acad Child Adolesc Psychiatry 39(10):1293–1299, 2000 11026184

Epstein RA Jr: Inpatient and residential treatment effects for children and adolescents: a review and critique. Child Adolesc Psychiatr Clin N Am 13(2):411–428, 2004 15062354

Friedman RM, Pinto A, Behar L, et al: Unlicensed residential programs: the next challenge in protecting youth. Am J Orthopsychiatry 76(3):295–303, 2006 16981808

Fujita M, Arnold V: Community residential programs, in Community Child and Adolescent Psychiatry: A Manual of Clinical Practice and Consultation. Edited by Petti TA, Salguero C. Washington, DC, American Psychiatric Publishing, 2006, pp 219–230

Furniss T, Müller JM, Achtergarde S, et al: Implementing psychiatric day treatment for infants, toddlers, preschoolers and their families: a study from a clinical and organizational perspective. Int J Ment Health Syst 7(1):12, 2013 23601961

Greene RW, Ablon JS, Martin A: Innovations: child & adolescent psychiatry: use of collaborative problem solving to reduce seclusion and restraint in child and adolescent inpatient units. Psychiatr Serv 57:610–612, 2006 16675751

Grizenko N: Outcome of multimodal day treatment for children with severe behavior problems: a five-year follow-up. J Am Acad Child Adolesc Psychiatry 36(7):989–997, 1997 9204678

Henggeler SW, Rowland MD, Randall J, et al: Home-based multisystemic therapy as an alternative to the hospitalization of youths in psychiatric crisis: clinical outcomes. J Am Acad Child Adolesc Psychiatry 38(11):1331–1339, 1999 10560218

Herpertz-Dahlmann B, Schwarte R, Krei M, et al: Day-patient treatment after short inpatient care versus continued inpatient treatment in adolescents with anorexia nervosa (ANDI): a multicentre, randomised, open-label, non-inferiority trial. Lancet 383(9924):1222–1229, 2014 24439238

Huey SJ Jr, Henggeler SW, Rowland MD, et al: Multisystemic therapy effects on attempted suicide by youths presenting psychiatric emergencies. J Am Acad Child Adolesc Psychiatry 43(2):183–190, 2004 14726725

Katz LY, Cox BJ, Gunasekara S, et al: Feasibility of dialectical behavior therapy for suicidal adolescent inpatients. J Am Acad Child Adolesc Psychiatry 43(3):276–282, 2004 15076260

Kiser L, Heston JD, Paavola M: Day treatment center/partial hospital setting, in Community Child and Adolescent Psychiatry: A Manual of Clinical Practice and Consultation. Edited by Petti TA, Salguero C. Washington, DC, American Psychiatric Publishing, 2006, pp 189–203

Kolko DJ: Short-term follow-up of child psychiatric hospitalization: clinical description, predictors, and correlates. J Am Acad Child Adolesc Psychiatry 31(4):719–727, 1992 1644736

Kutash K, Rivera VR: Effectiveness of children's mental health services: a review of the literature. Education and Treatment of Children 18(4):443–477, 1995

Leichtman M, Leichtman ML, Barber CC, et al: Effectiveness of intensive short-term residential treatment with severely disturbed adolescents. Am J Orthopsychiatry 71(2):227–235, 2001 11347363

Leon SC, Snowden J, Bryant FB, et al: The hospital as predictor of children's and adolescents' length of stay. J Am Acad Child Adolesc Psychiatry 45(3):322–328, 2006 16540817

Lieberman RE: Future directions in residential treatment. Child Adolesc Psychiatr Clin N Am 13(2):279–294, 2004 15062346

Lyons JS, McCulloch JR: Monitoring and managing outcomes in residential treatment: practice-based evidence in search of evidence-based practice. J Am Acad Child Adolesc Psychiatry 45(2):247–251, 2006 16429096

Lyons JS, Schaefer K: Mental health and dangerousness: characteristics and outcomes of children and adolescents in residential care. J Child Fam Stud 9(1):67–73, 2000

Lyons JS, Libman-Mintzer LN, Kisiel CL, et al: Understanding the mental health needs of children and adolescents in residential treatment. Prof Psychol Res Pr 29(6):582–587, 1998

Lyons JS, Terry P, Martinovich Z, et al: Outcome trajectories for adolescents in residential treatment: a statewide evaluation. J Child Fam Stud 10(3):333–345, 2001

Manderscheid R, Atay JE, Male A, et al: Highlights of organized mental health services in 2000 and major national and state trends, in Mental Health in the United States, 2002. DHHS Publ No SMA-3938. Edited by Manderscheid RW, Henderson MJ. Rockville, MD, Center for Mental Health Services, Substance Abuse and Mental Health Services Administration, 2004, pp 243–279

Masters KJ: A CBT approach to inpatient psychiatric hospitalization. J Am Acad Child Adolesc Psychiatry 44(7):708–711, 2005 15968240

Masters KJ: Modernizing seclusion and restraint, in For Our Own Safety: Examining the Safety of High-Risk Interventions for Children and Young People. Edited by Nunno MA, Day DM, Bullard LB. Washington, DC, Child Welfare League of America, 2007, pp 45–66

Milazzo-Sayre LJ, Henderson MJ, Manderscheid RW, et al: Persons treated in specialty mental health programs, United States, 1997, in Mental Health, United States, 2000. Edited by Manderscheid RW, Henderson MJ. Rockville, MD, Center for Mental Health Services, 2000, pp 172–217

Milne L, Collin-Vézina D: Disclosure of sexual abuse among youth in residential treatment care: a multiple informant comparison. J Child Sex Abuse 23(4):398–417, 2014 24640965

Mohr WK, Martin A, Olson JN, et al: Beyond point and level systems: moving toward child-centered programming. Am J Orthopsychiatry 79(1):8–18, 2009 19290721

Nunno MA, Day DM, Bullard LB (eds): For Our Own Safety: Examining the Safety of High-Risk Interventions for Children and Young People. Washington, DC, Child Welfare League of America, 2007

Pappadopulos E, Macintyre Ii JC, Crismon ML, et al: Treatment recommendations for the use of antipsychotics for aggressive youth (TRAAY). Part II. J Am Acad Child Adolesc Psychiatry 42(2):145–161, 2003 12544174

Parmelee DX, Nierman P: Transitions from institutional to community systems of care, in Community Child and Adolescent Psychiatry: A Manual of Clinical Practice and Consultation. Edited by Petti TA, Salguero C. Washington, DC, American Psychiatric Publishing, 2006, pp 249–257

Petti TA: Future directions, in Community Child and Adolescent Psychiatry: A Manual of Clinical Practice and Consultation. Edited by Petti TA, Salguero C. Washington, DC, American Psychiatric Publishing, 2006, pp 269–275

Petti TA, Stigler KA, Gardner-Haycox J, et al: Perceptions of P.R.N. psychotropic medications by hospitalized child and adolescent recipients. J Am Acad Child Adolesc Psychiatry 42(4):434–441, 2003 12649630

Petti TA, Blitsch M, Blix S, et al: Deliberate foreign body ingestion in hospitalized youth: a case series and overview. Adolesc Psychiatry 29:249–287, 2005

Pogge DL, Stokes J, Buccolo ML, et al: Discovery of previously undetected intellectual disability by psychological assessment: a study of consecutively referred child and adolescent psychiatric inpatients. Res Devel Disabilities 35(7):1705–1710, 2014 24679700

Pottick K, Warner L, Isaacs M, et al: Children and adolescents admitted to specialty mental health care in the United States, 1986 and 1997, in Mental Health in the United States, 2002. DHHS Publ No SMA-3938. Edited by Manderscheid RW, Henderson MJ. Rockville, MD, Center for Mental Health Services, Substance Abuse and Mental Health Services Administration, 2004, pp 314–326

Ringle JL, Huefner JC, James S, et al: 12-month follow-up outcomes for youth departing and integrated residential continuum of care. Child Youth Serv Rev 34(4):675–679, 2012 24273362

Rosato NS, Correll C, Pappadopulos E, et al: Treatment of maladaptive aggression in youth: CERT guidelines II. Treatment and ongoing management. Pediatrics 129(6):e1577–e1586, 2012

Sanislow CA, Grilo CM, Fehon DC, et al: Correlates of suicide risk in juvenile detainees and adolescent inpatients. J Am Acad Child Adolesc Psychiatry 42(2):234–240, 2003 12544184

Sharp C, Williams LL, Ha C, et al: The development of a mentalization-based outcomes and research protocol for an adolescent inpatient unit. Bull Menninger Clin 73(4):311–338, 2009 20025427

Snowden JA, Leon SC, Bryant FB, et al: Evaluating psychiatric hospital admission decisions for children in foster care: an optimal classification tree analysis. J Clin Child Adolesc Psychol 36(1):8–18, 2007 17206877

Stroup A, Witkin M, Atay J, et al: Residential Treatment Centers for Emotionally Disturbed Children 1983 (Mental Health Statistical Note No 188). Rockville, MD, National Institute of Mental Health, 1988

Subramaniam GA, Stitzer MA, Clemmey P, et al: Baseline depressive symptoms predict poor substance use outcome following adolescent residential treatment. J Am Acad Child Adolesc Psychiatry 46(8):1062–1069, 2007 17667484

Sukhodolsky DG, Cardona L, Martin A: Characterizing aggressive and noncompliant behaviors in a children's psychiatric inpatient setting. Child Psychiatry Hum Dev 36(2):177–193, 2005 16228146

Teich JL, Ireys HT: A national survey of state licensing, regulating, and monitoring of residential facilities for children with mental illness. Psychiatr Serv 58(7):991–998, 2007 17602017

Tse J: Research on day treatment programs for preschoolers with disruptive behavior disorders. Psychiatr Serv 57(4):477–486, 2006 16603742

Whittaker JK: The re-invention of residential treatment: an agenda for research and practice. Child Adolesc Psychiatr Clin N Am 13(2):267–278, 2004 15062345

Whitted BR: Legal issues in residential treatment. Child Adolesc Psychiatr Clin N Am 13(2):295–307, 2004 15062347

PART VII

Consultation

CHAPTER 48

School-Based Interventions

Heather J. Walter, M.D., M.P.H.

The substantial gap between children's mental health service needs and available resources has been well documented in the United States. Although more than 10% of all children and adolescents have a psychiatric disorder associated with significant functional impairment and an estimated 25%–50% of youth engage in risky behaviors such as unprotected sexual activity, substance use, and aggression, only 20% of children and adolescents in need of mental health services receive them (President's New Freedom Commission on Mental Health 2003).

Lack of access to services poses a major barrier to meeting the mental health needs of young people. Providing mental health services in schools increasingly is considered a logical way to surmount this barrier, as schools require attendance, are highly accessible to children and their families, comprise a milieu that can be structured to generalize and maintain therapeutic outcomes, provide opportunities for prevention and early intervention, employ professionals capable of providing a spectrum of services in a setting that may be less stigmatizing than clinics or hospitals, and provide more ecologically grounded roles for clinicians. School-based mental health services have been shown to have a positive impact on a number of student, family, and school outcomes, including decreased emotional and behavioral problems, increased prosocial behavior, increased family engagement, improved school climate, and fewer special education and disciplinary referrals (Stephan et al. 2007). Accordingly, strong support for the expansion of school mental health services has been expressed in policy statements from the federal government (e.g., President's New Freedom Commission on Mental Health 2003; U.S. Department of Health and Human Services 1999; U.S. Public Health Service 2000) and from professional organizations (e.g., Taras and American Academy of Pediatrics Committee on School

Health 2004; Tolan et al. 2001; Walter et al. 2005). These statements converge in their recommendation that schools provide a broad range of preventive, early intervention, and clinical mental health services for enrolled students.

History

For more than a century, clinicians have collaborated with school personnel to improve the mental health of students. Since the 1950s, a number of psychiatrists have made seminal contributions to the interface between psychiatry and education, notably Caplan (1970), Berlin (1975), Comer (1992), and Berkovitz (2001). During this time, mental health consultation and service to schools underwent five major periods of expansion that were stimulated by broad sociocultural movements. First, the community mental health movement after World War II advanced the idea that schools were appropriate community-based sites for the delivery of mental health services. Second, the civil rights movement in the 1960s led to educational rights legislation prohibiting discrimination against and providing services to students with mental disabilities. Third, the dramatic change in social mores in the 1960s through the 1980s led to students' increased involvement in risky behaviors and pressure on schools to intervene with preventive interventions. Fourth, the growth of the school-based health clinic movement in the 1990s led to recognition of the high prevalence of mental health problems among students attending the clinics and the corresponding need for increased mental health services. Most recent is the move toward greater academic accountability in the school setting, which has led to a call for parallel accountability in the social-emotional domain of education.

Over time, schools have attempted to respond to the need for broader mental health services by gradually expanding the array of programs available on site. According to a recent national School Health Policies and Practices Study (U.S. Department of Health and Human Services and Centers for Disease Control and Prevention 2012), the prevalence of school mental health services in school districts nationwide was as follows: individual counseling (49%), case management (48%), assessment (42%), family counseling (39%), and group counseling (35%). Even higher was the prevalence of teacher training in the following topic areas: making appropriate mental health referrals (79% of districts); managing students with emotional or behavioral problems (81%); and recognizing signs and symptoms of bullying, depression and suicidality, physical or sexual abuse, and substance abuse (91%, 70%, 71%, and 61%, respectively). Yet despite what appears to be an encouraging array of services, funding constraints, competing academic priorities, limited availability of service providers, and lack of program coordination continue to perpetuate the marginalization and fragmentation of mental health and social services in the school setting (Taylor and Adelman 2000).

Models of School Consultation and Direct Service

Consultation

Case Consultation

In this model, clinicians advise school personnel about appropriate educational and/or therapeutic approaches to and/

or services for individual students with developmental, cognitive, emotional, behavioral, or social problems. The consultation may be direct or indirect. In direct consultation, the clinician assesses the student and suggests to school personnel appropriate interventions that are typically provided by professionals other than the consultant. In indirect consultation, the clinician does not assess the student but rather assesses a student issue (e.g., behavioral, social) articulated by school personnel and makes general recommendations to school personnel about resolving the problem. Because in this model the clinician typically is engaged by the school to provide consultative services to school personnel, role, boundary, and confidentiality issues must be clarified at the outset to protect all involved parties and conform to federal, state, and local regulations.

Systems Consultation

In this model, clinicians are engaged by the school to advise school personnel about the creation of a milieu that is conducive to learning. Individual students' needs typically are not addressed in this type of consultation; rather, the focus of consultation may include creating programs that foster, for example, a positive school environment, school connectedness among students and parents, teacher and staff competency and morale, and mental health among students.

Direct Service

School-Based Health Centers

In this model, mental health services are delivered in the context of a school-based health center (SBHC). Initially developed to address reproductive health needs, SBHCs increasingly have developed services to address mental health needs, which can comprise the majority of presentations (e.g., Walter et al. 1995a). Of the approximately 2,000 SBHCs located in 46 of 50 states (Lofink et al. 2013), about two-thirds are staffed by both primary care and mental health practitioners. Centers with mental health practitioners provide a broad range of mental health services including crisis intervention (78% of centers), individual evaluation/treatment (73%), case management (69%), classroom behavior support (62%), and medication management (39%), as well as programs addressing mental health promotion and risky behavior reduction. However, the evidence supporting the effectiveness of this model on mental health outcomes remains sparse. Although early pilot studies were promising (Armbruster and Lichtman 1999; Weist et al. 1996), a recent systematic review of 27 studies of school-based health centers (Mason-Jones et al. 2012) noted that there are no randomized controlled trials addressing mental health outcomes. Most of the research has been descriptive, demonstrating, for example, that girls and students with greater sociodemographic disadvantage and higher levels of mental health difficulties (particularly internalizing problems) are more likely to initiate and use services (e.g., Armbruster et al. 1997; Walter et al. 1996; Weist et al. 1999). Although ease of access was cited by Mason-Jones et al. (2012) as the most frequent reason for service use, significant barriers were endorsed, including students' perceptions of being healthy and not needing services, already having a physician, and concerns about confidentiality.

School-Linked Health Centers

In this model, schools are linked with hospitals or community clinics that are contracted to provide medical and mental health services to students at convenient locations off site from the school. In some settings, this model better suits the community's needs and preferences and can be more cost-effective and therefore sustainable because of greater fee-for-service billing capability (Jennings et al. 2000).

Expanded School Mental Health Programs

The notion of expanded school mental health (ESMH) arose in response to the report from the President's New Freedom Commission on Mental Health (2003), which recognized the importance of providing a full continuum of mental health services to children in communities and recommended that schools "improve and expand school mental health programs." According to Weist and Christodulu (2000), ESMH is a framework that creates a partnership between schools and community agencies and programs to move toward a full continuum of mental health services. The key elements of ESMH programs are 1) school-family community agency partnerships; 2) a commitment to a full continuum of mental health education, mental health promotion, assessment, problem prevention, early intervention, and treatment; and 3) services for all youth, including those in general and special education (Weist et al. 2005). The ESMH movement remains influential but small, with only 10% of the nation's schools estimated to have implemented this model (Brener et al. 2001).

Educational Rights of Students With Mental Disabilities

The foundation for all legislation pertaining to the educational rights of children with disabilities, including mental disabilities, rests in the Fourteenth Amendment to the U.S. Constitution, which prohibits discrimination through its equal protection clause. Despite this federal protection, through the first half of the twentieth century, many states either completely excluded children with disabilities from public school systems and placed them in institutions or relegated them to segregated classes in schools where they received little attention. The U.S. Supreme Court decision in *Brown v. Board of Education of Topeka* (347 U.S. 483 [1954]) rectified this inequity, asserting that education is a "right that must be made available to all on equal terms." Throughout the next four decades, the U.S. Congress took steps to end discrimination in schools against children with disabilities, guided by the principle that all such children must receive a "free and appropriate public education" in the "least restrictive environment."

Americans With Disabilities Act and Section 504 of the Rehabilitation Act

The Americans With Disabilities Act prohibits the denial of educational services to students with disabilities and prohibits discrimination against such students once enrolled. If parents suspect their child has a disability, they can request an evaluation to see what accommodations might be helpful. *Accommodations* are environmental changes designed to overcome impediments to learning posed by the disability. Accommodations can be formalized in a written 504 plan. This type of plan derives from Section 504 of the Rehabilitation Act (P.L. 93-112, 93rd Congress, H. R. 8070, September 26, 1973), which mandates inclusion without discrimination for any person who has a "physical or mental impairment that substantially limits a major life activity." Typical accommodations relevant to common psychiatric disorders are suggested at http://www2.massgeneral.org/schoolpsychiatry/classroom_interventions.asp. A behavioral intervention plan (BIP) can be written into a 504 plan for students with disruptive behavior. A BIP derives from the findings of a functional behavioral assessment, which identifies the disruptive behaviors with their precipitants, functions, and settings. The BIP specifies 1) behavioral goals based on functional alternatives to disruptive behaviors and 2) behavioral interventions designed to help the student achieve the behavioral goals. Table 48–1 presents a sample functional behavioral assessment and BIP.

Individuals With Disabilities Education Act

The Education for All Handicapped Children Act (EAHCA, P.L. 94-142 [1975]) mandated the provision of special education and related services to meet the unique needs of children with physical or mental disabilities. Although Section 504 had established the principle of educational inclusion on civil rights grounds, for the first time the EAHCA provided federal funds to support the efforts of states to develop individualized special education programs. A number of amendments have been made to the EAHCA since its passage. Whereas EAHCA had applied only to youth between 6 and 21 years old, initial amendments extended the protections to children younger than age 6 years. Subsequent amendments expanded the list of protected disabilities, specifically defined special education and related services, and increased early intervention services for young children. The most recent amendments provide for increased related services, delineate specific guidelines for school-based discipline of children with disabilities, and expand parental rights in the special education process. There can be considerable local variation in the interpretation of the federal educational rights legislation.

According to the provisions of the Individuals With Disabilities Education Act (IDEA), a child is eligible for special education services if he or she meets criteria for one or more categories of disability (Table 48–2) and if the disability substantially interferes with his or her educational progress. States have a responsibility to actively "find" children with suspected disabilities, who can be identified by their parents, by teachers or other professionals, or through school-based global screening (e.g., vision/hearing tests, group achievement tests). Checklists have been developed to help parents assess whether their child has learning difficulties (e.g., National Center for Learning Disabilities Learning Disabilities Checklist, accessible at http://childdevelopmentinfo.com/wp-content/uploads/2014/12/ldchecklist.pdf). A number of psychiatric disorders correspond to IDEA disability designations (see Table 48–2).

A child with a suspected disability may benefit from prereferral interventions that attempt to improve learning prior to a referral for formal special education evaluation. Teachers may initiate such interventions when they observe a struggling student, or parents with concerns about their child's academic progress can discuss potential interventions with their child's teacher. Many schools use the response to intervention (RTI) framework to organize their prereferral interventions. RTI is a multi-tiered approach to providing services based on progress monitoring and data analysis to students who struggle with learning at

TABLE 48–1. Functional behavioral assessment and behavioral intervention plan for disruptive behavior

Functional behavioral assessment

- Define behavior (physical aggression)
- Describe behavior (e.g., Brian pushes, hits, trips other students, usually smaller students, especially when no adults are watching)
- Describe antecedents (unstructured time in hallways, when unsupervised, when around students who provoke him)
- Describe consequences (teacher and peer attention, verbal reprimand, after-school detention, in-school suspension)
- Hypothesize function of behavior (power seeking, expression of anger, retribution)
- Related information (low grades, few friends, disrupted family life)

Behavioral intervention plan

- Specify goal (e.g., Brian will decrease aggressive incidents toward peers)
- Specify interventions
  - Remediate skills deficits (model, practice, and reinforce the following: anger recognition and management skills, problem-solving skills, communication skills, friendship skills, personal space skills)
  - Remediate performance deficits (teach importance of personal safety, provide rewards [praise, tokens, privileges] for control of aggression)
  - Manipulate antecedents (pair with adult in hallways, monitor and intervene with provocations)
  - Provide other supports (skill-building services from school social worker, speech pathologist; daily home-school report card)
- Specify persons responsible (teachers, social worker, speech pathologist)
- Evaluate outcome (criterion: no fighting in next 6 weeks)

increasing levels of intensity. The essential components of RTI include 1) monitoring a student's academic progress using screening or tests; 2) implementing a scientifically proven intervention for struggling students; 3) monitoring how the student responds to the intervention; and 4) on the basis of the student's response to intervention, determining the level of support a student needs in order to be successful.

If prereferral interventions are ineffective, the student should undergo a special education evaluation to determine his or her eligibility for special education services. A special education evaluation is a comprehensive individual analysis of all suspected areas of disability conducted by a multidisciplinary team of school-based professionals (Table 48–3). The request for a special education evaluation should be made in writing and may specify the reasons for the request (e.g., child is performing below grade level academically or is having attention, behavioral, social, emotional, developmental, or communication problems). Although requests from parents or professionals outside the school do not guarantee an evaluation, the "child find" requirement makes it difficult for a school to refuse such a request. If the school does refuse, it must explain why it refuses to take action and provide a description of all student information used as a basis for the decision. Under the Procedural Safeguards provision of IDEA, parents must be provided with a procedural safeguards notice at specific points: 1) on parental request for evaluation, 2) once each

TABLE 48–2. Individuals With Disabilities Education Act (IDEA) disability designations and examples of corresponding psychiatric disorders

IDEA	Diagnostic and Statistical Manual of Mental Disorders, Fifth Edition (DSM-5)
Autism	Autism spectrum disorder
Deaf-blindness	NA
Deafness	NA
Developmental delay	Global developmental delay
Emotional disturbance[a]	Bipolar; depressive; anxiety; disruptive, impulse-control, and conduct; schizophrenia spectrum; obsessive-compulsive; trauma- and stressor-related; dissociative; somatic symptom; feeding and eating; and elimination disorders
Hearing impairment	NA
Intellectual disability	Intellectual disability
Multiple disabilities	NA
Orthopedic impairment	NA
Other health impairment[b]	Attention-deficit/hyperactivity disorder
Specific learning disability	Specific learning disorder (reading, written expression, mathematics)
Speech-language impairment	Communication disorders
Traumatic brain injury	NA
Visual impairment	NA

Note. NA=not applicable.
[a]One or more of the following characteristics are exhibited to a marked degree over an extended period of time that adversely affect a child's educational performance: 1) an inability to learn that cannot be explained by intellectual, sensory, or health factors; 2) an inability to build or maintain satisfactory interpersonal relationships with peers and teachers; 3) inappropriate types of behavior or emotions under normal circumstances; 4) a pervasive mood of unhappiness or depression; or 5) a tendency to develop physical symptoms or fears associated with personal or school problems. The term does not apply to children who are socially maladjusted, unless it is determined that they have an emotional disturbance.
[b]An acute or chronic health problem, including a heightened alertness to environmental stimuli, that results in limited alertness with respect to the educational environment and adversely affects a child's educational experience.

school year for students eligible for IDEA services, 3) when parents first file a complaint, 4) when the student is removed from his or her current education placement because of a violation of a code of conduct, and 5) on request by the parent. The procedural safeguards notice must contain information about parents' rights to 1) obtain independent educational evaluations, 2) receive prior written notice any time the school district plans to evaluate the student or schedules a meeting, 3) consent to evaluations, 4) have access to their child's educational records, and 5) present and resolve a complaint through due process (Table 48–4).

Informed consent for the special education evaluation must be sought by the school from the student's parents. If the school conducts a special education evaluation, it must be completed within a specified time period (the federal guideline is 60 calendar days after receiving parent consent). The team conducting the evaluation includes the student's parents; at least one regular and one special education teacher; a special education representative of the school district;

TABLE 48–3. Typical components of a special education evaluation

Usual components
Cognitive abilities
Communication abilities
Academic performance
Social/emotional status
Medical history/current health status
Vision/hearing screenings
Motor abilities
Additional components as indicated
Intelligence testing
Speech/language testing
Achievement testing
Neuropsychological testing
Physical examination
Occupational therapy evaluation
Physical therapy evaluation
Psychiatric assessment

an individual who can interpret the implications of evaluation results; any individuals who have knowledge of the student; and, when appropriate, the student. When the evaluation has been completed, the school-based team will schedule an eligibility meeting to present the findings to the parents. Students must meet both of "two prongs" to be eligible for special education services: 1) the student must be determined to have one or more disabilities listed in IDEA, and 2) the student must, as a result of the disability, need special education in order to make progress in school. If there is disagreement about the findings from the evaluation, then the parents may use appeal options that are available for conflict resolution (see Table 48–4).

If the findings from the special education evaluation indicate that the child has a disability and would benefit from special education, the school-based team will develop a written individualized education program (IEP) for the child in collaboration with his or her parents (Table 48–5) within a specified time period (the federal guideline is 30 calendar days). In addition to special education (i.e., instructional) services, the IEP may specify relevant modifications and accommodations and/or related services, as well as the setting in which they will be provided (Table 48–6). Specific accommodations (e.g., environmental changes designed to overcome impediments to learning caused by the disability) and/or related services (e.g., noninstructional services required to assist a child with a disability to benefit from special education) may be recommended for inclusion in the IEP. Modifications (e.g., curricular changes that can reduce learning expectations) should be recommended only with caution, as they may have the unintended consequence of reducing the child's opportunity to learn critical instructional content. According to the provisions of IDEA, the educational setting must be both appropriate to the child's needs and least restrictive of his or her interactions with peers without disabilities. If the parents disagree with the educational program proposed in the IEP, they can appeal as outlined previously (Table 48–4). The child remains in the current placement until the disagreement is resolved.

The IEP is reviewed and revised annually; however, if the parents believe that the child is not progressing adequately, they may request an IEP review at any time to consider changes in services. Every 3 years, a comprehensive reevaluation is conducted by the school-based team to determine whether the child continues to meet eligibility criteria for special education services and what services should be provided.

Children with an IEP are afforded special disciplinary considerations. Students

TABLE 48–4. Typical appeal options for Individuals With Disabilities Education Act conflict resolution

Discuss the issue informally with the school staff, principal, superintendent, and/or director of special education.
Request impartial mediation with a qualified mediator appointed at no cost by the state board of education.
File a written complaint with the state education agency. A full investigation must follow. If the parent disagrees with the findings of the investigation, he or she can request a review by the U.S. Department of Education.
Request a due process hearing with a hearing officer appointed by the state education agency. The parent has the right to legal counsel at his or her own expense; the officer may award attorneys' fees should the parent prevail in the decision.
File a civil lawsuit. The court may award attorneys' fees should the parent prevail in the decision.

whose disruptive behavior is a manifestation of their disability should have a BIP (see Table 48–1) written into their IEP, with the goal of preventing suspensions or expulsions. A student with a disability who has an IEP in place can be disciplined, like any other student, for 10 consecutive school days if he or she violates the school's code of conduct. For students with a disability whose disciplinary actions exceed 10 consecutive days in the same school year or when disciplinary actions exceed 10 nonconsecutive days in a school year and clearly indicate a pattern, then a manifestation determination review (MDR) must be conducted by the school to determine whether the behavior resulting in the suspensions was related to the child's disability. If the behavior was related to the child's disability, then the IEP and BIP must be revised to address the behavior problem. If the behavior was not related to the child's disability, the child may be excluded for more than 10 days, provided that he or she receives a free and appropriate public education during the removal period. The IEP must be revised to document this change in services. If the parents disagree with the decision of the MDR, they may appeal the decision (Table 48–4). Children suspected of having disabilities who become subject to discipline before they have been evaluated for special education services are entitled to the same protections as children already found eligible.

A student with a disability may be expelled and transferred to a temporary alternative placement for up to 45 days under several conditions: 1) if the student carries a weapon to school or a school function; possesses, uses, or sells illegal drugs or controlled substances at school or a school function; or has inflicted serious bodily injury on another person while at school or a school function; 2) if the hearing officer determines that maintaining the current placement is substantially likely to result in injury to the child or others; and 3) if the student commits violations of school policies other than those listed previously if students without disabilities are subject to the same disciplinary measures.

Interventions in the School Setting

Increasingly, schools are considered to be an ideal context for contributing to the transformation of mental health services according to a public health framework

TABLE 48–5. Typical components and related services of an individualized education program

Usual components	Comments
Present level of educational performance	Can include social/emotional/behavioral performance
Educational goals and objectives with measurable benchmarks	Can include social/emotional/behavioral goals with measurable benchmarks
Educational modifications and accommodations	Should address social/emotional/behavioral barriers to learning
Special education	Should be of sufficient intensity to meet educational goals
Placement and participation specifications	Placement should be least restrictive setting; mental health problems may preclude participation in standardized testing
Transition services planning	Posteducational planning process should consider student's mental health needs
Transfer of rights planning	Student must be apprised of rights when reaching age of majority
Related services as indicated	Can include speech/language, psychological, and counseling services
Adapted physical education	—
Assistive technology	Can include keyboarding devices for communication or students with motor impairments
Audiology	—
Behavioral intervention plan	See Table 48–1
Counseling services	For transition or transfer of rights planning
Extended school-year services	To prevent academic regression in students with cognitive impairments
Home-based support	—
Medical services	—
Occupational therapy	Can include training in penmanship, activities of daily living; may also include special cushions, devices, or techniques to address sensory sensitivities
Orientation/mobility services	—
Parent counseling/training	To enhance parent-teacher collaboration
Physical therapy	Can include development of gross and fine motor skills
Psychological services	For specialized testing

TABLE 48–5. Typical components and related services of an individualized education program *(continued)*

Usual components	Comments
Recreation	To enhance social skills
School health services	For medication administration, vital sign or other checks, nutrition services
School social work services	For individual, group, or family therapy
Speech/language services	For testing and therapy (pragmatics as well as articulation)
Transportation services	For students incapable of using school bus or public transportation

TABLE 48–6. Typical educational placement options (least to most restrictive)

Regular classroom
Regular classroom with consultative services to teacher
Regular classroom with modifications/accommodations/supports
Regular classroom with pull-out resource services
Special education classroom with some pull-out regular education
Special education classroom
Special (therapeutic) school
Home/hospital services

(Weist 2005). In this framework, mental health services are targeted at specific segments of the population according to risk status. *Universal preventive* interventions are intended to promote mental health and as such are targeted at all students, regardless of risk status. *Selective preventive* interventions are intended to prevent the development of symptoms in high-risk students and as such are targeted at students exhibiting risk factors for psychiatric disorders. *Indicated preventive* interventions are intended to prevent the escalation of subsyndromal symptoms of psychiatric disorders to syndromal disorders and as such are targeted at students exhibiting symptoms. *Clinical* interventions are intended to treat psychiatric disorders and are targeted at students with psychiatric diagnoses.

A number of strategies have been highlighted by Weist et al. (2005) to address perceived barriers to implementing school-based interventions, including 1) ensuring strong coordination and collaboration among families, school administrators, and mental health program leaders as programs are being planned; 2) ensuring that school mental health providers are well trained and closely supervised and that they understand the culture of schools and how to work as collaborators; 3) ensuring the high quality and empirical support of services; 4) framing services as effective means for reducing barriers to learning; and 5) documenting that services lead to outcomes valued by youth, families, and schools.

Preventive Interventions

Extant literature supports the overall effectiveness of rigorously evaluated school-based preventive interventions. In a systematic review of reviews of the outcomes of universal, selective, and indicated preventive interventions (Weare and Nind 2011), 50 of 52 reviews concluded that one or more of the interventions had at least small effects, and only four minor examples of apparent adverse effects were reported across hundreds of interventions reviewed.

This finding was congruent with those from a recent meta-analysis of the outcomes from 399 universal, selective, and indicated preventive interventions (Wilson and Lipsey 2007), in which the overall mean effect size was in the 0.20–0.35 range. For internalizing outcomes (e.g., depression, anxiety), the mean effect size ranged from 0.10 to 1.70, rising to 2.46 in higher-risk students. For externalizing outcomes (e.g., aggression/disruptive behavior), the mean effect size averaged 0.10, rising to 0.21–0.35 for higher-risk students. For social-emotional competency outcomes, the mean effect size ranged from 0.15 to 0.37. The following themes emerged from the findings: 1) interventions across the entire range of outcomes were consistently shown to have a stronger effect on higher-risk students; 2) the more effective interventions included a similar mix of cognitive-behavioral and social skills training for students and behavior management training for parents and teachers; 3) active teaching modalities (e.g., games, role plays, small group discussions) were more effective than didactic modalities; 4) intervention impact was significantly enhanced by having a qualified intervention agent (e.g., mental health professional) and involving parents; and 5) the balance of evidence supported beginning interventions in the early school years, with supportive "booster" interventions implemented later.

An important first step in the development of school-based interventions is a needs assessment, which can identify the primary mental health needs within a school and feasible, acceptable ways to meet those needs (e.g., Walter et al. 2006, 2011). Information can be gathered from all key constituent groups, including school personnel, school board members, special education administrators, students, parents, and community leaders, and can be acquired informally, through group discussions and individual interviews, or formally, through a survey.

Universal Preventive Interventions

General Interventions

School climate and connectedness. The milieu of a school is a key factor influencing the desirability and effectiveness of mental health interventions. The milieu derives from several interrelated components (Brookover et al. 1979), including the sociodemographic composition of the student body and school personnel (social inputs); the size, structure, and processes of the school (social structure); and attitudinal characteristics, such as the norms, expectations, and feelings about the school shared by students and staff (social climate). The school climate literature supports several key components of a positive climate, including a supportive, welcoming atmosphere; respectful peer and adult relationships; a variety of learning experiences; high expectations for achievement and self-regulation; fair and effective discipline; participation in extracurricular activities; and parent/community involvement (Jamal et al. 2013; Libbey 2004).

Perceptions of a positive school climate have been strongly associated with a sense of connectedness to the school—that is, the sense of bonding and commitment a student feels as a result of perceived caring from teachers and peers (Thompson et al. 2006). School connectedness, grounded in attachment, social control, and social development theories, has been shown to predict a variety of positive health outcomes, including higher levels of emotional well-being, less substance abuse, less aggression and victimization, better health, decreased levels of suicidal ideation, decreased depressive symptoms, and decreased deviant behavior and teen pregnancy (Bond et al. 2007; Catalano et al. 2004; McNeely and Falci 2004; Wilson 2004). Connectedness also has been shown to exert protective effects in the context of a negative school climate; that is, highly connected students in either positive or negative school climates engage in fewer risky behaviors (Wilson 2004).

Two examples of universal interventions designed to improve school climate and foster school connectedness are the Seattle Social Development Project (SSDP) and the Gatehouse Project. The SSDP (Catalano et al. 2004; Hawkins et al. 2008) targeted elementary school students and focused on teacher training, child skill development, and parent training. By twelfth grade, students in the intervention condition reported more school commitment, school attachment, and school achievement; fewer disciplinary actions; and lower levels of alcohol use, violence, and risky sexual behavior. By age 27, adults who had participated in the intervention as students reported better educational and economic attainment, mental health, and sexual health. The Gatehouse Project (Bond et al. 2004) targeted high school students and focused on developing cognitive and interpersonal skills and creating an environment that enhanced connectedness. By tenth grade, students with good school and social connectedness were less likely to experience mental health problems, less likely to be involved in risky behaviors, and more likely to have good educational outcomes (Bond et al. 2007).

Social-emotional skills. Key social-emotional skills include self-awareness, self-regulation, interpersonal skills, and decision making (Elias and Arnold 2006). A large body of evidence links social-emotional competencies to improved school-related attitudes (e.g., motivation, connectedness to school), behaviors (e.g., attendance, disciplinary actions), and performance (e.g., grades, test scores, graduation rates), as well as to reduction in risky behaviors and improved mental health (Zins et al. 2004).

Catalano et al. (2002) examined a database of 161 universal social-emotional skills curricula and ultimately designated 22 school-based programs as effective. Favorable results included improvements in interpersonal skills, quality of peer and adult relationships, and academic achievement, as well as reductions in problem behaviors such as school misbehavior and truancy, alcohol and drug use, high-risk sexual behavior, and violence and aggression.

Positive behavior. Disruptive behavior has been shown to be one of the biggest problems facing teachers (e.g., Walter et al. 2006) and constitutes a major barrier to teaching and learning. Examples of universal interventions designed to foster positive behavior include the Good Behavior Game (Dolan et al. 1989) and School-Wide Positive Behavioral Interventions and Supports (SWPBIS; https://www.pbis.org). The Good Behavior Game, developed by Barrish et al. (1969), is a classroom-wide, teacher-delivered intervention in which teachers in early elementary grades model and reinforce student behaviors identified by the schools as promoting a positive learning environment. The promise of this intervention suggested in multiple small studies (see Mackenzie et al., supplementary material, in Kellam et al. 2008) led to a large randomized trial, the results of which have been reported in multiple publications (Dolan et al. 1993; Kellam et al. 1994, 2008, 2014; Wilcox et al. 2008). These findings, generally replicated in other studies in the United States and abroad (Mackenzie et al. 2008), suggested the effectiveness of the program in reducing aggressive and disruptive behavior among males through elementary and middle school and in reducing drug use, high-risk sexual behaviors, incarceration for violence, and suicide in young adulthood, particularly among males who were aggressive and disruptive at study initiation.

Similar to the Good Behavior Game, SWPBIS posits that continual behavioral coaching combined with acknowledgment of positive student behavior will reduce unnecessary disciplinary actions and promote a climate of greater productivity, safety, and learning. A 5-year randomized controlled trial of SWPBIS (Bradshaw et al. 2010) demonstrated the effectiveness of the model in reducing suspensions, office referrals, bullying, and peer rejection and improving staff members' perceptions of the schools' organization health.

Specific Interventions

Suicide. According to a Cochrane review of school-based suicide prevention curricula targeted at general populations of students (Guo and Harstall 2002), there is insufficient evidence to either support or refute these programs. A subsequent review (Gould et al. 2003) went beyond curricula to examine the effects of other approaches to suicide prevention and intervention, including screening. The authors concluded that screening for suicidality is fraught with problems related to low specificity of the screening instrument, poor acceptability among school administrators, and paucity of referral sites; gatekeeper training is effective in improving skills among school personnel and is highly acceptable to administrators but has not been shown to prevent suicide; peer helpers have not been shown to be either efficacious or safe; and postvention is promising but underinvestigated.

A more recent review (Katz et al. 2013) of 16 school-based suicide prevention programs found that most studies were limited to knowledge and attitudes outcomes rather than suicidal behavior. Signs of Suicide (Aseltine and DeMartino 2004; Aseltine et al. 2007) and the Good Behavior Game (Wilcox et. al. 2008) were the only programs found to reduce suicide attempts. The Sources of Strength program (Wyman et al. 2010) was found to improve gatekeeper behavior, attitudes, and knowledge about suicide. A randomized trial of the effects of the intervention on suicidal behavior is under way.

Aggressive behavior. According to a meta-analysis of 77 studies of school-based programs targeted at aggressive behavior (Wilson and Lipsey 2007), the overall mean effect size was 0.21. Cognitively oriented programs (i.e., those focused on changing thinking and problem solving) were the most often used modality, but other modalities were also employed (e.g., behavioral strategies, social skills training, psychotherapy, peer mediation, parent training). None of the treatment modalities was superior to the others. In subgroup analyses, younger students showed larger effects than older students, and students of low socioeconomic status showed larger effects than their middle-class peers.

Substance use. According to a Cochrane review (Faggiano et al. 2005) of 32 school-based substance use prevention programs, skill-based programs (e.g., decision making, peer pressure resistance) appear to be effective in deterring early stage drug use. However, for school-based alcohol prevention, the results of a Cochrane review (Foxcroft and Tsertsvadze 2011) for both alcohol-specific and general social skills programs were mixed, with the strongest effects observed for drunkenness and binge drinking. A Cochrane review (Thomas et al. 2013) of 49 school-based cigarette smoking prevention studies found an average 12% reduction in smoking initiation at long-term follow-up compared with control groups. Combined social competence and social influences interventions showed the strongest effects; social influences approaches alone and information approaches alone were ineffective.

Early/unprotected sexual activity. Interventions for preventing unintended pregnancy and sexually transmitted diseases have included abstinence-oriented programs that target the delay of sexual debut by teaching students how to avoid situations in which they are vulnerable to having unintended intercourse and how to refuse offers to engage in intercourse if they do not feel ready and safe sex–oriented programs that target correct, consistent condom use by teaching students how to refuse intercourse if barrier protection is unavailable and how to use barrier protection correctly (e.g., Walter and Vaughan 1993). A Cochrane review (Oringanje et al. 2009) of such programs conducted in a variety of settings including schools concluded that both educational and skills-building interventions were effective in lowering the rate of unintended pregnancy, but the effect on initiation of sexual intercourse and on sexually transmitted diseases was inconclusive.

Depression. In a meta-analysis (Horowitz and Garber 2006) of the findings from 12 school-based depression prevention programs, the effect size was found to be 0.12 and 0.02 at postintervention and follow-up, respectively. This finding was echoed in more recent systematic reviews. Calear and Christensen (2010) found that only 39% of 23 universal trials showed reductions in depression symptoms at posttest, with effect sizes ranging from 0.30 to 1.40. Only 9% of universal trials reported significant effects at both postintervention and follow-up. Merry et al. (2011) reviewed 16 studies of psychological and educational depression prevention interventions and found that the risk of having a depressive disorder postintervention was significantly reduced immediately and up to 12 months later compared with no intervention. There was no evidence of effectiveness at 24 months postintervention.

Anxiety. In a meta-analysis of 16 school-based anxiety prevention programs, Neil and Christensen (2009) found significant differences between intervention and control conditions at posttest (effect size 0.31–1.37) for 69% of trials. Three of six trials (50%) reported significant effects at follow-up (effect size 0.22–0.70), while two (33%) reported significant effects at both posttest and follow-up. Overall, significant effects did not depend on the type of intervention (cognitive-behavioral therapy vs. others), type of program leader (teacher vs. others), or type of control group (attention vs. others).

Multiple risk factors. On the basis of the premise that risky behaviors such as smoking, drinking, illicit drug use, sexual risk, and aggressive behavior are all mutually predictive (e.g., Guilamo-Ramos et al. 2005; Walter et al. 1995b), there is growing interest in preventive interventions targeted at multiple risk factors. In a systematic review (Hale et al. 2014) of 44 studies evaluating 32 school-based interventions targeted at multiple health risk behaviors, 18 interventions (56%) showed a significant effect for two of three substances (tobacco, alcohol, drugs), and 9 (28%) had a positive effect for all three. Four interventions (Positive Action Program, Project PATHS, Social Development Curriculum, Life Skills Training) reported significant effects for all risk behaviors targeted (smoking, drinking, drug use, sexual risk, aggression) (Beets et al. 2009; Flay et al. 2004; Griffin et al. 2006; Li et al. 2011; Shek and Yu 2011). Nearly all interventions targeted individual attributes and skills (e.g., self-efficacy, problem solving, decision making, stress management) and social competencies (e.g., prosocial peer relationships, school connectedness).

Selective Preventive Interventions

Selective preventive interventions target students who are at high risk for developing emotional, behavioral, or social problems. School personnel must be able to identify vulnerable students, who can then be screened for underlying psychopathology and provided with appropriate services (Mattison 2000). Specially trained teachers, social workers, guidance counselors, and nurses can play key roles in this gatekeeping process. High-risk students fall into several categories: students who are performing poorly in school because of excessive absenteeism, frequent referrals for disciplinary actions, or academic failure; students who are engaging in multiple risky behaviors; and students who are exposed to psychosocial adversity. Undetected psychiatric disorders often underlie the overt presentation in high-risk students (see review by Mattison 2000).

Screening

The process of universally screening within a school to determine risk status and early intervention needs is gaining momentum (Dowdy et al. 2010). In a multiple gating screening, all students within a school are screened (first gate) to identify those at potential risk, and those students who screen positively are provided with focused assessment (second gate) to confirm risk. Students at confirmed risk are then comprehensively assessed to determine level of risk and need for services. Widely used examples of first-gate screening instruments include the Strengths and Difficulties Questionnaire (Bourdon et al. 2005; Goodman 1997), the Behavioral and Emotional Screening System (Kamphaus and Reynolds 2007), and the Pediatric System Checklist (Gall et al. 2000; Vogels et al. 2009); examples of second-gate instruments are the Behavior Assessment System for Children–Second Edition (Reynolds and Kamphaus 2004) and the Vanderbilt Parent and Teacher Rating Scales (Bard et al. 2013; Wolraich et al. 2013). Several protocols should be in place before the implementation of a screening program: training of gatekeepers to understand and appropriately use the screening instruments; obtaining parental consent and notifying parents of screening results; protecting the confidentiality of students' responses; initiating appropriate school-based assessment and early intervention if indicated; and providing appropriate, timely, and convenient links to external service providers for students who are in need of additional evaluation and treatment.

In a national survey of adolescent mental health (Green et al. 2013), school-based early identification was significantly associated with mental health service use for adolescents with mild to moderate mental health disorders. Yet less than 2% of schools currently use systematic screening. Barriers to screening include high costs, legal concerns, and beliefs that mental health screening is not the role of schools.

Indicated Preventive Interventions

Indicated preventive interventions target students who exhibit symptoms of emotional, behavioral, or social problems but do not meet the full diagnostic criteria for a specific disorder. Most of the programs of this type have targeted students with symptoms of aggression, depression, anxiety, or trauma and were designed for delivery in group settings by trained school personnel in collaboration with clinicians. Only a small number of such programs have been rigorously evaluated.

The largest body of evidence pertains to school-based violence prevention programs for aggressive students. A Cochrane review (Mytton et al. 2006) of 56 randomized controlled trials of these programs suggested that they appear to produce meaningful reductions in aggressive and violent behaviors, especially those interventions designed to improve relationships or social skills. According to a recent meta-analysis of 108 studies conducted by Wilson and Lipsey (2007), the overall mean effect size for selected/indicated programs targeted at aggression was 0.29. Although the most common programs were cognitively oriented, behavioral strategies, social skills training, and therapy were well represented. Higher-risk students showed larger effect sizes than lower-risk students, and behavioral strategies produced significantly greater reductions in aggressive/disruptive behavior than the other intervention modalities.

The evidence of the effectiveness of interventions targeting mood, anxiety, or trauma symptoms is more limited. In a meta-analysis of the findings from eight indicated depression prevention programs, Horowitz and Garber (2006) found the mean effect size to be 0.18 and 0.25 at postintervention and follow-up, respectively, suggesting the promise of these programs in improving subsyndromal depression. This conclusion was echoed in a more recent meta-analysis (Calear and Christensen 2010), which found that 60% of indicated depression prevention trials exhibited significant differences in depression symptoms between intervention and control conditions postintervention (effect sizes ranging from 0.25 to 1.35). Moreover, 67% of trials reported significant effects at follow-up (effect sizes ranging from 0.33 to 1.00). The most effective programs were based on cognitive-behavioral themes (e.g., positive thinking styles, emotional recognition and regulation, coping and personal effectiveness skills) rather than supportive or interpersonal therapy, were delivered by mental health rather than school professionals, and had a duration of 8–12 sessions.

In a meta-analysis of the findings from eight indicated anxiety prevention programs (Neil and Christensen 2009), four showed reductions in anxiety symptoms at posttest (effect size range 0.20–0.76). Five of six trials (83%) found significant effects at follow-up (effect size range 0.19–1.03). Two of eight trials found significant effects at both posttest and follow-up.

The effects of 19 programs targeted at students with symptoms of posttraumatic stress disorder were assessed in a meta-analysis (Rolfsnes and Idsoe 2011). Of the 19 studies, 14 (74%) had effect sizes in the medium to large range, with a mean effect size of 0.68. Most studies used an approach based on cognitive-behavioral therapy, and these programs demonstrated the strongest effect. However, interventions based on play/art, eye movement desensitization and reprocessing, and mind-body skills were also promising on the basis of individual studies. An important finding from one of the studies included in the analysis (Jaycox et al. 2010) was that the school setting led to considerably more students accessing and completing treatment than the clinical setting (91% vs. 15%, respectively).

Clinical Interventions

Clinical interventions target students who are found on clinical assessment to meet diagnostic criteria for specific psychiatric disorders. The literature regarding effective programs is limited, focusing primarily on the treatment of attention-deficit/hyperactivity disorder (ADHD).

The effects of school-based, nonpharmacological interventions for the treatment of ADHD were examined by DuPaul and Eckert (1997) in a meta-analysis of 63 outcome studies. They concluded that contingency management and tutoring were more effective than cognitive-behavioral strategies in reducing ADHD behaviors and enhancing academic performance. Herzig-Anderson et al. (2012) reviewed controlled trials of four school-based treatments for anxiety disorders (including trauma-related disorders). They concluded that although these programs had promise, a significant barrier to wider implementation is the reliance on specialized mental health clinicians to deliver the interventions, which is costly and resource intensive. In an older study, Mufson et al. (2004) suggested the potential of school-based programs for the treatment of depression.

Expanded Mental Health Interventions

An early example of ESMH services is described by Walrath et al. (2004). To date, investigations of this model are limited but promising. Bruns et al. (2004) tested ESMH services in elementary schools and found that schools providing ESMH services had better school mental health climate ratings from teachers and fewer student referrals to special education services. Walter et al. (2011) demonstrated that elementary school students participating in ESMH services had significantly fewer mental health problems and improved function and behavior, while teachers improved their proficiency in managing mental health problems in their classrooms. Ballard et al. (2014) found that students receiving ESMH services had fewer suspensions and higher attendance compared with matched students not receiving services and also had improvements in total mental health difficulties.

Telepsychiatry

Telepsychiatry with children and adolescents (Myers et al. 2008) has the potential to improve access to mental health services by addressing logistical, economic, capacity, and stigma-related barriers to care. Young (2004) described several possible uses of telepsychiatry in schools, including diagnostic assessments, ongoing individual and family therapy, medication management, teacher consultations, and continuing education. An early systematic review of telepsychiatry with children and adolescents (Pesämaa et al. 2004) suggested that despite communication barriers and challenges with audiovisual quality, the provision of telepsychiatry services improved access to care and resulted in savings related to time, cost, and travel. More recently, Grady et al. (2011) reviewed clinical, educational, and administrative/programmatic roles for telepsychiatry in schools and concluded that telehealth technology has demonstrated acceptance, expands educational opportunities for school personnel, and has a positive impact on the attitudes of teachers and other school personnel. Congruently, Cunningham et al. (2013) reported on the perspectives of psychiatrists who provide teleconsultation services to schools. Results indicated positive provider experiences with telepsychiatry, including reports that students were more likely to disclose clinical information via video compared with face-to-face contact. However, concerns regarding technological difficulties, logistics, and information sharing were endorsed by some of the psychiatrists—concerns that the authors suggested could be alleviated by increased training, supervision, and communication.

Crisis Intervention

A crisis at school occurs when the integrity of the school environment is threatened by an event to such a degree that the school's internal resources are deemed insufficient or exhausted (Arroyo 2001). Events that may precipitate a crisis include the suicide of a student or school staff member, a natural disaster, or violence that directly affects the school community.

The primary goals when creating a plan to effectively manage a crisis are to help the school resume a normal routine as quickly as possible and address the needs of students and staff beyond the immediate crisis period. Successful plans involve collaborations with organizations beyond the school, such as departments of health and mental health, law enforcement agencies, and other organizations skilled in crisis response. Crisis response plans should be highly organized and centralized in the school or district administrative office. The roles, responsibilities, and required training of both school staff and other collaborators should be specified in the plan, and the plan should contain a framework for the coordination of and communication with all of the collaborative entities. It also should contain guidelines for interacting with the media.

As described in the American Academy of Child and Adolescent Psychiatry Practice Parameter on Disaster Preparedness (Pfefferbaum et al. 2013), disaster-focused interventions can be conceptualized along a timeline including impact, immediate postimpact, intermediate postimpact, and recovery phases. During the impact and immediate postimpact phases, interventions should focus on providing "psychological first aid," including the provision of accurate and timely information about disaster reactions and available resources, social and emotional support to students and school personnel, and ongoing assessment and triage. Subsequently, in the intermediate postimpact phase, specific therapeutic techniques can be deployed, including family outreach, psychoeducation, screening, anxiety reduction, and ongoing social support. In the recovery phase, students exhibiting psychological difficulties should be referred for clinical assessment and evidence-based treatment as indicated.

Useful Web Sites

The following are some useful Web sites with information on school-based interventions:

School Psychiatry Program and MADI Resource Center, Massachusetts General Hospital: www.schoolpsychiatry.org

U.S. Department of Education, Building the Legacy: IDEA 2004: http://idea.ed.gov

University of Maryland School of Medicine Center for School Mental Health: http://csmh.umaryland.edu

Collaborative for Academic, Social, and Emotional Learning: www.casel.org

Substance Abuse and Mental Health Services Administration's National Registry of Evidence-Based Programs and Practices: http://nrepp.samhsa.gov

Summary Points

- The educational rights of children with mental disabilities are protected by federal law.
- Students with psychiatric disorders may be eligible for classroom accommodations, curricular modifications, special education, and related services to overcome impediments to learning imposed by their mental disabilities.
- Students with problems at school often have undetected, untreated psychiatric disorders.
- Students can be effectively screened with standardized rating scales for the presence of psychiatric disorders.
- There are effective school-based interventions for the promotion of social-emotional competency and school connectedness and the prevention of aggressive/disruptive behavior, substance use, early or unprotected sexual activity, and multiple risky behaviors.
- There are effective school-based interventions for the treatment of subsyndromal and syndromal disruptive behavior, mood, anxiety, and posttraumatic stress disorders.

References

Armbruster P, Lichtman J: Are school based mental health services effective? Evidence from 36 inner city schools. Community Ment Health J 35(6):493–504, 1999 10863986

Armbruster P, Gerstein SH, Fallon T: Bridging the gap between service need and service utilization: a school-based mental health program. Community Ment Health J 33(3):199–211, 1997 9211040

Arroyo W: School crisis consultation. Child Adolesc Psychiatr Clin N Am 10(1):55–66, 2001 11214420

Aseltine RH Jr, DeMartino R: An outcome evaluation of the SOS suicide prevention program. Am J Public Health 94(3):446–451, 2004 14998812

Aseltine RH Jr, James A, Schilling EA, et al: Evaluating the SOS suicide prevention program: a replication and extension. BMC Public Health 7:161, 2007 17640366

Ballard KL, Sander MA, Klimes-Dougan B: School-related and social-emotional outcomes of providing mental health services in schools. Community Ment Health J 50(2):145–149, 2014 24337471

Bard DE, Wolraich ML, Neas B, et al: The psychometric properties of the Vanderbilt attention-deficit hyperactivity disorder diagnostic parent rating scale in a community population. J Dev Behav Pediatr 34(2):72–82, 2013 23363972

Barrish HH, Saunders M, Wolf MM: Good behavior game: effects of individual contingencies for group consequences on disruptive behavior in a classroom. J Appl Behav Anal 2(2):119–124, 1969 16795208

Beets MW, Flay BR, Vuchinich S, et al: Use of a social and character development program to prevent substance use, violent behaviors, and sexual activity among elementary-school students in Hawaii. Am J Public Health 99(8):1438–1445, 2009 19542037

Berkovitz IH (ed): School Consultation/Intervention: Child and Adolescent Psychiatric Clinics of North America. Philadelphia, PA, WB Saunders, 2001

Berlin IN: Psychiatry and the school, in Comprehensive Textbook of Psychiatry II. Edited by Freedman AM, Kaplan HI, Sadow BJ. Baltimore, MD, Williams and Wilkins, 1975, pp 2253–2255

Bond L, Patton G, Glover S, et al: The Gatehouse Project: can a multilevel school intervention affect emotional wellbeing and health risk behaviours? J Epidemiol Community Health 58(12):997–1003, 2004 15547059

Bond L, Butler H, Thomas L, et al: Social and school connectedness in early secondary school as predictors of late teenage substance use, mental health, and academic outcomes. J Adolesc Health 40:357, 2007 17367730

Bourdon KH, Goodman R, Rae DS, et al: The Strengths and Difficulties Questionnaire: U.S. normative data and psychometric properties. J Am Acad Child Adolesc Psychiatry 44(6):557–564, 2005 15908838

Bradshaw CP, Mitchell MM, Leaf PJ: Examining the effects of school-wide positive behavioral interventions and supports on student outcomes: results from a randomized controlled effectiveness trial in elementary schools. Journal of Positive Behavioral Interventions 12(3):133–148, 2010

Brener ND, Martindale J, Weist MD: Mental health and social services: results from the School Health Policies and Programs Study 2000. J Sch Health 71(7):305–312, 2001 11586873

Brookover WB, Beady C, Flood P, et al: School Social Systems and Student Achievement: Schools Can Make a Difference. New York, Praeger, 1979

Bruns EJ, Walrath C, Glass-Siegel M, et al: School-based mental health services in Baltimore: association with school climate and special education referrals. Behav Modif 28(4):491–512, 2004 15186512

Calear AL, Christensen H: Systematic review of school-based prevention and early intervention programs for depression. J Adolesc 33(3):429–438, 2010 19647310

Caplan G: The Theory and Practice of Mental Health Consultation. New York, Basic Books, 1970

Catalano RF, Berglund ML, Ryan JAM, et al: Positive youth development in the United States: research findings on evaluations of positive youth development programs. Prevention & Treatment 5(1):15, 2002

Catalano RF, Haggerty KP, Oesterle S, et al: The importance of bonding to school for healthy development: findings from the Social Development Research Group. J Sch Health 74(7):252–261, 2004 15493702

Comer JP: School consultation, in Psychiatry, Vol 2. Edited by Michels R, Cooper AM, Guze SB. Philadelphia, PA, Lippincott, 1992, pp 1–10

Cunningham DL, Connors EH, Lever N, et al: Providers' perspectives: utilizing telepsychiatry in schools. Telemed J E Health 19(10):794–799, 2013 23980938

Dolan LJ, Jaylan T, Werthamer L, et al: The Good Behavior Game Manual. Baltimore, MD, Johns Hopkins Prevention Research Center, 1989

Dolan LJ, Kellam SG, Brown CH, et al: The short-term impact of two classroom-based preventive interventions on aggressive and shy behaviors and poor achievement. J Appl Dev Psychol 14(3):317–345, 1993

Dowdy E, Ritchey K, Kamphaus RW: School-based screening: a population-based approach to inform and monitor children's mental health needs. School Ment Health 2(4):166–176, 2010 21088687

DuPaul GJ, Eckert TL: The effects of school-based interventions for attention-deficit/hyperactivity disorder: a meta-analysis. School Psych Rev 26(1):5–27, 1997

Elias MJ, Arnold H: The Educator's Guide to Emotional Intelligence and Academic Achievement: Social-Emotional Learning in the Classroom. Thousand Oaks, CA, Corwin, 2006

Faggiano F, Vigna-Taglianti FD, Versino E, et al: School-based prevention for illicit drugs' use. Cochrane Database Syst Rev 2(2):CD003020, 2005 15846647

Flay BR, Graumlich S, Segawa E, et al: Effects of 2 prevention programs on high-risk behaviors among African American youth: a randomized trial. Arch Pediatr Adolesc Med 158(4):377–384, 2004 15066879

Foxcroft DR, Tsertsvadze A: Universal school-based prevention programs for alcohol misuse in young people. Cochrane Database Syst Rev 5(5):CD009113, 2011 21563171

Gall G, Pagano ME, Desmond MS, et al: Utility of psychosocial screening at a school-based health center. J Sch Health 70(7):292–298, 2000 10981284

Goodman R: The strengths and difficulties questionnaire: a research note. J Child

Psychol Psychiatry 38(5):581–586, 1997 9255702

Gould MS, Greenberg T, Velting DM, et al: Youth suicide risk and preventive interventions: a review of the past 10 years. J Am Acad Child Adolesc Psychiatry 42(4):386–405, 2003 12649626

Grady BJ, Lever N, Cunningham D, et al: Telepsychiatry and school mental health. Child Adolesc Psychiatr Clin N Am 20(1):81–94, 2011 21092914

Green JG, McLaughlin KA, Alegría M, et al: School mental health resources and adolescent mental health service use. J Am Acad Child Adolesc Psychiatry 52(5):501–510, 2013 23622851

Griffin KW, Botvin GJ, Nichols TR: Effects of a school-based drug abuse prevention program for adolescents on HIV risk behavior in young adulthood. Prev Sci 7(1):103–112, 2006 16604429

Guilamo-Ramos V, Litardo HA, Jaccard J: Prevention programs for reducing adolescent problem behaviors: Implications of the co-occurrence of problem behaviors in adolescence. J Adolesc Health 36(1):82–86, 2005 15661605

Guo B, Harstall C: Efficacy of Suicide Prevention Programs for Children and Youth. Edmonton, Canada, Alberta Heritage Foundation for Medical Research, 2002

Hale DR, Fitzgerald-Yau N, Viner RM: A systematic review of effective interventions for reducing multiple health risk behaviors in adolescence. Am J Public Health 104(5):e19–e41, 2014 24625172

Hawkins JD, Kosterman R, Catalano RF, et al: Effects of social development intervention in childhood 15 years later. Arch Pediatr Adolesc Med 162(12):1133–1141, 2008 19047540

Herzig-Anderson K, Colognori D, Fox JK, et al: School-based anxiety treatments for children and adolescents. Child Adolesc Psychiatr Clin N Am 21(3):655–668, 2012 22801000

Horowitz JL, Garber J: The prevention of depressive symptoms in children and adolescents: a meta-analytic review. J Consult Clin Psychol 74(3):401–415, 2006 16822098

Jamal F, Fletcher A, Harden A, et al: The school environment and student health: a systematic review and meta-ethnography of qualitative research. BMC Public Health 13:798, 2013 24007211

Jaycox LH, Cohen JA, Mannarino AP, et al: Children's mental health care following Hurricane Katrina: a field trial of trauma-focused psychotherapies. J Trauma Stress 23(2):223–231, 2010 20419730

Jennings J, Pearson G, Harris M: Implementing and maintaining school-based mental health services in a large, urban school district. J Sch Health 70(5):201–205, 2000 10900598

Kamphaus RW, Reynolds CR: Behavioral Assessment System for Children-Second Edition (BASC-2): Behavioral and Emotional Screening System (BESS). Bloomington, MN, Pearson, 2007

Katz C, Bolton SL, Katz LY, et al: A systematic review of school-based suicide prevention programs. Depress Anxiety 30(10):1030–1045, 2013 23650186

Kellam SG, Rebok GW, Ialongo N, et al: The course and malleability of aggressive behavior from early first grade into middle school: results of a developmental epidemiologically based preventive trial. J Child Psychol Psychiatry 35(2):259–281, 1994 8188798

Kellam SG, Brown CH, Poduska JM, et al: Effects of a universal classroom behavior management program in first and second grades on young adult behavioral, psychiatric, and social outcomes. Drug Alcohol Depend 95(suppl 1):S5–S28, 2008 18343607

Kellam SG, Wang W, Mackenzie ACL, et al: The impact of the Good Behavior Game, a universal classroom-based preventive intervention in first and second grades, on high-risk sexual behaviors and drug abuse and dependence disorders into young adulthood. Prev Sci 15(suppl 1):S6–S18, 2014 23070695

Li KK, Washburn I, DuBois DL, et al: Effects of the Positive Action programme on problem behaviours in elementary school students: a matched-pair randomised control trial in Chicago. Psychol Health 26(2):187–204, 2011 21318929

Libbey HP: Measuring student relationships to school: attachment, bonding, connectedness, and engagement. J Sch Health 74(7):274–283, 2004 15493704

Lofink H, Kuebler J, Juszczak L, et al: 2010–2011 School-Based Health Alliance Census Report. Washington, DC, School-Based Health Alliance, 2013. Available at: http://www.sbh4all.org/wp-content/uploads/2015/02/CensusReport_2010-11CensusReport_7.13.pdf. Accessed July 6, 2015.

Mason-Jones AJ, Crisp C, Momberg M, et al: A systematic review of the role of school-based healthcare in adolescent sexual, reproductive, and mental health. Syst Rev 1:49–60, 2012 23098138

Mattison RE: School consultation: a review of research on issues unique to the school environment. J Am Acad Child Adolesc Psychiatry 39(4):402–413, 2000 10761341

McNeely C, Falci C: School connectedness and the transition into and out of health-risk behavior among adolescents: a comparison of social belonging and teacher support. J Sch Health 74(7):284–292, 2004 15493705

Merry SN, Hetrick SE, Cox GR, et al: Psychological and educational interventions for preventing depression in children and adolescents. Cochrane Database Syst Rev 12(12):CD003380, 2011 22161377

Mufson L, Dorta KP, Wickramaratne P, et al: A randomized effectiveness trial of interpersonal psychotherapy for depressed adolescents. Arch Gen Psychiatry 61(6):577–584, 2004 15184237

Myers K, Cain S, Work Group on Quality Issues, et al: Practice parameter for telepsychiatry with children and adolescents. J Am Acad Child Adolesc Psychiatry 47(12):1468–1483, 2008 19034191

Mytton J, DiGuiseppi C, Gough D, et al: School-based secondary prevention programmes for preventing violence. Cochrane Database Syst Rev 3(3):CD004606, 2006 16856051

Neil AL, Christensen H: Efficacy and effectiveness of school-based prevention and early intervention programs for anxiety. Clin Psychol Rev 29(3):208–215, 2009 19232805

Oringanje C, Meremikwu MM, Eko H, et al: Interventions for preventing unintended pregnancies among adolescents. Cochrane Database Syst Rev 4(4):CD005215, 2009 19821341

Pesämaa L, Ebeling H, Kuusimäki ML, et al: Videoconferencing in child and adolescent telepsychiatry: a systematic review of the literature. J Telemed Telecare 10(4):187–192, 2004 15273027

Pfefferbaum B, Shaw JA, American Academy of Child and Adolescent Psychiatry (AACAP) Committee on Quality Issues: Practice parameter on disaster preparedness. J Am Acad Child Adolesc Psychiatry 52(11):1224–1238, 2013 24157398

President's New Freedom Commission on Mental Health: Achieving the Promise: Transforming Mental Health Care in America. Final Report (DHHS Publ No SMA-03-3832). Rockville, MD, U.S. Department of Health and Human Services, 2003

Reynolds CR, Kamphaus RW: Behavior Assessment System for Children, 2nd Edition (BASC-2). Circle Pines, MN, AGS, 2004

Rolfsnes ES, Idsoe T: School-based intervention programs for PTSD symptoms: a review and meta-analysis. J Trauma Stress 24(2):155–165, 2011 21425191

Shek DTL, Yu L: Prevention of adolescent problem behavior: longitudinal impact of the Project P.A.T.H.S. in Hong Kong. ScientificWorldJournal 11:546–567, 2011 21403974

Stephan SH, Weist M, Kataoka S, et al: Transformation of children's mental health services: the role of school mental health. Psychiatr Serv 58(10):1330–1338, 2007 17914011

Taras HL, American Academy of Pediatrics Committee on School Health: School-based mental health services. Pediatrics 113(6):1839–1845, 2004 15173522

Taylor L, Adelman HS: Toward ending the marginalization and fragmentation of mental health in schools. J Sch Health 70(5):210–215, 2000 10900600

Thomas RE, McLellan J, Perera R: School-based programmes for preventing smoking. Cochrane Database Syst Rev 4:CD001293, 2013 23633306

Thompson DR, Iachan R, Overpeck M, et al: School connectedness in the health behavior in school-aged children study: the role of student, school, and school neighborhood characteristics. J Sch Health 76(7):379–386, 2006 16918872

Tolan PH, Anton BS, Culbertson JL, et al: Developing Psychology's National Agenda for Children's Mental Health. Report of the APA Working Group on Children's Mental Health to the Board of Directors. Washington, DC, American Psychological Association, 2001

U.S. Department of Health and Human Services: Mental Health: A Report of the Surgeon General. Executive Summary. Rockville, MD, U.S. Department of Health and Human Services, Substance Abuse and Mental Health Services Administration, Center for Mental Health Services, National Institute of Health, National Institute of Mental Health, 1999

U.S. Department of Health and Human Services, Centers for Disease Control and Prevention: Results from the School Health Policies and Practices Study, 2012. Available at http://www.cdc.gov/healthyyouth/shpps/2012/pdf/shpps-results_2012.pdf. Accessed March 26, 2015.

U.S. Public Health Service: Report of the Surgeon General's Conference on Children's Mental Health: A National Action Agenda. Rockville, MD, U.S. Department of Health and Human Services, Substance Abuse and Mental Health Services Administration, Center for Mental Health Services, National Institute of Health, National Institute of Mental Health, 2000

Vogels AG, Crone MR, Hoekstra F, et al: Comparing three short questionnaires to detect psychosocial dysfunction among primary school children: a randomized method. BMC Public Health 9:489, 2009 20035636

Walrath CM, Bruns EJ, Anderson KL, et al: Understanding expanded school mental health services in Baltimore City. Behav Modif 28(4):472–490, 2004 15186511

Walter HJ, Vaughan RD: AIDS risk reduction among a multiethnic sample of urban high school students. JAMA 270(6):725–730, 1993 8336374

Walter HJ, Vaughan RD, Armstrong B, et al: School-based health care for urban minority junior high school students. Arch Pediatr Adolesc Med 149(11):1221–1225, 1995a 7581753

Walter HJ, Vaughan RD, Armstrong B, et al: Sexual, assaultive, and suicidal behaviors among urban minority junior high school students. J Am Acad Child Adolesc Psychiatry 34(1):73–80, 1995b 7860462

Walter HJ, Vaughan RD, Armstrong B, et al: Characteristics of users and nonusers of health clinics in inner-city junior high schools. J Adolesc Health 18(5):344–348, 1996 9156547

Walter HJ, Berkovitz IH, American Academy of Child and Adolescent Psychiatry: Practice parameter for psychiatric consultation to schools. J Am Acad Child Adolesc Psychiatry 44(10):1068–1083, 2005 16175112

Walter HJ, Gouze K, Lim KG: Teachers' beliefs about mental health needs in inner city elementary schools. J Am Acad Child Adolesc Psychiatry 45(1):61–68, 2006 16327582

Walter HJ, Gouze K, Cicchetti C, et al: A pilot demonstration of comprehensive mental health services in inner-city public schools. J Sch Health 81(4):185–193, 2011 21392010

Weare K, Nind M: Mental health promotion and problem prevention in schools: what does the evidence say? Health Promot Int 26(suppl 1):i29–i69, 2011 22079935

Weist MD: Fulfilling the promise of school-based mental health: moving toward a Public Mental Health Promotion approach. J Abnorm Child Psychol 33(6):735–741, 2005 16328748

Weist MD, Christodulu KV: Expanded school mental health programs: advancing reform and closing the gap between research and practice. J Sch Health 70(5):195–200, 2000 10900597

Weist MD, Paskewitz DA, Warner BS, et al: Treatment outcome of school-based mental health services for urban teenagers. Community Ment Health J 32(2):149–157, 1996 8777871

Weist MD, Myers CP, Hastings E, et al: Psychosocial functioning of youth receiving mental health services in the schools versus community mental health centers. Community Ment Health J 35(1):69–81, 1999 10094511

Weist MD, Paternite CE, Adelsheim S: School-based mental health services. Commissioned report for the Institute of Medicine, Board of Health Care Services, Crossing the Quality Chasm: Adaptation to Mental Health and Addictive Disorders Committee, Washington, DC, 2005

Wilcox HC, Kellam SG, Brown CH: The impact of two universal randomized first- and second-grade classroom interventions on young adult suicide ideation and attempts. Drug Alcohol Depend 95(suppl 1):S60–S73, 2008 18329189

Wilson D: The interface of school climate and school connectedness and relationships with aggression and victimization. J Sch Health 74(7):293–299, 2004 15493706

Wilson SJ, Lipsey MW: School-based interventions for aggressive and disruptive behavior: update of a meta-analysis. Am J Prev Med 33(2 suppl):S130–S143, 2007 17675014

Wolraich ML, Bard DE, Neas B, et al: The psychometric properties of the Vanderbilt attention-deficit hyperactivity disorder diagnostic teacher rating scale in a community population. J Dev Behav Pediatr 34(2):83–93, 2013 23363973

Wyman PA, Brown CH, LoMurray M, et al: An outcome evaluation of the Sources of Strength suicide prevention program delivered by adolescent peer leaders in high schools. Am J Public Health 100(9):1653–1661, 2010 20634440

Young TL: Telepsychiatry's potential in schools: psychiatric services can be delivered to children in underserved areas with phone- and/or internet based technologies. Behavioral Health Management 24(4):21–24, 2004

Zins JE, Bloodworth MR, Weissberg RP, et al: The scientific base linking social and emotional learning to school success, in Building Academic Success on Social and Emotional Learning: What Does the Research Say? Edited by Zins JE, Weissberg RP, Wang MC, et al. New York, Teachers College Press, 2004, pp 3–22

CHAPTER 49

Collaborating With Primary Care

L. Read Sulik, M.D.
Barry Sarvet, M.D.

Each year, one in four Americans will develop a mental illness or substance use disorder, while nearly half will develop a mental illness or substance use disorder during their lifetime, and most will have a co-occurring chronic physical health condition (Kessler et al. 2005). Health reform, spurred largely by the Patient Protection and Affordable Care Act (PPACA), commonly called the Affordable Care Act (P.L. 111-148, 124 Stat. 119; March 23, 2010), leading to expansion of health insurance and mental health parity, which requires improved coverage of behavioral health treatment, calls for increased provider accountability to improve access to and the experience of care and quality of care provided, at significant cost savings. The Institute for Healthcare Improvement has called these three aims of health reform the Triple Aim. Health systems and health plans are initiating changes to transform care delivery in order to align outcomes with the goals of the Triple Aim (Berwick et al. 2008).

The cost of care for treating a medical condition increases at least two to three times if the individual has a co-occurring mental illness or substance use disorder (Melek et al. 2014). While much of the focus on the cost of health care in the United States has been on adults, among children and adolescents, behavioral health disorders are the fourth leading cause for hospitalization, the highest cost setting in the spectrum of care (Yu et al. 2011).

Initiatives are under way that call for improved integration of behavioral health within primary care in response to the demand to improve the coordination of care and the efficiency and effectiveness of care. A goal is to achieve cost savings through the reduction of hospital admissions with the formation of accountable care organizations and patient-centered medical homes (Katon and Unützer 2011; Russell 2010). Models of integration range from the identification and treatment of mental disorders in primary care settings to addressing chronic medical conditions in patients with serious mental illness cared for in public mental health settings (Raney et al. 2013).

The terms *collaborative care* and *integrated care* are often used interchangeably. However, the former typically refers to the development of alliances and partnerships between various providers and/or agencies in order to provide effective care coordination across behavioral health and primary care. Collaborative care has typically included the availability of consultation by a psychiatrist or child psychiatrist to a primary care clinician who is treating a patient with a behavioral health condition. Integrated care typically involves a team of primary care and behavioral health clinicians, working together with patients and families (Peek and National Integration Academy Council 2013). The clinical and financial effectiveness of collaborating between or integrating behavioral health and primary care has been demonstrated repeatedly. A recent review by the Cochrane Collaboration of 79 worldwide randomized controlled trials, including 24,308 patients of all ages, found that collaborative care for the treatment of depression and/or anxiety, when compared with routine care, is more effective and leads to improved patient engagement and treatment adherence with increased patient satisfaction and quality of life (Archer et al. 2012).

Child and adolescent psychiatrists are in great demand in every community throughout the United States. The number of children and adolescents requiring access to mental health care continues to increase, while the number of child and adolescent psychiatrists practicing in the United States has grown little in the last two to three decades. There is great disparity across the United States in the availability of child psychiatrists, with rural and poor populations having the greatest shortage and therefore the worst access to care (Thomas and Holzer 2006). The shortage of child mental health professionals of all disciplines is a likely contributing factor to the Surgeon General's estimate that only 20% of the children with mental illness obtain any mental health care at all (U.S. Public Health Service 2000).

As the role of the pediatrician has expanded to include the identification and treatment of common mental health disorders, most pediatricians report that they do not feel prepared to address the psychosocial problems and mental health needs of their patients, citing inadequate training and experience as well as the lack of referral resources as the greatest barriers for providing mental health care in their clinics (Horwitz et al. 2007; Trude and Stoddard 2003). In recent years, toolkits for primary care physicians (PCPs) to improve their ability to identify, assess, diagnose, and treat mental illness and other psychosocial problems have been established (Cheung et al. 2007; Foy and American Academy of Pediatrics Task Force on Mental Health 2010a, 2010b; Foy et al. 2010a, 2010b; Zuckerbrot et al. 2007). Much work has also been done to provide guidance to child and adolescent psychiatrists in collaborating with primary care (DeMaso et al. 2010; Sarvet et al. 2011) and in integrating into the *medical home* (Martini et al. 2012).

Over the past decade, population-based systems, termed *child psychiatry access programs* (CPAPs), have been developed to provide a range of collaborative child and adolescent psychiatry services for pediatric primary care teams. These programs have aimed to enhance the ability of PCPs to address mental health needs of children and adolescents by setting up teams of child psychiatrists and other mental health professionals who deliver immediate telephone consultation, expedited in-person child psychiatry consultation, and care coordination services for a defined set of primary care providers across a geographic region. The first large-scale implementation of this model was undertaken in Massachusetts and has experienced robust use by pediatric PCPs, resulting in significant improvement in their self-reported ability to meet the mental health needs of children in their practices (Sarvet et al. 2010). The CPAP model has been replicated in many states across the United States (www.nncpap.org; Gadomski et al. 2014; Hilt et al. 2013). A majority of the programs serve children regardless of insurance. In addition to consultation and care coordination, the programs include strategies for education and professional development of pediatricians to increase expertise in and comfort with primary care child psychiatry, including mental health screening, knowledge of best practices in evaluation and management of common mental health presentations, and systems-based practices for the coordination of needed specialized mental health resources.

As pediatricians, family physicians, and advanced practice nurses (APNs) become more involved in providing mental health services, protocols and algorithms for assessment and treatment become as critical as in other areas of medicine (Foy et al. 2010d). Earlier identification and intervention by implementing evidence-based protocols for care should lead to improved clinical outcomes and reduced use of expensive inpatient hospitalization, emergency room visits, and out-of-home placements. Bringing mental health services into the primary care clinic in a more integrated manner improves access to care (Jayabarathan 2004). PCPs can provide "primary" mental health care services, such as anticipatory guidance, mental health screening, earlier identification, and earlier intervention (Jellinek 1997).

Expectations for the role of primary care in the mental health care of children include the following:

1. As part of the care of the well child and routine health maintenance, the PCP will provide anticipatory guidance to promote mental health and draw attention to early warning signs of mental health problems.
2. The PCP will screen for and identify signs and symptoms of and risks for mental health problems.
3. Mental health evidence-based assessment and diagnosis will be provided in the primary care setting by PCPs skilled in mental health diagnosis or in collaboration with co-located mental health care professionals.
4. Children and adolescents in need of mental health care will be able to receive evidence-based mental health treatment in the primary care clinic.
5. As part of evidence-based mental health treatment protocols, the PCP will be involved in follow-up care and monitoring for treatment effectiveness (symptom change and improvement in functioning).
6. The PCP will be able to monitor for patient safety (assessing for suicide risk) and for the safety of treatments prescribed (monitoring for adverse events associated with medications or other interventions).
7. The PCP will be part of a multidisciplinary team providing an integrated approach to the mental health care of the child.

8. The primary care clinic is the overall medical home as well as the mental health home for children and adolescents, where services involving various mental health and medical specialists can be coordinated.
9. The degree of collaboration between PCPs and child and adolescent psychiatrists and other mental health clinicians exists on a continuum according to the level of acuity of the patient. This may range from the PCP primarily managing the mental health care of the child to the other end of the spectrum in more severely ill patients, where the mental health care is primarily managed by the mental health specialists.

With these increased expectations, PCPs not only must seek additional training and education to improve their own skill sets but must also develop the ability to work collaboratively with child and adolescent psychiatrists, psychologists, and other mental health professionals (Committee on Psychosocial Aspects of Child and Family Health and Task Force on Mental Health 2009). This expanded role of the pediatrician and family physician in the delivery of mental health care to children requires the role of the child and adolescent psychiatrist to expand beyond the provision of direct clinical care. The child and adolescent psychiatrist will need to have improved skills in consultation, collaboration, teaching, and mentorship so that our primary care colleagues continue to improve their knowledge, experience, and comfort in 1) recognition of signs and symptoms, 2) assessment, 3) appropriate indications for and use of psychotropic medications, and 4) referral for psychotherapy and other treatment interventions. Child psychiatrists must assist PCPs in triaging and referring patients at higher levels of acuity, including helping PCPs to know which patients they should be able to manage and when and how to consult with a child and adolescent psychiatrist or other mental health professional. The child and adolescent psychiatrist must become much more aware of the culture and needs of the primary health care setting and have realistic expectations of what can and cannot be appropriately identified and treated in an outpatient primary care clinic.

Understanding the Primary Care Clinic Setting

Case Example

Jack is a 13-year-old who was seen along with his mother in the pediatric clinic by Dr. Rosen because of concerns about school. He was scheduled for a 15-minute appointment, and Dr. Rosen was already almost 60 minutes behind schedule. As Dr. Rosen was about to enter the room, his nurse walked by and stated, "That mom has called three times today, so make sure you see the note I left you in the chart before you go in there."

In the electronic health record was a provider alert note from the nurse that said, "The mom wants to see you without the patient first and wants a drug screen done today." Dr. Rosen noticed in the record that Jack had been seen in the clinic six times during the last year by several different partners for a variety of vague complaints.

Dr. Rosen put his head in the door and asked the mom to step out into the hall. She told him that Jack was completing the seventh grade but might be at risk of failing; he missed more than 30 days of school this year. She now cannot seem to get him to go to school at all, he does not do his homework, and "he has stopped caring about anything at all." She worried that he was using drugs and said, "I just don't want him to go down the same path as his brother" (who used drugs and dropped out of school).

Dr. Rosen walked into the examination room with Jack's mother. Jack did not look up or make eye contact, despite attempts to ask Jack about school. He then proceeded to say "I don't know" to most of the things that Dr. Rosen asked during the visit.

Dr. Rosen's nurse rang the phone in the exam room to let him know he was now 70 minutes behind and two patients were still waiting in rooms. Dr. Rosen excused the mom from the room and asked to talk to Jack briefly. Jack said that he was living at home with his mom, his older unemployed brother, his younger sister (who fought with him all the time), and his stepfather. He said, "I can't stand him," and stated that he and his stepfather fought "constantly." Jack stated that he cannot concentrate at school and that he received As and Bs through elementary school but is now "failing almost everything." Dr. Rosen asked if Jack was feeling depressed, and Jack said, "No. I'm not depressed," adamantly and angrily. Dr. Rosen asked Jack, "Do you ever have any suicidal thoughts?" and Jack replied, "Doesn't everybody?"

Dr. Rosen stepped out of the office and stated to his nurse, "Let's get a urine drug screen and get him in to see child psychiatry." Jack and his mother were instructed to wait in the room while the nurse tried to secure an appointment. After calls to the four child psychiatrists in the community and six other child psychiatry offices within a 2-hour radius, she learned that no one could see Jack. She found most were not taking new patients and only one would even schedule an intake appointment, with the next available appointment more than 3 months from now.

As this case exemplifies, the PCP is often caught off guard by the presentation of mental health concerns. Referring a patient for assessment and care is often not an immediate option. The role of the PCP involves prevention, screening, education, assessment, treatment, monitoring, and referral. Now many PCPs must initiate assessment and treatment but should be doing this in consultation and collaboration with mental health professionals. Collaborative models are not usually taught in either primary care or psychiatric training programs. Child and adolescent psychiatrists involved in collaboration with primary care clinics may be in the role of consulting not only on cases but also on clinic policies and procedures, such as on protocols for phone triage for clinic nurses or for assessments of attention-deficit/hyperactivity disorder.

In the case example, mental health screening at routine and acute visits might have helped identify problems much earlier. Also, clinic protocols in place for nurses and physicians would assist them in knowing how to schedule patients when a mental health concern is identified and also what tools to have available for the physician to help with a clinic-based mental health assessment. PCPs may need assistance in knowing how to screen, what screening tools to use, how to interpret self-report and parent-report questionnaires, and how to assimilate the information into an appropriate diagnostic formulation. Most PCPs have traditionally not received training on the diagnostic formulation and would benefit from assistance in identifying the patient's contributing biological, psychological, and social factors. PCPs do not typically feel comfortable or have the skills to interview patients or even parents in regard to mental health concerns and therefore may need mentoring, teaching, and even modeling of interview skills (Foy et al.

2010b). In addition, the entire clinic staff may need education and training on interacting and working with families of children with mental illness.

If a child and adolescent psychiatrist were not available to immediately evaluate this patient, the pediatrician could be guided by a consultant in the approach to assessment and initiation of treatment. If the pediatrician knew he could contact his consulting child and adolescent psychiatrist, perhaps at a predetermined time when the consultant would be available, the case could be discussed over the telephone, and an approach to evaluation could be determined. Once the diagnosis is made clear, further consultation might allow the pediatrician to initiate care so that the patient does not decompensate further while awaiting a referral appointment. Finally, with consultation availability, the pediatrician may be able to monitor the patient more effectively, knowing when to bring the patient back for follow-up visits and what to do at those follow-up visits.

Approaches to Education and Improving Skills of the Primary Care Physician

How can the child and adolescent psychiatrist assist the PCP in improving skills needed to provide mental health care to children? Improving knowledge and skills in order to create a change in physician behavior and clinical practice requires more than attending continuing medical education lectures or reading a journal article or textbook chapter. It is critical to develop training, consultation, and mentoring models with child psychiatrists and other mental health professionals. Collaborative models of care allow for ongoing access to child psychiatrists not only for case consultation but also for ongoing education and mentoring (DeMaso et al. 2010; Martini et al. 2012).

Collaborative Care

Optimal mental health care requires collaboration between the PCP and mental health specialists such as the child and adolescent psychiatrist, child psychologist, and APN and psychotherapists such as licensed clinical social workers, case managers, schoolteachers, and school-based mental health professionals. At the time of a mental health assessment in a primary care clinic, the physician must determine the acuity of the patient so that the appropriate level of care can be determined. If a PCP determines that he or she can manage the patient initially, adequate follow-up and monitoring will provide the opportunity for reassessment of the need for a higher level of care. Collaborative mental health care can be considered along a spectrum of five levels.

1. *Primarily primary care:* The pediatrician or family physician identifies and treats the child with a less severe psychiatric problem. In this situation, the primary care clinic is the primary site for the mental health care of the patient. The PCP educates the child and family, manages the overall care, prescribes any treatments, and monitors the treatments prescribed. An example would be a child with ADHD who is responsive to stimulant medications and who is without diagnostic or psychosocial complexities.
2. *Primarily primary care with consultation:* The PCP consults with a child psychiatrist or a psychologist regard-

ing approaches to assessment, diagnosis, and treatment. The psychiatrist may be consulted to inquire about medications: which ones to consider, when to consider them, appropriate dosing and titration, recommended length of treatment, and how to appropriately monitor. Consultation can occur at the assessment, at the initiation of treatment, or any time during the course of treatment, such as in a child with ADHD who is unresponsive to initial medication trials or in a child with exacerbation of a previously controlled depression.

3. *Shared care:* The PCP identifies, assesses, and then refers for an emergency consultation with a child and adolescent psychiatrist but then shares in the ongoing care of the patient. Communication is critical when a patient is shared. Additional mental health specialists such as psychologists and other therapists may be consulted and may share in the care of the patient. Sharing care implies that the required ongoing monitoring of the symptoms of the mental illness and the response to medications and therapy is a responsibility of *all* the providers involved and that there is ongoing communication about the patient among the providers. Examples here might be a child with depression comanaged for cognitive-behavioral therapy, a child requiring psychiatry evaluation because of inadequate response to medications, or a child with increased suicidal risk.
4. *Shared care and higher levels of care:* The patient may require a higher level of care, such as more frequent follow-up visits, closer monitoring, and even hospitalization, partial hospitalization (day treatment), or intensive outpatient treatment. Additional community support services may be required, such as a mental health case manager. In this situation, the responsibility for management is shifted to the mental health specialists, but the primary care provider is still actively involved as a treatment team member and shares in the overall care, as in a patient with depression following hospital discharge.
5. *Primarily mental health care:* The patient is referred to mental health specialty care for ongoing treatment and management. The child and adolescent psychiatrist is the primary medical provider managing the child's mental illness because of the level of severity, the level of complexity of the individual and family problems, higher levels of concern regarding safety, and/or the coexistence of other complicating conditions. The responsibility for ongoing care and management is with the child and adolescent psychiatrist and other mental health specialty team members, but the PCP is included in communication and is informed of changes in level of care (e.g. hospitalization), changes in medications, or other treatment plan changes. Examples would be children with bipolar disorder, schizophrenia, or severe ADHD unresponsive to usual medications.

Essential Skills for the Collaborating and Consulting Child and Adolescent Psychiatrist

1. Interpersonal communication: The child and adolescent psychiatrist must have an open and collaborative style of communication to facilitate rapport building that leads to effec-

tive partnerships with pediatric primary care colleagues.

2. Collaboration: The child and adolescent psychiatrist must be able to collaborate effectively as a member of a patient-centered health care team and be accessible effectively to other team members.
3. Consultation: The child and adolescent psychiatrist must be able to provide meaningful and effective case consultation to primary care colleagues, developing comfort in listening to brief case presentations, asking pertinent questions, and guiding the primary care clinician. Skills required to provide effective consultation will vary depending on whether the consultation is face to face, via telephone, via televideo, or in a small group in-person format.
4. Care planning and coordination: The child and adolescent psychiatrist must be able to collaboratively create and implement treatment plans and assist in the communication and coordination of the care plan with team members, patients, and families.
5. Teaching and mentoring: The child and adolescent psychiatrist must have knowledge and experience to develop a comfort with and ability to teach and mentor other health care team members about the following:
    a. Screening—the use of evidence-based and developmentally appropriate screening tools to improve the identification of children and adolescents with clinical symptoms and impairment in functioning
    b. Assessment—the use of evidence-based strategies in the assessment of common mental health problems, behavior problems, and safety risk
    c. Triaging—effective triage and referral of patients if indicated for a more comprehensive assessment or to specialized resources or higher levels of care on the basis of the assessment of the patient's acuity and complexity
    d. Clinical interventions—psychotherapies, behavioral interventions, and appropriate use of medications as well as the appropriate approach to monitoring for the safety and effectiveness of the various treatments prescribed
    e. Care planning and coordination—specific treatment goals and the coordination of care with other team members, patients, and families

Core Principles of Collaborative Care

The resources available to assist the PCP vary across communities. Providing mental health care in the primary care clinic requires that the pediatrician or family physician do the following:

1. Establish local or regional connections with mental health professionals to participate as team members in the patient's care. Some access to child and adolescent psychiatrists and clinical psychologists or licensed clinical social workers is necessary. Additional professionals, when indicated, may include county social services mental health case managers, school psychologists, special education teachers and educational case managers, school nurses, chemical dependency counselors, and possibly inpatient psychiatric treatment staff. Most primary care clinics do

not employ their own mental health professionals, and therefore clinics must have a consultative and collaborative relationship with professionals who are practicing independently or who are employed by a hospital or community agency.
2. Establish clear and regular communication, preferably via a common electronic medical record, so that real-time clinical information is readily available to the emergency department staff, mental health clinicians, and PCP.
3. Locate a mental health professional in the clinic to provide triage assessments, crisis counseling, case management services, and patient and family education. This has several important benefits, including removing some of the burden from the practicing physician, ensuring that referrals are properly made, and having more flexible time to deal with crises than is possible for the PCP.
4. Establish screening protocols, triage and referral processes, and treatment and monitoring pathways so that all providers consistently follow similar standards of care.
5. Have continuing education, in either lecture or case discussion format, to provide ongoing connection among psychiatrists, psychologists, social workers, APNs, and the PCP.

Components of Collaborative and Consultative Care in the Primary Care Setting

Screening

Collaborative child psychiatry consultants may have a critical role to play in the implementation of an effective screening process in the primary care setting through providing technical support in the selection of appropriate screening instruments and screening methodology and assisting in the follow-up assessment of patients with positive screens. Screening without well-planned follow-up strategies and resources results in unsatisfactory experiences with and lack of maintenance of screening. Although administration of the screening tool is ordinarily performed by paraprofessional office staff, interpretation and review of the completed screen with the patient and/or the parent involves clinical sensitivity and expertise. Consultation by a child and adolescent psychiatrist in the planning of the screening activity and subsequently as needed can facilitate the development of such competency.

Informal Consultation

A good relationship with good communication is essential. The informal or "curbside" consultation requires familiarity and trust between the clinicians. PCPs can begin the process of creating relationships with child and adolescent psychiatrists and psychologists by inviting local or regional potential colleagues to meet to discuss the process. In some settings, clinical case or roundtable discussions are held monthly between a child and adolescent psychiatrist and a group of pediatricians, with continuing medical education credit provided. Although this may be limited to 1 hour every month or even less, the relationship may be established for the continuation of informal consultations to continue to support the pediatrician. The PCP should document in the patient's chart the results of an informal consultation with a child and adolescent psychiatrist or psychologist. The notation includes the name of the professional consulted, the reason for the consultation, a reference to the case being summarized, and the resulting discussion of the diagnosis and recommendations for treatment. In integrated health systems with a shared electronic health record, the note is also available to the consulting child psychiatrist. If the informal child psychiatry consultant does not have an established relationship with the patient, the production of an official psychiatric record documenting the consultation may not be feasible. In this case, a telephone log for recording basic elements of the consultation for future reference is a desirable practice.

Formal Consultation

Psychiatric evaluation of patients referred by a PCP in a timely manner and the production of a succinct and prompt written report are an essential component of collaborative care. These consultations serve the purpose of helping to clarify ambiguous clinical presentations, confirm provisional diagnoses by PCPs with limited diagnostic experience and confidence, and identify clinical strategies for patients who are not responding favorably to treatment. An evaluation by a collaborating child psychiatrist may contribute powerfully to the PCP's learning process, particularly in the case of confirmatory consultations. Consultation letters should contain essential elements of history, examination, impression, and recommendations tailored to address the learning needs of the PCP.

Communication

Consent for release of information should be obtained during the initial mental health evaluation so that all providers can communicate with one another. The PCP who is prescribing psychotropic medications and is sharing the care of the patient with a therapist must have ongoing communication with the therapist to ensure optimal coordination of care. Physicians need to communicate to the therapist that ongoing communication is desired and is expected but also commit to communicating regularly with the therapist. Physicians may consider using a communication document that summarizes important information to be shared. When the PCP is sharing care with a child and adolescent psychiatrist, communication on medication changes is also critically important.

Triage

In order for the collaborative spectrum of care to be effective, the patient must be assessed for acuity so that the appropriate level of collaborative care can be provided. An acuity assessment allows the physician to determine what additional resources will be necessary in the care of the patient. Acuity is determined on the basis of the severity of symptoms, the degree of impairment in functioning, and a determination of safety. Acuity is assessed not only during an initial evaluation but also throughout the course of treatment because the level of acuity may change and the patient may move to a different level of care as a result.

Follow-Up

Frequently, the pediatrician calls the child and adolescent psychiatrist for a follow-up consultation after initiating treatment or to provide an update to determine if there are any other treatment modalities needed. During these consultations, the psychiatrist guides the pediatrician on how often to see a patient for follow-up, what to assess, and what information to provide at the follow-up visits. The PCP must communicate clearly with other team members regarding follow-up plans. The treatment team should agree on who will see the patient and how often the patient will be seen.

Financial Viability

As health care reform drives changes in payment methodologies toward pay-for-performance and total cost of care shared savings, the viability of collaborative and integrated care will be folded into the total cost of achieving these newly emphasized financial and clinical outcomes. Until that transformation in how clinicians are paid is complete, the support of collaboration and integration is still dependent on achieving payments for separate components such as screening, assessments, and consultations. The multiple state-funded child psychiatry consultation services now in existence are bridging this gap by paying for child psychiatrists to be available to consult with primary care clinicians (Gadomski et al. 2014; Hilt et al. 2013; Sarvet et al. 2010; Straus and Sarvet 2014; www.nncpap.org).

Summary Points

- Primary care physicians (PCPs) are increasingly expected to conduct mental health screening and provide mental health assessments and mental health treatment in the primary care clinic.
- Child and adolescent psychiatrists are increasingly involved in teaching, mentoring, and providing consultation to PCPs in order to improve access to mental health care for children and adolescents.
- Collaborative care includes mental health screening, mental health diagnostic assessments, and determination of where on a collaborative care continuum the child falls.
- The level of collaborative care is determined by the patient's acuity and can range from primary management of the patient by the PCP to a sharing of care between the PCP and the child and adolescent psychiatrist and other mental health specialists. Some patients' mental health care is managed primarily by the mental health specialists.
- PCPs and primary care clinic staff need to improve their understanding of mental health issues in children and adolescents and skills needed to identify and treat mental health disorders in the primary care clinic.
- Child and adolescent psychiatrists need to improve their understanding of the primary care setting and recognize how to provide support to PCPs and their staff.
- Improved collaboration between PCPs and child and adolescent psychiatrists can increase access to mental health care for children and reduce 1) the use of more intensive levels of mental health services and 2) overall cost in providing improved care because of earlier identification and earlier intervention.

References

Archer J, Bower P, Gilbody S, et al: Collaborative care for depression and anxiety problems. Cochrane Database Syst Rev 10(10):CD006525, 2012 23076925

Berwick DM, Nolan TW, Whittington J: The triple aim: care, health, and cost. Health Aff (Millwood) 27(3):759–769, 2008 18474969

Cheung AH, Zuckerbrot RA, Jensen PJ, et al: Guidelines for Adolescent Depression in Primary Care (GLAD-PC): II. Treatment and ongoing management. Pediatrics 120(5):e1313–e1326, 2007 DOI: 10.1542/peds.2006-1395 17974724

Committee on Psychosocial Aspects of Child and Family Health and Task Force on Mental Health: Policy statement: the future of pediatrics: mental health competencies for pediatric primary care. Pediatrics 124(1):410–421, 2009 19564328

DeMaso D, Martini R, Sulik LR, et al: A Guide to Building Collaborative Mental Health Care Partnerships in Pediatric Primary Care. Washington, DC, American Academy of Child and Adolescent Psychiatry Committee on Collaboration with Medical Professionals. June 2010

Foy JM, American Academy of Pediatrics Task Force on Mental Health: Enhancing pediatric mental health care: algorithms for primary care. Pediatrics 125(suppl 3):S109–S125, 2010a 20519563

Foy JM, American Academy of Pediatrics Task Force on Mental Health: Enhancing pediatric mental health care: report from the American Academy of Pediatrics Task Force on Mental Health. Introduction. Pediatrics 125(suppl 3):S69–S74, 2010b 20519564

Foy JM, Perrin J, American Academy of Pediatrics Task Force on Mental Health: Enhancing pediatric mental health care: strategies for preparing a community. Pediatrics 125(suppl 3):S75–S86, 2010a 20519565

Foy JM, Kelleher KJ, Laraque D, et al: Enhancing pediatric mental health care: strategies for preparing a primary care practice. Pediatrics 125(suppl 3):S87–S108, 2010b 20519566

Gadomski AM, Wissow LS, Palinkas L, et al: Encouraging and sustaining integration of child mental health into primary care: interviews with primary care providers participating in Project TEACH (CAPES and CAP PC) in NY. Gen Hosp Psychiatry 36(6):555–562, 2014 24973125

Hilt RJ, Romaire MA, McDonell MG, et al: The Partnership Access Line: evaluating a child psychiatry consult program in Washington State. JAMA Pediatr 167(2):162–168, 2013 23247331

Horwitz SM, Kelleher KJ, Stein RE, et al: Barriers to the identification and management of psychosocial issues in children and maternal depression. Pediatrics 119(1):e208–e218, 2007 17200245

Jayabarathan A: Shared mental health care. Bringing family physicians and psychiatrists together. Can Fam Physician 50:341–346, 2004 15318666

Jellinek MS: DSM-PC: bridging pediatric primary care and mental health services. J Dev Behav Pediatr 18(3):173–174, 1997 9213234

Katon W, Unützer J: Consultation psychiatry in the medical home and accountable care organizations: achieving the triple aim. Gen Hosp Psychiatry 33(4):305–310, 2011 21762825

Kessler RC, Chiu WT, Demler O, et al: Prevalence, severity, and comorbidity of 12-month DSM-IV disorders in the National Comorbidity Survey Replication. Arch Gen Psychiatry 62(6):617–627, 2005 15939839

Martini R, Hilt R, Marx L, et al: Best Principles for Integration of Child Psychiatry Into the Pediatric Health Home. Washington, DC, American Academy of Child and Adolescent Psychiatry, 2012

Melek, S, Norris, D, Paulus J: Economic Impact of Integrated Medical-Behavioral Healthcare: Implications for Psychiatry. Prepared for American Psychiatric Association. Denver, CO, Milliman, 2014

Peek CJ, National Integration Academy Council: Lexicon for Behavioral Health and Primary Care Integration: Concepts and Definitions Developed by Expert Consensus (AHRQ Publication No. 13-IP001-EF). Rockville, MD, Agency for Healthcare Research and Quality, 2013

Raney L, Kathol R, Summergrad P: Collaborative Care Models for Comorbid Medical and Behavioral Health Conditions. Focus 11(4):501–508, 2013

Russell L: Mental Health Care Services in Primary Care: Tackling the Issues in the Context of Health Care Reform. Washington, DC, Center for American Progress, 2010

Sarvet B, Gold J, Bostic JQ, et al: Improving access to mental health care for children: the Massachusetts Child Psychiatry Access Project. Pediatrics 126(6):1191–1200, 2010 21059722

Sarvet B, Gold J, Straus JH: Bridging the divide between child psychiatry and primary care: the use of telephone consultation within a population-based collaborative system. Child Adolesc Psychiatr Clin N Am 20(1):41–53, 2011 21092911

StrausJH, Sarvet B: Behavioral health care for children: the Massachusetts Child Psychiatry Access Project. Health Aff (Millwood) 33:2153–2161, 2014

Thomas CR, Holzer CE III: The continuing shortage of child and adolescent psychiatrists. J Am Acad Child Adolesc Psychiatry 45(9):1023–1031, 2006 16840879

Trude S, Stoddard JJ: Referral gridlock: primary care physicians and mental health services. J Gen Intern Med 18(6):442–449, 2003 12823651

U.S. Public Health Service: Report of the Surgeon General's Conference on Children's Mental Health: A National Action Agenda. Washington, DC, Department of Health and Human Services, 2000

Yu H, Wier LM, Elixhauser A: Hospital Stays for Children, 2009 (HCUP Statistical Brief No. 118). Rockville, MD, Agency for Healthcare Research and Quality, August 2011. Available at: http://www.hcup-us.ahrq.gov/reports/statbriefs/sb118.jsp Accessed May 14, 2015.

Zuckerbrot RA, Cheung AH, Jensen PS, et al: Guidelines for Adolescent Depression in Primary Care (GLAD-PC): I. Identification, assessment, and initial management. Pediatrics 120(5):e1299–e1312, 2007 17974723

Index

Page numbers printed in **boldface** *type refer to figures or tables.*